Stedman's

GI & GU

WORDS

INCLUDES
NEPHROLOGY

THIRD EDITION

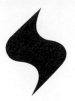

Stedman's

GI & GU
WORDS

INCLUDES
NEPHROLOGY

THIRD EDITION

LIPPINCOTT
WILLIAMS
& WILKINS

Publisher: Rhonda M. Kumm
Senior Manager: Julie K. Stegman
Associate Managing Editor: Trista A. DiPaula
Associate Managing Editor: William A. Howard
Art Director: Jennifer Clements
Production Coordinator: Kevin Iarossi
Typesetter: Peirce Graphic Services, Inc.
Printer & Binder: Malloy Litho

Printed in the United States of America

2002

Library of Congress Cataloging-in-Publication Data

Stedman's GI & GU words : includes nephrology.—3rd ed.
    p. cm.
    Rev. ed. of Stedman's GI & GU words. 2nd ed.
    C 1996
    ISBN 0-7817-3058-9 (alk. paper)
    1. Gastroenterology—Terminology. 2. Urology—Terminology. I. Title: Stedman's
GI and GU words. II. Title: GI & GU words. III. Stedman, Thomas Lathrop, 1853–1938.
    [DNLM: 1. Gastrointestinal Diseases—terminology. 2. Gastroenterology—
terminology. 3. Urogenital Diseases—terminology. 4. Urologic Diseases—
terminology. 5. Nephrology—terminology.]
RC802 .S68 2001
616.3'3'0014—dc21

2001050350

02 03
2 3 4 5 6 7 8 9 10

Contents

Acknowledgments

An important part of our editorial process is the involvement of medical transcriptionists—as advisors, reviewers, and/or editors.

We extend special thanks to Jeanne Bock, CSR, MT; and Kathryn C. Mason, CMT, for editing the manuscript, helping resolve many difficult questions, and contributing material for the appendix sections. We are grateful to our MT Editorial Advisory Board members, including Marty Cantu, CMT; Ava George; Kathy Hess, CMT; Nancy Hill, MT; Robin Koza; Tracy Vasquez; and, Sandra Wideburg, CMT, who were instrumental in the development of this reference. They recommended sources and shared their valuable judgment, insight, and perspective.

We also extend thanks to Marty Cantu, CMT, and Jeanne Bock, CSR, MT, for working on the appendix. Additional thanks goes to Helen Littrell for performing the final prepublication review. Other important contributors to this edition include Shemah Fletcher; Deborah B. Hahn, CMT; Sandy Kovacs, CMT; Cheryl A. Letner, CMT; Wendy Ryan, RHIT; Tina Whitecotton, MT; and, Mary Chiara Zaratkiewicz.

And, as always, Barb Ferretti played an integral role in the process by reviewing the content files for format, updating the database, and providing a final quality check.

As with all our *Stedman's* word references, this resource incorporates the suggestions and expertise of our many contacts in the medical transcriptionist community. Thanks to all of our advisory board participants, reviewers, and editors; AAMT meeting attendees; and others who have written us with requests and comments—keep talking, and we'll keep listening.

Editor's Preface

We all have favorite books. If a group of people were asked to name their favorite book, the responses in the group would be as diverse as the people in the group. One person might name a historical novel, another a biography, while a third person might name a much-loved romance novel. We could all name favorite books.

As a medical language specialist, I have favorite reference books. I feel great affection for some of the books in my library. Though they may have lost their new-book smell and no longer have crisp pages, they are special to me. One book in my library that I have always loved is *Stedman's GI & GU Words, Second Edition*. Consequently, you can imagine my excitement and pleasure when asked to edit *Stedman's GI & GU Words, Third Edition*. I was given the opportunity to enhance a book I consider the best in the specialty it represents.

The book is completed, and I am very pleased with the result. In this third edition you will find terms you most likely highlighted for easy reference in the second edition of *Stedman's GI & GU Words:* gastrointestinal, genitourinary, and nephrology terms. You will also find a plethora of new entries taken from the most current journals, websites, and textbooks.

That's what you'll find in the A-Z portion of the book, and if we had stopped there, this would be a fantastic resource. In addition, though, you will find a large and extensive appendix. The appendix includes anatomic illustrations, lab values, GI/GU drugs referred to in medical dictation, herbs used to treat gastrointestinal and genitourinary conditions, and sample reports with listings of common terms found in those sample reports.

My thanks go to Lippincott Williams and Wilkins for continually striving to provide the most inclusive and complete books in the marketplace. I also thank Kathryn Mason for working with me in the editing of the manuscript and Barb Ferretti for being an unflagging and invaluable resource during the editing process.

Jeanne Bock, CSR, MT

Publisher's Preface

Stedman's GI & GU Words, Third Edition, offers an authoritative assurance of quality and exactness to the wordsmiths of the healthcare professions—medical transcriptionists, medical editors and copyeditors, health information management personnel, court reporters, and the many other users and producers of medical documentation.

The specialties of gastroenterology, urology, and nephrology have evolved significantly over the past several years. Gastroenterology-related terminology includes: GI endoscopy, hepatology, and clinical nutrition. Urology-related terminology includes: genitourinary surgery, laparoscopic urology, endourology, urolithology and lithotripsy, renography, ultrasonography, male infertility, urogynecology, and fluorodynamics.

In *Stedman's GI & GU Words, Third Edition,* users will find thousands of words as they relate to the specialties of gastroenterology, urology, and nephrology. Users will also find terms for protocols, diagnostic and therapeutic procedures, new techniques, lab tests, clinical research terms, as well as equipment names, and abbreviations with their expansions. The appendix sections provide anatomical illustrations with useful captions and labels, sample reports, and common terms by procedure.

This compilation of more than 100,000 entries, fully cross-indexed for quick access, was built from a base vocabulary of approximately 66,000 medical words, phrases, abbreviations, and acronyms. The extensive A-Z list was developed from the database of *Stedman's Medical Dictionary, 27th Edition,* and supplemented by terminology found in current medical literature (please see list of References on page xiv).

We at Lippincott Williams & Wilkins strive to provide you with the most up-to-date and accurate word references available. Your use of this word book will prompt new editions, which we will publish as often as updates and revisions justify. We welcome your suggestions for improvements, changes, corrections, and additions—whatever will make this *Stedman's* product more useful to you. Please complete the postpaid card at the back of this book, and send your recommendations care of "Stedman's" at Lippincott Williams & Wilkins.

Explanatory Notes

Medical transcription is an art as well as a science. Both approaches are needed to correctly interpret the dictation of a physician, whose language is a product of education, training, and experience. This variety in medical language means that there are several acceptable ways to express certain terms, including jargon. *Stedman's GI & GU Words, Third Edition,* provides variant spellings and phrasings for many terms. These elements, in addition to complete cross-indexing, make *Stedman's GI & GU Words, Third Edition,* a valuable resource for determining the validity of terms as they are encountered.

Alphabetical Organization

Alphabetization of main entries is letter by letter as spelled, ignoring punctuation, spaces, prefixed numbers, or other characters. For example:

O'Hara forceps
25(OH)D3
OHS

Terms beginning with Greek letters show the Greek letters spelled out and listed alphabetically. For example:

alpha, α
    a. blockade
    estrogen receptor a. (ER alpha)
    a. gene

In subentry alphabetization, the abbreviated singular form or the spelled-out plural form of the noun main entry word is ignored.

Format and Style

All main entries are in **boldface** to expedite locating a sought-after term, to enhance distinction between main entries and subentries, and to relieve the textual density of the pages.

Irregular plurals and variant spellings are shown on the same line as the singular or preferred form of the word. For example:

necrosis, pl. **necroses**
NCAM, N-CAM

Hyphenation

As a rule of style, multiple eponyms (e.g., Mears-Rubash approach) are hyphenated. Also, hyphens have been added between a manufacturer and one or more eponyms (e.g., Vital-Metzenbaum dissecting scissors). Please note that in many cases, hyphenation is a question of style, not of accuracy, and thus is a matter of choice.

Possessives

Possessive forms have been dropped in this reference for the sake of consistency and conformance with the guidelines of the American Association for Medical Transcription (AAMT) and other groups. Please note, however, that in many cases, retaining the possessive, like hyphenating, is a question of style, not of accuracy, and thus is a matter of choice. To form the possessive of a word, simply add the apostrophe or apostrophe "s" to the end of the word.

Cross-indexing

The word list is in an index-like main entry-subentry format that contains two combined alphabetical listings:

(1) A *noun* main entry-subentry organization, which is typical of the A-Z section of medical dictionaries like *Stedman's:*

matrix
  m. calculus
  extracellular m.
  m. urinary lithiasis

phosphate
  aluminum p.
  p. binder therapy
  p. enema

(2) An *adjective* main entry-subentry organization, which lists words and phrases as you hear them. The main entries are the adjectives or modifiers in a multiword term. The subentries are the nouns around which the terms are constructed and to which the adjectives or modifiers pertain:

proximal
  p. gastrectomy
  p. muscle weakness
  p. pouch leak
  p. venous plexus

resting
  r. anal sphincter pressure
  r. membrane potential
  r. tremor
  r. urethral pressure profile

This format provides the user with more than one way to locate and identify a multiword term. For example:

Linton
    L. shunt

shunt
    Linton s.

anastomosis
    Pagano ureteral a.
    pancreaticogastric a.

Pagano
    P. technique ureterocolonic anastomosis
    P. ureteral anastomosis

It also allows the user to see together all terms that contain a particular descriptor, as well as all types, kinds, or variations of a noun entity. For example:

aspiration
    a. biopsy
    corporeal a.
    fine-needle a.
    Levin tube a.

complex
    c. enterocele
    Eshmun c.
    c. hypospadias
    migrating motor c.

Wherever possible, abbreviations are separately defined and cross-referenced. For example:

EMD
    esophageal motility disorder

esophageal
    e. motility disorder (EMD)

disorder
    esophageal motility d. (EMD)

References

In addition to the manufacturers' literature we gather at various medical meetings, scientific reports from hospitals, and the lists of our MT Editorial Advisory Board members (from their daily transcription work), we used the following sources for new terms in *Stedman's GI & GU Words, Third Edition.*

Books

Blumenthal M, Goldberg A, Brinckmann J. Herbal Medicine: Expanded Commission E Monographs. Newton, MA: Integrative Medicine Communications, 2000.

Drake E. Sloane's Medical Word Book, 4th Edition. Philadelphia: Saunders, 2001.

Eastwood G, Avunduk C. Manual of Gastroenterology, 2nd Edition. Baltimore: Lippincott Williams & Wilkins, 1994.

Gilinsky NH, Forbes A. Self-Assessment Color Review of Gastroenterology. Baltimore: Lippincott Williams & Wilkins, 1999.

GI Words and Phrases. Modesto, CA: Health Professions Institute, 1989.

Gomella LG. The 5-Minute Urology Consult. Baltimore: Lippincott Williams & Wilkins, 2000.

Graham SD, Jr. Glenn JF. Glenn's Urologic Surgery, 5th Edition. Philadelphia: Lippincott Williams & Wilkins, 1998.

Peters DC. Treatment Options in Gastroenterology. Baltimore: Lippincott Williams & Williams, 2000.

Massry SG, Glassock RJ. Massry and Glassock's Textbook of Nephrology, 4th Edition. Baltimore: Lippincott Williams & Wilkins, 2000.

Lance LL. 2001 Quick Look Drug Book. Baltimore: Lippincott Williams & Wilkins, 2000.

Pyle V. Current Medical Terminology, 8th Edition. Modesto: Health Professions Institute, 2000.

Schrier RW. Manual of Nephrology, 5th Edition. Baltimore: Lippincott Williams & Wilkins. 1999.

Seldin DW, Giebisch G. The Kidney: Physiology and Pathophysiology, 3rd Edition. Baltimore: Lippincott Williams & Wilkins, 2000.

Stedman's GI & GU Words, 2nd Edition. Baltimore: Lippincott Williams & Wilkins, 1996.

Stedman's Medical Dictionary, 27th Edition. Baltimore: Lippincott Williams & Wilkins, 2000.

Tessier C. The AAMT Book of Style. Modesto: AAMT, 1995.

Walsh PC, Retik AB, Vaughan ED, Wein AJ. Campbell's Urology, 7th Edition. Philadelphia: Saunders, 1998.

Journals

American Journal of Gastroenterology. Baltimore: Lippincott Williams & Wilkins, 1998, 2000–2001.

AUA News. Baltimore: Lippincott Williams & Wilkins, 1996–2000.

Contemporary Dialysis and Nephrology. Philadelphia: Lippincott Williams & Wilkins, 1996.

Contemporary Gastroenterology. Philadelphia: Lippincott Williams & Wilkins, 1999–2000.

Contemporary Urology. Philadelphia: Lippincott Williams & Wilkins, 1996, 1999–2000.

Current Opinion in Gastroenterology. Philadelphia: Lippincott Williams & Wilkins, 1999–2001.

Current Opinion in Nephrology and Hypertension. Philadelphia: Lippincott Williams & Wilkins, 1999–2001.

Current Opinion in Urology. Philadelphia: Lippincott Williams & Williams, 1999–2001.

Dialysis & Transplantation. Van Nuys, CA: Creative Age Publications, Inc., 1996.

Diseases of the Colon & Rectum. Philadelphia: Lippincott Williams & Wilkins, 1999–2001.

Gastroenterology Nursing. Philadelphia: Lippincott Williams & Wilkins, 1996.

Gastrointestinal Endoscopy. St. Louis: Mosby-Yearbook, Inc., 1996–2001.

Inflammatory Bowel Disease. Philadelphia: Lippincott Williams & Wilkins, 1999–2001.

Journal of Clinical Gastroenterology. Philadelphia: Lippincott Williams & Wilkins, 1999–2001.

Journal of the American Society of Nephrology. Philadelphia: Lippincott Williams & Wilkins, 1996–2001.

Journal of Urology. Baltimore: Lippincott Williams & Wilkins, 1997–2001.

The Latest Word. Philadelphia: Saunders, 1999–2001.

Ostomy/Wound Management. Wayne, PA: HMP Communications, 1999–2000.

Techniques in Urology. Philadelphia: Lippincott Williams & Wilkins, 1999–2000.

Urology Times. Cleveland: Advanstar Communications, 1996.

CDs

UpToDate Clinical Reference Library on CD, Version 8:3. Wellesley, MA: UpToDate, 2000.

Yamada T, Alpers DH, Laine L, Owyang C, Powell DW. Textbook of Gastroenterology, 3rd Edition on CD-ROM. Philadelphia: Lippincott Williams & Wilkins, 1999.

Websites

http://gastroenterology.medscape.com/Home/Topics/gastroenterology/gastroenterology.html

http://urology.medscape.com/Home/Topics/urology/urology.html

http://www.acg.gi.org/

http://www.asge.org/index.jsp

http://www.asn-online.com/

http://www.centerwatch.com/

http://www.duj.com/

http://www.fascrs.org/

http://www.gastro.org/

http://www.hpisum.com

http://www.kidney.org

http://www.mtdaily.com

http://www.mtdesk.com

http://www.niddk.nih.gov/

http://www.virtualdrugstore.com/druglist.html

A

A antigen
A Bayesian nomogram
A bile
A ring
A ring of esophagus

A_4

leukotriene A_4

A2008 ABGII hemodialysis machine
A28 immunological study
A-4 protein
AAA

abdominal aortic aneurysm
aromatic amino acid

AA amyloid
AAC

antibiotic-associated colitis

AAD

antibiotic-associated diarrhea

AAG

antral atrophic gastritis

Aagenaes syndrome
A-a gradient
AAII

atypical adenomatous hyperplasia

AAL

anterior axillary line

AAPBDS

anomalous arrangement of
pancreaticobiliary ductal system

AAPC

antibiotic-associated pseudomembranous
colitis

AAPMC

antibiotic-associated pseudomembranous
colitis

Aaron sign
Aarskog-Scott syndrome
Aarskog syndrome
AAS

acute abdominal series

AASK

African-American Study of Kidney
Disease and Hypertension

AASLD

American Association for the Study of
Liver Diseases

AAT

androgen ablation therapy

AATD

alpha-1-antitrypsin disease

AATD-related emphysema
AAV

adenoassociated virus

AAWC

American Academy of Wound
Management

abacterial pyuria
Abadie enterostomy clamp
Abarelix-D
Abarelix-Depot-F
Abbe

A. intestinal anastomosis
A. small bowel operation

Abbott

A. esophagogastroscopy
A. esophagogastrostomy
A. HCV EIA 2nd generation kit
A. HCV 2.0 test kit
A. IMx PSA assay
A. LifeCare pump
A. Lifeshield needleless system
A. TDx monoclonal fluorescence
polarization immunoassay
A. tube

Abbott-Miller tube
**Abbott-Rawson double-lumen
gastrointestinal tube**
ABC

avidin-biotin complex
ABC reagent

ABD

adynamic bone disease

abdomen

acute surgical a.
boardlike rigidity of a.
boat-shaped a.
carinate a.
diffusely tender a.
distended a.
doughy a.
exquisitely tender a.
flabby a.
flat a.
flat plate of a.
hyperresonant a.
navicular a.
nondistended a.
a. obstipum
pendulous a.
plain film of a.
protuberant a.
resonant a.
rigid a.
rotund a.
scaphoid a.
silent a.
soft a.
splinting of a.

abdomen *(continued)*
    surgical a.
    tight a.
    tympanitic a.
abdominal
    a. abscess
    a. angina
    a. aortic aneurysm (AAA)
    a. aortography
    a. apoplexy
    a. apron
    a. ballottement
    a. bruit
    a. canal
    a. cavity
    a. circumference (AC)
    a. colectomy
    a. compartment syndrome (ACS)
    a. compression (AC)
    a. compression belt
    a. content
    a. crisis
    a. cryptorchidism
    a. cutaneous nerve entrapment syndrome
    a. decompression
    a. desmoid tumor
    a. distention
    a. dropsy
    a. ectopic pregnancy
    a. esophagus
    a. fasciocutaneous flap
    a. fat
    a. fat pad
    a. fistula
    a. fluid wave
    a. fullness
    a. ganglion block
    a. girth
    a. guarding
    a. incision dehiscence
    a. inguinal ring
    a. kidney
    a. laparotomy pad
    a. lavage
    a. leak-point pressure (ALPP)
    a. migraine
    a. muscle deficiency syndrome
    a. nephrectomy
    a. nephrotomy
    a. pain
    a. paracentesis
    a. partitioning
    a. patch electrode
    a. peritoneum
    a. pool
    a. pressure
    a. pressure technique

    a. procedure
    a. pulse
    a. rectopexy
    a. retropexy
    a. rigidity
    a. section
    a. situs inversus
    a. stoma
    a. tap
    a. testis
    a. tomodensitometric examination
    a. tympany (AT)
    a. typhoid
    a. ultrasonography
    a. ureter
    a. vascular accident
    a. viscus
    a. wall
    a. wall hernia
    a. wall mass
    a. wall venous pattern
    a. zone
abdominalgia
    periodic a.
abdominalis
    angina a.
    facies a.
    pulsus a.
    purpura a.
abdominal-wall lift technique
abdominis
    angina a.
    diastasis rectus a.
    hydrops a.
    rectus a.
abdominocentesis
abdominogenital
abdominopelvic orocecal transit time
abdominoperineal
    a. excision
    a. resection (APR)
abdominoplasty
    Ehrlich a.
    Monfort a.
    Randolph a.
abdominosacral resection
abdominoscopy
abdominoscrotal hydrocele
abdominovesical pouch
abenteric
aberrans
    vas a.
    vasculum a.
aberrant
    a. crypt focus (ACF)
    a. mRNA splicing
    a. obturator vein
    a. pancreas

a. suprarenal cortex
a. umbilical stomach
a. ureter

aberrantes
ductuli a.

aberration

aberratio testis

abetalipoproteinemia

ABG
arterial blood gas

ABH blood group

ability
impaired urinary concentrating a.
renal autoregulatory a.

Ablaser laser delivery catheter

ablate-and-chip method

Ablatherm HIFU system

ablation
androgen a.
carbon dioxide laser plaque a.
cold forceps a.
cold snare a.
cryogenic a.
cryosurgical a.
endoscopic thermal a.
homogeneous a.
laser a.
neoadjuvant total androgen a.
photochemical a.
photothermal laser a.
prostate gland needle a.
sphincter of Oddi a.
thermal a.
transurethral needle a. (TUNA)
tumor a.
valve a.
visual laser a.

ablative
a. adrenalectomy
a. laser therapy

ABM
adjusted body mass

abnormality
amino acid a.
atherosclerotic a.
CHARGE a.'s
chromosomal a.
clotting a.
coloboma, heart disease, atresia
choanae, retarded growth, genital
hypoplasia, and ear a.'s
(CHARGE)

congenital urologic a.
crystallization a.
diminished branching a.
electrolyte a.
hematologic a.
hepatic a.
a. of hepatic artery
immunologic a.
laboratory a.
mucosal a.
ocular a.
OEIS a.'s
omphalocele, exstrophy of the
bladder, imperforate anus, and
spinal a.'s
platelet a.
pruning a.
rectosphincteric a.
spinal cord injury without
radiographic a. (SCIWOA)
vascular a.

ABO
ABO barrier
ABO blood group
ABO incompatible

Abocide disinfectant

aboral migration

AB/PAS
Alcian blue and periodic acid-Schiff

Abrams-Griffith nomogram

abrasion
mucosal a.

Abrikosov tumor

abrogate

abrupt pulse

abscess
abdominal a.
amebic liver a.
anal a.
anorectal a.
appendiceal a.
bile duct a.
biliary a.
cavernosal a.
cholangitic a.
cortical a.
crypt a.
cuff a.
deep interloop a.
diaphragmatic a.
distant a.
diverticular a.

NOTES

3

abscess *(continued)*
Douglas a.
echinococcal liver a.
endoscopic transpapillary drainage of pancreatic a.
entamebic a.
Entamoeba histolytica a.
enteroperitoneal a.
epididymal a.
epiploic a.
fecal a.
filarial a.
a. formation
fungal liver a.
gallbladder wall a.
gas a.
gas-forming liver a.
helminthic a.
hepatic a.
high intermuscular a.
horseshoe a.
interloop a.
intermesenteric a.
intersphincteric perirectal a.
intraabdominal a.
intrahepatic a.
intramesenteric a.
intraperitoneal a.
ischiorectal perirectal a.
kidney a.
lacunar a.
liver a.
midabdominal a.
non-gas-forming liver a.
pancreatic pseudocyst a.
paracolic a.
parafrenal a.
paranephric a.
pararectal a.
pelvic a.
pelvirectal a.
percutaneous drainage of epididymal a.
perianal fistula a.
pericecal a.
pericholecystic a.
pericolic a.
perineal a.
perinephric a.
perirectal a.
perirenal a.
peritoneal cavity a.
periureteral a.
periurethral a.
phlegmonous a.
pilonidal perirectal a.
postcecal a.
postoperative a.

preperitoneal a.
prostatic a.
protozoal a.
psoas a.
pyogenic liver a.
rectal a.
renal cortical a.
retrocecal a.
retroesophageal a.
retroperitoneal a.
retroperitoneal-iliopsoas a.
seminal vesicle a.
spermatic a.
splenic a.
stercoraceous a.
stercoral a.
sterile a.
subacute a.
subaponeurotic a.
subcapsular hepatic a.
subdiaphragmatic a.
subhepatic a.
subperitoneal a.
subphrenic a.
suprahepatic a.
supralevator perirectal a.
testicular a.
tympanitic a.
urachal a.
urethral a.
urinary a.
urinous a.

absence
enuretic a.
protein in vitamin K a. (PIVKA)

absent
a. ankle jerk
a. bowel sounds
a. gag reflex
a. peristalsis

Absidia
A. capillata
A. corymbifera
A. ramosum

absolute
a. alcohol
a. alcohol sclerosant
a. diet
a. erythrocytosis
a. sterility

absorbable
a. clip
a. gelatin sponge
a. staple
a. suture

absorbent padding

absorptiometer
QDR 1000 densitometer a.

absorptiometry
dual-energy x-ray a. (DEXA, DXA)
dual-photon a.
absorption
alcohol a.
fluorescent treponemal antibody a. (FTA-ABS)
gastrointestinal a.
impaired gastric a.
oxalate intestinal a.
paracetamol a.
reservoir mucosal a.
transcellular a.
xenobiotic a.
absorptive
a. cell
a. hypercalciuria
a. hyperoxaluria
abstinence
abuse
alcohol a.
ethanol a.
intravenous drug a.
ipecac a.
laxative a.
phencyclidine a.
salicylate a.
sexual a.
substance a.
ABV
doxorubicin, bleomycin sulfate, vinblastine
ABVD
doxorubicin, bleomycin sulfate, vinblastine, dacarbazine
ABW
actual body weight
AC
abdominal circumference
abdominal compression
activated charcoal
acute cholecystitis
adenylate cyclase
alcoholic cirrhosis
Pepcid AC
ACA
adenocarcinoma
anticardiolipin antibody
anticentromere autoantibody
acalculous
a. cholecystitis

a. cholesterolosis
a. gallbladder disease
Acanthocephala
acanthocytosis
acanthosis
glycogenic a.
a. nigricans
acarbose
Ac-5-ASA
N-acetyl-5-ASA
Acationox
ACBE
air-contrast barium enema
accelerated
a. hypertension
a. senescence
a. transplant rejection
acceleration
cavernous artery blood flow a.
accelerator
serum thrombotic a.
access
a. papillotomy
peritoneal a.
vascular a.
accessorium
pancreas a.
accessorius
ductus pancreaticus a.
lien a.
accessory
a. adrenal
Assura irrigation a.
a. duct of Luschka
a. obturator artery
a. pancreas
a. pancreatic duct
a. phallic urethra
a. portal system of Sappey
a. sex gland
a. spleen
a. trocar
a. vessel
accident
abdominal vascular a.
accidental acetaminophen
accordion-like bunching
accordion sign
Accu-Chek III
Accu-Dx test
AccuMeter
ChemTrak A.

NOTES

accumulation
gamma-aminobutyric acid a.
glycoprotein a.
lysosomal a.
tubular iron a.
Accurate catheter
Accuratome pre-curved papillotome
AccuSharp endoscope
Accuson-128 color flow Doppler machine
Accutorr oscillometric device
ACD
adult celiac disease
ACE
angiotensin-converting enzyme
antegrade colonic enema
antegrade continence enema
BICAP silver ACE
ACE gene polymorphism
ACE inhibitor
ACEI
angiotensin-converting enzyme inhibitor
acetabulum
acetaldehyde (Ach)
acetaminophen
accidental a.
a. hepatotoxicity
a. overdose
a. toxicity
acetate
anaritide a.
buserelin a.
calcium a.
chlormadinone a.
cortisone a.
cyproterone a. (CPA)
desmopressin a.
free a.
goserelin a.
hydrocortisone a.
Hydrocortone A.
leuprolide a.
mafenide a.
medroxyprogesterone a.
megestrol a.
methylprednisolone a.
octreotide a.
phorbol myristate a. (PMA)
roxatidine a.
uranyl a.
acetazolamide
acetic acid
acetohydroxamic
a. acid
a. acid irrigation
acetomorphine
acetonemic
acetonitrile eluate

acetonuria
acetowhite lesion
acetylation
acetylcholine
acetylcholinesterase
acetyl coenzyme hypoglycin A
acetylcysteine
acetylsalicylic
a. acid
5-a. acid
acetylsulfadiazine
acetylsulfaguanidine
acetylsulfathiazole
***N*-acetyltransferase 2**
acetyltriglycine renal scan
ACF
aberrant crypt focus
ACG
American College of Gastroenterology
Ach
acetaldehyde
achalasia
a. balloon dilation
a. cardia
classic a.
cricopharyngeal a.
a. dilator
esophageal a.
idiopathic a.
pelvirectal a.
secondary a.
sphincteral a.
vigorous a.
achalasia-like esophagus
achiever
A. balloon dilation catheter
A. balloon dilator
achlorhydria
a. apepsia
gastric a.
histamine-resistant a.
medically induced a.
acholangic
a. biliary cirrhosis
a. biliary fibrosis
acholia
acholic stool
acholuria
acholuric jaundice
achoresis
achromaturia
Achromycin
A. V
achylia
a. gastrica
a. gastrica haemorrhagica
a. pancreatica
achylous

achymia

acid

acetic a.
acetohydroxamic a.
acetylsalicylic a.
5-acetylsalicylic a.
amino a.
aminocaproic a.
aminolevulinic a. (ALA)
5-aminolevulinic a. (5-ALA)
4-aminosalicylic a. (4-ASA)
5-aminosalicylic a. (5-ASA)
amoxicillin-clavulanic a.
anti-double-stranded
  deoxyribonucleic a. (anti-dsDNA)
arachidonic a.
aromatic amino a. (AAA)
ascorbic a.
a. base imbalance
benzoic a.
benzoyl-tyrosyl-paraaminobenzoic a.
  (BT-PABA)
7-beta-epimer of
  chenodeoxycholic a.
bile a. (BA)
branched-chain amino a. (BCAA)
caustic a.
a. cell
chenodeoxycholic a. (CDA, CDCA)
choleic a.
cholic a. (CA)
cinnamic a.
citric a.
clavulanic a.
a. clearance test (ACT)
cocarcinogenic fecal bile a.
complementary deoxyribonucleic a.
  (cDNA)
conjugated bile a.
cyclooxygenase messenger
  ribonucleoprotein a. (COX mRNA)
cysteinesulfinic a.
delta-aminolevulinic a. (d-ALA)
deoxycholic a.
deoxyribonucleic a. (DNA)
Diagnex Blue test for gastric a.
diatrizoic a.
diethylenetriamine pentaacetic a.
  (DTPA)
dihydroxyeicosatrienoic a.
diisopropyliminodiacetic a. (DISDA,
  DISIDA)

dimercaptosuccinic a. (DMSA)
a. dyspepsia
eicosapentaenoic a. (EPA)
epoxyeicosatrienoic a. (EET)
epsilon-aminocaproic a.
essential amino a.
essential fatty a. (EFA)
esterified fecal a.
ethacrynic a.
ethylenediamine tetraacetic a.
  (EDTA)
ethylene glycol tetraacetic a.
  (EGTA)
fatty a.
fecal bile a. (FBA)
folic a.
folinic a.
free fatty a.
free fecal bile a.
gamma-aminobutyric a.
gastric a.
genomic deoxyribonucleic a.
glutamic a.
a. guanidine thiocyanate-phenol-
  chloroform method
a. hematin method
a. hemolysis test
hepatoiminodiacetic a. (HIDA)
hippuric a.
homovanillic a. (HVA)
hyaluronic a.
hydrochloric a. (HCl)
hydroxyeicosatetraenoic a. (HETE)
20-hydroxyeicosatetraenoic a.
hydroxyindoleacetic a. (HIAA)
5-hydroxyindoleacetic a. (5-HIAA)
a. hypersecretion
hypervariable deoxyribonucleic a.
iminodiacetic a. (IDA)
a. indigestion
a. infusion
a. ingestion
a. injury
intravesical hyaluronic a.
iocetamic a.
iopanoic a.
iothalamic a.
^{131}I para-aminohippuric a.
isovaleric a.
keto a.
a. labile
lactic a.

NOTES

acid *(continued)*
    Lewis a.
    linoleic a.
    lithocholic a. (LCA)
    long-chain fatty a. (LCFA)
    luminal a.
    mandelic a.
    medium-chain fatty a. (MCFA)
    mefenamic a.
    2-mercaptoethanesulfonic a. (mesna)
    messenger ribonucleic a. (mRNA)
    methylaminoisobutyric a. (MeAIB)
    2-methylcitric a.
    methylmalonic a.
    a. microclimate
    mucosal fatty a.
    nalidixic a. (NA)
    N-benzoyl-L-tyrosyl-P-
        aminobenzoic a.
    nitroblue tetrazolium-
        paraaminobenzoic acid (NBT-
        PABA)
    nonsulfated bile a.
    Novamine amino a.
    nucleic a.
    oleic a.
    oral bile a. (OBA)
    oxalic a.
    PAH a.
    pantothenic a.
    paraaminobenzoic a. (PABA)
    paraaminohippuric a.
    paraisopropyliminodiacetic a.
        (PIPIDA)
    a. peptic ulcer
    a. perfusion test
    phenazopyridine hydrochloric a.
    a. phosphate osteoclast
    polyglycolic a.
    polyprenoic a.
    pteroylglutamic a.
    a. reflux
    a. reflux test
    a. regurgitation
    renal excretion of a.
    renal messenger ribonucleic a.
    reptilase a.
    retinoic a.
    ribonucleic a. (RNA)
    saponifiable fecal bile a.
    saturated fatty a. (SFA)
    secondary bile a.
    a. secretion
    a. secretory disorder
    seminal plasma citric a.
    serum hyaluronic a.
    serum uric a.
    short-chain fatty a. (SCFA)

    sialic a.
    sulfuric a.
    a. suppression
    tannic a.
    taurocholic a.
    technetium-99m diethylenetriamine
        pentaacetic a. (^{99m}Tc-DPTA)
    technetium-99m pentetic a.
    technetium-99m (Tc-99m)
        iminodiacetic a.
    total bile a. (TBA)
    tranexamic a.
    Travasol amino a.
    tricarboxylic a. (TCA)
    trichloroacetic a. (TCA)
    trihydrocoprostanic a. (TCA)
    unsaturated fatty a.
    uric a.
    ursodeoxycholic a. (UDCA)
    valproic a.
    vanillacetic a. (VLA)
    vanillylmandelic a. (VMA)
acid-ash diet
acid-base
    a.-b. balance
    a.-b. disorder
    a.-b. disturbance
    a.-b. equilibrium
    a.-b. map
acidemia
    isovaleric a.
acid-fast bacillus (AFB)
acidic
    a. environment
    a. epididymal glycoprotein
    a. fibroblast growth factor
    a. sialomucin
    a. sulfomucin
acidification
    a. defect
    duodenal a.
    a. of stool test
    urine a.
acid-inhibitory factor
acidity
    circadian gastric a.
    gastric a.
    intracellular a.
    intragastric a.
    titratable a.
    urinary a.
acid-neutralizing capacity (ANC)
acidopathy
    specific organic a.
acidophilic
    a. body
    a. PAS-positive granule

acidophilus
>a. capsule
>*Lactobacillus a.*
>a. milk

acidosis
>acute a.
>a. after urinary intestinal diversion
>anion gap a.
>bicarbonate wastage renal
>>tubular a.
>
>carbon dioxide a.
>chronic metabolic a.
>congenital lactic a.
>distal renal tubular a. (dRTA)
>high anion gap metabolic a.
>hyperchloremic metabolic a.
>hypokalemic renal tubular a.
>lactic a.
>metabolic a.
>non-anion-gap metabolic a.
>renal tubular a. (RTA)
>renal tubular a. I (RTA-I)
>renal tubular metabolic a.
>renal tubular a. (type I–IV)
>respiratory a.
>uremic a.
>winter a.

acidotic
acid-pepsin reflux esophagitis
acid-peptic
>a.-p. disease
>a.-p. esophagitis
>a.-p. juice

acid-provoked spasm
acid-related disorder (ARD)
acid-Schiff
>Alcian blue and periodic a.-S.
>>(AB/PAS)
>
>periodic a.-S. (PAS)
>a.-S. stain

acid-suppressed stomach
acid-suppression therapy
Acidulin
aciduria
>L-glyceric a.
>3-hydroxy 3-methylglutaric a.

acification
>intracellular a.

acinar
>a. cell
>a. cell carcinoma
>a. defect

>a. gradient
>a. hepatocellular carcinoma
>a. tissue

acinarization of pancreas
Acinetobacter calcoaceticus
acini (*pl. of* acinus)
aciniform
acinitis
acinose
acinotubular
acinous
>a. adenoma
>a. cell

acinus, pl. acini
>liver a.
>pancreatic a.

Aciphex
acipimox
acivicin
ACKD
>acquired cystic kidney disease

ackee fruit poisoning
ACL
>anal canal length

ACLA
>anticardiolipin antibody

aclacinomycin A
Acme One Time enteral feeding bag
ACMI
>ACMI cystourethroscope
>ACMI endoscope
>ACMI fiberoptic colonoscope
>ACMI fiberoptic esophagoscope
>ACMI fiberoptic
>>proctosigmoidoscope
>
>ACMI gastroscope
>ACMI Martin endoscopy forceps
>ACMI monopolar electrode
>ACMI T-915, TX-915 fiberoptic
>>sigmoidoscope
>
>ACMI ulcer measuring device

acnes
>*Propionibacterium a.*

acne vulgaris
aconitine
acontractile detrusor
acontractility
>bladder a.
>detrusor a.

aconuresis
acoprosis
acoprous

NOTES

9

acorn-tipped
    a.-t. bougie
    a.-t. catheter
acorn treatment
acoustically transparent cradle
acoustic blink
acquired
    a. chordee
    a. cystic kidney disease (ACKD)
    a. diverticulosis
    a. functional megacolon
    a. gastric ectopy
    a. hyperlipoproteinemia
    a. hyperoxaluria
    a. immunity
    a. immunodeficiency
    a. immunodeficiency syndrome
      (AIDS)
    a. lactose deficiency
    a. neutrophil chemotaxis defect
    a. pancreatitis
    a. renal artery aneurysm
    a. renal cystic disease (ARCD)
    a. ureteropelvic junction obstruction
acquisita
    epidermolysis bullosa a.
    hypertrichosis lanuginosa a.
acraturesis
acrobystia
acrobystiolith
acrobystitis
acrocephalopolydactylous dysplasia
acrochordon
acrocyanosis
acrodermatitis enteropathica
acrolein
acromegalic
acromphalus
acrophase
acroposthitis
acrosin
acrosome
    a. reaction
    a. reaction assay
acrosome-reacted spermatozoa
acrylate
ACS
    abdominal compartment syndrome
ACT
    acid clearance test
ACTH
    adrenocorticotropic hormone
Acticoat
    A. composite dressing
    A. foam dressing
Acticon neosphincter
Actidose-Aqua
Actigall

actin
    a. filament
    smooth muscle isoform a.
Actinomyces naeslundii
actinomycin C, D
actinomycosis
    biliary a.
    gastric a.
actinomycotic
    a. appendicitis
    a. esophageal disease
actinomycotica
    perityphlitis a.
action
    cytolytic a.
    immunomodulatory a.
    snake venom converting enzyme
      inhibiting a.
    virus-like a. (VLA)
Action-II
Actis venous flow controller (VFC)
activated
    a. alkaline glutaraldehyde
    a. charcoal (AC)
    a. partial thromboplastin time
      (aPTT)
    a. protein C resistance (APCR)
    a. thromboplastin time
activation
    B-lymphocyte a.
    complement a.
    nuclear transcriptional a.
    platelet a.
    selective bladder a.
    T-cell a.
    T-lymphocyte a.
    very late a. (VLA)
activator
    plasminogen a. (PA)
    tissue plasminogen a. (TPA, tPA)
    tissue-type plasminogen a.
    urokinase plasminogen a.
    vascular plasminogen a. (v-PA)
active
    a. bowel sounds
    bowel sounds a. (BSA)
    bowel sounds normal and a.
      (BSNA)
    a. chronic hepatitis
    a. congestion
    a. duodenal ulcer
    A. Living incontinence pad
    A. Living incontinence shield
    a. renin
    a. schistosomiasis
    a. source of bleeding
    a. systemic bacterial infection
    a. transport

actively bleeding varix
activin
    a. A
activity
    adenosine deaminase a.
    a. assay
    ATPase a.
    beta galactosidase a.
    brush-border disaccharidase
      specific a.
    brush-border enzyme a.
    brush-border hydrolase a.
    complement hemolytic a.
    disaccharidase enzyme a.
    efferent renal sympathetic nerve a.
      (ERSNA)
    endogenous peroxidase a.
    fibrinolytic a.
    gastric myoelectrical a.
    gastric urease a.
    hepatic uroporphyrinogen
      decarboxylase a.
    hyaluronidase a.
    intrinsic enzymatic a.
    Knodell criteria for histology a.
    mitotic a.
    motor a.
    muscarinic a.
    myoelectric a.
    NA+/H+ antiporter a.
    Na/K-ATPase a.
    necroinflammatory a.
    opsonic a.
    oxidoreductase a.
    phasic contractile a.
    phospholipase A2 catalytic a.
    plasma renin a. (PRA)
    postheparin lipolytic a. (PHLA)
    protein serine/threonine kinase a.
    PyNPase a.
    renal sympathetic a.
    renal vein renin a. (RVRA)
    renal xanthine oxidase-xanthine
      dehydrogenase a.
    respiratory burst a.
    a. score
    serum cholinesterase a.
    single potential analysis cavernous
      electrical a.
    specific a.
    spike-burst electrical a.
    succinate dehydrogenase a. (SDH)

    sympathetic nervous system a.
    thermic effect of physical a.
      (TEPA)
    tumorigenesis a.
    tyrosine kinase a.
Actril disinfectant
actual
    a. body weight (ABW)
    a. intraprostatic temperature
    a. weight (AW)
Acucise
    A. balloon
    A. balloon catheter
    A. balloon cutting device
    A. endopyelotomy
    A. endopyelotomy catheter
    A. retrograde procedure
    A. RP outpatient procedure
AcuClip endoscopic multiple clip
    applier
acuity
acuminatum, pl. **acuminata**
    condyloma a.
    esophageal condyloma a.
    giant anorectal condyloma a.
acupuncture
AcuSnare polypectomy device
acute
    a. abdominal series (AAS)
    a. abdominal vascular disease
    a. acalculous cholecystitis
    a. acidosis
    a. alcoholic hepatitis
    a. appendicitis
    a. cellular rejection
    a. cholecystitis (AC)
    a. colonic pseudoobstruction
    a. corrosive esophagitis
    a. cystitis
    a. diverticulitis
    a. drug-induced cholestasia
    a. edematous pancreatitis (AEP)
    a. epididymitis
    a. erosive gastritis (AEG)
    a. esophageal food impaction
      (AEFI)
    a. extrarenal obstruction
    a. fatty liver
    a. fatty liver of pregnancy (AFLP)
    a. febrile neutrophilic dermatosis
    a. flank pain
    a. flank pain syndrome

NOTES

acute *(continued)*
a. focal bacterial nephritis (AFBN)
a. gallstone pancreatitis (AGP)
a. gastric anisakiasis
a. gastric ischemia
a. gastric mucosal lesion
a. gastroenteritis (AGE)
a. glomerulonephritis (AGN)
a. graft-versus-host disease
a. hemorrhagic cystitis (AHC)
a. hemorrhagic gastritis
a. hemorrhagic pancreatitis
a. hepatic coma
a. hepatic failure
a. hepatic rupture
a. hepatic toxicity
a. hepatitis (AH)
a. hepatocellular degeneration
a. hydramnios
a. hypokalemic nephropathy
a. idiopathic inflammatory bowel disease
a. infectious colitis
a. infectious diarrhea
a. infectious nonbacterial gastroenteritis
a. infundibulopelvic angle
a. intermittent porphyria (AIP)
a. interstitial nephritis (AIN)
a. intrinsic renal failure
a. juvenile cirrhosis
a. lead poisoning
a. leukopenia
a. liver failure (ALF)
a. lymphoblastic leukemia
a. lymphocytic leukemia
a. megacolon
a. mercury poisoning
a. mesangial proliferative glomerulonephritis
a. methanol intoxication
a. mononucleosis-like hepatitis
a. MVT
a. myelomonocytic leukemia
a. necrotizing esophagitis
a. nephrosis
a. nonobstructive pyelonephritis
a. nonocclusive bowel infarction
a. nonvariceal upper gastrointestinal hemorrhage
a. obstructive cholangitis
a. obstructive suppurative cholangitis (AOSC)
a. occlusive mesenteric ischemia
a. on chronic liver disease (AOCLD)
a. parenchymatous hepatitis
a. phase protein

a. physiology, age and chronic health evaluation (APACHE)
a. polycystic disease
a. porphyria
a. poststreptococcal glomerulonephritis (APSGN)
a. proctitis
a. recurrent pancreatitis (ARP)
a. rejection of liver transplant
a. relapsing pancreatitis
a. renal failure (ARF)
a. renal insufficiency (ARI)
a. renal transplant vasculopathy
a. schistosomiasis
a. sclerosing hyaline necrosis (ASHN)
a. scrotum
a. self-limited colitis (ASLC)
a. self-limited hepatitis
a. serum sickness nephritis
a. suppurative cholangitis (ASC)
a. surgical abdomen
a. tubular necrosis (ATN)
a. tubular necrosis backleak
a. urate nephropathy
a. ureteric colic
a. urethral syndrome
a. urethritis
a. urinary retention (AUR)
a. vascular rejection
a. viral hepatitis (AVH)
a. yellow atrophy
acute-phase response element (APRE)
AcuTrainer hand-held electronic device
Acutrim
acyclovir sodium
acylic retinoid
acyltransferase
lecithin-cholesterol a. (LCAT)
acystia
acystinervia
acystineuria
ADA
American Diabetes Association
ADA diet
Adair-Allis forceps
Adalat CC
Adamantiades-Behçet syndrome
Adapin
adaptation
failed a.
intestinal a.
adapter, adaptor
camera a.
C-mount a.
Cook plastic Luer lock a.
friction-fit a.
Olympus a.

Polaroid SX-70 with ACMI a.
Ralks a.
swivel a.
Tuohy-Borst a.
Y a.

adaptic
    a. colitis
    A. dressing
    A. packing

adaptive
    a. gastroprotection
    a. immunity
    a. relaxation
    a. thermogenesis (AT)

adaptor (*var. of* adapter)

ADC
    antral diverticulum of the colon

ADCC
    antibody-dependent cell-mediated
      cytotoxicity
    antibody-dependent cellular cytotoxicity

Adcon-P adhesion barrier solution

ADD
    angled delivery device

Add-A-Cath
    Lawrence A.-A-C.

add-back treatment

Addis method

Addison
    A. crisis
    A. disease
    A. plane
    A. point
    A. syndrome

addisonian syndrome

addisonii
    melasma a.

additional unproven role

addressin

ADD'Stat laser

adduction
    arytenoid a.

adductor
    a. brevis muscle
    a. longus muscle

ADE
    apparent digestive energy

adelomorphous cell

adenasthenia gastrica

adenemphraxis

Aden fever

adenine
    a. phosphoribosyltransferase (APRT)
    a. phosphoribosyltransferase
      deficiency

adenitis
    mesenteric a.
    phlegmonous a.
    syphilitic inguinal a.

adenoacanthoma

adenoassociated virus (AAV)

adenocarcinoma (ACA)
    annular a.
    appendiceal a.
    bladder mesonephric a.
    clear cell a.
    colloid-producing a.
    colonic a.
    colorectal a.
    duodenal a.
    esophageal a.
    exophytic a.
    flat rectal a.
    gastric a.
    giant cell a.
    hepatoid a.
    a. of infantile testis
    infiltrating a.
    invasive a.
    metachronous small bowel a.
    metastatic a.
    mucinous a.
    mucin-producing a.
    mucosal a.
    papillary a.
    Paris renal a.
    peritoneal a.
    prostatic a.
    renal a.
    rete testis a.
    scirrhous a.
    seminal vesicle a.
    a. in situ
    testicular a.
    ulcerating a.
    urachal a.

adenofibromyoma
    testicular a.

adenohypersthenia gastrica

adenoid cystic carcinoma

adenolelomyofibroma

adenolysis

NOTES

13

adenoma
    acinous a.
    adrenal cortex a.
    adrenocortical a.
    aggressive a.
    aldosterone a.
    bile duct a. (BDA)
    bladder nephrogenic a.
    Brunner gland a.
    carcinoma ex pleomorphic a.
    chromophobe a.
    colonic a.
    colorectal villous a.
    cortical a.
    depressed a.
    a. destruens
    duodenal a.
    embryonal a.
    flat a.
    hepatic a.
    hepatocellular a. (HCA)
    incidental a.
    islet cell a.
    kidney a.
    Leydig cell a.
    liver cell a. (LCA)
    mesonephric a.
    metachronous a.
    moderately differentiated a.
    mucinous a.
    nephrogenic a.
    nonhyperfunctioning
      adrenocortical a.
    nonpolypoid a.
    papillary a.
    periampullary a. (PAA)
    Pick tubular a.
    pituitary a.
    poorly differentiated a.
    prostatic a.
    rectal villous a.
    renal cortical a.
    a. sebaceum
    serrated a.
    sessile a.
    sheet-like a.
    synchronous a.
    testicular tubular a.
    tubulovillous a.
    undifferentiated a.
    villoglandular a.
    villous colorectal a.
    well-differentiated a.
adenoma-associated antigen
adenoma-carcinoma sequence
adenoma-hyperplastic polyp ratio
adenoma-nonadenoma ratio
adenomatoid tumor

adenomatosis
    multiple endocrine a. type I
      (MEA-I)
    multiple endocrine a. type II
      (MEA-II)
adenomatous
    a. colorectal polyp
    a. epithelium
    a. gastric polyp
    a. hyperplasia (AH)
    a. polyp (AP)
    a. polyp-cancer sequence
    a. polyposis
    a. polyposis coli (APC)
    a. polyposis coli gene
adenomucinosis
    disseminated peritoneal a.
adenomyoepithelioma of stomach
adenomyoma of gallbladder
adenomyomatosis
    gallbladder a.
adenomyosarcoma
adenomyosis
adenopapillomatosis
    gastric a.
adenopathy
    axillary a.
    inguinal a.
    lymph node a.
    palpable a.
    paraductal a.
adenosarcoma
    embryonal a.
adenosine
    a. deaminase
    a. deaminase activity
    a. diphosphatase (ADPase)
    a. diphosphate (ADP)
    a. monophosphate (AMP)
    a. nucleotide
    a. signal
    a. triphosphatase (ATPase)
    a. triphosphate (ATP)
adenosis
    sclerosing a.
adenosquamous cell carcinoma
adenovirus
    a. colitis
    enteric a.
    human a. 12
    a. infection
adenovirus-12 viral protein
adenylate
    a. cyclase (AC)
    a. cyclase complex
adenyl cyclase stimulation
adequacy
    dialysis a.

a. issue
urea a.
ADF
aortoduodenal fistula
ADH
alcohol dehydrogenase
antidiuretic hormone
adherence
a. assay
bacterial a.
adherent clot
adhesin
bacterial a.
adhesion
antigen-independent a.
attic a.
bacterial a.
banjo-string a.
cell-cell a.
coronal a.
dense a.
a. dyspepsia
filmy a.
a. formation
freeing up of a.
hard a.
hepatic a.
intraabdominal a.
intraperitoneal a.
lysis of a.
mannose-specific a.
a. molecule
omental a.
pelvic a.
perihepatic a.
peritoneal a.
postcholecystitis a.
postoperative a.
preputial a.
taking down of a.
T-cell a.
thick a.
thin a.
tight perirectal a.
tuft a.
violin-string a.
adhesive
a. band
Comfeel skin a.
a. dressing
fibrin tissue a.
a. ileus

Indermil a.
Mastisol liquid surgical a.
a. protein receptor
a. tape
Uro-Bond skin a.
ADHF
American Digestive Health Foundation
Adipex-P
adiphenine
adipocele
adipohepatic
adipolytic
adipopectic
adipopexis
adipose tissue
adiposis
a. hepatica
a. orchalis
adiposogenital dystrophy
adiposum
hepar a.
adiposuria
adiposus
ascites a.
adjunctive nephrectomy
adjustable silicone gastric banding (ASGB)
adjusted body mass (ABM)
adjustment
risk a.
adjuvant
a. alpha blockade
anesthesia a.
a. drug therapy
Freund a.
a. hepatic arterial infusion chemotherapy
a. nephrectomy
a. treatment
administration
intravesical electromotive drug a. (EMDA)
percutaneous bacille Calmette-Guérin a.
adnexal
a. fullness
a. mass
a. tenderness
a. torsion
a. tumor
adolescent
a. genitalia

NOTES

adolescent *(continued)*
  a. genitourinary examination
  a. incontinence
  a. penis
  a. spina bifida
  a. stress hematuria
  a. urologic evaluation
adoptive immunotherapy
ADP
  adenosine diphosphate
ADPase
  adenosine diphosphatase
ADPKD
  autosomal dominant polycystic kidney
    disease
    oligosymptomatic ADPKD
ADPKD1
  ADPKD1 gene
  ADPKD1 genotype
ADPKD2 genotype
ADR
  Adriamycin
adrenal
  accessory a.
  a. artery
  a. catecholamine
  a. cortex
  a. cortex adenoma
  a. cortex androgen
  a. cortex carcinoma
  a. cortex estrogen-secreting tumor
  a. cortex fine-needle biopsy
  a. cortex ganglioneuroma
  a. cortex hyperfunction
  a. cortex testosterone-secreting
    tumor
  a. cortex zone
  a. corticoadenoma
  a. crisis
  a. cryptococcosis
  a. disease
  a. gland
  a. gland atrophy
  a. gland composition
  a. gland cyst
  a. gland incidentaloma
  a. gland innervation
  a. gland laparoscopic excision
  a. gland mass
  a. gland melanoma
  a. gland metastatic tumor
  a. gland microscopic section
  a. gland myelolipoma
  a. hemorrhage
  a. hirsutism
  a. insufficiency
  Marchand a.'s
  a. medulla

  a. rest
  a. rest tumor
  a. scintigraphy
  a. steroid
  a. tuberculosis
  a. vein
  a. vein aldosterone sampling
  a. venography
  a. virilism
  a. zona glomerulosa hyperplasia
adrenalectomy
  ablative a.
  endoscopic a.
  flank approach a.
  ipsilateral a.
  laparoscopic a.
  needlescopic a.
  open a.
  partial a.
  retroperitoneoscopic a.
  transperitoneal laparoscopic a.
    (TLA)
adrenalin
  a. chloride
  a. injection
  a. injection therapy
adrenalinuria
adrenal-sparing surgery
adrenergic
  a. neuron
  a. receptor
  a. signal
adrenergic-cholinergic agonist
adrenoceptive
adrenocortical
  a. adenoma
  a. macrocyst
adrenocorticohyperplasia
adrenocorticotropic
  a. hormone (ACTH)
  a. hormone infusion test
adrenogenital syndrome
adrenomedullin 52-amino acid peptide
adrenoreceptor
  alpha-1 a.
adrenostatic
adrenotoxin
adrenotropic
adrenotropin
adrenotropism
Adriamycin (ADR)
  cisplatin, cyclophosphamide, A.
    (CISCA)
  A. glomerulopathy
  A. nephropathy
  A. PFS
Adriamycin-induced nephrosis
Adrucil

Adson
  A. clamp
  A. dissecting hook
  A. needle holder
  A. suction tube
  A. tissue forceps
Adson-Brown tissue forceps
adsorption
adult
  a. celiac disease (ACD)
  a. familial hyaline membrane
    disease
  a. hypolactasia
  a. lactase deficiency
  a. phimosis
  a. polycystic disease (APCD)
  a. polycystic kidney disease
    (APKD)
  a. polycystic liver disease (APLD)
  a. respiratory distress syndrome
  a. sigmoidoscope
adult-onset
  a.-o. enuresis
  a.-o. obesity
advance
  A. formula
  a. to regular diet
advanced
  A. Care cholesterol test
  a. glycation end (AGE)
  A. surgical suture applier
  a. therapeutic endoscopy
advancement
  Duckett meatal a.
  Glenn-Anderson a.
  meatal a.
  a. of rectal flap
  sleeve a.
  a. sleeve flap
Advanta bed
advantage
  GE RT 3200 A. II
Advantx digital system
adventitia
  fibrofatty a.
  tunica a.
adventitial fibroplasia
adventitious
  a. albuminuria
  a. cyst
adverse prognostic factor

advice
  dietary a.
adynamic
  a. bone
  a. bone disease (ABD)
  a. ileus
  a. intestinal obstruction
adysplasia
  kidney a.
Adzorbstar
AEC
  American Endosonography Club
  AEC Study
AEFI
  acute esophageal food impaction
AEG
  acute erosive gastritis
AELT
  ascites euglobulin lysis time
AEP
  acute edematous pancreatitis
AER
  albumin excretion rate
  automatic endoscopic reprocessor
AERD
  atheroembolic renal disease
aerobic
  a. culture
  a. glycolysis
aerobilia
Aerochamber pediatric spacer device
Aerococcus
aerocystography
aerocystoscope
aerocystoscopy
aerogastria
  blocked a.
aerogenes
  Enterobacter a.
aerogenosum
  sputum a.
Aeromonas
  A. *caviae*
  A. *diarrhea*
  A. *hydrophila*
  A. *liquefaciens*
  A. *punctata*
  A. *salmonicida*
  A. *sobria*
Aeromonas-**associated enterocolitis**
aeroperitonia
aerophagia, aerophagy

NOTES

aerosialophagy
aerosis
aerosol
>hydrocortisone acetate rectal a.
>inhalation a.
>^{99m}Tc DTPA a.

aerourethroscopy
aeruginosa
>*Pseudomonas a.*

AES
>anal endosonography
>anterior esophageal sensor

AESOP
>automated endoscopic system for optimal positioning
>AESOP ReView feature

aethoxysclerol
AFB
>acid-fast bacillus

AFBN
>acute focal bacterial nephritis

afferent
>a. arteriolar vasoconstriction
>a. fiber
>a. glomerular arteriole
>a. ileal limb
>a. innervation
>a. limb nipple stenosis
>a. loop
>a. loop syndrome
>mechanosensitive a.
>a. neuron
>a. projection
>a. renal nerve
>splanchnic primary a.
>a. terminal
>a. tubular isoperistaltic segment

afferentia
>vasa a.

affinity
affinity-avidity hypothesis
AFIP
>Armed Forces Institute of Pathology

aflatoxin
AFLP
>acute fatty liver of pregnancy

AFP
>alpha fetoprotein

African
>A. hemochromatosis
>A. iron overload

African-American
>A.-A. Study of Kidney Disease
>A.-A. Study of Kidney Disease and Hypertension (AASK)

africanum
>*Pygeum a.*

AFTP
>ascitic fluid total protein

AGA
>American Gastroenterological Association
>antigliadin antibody
>IgG AGA
>>immunoglobulin G antigliadin antibody

agalactiae
>*Streptococcus a.*

agalactosuria
agammaglobulinemia
>Bruton-type a.
>X-linked infantile a.

aganglionic
>a. bowel
>a. megacolon
>a. segment of colon

aganglionosis
>congenital intestinal a. (CIA)

agar
>brain-heart infusion a.
>a. bridge
>a. dilution
>EMB a.
>eosin-methylene blue a.
>a. gel
>MacConkey a.
>phenylethyl alcohol a.
>Sabouraud glucose a.
>sorbitol-MacConkey a.
>thiosulfate-citrate-bile salts-sucrose a. (TCBS)
>vancomycin/nalidixic acid a.
>Wilkins-Chalgren a.

agarose
>a. gel
>a. gel electrophoresis

agastria
agastric
AGE
>acute gastroenteritis
>advanced glycation end

agency
>Regional Organ Procurement A. (ROPA)

agenesis
>bladder a.
>corpus callosum a.
>kidney a.
>renal a.
>sacral a.
>scrotal a.
>seminal vesicle a.

agenitalism
agenosomia

agent
Albunex imaging/contrast a.
antiadhesive a.
anticholinergic a.
antidiarrheal a.
antidiuretic hormone-like a.
antifungal a.
antihypertensive a.
antimicrobial a.
antimotility a.
antimuscarinic a.
antisecretory a.
antispasmodic a.
5-ASA a.
azole antifungal a.
benzamide prokinetic a.
beta-sympathomimetic tocolytic a.
bulk a.
bulking a.
carbon dioxide trapping a.
central adrenergic a.
contrast a.
cyanocobalamin radioactive a.
cytotoxic a.
distal tubular acting a.
Durasphere injectable bulking a.
embolic a.
gallstone-solubilizing a.
gastrokinetic a.
Hawaii a.
hemostatic a.
imidoacetic acid radioactive a.
interleukin-2 receptor-blocking a.
iodinated contrast a.
iopamidol contrast imaging a.
Levovist contrast a.
Macroplastique soft tissue synthetic
  bulking a.
motility a.
mucolytic a.
nonsteroidal antiinflammatory a.
  (NSAIA)
Norwalk a.
parasympathomimetic a.
peripheral adrenergic a.
periurethral bulking a.
pharmacological a.
progesteronal a.
prokinetic a.
Racobalamin-57 radioactive a.
Robengatope radioactive a.

rose bengal sodium ^{131}I
  radioactive a.
Rubratope-57 radioactive a.
sclerosing a.
selenomethionine radioactive a.
Sethotope radioactive a.
test-yolk buffer cryopreservation a.
thrombolytic a.
vanilloid a.
virucidal a.
age-related nocturia
ageusia
ageusic
agglutination test
agglutinin
peanut a. (PNA)
aggregate
lymphoid a.
aggregati
folliculi lymphatici a.
aggregation
bile salt a.
erythrocyte a.
familial a.
aggressive
a. adenoma
a. fibromatosis
a. therapeutic trial
agilis
Lactobacillus a.
aging
chemoprevention of a.
aglomerular
AGM1470
AGN
acute glomerulonephritis
agona
Salmonella a.
agonadal
agonadism
agonic intussusception
agonist
adrenergic-cholinergic a.
alpha-1 a.
alpha-adrenergic a.
alpha-2-adrenergic a.
Bay K 8644 channel a.
beta-2 a.
beta-3 a.
beta-adrenergic a.
cholinergic a.
dopamine a.

NOTES

19

agonist *(continued)*
 dopaminergic a.
 5-HT4 a.
 kappa receptor opioid a.
 muscarinic cholinergic a.
 nicotinic a.
 nonpeptidyl a.
 opioid receptor a. (ORA)
Agoral
AGP
 acute gallstone pancreatitis
agranulocytic ulcer
AGUS
 atypical glandular cells of unknown
  significance
AH
 acute hepatitis
 adenomatous hyperplasia
 alcoholic hepatitis
ahaustral
AHC
 acute hemorrhagic cystitis
AHLT
 auxiliary heterotopic liver transplantation
AHO
 Albright hereditary osteodystrophy
AHS
 antiepileptic drug hypersensitivity
AID
 artificial insemination donor
AIDS
 acquired immunodeficiency syndrome
AIDS-related complex (ARC)
AIH
 artificial insemination husband
 autoimmune hepatitis
AIN
 acute interstitial nephritis
 anal intraepithelial neoplasia
AIO
 all-in-one
  AIO parenteral solution
AIP
 acute intermittent porphyria
 aldosterone-induced protein
AIPRI
 Angiotensin-Converting Enzyme
  Inhibition in Progressive Renal
  Insufficiency
  AIPRI trial
air
 biliary a.
 blood gas on room a.
 a. cushion
 a. cyst
 a. cystogram
 a. embolism
 free a.

 a. insufflation
 intramural colonic a.
 intraperitoneal a.
 a. pressure enema reduction
 a. pyelography
 a. swallowing
 a. thermometer
 a. tightness test
air-contrast barium enema (ACBE)
air-filled
 a.-f. balloon
 a.-f. loop
airflow obstruction
air-fluid level
airfuge
 Beckman a.
airway
 double-lumen gastric laryngeal
  mask a.
 a. epithelium
 esophageal gastric tube a. (EGTA)
 esophageal obturator a. (EOA)
 gastric laryngeal mask a. (GLMA)
 a. obstruction
 patent a.
airway-arterial fistula
AJCC TNM tumor classification
AJCC/UICC
 American Joint Committee on
  Cancer/International Union Against
  Cancer
  AJCC/UICC staging system
Ajmalin
 A. liver disease
 A. liver injury
AJPBD
 anomalous junction of pancreaticobiliary
  ducts
Akerlund
 A. deformity
 diverticulum of A.
akinesia
 rectal a.
ALA
 aminolevulinic acid
5-ALA
 5-aminolevulinic acid
Alagille syndrome
Alagille-Watson syndrome
AL amyloid
alanine aminotransferase (ALT)
alanine-glyoxylate aminotransferase
alarm
 bed-wetting a.
 a. clock voiding
 enuresis a.
 glutaraldehyde a.

a. symptom
a. therapy
Alaxin
Alazide
alba
linea a.
Albarran
A. deflecting level
A. disease
A. gland
A. laser cystoscope
A. mechanism
A. reflecting bridge
A. test
A. tubule
albendazole
albensis
Vibrio cholerae biotype *a.*
Albert-Lembert suture
Albert suture
albicans
Candida a.
albiduria
Albright
A. hereditary osteodystrophy (AHO)
A. solution
A. syndrome
Albuferon
albuginea
a. penis
a. testis
tunica a.
albugineotomy
albugineous
albuginitis
albumin
^{125}I-a.
Bence Jones a.
bovine serum a. (BSA)
diethylenetriamine-pentaacetic acid-galactosyl-human serum a. (technetium GSA)
a. excretion rate (AER)
fatty acid-free bovine serum a.
glycated a.
a. gradient
human a.
human serum a.
intravenous a.
macroaggregated a. (MAA)
a. messenger RNA
a. metabolism

nonglycated a.
plasma a.
a. plasma concentration
serum a.
sonicated a.
a. synthesis
technetium-99m galactosyl-human serum a. (^{99m}Tc-GSA)
technetium-99m macroaggregated a. (^{99m}Tc-MAA)
albuminaturia
albumin-coated resin hemoperfusion
albuminocholia
albuminorrhea
albuminous nephritis
albuminuria
adventitious a.
Bamberger hematogenic a.
globular a.
nephrogenous a.
postrenal a.
residual a.
albuminuric retinitis
albumosuria
Bence Jones a.
Albunex
A. imaging/contrast agent
A. injection
albus
Staphylococcus a.
Albustix test
albuterol
alcalifaciens
Providencia a.
Alcian
A. blue
A. blue dye
A. blue and periodic acid-Schiff (AB/PAS)
A. blue stain
Alcock
A. canal
A. syndrome
Alcock-Timberlake obturator
alcohol
absolute a.
a. absorption
a. abuse
a. consumption
a. cooling bath
a. dehydrogenase (ADH)
a. dehydrogenase inhibition

NOTES

alcohol *(continued)*
   a. diuresis
   ethyl a.
   graded a.
   a. injection of tumor
   a. intoxication
   isoamyl a.
   polyvinyl a.
   a. potentiation
   a. sclerosis
   a. thermometer
alcohol-fixed gastric biopsy
alcoholic
   a. cirrhosis (AC)
   a. diarrhea
   a. fatty liver
   a. fibrosis
   a. hemorrhagic gastritis
   a. hepatitis (AH)
   a. hyalin
   a. liver disease (ALD)
   a. pancreatitis
   a. prognostic factor
   a. varix
alcohol-induced
   a.-i. extracellular volume
     contraction
   a.-i. gastric injury
   a.-i. gastrointestinal symptom
   a.-i. hypoglycemia
   a.-i. pancreatitis
alcoholuria
Alconefrin
ALD
   alcoholic liver disease
Aldactazide
Aldactone
Aldara
aldehyde dehydrogenase (ALDH)
Alden loop gastric bypass
aldesleukin
   Proleukin a.
ALDH
   aldehyde dehydrogenase
Aldoclor
aldolase
   fructose a.
Aldomet
Aldoril
aldose reductase (AR)
aldosterone
   a. adenoma
   a. deficiency
   a. synthase
   a. synthase polymorphism
aldosterone-induced protein (AIP)
aldosterone-sensitive distal nephron
aldosterone-to-renin ratio

aldosteronism
aldosteronoma
aldosteronopenia
aldosteronuria
Aldrich-Mees line
Aldridge operation
alendronate
Aleo meter
alert
   Sears Wee A.
Alexander-Adams operation
Alexander elevator
alexandrite
   a. laser
   a. laser lithotripsy
   a. and rhodamine
alexithymia
aleydigism
ALF
   acute liver failure
   American Liver Foundation
alfa
   epoetin a.
alfa-2a
   interferon a.-2a
   PEG-interferon a.-2a
   recombinant interferon a.-2a
   teceleukin and interferon a.-2a
alfa-2b
   interferon a.-2b
alfacon-1
   interferon a.
alfa-n1
   interferon a.-n.
alfa-n3
   interferon a.-n.
alfaxalone
alfentanil
Alferon
   A. N
alfuzosin
Algenic Alka
algesimeter
   Boas a.
Al-Ghorab
   A.-G. modification
   A.-G. modification shunt
   A.-G. procedure
Algicon
algidicarnis
   Clostridium a.
algid malaria
alginate spray
alginolyticus
   Vibrio a.
alginuresis
Alglucerase
algoid cell

algorithm
    current a.
    management a.
    specific a.
Alibra
alimentary
    a. apparatus
    a. bolus
    a. canal
    a. diabetes
    a. edema
    a. glycosuria
    a. hyperinsulinism
    a. obesity
    a. system
    a. therapy
    a. tract
    a. tract duplication
alimentation
    central venous a.
    enteral a.
    forced a.
    parenteral a.
    peripheral intravenous a.
    rectal a.
    total parenteral a.
Alimentum
aliquot
AlitraQ
Alka
    Algenic A.
alkali
    caustic a.
    a. ingestion
alkaline
    a. citrate therapy
    a. injury
    a. milk drip
    a. phosphatase (ALP, AP)
    a. phosphatase antialkaline
      phosphatase (APAAP)
    a. phosphatase isoenzyme
    a. phosphatase test
    a. reflux esophagitis
    a. reflux gastritis
alkaline-ash diet
alkalinity
alkalinization
    a. test
    urinary a.
alkalitherapy

alkaloid
    ergot a.
    indolalkylamine a.
    Veratrum a.
alkalosis
    hypochloremic hypokalemic
      metabolic a.
    hypokalemic metabolic a.
    metabolic a.
    respiratory a.
    watery diarrhea with
      hypokalemic a. (WDHA)
Alka-Mints
alkane
    breath a.
alkaptonuria
Alka-Seltzer
Alken approach
Alkets
allantoic
    a. cyst
    a. tract
allantois
allele
    HLA-DP a.
    I1307K a.
allelic
    DC locus a.
allelotyping
    p53 a.
Allemann syndrome
Allen
    A. anastomosis clamp
    A. intestinal clamp
    A. intestinal forceps
    A. stirrups
    A. strap
    A. test
Allen-Brown shunt
Allen-Kocher clamp
Allen-Masters syndrome
allergen
    food a.
allergic
    a. colitis
    a. cystitis
    a. dermatitis
    a. enteropathy
    a. interstitial nephritis
    a. proctitis
    a. reaction
    a. vasculitis

NOTES

allergy
>cow's milk a. (CMA)
>cow's milk protein a.
>food a.
>gastrointestinal a.
>latex a.
>medication a.

all four quadrants
ALLHAT
>Antihypertensive and Lipid-Lowering Treatment to Prevent Heart Attack Trial

Alliance integrated inflation system
alligator jaws Olympus FG 6L grasping forceps
alligator-type grasping forceps
Allingham
>A. colotomy
>A. fissure
>A. operation
>A. rectum excision
>A. ulcer

all-in-one (AIO)
Allis
>A. catheter
>A. clamp
>A. forceps
>A. inhaler
>A. tooth grasper

Alliston GE reflux repair
allium vegetable
alloantigen response
allocating cadaveric kidney
allocation
>Eurotransplant kidney a.

allochezia, allochetia
allodynia
allogeneic
>a. mixed leukocyte culture
>a. MLC

allogenic
>a. kidney transplant
>a. liver perfusion

allograft
>clinically stable human renal a.
>hepatic a.
>human leukocyte antigen renal a.
>kidney a.
>nephrectomy a.
>a. parenchyma
>a. rejection
>renal a.
>Repliform dermal a.
>a. survival
>a. survival rate

allograft-mediated hypertension
alloplast
>bioactive antimicrobial coated solid a.

alloplastic
>a. biomaterial
>a. prostatic bladder
>a. spermatocele

allopurinol
allotransplantation
allowance
>recommended daily a. (RDA)

alloy
>shape memory a. (SMA)

All-Silicone Side-Eye EPT feeding tube
allylamine
Allyn stirrups
Almacone
>A. II

AlmethaPred
aloe
>cascara sagrada and a.

Aloka MP-PN ultrasound probe
alopecia
alosetron hydrochloride
ALP
>alkaline phosphatase

alpha
>estrogen receptor a. (ER alpha)
>a. fetoprotein (AFP)
>a. gene
>a. glycerylphosphorylcholine
>a. heavy-chain disease
>A. I inflatable penile prosthesis
>a. interferon
>interferon a.
>a. interferon treatment
>a. ketoglutaramate
>a. motor neuron
>a. sigmoid loop
>a. sympathetic blockade

alpha-1
>a.-1 adrenoreceptor
>a.-1 agonist
>a.-1 blocker

alpha-2
>a.-2 globulin

alpha-1-acid glycoprotein
alpha-1-adrenoceptor antagonist
alpha-21 antiplasmin
alpha-3-beta-1 integrin
alpha-5-beta-1 integrin
alpha-adducin
alpha-adrenergic
>a.-a. agonist
>a.-a. antagonist
>a.-a. receptor

alpha-2-adrenergic
>a.-2-a. agonist
>a.-2-a. receptor

alpha-1-adrenergic receptor

alpha-amylase
    pancreatic a.-a.
5-alpha-androstane-3-alpha, 17-beta-diol
5-alpha-androstanc-3-beta, 17-beta-diol
alpha-1-antitrypsin
    a.-1-a. deficiency
    a.-1-a. deficiency disease
    a.-1-a. disease (AATD)
    a.-1-a. disease-related emphysema
    a.-1-a. globulin
    a.-1-a. level
alpha-2b
    interferon a.
alpha-2-beta-1 integrin cell-surface
  collagen
alpha-blocker
    a.-b. therapy
    a.-b. treatment
alpha-chain disease
alpha-delta-mannosidase
alpha-dextrinase
alpha-fetoprotein level
9-alpha-fluorohydrocortisone
alpha-galactosidase A
alpha-gliadin fraction
alpha-glucosidase inhibitor
alpha-1-glycero-monooctanoin
alpha-hemolytic Streptococcus
alpha-interferon therapy
alpha-ketoacid dehydrogenase
alpha-loop maneuver
alpha-methylparatyrosine
Alphamul
alphaprodine
alpha-receptor
    a.-r. antagonist
    a.-r. blockade therapy
5-alpha-reductase
    5-a.-r. inhibition
    5-a.-r. inhibitor
alpha *Streptococcus viridans*
alpha-TGI
Alport syndrome
ALPP
    abdominal leak-point pressure
alprazolam
alprostadil/prazosin HCl
alprostadil urethral suppository
Alprox-TD
ALR cystoresectoscope
Alseroxylon-Alkavervir
Alstrom disease

Alstrom-Edwards syndrome
ALT
    alanine aminotransferase
    ALT test
Altace
Altemeier
    A. perineal rectosigmoidectomy
    A. repair
alteplase
alteration
    genetic a.
    molecular genetic a.
    nuclear matrix a.
altered sperm motility
ALternaGEL
alternate-day treatment
alternate mRNA splicing
alternating calculus
alternative cell attachment domain
Altertome
    Microvasive A.
Althausen test
Altmann pulse
Altracin
ALTRA-FLUX hemodialyzer
ALT-RCC
    autolymphocyte-based treatment for renal
    cell carcinoma
altretamine
Alu-Cap
Aludrox
alum
    a. curd
    intravesical a.
aluminum
    a. carbonate
    a. hydroxide
    a. hydroxide, magnesium hydroxide,
    and simethicone
    a. hydroxide and magnesium
    trisilicate
    a. phosphate
    a. toxicity
Alupent
Alutabs
alvei
    Hafnia a.
alveolar
    a. hydatid cyst
    a. hydatid disease
    a. rhabdomyosarcoma

NOTES

25

AlveoSampler
    Quintron A.
alverine citrate
alvi
    incontinentia a.
alvine calculus
alvus
Alzer Model 2001 osmotic minipump
AMA
    antimitochondrial antibody
    AMA inflatable cylinder
Amadori product
AMAG
    autoimmune metaplastic atrophic gastritis
amalonaticus
    Citrobacter a.
Amanita
    Amanita mushroom
    Amanita mushroom hepatotoxicity
    Amanita phalloides mushroom
      poisoning
amantadine
Amaryl
amasesis
amastigote
amatoxin
amaurosis
    Leber a.
ambenonium chloride
Ambicor penile prosthesis
ambigua
    Shigella a.
ambiguous external genitalia
ambiguus
    nucleus a.
Ambilhar
AmB-induced reduction GFR
ambiothermic
amblygeustia
ambulation
ambulatory
    a. blood pressure
    a. hemorrhoidectomy
    a. intraesophageal bilirubin
      monitoring
    a. intraesophageal pH monitoring
    a. manometry
    a. probe
    a. urodynamic monitoring
    a. urodynamics
amebiasis
    a. of bladder
    hepatic a.
    indigenous a.
amebic
    a. appendicitis
    a. colitis
    a. dysentery

    a. granuloma
    a. hepatitis
    a. lectin antigen
    a. liver abscess
    a. ulcer
amebicidal
ameboma
ameliorate
ameliorated vasodilating response
America
    Crohn and Colitis Foundation
      of A. (CCFA)
American
    A. Academy of Wound
      Management (AAWC)
    A. ACMI (S3565, TX-915) flexible
      fiberoptic sigmoidoscope
    A. Anorexia/Bulimia Association
    A. Association for the Study of
      Liver Diseases (AASLD)
    A. College of Gastroenterology
      (ACG)
    A. Diabetes Association (ADA)
    A. Digestive Health Foundation
      (ADHF)
    A. Dilation System dilator
    A. Endoscopy automatic reprocessor
    A. Endoscopy dilator
    A. Endoscopy mechanical
      lithotriptor
    A. Endosonography Club (AEC)
    A. Endosonography Club Study
    A. Gastroenterological Association
      (AGA)
    A. Joint Committee on
      Cancer/International Union Against
      Cancer (AJCC/UICC)
    A. Liver Foundation (ALF)
    A. Society for Gastrointestinal
      Endoscopy (ASGE)
    A. trypanosomiasis
    A. type culture collection
    A. Urological Association (AUA)
    A. Urological Association symptom
      index
americanus
    Necator a.
Amerlex-M second antibody
Ames
    A. Hemastix reagent strip
      semiquantitative agglutination
      SERA-TEK A.
    A. test
AMF
    autocrine motility factor
Amicar
Amicon D-20 filter
amicrobic cystitis

amicrofilaremic filariasis
amidation
> carboxyl-terminal a.

amifloxacin
amifostine
amikacin
Amikin
amiloride hydrochloride
amiloride-sensitive, electroneutral Na+/H+ antiporter
Amin-Aid powdered feeding
amine
> aromatic a.
> biogenic a.
> a. precursor uptake and decarboxylation (APUD)
> a. precursor uptake and decarboxylation cell

amino
> a. acid
> a. acid abnormality
> a. acid-based dialysate solution
> a. acid excretion in neonate
> a. acid-glucose mixture
> 28-a. acid peptide
> A. Mel Hepa
> a. terminus

aminoacetate
> dihydroxyaluminum a.

aminoacidopathy
> dibasic a.

aminoaciduria
> hyperdibasic a.
> imidazole a.
> a. in neonate
> overflow a.
> renal a.
> transport a.

aminobenzoate
> butyl a.
> a. potassium

4-aminobiphenyl
aminobiphosphonate gastrotoxic drug
aminocaproic acid
Aminofusin L Forte amino acid solution
aminoglutethimide
aminoglycoside
aminoguanidine
aminoisobutyricaciduria
> beta a.

5-aminolevulinic
> 5-a. acid (5-ALA)
> 5-a. acid-induced fluorescence endoscopy

aminolevulinic acid (ALA)
aminonucleoside
> glomerular epithelial cell toxin puromycin a.
> puromycin a.

aminopeptidase
> leucine a. (LAP)

aminophylline
aminopropionitrile
> beta a.

aminopyrine
> a. breath test
> a. clearance

aminorex
aminosalicylate
5-aminosalicylic
> 5-a. acid (5-ASA)
> 5-a. acid enema

4-aminosalicylic acid (4-ASA)
amino-terminal undecapeptide
aminothiol concentration
aminotransferase
> alanine a. (ALT)
> alanine-glyoxylate a.
> aspartate a. (AST)

amiodarone
Amipaque
Amitone
amitriptyline hydrochloride
AML
> angiomyolipoma

amlodipine besylate
ammonia (N)
> arterial a.
> blood a.
> a. level
> plasma a.
> a. production
> serum a.
> a. toxicity

ammonia-13 (^{13}N)
ammoniagenesis
ammoniagenic coma
ammonium
> a. acid urate calculus
> a. acid urate urinary lithiasis
> a. hydroxide

NOTES

amnesia
>antegrade a.
>procedural a.
>retrograde a.

amnion

amodiaquine

amoeba

Amogel PG

amorphous filling defect

amoxicillin
>luminal a.
>a. trihydrate

amoxicillin-clavulanate

amoxicillin-clavulanic acid

amoxicillin-omeprazole treatment

amoxicillin-tinidazole-ranitidine therapy

Amoxil

AMP
>adenosine monophosphate
>AMP level
>urinary cyclic AMP

amperage

amphetamine

amphibolic fistula

amphibolous fistula

amphiregulin

Amphojel

amphotericin
>a. B
>a. B-induced reduction glomerular filtration rate (AmB-induced reduction GFR)
>a. B nephropathy
>a. B resistance
>a. B therapy

ampicillin

Ampicin

Amplatz
>A. catheter
>A. fascial dilator
>A. sheath
>A. Super Stiff guidewire
>A. TractMaster system

amplification refractory mutation system-polymerase chain reaction (ARMS-PCR)

amplitude
>a. coded-color Doppler sonography esophageal body contraction a.
>mean distal contraction a. (MDCA)

amplitude-acrophase vector

ampulla, pl. **ampullae**
>a. ductus deferentis
>Henle a.
>a. hepatopancreatica
>invagination of the a.
>Lieberkühn a.
>rectal a.

>a. of vas deferens
>a. of Vater

ampullary
>a. ablative therapy
>a. carcinoma
>a. granulation tissue
>a. hamartoma
>a. lesion
>a. stenosis
>a. stone
>a. tumor

ampullectomy
>endoscopic snare a.

ampulloma

ampullopancreatic carcinoma

amputation
>penile a.

AMS
>AMS artificial sphincter
>AMS controlled expansion penile prosthesis cylinder
>AMS 700CX penile prosthesis cylinder
>AMS Hydroflex penile prosthesis
>AMS 700 inflatable penile prosthesis
>AMS 600 malleable penile prosthesis
>AMS 700-series double-cuff Silastic artificial urinary sphincter
>AMS 800-series double-cuff Silastic artificial urinary sphincter
>AMS three-piece inflatable penile prosthesis
>AMS Ultrex penile prosthesis

AMSA
>amsacrine

amsacrine (AMSA)

Amsterdam
>A. biliary stent
>A. criteria
>A. criteria for hereditary nonpolyposis colorectal cancer

Amsterdam-type prosthesis

Amussat
>A. incision
>A. operation
>A. valve
>A. valvula

amygdala

amylacea
>corpora a.

amylase
>ascitic a.
>a. concentration
>pancreatic a.
>P-type a.
>salivary a.

serum a.
S-type a.
a. unit
urinary a.
amylase/creatinine clearance ratio
amylase-resistant starch (ARS)
amylin
amyl nitrite
amylo-1,6-glucosidase deficiency
amyloglucosidase
amyloid
AA a.
AL a.
a. kidney
a. nephropathy
a. nephrosis
serum a. P (SAP)
amyloid-like glomerulopathy
amyloidoma
amyloidosis
a. of the bladder
cutaneous lichen a.
hepatic a.
kidney a.
localized a.
rectal a.
renal a.
secondary a.
systemic a.
a. type AA
type IV a.
amyloidotic glomerulus
amylopectinosis
amylorrhea
AN
anorexia nervosa
AN69 membrane dialyzer
ANA
antinuclear antibody
anabolic
a. steroid
a. steroid spermatogenesis
impairment
a. steroid treatment
Anacardium occidentale L
anacidic stomach
anacidity
ANAD
anorexia nervosa and associated disorder
anacrobe
obligate a.

anaerobic
a. culture
a. glycolysis
anal
a. abscess
a. anastomosis
a. atresia
a. bulging
a. canal
a. canal hypertonia
a. canal length (ACL)
a. column
a. condyloma
a. crypt
a. dilation
a. dilator
a. discharge
a. disk
a. effluent
a. electrical stimulation
a. EMG PerryMeter sensor
a. encirclement
a. endoscopy
a. endosonography (AES)
a. epidermoid carcinoma
a. fascia
a. fibrosis
a. fissure
a. fistula
a. foreign body
a. ileostomy with preservation of
sphincter
a. incontinence
a. intersphincteric groove
a. intraepithelial neoplasia (AIN)
a. intramuscular gland
a. mapping
a. margin
a. neoplasm
a. pecten
a. pit
a. pitting
a. plate
a. pouch
a. procidentia
a. prolapse
a. protrusion
a. reflex
a. sepsis
a. sinus
a. sphincter (AS)
a. sphincter contraction

NOTES

anal *(continued)*
    a. sphincter dysfunction
    a. sphincter function
    a. sphincter reconstruction
    a. sphincter repair
    a. sphincter squeeze pressure
    a. sphincter tone
    a. squamous dysplasia
    a. squamous intraepithelial lesion
    a. stenosis
    a. stricture
    a. surgery
    a. transitional zone (ATZ)
    a. transitional zone dysplasia
    a. triangle
    a. ulceration
    a. valve
    a. vector manometry
    a. verge
    a. wart
    a. wink
    a. wound
analeptic enema
anales
    columnae a.
    sinus a.
    valvulae a.
analgesia
    patient a.
analgesic
    narcotic a.
    a. nephropathy
    a. requirement
analgesic-antipyretic
analgosedation
analis
    pecten a.
analog, analogue
    arginine a.
    prostaglandin a.
    somatostatin a.
Analpram-HC anorectal cream
analysis
    anthropometric a.
    bioelectrical impedance a. (BIA)
    Bland-Altman a.
    body composition a.
    CFTR gene a.
    cineradiographic a.
    contexture a.
    cosinor a.
    cost-effectiveness a.
    cytogenetic a.
    cytometric a.
    Diacyte DNA ploidy a.
    DNA ploidy a.
    electrophoresis immunoblot a.
    encrustation a.

    energy dispersive x-ray a.
    enzymatic spectrophotometric a.
    fecal a.
    flow cytometric a.
    fluid a.
    fluorescent image a.
    Fourier transform a.
    gastric a.
    gene-linkage a. (GLA)
    heteroduplex a.
    histochemical-ultrastructural a.
    image a.
    Kaplan-Meier a.
    logistic regression a.
    monoclonality by genetic a.
    Northern blot a.
    pentagastrin stimulated a.
    ploidy a.
    prefreeze semen a.
    pressure flow a.
    p53 tumor suppressor gene a.
    pulse-width a.
    real-time spectral a.
    reflectance a.
    regression a.
    renal morphometric a.
    semen a.
    sequencing a.
    serum cytokine a.
    single-parameter DNA a.
    single strand conformation
      polymorphism a.
    Southern blot a.
    spectral a.
    spectrophotometric a.
    step-wise regression a.
    survival a.
    trace-gas a.
    two-dimensional flow cytometric a.
    univariate a.
    urine cytokine a.
    Vindelov method flow cytometry a.
    Western blot a.
    x-ray a.
analyzer
    automatic chemical a.
    Beckman ion-selective a.
    Cell Soft 2000 semen a.
    C-Trak a.
    GastrograpH Mark III pH a.
    Hamilton-Thorn motility a.
    Hitachi 717 a.
    Menuet Compact primary
      urodynamic a.
    MicroLyzer Gas a.
    Olympus SP-series image a.
    Orion model AE 940 ion a.
    Packard Auto-Gamma 5650 a.

reflectance TS-200 spectrum a.
RJL Model 10 bioelectrical
  impedance a.
sequential multiple a. (SMA)
Siemens Somatom DRH CT a.
SYNCHRON CX-5, CX-7
  automated a.
Ultrasound Bone A.
Anandron
anaphylactic reaction
anaphylactoid
  a. food sensitivity
  a. purpura
  a. purpura nephritis
anaphylaxis
anaplasia
anaplastic
  a. malignant teratoma
  a. seminoma
  a. Wilms tumor
Anaprox
anaritide   acetate
anasarca
anascitic
Anaspaz
anastalsis
anastomose
anastomosis, pl. **anastomoses**
  Abbe intestinal a.
  anal a.
  antecolic a.
  antiperistaltic a.
  aseptic a.
  biliary-enteric a.
  Billroth I, II a.
  bladder neck-to-urethra a.
  Brackin ureterointestinal a.
  Braun a.
  Carrel aortic patch a.
  cervical esophagogastric a.
  choledococaval a. (CDCA)
  circular stapled a.
  a. clamp
  Coffey ureterointestinal a.
  coloanal a. (CAA)
  colocolonic a.
  colorectal a.
  Cordonnier technique
    ureterocolonic a.
  Couvelaire ileourethral a.
  crunch stick a.
  curved end-to-end a. (CEEA)

Daines-Hodgson a.
delayed a.
dismembered a.
dog-ear of a.
double-stapled ileal pouch-anal a.
end-to-end a. (EEA)
end-to-side a.
enteroenteric a.
esophagocolic a.
esophagojejunal a.
extracorporeal a.
extravesical a.
fishmouth a.
Furniss ureterointestinal a.
Gambee a.
Goodwin technique
  ureterocolonic a.
Halsted a.
handsewn a.
hepaticojejunal a.
Higgins ureterointestinal a.
Hofmeister a.
homocladic a.
Horsley a.
H-shaped ileal pouch-anal a.
ileal pouch-anal a. (IPAA)
ileal pouch-distal rectal a.
ileoanal a.
ileocolic a. (ICA)
ileorectal a. (IRA)
ileosigmoid a.
ileotransverse colon a.
ileovesical a.
intestinal a.
intracorporeal a.
intravesical a.
isoperistaltic a.
J-shaped ileal pouch-anal a.
Kocher a.
Leadbetter and Clarke ureteral a.
LeDuc ureteral a.
Lich-Gregoire a.
low anterior resection in
  combination with coloanal a.
  (LAR/CAA)
low coloanal a.
mechanical a.
mesocaval a.
mucosa-to-mucosa a.
Navy single-layer everting a.
neobladder-urethra a.
Nesbit technique ureterocolonic a.

NOTES

anastomosis *(continued)*
    nondismembered a.
    Pagano technique ureterocolonic a.
    Pagano ureteral a.
    pancreaticogastric a.
    Parks ileoanal a.
    peristaltic a.
    Politano-Leadbetter a.
    Pólya a.
    portacaval a.
    pouch-anal a.
    primary a.
    pyeloileocutaneous a.
    rectosigmoid a.
    reniportal a.
    retrocolic a.
    right-angled end-to-side a.
    Roux-en-Y a.
    Roux-type gastroduodenal a.
    Schoemaker a.
    side-to-side a.
    single-layer continuous intestinal a.
    small bowel a.
    spatulated overlap a.
    splenorenal venous a.
    S-shaped ileal pouch-anal a.
    stapled end-to-end ileoanal a.
    stapled intestinal a.
    stapled pouch-anal a.
    State end-to-end a.
    Strickler technique ureterocolonic a.
    Strickler ureteral a.
    sutureless bowel a.
    tension-free a.
    transanal a.
    transureteroureteral a.
    two-layer interrupted intestinal a.
    ultralow a.
    ureteral a.
    ureterocolonic a.
    ureteroileal a.
    ureterointestinal a.
    ureterosigmoid a.
    ureterotubal a.
    ureteroureteral a.
    urethrovesical a.
    vascular a.
    vesicourethral a.
    Von Haberer-Finney a.
    Wallace a.
    wide elliptical a.
    wide-lumen stapled a.
    W-shaped ileal pouch-anal a.
    Z-plasty a.
anastomotic
    a. complication
    a. leak
    a. leakage
    a. material
    a. recurrence
    a. stoma
    a. stricture
    a. suture
    a. ulcer
    a. ulceration
    a. urethroplasty
anastomotic-stomal ulcer
anatomical
    a. anomaly
    a. radical retropubic prostatectomy
anatomic stress incontinence
anatomy
    anomalous a.
    aortoiliac a.
    Billroth II a.
    congenitally altered a.
    peritoneal a.
Anatrast barium sulfate paste
anatrophic
    a. nephrolithotomy
    a. nephroscopy
    a. nephrotomy
ANC
    acid-neutralizing capacity
ANCA
    antineutrophil cytoplasmic antibody
ANCA-associated systemic vasculitis
Ancalixir
ANCA-SVV
    antineutrophilic cytoplasmic
      autoantibody-small vessel vasculitis
Ancef
anchor
    Cope viscerotomy a.
    esophageal Z stent with a.
    Mainstay urologic soft tissue a.
    Mitek bone a.
anchoring
    a. balloon
    a. suture
**Ancure abdominal aortic aneurysm
system**
Ancylostoma duodenale
ancylostomiasis
Andersen
    A. disease
    A. syndrome
    A. triad
Anderson
    A. classification
    A. gastric tube
**Anderson-Hynes dismembered
pyeloplasty**
Andractim
Andresen diet

Andrews
>A. operation
>A. suction tip

androblastoma

Androderm testosterone transdermal patch

Androgel

androgen
>a. ablation
>a. ablation therapy (AAT)
>a. ablative monotherapy
>adrenal cortex a.
>a. blockade
>a. deficiency
>a. deprivation
>a. deprivation therapy
>exogenous a.
>a. gonadotropin feedback control
>a. insensitivity syndrome
>plasma a.
>a. precursor
>a. priming
>a. receptor
>a. receptor element
>a. suppression
>a. withdrawal endocrine therapy

androgen-binding protein

androgen-independent prostate cancer

androgenital syndrome

androgenization

androgenize

andrology

andropause

androstenedione
>basal a.

androstenedione-to-testosterone ratio

androsterone

anechoic

anejaculation

anemia
>autoimmune hemolytic a.
>B_{12} a.
>Banti splenic a.
>a. of chronic renal failure
>copper-deficiency a.
>deficiency a.
>Faber a.
>febrile pleomorphic a.
>folate a.
>hemodialysis associated a.
>hemolytic a.
>homozygous sickle cell a.

>hypochromic microcytic a.
>hypovolemic a.
>iron-deficiency a.
>macroangiopathic hemolytic a.
>megaloblastic a.
>pernicious a.
>posthepatitis aplastic a.
>refractory sideroblastic a.
>sickle cell a.

anemic urine

anephric

anepiploic

Anergan

anergy
>clonal a.

aneroid manometry

Anestacon 2% lidocaine hydrochloride jelly

anesthesia
>a. adjuvant
>general a.
>general endotracheal a. (GETA)
>local a.
>methoxyflurane a.
>pharyngeal a.
>Ponka technique herniorrhaphy a.
>Ponka technique for local a.
>preperitoneal a.
>spinal a.
>topical a.
>topical oropharyngeal a. (TOPA)

anesthetic
>Cetacaine topical a.
>EMLA a.
>eutectic mixture of local a.'s (EMLA)
>a. hepatitis
>a. hepatotoxicity
>lidocaine topical a.
>topical a.
>Xylocaine topical a.

aneuploid cell

aneuploidy
>DNA a.
>mucosal a.

AneuRx stent graft system

aneurysm
>abdominal aortic a. (AAA)
>acquired renal artery a.
>aortic a.
>arterial a.
>arteriosclerotic a.

NOTES

aneurysm *(continued)*
    berry a.
    bilobate false a.
    cirsoid a.
    congenital renal artery a.
    cricoid a.
    Dieulafoy cirsoid a.
    dissecting abdominal a.
    dissecting renal artery a.
    embolization of a.
    extravisceral a.
    false a.
    fusiform renal artery a.
    gastric a.
    GDA a.
    hepatic artery a.
    hypogastric artery a.
    iliac artery a.
    intramural a.
    intrarenal renal artery a.
    mycotic a.
    perforating a.
    renal artery a.
    ruptured abdominal aortic a.
      (RAAA)
    saccular a.
    splenic artery a. (SAA)
    thoracoabdominal aortic a. (TAAA)
aneurysmal dilation
aneurysmatic
aneurysmectomy
ANF
    atrial natriuretic factor
Angelchik
    A. antireflux prosthesis
    A. ring prosthesis
Anger scintillation camera
angiitis
    hypersensitivity a.
angina
    abdominal a.
    a. abdominalis
    a. abdominis
    a. dyspeptica
    intestinal a.
    Schultz a.
anginal attack
anginiform
anginose, anginous
angioblast
angiocatheter
Angiocath PRN catheter
angiocholecystitis
angiocholitis proliferans
Angiocol
angiodysplasia
    bleeding colonic a.
    diffuse a.

    submucosal endothelial a.
    submucosal fibromuscular a.
angiodysplastic lesion
angioectasia
angioedema
    hereditary a. (HAE)
angiofibroma
    nasopharyngeal a.
    a. of penis
angiogenesis
    tumor a.
angiogenic factor
Angiografin
angiogram
    celiac a.
    cystic duct a.
    mesenteric a.
    splenic a.
angiographic
    a. assessment
    a. end hole catheter
    a. intervention
    a. portacaval shunt
    a. variceal embolization
angiographically
angiography
    biliary a.
    a. catheter
    celiac a.
    computed tomographic a. (CTA)
    computerized tomographic
      hepatic a. (CTHA)
    3-D gadolinium-enhanced MR a.
    diagnostic a.
    digital subtraction a.
    digital venous subtraction a. (DSA)
    Doppler ultrasonography a.
    dynamic fluorescein a.
    fluorescence a.
    intraarterial digital subtraction a.
    intraoperative a.
    intravenous renal a.
    magnetic resonance a. (MRA)
    mucosal a.
    quantitative a.
    renal a.
    selective mesenteric a.
    subtraction a.
    superior mesenteric a.
    therapeutic a.
    visceral a.
    Wilms tumor a.
angioinfarction
AngioJet Xpeedior catheter
angiokeratoma
    a. corporis diffusum
    a. corporis diffusum universale
    diffuse a.

a. of Fordyce
scrotal a.
a. of scrotum
angioma, pl. **angiomata**
bleeding a.
cherry a.
gastric a.
littoral cell a.
petechial a.
spider a.
telangiectatic a.
testicular a.
umbilicated a.
upper gastrointestinal a.
angiomatoid tumor
angiomatosis
hepatic a.
angiomatous lymphoid hamartoma
Angiomed
A. blue stent
A. Puroflex stent
angiomyolipoma (AML)
gastric a.
kidney a.
renal a.
tuberous sclerosis a.
angioneurectomy
angioneurotic
a. anuria
a. edema
a. hematuria
angioplasia
angioplasty
a. balloon
a. balloon catheter
balloon percutaneous transluminal a.
percutaneous transluminal a. (PTA)
percutaneous transluminal balloon a.
percutaneous transluminal renal a.
(PTRA)
renal percutaneous transluminal a.
angiosarcoma
bladder a.
hepatic a.
radiation-induced a.
angiosclerosis
radiation-induced a.
angiosclerotica
dyspragia a.
angiostatin
AngioStent
angiostrongyliasis

angiotensin
a. I-converting enzyme
insertion/deletion polymorphism
a. I, II, III
a. II infusion test
a. II receptor
a. receptor blocker (ARB)
angiotensin-converting
a.-c. enzyme (ACE)
a.-c. enzyme gene
a.-c. enzyme gene polymorphism
A.-c. Enzyme Inhibition in
Progressive Renal Insufficiency
(AIPRI)
A.-c. Enzyme Inhibition in
Progressive Renal Insufficiency
trial
a.-c. enzyme inhibitor (ACEI)
angiotensin-dependent hypertension
angiotensinogen
Angiovist
AngioZyme
angle
acute infundibulopelvic a.
anopouch a.
anorectal a.
Camper a.
cardiohepatic a.
duodenojejunal a.
epigastric a.
hepatorenal a.
a. of His
a. of incidence
infundibulopelvic a.
LIP a.
lower infundibulopelvic a.
mesangial a.
splenorenal a.
angled
a. delivery device (ADD)
a. dissecting forceps
angle-tip Glidewire
angular
a. notch of stomach
a. velocity
angularis
a. body
incisura a.
angulation
angulus, pl. **anguli**
a. on the lesser curve
a. of stomach

NOTES

anhaustral colonic gas pattern
anhemolytic Streptococcus
anhepatic stage of liver transplantation
anhydrase
    carbonic a. (CA)
    carbonic a. II
anhydrosis
anhydrous
    sodium phosphate dibasic a.
ani (*pl. of* anus)
anicteric
    a. sclerae
    a. skin
    a. viral hepatitis
anileridine
anion
    a. exchange resin
    a. gap
    a. gap acidosis
anionic
    a. ferritin
    a. IgG 4 fraction
aniridia
anisakiasis
    acute gastric a.
    gastric a.
Anisakis marina
anismus
anisocoria
anisokaryosis
anisotropine methylbromide
anisoylated plasminogen streptokinase
  activator complex
anistreplase
anitidine
ankle jerk
ankyloproctia
ankylosing spondylitis
ankylostomiasis
ankylurethria
anlage
    a. of pancreas
    splenic a.
anlagen
    prepancreatic a.
Ann
    A. Arbor cancer staging
    A. Arbor classification
ANNA
  antineuronal nuclear antibody
annexin
annular
    a. adenocarcinoma
    a. esophageal stricture
    a. pancreas
annulus urethralis

ano
    fissure in a.
    fistula in a.
anococcygeal raphe
anococcygeus
anocutaneous
    a. line
    a. reflex
    a. stimulation
anoderm
Anogesic
anomalotrophy
anomalous
    a. anatomy
    a. arrangement of pancreaticobiliary
      ductal system (AAPBDS)
    a. calix
    a. genitalia
    a. junction of pancreaticobiliary
      ducts (AJPBD)
    a. pancreaticobiliary communication
    a. pancreaticobiliary duct (APBD)
    a. pancreaticobiliary ductal union
      (APBDU)
    a. pancreaticobiliary union (APBU)
    a. pancreatobiliary duct junction
      (APBDJ)
anomaly
    anatomical a.
    Cruveilhier-Baumgarten a.
    Dieulafoy a.
    DiGeorge a.
    duplication a.
    fixation a.
    pan-bud a.
    ureter duplication a.
    urinary tract a.
    urogenital sinus a.
    vitelline duct a.
    a. of Zahn
anoplasty
    cutback a.
    dermal island-flap a.
    House advancement a.
    Martin a.
    a. treatment
    Y-V a.
anopouch angle
anorchia
    bilateral a.
anorchism
anorectal
    a. abscess
    a. angle
    a. atresia
    a. band
    a. carcinoma
    a. disease

a. dressing (ARD)
a. dysgenesis
a. endosonography
a. examination
a. fistula
a. flexure
a. foreign body
a. function test
a. herpes
a. imaging
a. junction
a. line
a. malformation
a. manometry
a. measurement
a. mobilization
a. myectomy
a. nomenclature
a. physiology
a. physiology testing
a. ring
a. sensorimotor dysfunction
a. sepsis
a. space
a. sphincter
a. stenosis
a. surgery
a. syphilis
a. varix
anorectic, anoretic
a. drug
anorectitis
anorectocolonic
anorectoplasty
Laird-McMahon a.
posterior sagittal a.
anorectum
anoretic (*var. of* anorectic)
anorexia
a. nervosa (AN)
a. nervosa and associated disorder (ANAD)
anorexia-cachexia syndrome
anorexiant
anorexic
anorexigenic
anorgasmia
anorgasmy
anoscope
Bacon a.
Boehm a.
Brinkerhoff a.

Buie-Hirschman a.
Ferguson a.
Hirschmann a.
Otis a.
Pratt a.
Pruitt a.
Sims a.
slotted a.
anoscopic
anoscopy
anosigmoidoscopy
anospinal center
anovaginal fistula
anovesical
anoxia
chemical a.
gastric a.
ANP
atrial natriuretic peptide
ANP receptor
ANS
autonomic nervous system
ansa
a. pancreatica
a. pancreaticus
Ansaid
Anson-McVay femoral herniorrhaphy
antacid
liquid a.
Remegel Soft Chewable A.
Anta-Gel
antagonist
alpha-adrenergic a.
alpha-1-adrenoceptor a.
alpha-receptor a.
beta-adrenergic a.
BQ123 receptor a.
calcium a.
calcium channel a. (CCA)
CCK a.
cholecystokinin a.
cytokine a.
dopamine a.
endothelin a.
EtA, EtB a.
histamine H2 a.
histamine H2-receptor a.
histamine-2 receptor a. (H2RA)
hormone a.
H2 receptor a. (H2RA)
$5-HT_3$ a.
$5-HT_4$ a.

NOTES

antagonist *(continued)*
    5HTM3 receptor a.
    interleukin-1 receptor a.
    intravenous H2 receptor a.
      (IVH2RA)
    KSG-504 CCK a.
    L-364,781 CCK a.
    L-365,260 CCK a.
    luteinizing hormone-releasing
      hormone a.
    opiate a.
    opioid a.
    PIVKA-II a.
    platelet glycoprotein 2b3a
      receptor a.
    potassium-canrenoate a.
    serotonin receptor a.
    TxA2 receptor a.
antagonistic drug
antagonist-II
    prothrombin induced by vitamin K
      absence or a.-I. (PIVKA-II)
antalgic gait
antecedent pancreatic injury
antecolic
    a. anastomosis
    a. gastrectomy
    a. long-loop isoperistaltic
      gastrojejunostomy
antecubital arteriovenous fistula
anteflexed uterus
antegrade
    a. amnesia
    a. approach
    a. colonic enema (ACE)
    a. continence enema (ACE)
    a. continence enema procedure
    a. contrast study
    a. cystography
    a. ejaculation
    a. endopyelotomy
    a. nephroscopy
    a. pyelogram
    a. pyelography
    a. pyeloureterography
    a. scrotal sclerotherapy
    a. ureteral drainage
    a. urography
Antegren
antepartum constipation
anterior
    a. abdominal wall
    a. abdominal wall syndrome
    a. approach
    arteria caecalis a.
    arteria pancreaticoduodenalis
      superior a.
    a. axillary line (AAL)

    a. band of colon
    a. cecal artery
    a. cord syndrome
    a. duodenal ulcer
    a. esophageal sensor (AES)
    a. extremity
    a. fecal incontinence
    a. fissure
    a. fistula
    a. hemiblock
    a. horn
    a. hypospadias
    a. innominate osteotomy
    a. nephrectomy
    a. pelvic exenteration
    a. perineum
    a. and posterior (A&P)
    a. rectopexy
    a. rectus fascia
    a. rectus sheath
    a. renal fascia
    a. resection
    a. rib impingement syndrome
    a. scrotal nerve
    a. spinal artery syndrome
    a. superior pancreaticoduodenal
      (ASPD)
    a. superior pancreaticoduodenal
      artery
    a. transabdominal approach
    a. urethra
    a. urethral valve
    a. wall antral ulcer
anterior-posterior cystoresectoscope
anterolateral thoracotomy incision
anterooblique position
anteverted uterus
antevesical hernia
anthracene glycoside
anthracene-type laxative
anthraquinone laxative
anthrax
    intestinal a.
anthrone
    a. colorimetric technique
    a. method
    Rhein a.
anthropometric
    a. analysis
    a. calculation
    a. marker
    a. measurement
anthropometry
anthropomorphic parameter
anti-40 kDa colonic antigen
anti-ABO antibody
antiactin antibody
antiadhesive agent

anti-alpha-fetoprotein
  ^{99m}Tc-labeled a.-a.-f.
antiandrogen withdrawal syndrome
antibasement membrane antibody
antibiotic
  beta-lactam a.
  broad-spectrum a.
  long-term a.
  macrolide a.
  a. management
  perioperative a.
  preoperative a.
  prophylactic a.
  a. prophylaxis
  a. therapy
  topical a.
antibiotic-associated
  a.-a. colitis (AAC)
  a.-a. diarrhea (AAD)
  a.-a. pseudomembranous colitis
    (AAPC, AAPMC)
antibiotic-coated stent
antibiotic-induced
  a.-i. diarrhea
  a.-i. enterocolitis
antibody
  Amerlex-M second a.
  anti-ABO a.
  antiactin a.
  antibasement membrane a.
  antibrush border a.
  anticardiolipin a. (ACA, ACLA)
  anticentromere a.
  anticolonic a.
  anticytokeratin monoclonal a.
  anti-DCP monoclonal a.
  antidelta IgM a.
  antidesmin monoclonal a.
  anti-double-stranded deoxyribonucleic
    acid a.
  antiendomysial a. (anti-EMA)
  antiendomysium a.
  antiendothelial a.
  antienterocyte a.
  antiepithelial membrane antigen a.
  antiextractable nuclear a. (anti-
    ENA)
  anti-GBM a.
  antigliadin a. (AGA)
  antiglomerular basement
    membrane a.
  anti-HA a.

anti-HAV IgM a.
anti-HB a.
anti-HBc IgM a.
anti-HBe a.
anti-HBs a.
anti-HCV core a.
anti-HD a.
anti-HGF a.
antihuman leukocyte antigen a.
antiidiotype a.
anti-interleukin-2 receptor alpha
  monoclonal a.
antilymphocyte a.
antimicrosomal a.
antimitochondrial a. (AMA)
antineuronal nuclear a. (ANNA)
antineutrophil cytoplasmic a.
  (ANCA)
antineutrophil cytoplasmic IgG a.
antinuclear a. (ANA)
anti-PCNA/cyclin monoclonal a.
antiphospholipid a. (APA)
antiphospholipid-anticardiolipin a.
anti-RAP a.
anti-RAP-GST a.
antireticulin a.
anti-RNA polymerase a.
antirotavirus a.
anti-Saccharomyces cerevisiae a.
  (ASCA)
antismooth muscle a.
antisomatostatin a.
antisperm a.
anti-TBM a.
anti-Thy-1 a.
antithyroglobulin a. (ATA)
anti-TNF-alpha a.
antivimentin a.
ATGAM polyclonal a.
basal cell-specific anticytokeratin a.
bladder a.
4B4 monoclonal a.
19B7 monoclonal a.
B72.3 murine monoclonal a.
a. to bromodeoxyuridine
cagA a.
CD14 monoclonal a.
CM1 polyclonal a.
a. to core peptide 9 (anti-CP9)
a. to core peptide 10 (anti-CP10)
a. to c100 protein
cytophilic a.

NOTES

antibody *(continued)*
    cytotoxic a.
    a. directed cytotoxic response
    eluted a.
    a. to EMA
    endomysial a. (EMA)
    endomysium a.
    endotoxin a.
    enzyme-conjugated anti-IgA a.
    fibronectin monoclonal a.
    fluorescein isothiocyanate-
      conjugated a.
    fluorescein isothiocyanate-labeled
      monoclonal a.
    fluorescent antinuclear a. (FANA)
    Fx1A a.
    a. to GOR (anti-GOR)
    a. to GOR epitope
    HBe a.
    HBeAb a.
    HCV a.
    a. to hepatitis-associated antigen
      (anti-HAA)
    a. to hepatitis A virus (anti-HAV)
    hepatitis B core a. (HBcAb)
    hepatitis Be a. (HBeAb, HbeAb)
    hepatitis B surface a. (HBsAb)
    a. to hepatitis C virus (anti-HCV)
    a. to hepatitis D virus (anti-HDV)
    heterologous anti-GBM a.
    Heymann a.
    HMB-45 monoclonal a.
    a. to HTLV-I (anti-HTLV-I)
    humanized monoclonal a.
    hybridoma-derived monoclonal a.
    IgG2a a.
    IgG alpha-gliadin a.
    IgG reticulin a.
    IgM anti-HAV a.
    IgM anti-HBc a.
    IgM-HA a.
    immunoglobulin A endomysial a.
    immunoglobulin A
      transglutaminase a. (IgA tTG)
    immunoglobulin G2a a.
    immunoglobulin G antigliadin a.
      (IgG AGA)
    indium-111 murine anti-CEA
      monoclonal a.
    infectious mononucleosis
      heterophil a.
    IOT29, clone K20 monoclonal a.
    islet cell a. (ICA test)
    4KB5 monoclonal a.
    a. to keratin
    LDP-02 a.
    a. to Leu M1
    liver-kidney microsomal a.

    lymphocytotoxic a.
    M a.
    microsome a. (MCHA)
    milk protein a.
    mitochondrial a.
    monoclonal a. (MAb, mAb, MoAb)
    MU-3 monoclonal a.
    mycelial a.
    mycobacterial a.
    OKT3 anti-T-cell a.
    OKT3 monoclonal a.
    p53 a.
    PAb 1801 monoclonal a.
    panel-reactive a. (PRA)
    para-ANC a.
    PBC-associated a.
    PC10 monoclonal a.
    perinuclear antineutrophil
      cytoplasmic a. (p-ANCA)
    phosphotyrosine a.
    polyclonal epidermal growth
      factor a.
    protein a. (PAb)
    recipient-derived anti-HLA a.
    serum virus a.
    smooth muscle a. (SMA)
    thyroglobulin a. (TGHA)
    thyroid microsomal a.
    a. to B72.3
    a. to c100 (anti-c100)
    a. to C22-3
    UCHL-1 monoclonal a.
    xenoreactive a.
    ZCE 025 a.
antibody-dependent
    a.-d. cell-mediated cytotoxicity
      (ADCC)
    a.-d. cellular cytotoxicity (ADCC)
anti-BrDu
    anti-bromodeoxyuridine
anti-bromodeoxyuridine (anti-BrDu)
antibrush border antibody
anti-c100
    antibody to c100
anticardiolipin
    a. antibody (ACA, ACLA)
    a. antibody syndrome
anti-CD3
anti-CD45
anticentromere
    a. antibody
    a. autoantibody (ACA)
anticholinergic
    a. agent
    a. drug
    a. medication
    a. medicine therapy

anticholinesterase
    parasympathomimetic a.
antichymotrypsin
    prostate-specific antigen bound to
      alpha-1 a. (PSA-ACT)
anti-class II MAb
anti-CMV antiserum
anticoagulant
    lupus a. (LA)
anticoagulant-induced hematuria
anticoagulation therapy
anticodon
anticolonic antibody
anticonvulsant agent hepatotoxicity
anti-CP9
    antibody to core peptide 9
anti-CP10
    antibody to core peptide 10
anticytokeratin
    a. monoclonal antibody
anticytokine
anti-DCP monoclonal antibody
antidelta IgM antibody
antidepressant
    a. drug hepatotoxicity
    tricyclic a.
antidesmin monoclonal antibody
antidiabetic agent hepatotoxicity
antidiarrheal
    a. agent
    opioid a.
antidiuretic
    a. arginine vasopressin V2 receptor
      (AVPR2)
    a. hormone (ADH)
    a. hormone-like agent
anti-DNA immunological study
antidopaminergic
anti-double-stranded
    a.-d.-s. deoxyribonucleic acid (anti-
      dsDNA)
    a.-d.-s. deoxyribonucleic acid
      antibody
anti-dsDNA
    anti-double-stranded deoxyribonucleic
      acid
antidysenteric
anti-E2
    envelope 2 antigen
antielastase
anti-EMA
    antiendomysial antibody

antiemetic drug
anti-ENA
    antiextractable nuclear antibody
anti-ENA immunological study
antiendomysial
    a. antibody (anti-EMA)
    a. antibody test
antiendomysium antibody
antiendothelial antibody
antiendotoxin measure
antienterocyte antibody
antiepileptic drug hypersensitivity (AHS)
antiepithelial membrane antigen
  antibody
antiestrogen
antiextractable nuclear antibody (anti-
  ENA)
antifilarial
antifol
    Baker a.
antifolate
    multitargeted a.
antifungal
    a. agent
    a. esophageal infection
antifungal-resistant opportunistic
  infection
anti-GBM
    a.-GBM antibody
    a.-GBM disease
    a.-GBM glomerulonephritis
antigen
    A a.
    adenoma-associated a.
    amebic lectin a.
    antibody to hepatitis-associated a.
      (anti-HAA)
    anti-40 kDa colonic a.
    antineutrophil cytoplasmic a.
    antismooth muscle a. (ASMA)
    antiviral capsid a. (VCA)
    Australian a.
    B a.
    basement membrane a.
    bladder tumor a. (BTA)
    blood group a.
    C100-3 a.
    Ca50 a.
    cancer a. 125 (CA-125, CA125)
    cancer-associated sialyl-Lea a.
    carbohydrate a. 19-9 (CA19-9)

NOTES

antigen *(continued)*
carcinoembryonic a. (CEA)
CD25 a.
cell membrane epithelial a.
circulating tumor-associated a.
class I, II a.
a. DD23
DD23 a.
delta a.
endogenous renal a.
endomysium a.
enterobacterial common a. (ECA)
envelope 2 a. (anti-E2)
epithelial membrane a.
ethylchlorformate polymerized a.
extracted nuclear a. (ENA)
extrarenal a.
factor VIII a.
fetal sulfoglycoprotein a. (FSA)
free prostate-specific a.
gastrointestinal cancer-associated a.
  (GICA)
HBeAg a.
hepatitis-associated a. (HAA)
hepatitis B a. (HBAg)
hepatitis B core a. (HBcAg)
hepatitis Be a.
hepatitis B early a. (HBeAg,
  HbeAg)
hepatitis B surface a. (HBsAg)
hepatitis B virus-encoded a.
hepatitis D a. (HDAg)
hidden a.
histocompatibility a.
HIV P24 a.
HLA-DR a.
human leukocyte a. (HLA)
immunobead-reacting a.
jejunum a.
K a.
40-kDa colonic a.
leukocyte common a.
Lewis A blood group a.
Lewis B, X, Y a.
liver membrane a.
liver-specific a.
M344 a.
a. M344
a. marker
MHC class I, II a.
monoclonal a.
nephritogenic a.
nuclear protein cyclin proliferating
  cell nuclear a.
O a.
P24 a.
486p 3/12 a.

pancreatic oncofetal a. (POA)
pHCV31 a.
pHCV34 a.
polysaccharide a.
proliferating cell nuclear a.
  (PCNA)
prostate gland prostate-specific
  membrane a.
prostate-specific a. (PSA)
prostate-specific membrane a.
  (PSMA)
recombinant hepatitis C a.
reticulin a.
sialosyl-Tn a.
sialyl Lewis A a.
sialyl-Tn a.
solubilized human leukocyte a.
  (solubilized HLA)
soluble egg a. (SEA)
soluble liver a. (SLA)
a. specific
squamous cell carcinoma a.
stage-specific embryonic a.
a. stimulation
a. stool detection test
T a.
T138 a.
Thomsen-Friedenreich a.
tissue polypeptide a.
a. to total prostate-specific a. (F:T
  PSA, FTPSA, F:T PSA)
transplantation a.
tumor-associated a. (TAA)
tumor-rejection a.
Ulex europeus I a.
antigen-antibody system
antigen-dependent pathway
antigenemia
PP65 a.
antigenic
a. determinant
a. modulation
a. phenotype
antigen-independent
a.-i. adhesion
a.-i. pathway
antigen-presenting cell
antigen-specific
nucleocapsid a.-s.
antigliadin
a. antibody (AGA)
luminal a.
antiglomerular
a. basement membrane
a. basement membrane antibody
a. basement membrane antibody
  nephritis

a. basement membrane disease
a. basement membrane
  glomerulonephritis
a. basement membrane-negative
  crescentric glomerular nephritis
anti-GOR
  antibody to GOR
anti-gp330 immunoglobulin G
anti-HAA
  antibody to hepatitis-associated antigen
anti-HA antibody
anti-HAV
  antibody to hepatitis A virus
  IgM anti-HAV
  anti-HAV IgM antibody
anti-HAV-positive
  IgG a.-HAV-p.
anti-HB antibody
anti-HBc
  a.-HBc IgM antibody
  monoclonal a.-HBc
anti-HBe
  a.-HBe antibody
anti-HBs
  a.-HBs antibody
anti-HCV
  antibody to hepatitis C virus
  anti-HCV antibody 3rd generation
  anti-HCV core antibody
anti-HD antibody
anti-HDV
  antibody to hepatitis D virus
anti-*Helicobacter*
  a.-*H.* pylori IgM
  a.-*H.* pylori treatment
antihepatitis A-IgM immunological study
anti-HGF antibody
antihistamine
anti-HSV IgM Ab titer
anti-HTLV-I
  antibody to HTLV-I
antihuman leukocyte antigen antibody
anti-Hu test
antihydropic
antihypertensive
  a. agent
  A. and Lipid-Lowering Treatment
    to Prevent Heart Attack Trial
    (ALLHAT)
antiicteric
antiidiotype antibody
antiincontinence procedure

antiinfective biomaterial
antiinflammatory cytokine
antiinhibin
**anti-interleukin-2 receptor alpha
  monoclonal antibody**
antilipemic drug
antilithic
antiliver microsomal antibody detection
antilymphocyte
  a. antibody
  a. globulin
  a. heteroconjugate
  a. therapy
anti-M2 antimitochondrial antibody level
antimajor histocompatibility complex
antimegalin antiserum
antimesenteric
  a. border
  a. border of distal ileum
  a. enterotomy
  a. fat pad
  a. surface
antimesocolic side of the cecum
antimicrobial
  a. agent
  macrolide a.
  a. prophylaxis
  a. resistance
  a. therapy
antimicrosomal antibody
Antiminth
antimitochondrial antibody (AMA)
antimony
  a. monocrystalline electrode
  a. pH electrode
antimotility
  a. agent
  a. drug
antimüllerian derivative syndrome
antimuscarinic
  a. agent
  a. drug
antimycobacterial drug
antinatriuresis
antinauseant
antineoplastic drug hepatotoxicity
antinephrocalcin antiserum
antineuronal
  a. enteric antibody test
  a. nuclear antibody (ANNA)
antineutrophil
  a. cytoplasmic antibody (ANCA)

NOTES

antineutrophil *(continued)*
    a. cytoplasmic antibody titer
    a. cytoplasmic antigen
    a. cytoplasmic autoantibody
    a. cytoplasmic IgG antibody
antineutrophilic cytoplasmic autoantibody-small vessel vasculitis (ANCA-SVV)
antinociceptive effect
antinuclear
    a. antibody (ANA)
    a. antibody immunological study
antioncogene therapy
antioxidant
    endogenous lipophilic a.
    A. Polyp Prevention Trial
anti-PCNA/cyclin monoclonal antibody
antiperistalsis
antiperistaltic
    a. anastomosis
    a. reflux
    a. technique
antiphospholipid
    a. antibody (APA)
    a. syndrome
antiphospholipid-anticardiolipin antibody
antiplasmin
    alpha-21 a.
antiporter
    Na+/H+ a.
antiproteinuric effect
antiprotozoal
antipsychotic drug hepatotoxicity
antipyrine clearance
anti-RAP antibody
anti-RAP-GST antibody
antireflux
    a. double-J stent
    a. flap-valve mechanism
    a. nipple
    a. operation
    a. procedure
    a. prosthesis
    a. regimen
    a. surgery
    a. therapy
    a. ureteral implantation technique
    a. valve
    a. wrap
antirefluxing
    a. colonic conduit
    a. nipple
antireticulin antibody
anti-RNA polymerase antibody
antirotavirus antibody
antiruminant
anti-*Saccharomyces cerevisiae* antibody (ASCA)

antisarcoma chemotherapy
anti-Schiff stain
antischistosomal
antisecretory
    a. agent
    a. drug
    a. opioid
    a. therapy
antisense
    a. DNA inhibition
    a. oligonucleotide
    a. RNA probe
    a. strategy
antiseptic
    Avagard instant hand a.
    a. dressing
    a. impregnated central venous catheter
antiserum, pl. **antisera**
    anti-CMV a.
    antimegalin a.
    antinephrocalcin a.
    galanin a.
    nephrotoxic a.
    VIP a.
anti-SLA test
antismooth
    a. muscle antibody
    a. muscle antigen (ASMA)
antisomatostatin antibody
Antispas
antispasmodic
    a. agent
    a. drug
antisperm antibody
anti-SSA immunological study
anti-SSB immunological study
antistreptolysin-O
    a.-O titer
anti-Tamm-Horsfall protein
anti-TBM antibody
antithrombin III deficiency
anti-Thy-1
    a.-T.-1 antibody
    a.-T.-1 nephritis
antithymocyte
    a. antibody-induced glomerulonephritis
    a. gammaglobulin (ATGAM)
    a. globulin (ATG)
antithyroglobulin antibody (ATA)
antithyroid
    a. autoantibody
    a. drug hepatotoxicity
anti-TNF-alpha antibody
antitopoisomerase-I autoantibody
antitubular basement membrane
antiulcer

Antivert
antivimentin antibody
antiviral
    a. capsid antigen (VCA)
    a. chemotherapy
antiviral capsid antigen (VCA)
Antizol for injection
Antopol-Goldman lesion
antra (*pl. of* antrum)
antral
    a. atrophic gastritis (AAG)
    a. biopsy
    a. cancer
    a. D-cell
    a. diverticulum of the colon
      (ADC)
    a. EC-cell
    a. edema
    a. gastric cell
    a. gastrin
    a. gastrin cell hyperfunction
    a. G-cell hyperplasia
    a. manometry
    a. membrane
    a. mucosa
    a. nodularity
    a. peptide
    a. pcristalsis
    a. polyp
    a. pressure transducer
    a. resection
    a. scintigraphy
    a. somatostatin
    a. stasis
    a. stenosis
    a. stricture
    a. ulcer
    a. vascular ectasia
    a. web
antralization
antral-predominant gastritis
antral-type mucosa
antrectomy
    Roux-en-Y biliary bypass with a.
Antrenyl
Antrocol
antroduodenal
    a. manometry
    a. ulcer
antroduodenectomy
antroduodenojejunal manometry
antrofundal mucosa

Antron catheter
antropyloric
antropyloroduodenal
    a. common chamber (APDCC)
    a. region
antrostomy
antrotomy
antrum, pl. antra
    cardiac a.
    duodenal a.
    gastric a.
    a. gastritis
    prepyloric a.
    a. pyloricum
    retained a.
    a. of stomach
    a. of Willis
anucleate fragment
anulus, pl. anuli
anum
    per a.
anuresis
anuretic
anuria
    angioneurotic a.
    calculous a.
    compression a.
    flash pulmonary edema with a.
    obstructive a.
    postrenal a.
    prerenal a.
    renal a.
    suppressive a.
anuric
anus, pl. ani
    arcus tendineus musculi levatoris
     ani
    artificial a.
    atresia ani
    ectopic a.
    imperforate a.
    levator ani
    a. malformation
    patulous a.
    preternatural a.
    pruritus ani
    rosette appearance of a.
    Rusconi a.
    a. vesicalis
    a. vestibularis
    vulvovaginal a.
anusitis

NOTES

Anusol HC
anvil portion of EEA stapler
Anxanil
anxiety-related diarrhea
anxiolytic sedative
Anzemet
AOCLD
    acute on chronic liver disease
AOM
    azoxymethane
aorta
    supraceliac a.
aortic
    a. aneurysm
    a. dissection
    a. graft
    a. hiatus
    a. patch
    a. punch
    a. valvular stenosis
aortica
    dysphagia a.
aortic-superior mesenteric artery bypass
aortoduodenal fistula (ADF)
aortoenteric
    a. fistula
    a. graft
aortoesophageal fistula
aortogastric fistula
aortograft duodenal fistula
aortography
    abdominal a.
    biplanar a.
aortohepatic arterial graft
aortoiliac anatomy
aortoostial lesion
aortorenal
    a. bypass
    a. bypass graft
    a. reimplantation
aortosigmoid fistula
aortotomy
AOSC
    acute obstructive suppurative cholangitis
AP
    adenomatous polyp
    alkaline phosphatase
        AP marker enzyme
AP1
    transcription factor AP1
A&P
    anterior and posterior
APA
    antiphospholipid antibody
APAAP
    alkaline phosphatase antialkaline
     phosphatase

APACHE
    acute physiology, age and chronic health
     evaluation
        APACHE-II, -III scoring system
APACHE-II
    A.-II point
    A.-II score
apancreatic
apatite
    a. calculus
    carbonate a.
APBD
    anomalous pancreaticobiliary duct
APBDJ
    anomalous pancreatobiliary duct junction
APBDU
    anomalous pancreaticobiliary ductal
     union
APBU
    anomalous pancreaticobiliary union
APC
    adenomatous polyposis coli
    argon plasma coagulation
    argon plasma coagulator
        APC 300
        APC tumor suppressor gene
APCD
    adult polycystic disease
APCR
    activated protein C resistance
APD
    automated peritoneal dialysis
APDCC
    antropyloroduodenal common chamber
apellous
apenteric
apepsia
    achlorhydria a.
apepsinia
aperistalsis
aperistaltic esophagus
Apert syndrome
aperture
    stomal a.
apex, pl. apices
    a. of duodenal bulb
    a. of external ring
aphallia
aphasia
apheresis
Aphrodyne
aphtha, pl. aphthae
aphthoid
    a. proctocolitis
    a. ulcer
aphthous
    a. erosion
    a. gastropathy

a. stomatitis
a. ulcer
aphthous-type lesion
apical
a. biopsy status
a. canaliculus
a. duodenal ulcer
a. polar nephrectomy
a. sound
a. thickening
apices (*pl. of* apex)
APKD
adult polycystic kidney disease
aplasia
bone marrow a.
kidney a.
pure red cell a. (PRCA)
seminal vesicle a.
aplastic bone disease
APLD
adult polycystic liver disease
apnea
obstructive sleep a.
apo
apolipoprotein
apo A-I
apo A-IV
apo B
apo B-48
Apo-Amitriptyline
Apo-Amoxi
APOB **gene**
Apo-Chlorax
Apo-Chlordiazepoxide
Apo-Cimetidine
Apo-Erythro
Apo-Erythro-ES
Apo-Hydroxyzine
apolipoprotein (apo)
a. B-containing lipoprotein
a. B gene
a. CII-CIII ratio
a. synthesis
APOLT
auxiliary partial orthotopic liver
transplantation
Apo-Metronidazole
apomorphine
aponeurosis
buccopharyngeal a.
external oblique a.
a. of external oblique

a. of internal oblique
ischiorectal a.
superficial perineal a.
apoplexy
abdominal a.
mesenteric a.
urethral a.
apoprotein
apoptosis
crypt cell a.
enterocyte a.
apoptotic
a. index
a. response
Apo-Ranitidine
Apo-Sulfatrim
Apo-Tetra
Apo-Tolbutamide
Apo-Trimip
apparatus, pl. **apparatus**
alimentary a.
biliary a.
contractile a.
digestive a.
a. digestorius
GIA autosuture a.
Golgi a.
juxtaglomerular a.
Manifold II slot-blot a.
Von Petz suturing a.
Wangensteen suction a.
apparent
a. digestive energy (ADE)
a. mineral corticoid excess
syndrome
appearance
beaklike a.
bird-beak a.
bull's eye a.
cloverleaf a.
cobblestone a.
coiled-spring a.
corkscrew a.
ground-glass a.
lead-pipe a.
leafless tree a.
mushroom-and-stem a.
normalized protein nitrogen a.
(nPNA)
picket fence a.
pinwheel a.
pseudo-Billroth I a.

NOTES

appearance *(continued)*
    pseudotumor a.
    sausagelike a.
    sawtoothed a.
    soap-sudsy a.
    spiculated a.
    stack-of-coins a.
    string-of-beads a.
    tadpole-like a.
    target a.
    through-and-through a.
    tigroid a.
    toxic a.
    wind-sock a.
Appedrine
appendage
    cecal a.
    epiploic a.
    torsion of a.
    vermicular a.
appendagitis
appendalgia
appendectomy (appy)
    colonoscopic a.
    emergency a.
    emergent a.
    incidental a.
    interval a.
    inversion a.
    inversion-ligation a.
    laparoscopic a.
    a. tape
appendiceal
    a. abscess
    a. adenocarcinoma
    a. intussusception
    a. Kaposi sarcoma
    a. mass
    a. mucocele
    a. opening
    a. orifice
    a. perforation
    a. stump
appendicealgia
appendicectasis
appendicectomy
appendices (*pl. of* appendix)
appendicism
appendicitis
    actinomycotic a.
    acute a.
    amebic a.
    chronic a.
    a. by contiguity
    foreign-body a.
    fulminating a.
    gangrenous a.
    a. granulosa

    helminthic a.
    a. larvata
    left-sided a.
    lumbar a.
    myxoglobulosis a.
    necropurulent a.
    nonperforated a.
    a. obliterans
    obstructive a.
    pelvic a.
    perforated a.
    purulent a.
    recurrent a.
    relapsing a.
    retrocecal a.
    retroileal a.
    segmental a.
    skip a.
    stercoral a.
    subperitoneal a.
    suppurative a.
    syncongestive a.
    traumatic a.
    verminous a.
appendiclausis
appendicocecostomy
appendicocele
appendicocystostomy
    continent cutaneous a.
    dismembered reimplanted a.
    nonplicated a.
    orthotopic a.
    plicated a.
    reversed reimplanted a.
appendicoenterostomy
appendicolithiasis
appendicolysis
appendicopathia
appendicopathy
appendicosis
appendicostomy
    Malone continent a.
appendicoumbilical stoma
appendicovesicostomy
    Mitrofanoff a.
appendicular
    a. artery
    a. colic
    a. dyspepsia
appendicularis
    arteria a.
appendilothiasis
appendix, pl. **appendices**
    base of a.
    cecal a.
    a. dyspepsia
    a. epididymis
    epiploic a.

a. fibrosa
gangrenous a.
hot a.
indurated a.
inflamed a.
Morgagni a.
nonperforated a.
normal a.
paracecal a.
perforated a.
retrocccal a.
retroileal a.
ruptured a.
subcecal a.
suppurative a.
a. testis
a. testis torsion
vermiform a.
xiphoid a.
appendolithiasis
appetite
a. disorder
perverted a.
voracious a.
apple
cashew a.
apple-core lesion
apple-peel bowel syndrome
appliance
external cooling a.
Gentle Touch colostomy a.
Karaya ring ileostomy a.
ostomy a.
application
laparoscopic clip a.
research a.
applicator
Betadine PrepStick Plus a.
Mick TP-200 a.
microwave a.
Multifire clip a.
multiload occlusive clip a.
resorbable thread clip a.
Applied Biosystems 340A nucleic acid extractor
applier
AcuClip endoscopic multiple clip a.
Advanced surgical suture a.
clip a.
cotton-tipped a.

Endoclip a.
multiloaded clip a.
Stone clamp a.
Appolito suture
approach
Alken a.
antegrade a.
anterior a.
anterior transabdominal a.
Bianchi a.
case-by-case a.
choledochofiberscopic a.
consortial a.
extrasphincteric a.
fascial sling a.
flank a.
Framingham risk-factor a.
gasless laparoscopic a.
Henry a.
Kraske parasacral a.
laparoscopic-assisted a.
microbial a.
minilaparatomy a.
percutaneous transhepatic a.
peroral a.
posterior lumbar a.
preperitoneal a.
Redman a.
retrograde a.
retroperitoneal a.
supraduodenal a.
thoracoabdominal extrapleural a.
thoracoabdominal intrapleural a.
transduodenal a.
transmural a.
transpapillary a.
vaginal wall a.
ventral transperitoneal
laparoscopic a.
wait-and-see a.
Appropriate Use of Gastrointestinal Endoscopy guideline
approximation
a. suture
tissue a.
wound a.
approximator clamp
appy
appendectomy
APR
abdominoperineal resection

NOTES

apraxia
    constructional a.
    swallow a.
APRE
    acute-phase response element
Apresoline
aprindine
aproctia
apron
    abdominal a.
    fatty omental a.
    a. skin incision
aprotinin
APRT
    adenine phosphoribosyltransferase
        APRT deficiency
APS
    arterioportal vein shunting
APS-1
    autoimmune polyglandular syndrome
       type 1
APSGN
    acute poststreptococcal
       glomerulonephritis
APT-Downey alkali denaturation test
Aptosyn
aPTT
    activated partial thromboplastin time
APUD
    amine precursor uptake and
       decarboxylation
       APUD cell
Aquachloral
AquaMEPHYTON
aquaporin
aquaporin-1
**AquaSens FMS 1000 fluid monitoring
  system**
Aquatag
aquaticus
    Thermus a.
aquatosis coli
Aquazide-H
aqueous
    A. Charcodote
    a. phenol
AR
    aldose reductase
       AR mRNA
arabinotarda
    Shigella a. type A, B
arachidonic
    a. acid
    a. acid metabolite
    a. acid oxidation
arachis oil
arachnoid fibrosis
Aralen

Aramine
Arandel cell harvester
Arantius ligament
ARB
    angiotensin receptor blocker
arbaprostil
arbitrary unit (AU)
arborization of ducts
ARC
    AIDS-related complex
arc
    sacral reflex a.
    tendinous a.
arcade
    gastroepiploic a.
ARCD
    acquired renal cystic disease
arch
    arterial a.
    cortical a.
    fallopian a.
    pubic a.
    Treitz a.
archaea
    methanogenic a.
architecture
    crypt a.
    distorted crypt a.
    hepatic a.
    intestinal villous a.
    lobular a.
arcuate
    a. artery
    a. line
    a. vein
arcus
    a. tendineus fascia pelvis
    a. tendineus musculi levatoris ani
ARD
    acid-related disorder
    anorectal dressing
ardor urinae
area, pl. **areae**
    cell surface a.
    choledochoduodenal a.
    a. gastrica
    areae gastricae
    gastrohepatic bare a.
    high-echoic a.
    intermicrovillar a.
    medial preoptic a.
    midepigastric a.
    midrectal a.
    a. nuda hepatis
    Paget disease of perianal a.
    perianal a.
    pericolostomy a.
    peripancreatic a.

periportal a.
peristomal a.
postcricoid a.
a. postrema
punctate a.
retroperitoneal a.
skip a.
subhepatic a.
target a.
a. under pH4 (AU4)
watershed a.
areflexia
detrusor a.
areflexic bladder
ARF
acute renal failure
mercuric chloride-induced ARF
argentaffin
a. cell
a. reaction test
a. stain
arginase deficiency
arginine
a. analog
a. vasopressin (AVP)
arginosuccinate
argon
a. beam coagulator
A. Beamer 2 device
a. beam plasma coagulation
a. ion laser
a. ion plasma coagulation
a. laser therapy
a. plasma coagulation (APC)
a. plasma coagulator (APC)
argon-pumped dye laser
argyle
A. chest tube
A. Ingram trocar catheter
A. Medicut R catheter
Argyle-Salem sump tube
argyrophilia
cytoplasmic a.
argyrophilic
a. and argyophobic neuron
a. cell
ARI
acute renal insufficiency
Arias syndrome
Aristocort
ARKD
autosomal recessive kidney disease

arm
cell-mediated a.
humoral a.
Leonard A.
armamentarium
Armanni-Ebstein lesion
Armanni-Ehrlich degeneration
Armed Forces Institute of Pathology (AFIP)
armillatus
Armillifer a.
Armillifer armillatus
ARMS-PCR
amplification refractory mutation system-polymerase chain reaction
Army-Navy retractor
Arndorfer
A. capillary perfusion system
A. pneumohydraulic capillary infusion system
aromatase inhibitor
aromatic
a. amine
a. amino acid (AAA)
Aronson esophageal retractor
ARP
acute recurrent pancreatitis
ARPKD
autosomal recessive polycystic kidney disease
array
DNA a.
arrest
spermatogenic a.
Arrestin
arrhythmogenicity
arrow
A. Raulerson syringe
A. UserGard injection cap system
ARROWgard Blue hemodialysis catheter
arrowhead sign
ARS
amylase-resistant starch
Artane
artefacta
dermatitis a.
arteria, pl. arteriae
a. appendicularis
a. caecalis anterior
a. caecalis posterior
a. caudae pancreatis
a. colica dextra

NOTES

arteria *(continued)*
a. colica media
a. epigastrica inferior
a. epigastrica superficialis
a. epigastrica superior
a. gastrica dextra
arteriae gastricae breves
a. gastrica posterior
a. gastrica sinistra
a. gastroomentalis dextra
a. gastroomentalis sinistra
a. hepatica communis
a. hepatica propria
arteriae ilei
a. ileocolica
arteriae intestinales
arteriae jejunales
a. lienalis
a. lusoria
a. mesenterica inferior
a. mesenterica superior
a. pancreatica dorsalis
a. pancreatica inferior
a. pancreatica magna
arteriae pancreaticoduodenales inferiores
a. pancreaticoduodenalis superior anterior
a. pancreaticoduodenalis superior posterior
a. rectalis inferior
a. rectalis media
a. rectalis superior
arteriae sigmoideae
a. splenica

arterial
a. ammonia
a. aneurysm
a. arch
a. blood gas (ABG)
a. blood sample
a. circulation
a. embolization
a. line
a. oxygen desaturation
a. portography
a. priapism
a. saturation
a. spider
a. steal
a. stimulation venous sampling (ASVS)
a. thrombosis
a. underfilling

arterial-enteric fistula
arterialization of portal vein
arteriogenic impotence

arteriogram
hepatic a.
superior mesenteric a.
arteriographic embolization
arteriography
celiac a.
celiomesenteric a.
gastric a.
hepatic a.
mesenteric a.
pancreaticoduodenal a.
penile a.
renal a.
selective left gastric a.
superselective a.
visceral a.
arteriohepatic dysplasia
arteriolar
a. hyalinosis
a. nephrosclerosis
arteriole
afferent glomerular a.
efferent glomerular a.
glomerular a.
Isaacs-Ludwig a.
juxtamedullary a.
postglomerular a.
preglomerular a.
renal a.
arteriolopathy
cyclosporine a.
arterioportal
a. fistula
a. vein shunting (APS)
a. venous shunt
arterioportographical examination
arterioportography
arteriosclerosis obliterans
arteriosclerotic
a. aneurysm
a. renal artery disease (ASO-RAD)
arteriotomy
end-to-side a.
arteriovenous (AV)
a. catheter
a. fistula (AVF)
a. hemofiltration
a. malformation (AVM)
a. shunt
arteritis
radiation-induced obliterative a.
Takayasu a.
villous a.
artery
abnormality of hepatic a.
accessory obturator a.
adrenal a.
anterior cecal a.

anterior superior
  pancreaticoduodenal a.
appendicular a.
arcuate a.
ascending ileocolic a.
ASPD a.
atherosclerotic renal a.
bladder a.
bulbar a.
bulbourethral a.
caliber-persistent a.
capsular a.
carotid a.
caudal pancreatic a.
cavernosal a.
colic a.
common hepatic a. (CHA)
common iliac a.
common penile a.
cremasteric a.
cystic a.
deep a.
deferential a.
dorsal pancreatic a.
dorsal penile a.
a. of Drummond
epigastric a.
external iliac a.
femoral a.
gastric a.
gastroduodenal a. (GDA)
gastroepiploic a. (GEA)
gluteal a.
gonadal a.
great pancreatic a.
helicine a.
hepatic a.
high transection of the inferior
  mesenteric a.
hypogastric a.
ileal a.
ileocolic a.
iliac a.
inferior hemorrhoidal a.
inferior mesenteric a. (IMA)
inferior pancreatic a.
inferior pancreaticoduodenal a.
inferior phrenic a.
interlobar renal a.
internal iliac a.
internal pudendal a.
left gastroomental a.

lienal a.
lumbar a.
lusorian a.
mesenteric a.
middle colic a. (MCA)
middle hemorrhoidal a.
obturator a.
ovarian a.
pancreatica magna a.
penile a.
phrenic a.
piriformis a.
polar a.
posterior superior
  pancreaticoduodenal a.
preureteral iliac a.
proper hepatic a.
prostatic a.
proximal superior mesenteric a.
pudendal a.
rectal a.
renal a. (RA)
retroduodenal a.
retrograde vascularization of
  superior mesenteric a.
right gastroomental a.
sacral a.
scrotal-perineal a.
spermatic a.
splenic a.
submucosal a.
superior hemorrhoidal a.
superior mesenteric a. (SMA)
superior vesical a.
testicular a.
umbilical a.
urethral a.
uterine a.
vesical a.
vesiculodeferential a.
a. weld strength
arthralgia
arthritis, pl. **arthritides**
colitic a.
dysenteric a.
enteropathic reactive a.
peripheral a.
reactive a.
rheumatoid a.
temporomandibular a.
urethral a.
villous a.

NOTES

arthropathy
    psoriatic a.
arthroplasty
arthrosia
    exanthesis a.
Articulator injection needle
artifact
    barium a.
    mirror-image a.
    pellet a.
    reverberation a.
artificial
    a. anus
    a. bezoar
    a. erection
    a. erection test
    a. genitourinary sphincter
    a. genitourinary sphincter
      implantation
    a. gut
    a. hepatic support
    a. insemination donor (AID)
    a. insemination husband (AIH)
    a. kidney
    a. organ
    a. urethral sphincter (AUS)
    a. urinary sphincter
    a. urinary sphincter implantation
aryepiglottic
    a. fold
    a. muscle
arylamine
arytenoid
    a. adduction
    a. cartilage
AS
    anal sphincter
AS-800
    AS-800 artificial sphincter
    AS-800 balloon
    AS-800 cuff
    AS-800 male bulbous urethra
4-ASA
    4-aminosalicylic acid
5-ASA
    5-aminosalicylic acid
    5-ASA agent
    5-ASA enema
Asacol delayed-release tablet
ASA-induced gastric ulceration
ASAP
    atypical small acinar proliferation of
      prostate
    ASAP channel cut automated
      biopsy needle
    ASAP prostate biopsy needle
    ASAP Stacker automated multi-
      sample biopsy system

asbestos
ASC
    acute suppurative cholangitis
ASCA
    anti-*Saccharomyces cerevisiae* antibody
ascariasis
    biliary a.
    endobiliary a.
    intrahepatic a.
    pancreatic a.
ascaricidal
ascaricide
ascarid
ascarides (*pl. of* ascaris)
ascaridiasis
ascaridosis
ascariosis
Ascaris
    A. infestation
    A. lumbricoides
ascaris, pl. **ascarides**
ascendens
    colon a.
ascending
    a. cholangitis
    a. colon
    a. ileocolic artery
    a. limb
    a. pyelography
    a. pyelonephritis
    a. urethrogram
ascent
    kidney a.
ascites
    a. adiposus
    bile a.
    biliary a.
    blood-tinged a.
    bloody a.
    chyliform a.
    chylous a., a. chylosus
    cirrhotic a.
    cloudy a.
    culture-negative neutrocytic a.
      (CNNA)
    demeclocycline-induced a.
    dialysis-related a.
    a. drainage tube
    eosinophilic a.
    a. euglobulin lysis time (AELT)
    exudative a.
    fatty a.
    gelatinous a.
    hemodialysis-associated a.
    hemorrhagic a.
    hydremic a.
    idiopathic a.
    malignant a.

A

milky a.
myxedema a.
narrow albumin gradient a.
nephrogenic a.
nephrogenous dialysis a.
neutrocytic a.
nonchylous a.
pancreatic a.
pseudochylous a.
refractory a.
resistant a.
straw-colored a.
tense a.
transudative a.
urinary a.
urine a.
wide albumin gradient a.

ascitic
a. amylase
a. fluid
a. fluid total protein (AFTP)
a. tumor fluid (ATF)

ascitogenous
ascorbic acid
Ascriptin A/D
ASCUS
atypical squamous cells of undetermined significance

asecretory
Aselli pancreas
aseptic
a. anastomosis
a. technique
a. wound

Asepti-steryl disinfectant
Asepto irrigation syringe
ASGB
adjustable silicone gastric banding

ASGE
American Society for Gastrointestinal Endoscopy

Asherson syndrome
Ashkenazi Jewish community
ASHN
acute sclerosing hyaline necrosis

Ashton
A. brief
A. pants

ASI
ASI prostatic stent
ASI Titan stent

asialia

asialoglycoprotein
a. receptor

Asiatic
A. cholera
A. schistosomiasis

ASID Bonz PP infusion pump
asitia
Ask-Upmark
A.-U. kidney
A.-U. renal segment

ASLC
acute self-limited colitis

ASMA
antismooth muscle antigen

Asopa
A. hypospadias repair
A. procedure

ASO-RAD
arteriosclerotic renal artery disease

asparaginase
asparagine
aspartate
a. aminotransferase (AST)
a. transferase

aspartyl protease-mediated cleavage
A-Spas
ASPD
anterior superior pancreaticoduodenal
ASPD artery

aspect
paraspinous a.
spinous a.

aspergillosis esophagitis
Aspergillus
A. bezoar
A. *flavus*
A. *fumigatus*
A. infection

Aspergum
aspermatism
aspermatogenesis
aspermatogenic sterility
aspermia
asphyxiating thoracic dystrophy
aspirate
gastric a.
heme-positive NG a.
nasogastric a.

aspirated sample
aspirating needle
aspiration
a. biopsy

NOTES

aspiration *(continued)*
    a. biopsy cytology
    a. catheter
    corporeal a.
    CT-guided fine-needle a.
    diagnostic a.
    a. and dissection tube
    endoscopic transesophageal fine-
        needle a.
    endoscopic ultrasound-guided fine-
        needle a. (EUS-FNA)
    epididymal sperm a. (ESA)
    EUS-guided fine-needle a.
    fetal bladder a.
    fine-needle a. (FNA)
    gastric a.
    Iglesias method of a.
    Levin tube a.
    lymphocele a.
    microepididymal sperm a. (MESA)
    microscopic epididymal sperm a.
    microsurgical epididymal sperm a.
        (MESA)
    a. mucosectomy
    percutaneous balloon a.
    percutaneous CT-guided a.
    percutaneous epididymal sperm a.
    percutaneous needle a.
    peritoneal a.
    a. pneumonia
    pulmonary a.
    real-time endoscopic ultrasound-
        guided fine-needle a.
    real-time fine-needle a. (RTFNA)
    seminal vesicle a.
    silent a.
    sonography-guided a.
    sperm a.
    suprapubic a.
    a. syringe
    tracheobronchial a.
aspirator
    Cavitron Ultrasonic Surgical A.
        (CUSA)
    Thorek gallbladder a.
aspirin
    enteric-coated a.
aspirin-induced gastritis
Aspisafe nasogastric tube
asplenia syndrome
AS-800 pump
Assam fever
assay
    Abbott IMx PSA a.
    acrosome reaction a.
    activity a.
    adherence a.
    Aura-Tek FDP a.

Ausab EIA a.
Behring OPUS Plus
    immunofluorescence a.
Bioclot protein S a.
Bio-Rad protein a.
BioWhittaker a.
bladder tumor a.
calprotectin a.
^{14}C glucose uptake a.
Ciba-Corning ACS PSA a.
Clostridium difficile toxin a.
competition-binding a.
competitive protein binding a.
cytotoxin a.
disaccharidase a.
electroimmunodiffusion a.
ELISA-like a.
enhanced reverse transcriptase
    polymerase chain reaction a.
enzyme-linked immunosorbent a.
    (ELISA)
enzyme-linked immunosorbent a. I
    (ELISA-I)
enzyme-linked immunosorbent a. II
    (ELISA-II)
erythrocyte lysis a.
estrogen receptor a. (ERA)
fibroblast ECM adhesion a.
fibroblast PMN adhesion a.
Galacto-Light a.
gastric-juice ammonia a.
heme-porphyrin a.
hemizona a.
HemoQuant a.
Hybritech Tandem prostate specific
    antigen a.
Hybritech Tandem-R PSA a.
IgA tTG a.
immunobead a.
immunoradiometric a. (IRMA)
IMX Hg a.
indirect immunofluorescence a.
inhibition a.
Inno-LiPA a.
intact hormone a.
latex agglutination a.
limiting dilution a.
liquid chromatographic a.
p53 a.
PMN chemotaxis a.
PP65 antigenemia a.
Pros-Check PSA a.
protein-protein a.
PTH-rP by immunoradiometric a.
Pyrilinks-D urinary a.
qualitative microculture a.
radioenzymatic a.
radioimmunoinhibition a.

radioimmunoprecipitation a.
recombinant immunoblot a. (RIBA)
recombinant tissue transglutaminase
  radioligand a.
recombinant tTG radioligand a.
renal vein renin a. (RVRA)
second-generation recombinant
  immunoblot a.
solution hybridization RNAse
  protection a.
sperm penetration a. (SPA)
stool antigen a.
stool toxin a.
Tandem-E-PSA
  immunoenzymetric a.
Tandem-ERA PSA
  immuenzymetric a.
tandem PSA a.
Tandem-R PSA a.
tissue culture a.
TNF-alpha a.
Tosoh a.
toxin a.
transcriptase polymerase chain
  reaction a.
tumor necrosis factor alpha a.
urine-based enzyme linked
  immunosorbent a.
UroVysion a.
Yang polyclonal a.
Yang Pros-Check PSA a.

assay-2
recombinant immunoblot a.-2

assemble
sleeve-multiple sidehole
  manometric a.

assembly
dilating catheter-gastrostomy tube a.
Konigsberg 5-channel solid-state
  catheter a.
8-lumen catheter a.

assessment
angiographic a.
blood flow a.
endoscopic color Doppler a.
extrapyramidal function a.
integrated a.
nutritional a.
outcome and process a.
penile vascular function a.
urodynamic a.

ASSI
ASSI laparoscopic electrode
ASSI METE-5168 (end-to-end)
  vasoepididymostomy
ASSI METS-3668 Microspike
  approximator clamp
ASSI MKCV-2040 Microspike
  approximator clamp
ASSI MSPK-3678 Microspike
  approximator clamp

assistant
gastrointestinal a.

assisted
a. reproduction
a. reproductive technique

association
American Anorexia/Bulimia A.
American Diabetes A. (ADA)
American Gastroenterological A.
  (AGA)
American Urological A. (AUA)
Internal Ostomy A. (IOA)
megacystis-megaureter a.
MURCS a.
United Ostomy A. (UOA)

Assura
A. closed mini pouch
A. convex drainable pouch
A. convex urostomy pouch
A. deluxe irrigation set
A. economy irrigation set
A. irrigation accessory
A. irrigation sleeve
A. pediatric pouch
A. pediatric skin barrier flange
A. standard drainable pouch
A. stoma cap
A. stomy belt

AST
aspartate aminotransferase
AST test

AST/ALT ratio
astemizole
asterixis
asteroid body
asthenospermia
asthenospermic
asthenoteratospermia
asthenozoospermia
asthma

NOTES

Astler-Coller
    A.-C. classification (A, B1, B2, C1, C2)
    A.-C. modification of Dukes classification
ASTRA
    ASTRA profile
    ASTRA profile test
Astra/Merck Group
Astramorph
astrovirus gastroenteritis
Astwood-Coller staging system for carcinoma
ASVS
    arterial stimulation venous sampling
asymmetrical
asymmetric pupils
asymmetry
asymptomatic
    a. bacteriuria
    a. gallstone
    a. hemodialysis patient
    a. hypocalcemia
    a. mass
    a. proteinuria
    a. pyelonephritis
    a. urinary lithiasis
    a. urinary tract infection (AUTI)
    a. urolithiasis
asystole
    lavage-induced cardiac a.
AT
    abdominal tympany
    adaptive thermogenesis
ATA
    antithyroglobulin antibody
Atabrine
Atarax
ataxia
    cerebellar a.
    late-onset a.
ataxic gait
atelectasis
atelectatic
atenolol
ATF
    ascitic tumor fluid
ATG
    antithymocyte globulin
ATGAM
    antithymocyte gammaglobulin
    ATGAM polyclonal antibody
atheroembolic renal disease (AERD)
atheroembolism
atheroembolus
atherogenesis
atheromatous

atherosclerosis
    graft a.
    ostial artery a.
atherosclerosis-induced cavernosal ischemia
atherosclerotic
    a. abnormality
    a. plaque
    a. renal artery
    a. renal artery stenosis
    a. renovascular disease
Ativan
Atkins diet
Atkinson
    A. introducer
    A. prosthesis
    A. scoring system for dysphagia
    A. silicone rubber tube
Atlantic ileostomy catheter
ATN
    acute tubular necrosis
atomic absorbance spectrophotometer
atonic
    a. bladder
    a. constipation
    a. dyspepsia
    a. esophagus
atony
    chronic intestinal a.
    gastric a.
    intestinal a.
    sphincter a.
    ureteral a.
atopic
    a. dermatitis
    a. eczema
atorvastatin
atovaquone
ATP
    adenosine triphosphate
ATP7A **gene**
ATPase
    adenosine triphosphatase
    ATPase activity
    ATPase inhibitor
atracurium
atraumatic
    a. clamp
    a. grasper
    a. locking/grasping forceps
    a. suture
atresia
    anal a.
    a. ani
    anorectal a.
    bile duct a.
    biliary a.
    congenital biliary a.

congenital duodenal a.
duodenal a.
esophageal a.
extrahepatic bile duct a. (EHBDA)
extrahepatic biliary a. (EBA)
follicular a.
gastric a.
Gauthier classification for
  extrahepatic bile duct a.
ileal a.
intestinal a.
intrahepatic a. (IHA)
jejunoileal a.
Kasai classification for extrahepatic
  bile duct a.
meatal a.
prepyloric a.
pyloric a.
suprapubic cystotomy tract
  urethral a.
urethral a.
vaginal a.

atretogastria
atrial
a. liver pulse
a. natriuretic factor (ANF)
a. natriuretic peptide (ANP)

Atrigel
atrium
Atrocholin
atrophia
atrophic
a. cirrhosis
a. gastritis
a. pangastritis
a. urethritis
a. vagina

atrophicus
lichen sclerosus et a.

atrophy
acute yellow a.
adrenal gland a.
crypt a.
familial microvillus a.
fundic gland a.
gastric mucosal a.
healed yellow a.
intestinal a.
lobar a.
mucosal a.
multiple system a.
muscle a.

parenchymal a.
partial villous a. (PVA)
proliferative inflammatory a.
sclerotic a.
seminal vesicle a.
skin a.
splenic a.
subtotal villous a. (SVA)
Sudeck a.
tubular a.
villous a.
white a.
yellow a. of the liver

atropine
a. derivative
a. infusion
a. methylnitrate
a. sulfate

Atrovent
ATS
autotransfusion
ATS canister

attachment
mesenteric a.
peritoneal a.

attack
anginal a.
Gowers a.

Attain tube feeding formula
attapulgite
attenuated adenomatous polyposis coli
attenuation
attic adhesion
atubular glomerulus
atypia
cellular a.
hepatocellular a.

atypical
a. adenomatous hyperplasia (AAH)
a. distribution of disease
a. ductular cell
a. gallbladder disease
a. glandular cells of unknown
  significance (AGUS)
a. small acinar proliferation of
  prostate (ASAP)
a. squamous cells of undetermined
  significance (ASCUS)

ATZ
anal transitional zone

AU
arbitrary unit

NOTES

AU4
area under pH4
¹⁹⁸Au
gold-198
AUA
American Urological Association
AUA Symptom Index
Aub-Dubois
A.-D. standard
A.-D. table
Auerbach
A. and Meissner plexus
A. mesenteric plexus
augmentation
bladder a.
a. cystoplasty
demucosalized a.
gastroileac a.
ileocecocystoplasty bladder a.
Mainz pouch a.
orthotopic bladder a.
a. plaque
rectal a.
ureteral bladder a.
augmented
a. biofeedback
a. bladder
a. valved rectum
Augmentin
Ault intestinal occlusion clamp
AUR
acute urinary retention
auranofin
Aura-Tek
A.-T. FDP assay
A.-T. FDP test
aureus
methicillin-resistant
Staphylococcus a. (MRSA)
Staphylococcus a.
Auriculin
AUS
artificial urethral sphincter
Ausab EIA assay
auscultation of bowel sounds
auscultatory
a. sign
a. sound
Ausonics OPUS-1
Australian antigen
autacoid
autemesia
authority
United Kingdom Transplant Support
Service A. (UKTSSA)
AUTI
asymptomatic urinary tract infection

auto
A. Suture Multifire Endo GIA 30
stapler
A. Suture Premium CEEA stapler
autoanalyzer
Beckman 2 a.
Hitachi 737 a.
autoantibody
anticentromere a. (ACA)
antineutrophil cytoplasmic a.
antithyroid a.
antitopoisomerase-I a.
circulating a.
a. production
ScI-70 a.
autoaugmentation
bladder a.
a. cystoplasty
laparoscopic laser-assisted a.
autocholecystectomy
autoclave
heat-sterilized by a.
steam a.
a. sterilized
autoclaved India ink
autoclaving
autocoid
autocrine
a. motility factor (AMF)
a. regulation
autocystoplasty
autodigestion
autoerotic rectal trauma
autofluorescent endsocopic system
autogenous
a. spermatocele
a. tunica vaginalis graft
autografting
autoimmune
a. cholangitis
a. cirrhosis
a. connective tissue disorder
a. deficiency syndrome
a. hemolytic anemia
a. hepatitis (AIH)
a. immunoglobulin mediation
a. interstitial nephritis
a. metaplastic atrophic gastritis
(AMAG)
a. polyglandular syndrome type 1
(APS-1)
a. sensorineural hearing loss
a. thyroid disease
a. thyroiditis
autoimmunity
thyroid a.
autointoxicant
autointoxication

autolavage
autologous
    a. chondrocyte
    a. fat
    a. HBcAg-specific CD4+
    a. liver cell
    a. rectus fascia sling
    a. transfusion
autolymphocyte-based treatment for renal cell carcinoma (ALT-RCC)
autolymphocyte therapy
automated
    a. endoscopic system for optimal positioning (AESOP)
    a. peritoneal dialysis (APD)
automatic
    a. chemical analyzer
    a. endoscopic reprocessor (AER)
    a. needle driver
    a. titration system
autonephrectomy
    silent a.
autonomic
    a. dysfunction
    a. dysreflexia
    a. hyperreflexia
    a. nerve fiber
    a. nerve-preserving three-space dissection
    a. nervous system (ANS)
    a. neurogenic bladder
    a. neuropathy
autopepsia
autophosphorylation
autoplasty
    peritoneal a.
autopoisonous
autoradiogram
autoradiography
autoreactivity
    liver-directed a.
autoregressive
autoregulation
    renal a.
autosomal
    a. dominant disorder
    a. dominant polycystic kidney disease (ADPKD)
    a. recessive kidney disease (ARKD)
    a. recessive mode

    a. recessive polycystic kidney disease (ARPKD)
autosomally
    a. inherited forms of nephrolithiasis
    a. recessively inherited disease
autosomal-recessive Alport syndrome
autosplenectomy
autostapling device
autosuture technique
autotoxic
autotoxicosis
autotoxin
autotransfusion (ATS)
autotransplantation
    colostomy pyloric a.
    posttraumatic a.
    pyloric a.
    renal a.
    a. of splenic fragment
auxiliary
    a. heterotopic liver transplantation (AHLT)
    a. liver transplantation
    a. partial orthotopic liver transplantation (APOLT)
    a. partial orthotopic living donor transplantation
    a. transplant
AV
    arteriovenous
    AV fistula
    AV shunt
Avagard instant hand antiseptic
avascular
    a. cuff technique
    a. necrosis
avenolith
Aventyl
average flow rate
AVF
    arteriovenous fistula
AVF-induced renal ischemia
AVH
    acute viral hepatitis
avian myeloblastosis virus reverse transcriptase
avidin-biotin complex (ABC)
avidin-biotin-peroxidase
    a.-b.-p. complex
    a.-b.-p. complex method
Avihepadnavirus
Avitene

NOTES

avium
    Mycobacterium a.
avium-intracellulare
    Mycobacterium a.-i. (MAI)
AVM
    arteriovenous malformation
avoidance maneuver
AVP
    arginine vasopressin
AVPR2
    antidiuretic arginine vasopressin V2
     receptor
avulsion
    splenic a.
AW
    actual weight
axes (*pl. of* axis)
axial
    a. flap
    a. hiatal hernia
    a. image
Axid
axillary adenopathy
Axiom double sump tube
axis, pl. axes
    bowel a.
    brain-gut a.
    cardiopyloric a.
    celiac a.
    crypt-villus a.
    a. deviation
    enteroinsular a.
    hypertension resistance a.
    hypothalamic-pituitary a. (HPA)
    hypothalamic-pituitary-testicular-
     penile a.
    macrophage-TGF-beta a.
    neurohumoral-immune a.
    pituitary-gonadal a.
    renin-angiotensin-aldosterone a.
    reproductive a.
axoaxonic synapse
axonopathy
axon reflex
axoplasmic
Axxcess ureteral catheter

Aylett operation
Ayre brush
Azactam
azamethonium
azan stain
azapetine
Aza-Pred therapy
azasteroid inhibitor
azathioprine
azide
    sodium a.
azidothymidine (AZT)
azithromycin
Azlin
azlocillin
Azo
    A. Gantanol
    A. Gantrisin
azole
    a. antifungal agent
    a. therapy
azoospermatism
azoospermia
    excretory a.
    occlusive a.
    steroid-induced a.
    unreconstructable obstructive a.
Azo-Standard
azotemia
    extrarenal a.
    prerenal a.
azotemic osteodystrophy
azoturia
azoturic
azoxymethane (AOM)
AZT
    azidothymidine
Aztec two-step
aztreonam
Azulfidine
Azulfidine EN-tabs
azygos
    a. blood flow
    coronary a.
    a. vein

B

B antigen
B bile
B cell
B cell line
B lymphocyte
B ring
B ring of esophagus

B-48

apo B-48
plasma apo B48

B72.3

antibody to B72.3
B72.3 murine monoclonal antibody

B₆

vitamin B_6

1b

HCV genotype 1b

B-1

Dukes B-1

B2

bromobenzene

B₁₂

B_{12} anemia
vitamin B_{12}

B12 immunological study
b558 membrane-bound cytochrome
B5 tumor marker
BA

bile acid

Ba

barium

Babcock

B. clamp
B. intestinal forceps

Babinski

B. reflex
B. sign

baby

b. Balfour retractor
Clinical Risk Index for B.'s
(CRIB)
b. scope
b. soft diet (BSD)

BAC

benzalkonium chloride

bacampicillin
bacillary

b. dysentery
b. peliosis

bacille Calmette-Guérin (BCG, bCG)
bacillus, pl. **bacilli**

acid-fast b. (AFB)
Calmette-Guérin b.
B. cereus

coliform b.
curved b.
dysentery b.
Friedländer b.
Schmitz b.
Shiga b.
Sonne-Duval b.
Stanley b.

bacitracin
backflow

pyelolymphatic b.
pyelorenal b.
pyelosinus b.
pyelotubular b.
pyelovenous b.

background

experimental b.
mucosal b.

Backhaus

B. dilator
B. towel clamp
B. towel forceps

backleak

acute tubular necrosis b.

backwash ileitis
baclofen
Bacon anoscope
Bacon-Babcock rectovaginal fistula operation
bacterascites

monomicrobial nonneutrocytic b.
(MNB)
polymicrobial b.

bacteremia

Streptococcus bovis b.

bacteria (*pl. of* bacterium)
bacterial

b. adherence
b. adhesin
b. adhesion
b. biofilm
b. biofilm formation
b. cast
b. cholangitis
b. cirrhosis
b. cleavage
b. colitis
b. complication
b. culture
b. cystitis
b. endotoxin
b. enterocolitis
b. esophagitis
b. flora
b. food poisoning

bacterial *(continued)*
    b. host interaction
    b. infection
    b. metabolism in intestine
    b. mucosal infiltration
    b. nephritis
    b. overgrowth
    b. overgrowth syndrome
    b. pathogenesis
    b. peritonitis
    b. prostatitis
    b. toxigenic diarrhea
    b. vaginosis
    b. vector
    b. virulence factor
bactericidal
    b. function of phagocyte
    b. stomach environment
bactericide
bacteriocholia
bacteriology
bacteriospermia
bacteriostatically
bacteriostatic barrier
bacterium, pl. **bacteria**
    Chauveau b.
    coliform b.
    colonic b.
    gram-negative b.
    gram-positive b.
    human gut b.
    intestinal b.
    mesophilic b.
    pathogenic b.
    pyogenic b.
    spiral b.
    toxigenic b.
    urinalysis sediment microscopy
      bacteria
bacteriuria
    asymptomatic b.
    catheter-associated b.
Bacteroidaceae
Bacteroides
    B. distasonis
    B. eggerthii
    B. fragilis
    B. melaninogenicus
    B. ovatus
    B. praeacutus
    B. putredinis
    B. splanchnicus
    B. thetaiotaomicron
    B. uniformis
    B. ureolyticus
    B. vulgatus
bactibilia
Bactocill

Bactrim DS
baculovirus
baculum
BAD
    benign anorectal disease
BA-EDTA solution
Baehr-Lohlein lesion
Baermann
    B. stool filter
    B. stool test
bag
    Acme One Time enteral feeding b.
    Belly B.
    bile b.
    Biohazard b.
    bowel b.
    Coloplast b.
    colostomy b.
    Davol feeding b.
    DeRoyal Surgical grab b.
    Dobbhoff enteral feeding b.
    endo catch b.
    EndoMate grab b.
    Entri-Pak enteral feeding b.
    eXtract specimen b.
    1090 Gavage B.
    Hollister urostomy b.
    ileostomy b.
    intestinal b.
    Keofeed enteral feeding b.
    Lahey liver transplant b.
    Le B.
    Mikulicz b.
    Mosher b.
    nylon tissue biopsy b.
    ostomy b.
    perfusate b.
    Perry b.
    Petersen b.
    Plummer b.
    pneumatic b.
    Polar enteral feeding b.
    stomal b.
    Top-Fill enteral feeding b.
    Vacutainer b.
    Whitmore b.
BAGF
    brachioaxillary bridge graft fistula
Bagley helical basket
BAIBF
    bile acid-independent bile formation
Bainbridge
    B. intestinal clamp
    B. intestinal forceps
Bakamjian flap
Baker
    B. antifol

B. intestinal decompression tube
B. jejunostomy tube
Bakes
B. common duct dilator
B. probe
BAL
blood alcohol level
balance
acid-base b.
chloride b.
electrolyte b.
equal fluid b.
glomerulotubular b.
B. lavage solution
metabolic b.
negative nitrogen b.
nitrogen b.
positive nitrogen b.
potassium b.
sodium b.
vagosympathetic b.
water b.
balanced
b. diet
b. electrolyte solution
b. salt solution (BSS)
b. voiding dysfunction
balanic hypospadias
balanitic epispadias
balanitis
b. circinata
circinate b.
b. circumscripta plasmacellularis
b. diabetica
Follmann b.
b. gangraenosa
gangrenous b.
keratotic pseudoepitheliomatous b.
plasma cell b.
trichomonal b.
b. xerotica
b. xerotica obliterans (BXO)
yeast b.
b. of Zoon
balanoblennorrhea
balanocele
balanoplasty
balanoposthitis chronica circumscripta
plasma cellularis
balanoposthomycosis
balanopreputial
balanorrhagia

balanorrhea
balantidial
b. colitis
b. dysentery
balantidiasis
Balantidium coli **colitis**
balantidosis
balanus
Balch 1 broth medium
bald gastric fundus
Balfour
B. abdominal retractor
B. gastroenterostomy
B. self-retaining retractor
Balkan
B. nephrectomy
B. nephritis
B. nephropathy
ball
b. electrode
food b.
fungal b.
gastrointestinal fungal b.
hair b.
b. myoma
B. operation
B. procedure
ureteropelvic fungus b.
B. valve
wool b.
Ballance sign
Ballenger forceps
Ballobes gastric balloon
balloon
Acucise b.
air-filled b.
anchoring b.
angioplasty b.
AS-800 b.
Ballobes gastric b.
banana-shaped b.
barostat b.
barostatic b.
Bilisystem stone removal b.
Brandt cytology b.
b. catheter and basket-retrieval
technique
centering b.
b. cholangiogram
cylindrical b.
b. cystoscope
b. cytology

NOTES

balloon *(continued)*
    b. decompression
    b. defecation
    b. dilating catheter
    b. dilation
    b. dilation of the papilla
    b. dilator
    dissecting b.
    doughnut-shaped b.
    esophageal single b.
    b. expulsion test
    extraction b.
    Extractor XL triple-lumen
      retrieval b.
    fluid-filled b.
    Fogarty b.
    French Swan-Ganz b.
    Garren b.
    Garren-Edwards b.
    gastric b.
    Gau gastric b.
    Grüntzig b.
    Helmstein b.
    high-compliance latex b.
    hot wire b.
    hydrostatic b.
    intragastric b.
    Kaye nephrostomy tamponade b.
    b. kymography
    b. laser
    latex b.
    low-compliance b.
    MaxForce TTS b.
    mercury-containing b.
    Microvasive retrieval b.
    Microvasive Rigiflex through-the-
      scope b.
    occlusion b.
    b. occlusion cholangiography
    Percival gastric b.
    b. percutaneous transluminal
      angioplasty
    b. photodynamic therapy
    preperitoneal distention b. (PDB)
    b. proctogram
    Provocative sensitivity b.
    Quantum TTC biliary b.
    rectal b.
    b. reflex manometry
    retrieval b.
    Riepe-Bard gastric b.
    Rigiflex achalasia b.
    Rigiflex TTS b.
    scintigraphic b.
    Sengstaken-Blakemore esophageal b.
    silicone b.
    stone retrieval b.
    b. tamponade prosthesis

    Taylor gastric b.
    through-the-scope b.
    b. topogram
    treatment b.
    b. tube tamponade
    b. ureteral occlusion
    water displacing b.
    Wilson-Cook dilating b.
    Wilson-Cook esophageal b.
    Wilson-Cook gastric b.
    windowed esophageal b.
    wire-guided hydrostatic b.
ballooning
    b. of cell
    b. degeneration
    b. degeneration of hepatocyte
    eosinophilic b.
    b. esophagoscope
    hepatocellular b.
    b. of papilla
balloon-occluded retrograde transvenous
    obliteration (B-RTO)
ballottable liver
ballottement
    abdominal b.
    kidney b.
    b. tenderness
balm
Balneol
BALP
    bone-specific alkaline phosphatase
balsalazide disodium
Balser fatty necrosis
Balthazar grading system
BAM
    bile acid malabsorption
Bamberger hematogenic albuminuria
bamboo joint-like appearance of gastric
    body
Bamethan
banana
    b. peel effect
    b. plug dipolar generator
    b.'s, rice, cereal, applesauce, tea,
      and toast (BRATT)
    b.'s, rice, cereal, applesauce, and
      toast (BRAT)
banana-shaped balloon
bancrofti
    Wuchereria b.
band
    adhesive b.
    anorectal b.
    anterior b. of colon
    cholecystoduodenal b.
    dysgenetic fibrous b.
    b. form
    free b. of colon

B

genitomesenteric b.
Harris b.
Henle b.
hymenal b.
Ladd b.
Lane b.
b. ligation
Lyon ring-constrictive b.
Marlex b.
mesocolic b.
omental b.
pecten b.
peritoneal b.
b. placement
b. 3 protein
retention b.
silicone elastomer b.
snap gauge b.
b. and snare technique
Swedish Adjustable Gastric B. (SAGB)
WBC b.
bandage
Sureseal pressure b.
suspensory b.
T-b.
banded gastroplasty with a divided pouch
banding
adjustable silicone gastric b. (ASGB)
b. cylinder
esophageal b.
hemorrhoidal b.
laparoscopic adjustable gastric b.
laser adjustable silicone gastric b. (LASGB)
suction b.
variceal b.
Bandito single-band ligator
band-ligator device
band-snare technique
Banff classification
banjo-string adhesion
Bannayan-Zonana syndrome
Banocide
Banthine
Banti
B. disease
B. splenic anemia
B. syndrome

BAO
basal acid output
BAP
bone alkaline phosphatase
BAR
biofragmentable anastomotic ring
Valtrac BAR
bar
cricopharyngeal b.
intersymphyseal b.
leading b.
Mercier b.
symphyseal b.
barbed snare
barber pole sign
Barbidonna
B. No. 2
Barbita
barbital-acetate buffer
barbotage
Barcat
B. procedure
B. technique
Barcat-Redman hypospadias repair
Barcoo vomitus
Bard
B. alligator cup
B. automatic reprocessor
B. Biopty gun
B. Biopty instrument
B. BladderScan
B. BladderScan bladder volume instrument
B. BTA test
B. button
B. closed-end adhesive pouch
B. Companion papillotome
B. Director guidewire
B. drainage adhesive pouch
B. endoscopic suturing system
B. Extra Ileo B pouch
B. gastrostomy catheter
B. gastrostomy feeding tube
B. Integrale pouch
B. irrigation sleeve
B. Memotherm colorectal stent
B. oval cup
B. PEG
B. PEG tube
B. Precisor direct bite forceps
B. protective barrier
B. protective barrier film

NOTES

Bard (*continued*)
    B. regular one-piece
    B. security pouch
    B. Urolase
    B. Urolase fiber laser system
Bardet-Biedl syndrome
Bardex-Foley catheter
Bard-Parker
    B.-P. blade
    B.-P. knife
BardPort implanted port
Bard-Stiegmann-Goff variceal ligation kit
bare area of liver
bariatric
    b. operation
    b. surgery
Baricon contrast medium
barium (Ba)
    b. artifact
    b. bezoar
    b. burger
    b. contrast radiography
    double tracking of b.
    b. enema (BE)
    b. enema reduction
    b. enema with air contrast
    b. esophagram
    b. granuloma
    b. meal
    b. paste
    b. peritonitis
    residual b.
    retained b.
    b. retention
    b. sediment in urine
    b. study
    b. sulfate
    b. sulfate solution
    b. sulfate for suspension
    b. swallow
barium-impregnated marshmallow
Barnes common duct dilator
Barnett pouch
Baro-CAT
Baroflave contrast medium
barogenic perforation
Barophen
baroreceptor
    high-pressure arterial b.
    low-pressure cardiopulmonary b.
    renal b.
    sinoaortic b.
baroreceptor-mediated mesenteric arterial vasoconstriction
baroreflex
    cardiopulmonary b.
Barosperse contrast medium

barostat
    b. balloon
    electronic b.
    b. method
    rectal b.
barostatic balloon
barotrauma
Barr
    B. fistula hook
    B. fistula probe
    B. rectal retractor
    B. rectal speculum
Barracuda flexible cystoscopic hot biopsy forceps
barrel
    b. chest
    Opti-Vue plastic b.
Barrett
    B. carcinoma
    B. disease
    B. dysplasia
    B. epithelium
    B. esophagitis
    B. esophagus (BE)
    B. intestinal forceps
    B. metaplasia
    B. segment
    B. syndrome
    B. ulcer
Barrett-Clagett esophagogastrostomy
Barrett-Donovan-Mayo artificial bladder
Barrett-Murphy intestinal thumb forceps
barrier
    ABO b.
    bacteriostatic b.
    Bard protective b.
    blood-epididymis b.
    blood-liquor b.
    blood-testis b.
    blood-urine b.
    Coloplast skin b.
    Comfeel skin b.
    Dansac skin b.
    b. drape
    filtration b.
    gastric mucosal b.
    high-pressure antireflux b.
    Hollister Guardian F skin b.
    Interceed absorbable adhesion b.
    Nu-Hope Adhesive waterproof skin b.
    pectin-base skin b.
    ReliaSeal skin b.
    seminiferous tubule blood-testis b.
    Sween-A-Peel skin b.
    United XL 14 skin b.
Barrington third reflex

Barron
  B. ligation
  B. rubber band ligator
Barr-Shuford rectal speculum
Barsony-Polgar syndrome
Bartel cytotoxicity
Barth hernia
Bartholin
  B. cyst
  B. gland
Bartonella henselae
Bartter syndrome
bar-type esophageal varix
baruria
BAS-300 transurethral thermotherapy device
basal
  b. acid output (BAO)
  b. acid secretion
  b. anal canal pressure
  b. anal sphincter pressure
  b. androstenedione
  b. carbohydrate oxidation rate
  b. cell carcinoma
  b. cell nevus syndrome
  b. cell-specific anticytokeratin antibody
  b. diet
  b. ganglia
  b. granular cell
  b. interferon-gamma
  b. lamina
  b. metabolic rate (BMR)
  b. metabolism (BM)
  b. release of motilin
  b. renal excretion
  b. renal vascular resistance
  b. secretory flow rate (BSFR)
  b. secretory flow rate test
  b. testosterone
Basaljel
basaloid squamous cell carcinoma (BSCC)
bascule
  cecal b.
base
  b. of appendix
  crypt b.
  erythromycin b.
  b. excess
  b. of renal pyramid
  ulcer b.

baseball stitch
baseline
  delta over b. (DOB)
  b. tenting
  b. troponin T
basement
  b. membrane
  b. membrane antigen
  b. membrane protein
bas-fond
basic
  b. diet
  b. dye
  b. fibroblast growth factor (bFGF)
  b. fibroblastic growth factor
  b. gastrin (BG)
basidiobolomycosis
Basidiobolus ranarum
basiliximab
basket
  Bagley helical b.
  Dormia stone b.
  Eliminator stone extraction b.
  Ellik kidney stone b.
  b. extraction
  3.2F Cook N-Circle tipless stone b.
  b. forceps
  Gemini paired wire helical b.
  Glassman b.
  Helical b.
  laser lithotriptor b.
  mini-helical b.
  nitinol b.
  Olympus stone retrieval b.
  Positrap mini-retrieval b.
  b. procedure
  Pursuer CBD helical stone b.
  Pursuer mini-helical stone b.
  retrieval b.
  Segura b.
  Segura-Dretler laser b.
  six-wire spiral tip Segura b.
  sphincterotomy b.
  spiral b.
  stone retrieval b.
  trapped b.
basketing
  ureteral scoping b.
basket-type crushing forceps

B

NOTES

69

baso
> basophil

basolateral membrane (BLM)

basophil (baso)
> WBC b.

Bassen-Kornzweig
> B.-K. disease
> B.-K. syndrome

Bassini
> B. inguinal hernia repair
> B. inguinal herniorrhaphy
> B. needle
> B. operation

Bates-corrected beta

Bates operation

bath
> alcohol cooling b.
> sitz b.

bathroom privilege

battery
> button b.
> b. ingestion

battery-powered endoscope

battle
> B. incision
> B. operation
> B. sign

Battle-Jalaguier-Kammerer incision

bat-wing catheter

Bauhin
> valve of B.
> B. valve

Baumgarten
> B. cirrhosis
> B. syndrome

Baumrucker urinary incontinence clamp

Baxter
> B. CA-210 filter
> 1550 B. hemodialyzer
> B. Interline IV system

Bay K 8644 channel agonist

Baylor bleeding score

bayonet-stylet

bayonet-tip electrode

bayonet-type forceps

Bazex syndrome

BBDS
> benign bile duct stricture

B1, B2 integrin

BBM
> brush-border membrane

BBMV
> brush-border membrane vesicle

BBS
> brown bowel syndrome

BC
> biliary colic
> BC Cold Powder

BCAA
> branched-chain amino acid

BCAA/AAA plasma ratio

B-cell
> B-c. antigen CD20
> B-c. differentiation factor
> B-c. epitope
> B-c. PHSL

B-cellular phenotype

BCG, bCG
> bacille Calmette-Guérin
> BCG immunotherapy
> intravesical BCG
> BCG live intravesical injection
> *Mycobacterium bovis* BCG
> BCG vaccine

bcl-2

BCM
> body cell mass

BCNU
> carmustine

BCO
> biliary cholesterol output

BCR
> bulbocavernosus reflex

BDA
> bile duct adenoma

BDL
> bile duct ligation

bDNA
> branched chain DNA

BDNF
> brain-derived neurotrophic factor

BDP
> beclomethasone dipropionate

B-D Safety-Gard needle

BE
> barium enema
> Barrett esophagus

Beacon surgical line

bead
> b. chain cystography
> b. chain study
> Percoll b.
> PMMA b.
> Septopal b.

beaded hepatic duct

beading sign

beaker cell

beaklike appearance

Beale
> sacculi of B.

beam
> x-ray b.

Beamer
> B. ejection stent
> B. injection stent
> B. injection stent system

bear claw ulcer
Beardsley
  B. cecostomy trocar
  B. esophageal retractor
  B. intestinal clamp
  B. intestinal forceps
Bearn-Kunkel-Slater syndrome
Beasley-Babcock forceps
beaver
  B. blade
  B. dissector
  b. fever
BEB
  blind esophageal brushing
BEC
  biliary epithelial cell
becanechol
Beck
  B. abdominal scoop
  B. aorta forceps
  B. Depression Inventory
  B. gastrostomy
  B. method
Beck-Jianu gastrostomy
Beckman
  B. airfuge
  B. 2 autoanalyzer
  B. ion-selective analyzer
  B. 39042 pH probe
Beckwith-Wiedemann syndrome
Béclard hernia
beclomethasone dipropionate (BDP)
bed
  Advanta b.
  gallbladder b.
  graft b.
  hepatic b.
  liver b.
  nail b.
  b. pad
  portal vascular b.
  raw surface of liver b.
  stomach b.
  suburothelial vascular b.
  ulcer b.
Bedge
  B. antireflux mattress
  B. pillow
bedside drainage (BSD)
bed-wetting alarm
Beebe hemostatic forceps
beef tapeworm

Beelith
Beer nephroureterectomy
BEF
  bronchoesophageal fistula
B.E. Glass abdominal retractor
behavior
  binge-purge b.
behavioral treatment
Behçet
  B. colitis
  B. disease
  B. syndrome
Behrend cystic duct forceps
Behring OPUS Plus immunofluorescence
  assay
beigelli
  Trichosporon b.
belch
  silent b.
Belfield operation
bell
  b. clapper deformity
  B. law
  B. muscle
  B. suture
Belladenal
belladonna
  tincture of b.
Bellafoline
Bellalphen
Bellergal-S
belli
  Isospora b.
Bellini
  B. duct
  B. duct carcinoma
  B. ligament
  B. tubule
bellow response
bell-shaped orifice
belly
  B. Bag
  wooden b.
bellyache
BELS
  bioartificial extracorporeal liver support
  system
Belsey
  B. 270-degree fundoplication
  B. Mark IV antireflux operation
  B. Mark IV 240-degree
    fundoplication

B

NOTES

Belsey *(continued)*
    B. Mark IV procedure
    B. Mark IV repair
    B. Mark V operation
    B. partial fundoplication
    B. two-thirds wrap fundoplication
belt
    abdominal compression b.
    Assura stomy b.
    Coloplast ostomy b.
    B. technique
    b. test
Belt-Fuqua hypospadias repair
Belzer
    B. machine
    B. UW liver preservation solution
Benadryl
benazepril HCl
Bence
    B. Jones albumin
    B. Jones albumosuria
    B. Jones cylinder
    B. Jones globulin
    B. Jones protein
    B. Jones protein method
    B. Jones proteinuria
    B. Jones urine
bench
    b. surgery
    b. surgical technique
Benchekroun
    B. hydraulic ileal valve
    B. pouch
bend
    cautery b.
    iliac b.
bendroflumethiazide
Benedict
    B. and Franke method
    B. gastroscope
Benedict-Osterberg method
Benedict-Talbot body surface area method
Benelux Multicentre Trial Study Group
Benemid
Bengt-Johanson repair
benign
    b. adenomatous polyp
    b. anorectal disease (BAD)
    b. bile duct stricture (BBDS)
    b. biliary stricture
    b. cystic mesothelioma
    b. cystic teratoma
    b. duodenocolic fistula
    b. familial hematuria
    b. familial icterus
    b. familial pemphigus
    b. gastric ulcer

    b. hyperplastic gastropathy
    b. lymphoma
    b. mesenchymoma
    b. mesothelioma of genital tract
    b. mucous membrane pemphigoid (BMMP)
    b. neoplastic precursor
    b. nephrosclerosis
    b. papillary stenosis
    b. paroxysmal peritonitis
    b. pneumatic colonoscopy complication
    b. pneumoperitoneum
    b. postoperative cholestasis
    b. postoperative jaundice
    b. prostatic enlargement (BPE)
    b. prostatic hyperplasia (BPH)
    b. prostatic hyperplasia transurethral vaporization
    b. prostatic hypertrophy (BPH)
    b. prostatic obstruction (BPO)
    b. recurrent intrahepatic cholestasis (BRIC)
    b. tumor
    b. ulcer
Béniqué sound
Bennett operation
benoxaprofen
benserazide
Benson pylorus separator
bentiromide test
Bentle button
bent nail syndrome
bentonite flocculation test
Bentson floppy-tipped guidewire
Bentson-type Glidewire guidewire
Bentyl
Bentylol
Benzacot Injection
benzaldehyde dehydrogenase
benzalkonium chloride (BAC)
benzamide prokinetic agent
benzathine penicillin
benzidine
benzimidazole
    substituted b.
benzoate
benzocaine
benzodiazepine conscious sedation
benzodiazepine-induced hypoventilation
benzoic acid
benzoin
    tincture of b.
benzoyl-tyrosyl-paraaminobenzoic acid (BT-PABA)
benzphetamine
benzquinamide
benzthiazide

benztropine
benzydamine
benzyl chloride
benzylpenicillin
BEP
    bleomycin, etoposide, cisplatin
Beppu score
bepridil
Berci-Shore
    B.-S. choledochoscope
    B.-S. choledochoscopy
Berens esophageal retractor
Bergenhem operation
Berger
    B. disease
    B. nephropathy
Bergkvist grading system
Bergman sign
Beriplast fibrin sealant
Berkeley-Bonney retractor
Berlin
    B. blue
    B. blue staining
Bernard
    B. canal
    B. duct
    B. glandular layer
Bernard-Sergent syndrome
Bernard-Soulier syndrome
Bernstein
    B. acid perfusion test
    B. gastroscope
berry aneurysm
Bertin
    hypertrophy of column of B.
Bertrand method
berylliosis
Besnier-Boeck-Schaumann disease
BESP
    Bipolar EndoStasis probe
Bessauds-Hilmand-Augier syndrome
Bessey-Lowry unit for alkaline
  phosphatase
best
    B. bite block
    B. gallstone forceps
    B. operation
    B. right-angle colon clamp
bestatin
besylate
    amlodipine b.

beta
    b. adrenergic blocker
    b. aminoisobutyricaciduria
    b. aminopropionitrile
    Bates-corrected b.
    b. chain
    epoetin b.
    estrogen receptor b. (ER beta)
    b. fetoprotein
    b. galactosidase
    b. galactosidase activity
    growth factor b.
    b. inhibin
    interferon b.
    b. interferon
    b. microseminoprotein
    b. sitosterolemia
    transforming growth factor b.
     (TGF-beta)
beta-1
    b.-1 chain
    b.-1 chain integrin
beta-2
    b.-2 agonist
    b.-2 microglobulin control
    b.-2 test
beta-3 agonist
beta-actin
    b.-a. cDNA probe
    b.-a. mRNA
    b.-a. mRNA signal
beta-adrenergic
    b.-a. agonist
    b.-a. antagonist
    b.-a. blockade
    b.-a. receptor
beta-blocker
Beta-Cap
    B.-C. catheter closure
    B.-C. II closure
Betadine
    B. gel
    B. PrepStick Plus applicator
    B. scrub
17-beta-diol
    5-alpha-androstane-3-alpha, 17-b.-d.
    5-alpha-androstane-3-beta, 17-b.-d.
beta-endorphin
    b.-e. peptide YY
beta-fibroblastic growth factor
beta-galactose
Betagan

NOTES

beta-HCG, beta-hCG
> b.-HCG autocrine motility factor

beta-hemolytic Streptococcus
beta-hydroxyacyl-coenzyme A dehydrogenase
beta hydroxylase
> dopamine b.-h.

3-beta-hydroxysteroid
> 3-b.-h. dehydrogenase
> 3-b.-h. dehydrogenase deficiency

beta-lactam antibiotic
beta-lactamase-resistant penicillin
beta-lactam-associated diarrhea
betamethasone
> topical b.

beta-2-microglobulin
beta-oxidation
> mitochondrial fatty acid b.-o.
> b.-o. pathway

beta-pleated sheet formation
beta-subunit
> transmembrane b.-s.

beta-sympathomimetic tocolytic agent
betaxolol
betazole stimulation test
bethanechol
> b. chloride
> b. hydrochloride
> b. test

bethanidine
Bethesda System for cervicovaginal sample
Bethune shears
Bevan
> B. abdominal incision
> B. gallbladder forceps
> B. operation
> B. orchiopexy

Bevan-Rochet operation
bevel
> Menghini-type coring b.

beveled speculum
bezafibrate
bezoar
> artificial b.
> *Aspergillus* b.
> barium b.
> fungal b.
> gastric b.
> medication b.
> orange b.
> percutaneous removal of b.
> persimmon b.

BF
> bile flow

bFGF
> basic fibroblast growth factor

BFR
> blood flow rate

BG
> basic gastrin
> bicolor guaiac

B2 glycoprotein I
BGP
> brain-type glycogen phosphorylase

BGV
> bleeding gastric varix

Bi
> bismuth

BIA
> bioelectrical impedance analysis

Biafine wound dressing emulsion
Bianchi approach
Biaxin
BIB
> biliointestinal bypass

bibasilar
bicalutamide
> b. monotherapy
> b. withdrawal phenomenon

BICAP
> Bipolar Circumactive Probe
> > BICAP bipolar diathermy
> > BICAP bipolar hemostasis probe
> > BICAP coagulation
> > BICAP electrocoagulation probe
> > BICAP electrode probe
> > BICAP endoscopic probe
> > BICAP hemostatic system
> > BICAP II cautery
> > BICAP monopolar
> > BICAP silver ACE

bicarb
> bicarbonate

Bicarbolyte
bicarbonate (bicarb)
> b. buffer system
> b. dialysate
> b. electrolyte
> potassium b.
> saliva b.
> serum b.
> sodium b.
> urinary b.
> b. wastage renal tubular acidosis

bicarotid trunk
BiCart dialysis fluid
biceps femoris musculocutaneous unit
bicho
Bicitra
BiCNU
bicolor guaiac (BG)
bicornuate uterus
bicoudate catheter
bi-curved needle

B

bidigital rectal examination
bidirectional ligation
Biebl loop
bieneusi
    Enterocytozoon b.
Biermer disease
Biesiadecki fossa
bifid
    b. branches
    b. clitoris
    b. penis
    b. renal pelvis
    b. scrotum
    b. tongue
    b. ureter
bifida
    adolescent spina b.
    spina b.
Bifidobacterium
    B. bifidum
    B. brevis
    B. infantis
    B. longum
bifidum
    Bifidobacterium b.
bifidus
    Lactobacillus b.
bifocal multiplane rectal transducer
bifurcation
    b. of common bile duct
    hepatic b.
    tracheal b.
    b. tumor
Bigelow
    B. litholapaxy
    B. operation
bigeminy
biglycan
    proteoglycan b.
Biguanides
Bihrle
    B. dorsal clamp
    B. dorsal clamp-T-C needle holder
BII
    BPH impact index
bikunin
bilabe
Bilagog
bilaminar embryonic disk
Bilarcil
bilateral
    b. anorchia

    b. cryptorchidism
    b. hydronephrosis
    b. lithotomy
    b. nephrectomy
    b. nephroureterectomy
    b. pheochromocytoma
    b. pudendal artery embolization
    b. renal tumor
    b. renal vein thrombosis
    b. subcostal incision
    b. transabdominal incision
    b. ureteral obstruction (BUO)
    b. ureterostomy takedown
    b. vagotomy
    b. Wilms tumor
bilayer
    lipid b.
    phospholipid b.
Bilbao-Dotter tube
bile
    A b.
    b. acid (BA)
    b. acid binder
    b. acid breath test
    b. acid diarrhea (type 1,2)
    b. acid-EDTA solution
    b. acid-independent bile formation
      (BAIBF)
    b. acid malabsorption (BAM)
    b. acid pool
    b. acid sequestrant
    b. acid therapy
    b. acid tolerance test
    b. ascites
    B b.
    b. bag
    C b.
    canalicular b.
    clear b.
    cloudy b.
    b. concretion
    cystic b.
    b. duct
    b. duct abscess
    b. duct adenoma (BDA)
    b. duct atresia
    b. duct brushing
    b. duct canaliculus
    b. duct cancer
    b. duct cannulation
    b. duct carcinoma
    b. duct cyst

NOTES

bile *(continued)*
    b. duct dyskinesia
    b. duct epithelial cell
    b. duct hypoplasia
    b. duct ligation (BDL)
    b. duct lumen
    b. duct paucity
    b. duct pressure
    b. duct proliferation
    b. duct stenosis
    b. duct stone
    b. duct stricture
    b. duct trauma
    b. duct type cytokeratin
    b. ductular cholestasia
    extravasated b.
    b. flow (BF)
    b. infarct
    inspissated b.
    b. lake
    limy b.
    lithogenic b.
    milk-of-calcium b.
    b. papilla
    b. peritonitis
    b. phospholipid concentration (BPC)
    b. phospholipid output (BPO)
    b. pleuritis
    b. plug
    b. pulmonary embolism
    b. reflux
    b. reflux gastritis
    b. salt (BS)
    b. salt aggregation
    b. salt concentrate (BSC)
    b. salt deficiency
    b. salt diarrhea
    b. salt export pump (BSEP)
    b. salt injury
    b. salt-losing enteropathy
    b. salt metabolism (BSM)
    b. salt output (BSO)
    b. salt-phospholipid ratio
    b. salt-stimulated lipase (BSSL)
    b. secretory failure
    SI of b.
    b. solubility test
    stagnant b.
    b. stasis
    supersaturated b.
    thick b.
    b. thrombus
    turbid b.
    viscid b.
    viscous b.
    white b.
bile-laden macrophage
bile-salt binding resin

bile-stained
    b.-s. fluid
    b.-s. vomitus
bile-tinged fluid
Bilezyme
bilharzial
    b. bladder cancer syndrome
    b. dysentery
    b. worm
bilharziasis
bilharzioma
bili
    bilirubin
    bili light
    Bili mask
biliaris
    collum vesicae b.
    corpus vesicae b.
    ductus b.
    fossa vesicae b.
    fundus vesicae b.
    vesica b.
biliary
    b. abscess
    b. actinomycosis
    b. air
    b. angiography
    b. apparatus
    b. ascariasis
    b. ascites
    b. atresia
    b. balloon catheter
    b. balloon dilator
    b. balloon probe
    b. calculus
    b. cannulation
    b. carcinoma
    b. cholangitis
    b. cholesterol output (BCO)
    b. cholesterol secretion
    b. cirrhosis
    b. cirrhotic liver
    b. clonorchiasis
    b. colic (BC)
    b. cryptosporidiosis
    b. cycle
    b. cyst
    b. cystadenocarcinoma
    b. cystadenoma
    b. decompression
    b. dilation
    b. dilator catheter
    b. diverticulum
    b. drainage
    b. dyskinesia
    b. dyspepsia
    b. dyssynergia
    b. echinococcosis

B

b. endoprosthesis
b. endoprosthesis insertion
b. endoscopic sphincterotomy
b. epithelia hyperplasia
b. epithelial cell (BEC)
b. excretion
b. fibroadenomatosis
b. fibrosis
b. fistula
b. hypercholesterolemia
  xanthomatosis
b. immunoglobulin
b. infestation
b. instrumentation
b. leakage
b. lipid
b. lithotripsy
b. manometry
b. microhamartoma
b. mud
b. orifice
b. pain
b. pancreatitis
b. papillomatosis
b. passage
b. piecemeal necrosis
b. plexus
b. prosthesis
b. radicle
b. reconstruction
b. saturation index
b. scintiscan
b. sclerosis
b. sepsis
b. sludge
b. sphincter
b. sphincterotomy
B. Spiral Z stent
b. stasis
b. steatorrhea
b. stent
b. stenting
b. stent patency
b. structure
b. tract
b. tract disease
b. tract obstruction
b. tract pain (BTP)
b. tract pressure
b. tract stone
b. tract stricture
b. tract torsion

b. tract tumor
b. tree
b. tree duplication
biliary-bronchial fistula
biliary-cutaneous fistula
biliary-duodenal
  b.-d. fistula
  b.-d. pressure gradient
biliary-enteric
  b.-e. anastomosis
  b.-e. fistula
biliation
Bilibed
BiliBlanket Phototherapy System
BiliBottoms
BiliCheck test
bilicyanin
bilifaction, bilification
bilifer
  canaliculus b.
biliferi
  ductuli b.
  ductus b.
biliferous
bilification (*var. of* bilifaction)
biliflavin
bilifulvin
bilifuscin
biligenesis
biligenetic
biligenic
Biligrafin contrast medium
bilihumin
bilin
bilioduodenal prosthesis
bilioenteric
  b. bypass
  b. fistula
biliointestinal bypass (BIB)
biliopancreatic
  b. bypass (BPB)
  b. diversion
  b. obesity surgery
  b. shunt
bilious
  b. cholera
  b. colic
  b. diarrhea
  b. emesis
  b. flux
  b. leakage
  b. remittent fever

NOTES

bilious *(continued)*
    b. remittent malaria
    b. stool
    b. vomiting
biliousness
biliprasin
biliptysis
bilirachia
bilirubin (bili)
    conjugated b.
    delta b.
    direct b.
    b. encephalopathy
    b. ester conjugate
    fat-soluble b.
    fractionation of b.
    indirect b.
    b. infarct
    b. pigment gallstone
    b. protein conjugate
    serum b.
    b. test
    total b.
    unconjugated b. (UCB)
    urinary b.
    urine b.
    water-soluble b.
bilirubinate stone
bilirubinemia
bilirubinometer
    direct-reading b.
bilirubinuria
bilis
    vesicula b.
Biliscopin contrast medium
Bilisystem
    B. ERCP cannula
    B. stone removal balloon
    B. wire-guided papillotome
Bilitec 2000 intraluminal fiberoptic probe
bilitherapy
biliuria
biliverdin
Bilivist contrast medium
Billingham-Bookwalter rectal fenestrated blade
Billroth
    B. cord
    B. forceps
    B. gastroduodenoscopy
    B. gastroenterostomy (type I, II)
    B. gastrojejunostomy (type I, II)
    B. hypertrophy
    B. I gastroduodenostomy
    B. II anastomotic scar
    B. II anatomy
    B. I, II anastomosis

    B. I, II gastrectomy
    B. I, II reconstruction
    B. strand
    B. venae cavernosae
bilobar
    b. hyperplasia
    b. hypertrophy
bilobate false aneurysm
bilobed
    b. gallbladder
    b. polypoid lesion
bilocular stomach
biloma
Bilopaque contrast medium
Biloptin contrast medium
Biltricide
bimucosa
    fistula b.
binary factor
binder
    bile acid b.
    Dale abdominal b.
    T-b.
    b. test
binding
    phosphotyrosine-SH2 b.
    ryanodine b.
    sperm-immunobead b.
    vasoactive intestinal polypeptide b.
binge
bingeing and purging
binge-purge behavior
binucleate renal tubule epithelial cell
bioactive antimicrobial coated solid alloplast
bioartificial
    b. extracorporeal liver support system (BELS)
    b. liver support device
bioassay
    mink cell b.
bioavailability
biochanin A
biochemical marker
Bioclot protein S assay
biocompatibility
biocompatible membrane
Biodan Prostathermer
biodegradable microsphere
biodistribution of N-isopropyl-p-iodoamphetamine
bioeffect
bioelectrical impedance analysis (BIA)
Bio-Enzabead test
biofeedback
    augmented b.
    bladder b.
    cystometric b.

B

sensory b.
b. therapy
voiding b.

biofilm
bacterial b.
b. related encrustation
BioFIT Herbgels
Biofix stent
biofragmentable anastomotic ring (BAR)
BioGel P4
Biogenex antigen retrieval method
biogenic amine
Bio-Gen urine test strip
Bioglass
Biohazard bag
bioincompatible membrane
Biolab
Malakit *Helicobacter pylori* B.
biologic
b. collagen-based tissue-matrix graft
b. marker
b. response modifier (BMR)
b. response modifier therapy
BioLogic-DTPF system
BioLogic-DT system
biomarker
intermediate b.
biomaterial
alloplastic b.
antiinfective b.
encrustation of b.
b. surface
b. type
biomaterial-associated infection
biomedical
b. research
b. science
biomembrane
BIO101 MERmaid kit
biomodulation
Biomox
bio-occlusive dressing
Bioplastique
biopsy
adrenal cortex fine-needle b.
alcohol-fixed gastric b.
antral b.
aspiration b.
bite b.
bladder b.
blind percutaneous liver b.
bone marrow b.

borderline b.
brush b.
b. channel
CLO b.
cold cup b.
colonic b.
colonoscopic b.
colorectal b.
cone b.
contralateral testicular b.
core needle b.
corporal b.
corpus cavernosum b.
Crosby-Kugler capsule for b.
CT-guided liver b.
CT-guided needle-aspiration b.
cytologic b.
diathermic loop b.
digitally guided b.
direct vision liver b.
double bite b.
duodenal b.
endoluminal ultrasonography-guided
   fine-needle aspiration b.
endoscopic small bowel b.
endoscopic strip b.
endoscopic transpapillary b.
endourologic b.
ERCP-guided b.
esophageal b.
fine-needle aspiration b. (FNAB)
fine-needle capillary b.
b. forceps
four-quadrant jumbo b.
freehand b.
full-thickness b.
fundic b.
b. of gastric mucosa
grasp b.
guided transcutaneous b.
guillotine needle b.
b. gun
hot b.
ileal b.
incisional b.
b. instrument
intestinal b.
jejunal drainage and b.
jumbo b.
laparoscopic b.
large-forceps b.
large-particle b.

NOTES

biopsy *(continued)*
    laser-guided b.
    lift-and-cut b.
    liver b.
    Menghini technique for
      percutaneous liver b.
    mucosal b.
    multiple b.
    native renal b.
    needle aspiration b. (NABX)
    needle core b. (NCB)
    open b.
    paracollicular b.
    percutaneous fine-needle
      pancreatic b.
    percutaneous liver b. (PLB)
    percutaneous native renal b.
    percutaneous pancreas b.
    peritoneal b.
    peroral jejunal b.
    pinch b.
    plugged liver b.
    pouch b.
    prostate gland b.
    protocol b.
    PTC-guided b.
    punch b.
    b. punch
    random bladder b.
    rectal b.
    renal b.
    saucerized b.
    scan-directed b.
    shave b.
    skinny-needle b.
    small bowel b.
    snap-frozen b.
    snare excision b.
    snare loop b.
    sonoguided b.
    strip b.
    suction b.
    systematic sextant b.
    tangential b.
    targeted b.
    testicular b.
    transcutaneous b.
    transfemoral liver b.
    transgastric fine-needle aspiration b.
    transitional zone b.
    transjugular liver b.
    transpapillary b.
    transrectal ultrasonography-guided b.
    transrectal ultrasound-guided-
      sextant b.
    transvenous liver b.
    trephine b.
    Tru-Cut needle b.

    ultrasound-guided anterior subcostal
      liver b.
    ultrasound-guided systematic
      sextant b.
    b. urease test
    vaginal cone b.
    Vim-Silverman technique for
      liver b.
    Watson capsule b.
    wedge hepatic b.
biopsy-verified chronic
    glomerulonephritis
Biopty
    B. cut needle
    B. gun
Bio-Rad protein assay
bioresorbable stent
Biosafe PSA4 screen
Biosearch 7000 enteral feeding pump
BioSorb resorbable urology stent
biosynthesis
biota
    gastrointestinal b.
Biotel home screening test
biothesiometry
    penile b.
biotin
    b. deficiency
    endogenous b.
biotinylated DNA probe
Bio-Tract proprietary strain
biotransformation
BioWhittaker
    B. assay
    B. assay test
BIP
    BIP biopsy instrument
    BIP high-speed multi biopsy needle
biperiden
biphasic diurnal rhythm
4,5-biphosphate
    phosphatidylinositol-4,5-b.
biplanar aortography
biplane sector probe
bipolar
    b. bleeding
    b. cautery probe BP-7350A
    B. Circumactive Probe (BICAP)
    B. Circumactive Probe coagulation
    b. coagulating forceps
    b. coagulation
    b. electrocautery
    b. electrocoagulation (BPEC)
    B. EndoStasis probe (BESP)
    b. esophageal recording
    b. glass electrode
    b. hemostasis probe
    b. neuron

b. sphincterotome
b. TURP
b. urological loop
bird-beak
b.-b. appearance
b.-b. configuration
b.-b. narrowing
birefringence
Bisac-Evac
bisacodyl
Fleet B.
b. tannex
bisantrene
Bisco-Lax
Bishop-Koop ileostomy
Biskra button
bismuth (Bi)
b. benign bile duct stricture classification
b. compound
b., metronidazole, tetracycline (BMT)
b. nephropathy
b. salt
b. sclerotherapy
b. subsalicylate
b. triple monocapsule
b. triple regimen
B. tumor
b. type IV
bismuthate
bismuth-free triple therapy
Bisodol
bisoprolol
bisphosphonate
bistable
bistriazole
bitartrate
cysteamine b.
bite
b. biopsy
b. biopsy forceps
bithionol
Bitome
B. bipolar sphincterotome
B. bipolar system
B. catheter
Bittorf reaction
bivalve
bizarre leiomyoma
black
B. Beauty ureteral stent

b. clot
b. cohosh
b. esophagus
b. faceted stone
b. hairy tongue
b. jaundice
b. liver disease
b. pigment gallstone
b. pigment stone
b. sickness
b. silk suture (BSS)
b. tarry stool
b. urine
b. vomitus
Black-Draught
Black-Draught Lax-Senna
bladder
b. acontractility
b. agenesis
alloplastic prostatic b.
amebiasis of b.
amyloidosis of the b.
b. angiosarcoma
b. antibody
areflexic b.
b. artery
atonic b.
b. augmentation
augmented b.
b. autoaugmentation
autonomic neurogenic b.
Barrett-Donovan-Mayo artificial b.
b. biofeedback
b. biopsy
b. calculus
b. cancer
b. cancer angiogenic factor
b. *Candida* infection
b. capacity
b. carcinoma in situ
b. carcinosarcoma
b. chimney procedure
b. chondrosarcoma
b. choriocarcinoma
color Doppler imaging of ureteral jet into b.
compliance of b.
b. compliance
congenital bifid b.
b. congenital diverticulum
b. congenital megacystis
b. cooling reflex

NOTES

bladder *(continued)*
cord b.
b. cuff
b. decompensation
b. decompression
defunctionalized b.
b. denervation
b. descensus
distended b.
b. diverticulectomy
dome of b.
double b.
dropped b.
b. duplication
b. dysplasia
b. ear
embryonal transitory b.
b. emptying
encysted b.
b. enlargement
b. epithelium
b. examination
b. excision
b. exstrophy
fasciculate b.
fasciculated b.
b. filling
b. fistula
gastric b.
Gilchrist ileocecal b.
b. granular cell myoblastoma
b. hernia
high-riding b.
b. histology
b. hydrodistention
hyperreflexic b.
hypertonic b.
b. hypoplasia
hypotonic b.
ileal b.
ileocecal b.
ileocolonic b.
b. imaging
b. incontinence
b. inhibition
b. injury
b. innervation
b. intravesical pressure
inversion of b.
b. inverted papilloma
b. involuntary contraction
b. irrigation
irritable b.
kidneys, ureters, b. (KUB)
b. leiomyosarcoma
b. leukoplakia
b. liposarcoma
low-compliance b.

b. lymphohemangioma
b. lymphoma
b. malacoplakia
b. malignant melanoma
b. mapping
b. mast cell
Mayo b.
b. mesonephric adenocarcinoma
b. mucosal graft
b. muscarinic receptor
b. neck
b. neck closure (BNC)
b. neck contracture
b. neck detrusor muscle
b. neck dysfunction
b. neck hypermobility
b. neck obstruction
b. neck preserving technique
b. neck reconstruction
b. neck sphincteric function
b. neck support pessary
b. neck support prosthesis
b. neck suspension (BNS)
b. neck-to-urethra anastomosis
b. neck transurethral resection
b. neck tubularization
b. neck Y-V plasty
b. neoplasm
b. nephrogenic adenoma
nephroureterectomy with en bloc
  removal of cuff of b.
nervous b.
b. neurofibroma
neurogenic b.
neuropathic b.
b. neurosis
b. nonepithelial tumor
nonneurogenic neurogenic b.
orthotopic b.
b. osteosarcoma
b. outflow obstruction
b. outlet
b. outlet closure
b. outlet kinesiologic study
b. outlet obstruction (BOO)
b. outlet reconstruction
overactive b.
b. overdistention
b. pain
b. palpation
pancreatic b.
b. patch
b. perforation
b. pheochromocytoma
b. pillar block
pine cone appearance of b.
b. plasmacytoma
b. plate

poorly compliant b.
b. post-cystourethropexy instability
b. preservation
b. pressure (BP)
b. pressure sensor
b. prolapse
prosthetic b.
pseudoneurogenic b.
b. pseudosarcoma
psychologic nonneuropathic b.
b. reconstruction
reflex neurogenic b.
reflex neuropathic b.
b. regeneration
b. replacement
b. replacement urinary pouch
b. retraction
b. rhabdomyosarcoma
ruga of urinary b.
b. rupture
sacculated b.
b. sarcoma
b. schistosomiasis
b. sensation
b. small cell carcinoma
b. smooth muscle
b. spasm
spinning top deformity of the b.
b. squamous cell carcinoma
b. squamous metaplasia
stammering b.
b. stone
b. storage function
strangulation of b.
b. stress relaxation
b. substitution
summit of b.
b. support
suprapubic aspiration of the b.
teardrop b.
b. thimble
thimble b.
tic douloureux of the b.
trabeculated b.
b. training
b. transection
b. transitional cell carcinoma
transitional cell carcinoma of
  the b. (TCCB)
b. trauma
b. trigone

b. tuberculosis
tuberculosis of kidney and b.
b. tumor (BT)
b. tumor antigen (BTA)
b. tumor antigen test
b. tumor assay
b. ulcer
b. ultrasonography
uninhibited neurogenic b.
uninhibited overactive b.
unstable b.
ureteral jet into b.
urinary b.
uvula of b.
valve b.
b. vein
vertex of urinary b.
b. viscoelasticity
b. volume
b. washing
b. worm
b. xanthoma
b. yolk sac tumor
**BladderManager portable ultrasonic
  device**
BladderScan
  Bard B.
  B. ultrasound
blade
  Bard-Parker b.
  Beaver b.
  Billingham-Bookwalter rectal
    fenestrated b.
  Bookwalter-Cook anal rectal b.
  Bookwalter malleable retractor b.
  Bookwalter-Mayo b.
  Bookwalter-Parks anal sphincter b.
  Bovie b.
  Deaver-type b.
  knife b.
  malleable b.
  razor b.
  scalpel b.
Blair silicone drain
**Blaivas urinary incontinence
  classification**
Blake gallstone forceps
Blakemore-Sengstaken tube
Blakemore tube
Blalock pulmonary artery forceps
Blanchard hemorrhoid forceps

NOTES

blanching
>b. of lesion
>b. of mucosa

bland
>b. diet
>b. food
>b. pulmonary hemorrhage
>b. thrombosis

Bland-Altman analysis

blanket
>Gaymar water-circulating b.

blast
>b. cell
>b. injury
>refractory anemia with excess of b.'s (RAEB)
>white blood cell b.

blastema
>renal b.

blastocyst hatching

Blastocystis hominis

blastoid transformation

blastomere

Blastomyces dermatitidis

blastomycosis
>peritoneal b.

Blatin
>B. sign
>B. syndrome

bleb

bleed
>gastrointestinal b.
>GI b.
>herald b.
>postgastrectomy b.
>postpolypectomy b.

bleeder

bleeding
>b. acid-peptic disease
>active source of b.
>b. angioma
>bipolar b.
>b. colonic angiodysplasia
>colorectal variceal b.
>contact b.
>b. control
>diverticular b.
>b. diverticulosis
>b. diverticulum
>duodenal b.
>dysfunctional b.
>esophageal variceal b.
>esophagogastric variceal b.
>excessive b.
>functional b.
>gastric varix b.
>b. gastric varix (BGV)
>b. gastritis

>gastrointestinal b. (GIB)
>GI b.
>b. hemorrhoid
>jetlike b.
>b. lesion
>lower gastrointestinal b. (LGIB)
>lower GI b.
>minute b.
>mucosal b.
>occult gastrointestinal b.
>painless rectal b.
>pancreatitis-related b.
>peptic ulcer b.
>per anum b.
>b. per rectum
>b. pile
>b. point
>b. polyp
>b. proctitis
>rectal b.
>b. site
>b. site localization
>b. time
>b. tumor
>b. ulcer
>upper gastrointestinal b. (UGIB)
>vaginal b.
>variceal b.

blend
>b. waveform
>b. waveform desiccation

blended
>b. current
>b. cut
>b. electrocautery

blenderized diet

blennemesis

blennorrhagica
>keratoderma b.
>keratosis b.

blennuria

BLEO
>bleomycin

bleomycin (BLEO)
>carboplatin, etoposide, b. (CEB)
>b., etoposide, cisplatin (BEP)
>platinum, etoposide, b. (PEB)
>platinum, Velban, b. (PVB)
>b. sulfate
>b. toxicity
>Velban, actinomycin-D, b. (VAB)
>vinblastine, actinomycin D, b. (mini-VAB)

bleomycin-associated adult respiratory distress syndrome

blepharitis

blepharospasm

B

blind
    b. cautery
    b. enema
    b. esophageal brushing (BEB)
    b. fistula
    b. intestine
    b. limb
    b. lithotripsy
    b. loop
    b. loop syndrome (BLS)
    b. percutaneous liver biopsy
    b. stump
    b. subtotal colectomy
    b. technique
    b. upper esophageal pouch
blindgut
blindness
    river b.
blink
    acoustic b.
blinking reflex
BLL
    blood lead level
BLM
    basolateral membrane
bloc
    harvesting en b.
Blocadren
Bloch-Paul-Mikulicz operation
block
    abdominal ganglion b.
    Best bite b.
    bladder pillar b.
    caudal b.
    celiac plexus b.
    collision b.
    endoscopic ultrasound-guided celiac
      plexus b.
    Marcaine b.
    nerve b.
    neurolytic celiac plexus b.
    OB-10 Comfort bite b.
    periprostatic b.
    portal b.
    transitory b.
Block-Ace solution
blockade
    adjuvant alpha b.
    alpha sympathetic b.
    androgen b.
    beta-adrenergic b.
    cavernosal alpha b.

    combined androgen b. (CAB)
    differential neuroaxial b.
    lipoxygenase b.
    maximal androgen b. (MAB)
    muscarinic b.
    reversible b.
blockage
    complete hormonal b.
blocked aerogastria
blocker
    alpha-1 b.
    angiotensin receptor b. (ARB)
    beta adrenergic b.
    calcium channel b.
    calcium entry b.
    H2 b.
    nicotinic receptor b.
    proton pump b.
    RAS b.
    renin-angiotensin system b.
    starch b.
blocking
    electrical b.
    thermal b.
Blocksom vesicostomy
Blom-Singer
    B.-S. esophagoscope
    B.-S. tracheoesophageal fistula
blood
    b. admixed with stool
    b. agar plate
    b. alcohol level (BAL)
    b. ammonia
    bright red b.
    b. calculus
    b. cast
    b. clot
    clotted b.
    b. coagulation
    b. coagulation disorder
    b. collection
    crossmatched b.
    b. culture
    dark burgundy b.
    b. flow
    b. flow assessment
    b. flow rate (BFR)
    frank b.
    b. gas on oxygen
    b. gas on room air
    b. group antigen
    b. lead level (BLL)

NOTES

blood *(continued)*
    maroon b.
    nonhemolyzed b.
    nostril b.
    occult b.
    b. on surface of stool
    oozing b.
    b. passed with stool
    b. per rectum (BPR)
    b. pH
    b. pressure (BP)
    b. sample
    spurting b.
    b. in stool
    stool for occult b.
    b. stream infection (BSI)
    b. transfusion
    b. type
    typed b.
    b. urea concentration
    b. urea level
    b. urea nitrogen (BUN)
    b. vessel
    whole b.
blood-borne
    b.-b. non-A, non-B hepatitis
    b.-b. pathogen
    b.-b. transmission
blood-contactin catheter
blood-epididymis barrier
Bloodgood
    B. operation
    B. procedure
blood-liquor barrier
blood-streaked stool
blood-testis barrier
blood-testis-epididymis
blood-tinged ascites
blood-urine barrier
bloody
    b. ascites
    b. diarrhea
    b. discharge
    b. peritoneal fluid
    b. stool
    b. vomitus
blooming effect
blot
    Southern b.
    Western b.
blotting
    ECL Western b.
    enhanced chemiluminescence
      Western b.
    Western b.
Blount disease

blow-hole
    b.-h. cecostomy
    b.-h. ileostomy
blown pupil
BLQ
    both lower quadrants
BLS
    blind loop syndrome
blue
    Alcian b.
    Berlin b.
    carmine b.
    b. diaper syndrome
    b. dot sign
    eosin-methylene b. (EMB)
    Evans b.
    B. Max balloon catheter
    methylene b.
    b. navel
    periodic acid-Schiff-Alcian b. (PAS-
      AB)
    b. rubber bleb nevus syndrome
    b. toe syndrome
    toluidine b.
    Urolene B.
    b. varix
Bluemle pump
Blumberg
    inguinal ligament of B.
    B. sign
Blumer rectal shelf
blunt
    b. abdominal trauma
    b. liver trauma
    b. needle
    b. pancreatic trauma
    b. probe
    b. and sharp dissection
blunting
    costophrenic b.
    haustral b.
    b. of valve
blunt-tipped obturator
blush
    delayed b.
    immediate b.
B-lymphocyte
    B-l. activation
    B-l. system
BM
    basal metabolism
    bowel movement
BMD
    bone mineral densitometry
    bone mineral density
BMI
    body mass index

B

BMMP
  benign mucous membrane pemphigoid
B-mode
    B-m. imaging
    B-m. ultrasonography
    B-m. ultrasound image
BMR
  basal metabolic rate
  biologic response modifier
BMS
  burning mouth syndrome
BMT
  bismuth, metronidazole, tetracycline
  bone marrow transplantation
BNC
  bladder neck closure
BNO
  bowels not open
BNP
  brain natriuretic peptide
BNS
  bladder neck suspension
boardlike
    b. rigidity
    b. rigidity of abdomen
Boari
    B. bladder flap
    B. bladder flap procedure
    B. operation
    B. ureteral flap repair
Boari-Ockerblad
    B.-O. flap
    B.-O. principle
Boas
    B. algesimeter
    B. point
    B. sign
    B. test meal
boat-shaped abdomen
Bochdalek
    foramen of B.
    B. hernia
Bodansky unit
Boden-Gibb tumor staging
Bodenhammer rectal speculum
body
    acidophilic b.
    anal foreign b.
    angularis b.
    anorectal foreign b.
    asteroid b.

bamboo joint-like appearance of
  gastric b.
Call-Exner b.
b. cell mass (BCM)
CMV inclusion b.
cobblestone appearance of
  gastric b.
coccidian b.
colonic foreign b.
b. composition analysis
compressible cavernous b.
corneal foreign b.
Councilman b.
Cowdry type A inclusion b.
crescentic b.
Cyanobacterium-like b.
Donovan b.
duodenal foreign b.
embryoid b.
b. of epididymis
epithelial inclusion b.
esophageal foreign b.
esophageal Lewy b.
falciform b.
b. fluid osmolality
foreign b.
gastric foreign b.
b. habitus
Highmore b.
Howell-Jolly b.
inclusion b.
ingested foreign b.
intracytoplasmic CMV inclusion b.
intraepithelial b.
intranuclear CMV inclusion b.
Jaworski b.
juxtaglomerular b.
ketone b. (KB)
Lafora b.
lower GI tract foreign b.
Mallory hyaline b.
malpighian b.
b. mass index (BMI)
Michaelis-Gutmann b.
oval fat b.
penile b.
perineal b.
polar b.
b. position
b. of pubis
rectal foreign b.
retained foreign b. (RFB)

NOTES

body *(continued)*
    Savage perineal b.
    Schaumann b.
    Schiller-Duval b.
    S-shaped b.
    string-of-pearls appearance of
      gastric b.
    b. substance isolation (BSI)
    Symington b.
    upper GI tract foreign b.
    vaginal foreign b.
    vermiform b.
    viral inclusion b.
    b. water
    b. weight (BW)
Boeck sarcoma
Boehm
    B. anoscope
    B. proctoscope
    B. rectal diagnostic and treatment
      set
    B. sigmoidoscope
Boehringer kit
Boerema
    B. anterior gastropexy
    B. hernia repair
Boerhaave syndrome
Boettcher crystal
boggy prostate
Bogros space
Bohr effect
Bolande tumor
Boley vascular ectasia
bolster suture
bolus
    alimentary b.
    b. challenge test
    b. dressing
    b. extraction
    b. feeding
    food b.
    heparin b.
    b. hold-up
    marshmallow b.
    b. transport
bombesin receptor
bone
    adynamic b.
    b. alkaline phosphatase (BAP)
    b. densitometry
    b. disease
    b. formation
    innominate b.
    b. marrow aplasia
    b. marrow biopsy
    b. marrow-derived B cell
    b. marrow stem cell
    b. marrow transplantation (BMT)

    b. marrow transplantation-related
      problem
    b. mineral densitometry (BMD)
    b. mineral density (BMD)
    b. morphogenic protein
    b. scan
    b. turnover marker
**bone-specific alkaline phosphatase
  (BALP)**
Bonine
Bonney test
bony
    b. defect
    b. dysraphism
    b. landmark
    b. pelvis
    b. spicule
    b. tenderness
BOO
    bladder outlet obstruction
Bookler swivel-ball laparoscope holder
Bookwalter
    B. malleable retractor blade
    B. retractor system
    B. ring retractor
Bookwalter-Cook anal rectal blade
Bookwalter-Goulet retractor
Bookwalter-Hill-Ferguson rectal retractor
Bookwalter-Mayo blade
Bookwalter-Parks anal sphincter blade
**Bookwalter-St. Mark deep pelvic
  retractor**
**Boorman gastric cancer typing system
  (type 1–4)**
Boost Nutritional Energy Drink
boot
    Heelift smooth b.
BOR
    bowels open regularly
    branchio-oto-renal syndrome
borborygmus, pl. **borborygmi**
Borchardt triad
border
    antimesenteric b.
    brush b.
    b. cell
    fundopyloric mucosal b.
    intestinal brush b. (IBB)
    lobulated b.
    mucosal b.
    scalloped antimesenteric b.
    b. zone
borderline biopsy
bore
    magnetic b.
Borge clamp
boring pain
Boros esophagoscope

Borreliosis classification for advanced gastric cancer
Borrmann
    B. gastric cancer
    B. gastric cancer classification
    B. gastric carcinoma (types I–IV)
    B. scirrhous carcinoma
Bors ice water test
Bosniak
    B. classification
    B. criteria
    B. lesion (category I–IV)
bosselated surface
B&O suppository
both
    b. lower quadrants (BLQ)
    b. upper quadrants (BUQ)
Botkin disease
Botox
botryoid
    interlabial sarcoma b.
    b. sarcoma
Bottini operation
bottle
    McGaw plastic b.
    Nu-Hope urine collection b.
    b. operation
    Vacutainer b.
botulinum
    Clostridium b.
    b. toxin (BTX)
    b. toxin injection
botulism
Bouchard
    B. disease
    B. index
bougie
    acorn-tipped b.
    b. à boule
    bulbous b.
    Celestin dilator b.
    b. dilator
    elastic b.
    elbowed b.
    EndoLumina b.
    filiform b.
    following b.
    French b.
    Hegar intrarectal b.
    Hurst mercury b.
    Hurst-type b.
    Jackson esophageal b.

    Klebanoff common duct b.
    large-diameter b.
    Maloney b.
    mercury-weighted rubber b.
    polyvinyl b.
    Savary b.
    Savary-Gilliard Silastic flexible b.
    Savary-Gilliard wire-guided b.
    tapered rubber b.
    through-the-scope b.
    Trousseau esophageal b.
    Wales rectal b.
    wax-tipped b.
    wire-guided polyvinyl b.
bougienage
    esophageal b.
    Hurst b.
    peroral b.
    transgastric esophageal b.
bouillon
Bouin fixative solution
boulardii
    Saccharomyces b.
boule
    bougie à b.
bouquet fever
Bourne test
Bourneville disease
bouton en chemise
Bouveret
    B. syndrome
    B. ulcer
Bouveret-Duguet ulcer
Bovie
    B. blade
    B. cautery
    B. coagulation
    B. electrocautery
    B. electrocoagulation unit
    B. holder
bovied
bovine
    b. dermal collagen
    b. graft
    b. serum albumin (BSA)
    b. thrombin
    b. trypsin
bovis
    Cysticercus b.
    Moraxella b.
    Mycobacterium b.
    Streptococcus b.

NOTES

B

bowed sternum
bowel
> b. adherent to omentum
> aganglionic b.
> b. axis
> b. bag
> b. bypass
> b. bypass syndrome
> competent b.
> b. content
> b. continuity
> dead b.
> detubularized small b.
> dilated loops of b.
> b. dilation
> b. disease
> B. Disease Questionnaire
> b. displacement
> b. emptying regimen
> entrapment of b.
> fixed segment of b.
> fluid-filled small b.
> b. forceps
> b. function
> gangrenous b.
> b. gas
> b. grasper
> greedy b.
> b. habit
> incarcerated b.
> b. incontinence
> infarcted b.
> b. injury
> b. intussusception
> b. irrigation
> ischemic b.
> kink in b.
> Ladd correction of malrotation
>   of b.
> large b.
> b. loop
> b. lumen
> b. movement (BM)
> b. necrosis
> necrotizing vasculitis of b.
> Noble surgical plication of b.
> b.'s not open (BNO)
> b. obstruction
> b.'s open regularly (BOR)
> b. perforation
> b. plate
> pleating of small b.
> b. preparation
> b. preparation complication
> prolapsed b.
> b. pseudoobstruction
> b. refashioning procedure
> b. resection

> b. rest (BR)
> small b.
> b. sounds
> b. sounds active (BSA)
> b. sounds normal (BSN)
> b. sounds normal and active
>   (BSNA)
> b. stoma
> strangulated b.
> The B. Disease Questionnaire
> b. tone
> toxic dilatation of b.
> b. wall
> b. wall induration

Bowen
> B. disease
> B. papule
> B. patch

bowenoid papulosis
Bower PEG tube
bowler hat sign
Bowman
> B. capsule
> B. space
> B. space cyst

Boyarsky
> B. BPH symptom score
> B. symptom scoring system

Boyce
> longitudinal nephrotomy of B.
> B. modification of Sengstaken-
>   Blakemore tube
> B. sign

Boyce-Vest procedure
Boyden
> B. sphincter
> B. test
> B. test meal

boydii
> *Pseudallescheria b.*
> *Shigella b.*

Boyle and Goldstein saline test
Bozeman
> B. forceps
> B. operation

Bozeman-Fritsch catheter
Bozicevich test
BP
> bladder pressure
> blood pressure

BP-7350A
> bipolar cautery probe BP-7350A

BPB
> biliopancreatic bypass

BPC
> bile phospholipid concentration

BPE
> benign prostatic enlargement

B

BPEC
bipolar electrocoagulation
BPH
benign prostatic hyperplasia
benign prostatic hypertrophy
BPH impact index (BII)
BPO
benign prostatic obstruction
bile phospholipid output
BPR
blood per rectum
BQ123 receptor antagonist
BR
bowel rest
BR96
monoclonal antibody B.
Braasch
B. bulb
B. catheter
B. direct catheterization cystoscope
Braasch-Kaplan direct vision cystoscope
brachial pressure index
**brachioaxillary bridge graft fistula
(BAGF)**
brachioradialis
**brachiosubclavian bridge graft fistula
(BSGF)**
brachyesophagus
BrachySeed
B. brachytherapy seed
B. prostate cancer treatment
brachytherapy
interstitial b.
intracavitary application b.
salvage b.
transperineal b.
transperineal interstitial permanent
prostate b. (TIPPB)
Brackin
B. ureterointestinal anastomosis
B. ureterointestinal anastomosis
technique
Bradley
B. classification of voiding
dysfunction
B. disease
B. loop
bradyarrhythmia
bradycardia
reflex b.
sinus b.
bradygastria

bradykinin
bradypepsia
bradyphagia
bradyspermatism
bradystalsis
bradytrophia
bradytrophic
bradyuria
brain
b. metastasis
b. natriuretic peptide (BNP)
b. stem-sacral loop
b. tumor
**brain-derived neurotrophic factor
(BDNF)**
Brainerd diarrhea
brain-gut
b.-g. axis
b.-g. peptide
brain-heart infusion agar
**brain-type glycogen phosphorylase
(BGP)**
brake
duodenal b.
ileal b.
bran
branch
bifid b.'s
b. duct-type tumor
lateral b.
b. pancreatic duct
b. renal artery disease
side b.
branched
b. calculus
b. chain DNA (bDNA)
b. crypt
b. vascular graft
branched-chain
b.-c. alpha-ketoacid dehydrogenase
b.-c. amino acid (BCAA)
brancher
b. deficiency
b. deficiency glycogenosis
b. enzyme
b. glycogen storage disease
branching tubule formation
branchiogenous cyst
branchio-oto-renal syndrome (BOR)
Brandel cell harvester
Brandt cytology balloon

NOTES

brash
sour b.
water b.
weaning b.
brasiliensis
Nippostrongylus b.
Paracoccidioides b.
BRAT
bananas, rice, cereal, applesauce, and toast
BRAT diet
BRATT
bananas, rice, cereal, applesauce, tea, and toast
BRATT diet
Braun
B. anastomosis
B. enteroenterostomy
B. stent
Braune
B. muscle
B. valve
Braun-Jaboulay gastroenterostomy
BRBPR
bright red blood per rectum
BrDu, BrdU, BrdUrd
bromodeoxyuridine
BrDu staining
break
b. cluster homology gene
mucosal b.
breakage
intracorporeal needle b.
breakbone fever
breakfast
Ewald b.
test b.
Breakstone lithotriptor
breakthrough dose
breast
b. cancer
b. cancer-associated protein pS2 expression
breath
b. alkane
b. alkane testing
b. ethane level
b. hydrogen excretion test
b. isotope bacterial urease detection
liver b.
b. odor
b. pentane test
b. sound
uremic b.
breath-hold MR cholangiography
breathing
deep b.
diaphragmatic b.

intermittent positive pressure b. (IPPB)
Kussmaul b.
mouth b.
sleep-disordered b. (SDB)
Breisky-Navratil straight retractor
Brennemann syndrome
Brenner tumor
brequinar sodium
Brescia-Cimino
B.-C. fistula
B.-C. shunt
Breslow-Day test
Brethine
Bretschneider histidine tryptophan solution
bretylium
breves
arteriae gastricae b.
Brevibloc
brevis
Bifidobacterium b.
Brewer
B. infarct
B. point
BRIC
benign recurrent intrahepatic cholestasia
Bricanyl
Bricker
B. ileal conduit
B. operation
B. pouch
B. technique
B. ureteroileostomy
B. urinary diversion
bridge
agar b.
Albarran reflecting b.
colostomy b.
B. deep-surgery forceps
loop ostomy b.
mucosal b.
suture b.
B. X3 renal stent system
bridging
mucosal b.
b. necrosis
portal-to-portal b.
b. therapy
bridle
control b.
brief
Ashton b.
Holyoke b.
Kim Care contour b.
B. Male Sexual Function Inventory for Urology
Suretys incontinence b.

Brigham sling
bright
  B. disease
  b. red blood
  b. red blood per rectum (BRBPR)
  b. red vomitus
brim
  pelvic b.
Brinkerhoff
  B. anoscope
  B. rectal speculum
Brinton disease
Bristol nomogram for uroflowmetry
BRL 38227
broad-based
  b.-b. gait
  b.-b. polyp
broadening
  spectral b.
broad-spectrum antibiotic
Brödel line
Broder index
Brodie sign
Broesike fossa
broken stent retrieval device
bromelain
bromfenac
bromide
  cetyldimethylethyl ammonium b.
  clidinium b.
  emepronium b.
  ethidium b.
  hexamethonium b.
  mepenzolate b.
  methantheline b.
  methscopolamine b.
  propantheline b.
  valethamate b.
bromine-75
bromobenzene (B2)
bromocriptine dopaminergic medication
bromodeoxyuridine (BrDu, BrdU, BrdUrd)
  antibody to b.
  b. cell kinetics
5-bromodeoxyuridine
bromodiphenhydramine
Bromo Seltzer
brompheniramine
bromsulphalein (BSP)
  b. clearance

bronchia
bronchial
  b. carcinoid
  b. obstruction
  b. sound
bronchobiliary fistula
Broncho-Cath double-lumen endotracheal tube
bronchoesophageal fistula (BEF)
bronchoesophagology
bronchoesophagoscopy
bronchopancreatic fistula
bronchophony
bronchopulmonary
  b. dysplasia
  b. foregut malformation
bronchoscope
  Fujinon EB-410S b.
  Savary b.
bronchospasm
bronchus
Bronkosol
Brooke ileostomy
bropirimine
broth
  cysteine Brucella b.
  tryptic soy b.
Broviac
  B. catheter
  B. catheter cecostomy
brown
  b. bowel syndrome (BBS)
  B. dietary method for colon preparation
  b. pigment gallstone
  b. pigment stone
  b. stool
  B. and Wickham pressure profile method
Brown-Buerger cystoscope
Browne operation
brownian motion
Browning and Parks continence grading system (category A, B, C, D)
Brown-McHardy
  B.-M. pneumatic dilator
  B.-M. pneumatic mercury bougie dilation
Brown-Mueller
  B.-M. T-bar fastener
  B.-M. T-fastener

NOTES

Broyle
B. esophagoscope
B. retrograde cystoscope
B-RTO
balloon-occluded retrograde transvenous obliteration
Brucella melitensis
brucellosis
Brudzinski sign
Bruel-Kjaer
B.-K. axial transducer
B.-K. scanner
B.-K. 1846 ultrasound system
Bruening esophagoscope
Brugia
B. lymphatic obstruction
B. *malayi*
B. *timori*
bruisability
easy b.
bruit
abdominal b.
carotid b.
femoral b.
vascular b.
Brunings esophagoscope
Brunn epithelial nest
Brunner
B. gland
B. gland adenoma
B. gland of duodenum
B. gland hamartoma
B. gland hyperplasia
B. intestinal forceps
B. ligature set
B. tissue forceps
brunneroma of duodenum
Brunschwig operation
brush
Ayre b.
b. biopsy
b. border
b. catheter
Combo Cath wire-guided cytology b.
Cragg thrombolytic b.
b. cytology
cytology b.
Endovations disposable cytology b.
Glassman b.
Olympus cytology b.
scraping b.
sheathed cytology b.
Suction oral b.
brush-border
b.-b. digestion
b.-b. disaccharidase specific activity
b.-b. enzyme activity
b.-b. hydrolase activity
b.-b. marker enzyme
b.-b. membrane (BBM)
b.-b. membrane vesicle (BBMV)
brushing
bile duct b.
blind esophageal b. (BEB)
cytologic b.
b. urea breath test
brushite
Bruton disease
Bruton-type agammaglobulinemia
Bryan-Leishman stain
BS
bile salt
BSA
bovine serum albumin
bowel sounds active
BSA-induced overload proteinuria
BSC
bile salt concentrate
B-scanner
BSCC
basaloid squamous cell carcinoma
BSD
baby soft diet
bedside drainage
BSD-300 device
BSEP
bile salt export pump
BSFR
basal secretory flow rate
BSFR test
BSGF
brachiosubclavian bridge graft fistula
BSI
blood stream infection
body substance isolation
BSM
bile salt metabolism
BSN
bowel sounds normal
BSNA
bowel sounds normal and active
BSO
bile salt output
BSP
bromsulphalein
BSP retention
BSP test
BSS
balanced salt solution
black silk suture
BSSL
bile salt-stimulated lipase
BT
bladder tumor

B

BTA
    bladder tumor antigen
      BTA stat test
      BTA TRAK test
BTP
    biliary tract pain
BT-PABA
    benzoyl-tyrosyl-paraaminobenzoic acid
      BT-PABA test
BTX
    botulinum toxin
      BTX injection
bubble
    cavitation b.
    Garren-Edwards gastric b.
    Garren gastric b.
    gastric air b.
    GEG b.
    intragastric b.
    plasma b.
    b. therapy
bubo
    chancroidal b.
    gonorrheal b.
    indolent b.
    nonvenereal b.
    strumous b.
    venereal b.
bubonocele
buccal
    b. mucosa
    b. mucosal patch graft
    b. mucosal substitution urethroplasty
    b. mucosal urethral replacement
    b. smear
buccopharyngeal aponeurosis
bucket-handle incision
Buck fascia
buckling test
Bucladin-S
buclizine
bucrylate sclerosant
bud
    dorsal b.
    ureteral b.
    ureteric b.
    ventral b.
Budd
    B. cirrhosis
    B. disease
    B. jaundice

Budd-Chiari
    B.-C. disease
    B.-C. syndrome
BUD drainage catheter
budesonide
Buerhenne stone basket technique
buetschlii
    Iodamoeba b.
Buffaprin caplets/tablets
buffer
    barbital-acetate b.
    cacodylate b.
    guanidinium thiocyanate b.
    HEPES b.
    Krebs-Henseleit bicarbonate b.
     (KHB)
    Krebs-Ringer bicarbonate b.
    PBS-Tween b.
    Rapid-hyb b.
    b. solution
    b. system
buffered saline
Bufferin
    B. Arthritis Strength Caplets
    B. caplets/tablets
buffering
    intracellular b.
Bugbee
    B. electrocautery
    B. electrode
Buie
    B. biopsy forceps
    B. fistula probe
    B. fulguration electrode
    B. pile clamp
    B. pile forceps
    B. position
    B. rectal injection cannula
    B. rectal scissors
    B. rectal suction tip
    B. rectal suction tube
    B. sigmoidoscope
Buie-Hirschman anoscope
Buie-Smith retractor
Build Up enteral feeding
bulb
    apex of duodenal b.
    Braasch b.
    b. of corpus cavernosum
    b. deformity
    duodenal b.

NOTES

bulb *(continued)*
    genital end b.
    b. suction
bulbar
    b. artery
    b. colliculus
    b. peptic ulcer
    b. urethra
    b. urethral carcinoma
bulbi (*pl. of* bulbus)
bulbocavernosus
    b. fat pad
    b. reflex (BCR)
bulbocavernous reflex latency measurement
bulbomembranous
    b. stricture
    b. urethra
    b. urethral squamous cell carcinoma
bulbospongiosus muscle
bulbourethral
    b. artery
    b. gland
    b. stricture
bulbourethralis
    ductus excretorius glandulae b.
bulbous
    b. bougie
    b. urethral cuff implantation
bulb-tip
    b.-t. retrograde study
    b.-t. retrograde ureterogram
bulbus, pl. **bulbi**
    b. penis
    b. urethrae
bulgaricus
    Lactobacillus b.
bulge
    inguinal b.
    luminal b.
bulging
    anal b.
    b. flank
    b. papilla
    b. of the perineum
bulimia nervosa
bulimorexia
bulk
    b. agent
    b. laxative
bulking
    b. agent
    b. technique
bulk-producing laxative
bulky
    b. colonic pouch
    b. dressing

    b. malignancy
    b. stool
bulla, pl. **bullae**
bulldog
    b. clamp
    b. forceps
bullet probe
bullet-tip
    b.-t. catheter
    b.-t. dilator
bullosa
    epidermolysis b. (EB)
    Herlitz junctional epidermolysis b.
bullous
    b. edema
    b. edema vesica
    b. pemphigoid
bull's eye appearance
bull's eye lesion
bumetanide
Bumex
bumper
    Cloverleaf internal b.
    dome-shaped internal b.
    gastrostomy b.
    PEG b.
BUN
    blood urea nitrogen
bunching
    accordion-like b.
    b. maneuver
bundle
    coherent b.
    conjoined fiber b.
    fiber b.
    fiberoptic b.
    b. of His
    image guide b.
    b. of Itis
    light guide b.
    master IG b.
    microfilament b.
    neovascular b.
    vasa recta b.'s
BUN-to-creatinine ratio
BUO
    bilateral ureteral obstruction
bupivacaine hydrochloride
buprenorphine narcotic analgesic therapy
bupropion
BUQ
    both upper quadrants
bur
    ultrasonic oscillating b.
Burch
    B. iliopectineal ligament urethrovesical suspension

B. procedure
B. retropubic colposuspension
Burch-Cooper ligament sling
burden
stone b.
Burdwan fever
burger
barium b.
Bürger-Grütz syndrome
Burhenne steerable catheter
buried
b. bumper syndrome
b. penis
b. suture
Burkitt lymphoma
burn
genital b.
thermal b.
transmural b.
burned-out
b.-o. mucosa
b.-o. testis cancer
b.-o. tumor
burnetii
Coxiella b.
Burnett syndrome
burning
b. feet syndrome
b. mouth syndrome (BMS)
b. pain
b. sensation
Burnishine disinfectant
Burow vein
burp
burrowing incision
Burrow solution
bursa, pl. **bursae**
b. of Fabricius
infrapatellar b.
bursitis
omental b.
bursoscopy
supragastric b.
burst
oxidative b.
phagocyte respiratory b.
respiratory b.
bursula
Buschke-Löwenstein tumor
Busch umbilical scissors
Buselmeier shunt
buserelin acetate

bush tea
buski
Fasciolopsis b.
Busodium
Buspar
buspirone hydrochloride
busulfan
butabarbital
Butalan
butalbital
1-butanol
Butibel
Butisol
butorphanol
butter
b. meal
b. stool
Butterfield cystoscope
butterfly
b. hematoma
b. needle
b. rash
b.'s in the stomach
buttock
button
Bard b.
b. battery
b. battery ingestion
Bentle b.
Biskra b.
compression b.
b. drainage
b. of duodenum
b. electrode
b. gastrostomy
gastrostomy b.
Jaboulay b.
Murphy b.
One-Step gastric b.
B. One-Step gastrostomy device
peritoneal b.
Surgitek b.
b. suture
buttonhole
b. incision
b. preputial transposition
b. puncture technique
buttonpexy fixation of stomal prolapse
button-type G-tube
buttress
fascia lata b.
butyl aminobenzoate

B

NOTES

butylbromide
>   hyoscine b.

butyl-silane extraction column

butyrate

butyricum
>   *Clostridium b.*

BW
>   body weight

BXO
>   balanitis xerotica obliterans

Byars flap

Byclomine

Byler
>   B. disease
>   B. syndrome

bypass
>   Alden loop gastric b.
>   aortic-superior mesenteric artery b.
>   aortorenal b.
>   bilioenteric b.
>   biliointestinal b. (BIB)
>   biliopancreatic b. (BPB)
>   bowel b.
>   cardiopulmonary b.
>   duodenoileal b. (DIB)
>   gastric b. (GBP)
>   gastroduodenal-to-renal artery b.

>   b. graft
>   Greenville gastric b.
>   Griffen Roux-en-Y b.
>   Hallberg biliointestinal b.
>   hepatic-to-renal artery saphenous vein b.
>   hepatorenal b.
>   ileorenal b.
>   intestinal b.
>   jejunal b.
>   jejunoileal b. (JIB)
>   laparoscopic gastric b.
>   long-limb surgical b.
>   mesenterorenal b.
>   partial ileal b.
>   Payne-DeWind jejunoileal b.
>   percutaneous biliary b.
>   b. procedure
>   Roux-en-Y gastric b.
>   Scopinaro pancreaticobiliary b.
>   Scott jejunoileal b.
>   splenorenal b.
>   superior mesenterorenal b.
>   thoracic aortorenal b.
>   venovenous b.
>   b. wire

Bywaters syndrome

C
- C bile
- C graft
- C of Hosmer-Lemeshow ratio test

C3
- C3 convertase
- C3 deposit
- C3 immunological study
- C3 receptor
- seminal plasma C3

C_4
- leukotriene C_4

C100-3
- C100-3 antigen
- C100-3 hepatitis C marker

C-11
- carbon-11

C22-3
- antibody to C22-3

^{14}C
- ^{14}C glucose uptake assay
- ^{14}C UBT
- ^{14}C urea breath test (^{14}C UBT)

C3a
- plasma-activated complement 3
- C3a complement

C4a
- plasma-activated complement 4

C5a
- plasma-activated complement 5

c100
- antibody to c. (anti-c100)

C18 Sep-Pack column
C-1 esterase inhibitor
C1q nephropathy
C5 receptor
CA
- carbonic anhydrase
- cholic acid
  - CA cellulose acetate membrane hollow-fiber dialyzer
  - CA 1-18 tumor marker
  - CA 72-4 tumor marker

CA125 (*var. of* CA-125)
CA19-9
- carbohydrate antigen 19 9
  - CA19-9 test

Ca2+
- inositol 1,4,5-triphosphate Ca2+

CA110 dialyzer
CA-125, CA125
- cancer antigen 125

Ca50 antigen
CAA
- coloanal anastomosis

Ca^{2+}-activated K+
CAB
- combined androgen blockade

cable
- fiberoptic light c.
- internal fiberoptic c.
- leakage bypass c.
- light c.

Cabot-Nesbit orchiopexy
CaC3 crystal
Cacchi-Ricci
- C.-R. disease
- C.-R. syndrome

cachectic
- c. diarrhea
- c. fever

cachectin
cachexia
- c. aphthosa
- Grawitz c.
- malignant c.
- tumor c.
- urinary c.
- vascular c.

CaCo2 cell
cacodylate buffer
cadaver
- c. kidney
- c. renal preservation

cadaveric
- c. intestinal transplant
- c. renal transplant
- c. renal transplantation
- c. segmental graft

cadaveris
- *Clostridium* c.

caddy stool
cadmium-induced nephrotoxicity
cadmium nephropathy
caecalis
- fossa c.

caecus minor ventriculi
cafe
- c. coronary
- c. coronary syndrome

Cafergot
caffeine
- c., alcohol, pepper, spicy foods (CAPS)
- c. clearance
- c. gut

caffeinism
CAG
- cholangiogram
- chronic atrophic gastritis

C

cagA
> cytotoxin-associated gene A
>> cagA antibody
>> cagA gene
>> cagA protein

cagA-negative *Helicobacter pylori*
cagA-positive *Helicobacter pylori*
CAGEIN
> catheter-guided endoscopic intubation

CAH
> chronic active hepatitis
> chronic aggressive hepatitis
> congenital adrenal hyperplasia

CAI
> carbonic anhydrase inhibitor

Cajal
> interstitial cells of C. (ICC)

cake kidney
Calan
calbindin
> subserosal c.

calbindin-D9k
> vitamin D-dependent c.-D.

calcaneal ultrasound bone densitometry
calcareous
> c. pancreatitis
> c. renal calculus

Calcibind
Calcidrine syrup
calcific
> c. flocculate
> c. flocculus
> c. pancreatitis

calcification
> carbonate apatite c.
> dystrophic c.
> kidney c.
> laminated c.
> pancreatic c.
> retroperitoneal c.
> scrotal c.
> scrotum c.
> tram-line c.
> ureteric c.

calcified
> c. enterolith
> c. gallstone
> c. zone

calciform cell
calcifying pancreatitis
Calcijex
calcineurin
> c. inhibitor
> c. inhibitor toxicity

calcinosa
> ureteritis cystica c.

calcinosis
> c. cutis, Raynaud phenomenon, esophageal motility disorder, sclerodactyly, and telangiectasia (CREST)
> c. cutis, Raynaud phenomenon, sclerodactyly, and telangiectasia (CRST)
> tumoral c.

calciphylaxis
calcite
calcitonin
> c. gene-related peptide (CGRP)
> serum c.

calcitriol
Calcitrol
calcium
> c. acetate
> c. antagonist
> c. ATPase pump
> c. bilirubinate stone
> c. binding protein
> c. carbonate
> c. carbonate and simethicone
> c. channel
> c. channel antagonist (CCA)
> c. channel blocker
> c. chloride
> c. concentration
> cytosolic c.
> c. deficiency
> dietary c.
> c. electrolyte
> c. entry blocker
> c. excretion
> exogenous c.
> extracellular c.
> c. gluconate
> c. homeostasis
> c. hydrogen phosphate
> c. infusion test
> intracytoplasmic c.
> c. metabolism
> c. oxalate
> c. oxalate calculus
> c. oxalate crystallization
> c. oxalate dihydrate
> c. oxalate dihydrate stone
> c. oxalate monohydrate crystal
> c. oxalate monohydrate stone
> c. oxalate nephrolithiasis
> c. oxalate stone former
> c. oxalate urinary lithiasis
> c. oxaluria
> c. phosphate calculus
> c. phosphate nephrocalcinosis
> c. phosphate urinary lithiasis
> plasma ionized c.

renal absorption of c.
renal excretion of c.
serum c.
c. supplementation
urinary c.
calcium-activated potassium channel
calcium-calmodulin complex
calcium-creatinine ratio
calcium-free dialysate
calcium-phosphate homeostasis
calcium-regulated protein
calcium-rich gluten-free diet
calcium-specific binding protein
calcoaceticus
    Acinetobacter c.
calculation
    anthropometric c.
    c. of renal ammonium excretion
calculi (*pl. of* calculus)
calculosis
calculous
    c. anuria
    c. cholecystitis
    c. cirrhosis
    c. formation
    c. gallbladder disease
    c. pyelitis
calculus, pl. calculi
    alternating c.
    alvine c.
    ammonium acid urate c.
    apatite c.
    biliary c.
    bladder c.
    blood c.
    branched c.
    calcareous renal c.
    calcium oxalate c.
    calcium phosphate c.
    caliceal diverticular c.
    carbonate apatite c.
    cat's eye c.
    cholesterol c.
    combination c.
    common duct c.
    coral c.
    c. culture
    cysteine c.
    cystine c.
    decubitus c.
    dendritic c.
    2,8-dihydroxyadenine c.

c. disease
encysted c.
fibrin c.
fusible c.
gallbladder c.
gastric c.
gonecystic c.
hemp seed c.
hepatic c.
impacted c.
indigo c.
indinavir c.
infection c.
intestinal c.
intrarenal c.
matrix c.
metabolic c.
midureteral c.
c. migration
mulberry c.
nephritic c.
noncalcareous renal c.
nonstruvite c.
oxalate c.
pancreatic c.
pocketed c.
preputial c.
primary renal c.
prostatic c.
c. radiography
renal pelvis c.
salivary c.
secondary renal c.
seminal vesicle c.
silicate c.
spermatic c.
spurious c.
staghorn c.
stomach c.
struvite c.
submucosal c.
triamterene c.
upper urinary tract c.
urate c.
ureteric c.
urethral c.
uric acid c.
urinary c.
urostealith c.
vesical c.
vesicoprostatic c.
Volkmann spoon for pancreatic c.

NOTES

calculus *(continued)*
    weddellite c.
    whewellite c.
    xanthic c.
    xanthine c.
Calcutript
    C. electrohydraulic lithotriptor
    Karl Storz C.
CALD
    chronic active liver disease
caldesmon
Calglycine
Calgocide disinfectant
caliber
    loop c.
    c. probe
caliber-persistent
    c.-p. artery
    c.-p. artery of the stomach
    c.-p. vessel
calibrate
calibration of the cardia
calibrator serum
caliceal, calyceal
    c. diverticular calculus
    c. diverticulum
    c. drainage
    c. extension
    c. filling time
    c. fistula
    c. fornix
    c. infundibulum
    c. puncture
calicectasis
calicectomy
calices (*pl. of* calix)
calicine
Caliciviridae virus family
Calicivirus **gastroenteritis**
calicoplasty
calicotomy
Calicylic
caliectasis, calycectasis, calyectasis
caliectomy, calycectomy
calioplasty, calycoplasty, calyoplasty
caliorrhaphy, calyorrhaphy
caliotomy, calycotomy, calyotomy
caliper
    Lange skin-fold c.'s
calix, calyx, pl. **calices, calyces**
    anomalous c.
    c. clubbing
    c. elongation
    c. enlargement
    extrarenal c.
    kidney c.
    multiple calices
    c. obstruction

    c. orchid
    c. puncture
Callaway formula
Call-Exner body
Calmette-Guérin
    bacille C.-G. (BCG, bCG)
    Calmette-Gúerin bacillus
    intravesical bacillus C.-G.
calmodulin
Calmoseptine ointment
Calogen LCT emulsion
caloric
    c. intake
    c. supplement
calorie
    high c.
calorimeter
Calot
    C. operation
    C. triangle
calpain in acute tubular necrosis
calponin
Cal Power calorie supplement
calprotectin
    c. assay
    fecal c.
calretinin
Caluso PEG gastrostomy tube
calyceal (*var. of* caliceal)
calycectasis (*var. of* caliectasis)
calycectomy (*var. of* caliectomy)
calyces (*pl. of* calix)
calycoplasty (*var. of* calioplasty)
calycotomy (*var. of* caliotomy)
calyectasis (*var. of* caliectasis)
Calymmatobacterium granulomatis
calyoplasty (*var. of* calioplasty)
calyorrhaphy (*var. of* caliorrhaphy)
calyotomy (*var. of* caliotomy)
calyx (*var. of* calix)
CAM
    complementary and alternative medicine
CAM-1189
Camalox
Cambridge pancreatitis classification (I–IV)
camera
    c. adapter
    Anger scintillation c.
    charge-coupled device
      monochrome c.
    Circon-ACMI MicroDigital-I c.
    endoscopic c.
    field-of-view c.
    Fujinon FG-series endoscopic c.
    gamma scintillation c.
    Gammatone II gamma c.
    instant c.

motion picture c.
Olympus OM-1 reflex c.
Olympus OM-series endoscopic c.
Olympus OM-2 c. with SM-45
  enlarging adapter
Olympus OTV-S-series miniature c.
Olympus SCA-series endoscopic c.
Pen-F half-frame c.
Pentax endoscopic c.
Polaroid c.
positron c.
single-lens reflex c.
still c.
television c.
Urocam video c.

Cameron
C. electrosurgical unit
C. erosion
C. lesion
C. omniangle gastroscope
C. ulcer

Cameron-Miller
C.-M. electrocoagulation unit
C.-M. electrode
C.-M. monopolar probe
C.-M. suction-coagulator

Camey
C. enterocystoplasty
C. enterocystoplasty urinary
  diversion
C. I, II operation
C. ileocystoplasty
C. I orthotopic urinary diversion
C. neobladder
C. procedure
C. reservoir
C. urinary pouch

cAMP
cyclic adenosine monophosphate
5′-cyclic adenosine monophosphate
  vasopressin-induced cAMP

Campbell
C. procedure
C. sound
C. technique
C. trocar

camper
C. angle
C. chiasm
C. fascia
fascia of C.

C. ligament
C. plane
Camptosar injection
camptothecin
Campy-BAP culture medium
Campylobacter
  C. cinaedi
  C. coli
  C. fetus
  C. fetus colitis
  C. fetus enteritis
  C. hyointestinalis
  C. jejuni
  C. lari
  C. pylori
  C. pyloridis gastritis
  C. upsaliensis
Campylobacter-**like**
  C.-l. organism (CLO)
  C.-l. organism test (CLOtest)
Campylobacter **test**
Camwrap plastic covering
Canada-Cronkhite syndrome
Canadian Urology Oncology Group
  (CUOG)
canal
  abdominal c.
  Alcock c.
  alimentary c.
  anal c.
  Bernard c.
  femoral c.
  c. of Hering
  histologic anal c.
  inguinal c.
  c. of Nuck
  pancreatobiliary c.
  pecten of anal c.
  pleuroperitoneal c.
  portal c.
  pudendal c.
  pyloric c.
  Santorini c.
  c. stenosis
  suprazonal part of anal c.
  ventricular c.
  vesicourethral c.
  c. of Wirsung
canalicular
  c. bile
  c. bile plug

C

NOTES

canalicular *(continued)*
    c. cholestasia
    c. cryptorchidism
canaliculus, pl. **canaliculi**
    apical c.
    bile duct c.
    c. bilifer
    pili torti et c.
    pseudobile c.
    secretory c.
Canasa suppository
cancelling A's test
cancer
    American Joint Committee on
        Cancer/International Union
        Against C. (AJCC/UICC)
    Amsterdam criteria for hereditary
        nonpolyposis colorectal c.
    androgen-independent prostate c.
    c. antigen 125 (CA-125, CA125)
    antral c.
    bile duct c.
    bladder c.
    Borreliosis classification for
        advanced gastric c.
    Borrmann gastric c.
    breast c.
    burned-out testis c.
    c. cell growth
    c. cell heterogeneity
    clear cell renal c.
    colon c.
    colorectal c. (CRC)
    columnar cuff c.
    cryoablation for prostate c.
    de novo liver c.
    depressed c.
    depressed-type colorectal c.
    disseminated c.
    c. doubling time
    c. drug resistance
    duodenal c.
    early gastric c. (EGC)
    endocrine c.
    esophageal c.
    esophagogastric junction c.
    European Organization for Research
        and Treatment of C. (EORTC)
    exenterative surgery for pelvic c.
    extragonadal germ cell c.
    extrahepatic bile duct c.
    familial colon c.
    c. family syndrome
    gastric c.
    gastrointestinal c.
    GI c.
    hereditary nonpolyposis colon c.
        (HNPCC)

    hereditary nonpolyposis colorectal c.
    hereditary papillary renal c.
        (HPRC)
    high-grade synchronous colon c.
    hypoechoic c.
    hypopharyngeal c.
    incurable c.
    intraepithelial c.
    intramucosal c.
    Japanese classification of c.
    large bowel c.
    liver c.
    low-lying rectal c.
    lung c.
    Matritech NMP22 test for
        bladder c.
    metachronous colon c.
    metastatic c.
    Mostofi grade prostate c.
    mucin-producing c.
    nonfixed c.
    nonpolyposis colorectal c.
    obstructing c.
    ovarian c.
    pancreatic c. (PC)
    pancreatoduodenal c.
    papillary renal c.
    polypoid c.
    postgastrectomy c.
    primary colorectal c. (PCRC)
    prostate c. (PCa)
    C. of the Prostate Strategic
        Urologic Research Endeavor
    rectal c.
    rectosigmoid c.
    recurrent colorectal c. (RCRC)
    restaging of c.
    c. screening
    squamous cell c.
    staging of c.
    stenotic c.
    suburothelial infiltrative c.
    superficial bladder c.
    superficial depressed c.
    teratoma testicular c.
    testis c.
    transplanted c.
    urethral c.
    urologic system c.
    urothelial c.
    Whitmore classification prostate c.
cancer-associated sialyl-Lea antigen
cancerous erosion
Candela
    C. MDA-200 Lasertripter
    C. Miniscope
    C. Miniscope Plus

C. Model MDL 2000 laser
C. 405-nm pulsed dye laser
Candida
   C. *albicans*
   C. esophagitis
   C. *glabrata*
   C. *immitis*
   C. immunological study
   C. infection
   C. *krusei*
   C. *neoformans*
   C. peritonitis
   C. symptom
   systemic *C.*
   C. treatment
   C. *tropicalis*
   ureteral *C.*
   vaginal *C.*
candidal
   c. cellulitis
   c. cystitis
   c. esophagitis
   c. infection
   c. intertrigo
   c. overgrowth
candidemia
candidiasis
   esophageal c. (EC)
   vulvovaginal c.
candidosis
candidum
   Geotrichum *c.*
caninum
   Dipylidium *c.*
canis
   Toxocara *c.*
canister
   ATS c.
canker sore
cannon
   C. point
   C. ring
cannula
   Bilisystem ERCP c.
   Buie rectal injection c.
   contour ERCP c.
   double-lumen irrigation c.
   ERCP c.
   Flexicath silicone subclavian c.
   Fluoro Tip ERCP c.
   Franklin-Silverman biopsy c.
   Hasson open laparoscopy c.

Intraducer peritoneal c.
Jetco-spray c.
laparoscopic c.
large-bore c.
Makler c.
Mayo-Ochsner suction trocar c.
Medicut c.
Olympus monopolar c.
perfusion c.
polyethylene c.
portal c.
Ramirez Silastic c.
Tandem XL triple-lumen ERCP c.
Teflon ERCP c.
Veress c.
washout c.
c. with preloaded 0.35-inch
   guidewire
cannulation, cannulization
   bile duct c.
   biliary c.
   c. of the biliary tree
   c. catheter
   deep c.
   duct c.
   endoscopic retrograde c.
   endoscopic transpapillary c.
   ERCP c.
   ex vivo c.
   freehand c.
   postsphincterotomy ERCP c.
   retrograde c.
   selective ductal c.
   stricture c.
   transpapillary c.
cannulatome
   Cotton c.
Can-Opt
   C.-O. dual lumen ERCP system
   C.-O. stand-alone dual lumen
     ERCP catheter
C-ANP
   C-type atrial natriuretic peptide
Cantil
Cantlie line
Cantor tube
Cantwell-Ransley
   C.-R. epispadias repair
   C.-R. technique
   C.-R. urethroplasty
CAP
   carcinoma of prostate

C

NOTES

CAP *(continued)*
chronic alcoholic pancreatitis
continent anal cap
cap
Assura stoma c.
Coloplast flange mini c.
Coloplast stoma c.
continent anal c. (CAP)
ConvaTec Active Life stoma c.
duodenal c. (DC)
c. method
phrygian c.
c. polyposis
pyloric c.
Sur-Fit Natura flange c.
Sur-Fit stoma c.
capacitive coupling
capacity
acid-neutralizing c. (ANC)
bladder c.
cystometric bladder c.
fluid absorptive c.
functional bladder c.
galactose elimination c. (GEC)
gastric c.
iron-binding c. (IBC)
maximum bladder c.
maximum cystometric c.
peritoneal membrane solute
transport c.
PMN oxidative burst c.
pressure-specific bladder c.
rectal c.
total iron binding c. (TIBC)
capacity-limited kinetics
cap-assisted resection
CAPD
chronic ambulatory peritoneal dialysis
continuous ambulatory peritoneal dialysis
Capecitabine
Capener gouge
Cape Town technique
cap-fitted
c.-f. endoscope
c.-f. gastroscopy
c.-f. panendoscope
capillarectasia
Capillaria philippinensis
capillariasis
intestinal c.
capillaritis
pulmonary c.
capillaropathy
capillary
c. dilation
c. endothelial cell
glomerular c.
c. hemangioma
c. hyperfiltration
c. network
peritubular c.
c. permeability
c. refill
C. System slide holder
c. wall
capillary-leak phenomenon
capillary-lymphatic invasion
capillata
Absidia c.
capistration
capita (*pl. of* caput)
capitatum
Trichosporon c.
capitonnage
caplets
Bufferin Arthritis Strength C.
Therapy Bayer C.
Vanquish Analgesic C.
caplets/tablets
Buffaprin c.
Bufferin c.
Capmul 8210
capnography
capnometry
capotement
Capoten
Capozide
CAPPP
Captopril Prevention Project
capreomycin
CAPS
caffeine, alcohol, pepper, spicy foods
caps
stoma c.
ZE C.
capsaicin
intravesical c.
CAPS-free diet
capsid-encoding region
capsula
c. adiposa renis
c. fibrosa
c. fibrosa hepatitis
c. fibrosa perivascularis
c. fibrosa renis
c. glomerulus
c. pancreatitis
capsular
c. artery
c. blood vessel
c. cirrhosis of liver
c. flap pyeloplasty
c. nephritis
c. penetration
c. tear

capsulatum
  Histoplasma c.
capsule
  acidophilus c.
  Bowman c.
  Carey c.
  Crosby c.
  Detrol LA c.
  enteric-coated c.
  fascial c.
  c. flap technique
  Gerota c.
  Glisson c.
  hepatic c.
  hepatobiliary c.
  liver c.
  Max-EPA c.
  müllerian c.
  mycophenolate mofetil c.
  c. of pancreas
  pH-sensitive radiotelemetry c.
  polysaccharide c.
  prostatic c.
  pyxigraphic sampling c.
  radioisotope c.
  radiotelemetering c.
  renal c.
  Sitzmarks radiopaque marker in
    gelatin c.
  splenic c.
  Synalgos-DC C.'s
  tolterodine tartrate c.
  Watson c.
capsules/tablets
  Disalcid C./t.
capsulitis
  hepatic c.
capsuloma
capsuloplasty
capsulotomy
  renal c.
CapSure continence shield
Captiflex polypectomy snare
Captivator polypectomy snare
captivus
  penis c.
captopril
  c. plasma renin activity test
  C. Prevention Project (CAPPP)
  c. renogram
  c. renography

captopril-DTPA
  c.-DTPA scanning
captopril-enhanced renography
caput, pl. **capita**
  c. epididymis
  c. gallinaginis
  c. medusae
  c. pancreatis
Carafate
Cara-Klenz skin cleanser
carbachol
carbamazepine hepatotoxicity
carbamoyl phosphate synthetase
  deficiency
carbamylation
carbamylcholine
carbenicillin
carbenoxolone
Carbicarb
carbidopa dopaminergic medication
CarboFlex odor control dressing
carbohydrate
  c. antigen 19-9 (CA19-9)
  c. antigen 19-9
    immunohistochemical expression
carbohydrate-induced hyperlipidemia
carbohydraturia
carbolfuchsin stain
carbon
  c. dioxide acidosis
  c. dioxide insufflator
  c. dioxide laser
  c. dioxide laser plaque ablation
  c. dioxide trapping agent
  c. tetrachloride
  c. tetrachloride-induced liver
    regeneration
  c. tetrachloride nephropathy
carbon-11 (C-11)
carbon-14
  c. urea breath test
  c. urinary excretion test
carbon-13 urea breath test (^{13}C-UBT)
carbonate
  aluminum c.
  c. apatite
  c. apatite calcification
  c. apatite calculus
  c. apatite stone
  calcium c.
  dihydroxyaluminum sodium c.

C

NOTES

107

carbonate *(continued)*
 lanthanum c.
 magnesium c.
carbonic
 c. anhydrase (CA)
 c. anhydrase II
 c. anhydrase inhibitor (CAI)
carbonuria
carboplatin
 c., etoposide, bleomycin (CEB)
carboprost tromethamine
Carbowax
carboxamide
 dimethyltriazenoimidazole c. (DTIC)
carboxyamidotriazole
carboxykinase
 phosphoenolpyruvate c. (PEPCK)
carboxylic ester hydrolase (CEH)
carboxyl-terminal amidation
carboxymethylcellulose
carboxymethyl cellulose jelly
carboxypeptidase
 c. B-like enzyme
 porcine c. B
carboxyterminal
 c. noncollagenous domain
 c. PTH
carbuncle
 kidney c.
 renal c.
carbunculoid
carbuterol
Carcassonne perineal ligament
carcinoembryonic antigen (CEA)
carcinogenesis
 chemical c.
 colorectal c.
 oncogene-induced c.
carcinogenicity
carcinogenic nitrosamine
carcinoid
 bronchial c.
 duodenal c.
 c. flush
 gastric c.
 gastroduodenal c.
 hindgut c.
 c. secretory granule
 seminal vesicle c.
 c. syndrome
 testis c.
 c. tumor
carcinoma, pl. carcinomas, carcinomata
 acinar cell c.
 acinar hepatocellular c.
 adenoid cystic c.
 adenosquamous cell c.
 adrenal cortex c.

ampullary c.
ampullopancreatic c.
anal epidermoid c.
anorectal c.
Astwood-Coller staging system
 for c.
autolymphocyte-based treatment for
 renal cell c. (ALT-RCC)
Barrett c.
basal cell c.
basaloid squamous cell c. (BSCC)
Bellini duct c.
bile duct c.
biliary c.
bladder small cell c.
bladder squamous cell c.
bladder transitional cell c.
Borrmann gastric c. (types I–IV)
Borrmann scirrhous c.
bulbar urethral c.
bulbomembranous urethral squamous
 cell c.
cervical c.
cholangiocellular c. (CCC)
cholangitis c.
clear cell hepatocellular c.
clear cell c. of kidney
clear cell nonpapillary c.
collecting duct c.
colon c.
colorectal c. (CRC)
cystic renal cell c. (CRCC)
deleted in colorectal c. (DCC)
diffuse hepatocellular c.
Dukes classification of c.
Edmondson grading system for
 hepatocellular c.
embryonal cell c.
embryonal testicular c.
encapsulated renal cell c.
encephaloid gastric c.
endometrial c.
epidermoid c.
esophageal squamous cell c.
excavated gastric c.
c. ex pleomorphic adenoma
fibrolamellar hepatocellular c. (FL-
 HCC)
flat c.
flat-type c.
focal c.
gallbladder c.
gastric c.
genitourinary c.
germ cell c.
hepatocellular c. (HCC)
hereditary nonpolyposis colorectal c.
hilar c.

intramucosal c.
invasive c.
islet cell c.
Jass staging for rectal c.
Jewett classification of bladder c.
kidney c.
large bowel c.
laryngeal c.
linitis plastica c.
liver cell c.
medullary thyroid c.
metastatic prostatic c.
metastatic renal cell c. (MRCC)
microtrabecular hepatocellular c.
monofocal papillary c.
mucin-hypersecreting c.
mucinous c.
mucoepidermoid c.
mutated colorectal c. (MCC)
nodular transitional cell c.
non-germ-cell c.
nonseminomatous testicular c.
oat cell c.
obstructing rectosigmoidal c.
oropharyngeal c.
ovarian c.
pancreatic c. (PCA)
pancreatic acinar cell c.
pancreatic islet cell c.
papillary gastric c.
papillary renal cell c.
papillary transitional cell c.
pediatric c.
penile c.
perforated c.
periampullary c.
peritoneal c.
PIVKA-II EIA kit for
  hepatocellular c.
polypoid c.
primary transitional cell c.
c. of prostate (CAP)
prostate gland small cell c.
prostatic urethral transitional cell c.
protuberant c.
rectal c.
rectal linitis plastica colorectal c.
renal cell c. (RCC)
renal medullary c.
renal pelvic transitional cell c.
RLP colorectal c.
sarcomatoid squamous cell c.

scirrhous c.
sclerosing hepatic c. (SHC)
secondary metastatic c.
sessile nodular c.
sigmoid colon c.
signet-ring cell c.
signet-ring pattern of gastric c.
c. in situ (CIS)
c. in situ of the glans penis
splenic flexure c.
sporadic (nonfamilial) clear cell c.
squamous cell c. (SCC)
stage B, C c.
superficial esophageal c. (SEC)
superficial gastric c.
superficially spreading c.
supraglottic squamous cell c.
testicular c.
TNM classification of c.
transitional cell c.
transthoracic resection of
  esophageal c.
tubular c.
ulcerating c.
unresectable hepatocellular c.
ureteral c.
urethral c.
urothelial c.
verrucous c.
vulvar c.
yolk sac c.

carcinomatosis
peritoneal c.
c. peritonei

carcinosarcoma
bladder c.
gastric c.
kidney c.
polypoid exophytic nonulcerating c.
renal c.

card
Hemoccult II c.

cardia
achalasia c.
calibration of the c.
crescent gastric c.
gastric c.
c. intestinal metaplasia (CIM)
patulous c.
c. of stomach

cardiac
c. antrum

NOTES

C

109

cardiac *(continued)*
    c. beta-adrenoreceptor
    hyporesponsiveness
    c. beta receptor
    c. cirrhosis
    c. decompression
    c. glycoside
    c. impression on the liver
    c. output
    c. output/cardiac index (CO/CI)
    c. proteinuria
    c. sphincter
    c. stomach
    c. stomach mucosa
    c. sympathovagal tone
cardiac-type
    c.-t. gland
    c.-t. mucosa
cardiectomy
cardinal
    c. ligament
    c. suture
    c. vein
cardiochalasia
cardiodiosis
cardioesophageal
    c. junction (CE, CEJ)
    c. mucosal junction
    c. reflex
    c. relaxation
    c. sphincter
cardiofundic gastropathy
cardiohepatic
    c. angle
    c. triangle
cardiohepatomegaly
cardiomegaly
cardiomyopathy
    uremic c.
cardiomyotomy
    Heller c.
cardiopexy
    ligamentum teres c.
cardioplasty
cardiopulmonary
    c. baroreflex
    c. baroreflex dysfunction
    c. baroreflex function
    c. bypass
    c. complication
cardiopyloric axis
cardiorespiratory complication
cardiospasm
cardiotomy
cardiotoxicity
    ipecac-induced c.
cardiovascular
    c. complication

    c. disease
    c. disorder
    c. drug hepatotoxicity
    c. mortality
carditis
    gastric c.
Cardizem
Cardura
care
    surgical c.
caretaker gene
Carey capsule
Carey-Coons biliary endoprosthesis kit
Ca-Rezz moisture barrier cream
caribi
Carignan syndrome
carina, pl. **carinae**
carinate abdomen
carinii
    Pneumocystis c.
carious teeth
Carle analytic gas chromatograph
Carlesta
C-arm
    C-a. fluoroscope
    C-a. fluoroscopy
Carmalt
    C. clamp
    C. forceps
    C. hemostat
Carman-Kirklin
    C.-K. meniscus complex
    C.-K. meniscus sign
Carman sign
Carmel clamp
carminative
carmine
    c. blue
    contrast chromoscopy using
      indigo c. (CCIC)
    indigo c.
carmustine (BCNU)
Carnett sign
Carney
    C. complex
    C. syndrome
carnitine
Carnitor
carnosinuria
Carnot
    C. function
    C. test
Caroid
Caroli
    C. disease
    C. syndrome
Caroli-Sarles classification

carotene
    serum c.
carotenemia
carotid
    c. artery
    c. bruit
Carpenter syndrome
carphenazine
Carrel
    C. aortic patch
    C. aortic patch anastomosis
carrier
    Deschamps ligature c.
    Endo-Assist disposable ligature c.
    gene c.
    Goldwasser suture c.
    hepatitis c.
    nongene c.
    Pereyra ligature c.
    Raz double-prong ligature c.
    Semb ligature c.
Carson
    C. internal/external endopyelotomy
        stent
    C. Zero Tip balloon dilation
        catheter
cart
    Fujinon video endoscopy c.
carteolol
Carter-Horsley-Hughes syndrome
Carter-Thomason
    C.-T. port closure device
    C.-T. suture passer
cartilage
    arytenoid c.
cartridge
    Clark hemoperfusion c.
Cartrol
cartwheel configuration
caruncle
    Morgagni c.
    urethral c.
carvedilol
Cary-Blair medium
cascade
    clotting c.
    fibrogenic c.
    intrarenal matrix-degrading
        enzyme c.
    MAP kinase signaling c.
    metastatic c.

signaling c.
    c. stomach
cascara
    c. sagrada
    c. sagrada and aloe
case
    poor surgical risk c.
    C. Power protein supplement
caseating
    c. granuloma
    c. necrosis
caseation
case-by-case approach
Casec calcium supplement
casei
    Lactobacillus c.
casein refeeding
caseosa
    nephritis c.
caseous nephritis
cashew apple
CAS 200 image cytometer
CaSki cell line
Casodex
Casoni skin test
cast
    bacterial c.
    blood c.
    coarse granular c.
    erythrocyte c.
    esophageal c.
    fat c.
    fatty c.
    fine granular c.
    granular c. (GC)
    hematin c.
    hyaline c.
    c. nephropathy
    proteinaceous c.
    red blood cell c.
    c. syndrome
    urinalysis sediment microscopy c.
    urinary sediment c.
    white blood cell c.
Castellani paint
Castleman
    C. disease
    C. tumor
cast-like tube
Castoria
    Fletcher's C.
castor oil

C

NOTES

castrate
castration
    functional c.
    radiologic c.
catabolism
catalase
Catapres
catarrhal
    c. cholangitis
    c. cystitis
    c. dysentery
    c. dyspepsia
    c. gastritis
    c. jaundice
    c. nephritis
catatonic trypsinogen DNA screening
catecholamine
    adrenal c.
    plasma c.
    c. synthetic enzyme
    urinary c.
catecholaminergic
category
    NIH Classification C. (I–IV)
category-specific isolation
cat-eye syndrome
catgut
    chromic c.
catharsis
cathartic
    c. colitis
    c. colon
    osmotic c.
Cathelin segregator
catheter
    Ablaser laser delivery c.
    Accurate c.
    Achiever balloon dilation c.
    acorn-tipped c.
    Acucise balloon c.
    Acucise endopyelotomy c.
    Allis c.
    Amplatz c.
    Angiocath PRN c.
    angiographic end hole c.
    angiography c.
    AngioJet Xpeedior c.
    angioplasty balloon c.
    antiseptic impregnated central
      venous c.
    Antron c.
    Argyle Ingram trocar c.
    Argyle Medicut R c.
    ARROWgard Blue hemodialysis c.
    arteriovenous c.
    aspiration c.
    Atlantic ileostomy c.
    Axxcess ureteral c.

    balloon dilating c.
    Bardex-Foley c.
    Bard gastrostomy c.
    bat-wing c.
    bicoudate c.
    biliary balloon c.
    biliary dilator c.
    Bitome c.
    blood-contactin c.
    Blue Max balloon c.
    Bozeman-Fritsch c.
    Braasch c.
    Broviac c.
    brush c.
    BUD drainage c.
    bullet-tip c.
    Burhenne steerable c.
    cannulation c.
    Can-Opt stand-alone dual lumen
      ERCP c.
    Carson Zero Tip balloon
      dilation c.
    central venous c.
    Chemo-Port c.
    Cholangiocath c.
    c. cholangiogram
    cholangiographic c.
    Clay-Adams (PE-10, PE-50) c.
    coaxial c.
    cobra c.
    coil c.
    Coil-Cath c.
    c. coiling sign
    colon motility c.
    combination biliary brush c.
    Comfort Cath I, II c.
    condom c.
    cone-tip c.
    conical c.
    Cook TPN c.
    Cope loop nephrostomy c.
    coudé c.
    Councill c.
    CRE balloon c.
    Curl Cath c.
    decompression c.
    Dent sleeve c.
    de Pezzer c.
    dilating c.
    dilation c. (DC)
    Dormia stone basket c.
    Dotter c.
    double-J c.
    double-lumen balloon c.
    double-lumen injection c.
    Dow-Corning ileal pouch c.
    Dowd II prostatic balloon
      dilatation c.

drainage c.
dual-lumen c. (DLC)
Duo-Flow c.
DURAglide 3 stone balloon c.
eight-lumen esophageal
    manometry c.
elbowed c.
Eliminator balloon c.
end-hole ureteral c.
endoscopic retrograde
    cholangiopancreatography c.
EndoSound endoscopic
    ultrasound c.
Entract c.
epidural c.
ERCP c.
esophageal motility perfused c.
esophageal perfusion c.
exdwelling ureteral occlusion
    balloon c.
exit site of c.
external ureteral c.
Extractor three-lumen retrieval
    balloon c.
5F c.
female c.
femoral hemodialysis c.
fenestrated c.
fiberoptic c.
Flexxicon Blue dialysis c.
Flexxicon II PC internal jugular c.
Fogarty balloon biliary c.
Fogarty irrigation c.
Foley c.
four-lumen polyvinyl manometric c.
French Cope loop nephrostomy c.
French mushroom tip c.
French pigtail nephrostomy c.
French Teflon pyeloureteral c.
Gauder Silicon PEG c.
Glidex coated Percuflex c.
Glo-tip biliary c.
Gold Probe Direct bipolar
    hemostasis c.
Gold Probe electrohemostasis c.
Gore-Tex c.
Gouley c.
Graham c.
Greenfield caval c.
Grüntzig balloon c.
c. guide
guiding c.

Handi-Cath c. kit
Hemoject injection c.
Hickman c.
hooked c.
Howmedica slit c.
Hurwitz dialysis c.
Hydromer grafted c.
hydrostatic balloon c.
ILUS c.
indwelling urinary c.
injection c.
Inmed whistle tip urethral c.
intraarterial chemotherapy c.
intracholedochal manometric c.
intraductal imaging c.
intrathecal c.
intravascular ultrasound c.
c. irrigation
IVUS c.
Jackson-Pratt c.
Jelco c.
Kaye tamponade balloon c.
kidney internal splint/stent c.
Kish urethral illuminate c.
KISS c.
Konigsberg c.
Kumpe c.
Lane gastroenterostomy c.
large-bore c.
LeVeen c.
Lifemed c.
long-term indwelling c.
8-lumen c. assembly
lumen-seeking c.
Mahurkar c.
male c.
Malecot reentry c.
Malecot suprapubic c.
Mallinckrodt c.
manometry c.
Mark IV Moss decompression-
    feeding c.
MaxForce TTS biliary balloon
    dilatation c.
MaxForce TTS high performance
    balloon dilatation c.
measuring-mounting c.
Medicut c.
Medina ileostomy c.
Medi-Tech bipolar c.
Medi-Tech steerable c.
Memokath c.

C

NOTES

catheter *(continued)*
Mentor nonhydrophilic PVC c.
Mentor straight c.
metal ball-tip c.
metallic-tip c.
Mewissen infusion c.
microtip sensor c.
microtip transducer c.
Microvasive balloon c.
Millar urodynamic c.
MiniBard c.
Missouri c.
MM c.
MS Classique balloon dilatation c.
multifiber c.
multilumen manometric c.
mushroom c.
nasobiliary c. (NBC)
nasobiliary drainage c.
nasocystic c.
nasopancreatic c.
nasovesicular c.
needle tip c.
Nélaton c.
nephrostomy c.
10 o'clock selector c.
olive-tipped c.
Olympus PW-1L wash c.
On-Command c.
open-ended ureteral c.
oral suction c.
over-the-wire balloon c.
Passage biliary dilatation c.
Passport Balloon-on-a-Wire
  dilatation c.
PE-MV balloon dilatation c.
Percuflex c.
percutaneous femoral vein c.
percutaneous nephrostomy
  Malecot c.
percutaneous transhepatic biliary
  drainage c.
percutaneous transhepatic pigtail c.
peritoneal dialysis c. (PDC)
PermCath dual lumen c.
Pezzer c.
Phantom 5 Plus ST balloon
  dilatation c.
Phillips c.
pigtail c.
Pollack ureteral c.
polyethylene c.
polyurethane nasoenteric c.
polyvinyl chloride c.
Porges c.
Port-A-Cath c.
portal c.
c. probe

c. probe-assisted endoluminal
  ultrasonography (CP-EUS)
c. probe ultrasound
prostatic c.
PTHC c.
pulse spray c.
pusher c.
PVC c.
pyeloureteral c.
Quinton c.
Quinton-Mahurkar dual-lumen
  peritoneal c.
radiopaque ERCP c.
Ranfac cholangiographic c.
Reddick cystic duct
  cholangiogram c.
red rubber Robinson c.
retrograde occlusion balloon c.
Rigiflex ABD balloon dilatation c.
Rigiflex biliary balloon dilatation c.
Rigiflex esophageal TTS balloon c.
Rigiflex OTW balloon dilatation c.
Rigiflex TTS balloon dilatation c.
Ring biliary drainage c.
Robinson c.
ruler c.
Sacks QuickStick c.
Sacks Single-Step c.
self-drainage c.
self-retaining c.
shepherd's hook c.
Siegel-Cohen dilating c.
Silastic c.
silicone rubber Dacron-cuffed c.
silver c.
SIM 2 c.
Simmons c.
Simplastic c.
single-lumen Broviac silicone c.
Soehendra dilating c.
solid-state esophageal manometry c.
Sonicath endoluminal ultrasound c.
c. sonography
Spectrum silicone Foley c.
spiral tip c.
Stamey-Malecot c.
Stamey open tip ureteral c.
standard ERCP c.
stenting c.
subclavian c.
Suction Buster c.
Supra-Foley c.
surgically implanted hemodialysis c.
  (SIHC)
Surgitek c.
Swan-Ganz pulmonary artery c.
swan-neck Missouri c.
swan-neck pediatric Coil-Cath c.

SynchroMed infusion system
intraspinal c.
synthetic 5-channel, water-perfused
motility c.
Tandem thin-shaft transureteroscopic
balloon dilatation c.
tapered-tip hydrophilic-coated
push c.
taper-tip c.
Taut cystic duct c.
Teflon guiding c.
Tenckhoff peritoneal dialysis c.
Tenckhoff two-cuff c.
Texas style two-piece c.
three-way irrigating c.
toposcopic c.
Toronto-Western c.
torque c.
Trabucco double balloon c.
Trach-Eze closed suction c.
Tracker c.
transanal c.
transducer c.
translumbar inferior vena cava c.
Tratner c.
trial without c. (TWOC)
Trilogy low-profile balloon
dilatation c.
triple-lumen manometry c.
c. tunnel infection
Tyshak c.
Uldall subclavian hemodialysis c.
ureteral occlusion balloon c.
Urocath external c.
urodynamic c.
UroMax II high-pressure balloon c.
Uro-San Plus external c.
van Sonnenberg gallbladder c.
Von Andel dilating c.
VTC biliary c.
Vygon Nutricath S c.
washing c.
water-infusion esophageal
manometry c.
water-perfused c.
whistle-tip ureteral c.
Willscher c.
Wilson-Cook fine-needle-
aspiration c.
Wilson-Cook Quantum TTC
esophageal balloon dilatation c.
winged c.

Witzel enterostomy c.
Xpeedior c.
Z-Med c.
catheter-associated bacteriuria
catheter-based ultrasound probe
**catheter-guided endoscopic intubation
(CAGEIN)**
catheterization
clean intermittent c. (CIC)
clean intermittent bladder c.
cystic duct c.
hepatic vein c.
in-and-out c.
intermittent c.
c. pouch
c. pouch rupture
retrourethral c.
Seldinger cystic duct c.
selective c.
subclavian vein c.
c. test
transhepatic c.
transnasal bile duct c.
transpapillary c.
umbilical vein c.
ureteral c.
urethral c. (UC)
urinary c.
catheterize
**catheter-related bloodstream infection
(CR-BSI)**
Cath-Secure
C.-S. catheter holder
C.-S. tape
cation
c. exchange
c. exchanger
c. transport
cationic
c. colloidal gold (CCG)
c. dye
cationized ferritin
cat's eye calculus
Cattell T-tube
cauda
c. epididymidis
c. epididymis
c. equina
c. equina lesion
c. equina syndrome
caudal
c. block

C

NOTES

caudal *(continued)*
   c. mesonephros
   c. pancreatic artery
   c. pancreaticojejunostomy
   c. pole
   c. regression syndrome
   c. traction
caudate
   c. eminence of liver
   c. lobe
   c. lobe of liver
caustic
   c. acid
   c. alkali
   c. colitis
   c. esophagitis
   c. ingestion
   c. stricture
   c. substance
cauterization
   colon c.
cauterize
cautery
   c. bend
   BICAP II c.
   blind c.
   Bovie c.
   endoscopic laser c.
   c. knife
   looped c.
   c. pencil
   snare c.
cava *(pl. of* cavum)
caval-atrial shunt
caveola
caveolated cell
caveolin-1
Caverject
CaverMap
   C. procedure
   C. surgical device
cavernitis
   fibrous c.
cavernosae
   Billroth venac c.
cavernosal
   c. abscess
   c. alpha blockade
   c. alpha blockade technique
   c. artery
   c. nerve
   c. nerve-sparing radical
      prostatectomy
   c. systolic pressure
   c. vein
cavernositis
cavernosogram
cavernosography

cavernosometry
   dynamic infusion c.
   gravity c.
   Menuel c.
cavernosonography
   dynamic infusion cavernosometry
      and c.
cavernosorum
   tunica albuginea corporum c.
cavernospongiosum shunt
cavernostomy
cavernosum
   bulb of corpus c.
   fibrotic corpus c.
Cavernotome
cavernous
   c. artery blood flow
   c. artery blood flow acceleration
   c. artery dilation
   c. artery disease
   c. artery injury
   c. artery occlusion pressure
   c. autonomic nerve dysfunction
   c. fibrosis
   c. hemangioma
   c. nerve
   c. nerve mapping
   c. transformation of the portal vein
      (CTPV)
   c. vein
cavernovenous leakage
CAVH
   chronic active viral hepatitis
   continuous arteriovenous hemofiltration
CAVH-B
   chronic active viral hepatitis, type B
CAVHD
   continuous arteriovenous hemodialysis
CAVHDF
   continuous arteriovenous
      hemodiafiltration
CAVH-NAB
   chronic active viral hepatitis, non-A, non-
      B
caviae
   Aeromonas c.
Cavilon diabetes foot care kit
cavitas peritonealis
cavitating tuberculoma
cavitation
   c. bubble
   pulmonary c.
Cavitron Ultrasonic Surgical Aspirator
   (CUSA)
cavity
   abdominal c.
   Cutinova c.
   intraperitoneal c.

nephrotomic c.
peritoneal c.
retroperitoneal c.
tension-free closure of
   abdominal c.
cavography
synchronous inferior c.
synchronous superior c.
vena c.
cavotomy
CAVU
continuous arteriovenous ultrafiltration
cavum, pl. **cava**
inferior vena cava (IVC)
infrahepatic vena cava
c. pelvis
retrohepatic vena cava
c. retzii
suprahepatic vena cava
vena cava
c. vesicouterinum
cayetanensis
   Cyclospora c.
CBAVD
congenital bilateral absence of the vas
   deferens
CBC
complete blood count
C3b, C4b receptor
CBD
common bile duct
   CBD 2 choledochoscope
   CBD stone
CBDE
common bile duct exploration
CBDM
common bile duct microlithiasis
C-beta gene
CBH
chronic benign hepatitis
CBI
continuous bladder irrigation
^{13}C-bicarbonate breath test
CBP
chronic bacterial prostatitis
copper-binding protein
   CBP test
CBS
colloidal bismuth subcitrate
CC
creatinine clearance
   Adalat CC

CCA
calcium channel antagonist
CCC
cholangiocellular carcinoma
chronic calculous cholecystitis
cylindrical confronting cisterna
CCD
charge-coupled device
cortical collecting duct
   CCD endoscope
   CCD perfusion
CCE
cholesterol crystal embolization
CCFA
Crohn and Colitis Foundation of America
CCG
cationic colloidal gold
C-cholyl-glycine breath excretion test
CCIC
contrast chromoscopy using indigo
   carmine
CCK
cholecystokinin
   CCK antagonist
CCK-8
cholecystokinin octapeptide
CCK-LI
cholecystokinin-like immunoreactivity
CCKNOW
Crohn and Colitis Knowledge
   CCKNOW score
CCK-OP
cholecystokinin octapeptide
CCK-PZ
cholecystokinin-pancreozymin
CCl4-induced cirrhosis
CCL-64 cell
CCL-277 colon cancer cell
CCNU
   methyl CCNU
CCP
chronic calcifying pancreatitis
colitis cystica profunda
CCPD
continuous cycling peritoneal dialysis
CCUP
colpocystourethropexy
CD
Clostridium difficile
collecting duct
common duct
Crohn disease

C

NOTES

CD *(continued)*
   cystic duct
      CD activity index
CD2
CD3+
CD4+
      autologous HBcAg-specific CD4+
      CD4+ cell
      CD4+ T-cell count
CD4
      CD4 lymphocyte count
      CD4 molecule
      CD4 phenotype
      CD4 protein
      CD4 T cell
CD8+
      CD8+ cell
      CD8+ T lymphocyte
CD8
      CD8 lymphocyte
      CD8 lymphocyte count
      CD8 molecule
      CD8 phenotype
      CD8 protein
CD20
      B-cell antigen CD20
CD29
CD44
CD45
C&D
   cystoscopy and dilation
CD14 monoclonal antibody
CD23 enterocyte
CD25 antigen
CD2-associated protein
CD3 protein
CD3+T cell
CD3-T cell receptor complex
CD4+–CD8+ T-cell ratio
CDA
   chenodeoxycholic acid
CDAD
   Clostridium difficile-associated diarrhea
CDAI
   Crohn Disease Activity Index
CDC
   Centers for Disease Control and
     Prevention
   choledochocholedochostomy
   complement-dependent cytotoxicity
   Crohn disease of colon
CDC42 protein
CDCA
   chenodeoxycholic acid
   choledococaval anastomosis
CDE
   common duct exploration
   cystine dimethylester

CDEIS
   Crohn Disease Endoscopic Index of
     Severity
CDJ
   choledochojejunostomy
CD40L
cDNA
   complementary deoxyribonucleic acid
     HSP-70 cDNA
     cDNA probe
CDNF
   ciliary-derived neurotrophic factor
     receptor
CDP
   computerized dynamic posturography
CDP571
CD45RA
CD45RO
     CD45RO lymphocyte
CDS
   commercial dialysis solution
CDY
   cystoduodenostomy
CE
   cardioesophageal junction
   conjugated estrogen
CE-24 needle
CEA
   carcinoembryonic antigen
     CEA test
CE-AD gastric lesion staging by
endoscopy
CEAker colorectal cancer marker
CEA-Scan
CEB
   carboplatin, etoposide, bleomycin
ceca (*pl. of* cecum)
cecal
      c. appendage
      c. appendix
      c. bascule
      c. colonoscopy
      c. cystoplasty
      c. dilation
      c. diverticulitis
      c. diverticulum
      c. fissure
      c. fold
      c. gangrene
      c. haustrum
      c. hernia
      c. homogenate
      c. imbrication procedure
      c. mucosal nodule
      c. necrosis
      c. perforation
      c. sacculation
      c. serosa

c. ulcer
c. vascular ectasia
c. volvulus
cecectomy
Cecil
    C. operation
    C. procedure
    C. repair
    C. urethral stricture syndrome
    C. urethroplasty
cecitis
Ceclor
cecocolic intussusception
cecocolon
cecocolopexy
cecocolostomy
cecocystoplasty
cecofixation
cecoileal reflux
cecoileostomy
cecopexy
cecoplication
cecoproctostomy
cecoptosis
cecorrhaphy
cecosigmoidostomy
cecostomy
    blow-hole c.
    Broviac catheter c.
    ileal Malone c.
    Malone c.
    percutaneous catheter c.
    percutaneous endoscopic c.
    tube c.
cecotomy
cecoureterocele
cecum, pl. **ceca**
    antimesocolic side of the c.
    coned c.
    cone-shaped c.
    conical c.
    watermelon c.
CEEA
    curved end-to-end anastomosis
    CEEA stapler
CE-EUS
    contrast-enhanced endoscopic
    ultrasonography
cefaclor
cefadroxil monohydrate
cefamandole

CE-FAST
    contrast-enhanced fast sequence
cefazolin sodium
cefepime
cefixime
cefmenoxine
cefmetazole
Cefobid
cefonicid
cefoperazone
ceforanide
Cefotan
cefotaxime
cefotetan disodium
cefotiam
cefoxitin
cefpirome
cefpodoxime proxetil
cefprozil
cefsulodin
ceftazidime
ceftibuten
Ceftin
ceftizoxime
ceftriaxone
    c. pseudolithiasis
    c. sodium
cefuroxime
cEGF
    concentration epidermal growth factor
CEH
    carboxylic ester hydrolase
CEJ
    cardioesophageal junction
celandine
    greater c.
celecoxib
    C. Long-Term Arthritis Safety
    Study (CLASS)
celectome
Celestin
    C. dilator bougie
    C. endoprosthesis
    C. esophageal tube
    C. graduated dilator
    C. latex rubber tube
    C. prosthesis
Celestone
celiac
    c. angiogram
    c. angiography
    c. arteriography

C

NOTES

celiac *(continued)*
    c. axis
    c. axis compression
    c. dimple
    c. flux
    c. lymph node
    c. plexus
    c. plexus block
    c. plexus neurolysis (CPN)
    c. plexus reflex
    c. plexus sectioning
    c. rickets
    c. sprue
    c. sprue disease
    c. trunk
    c. tumor
celiacography
celiac-superior mesenteric ganglia
celiacus
    truncus c.
celiagra
celiectomy
celiocentesis
celioenterotomy
celiogastrostomy
celiogastrotomy
celiomesenteric arteriography
celiomyalgia
celiomyomotomy
celioparacentesis
celiopathy
celiorrhaphy
celioscope
celioscopy
celiotomy
    exploratory c.
    c. incision
    vaginal c.
    ventral c.
cell
    absorptive c.
    acid c.
    acinar c.
    acinous c.
    adelomorphous c.
    algoid c.
    amine precursor uptake and
      decarboxylation c.
    c. analysis system
    C. Analysis System 200 image
      cytometer
    aneuploid c.
    antigen-presenting c.
    antral gastric c.
    APUD c.
    argentaffin c.
    argyrophilic c.
    atypical ductular c.

    autologous liver c.
    B c.
    ballooning of c.
    basal granular c.
    beaker c.
    bile duct epithelial c.
    biliary epithelial c. (BEC)
    binucleate renal tubule epithelial c.
    bladder mast c.
    blast c.
    bone marrow-derived B c.
    bone marrow stem c.
    border c.
    CaCo2 c.
    calciform c.
    capillary endothelial c.
    caveolated c.
    CCL-64 c.
    CCL-277 colon cancer c.
    CD4+ c.
    CD8+ c.
    CD3+T c.
    CD4 T c.
    central c.
    centroacinar c.
    chalice c.
    chief c.
    chromaffin c.
    chromogranin A-immunoreactive c.
    COLO 320 colon cancer c.
    columnar-cuboidal
      adenocarcinoma c.
    c. count
    crypt c.
    c. culture transwell
    c. cycle marker
    cytotoxic T c.
    D c.
    Davidoff c.
    delomorphous c.
    dendritic reticular c.
    diploid c.
    DNA haploid c.
    donor dendritic c.
    Dukes signet c. (A, B, C)
    dysmorphic red blood c.
    dysplastic c.
    ECL c.
    effector c.
    endocrine c.
    endodermic c.
    endothelial c.
    enteric ganglion c.
    enterochromaffin c.
    enterochromaffin-like c.
    enteroendocrine c.
    epithelial c. (EC)
    epithelial endocrine c.

eumorphic red blood c.
exfoliative epithelial colonic c.
F9 c.
fat c.
fat-storing liver c.
fatty liver c. (FLC)
fetal liver-derived B c.
flare c.
flattened epithelial microfold c.
flexura hepatica c.
foam c.
G c.
gastric pacemaker c.
gastrin c.
gastrin-secreting c.
Gaucher c.
giant c.
glitter c.
glomerular contractile c.
glomerular epithelial c.
gluconeogenic-competent human
  proximal tubule c.
goblet c.
Grimelius-positive c.
ground-glass c.
GTL-16 gastric carcinoma c.
haploid c.
HBV-specific T c.
Heidenhain c.
HeLa c.
helper T c.
hematopoietic c.
hepatic stellate c. (HSC)
hepG2 c.
HGF-stimulated renal epithelial c.
histamine-producing mast c.
HLF c.
hobnailed c.
HT-29 c.
human cytotoxic T c.
human intestinal epithelial Coco-
  2 c.
human umbilical vein endothelial c.
  (HUVEC)
hypochromic red c.
IEC-6 c.
IEL T c.
IgA-producing c.
IgG-producing c.
intercalated c.
interstitial immunocompetent c.
interstitial mononuclear c.

intestinal endocrine c.
intestinal epithelial c. (IEL)
intraglomerular mesangial c.
IPEC-J2 c.
islet c.
Ito c.
JR-St c.
KATO-III c.
killer T c.
Kulchitsky c.
Kupffer c. (KC)
L c.
LAK c.
lamina propria lymphoid c.
Langerhans c.
Langhans c.
LE c.
Leydig c.
LIM 2537 c.
c. line
lipid-laden clear c.
littoral c.
liver-deprived epithelial clonic c.
LLC-PK1-FBPase+ c.
LLCPK renal tubular c.
lymphocyte-target c.
lymphokine-activated killer c.
lymphomononuclear c.
M c.
mast c.
MDCK epithelial c.
c. membrane
c. membrane epithelial antigen
memory T c.
mesangial c. (MC)
mesenchyma c.
microfold c.
MN c.
mucous neck c.
mucus-secreting c.
multinucleated giant c.
murine B16 c.
murine lymphoid c.
murine mesangial c. (MMC)
murine proximal tubule c.
myeloid dentritic c.
myenteric ganglion c.
natural killer c.
c. necrosis
neuroendocrine c.
NK c.

NOTES

cell *(continued)*

non-alpha, non-beta pancreatic
   islet c.
non-antigen-expressing target c.
noncleaved B c.
nonrosetted c.
nuclear-tagged c.
oat c.
OK c.
OKT4 c.
OKT8 c.
osteoclast-like giant c. (OCLG)
oxyntic c.
P c.
pacemaker c.
packed red blood c.'s
pale c.
pancreatic acinar c.
pancreatic islet c.
Paneth c.
PAP-HT25 c.
paracrine c.
parietal c.
peptic c.
percentage of hypochromic red c.
   (%HYPO)
peripheral blood mononuclear c.
   (PBMC)
peripheral T c.
perisinusoidal c.
peritubular myoid c.
phagocytic stellate c.
Pick c.
pigment-laden Kupffer c.
pit c.
plasma c.
PLC-PRF 5 c.
PMN c.
Pockel c.
polymorphonuclear c.
postreceptor signaling of parietal c.
PP-immunoreactive c.
primed c.
principal c. (PC)
proliferating tubular c.
c. proliferation
prostate gland stromal c.
ptyocrinous c.
pulpar c.
purified T c.
Q c.
C. Recovery System (CRS)
rectal epithelial c.
red blood c. (RBC)
renal collecting duct c.
renal cortical tubule c.
renal epithelial c.
renal proximal tubular c.

renal tubular c.
renal tubule epithelial c.
renomedullary interstitial c. (RMIC)
S c.
C. Saver
Schwann c.
schwannian spindle c.
secretory c.
semen round c.
seminiferous tubule Sertoli c.
senescent c.
c. separation technique
serotonin c.
Sertoli c.
Sertoli-Leydig c.
signet-ring c.
silver c.
sinusoidal endothelial c. (SEC)
sinusoid-lining c.
small granule c.
C. Soft 2000 semen analyzer
C. Soft system
somatostatin c.
spillage of tumor c.'s
spindle c.
squamous c.
stellate c.
stem c.
c. substratum
suppressor T c.
c. surface area
c. surface receptor
SW 480 c.
c. swelling
T c.
T84 c.
target c.
T effector c.
tetraploid c.
thymus-derived c.
tolerogenic dendritic c.
trans-blotting c.
transitional c.
triploid c.
Trypan blue-stained c.
tubular epithelial c.
tumor c.
c. type
undifferentiated c.
unit of packed red blood c.'s
   (UPRBC)
ureteral muscle c.
urinalysis sediment microscopy c.
urine glitter c.
van Hansemann c.
vascular permeation of tumor c.
vascular smooth muscle c. (VSMC)
villous tip c.

villus c.
von Hanseman c.
von Kupffer c.
white blood c. (WBC)
xanthoma c.
XL1-Blue c.
zymogenic c.
cell-adhesion molecule
cell-cell
c.-c. adhesion
c.-c. contact
c.-c. interaction
CellCept
cell-mediated
c.-m. arm
c.-m. cytotoxicity
c.-m. hepatic injury
c.-m. immunity
c.-m. immunohistological response
c.-m. mechanism
c.-m. suppression
cell-positive margin
Cell-Track
cellular
c. atypia
c. differentiation
c. electrophysiology
c. enzyme
c. immune response
c. immunity
c. infiltration
c. peptide
c. proliferation
cellularis
balanoposthitis chronica
circumscripta plasma c.
cellule
cellulitis
candidal c.
vaginal cuff c.
cellulosae
Cysticercus c.
cellulose
c. diacetate membrane
c. phosphate
cellulose-based membrane
celomic epithelium
celoscope
celoscopy
celotomy
Celsius thermometer

cement
latex-base skin c.
Torbot c.
Wacker Sil-Gel 604 silicone c.
CE-M gastric lesion staging by endoscopy
C-EMR
cutting endoscopic mucosal resection
center
anospinal c.
C.'s for Disease Control and Prevention (CDC)
free-standing ambulatory surgical c.
organized germinal c.
pontine micturition c. (PMC)
rectovesical c.
swallowing c.
vomiting c.
centering balloon
centigrade thermometer
centigray (cGy)
centimeter
joule per c. (J/cm)
centipoise
central
c. adrenergic agent
c. cell
c. cystocele
c. echogenicity
c. hyaline sclerosis
c. hyperalimentation
c. lacteal
c. necrosis
c. nervous system (CNS)
c. spot
c. vagal nerve stimulation
c. venous alimentation
c. venous catheter
c. venous pressure (CVP)
c. venous pressure line
centrifugal pump
centrifugation
density gradient c.
Ficoll-Hypaque gradient c.
Polyprep c.
centrifuge
Ficoll-Hypaque density gradient c.
centrifuged
centrilobular
c. acidophilic necrosis
c. cholestasia

C

NOTES

centrilobular *(continued)*
  c. pancreatitis
  c. region of liver
centrizonal necrosis
centroacinar cell
Century bicarbonate dialysis control unit
Ceo-Two
cephalad traction
cephalexin
cephalin-cholesterol flocculation test
cephalocyst
cephalosporin
    prophylactic c.
    second-generation c.
    third-generation c.
cephalothin
cephalotrigonal technique
cephradine
Cephulac
ceramidase deficiency
ceramide lactoside lipidosis
c-ErbB-2/NEU oncoprotein
cercaria
cercaricidal
cerclage
    McDonald c.
    Shirodkar cervical c.
cerebellar ataxia
cerebelloretinal hemangioblastomatosis
cerebral
    c. edema
    c. fluid shunt
    c. hemangioblastoma
    c. palsy
    c. perfusion pressure (CPP)
cerebral-brain stem circuit
cerebral-sacral loop
cerebrohepatorenal syndrome (CHRS)
cerebrooculofacial syndrome
cerebrospinal fluid (CSF)
cerebrotendinous xanthomatosis
cerebrovascular
    c. complication
    c. disease
Cerespan
Ceretec
cereus
    Bacillus c.
Cerezyme
cerivastatin
ceroid-laden macrophage
cerulein
    exogenous cholecystokinin or c.
ceruloplasmin
    serum c.
cerumen obstruction

cervical
  c. carcinoma
  c. discharge
  c. erosion
  c. esophagogastric anastomosis
  c. esophagus
  c. friability
  c. gastroesophagostomy
  c. inflammation
  c. intraepithelial neoplasia (CIN)
  c. irregularity
  c. lymphadenopathy
  c. motion tenderness
  c. mucus-sperm interaction
  c. neuroblastoma
  c. polyp
  c. position
  c. spasm
  c. ulcer
  c. wart
cervicitis
    mucopurulent c.
    schistosomal c.
cervicocolpitis
cervicovaginitis
CESD
    cholesterol ester storage disease
cesium
cesium-137 wire
CE-SM gastric lesion staging by endoscopy
Cestoda **tapeworm**
cestode
cestodiasis
Cetacaine topical anesthetic
cetirizine
CETP
    cholesterol ester transfer protein
cetrimidesuboptimal
cetyldimethylethyl ammonium bromide
Ceylon sore mouth
CF
    cystic fibrosis
    CF epithelia
CF-200Z Olympus colonoscope
CF-HM
    CF-HM endoscope
    CF-HM fiberscope
    CF-HM magnifying colonoscope
CF-LB3R colonoscope
C-Flex
    C-F. Amsterdam stent
    C-F. ureteral stent
c-fos **protooncogene**
CF100TL
    Olympus CF100TL

CFTR
    cystic fibrosis transmembrane
      conductance regulator
        CFTR gene analysis
CFU
    colony-forming unit
CF-UHM colonoscope
CF-UM3 echocolonoscope
CG
    chronic glomerulonephritis
[14]C-glycocholate breath test
C-glycocholic acid breath test
CGM
    coffee-ground material
cGMP
    cyclic guanosine monophosphate
    5'-cyclic guanosine monophosphate
cGMP-mediated relaxant
CGN
    chronic glomerulonephritis
CGRP
    calcitonin gene-related peptide
CGS
    computer graphic simulation
c-GVHD
    chronic graft-versus-host disease
CGY
    cystogastrostomy
cGy
    centigray
      cGy radiation measure
CH
    chronic hepatitis
CH-40 activated charcoal
CHA
    common hepatic artery
Chaffin-Pratt drain
Chagas-Cruz disease
Chagas disease
chagasi
    Leishmania donovani c.
Chagasic megaesophagus
chain
    alpha-3-c.
    alpha-4-c.
    alpha-5-c.
    beta c.
    beta-1 c.
    c. cystogram
    c. cystourethrography
    food c.
    gamma light c.

    J c.
    kappa light c.
    monoclonal light c.
    obturator lymphatic c.
    c. suture
    sympathetic c.
chain-of-lakes
    c.-o.-l. deformity
    c.-o.-l. filling defect
    c.-o.-l. sign
chain-terminating inhibitor
chair
    Hausted all-purpose c.
    Vess c.
chalasia
chalazion
chalice cell
challenge
    c. diet
    fluid c.
    food c.
    gluten c.
    jejunal gluten c.
    rectal gluten c.
    solid bolus c.
chamaedrys
    Teucrium c.
chamber
    antropyloroduodenal common c.
      (APDCC)
    deglutitive pharyngeal c.
    hyperbaric oxygen c.
    Makler counting c.
    Microcell c.
    10 Pa Amicon c.
    Sigma 34 monoplace hyperbaric c.
    Ussing c.
chancre
    hunterian c.
    Nisbet c.
chancroid
chancroidal bubo
chancrous
change
    degenerative c.
    ductal c.
    enzyme c.
    erosive prepyloric c.
    fibrocystic c.
    fractional weight c.
    large cell c. (LCC)
    mesenchymal c.

C

NOTES

change *(continued)*
    orthostatic c.
    pancreatic ductal morphological c.
    phlegmonous c.
    polyneuropathy, organomegaly, endocrinopathy, monoclonal (M-) protein, and skin c.'s (POEMS)
    postsurgical c.
    segmental c.
    sensorium c.
    spatial c.
    trophic c.
    ultrastructural basket-weave c.

channel
    biopsy c.
    calcium c.
    calcium-activated potassium c.
    chloride c.
    common c.
    detrusor muscle potassium c.
    epithelial sodium c. (ENaC)
    gastric c.
    ion c.
    ligand-gated c.
    lymph c.
    lymphatic c.
    Malone antegrade continent enema c.
    Mitrofanoff catheterizable c.
    pancreatic duct-choledochus c.
    pancreaticobiliary common c.
    potassium c.
    preputial transverse island flap and glans c.
    pyloric c.
    Sonotrode c.
    stomalike c.
    stretch-sensitive ion c.
    suction c.
    treatment c.
    urea c.
    voltage-gated c.
    water c.

chaparral leaf
chaperone
    retinoid c.
characteristic
    client patient c.
    receiver-operating c. (ROC)
c-Ha-ras gene
CharcoAid
charcoal
    activated c. (AC)
    CH-40 activated c.
    c. filter
    c. hemoperfusion
    hemoperfusion with c.

    mitomycin adsorbed onto activated c. (M-CH)
    C. Plus
    c. suspension
CharcoCaps
Charcodote
    Aqueous C.
Charcot
    C. cirrhosis
    C. intermittent fever
    C. syndrome
    C. triad
    C. triangle
Charcot-Boettcher crystals and filaments
Charcot-Leyden crystal
Chardonna-2
CHARGE
    coloboma, heart disease, atresia choanae, retarded growth, genital hypoplasia, and ear abnormalities
        CHARGE abnormalities
        CHARGE syndrome
charge
    c. selectivity
    urine net c. (UNC)
charge-coupled
    c.-c. device (CCD)
    c.-c. device endoscope
    c.-c. device monochrome camera
Charrière scale
Chassard-Lapiné projection
chasteberry
ChAT
    choline acetyl transferase
Chatillon
    C. Digital Force gauge
    C. dolorimeter
Chauffard point
Chauveau bacterium
Cheatle-Henry
    C.-H. hernia
    C.-H. incision
Cheatle slit
checklist
    Hopkins symptom c.
Cheek-Perry syndrome
cheesy
    c. necrosis
    c. nephritis
cheilitis
    granulomatous c.
cheilosis
chelate
    gadolinium c.
Chelidonium majus
Chelsea-Eaton anal speculum
Chemet

chemical
- c. anoxia
- c. carcinogenesis
- c. cholecystitis
- c. cystitis
- cystogenic c.
- c. gastritis
- c. gastropathy
- c. litholysis
- c. peritonitis
- c. prostatitis
- c. splanchnicectomy
- c. urinalysis

chemical-induced esophagitis
chemically defined diet
chemiluminescence
- enhanced c. (ECL)
- luminol-enhanced c.

chemise
- bouton en c.

chemistry
- phosphoramidite c.

chemoattractant
chemodissolution
chemoembolization
- transarterial c. (TACE)
- transcatheter arterial c. (TACE)

chemoimmunotherapy
chemokine-orchestrated chemotaxis
chemokine receptor
chemolysis
- intrarenal c.

Chemo-Port catheter
chemoprevention of aging
chemoprophylaxis
- long-term low-dose maintenance c.
- traveler's c.

chemoradiation
- neoadjuvant c.
- c. therapy (CRT)

chemoradiotherapy
chemoreceptor
chemosensitivity
chemosis
chemotactic
- c. factor
- c. peptide

chemotaxis
- chemokine-orchestrated c.
- c. of polymorphonuclear leukocyte

chemotherapeutic agent hepatotoxicity

chemotherapy
- adjuvant hepatic arterial infusion c.
- antisarcoma c.
- antiviral c.
- continuous infusion c.
- cytotoxic c.
- c. gonadotoxicity
- hepatic arterial infusion c.
- high-dose c. (HDC)
- intraarterial c.
- intraperitoneal c.
- intraperitoneal hyperthermic c. (IPHC)
- intrathecal c.
- intravesical c.
- IP c.
- neoadjuvant c.
- platinum-based consolidation c.
- polyantibiotic c.

chemotherapy-induced
- c.-i. nausea
- c.-i. nausea and emesis (CINE)
- c.-i. sterility
- c.-i. vomiting

Chemstrip
- C. bG reagent
- C. LN dipstick

ChemTrak
- C. AccuMeter
- C. AccuMeter screen

Chenix Tablet
chenodeoxycholate
chenodeoxycholic acid (CDA, CDCA)
chenodiol
Cherchevski disease
Cherney incision
cherry
- c. angioma
- c. red spot (CRS)
- c. sponge

Cherry-Crandall method for testing serum lipase
chest
- barrel c.
- flail c.
- c. pain
- c. physiotherapy
- c. tube
- c. tube scar

Chester-Winter procedure

NOTES

Chevalier
    C. Jackson esophagoscope
    C. Jackson gastroscope
chevron incision
chew-and-spit test
chewing gum diarrhea
CHF
    congenital hepatic fibrosis
CHI
    creatinine height index
Chiari
    C. disease
    C. malformation
chiasm
    Camper c.
Chiba
    C. needle
    C. percutaneous cholangiogram
Chibroxin
chief cell
Chilaiditi
    C. sign
    C. syndrome
child
    C. class (A,B,C)
    C. (class A,B,C) patient
    C. esophageal varix classification
    c. esophagoscope
    C. hepatic dysfunction classification
    C. intestinal forceps
    C. liver criteria
    C. liver disease classification
    C. operation
    C. pancreaticoduodenostomy
childhood
    extraordinary urinary frequency
      syndrome of c.
    c. visceral myopathy (CVM)
Child-Phillips bowel plication
Child-Pugh
    C.-P. class
    C.-P. classification
    C.-P. criteria
    C.-P. score
children's
    c. coma scale
    C. Hospital intestinal forceps
Childs-Phillips intestinal plication needle
Child-Turcotte classification (CTC)
chili-bean pseudopolyp
Chilomastix
China ink
Chinese restaurant syndrome (CRS)
chip
    prostatic c.
Chiron
    C. RIBA HCV test

    C. RIBA HCV test system second
      generation
chiufa
Chlamydia
    C. psittaci
    C. trachomatis
    C. trachomatis infection
chlamydia urethritis
chloracetic
chloral hydrate
chlorambucil
chloramphenicol
chlorazepate
chlordiazepoxide
chlorhydria
chloride
    adrenalin c.
    c. balance
    benzalkonium c. (BAC)
    benzyl c.
    bethanechol c.
    calcium c.
    c. channel
    choline c.
    c. concentration
    CYT-356 radiolabeled with 111
      indium c.
    c. electrolyte
    mercury c. (HgCl2)
    mivacurium c.
    oxybutynin c.
    polyvinyl c. (PVC)
    potassium c. (KCl)
    c. secretion
    serum c.
    c. shunt
    sodium c.
    strontium-89 c.
    tetramethyl ammonium c. (TEMAC)
    titanous c.
    tridihexethyl c.
    urinary c.
chloride-to-phosphate ratio
chloridorrhea
    familial c.
chlorisondamine
chlormadinone acetate
chloroazotemic nephritis
chlorodontia
chloroform toxicity
chlorohydrate
    linsidomine c.
chloroma
    gastric c.
Chloromycetin
chloroplast
chloroprocaine
chloroquine-induced damage

chloroquine phosphate
chlorothiazide
chlorotrianisene
chlorozotocin
chlorpheniramine
chlorphenoxamine
chlorpromazine
chlorpromazine-induced cholestasia
chlorprothixene
chlorthalidone
chlorzoxazone toxicity
choana, pl. choanae
chocolate agar medium
CHOD-PAP cholesterol reagent
Cho/Dyonics two-portal endoscope
choice
    Medi-Jector C.
Choice2 test
choking
Cholac
cholagogic
cholagogue
cholaneresis
cholangeitis
cholangiectasis
cholangioadenoma
cholangiocarcinoma
    hilar c.
    metastatic c.
    perihilar c.
    peripheral c. (PCC)
    peripheral intrahepatic c.
    type III c.
Cholangiocath catheter
cholangiocatheter
    cystic duct c.
    saline-filled c.
cholangiocellular carcinoma (CCC)
cholangiocholecystocholedochectomy
cholangiodrainage
    percutaneous transhepatic c. (PTCD)
cholangiodysplastic pseudocirrhosis
cholangioenterostomy
    intrahepatic c.
cholangiofibroma
cholangiofibromatosis
cholangiogastrostomy
cholangiogram, cholangiography (CAG)
    balloon c.
    catheter c.
    Chiba percutaneous c.
    common duct c.

    contrast selective c.
    cystic duct c.
    endoscopic retrograde c.
    fine-needle percutaneous c.
    fine-needle transhepatic c.
    intraoperative c.
    intravenous c. (IVC)
    occlusion c.
    operative c.
    percutaneous transhepatic c. (PTC, PTHC)
    pernasal c.
    serial c.'s
    thin-needle percutaneous c.
    transgastric c.
    transhepatic c.
    T-tube c. (TTC)
cholangiographic
    c. catheter
    c. finding
cholangiography
    balloon occlusion c.
    breath-hold MR c.
    cystic duct c.
    delayed operative c.
    direct percutaneous transhepatic c.
    drip infusion c. (DIC)
    endoscopic retrograde c. (ERC)
    fine-needle transhepatic c. (FNTC, FNTHC)
    intraoperative c. (IOC)
    intravenous c. (IVC)
    magnetic resonance c. (MRC)
    nasobiliary drain c.
    non-breath-hold MR c.
    operative c.
    percutaneous hepatobiliary c.
    percutaneous transhepatic c. (PTC, PTHC)
    postoperative c.
    retrograde c.
    transabdominal c.
    transhepatic c. (TC, THC)
    T-tube c.
cholangiograsper
    Storz c.
cholangiohepatitis
    Oriental c.
    recurrent pyogenic c. (RPC)
cholangiohepatoma
cholangiojejunostomy
    intrahepatic c.

C

NOTES

129

cholangiolar
cholangiole
cholangiolitic
   c. cirrhosis
   c. hepatitis
cholangiolitis
cholangioma
cholangiopancreatography
   endoscopic retrograde c. (ERCP)
   magnetic resonance c. (MRCP)
cholangiopancreatoscopy
   peroral c. (PCPS)
cholangiopathy
   destructive c.
   eosinophilic c.
cholangiophytiasis
cholangioscope
   Olympus CHF-Q10 c.
   prototype c.
cholangioscopy
   intraductal c.
   percutaneous transhepatic c. (PTCS)
   peroral c. (PCS)
cholangiostomy
cholangiotomy
cholangiovenous
   c. communication
   c. reflux
cholangitic
   c. abscess
   c. biliary cirrhosis
cholangitis
   acute obstructive c.
   acute obstructive suppurative c.
    (AOSC)
   acute suppurative c. (ASC)
   ascending c.
   autoimmune c.
   bacterial c.
   biliary c.
   c. carcinoma
   catarrhal c.
   chronic nonsuppurative
    destructive c.
   destructive c.
   fibrous obliterative c.
   granulomatous c.
   idiopathic autoimmune c.
   intrahepatic sclerosing c.
   c. lenta
   lymphoid c.
   nonsuppurative destructive c.
   obstructive c.
   pleomorphic destructive c.
   postendoscopic c.
   posttransplantation c.
   primary sclerosing c. (PSC)
   progressive suppurative c.

   pyogenic c.
   rejection c.
   sclerosing c.
   secondary sclerosing c.
   septic c.
   small-duct primary sclerosing c.
   suppurative c.
   transient c.
   viral c.
cholanopoiesis
cholanopoietic
cholascos
cholate
cholebilirubin
Cholebrine contrast medium
cholechromopoiesis
cholecyanin
cholecystagogic
cholecystagogue
cholecystalgia
cholecystatony
cholecystectasia
cholecystectomy
   endoscopic laser c.
   laparoscopic c. (LC)
   laparoscopic laser c. (LLC)
   minilaparoscope c.
   prophylactic c.
   c. treatment
   videolaseroscopy c.
cholecystendysis
cholecystenteric fistula
cholecystenteroanastomosis
cholecystenterostomy
cholecystenterotomy
cholecystic
cholecystis
cholecystitis
   acalculous c.
   acute c. (AC)
   acute acalculous c.
   calculous c.
   chemical c.
   chronic c.
   chronic calculous c. (CCC)
   c. cystica
   c. emphysematosa
   emphysematous c.
   erythromycin-induced c.
   follicular c.
   gangrenous c.
   gaseous c.
   c. glandularis proliferans
   perforated c.
   c. with cholelithiasis
   xanthogranulomatous c.
cholecystobiliary fistula
cholecystocele

cholecystocholangiography
cholecystocholedochal fistula
cholecystocholedocholithiasis
cholecystocolonic fistula
cholecystocolostomy
cholecystocolotomy
cholecystoduodenal
    c. band
    c. fistula
    c. ligament
cholecystoduodenocolic
    c. fistula
    c. fold
cholecystoduodenostomy
    Jenckel c.
cholecystoendoprosthesis
    endoscopic retrograde c. (ERCCE)
cholecystoenterostomy
cholecystoenterotomy
cholecystogastric
cholecystogastrostomy
cholecystogogic
    oral c.
cholecystogram
    oral c. (OCG)
cholecystography
    drip infusion c.
    intravenous c.
    oral c.
    post-fatty meal c.
cholecystoileostomy
cholecystointestinal
cholecystojejunostomy
cholecystokinetic food
cholecystokinin (CCK)
    c. antagonist
    c. cholescintigraphy
    c. octapeptide (CCK-8, CCK-OP)
    c. test
cholecystokinin-like immunoreactivity
  (CCK-LI)
cholecystokinin-pancreozymin (CCK-PZ)
cholecystolithiasis
cholecystolithotomy
    percutaneous c. (PCCL)
    percutaneous transhepatic c.
    (PCTCL)
cholecystolithotripsy
cholecystomy
cholecystonephrostomy
cholecystoparesis
    diabetic c.

cholecystopathy
cholecystopexy
cholecystoptosis
cholecystopyelostomy
cholecystorrhaphy
cholecystoscopy
    percutaneous transhepatic c. (PTCC)
cholecystosis
    hyperplastic c.
cholecystostomy
    laparoscopy-guided subhepatic c.
    percutaneous transhepatic c.
cholecystotomy
    transpapillary endoscopic c. (TEC)
cholecystoxeransis
choledochal
    c. basal pressure
    c. cyst (grades I, II, III, IV, IVa)
    c. region
    c. sphincter
    c. sphincterotomy
choledochectomy
choledochendysis
choledochiarctia
choledochitis
choledochocele
choledochocholedochostomy (CDC)
choledochocolonic fistula
choledochocyst
choledochocystostomy
choledochodochorrhaphy
choledochoduodenal
    c. area
    c. fistula
    c. fistulotomy
    c. junctional stenosis
choledochoduodenostomy
choledochoenteric fistula
choledochoenterostomy
choledochofiberoscopy
    T-tube tract c.
choledochofiberscope
    Olympus URF-P2
    translaparoscopic c.
choledochofiberscopic approach
choledochogram
choledochography
choledochohepatostomy
choledochoileostomy
choledochojejunostomy (CDJ)
    end-to-side c.
    loop c.

C

NOTES

choledochojejunostomy *(continued)*
   retrocolic end-to-side c.
   Roux-en-Y c.
choledocholith
choledocholithiasis
choledocholithotomy
choledocholithotripsy, choledocholithotrity
choledochopancreatic ductal junction
choledochoplasty
choledochorrhaphy
choledochoscope
   Berci-Shore c.
   CBD 2 c.
   flexible fiberoptic c.
   Hopkins rod-lens system for
      rigid c.
   Machida c.
   Olympus CHF-P20 c.
   Olympus XCHF-37 c.
   URF-P2 c.
choledochoscopic guidance
choledochoscopy
   Berci-Shore c.
   cystic duct c.
   jejunostomy tract c.
   operative c.
   percutaneous c.
   postoperative c.
   T-tube tract c.
choledochosphincterotomy
choledochostomy
choledochotomy
   c. incision
   longitudinal c.
choledochus
   ductus c.
choledococaval anastomosis (CDCA)
choleglobin
cholehepatic shunt pathway
choleic acid
cholelith
cholelithiasis
   cholecystitis with c.
   cholesterol c.
   intrahepatic c.
   c. prevalence
cholelithic dyspepsia
cholelitholysis
cholelithoptysis
cholelithotomy
cholelithotripsy, cholelithotrity
cholelithotrity
cholemesis
cholemia
   familial c.
   Gilbert c.
cholemic nephrosis

cholepathia
   c. spastica
choleperitoneum
choleperitonitis
cholepoiesis
cholepoietic
choleprasin
cholera
   Asiatic c.
   bilious c.
   c. morbus
   c. nostras
   pancreatic c.
   c. sicca
   summer c.
   c. toxin
   c. toxin-induced diarrhea
cholerae
   Vibrio c.
choleraesuis
   Salmonella c.
choleraic diarrhea
choleresis
choleretic
   c. effect
   c. enteropathy
choleriform enteritis
cholerigenic, cholerigenous
cholerine
choleroid
cholerrhagia
cholerrhagic
cholescintigram
cholescintigraphy
   cholecystokinin c.
   hepatobiliary c.
   morphine c.
   radionuclide c.
cholescintigraphy
Cholestabyl
cholestasia, cholestasis
   acute drug-induced c.
   benign postoperative c.
   benign recurrent intrahepatic c.
      (BRIC)
   bile ductular c.
   canalicular c.
   centrilobular c.
   chlorpromazine-induced c.
   contraceptive pill-induced c.
   drug-induced c.
   estrogen-induced c.
   extrahepatic c.
   familial c.
   hepatocanalicular c.
   hepatocellular c.
   high-grade c.
   intrahepatic c.

methyltestosterone-induced c.
neonatal c.
Norwegian c.
c. patient
pericentral c.
progressive familial intrahepatic c.
  (PFIC)
progressive intrahepatic c.
pure c.
recurrent c.
tolbutamide-induced c.
cholestatic
c. hypersensitivity
c. jaundice
c. liver disease
c. reaction
c. syndrome
c. viral hepatitis
cholesteatoma
cholesterol
c. calculus
c. cholelithiasis
c. crystal embolization (CCE)
dietary c.
c. embolism
c. emboli syndrome
c. embolus
c. ester
c. ester storage disease (CESD)
c. ester transfer protein (CETP)
high-density lipoprotein c. (HDL-C)
low-density lipoprotein c. (LDLC)
c. monohydrate crystal
c. polyp
radioactive c.
c. saturation index (CSI)
seminal plasma c.
serum c.
c. stone
very low density lipoprotein c.
VLDL c.
cholesterol-cholesteroloxidase-phenol 4-aminophenazone method
cholesterol-containing gallstone
cholesteroleresis
cholesterolosis
acalculous c.
c. of gallbladder
c. of mucosal surface
cholesteryl ester
cholestyramine therapy
Choletec

choletelin
choletherapy
choleverdin
cholic
c. acid (CA)
c. acid clearance
cholicele
choline
c. acetyl transferase (ChAT)
c. chloride
c. deficiency liver disease
seminal plasma c.
cholinergic
c. agonist
c. innervation
c. neuron
c. receptor
c. syndrome
cholochrome
chologenetic
Cholografin contrast medium
chololith
chololithiasis
chololithic
cholopoiesis
cholorrhea
choloscopy
Cholybar
cholyl-^{14}C-glycine
chondrocyte
autologous c.
chondrocyte-alginate gel
chondrodysplasia
Jansen-type metaphyseal c.
Chondrogel
chondrogenic differentiation
chondroitin
chondroitinuria
chondrosarcoma
bladder c.
Chooz
chorda, pl. **chordae**
c. gubernaculum
c. spermatica
chordee
acquired c.
congenital c.
c. correction
fibrous c.
lateral c.
residual c.
chordeic penis

C

NOTES

choreoathetosis
choriocarcinoma
    bladder c.
chorioepithelioma
chorionic
chorista
choristoma
choroid plexus cyst (CPC)
Christie gallbladder retractor
Christmas
    C. tree appearance of pancreas
    C. tree sign
Christopher-Williams overtube
chromaffin
    c. cell
    c. tissue
chromaffinoma
chromagranin
chromatofocusing pH range
chromatograph
    Carle analytic gas c.
    Quintron Microlyzer 12 c.
chromatography
    column c.
    gas c.
    gel filtration c.
    high-performance liquid c. (HPLC)
    high-pressure liquid c. (HPLC)
    ion c.
    solid-phase extraction c.
    stool c.
    thin-layer c. (TLC)
    Varian model 3600 gas c.
chromatopectic
chromatopexis
chromic
    c. catgut
    c. catgut suture
    c. gut suture
chromium
    c. deficiency
    51-c.-labeled
        ethylenediaminetetraacetate (^{51}Cr-
        EDTA)
    c. sesquioxide
51-chromium-labeled
  ethylenediaminetetraacetate (^{51}Cr-
  EDTA)
chromocystoscopy
chromoendoscope
chromoendoscopy
    Lugol c.
    magnification c.
    phenol red c.
chromogen
chromogranin
    c. A-immunoreactive cell
    c. stain

chromopectic
chromopexic
chromopexy
chromophobe
    c. adenoma
    c. cell tumor
chromophore enhanced laser welding
chromoscopy
    gastric c.
chromosomal
    c. abnormality
    c. marker
chromosome
    c. deletion
    human c. 6
    c. insertion
    c. instability (CIN)
    c. inversion
    c. karyotype
    c. marker
    marker c.
    c. morphology
    Philadelphia c.
    c. ploidy
    X c.
    Y c.
chromoureteroscopy
chronic
    c. abacterial prostatitis
    c. active gastritis
    c. active hepatitis (CAH)
    c. active liver disease (CALD)
    c. active pouchitis
    c. active viral hepatitis (CAVH)
    c. active viral hepatitis, non-A,
        non-B (CAVH-NAB)
    c. active viral hepatitis, type B
        (CAVH-B)
    c. aggressive hepatitis (CAH)
    c. alcoholic cirrhosis
    c. alcoholic pancreatitis (CAP)
    c. allograft nephropathy
    c. ambulatory peritoneal dialysis
        (CAPD)
    c. anoplasty treatment
    c. appendicitis
    c. atrophic duodenitis
    c. atrophic gastritis (CAG)
    c. autoimmune hepatitis
    c. bacterial enteropathy
    c. bacterial prostatitis (CBP)
    c. bacterial pyelonephritis
    c. benign hepatitis (CBH)
    c. calcifying pancreatitis (CCP)
    c. calculous cholecystitis (CCC)
    c. cholecystitis
    c. cholestatic liver disease
    c. cicatrizing enteritis

c. cystic gastritis
c. diarrhea
c. diverticulitis
c. erosion
c. erosive gastritis
c. fibrosing hepatitis
c. follicular gastritis
c. functional constipation
c. functional gastrointestinal
symptom
c. functional symptomatology
c. glomerular disease
c. glomerulonephritis (CG, CGN)
c. graft-versus-host disease (c-GVHD)
c. granulomatous disease
c. hepatitis (CH)
c. hepatitis B, C
c. hypokalemic nephropathy
c. idiopathic constipation
c. idiopathic intestinal
pseudoobstruction (CIIP)
c. idiopathic jaundice
c. inflammatory bowel disease
(CIBD)
c. inflammatory cell infiltrate
c. inflammatory disease
c. interstitial gastritis
c. interstitial hepatitis
c. intestinal atony
c. intestinal dysmotility (CID)
c. intestinal ischemic syndrome
c. intestinal pseudoobstruction (CIP,
CIPO)
c. intestinal pseudoobstruction
syndrome
c. ischemic colonic lesion caused
by phlebosclerosis (CICLP)
c. lead poisoning
c. liver disease
c. lobular hepatitis (CLH)
c. low-frequency electrical
stimulation
c. membranous glomerulonephritis
(CMGN)
c. mercury poisoning
c. metabolic acidosis
c. nonbacterial prostatitis (CNP)
c. nonimmune gastritis
c. nonsuppurative destructive
cholangitis

c. obstructive pulmonary disease
(COPD)
c. obstructive uropathy
c. pancreatitis (CP)
c. pancreatitis of Kasugai
c. parenchymal liver disease
c. pelvic pain syndrome (CPPS)
c. peptic esophagitis
c. periesophagitis
c. persistent hepatitis (CPH)
c. progressive hepatitis
c. progressive tubulointerstitial
disease
c. prostate pain syndrome (CPPS)
c. prostatitis/pelvic pain syndrome
(CPPS)
c. pyelonephritis (CP, CPN)
c. radiation proctitis
c. regurgitation
c. relapsing pancreatitis
c. renal failure (CRF)
c. renal failure glomerulonephritis
c. renal insufficiency (CRI)
c. sacral neuromodulation
c. sacral spinal nerve stimulation
c. sclerosing hyaline fibrosis
c. superficial gastritis (CSG)
c. transplant rejection
c. tubular damage
c. type B hepatitis
c. ulcer
c. ulcerative colitis (CUC)
c. ulcerative proctitis
c. urate nephropathy
c. urethral syndrome
c. urinary retention (CUR)
c. viral hepatitis
chronica
enteritis cystica c.
gastrorrhea continua c.
ileocolitis ulcerosa c.
chronically inflamed gallbladder
chronic-continuous type
chronicus
lichen simplex c.
chronobiological parameter
chronotropism
Chronulac
CHRP
coagulation and hemostatic resection of
the prostate

NOTES

CHRPE
congenital hypertrophy of the retinal
pigment epithelium
CHRS
cerebrohepatorenal syndrome
CHUK
conserved helix-loop-helix ubiquitous
kinase
Church deep surgery scissors
Churg-Strauss syndrome
Chwalla membrane
chylangioma
chylaqueous
chylectasia
chyle cyst
chyli
cisterna c.
receptaculum c.
urina c.
chylifaction
chylifactive
chyliferous vessel
chylification
chyliform ascites
chylocele
parasitic c.
chyloderma
chylomediastinum
chylomicron
c. core
c. production
c. retention disease
c. secretion
chyloperitoneum
chylophoric
chylopoiesis
chylopoietic disease
chylorrhea
chylosa
diarrhea c.
chylosis
chylothorax
chylous
c. ascites
c. ascitic fluid
c. fistula
c. leukemia
c. peritonitis
c. urine
chyluria
chylus
chyme
c. discharge
c. transport
Chymex
chymification
chymobilia
iatrogenic c.

chymopoiesis
chymorrhea
chymotrypsin
CI
confidence interval
CIA
congenital intestinal aganglionosis
Cialis
Ciba-Corning ACS PSA assay
cibalis
fistula c.
CIBD
chronic inflammatory bowel disease
cibenzoline
cibi
urina c.
CIC
clean intermittent catheterization
cicatricial
c. stricture
c. tissue
cicatrix
cicatrization
CICLP
chronic ischemic colonic lesion caused
by phlebosclerosis
CID
chronic intestinal dysmotility
Cidecin
Cidex
C. activated dialdehyde solution
C. Plus solution
cidofovir
cIEL
crypt intraepithelial lymphocyte
CIFN
consensus interferon
CIFN therapy
cigarette drain
cigar-shaped hyperchromatic nucleus
ciguatera
C-III
Testred C-III
CIIP
chronic idiopathic intestinal
pseudoobstruction
cilastin
**ciliary-derived neurotrophic factor
receptor (CDNF)**
ciliary dysentery
ciliate dysentery
Cillium
CIM
cardia intestinal metaplasia
cimetidine
Cimicifuga heracleifolia

CIN
cervical intraepithelial neoplasia
chromosome instability
cinaedi
Campylobacter c.
CINE
chemotherapy-induced nausea and emesis
cinedefecogram
cinedefecography
cine-esophagogram
cine-esophagoscope
cine-esophagoscopy
cinefluorographic study
cinefluorography
cinefluoroscopic method
cinegastroscopy
cine-loop memory function
cineradiographic analysis
cineurography
cinnamic acid
Cinobac Pulvules
cinoxacin
CIP
chronic intestinal pseudoobstruction
CIPO
chronic intestinal pseudoobstruction
Cipro
ciprofloxacin hydrochloride
circadian
c. gastric acidity
c. periodicity
c. rhythm
c. rhythmicity
c. testosterone pattern
circadian-shaped infusion
Circe device
circinata
balanitis c.
circinate balanitis
circle
c. needle
Pagenstecher c.
Circon-ACMI
C.-ACMI lithotriptor
C.-ACMI MicroDigital-I camera
C.-ACMI miniscope
C.-ACMI (MR-6, MR-9) ureteroscope
C.-ACMI uteroscope
circuit
cerebral-brain stem c.
enteric neuronal c.

enteric secretomotor c.
extracorporeal cardiopulmonary c.
circuitous
circular
c. anal dilator
c. dichroism
c. folds of Kerckring
c. muscle
c. muscle fiber
c. myotomy
c. stapled anastomosis
c. stapler
c. stapler donut
c. stapling device
c. suture
c. tape
c. vesicomyotomy (CVM)
circulares
plicae c.
circulating
c. autoantibody
c. enzyme
c. immunocomplexes immunological study
c. tumor-associated antigen
circulation
arterial c.
collateral abdominal c.
cutaneous collateral c.
enterohepatic c. (EHC)
hepatic c.
hyperdynamic c.
mesenteric c.
portal c.
portal-collateral c.
venous c.
circulatory embarrassment
circumanal
circumcaval ureter
circumcise
circumcised
circumcision
c. complication
contraindication to c.
meatal stenosis after c.
Plastibell c.
routine neonatal c.
sleeve-type c.
trapped penis after c.
circumductive
circumference
abdominal c. (AC)

NOTES

circumferential
c. fundoplication
c. margin
c. mucosal dissection
c. transanal sleeve advancement
flap
circumflex vein
circumintestinal
circumlocution
circumumbilical incision
cirrhogenous, cirrhogenic
cirrhosis
acholangic biliary c.
acute juvenile c.
alcoholic c. (AC)
atrophic c.
autoimmune c.
bacterial c.
Baumgarten c.
biliary c.
Budd c.
calculous c.
capsular c. of liver
cardiac c.
CCl4-induced c.
Charcot c.
cholangiolitic c.
cholangitic biliary c.
chronic alcoholic c.
compensated c.
congestive c.
CPH-CAH c.
Cruveilhier-Baumgarten c.
cryptogenic c.
decompensated alcoholic c.
decompensated liver c.
drug-induced c.
end-stage c.
fatty c.
focal biliary c.
frank c.
glabrous c.
Glisson c.
Hanot c.
hemochromatotic c.
hepatic c.
hepatitis C antiviral long-term
treatment to prevent c. (HALT-C)
histologic c.
hypertrophic c.
hypochlorhydric c.
incomplete c.
juvenile c.
Laënnec c.
liver c. (LC)
macronodular c.

Maixner c.
Mayo Clinic system test for
primary biliary c.
micronodular c.
mixed c.
multilobular c.
necrotic c.
nonazotemic c.
nutritional c.
obstructive biliary c.
periportal c.
pigmentary c.
pipestem c.
portal c.
posthepatic c.
postnecrotic c.
primary biliary c. (PBC)
progressive familial c.
secondary biliary c.
stasis c.
c. of stomach
syndrome of primary biliary c.
Todd c.
toxic c.
type C c.
unilobular c.
vascular c.
cirrhotic
c. ascites
c. gastritis
c. hydrothorax
c. liver
cirsocele
cirsoid aneurysm
cirsomphalos
CIS
carcinoma in situ
cisapride
rectal c.
cisapride-assisted lavage
CISCA
cisplatin, cyclophosphamide, Adriamycin
CISCA protocol
cis-diaminedichloroplatinum
cisplatin
bleomycin, etoposide, c. (BEP)
c., cyclophosphamide, Adriamycin
(CISCA)
c., doxorubicin, cyclophosphamide
etoposide, ifosfamide, c.
methotrexate, c. (MC)
c., methotrexate, Velban (CMV)
c., methotrexate, vinblastine (CMV)
methotrexate, vinblastine,
Adriamycin, c. (MVAC, M-VAC)

methotrexate, vinblastine, cpirubicin, c. (M-VEC)
c. nephropathy (CPN)

cisplatin-Lipiodol-Spongel (CLS)

cisterna, pl. **cisternae**
c. chyli
cylindrical confronting c. (CCC)

CIT
cold ischemia time

Citra Forte

citrate
clomiphene c.
c. infusion
lead c.
c. of magnesia
magnesium c.
c. metabolism
piperazine c.
potassium c.
ranitidine bismuth c. (RBC)
c. replacement fluid
seminal plasma c.
sildenafil c.
sodium c.
c. supplementation
c. synthase
c. test
urinary c.

citric
c. acid
c. acid bladder mixture

citrinum
Penicillium c.

Citrobacter
C. amalonaticus
C. diversus
C. freundii
C. intermedius

Citrocarbonate

Citroma

Citro-Mag

Citro-Nesia

Citrotein liquid feeding

Citrucel sugar-free

citrulline

citrullinemia

Civiale operation

CIXU
constant infusion excretory urogram

c-jun
c-jun protooncogene
c-jun oncogene

CK-MB
muscle-brain isoenzyme of creative kinase

CKPT
combined kidney and pancreas transplant

^{13}C-labeled cholesteryl octanoate breath test

C-lactose test

Clado ligament

cladribine

CLA echoendoscope

Claforan

Clagett-Barrett
C.-B. esophagogastroscopy
C.-B. esophagogastrostomy

Clagett esophagogastrostomy

clam
c. enterocystoplasty
c. ileocystoplasty

clamp
Abadie enterostomy c.
Adson c.
Allen anastomosis c.
Allen intestinal c.
Allen-Kocher c.
Allis c.
anastomosis c.
approximator c.
ASSI METS-3668 Microspike approximator c.
ASSI MKCV-2040 Microspike approximator c.
ASSI MSPK-3678 Microspike approximator c.
atraumatic c.
Ault intestinal occlusion c.
Babcock c.
Backhaus towel c.
Bainbridge intestinal c.
Baumrucker urinary incontinence c.
Beardsley intestinal c.
Best right-angle colon c.
Bihrle dorsal c.
Borge c.
Buie pile c.
bulldog c.
Carmalt c.
Carmel c.
Collins umbilical c.
Cope crushing c.
Cope modification of a Martel intestinal c.

C

NOTES

clamp *(continued)*
  Crawford c.
  Crile appendix c.
  Crile hemostatic c.
  Cunningham urinary incontinence c.
  curved Mayo c.
  Daniel colostomy c.
  Dardik c.
  Dean-MacDonald gastric
    resection c.
  DeBakey c.
  DeMartel appendix c.
  DeMartel-Wolfson anastomosis c.
  Dennis c.
  Dixon-Thomas-Smith c.
  Doyen intestinal c.
  Earle hemorrhoid c.
  Edna towel c.
  Fehland intestinal c.
  Fogarty c.
  Foss anterior resection c.
  Foss intestinal c.
  Furniss anastomosis c.
  Furniss-Clute duodenal c.
  Gant c.
  Glassman noncrushing
    gastrointestinal c.
  Goldblatt c.
  Goldstein Microspike
    approximator c.
  Gomco umbilical c.
  Haberer intestinal c.
  Harvey Stone c.
  Hayes anterior resection c.
  Hayes colon c.
  Heaney c.
  hemorrhoidal c.
  hemostatic c.
  Hendren c.
  Herrick kidney c.
  hilar c.
  Hirschmann pile c.
  Hunt colostomy c.
  Hurwitz esophageal c.
  Hurwitz intestinal c.
  intestinal c.
  Jarvis hemorrhoid c.
  Jarvis pile c.
  Kane umbilical c.
  Kapp-Beck colon c.
  Kelly c.
  Kelsey pile c.
  kidney pedicle c.
  Kleinschmidt appendectomy c.
  Kocher c.
  Lane gastroenterostomy c.
  Lane intestinal c.
  laparoscopic Allis c.
  Linnartz intestinal c.
  Linton tourniquet c.
  Madden intestinal c.
  Martel c.
  Masters intestinal c.
  Masters-Schwartz liver c.
  Mayo abdominal c.
  Mayo-Robson intestinal c.
  McCleery-Miller intestinal c.
  McDougal prostatectomy c.
  McLean pile c.
  Meeker gallbladder c.
  metal wing c.
  Microspike approximator c.
  microvascular c.
  Mikulicz c.
  Mixter c.
  Mogen c.
  Moreno gastroenterostomy c.
  mosquito hemostatic c.
  Moynihan c.
  Myles hemorrhoidal c.
  noncrushing bowel c.
  Nussbaum intestinal c.
  occlusive c.
  Ochsner c.
  O'Hanlon intestinal c.
  Olsen cholangiogram c.
  partial-occlusion c.
  Payr pyloric c.
  Péan c.
  pedicle c.
  Pemberton sigmoid c.
  penile c.
  Pennington c.
  Petz c.
  Phillips rectal c.
  Rankin c.
  Redo intestinal c.
  right-angle c.
  Roosevelt c.
  rubber-sheathed c.
  rubber-shod c.
  Satinsky c.
  Schwartz c.
  Scudder intestinal c.
  serrefine c.
  Shoemaker intestinal c.
  Singley intestinal ring c.
  slotted nerve c.
  Stetten intestinal c.
  Stille c.
  Stone-Holcombe intestinal c.
  Stone intestinal c.
  straight mosquito c.
  Strelinger colon c.
  tonsil c.
  tubing c.

vascular c.
von Petz c.
Wangensteen anastomosis c.
Wirthlin splenorenal c.
Wolfson intestinal c.
Wylie hypogastric c.
Zachary Cope-DeMartel c.
Zeppelin c.
Zipser penile c.
clamping
hyperglycemic c.
clamshell technique
clandestine intake
clapotage, clapotement
clarithromycin
lansoprazole, amoxicillin, c.
omeprazole, amoxicillin, c. (OAC)
omeprazole, metronidazole, c.
(OMC)
ranitidine bismuth citrate,
amoxicillin, c. (RAC)
c. triple therapy
Clark
C. common duct dilator
C. hemoperfusion cartridge
C. operation
C. sign
Clarke-Hadfield syndrome
Clarke-Reich knot pusher
CLASS
Celecoxib Long-Term Arthritis Safety
Study
class
c. I, II antigen
c. I, II MHC molecule
Child c. (A,B,C)
Child-Pugh c.
Classen-Demling papillotome
classic achalasia
classification
AJCC TNM tumor c.
Anderson c.
Ann Arbor c.
Astler-Coller c. (A, B1, B2, C1,
C2)
Astler-Coller modification of
Dukes c.
Banff c.
bismuth benign bile duct
stricture c.
Blaivas urinary incontinence c.
Borrmann gastric cancer c.

Bosniak c.
Cambridge pancreatitis c. (I–IV)
Caroli-Sarles c.
Child esophageal varix c.
Child hepatic dysfunction c.
Child liver disease c.
Child-Pugh c.
Child-Turcotte c. (CTC)
Correa c.
Cotton c.
Couinaud c.
Dagradi esophageal variceal c.
Dubin-Amelar varicocele c.
Dukes c. of carcinoma
Forrest c.
Fredrickson c.
gastric mucosal pattern c.
Hald-Bradley c.
IGCCCG c.
International Continence Society
voiding function c.
International Germ Cell Cancer
Collaborative Group c.
Japanese cancer c.
Jewett bladder carcinoma c.
Kasugai c.
Kelami c.
LA c.
Lapides c.
Lauren gastric carcinoma c.
Los Angeles c.
Lukes-Collins c.
Marseille pancreatitis c.
McNeer c.
megaureter c.
Ming gastric carcinoma c.
Mt. Sinai c.
Musshoff modification of the Ann
Arbor c.
NIH-CPSI prostatitis c.
Pugh c.
Ranson acute pancreatitis c.
Rappaport c.
reflux esophagitis c. (I–IV)
Santiani-Stone c.
Siurala c.
Solcia c.
Sonnenberg c.
Stamey c.
Sumikoshi c.
Sydney system gastritis c.
c. system

C

NOTES

classification *(continued)*
TNM carcinoma c.
UICC tumor c.
Visick dysphagia c.
voiding dysfunction c.
Whitehead c.
WHO gastric carcinoma c.
clathrin-coated pit
claudication
Clave needleless system
clavulanate
clavulanic acid
Clavulin
claw forceps
Clay-Adams (PE-10, PE-50) catheter
Claybrook sign
clay-colored stool
CLD
NBNC CLD
non-B, non-C chronic liver disease
CLE
columnar-lined esophagus
long-segment CLE
short-segment CLE
clean
c. intermittent bladder
catheterization
c. intermittent catheterization (CIC)
clean-catch urine specimen
cleaner
Endozime AW bacteriostatic
enzyme c.
cleaning
diathermic c.
cleanser
Cara-Klenz skin c.
Rediwash skin c.
UltraKlenz skin c.
cleansing
c. hypertonic phosphate enema
clean-voided specimen (CVS)
clear
c. bile
c. cell adenocarcinoma
c. cell carcinoma of kidney
c. cell hepatocellular carcinoma
c. cell nonpapillary carcinoma
c. cell renal cancer
c. cell sarcoma
c. discharge
enemas until c.
c. liquid diet
clearance
aminopyrine c.
antipyrine c.
bromsulphalein c.
caffeine c.
cholic acid c.

creatinine c. (CC, Crcl)
^{51}Cr-labeled albumin c.
dextran c.
equivalent residual renal urea c.
(eKru)
esophageal acid c.
fractional c.
hepatic c.
24-hour creatinine c.
hydrogen gas c.
ICG c.
I-125 iothalamate c.
immunoglobulin G c.
indocyanine green c. (ICG
clearance)
instantaneous c.
integrated c.
inulin c.
iodoantipyrine c.
iothalamate c.
kidney c.
lithium c. (CLi)
luminal acid c.
mucociliary c.
osmolar c.
PAH c.
paraaminohippurate c.
plasma c.
prescribed c.
renal c.
retinyl ester c.
stone c.
theophylline c.
urea c.
in vitro c.
in vivo c.
whole blood clearance and blood-
water c.
clearing
esophageal c.
cleavage
aspartyl protease-mediated c.
bacterial c.
embryonic c.
c. plane
cleaved extracellular domain
cleft palate
Cleocin
Cleveland
C. Clinic Incontinence Score
C. Clinic weighted scale of
endoscopic procedures
Clexane
CLH
chronic lobular hepatitis
CLi
lithium clearance

click
    intermittent c.
    prosthetic valve c.
    systolic c.
clidinium bromide
client patient characteristic
CLIM computer program
clindamycin
Clindex
clinic
    urology c.
clinical
    c. determinant
    c. hypergastrinemia
    c. implication
    c. monitoring
    c. parameter
    c. problem
    c. protocol
    c. rejection
    C. Risk Index for Babies (CRIB)
    c. sequela
    c. trial
clinically stable human renal allograft
clinicobiological criteria
clinicopathological
clinicopathologic staging
Clinifeed Iso enteral feeding
Clinitest-negative stool
Clinitest-positive stool
Clinitest stool test
Clinoril
Clinoxide
clip
    absorbable c.
    c. applier
    Heifitz c.
    Hulka c.
    Kifa skin c.
    laparoscopic tie c.
    Lapra-Ty c.
    metal c.
    Michel c.
    silver c.
    titanium c.
    towel c.
    von Petz suture c.
    Weck c.
Clipoxide
clipping
    endoluminal c.

    endoscopic c.
    laser c.
Clirans T-series dialyzer
clitoral
    c. index
    c. recession
clitoridis
    preputium c.
clitoris, pl. **clitorides**
    bifid c.
clitoroplasty
clitorovaginoplasty
CLO
    Campylobacter-like organism
    CLO biopsy
cloaca
    congenital c.
    persistent c.
    c. septation
cloacae
    Enterobacter c.
cloacal
    c. exstrophy
    c. exstrophy one-stage repair
    c. exstrophy two-stage repair
    c. malformation
    c. membrane
    c. plate
    c. remnant
    c. septum
cloacogenic polyp
clodronate
clofazimine
clofibrate
Clomid
clomiphene
    c. citrate
    c. test
clomipramine
clonal
    c. anergy
    c. deletion
    c. dilution
clonality
clonazepam
clone
    gliadin-specific T-cell c.
clonic contraction
clonidine suppression test
cloning
    molecular c.
clonogenic repopulation

C

NOTES

143

clonorchiasis
    biliary c.
clonorchiosis
Clonorchis sinensis
clonus
    left-sided c.
    right-sided c.
C-loop
    duodenal C-l.
    C-l. of duodenum
Cloquet
    C. hernia
    node of C.
clorazepate dipotassium
clortermine
closed
    c. afferent loop
    c. colon
    c. continuous lavage
    c. drainage
    c. duodenum
    c. efferent loop
    c. esophagus
    c. eyes sign
    c. hemorrhoidectomy
    c. injury
    c. morphology
    c. pylorus
    c. suction drain
    c. suction drainage system
    c. tubule fixation technique
closed-end ostomy pouch
closed-loop intestinal obstruction
closing pressure
Clostoban
clostridial nephritis
Clostridium
    C. *algidicarnis*
    C. *botulinum*
    C. *butyricum*
    C. *cadaveris*
    C. *coccoides*
    C. *difficile* (CD)
    C. *difficile*-associated diarrhea
    (CDAD)
    C. *difficile* enteritis
    C. *difficile* enterotoxin
    C. *difficile* toxin assay
    C. *fallax*
    C. *leptum*
    C. *perfringens*
    C. *ramosum*
    C. *tertium*
    C. *tetani*
    C. *welchii*
closure
    Beta-Cap catheter c.
    Beta-Cap II c.

    bladder neck c. (BNC)
    bladder outlet c.
    delayed primary c. (DPC)
    exstrophy c.
    Graham c.
    ileostomy c.
    muscularis tunnel c.
    primary c.
    pyelotomy c.
    secondary c.
    Smead-Jones c.
    stapled c.
    Sur-Fit Natura irrigation sleeve
      tail c.
    sutureless colostomy c.
    Tom Jones c.
    Witzel c.
    wound c.
clot
    adherent c.
    black c.
    blood c.
    c.'s and debris
    fresh c.
    fundic c.
    hematuria with c.'s
    intraluminal c.
    nonadherent c.
    overlying c.
    sentinel c.
CLOtest
    Campylobacter-like organism test
clot-induced urinary tract obstruction
clotrimazole
clotted blood
clotting
    c. abnormality
    c. cascade
    c. factor
    c. parameter
    c. time
cloud
    c. phenomenon
    plasma c.
cloudy
    c. ascites
    c. bile
    c. fluid
cloverleaf
    c. appearance
    c. deformity
    c. excision of hemorrhoid
    C. internal bumper
cloxacillin-induced cholestatic jaundice
Cloxapen
CLS
    cisplatin-Lipiodol-Spongel

club

American Endosonography C. (AEC)

clubbed

c. common bile duct

c. finger

c. penis

clubbing

calix c.

finger c.

c. of the fingers and toes

clustered

c. jejunal waves

c. waves (CW)

cluster of grapelike cysts

clusterin mRNA

CLVP

contact laser vaporization of the prostate

clysis

clysma

Clysodrast

clyster

CM-101

CM1 polyclonal antibody

CMA

cow's milk allergy

c-met

c-met oncogene

c-met receptor

c-MET protein

CMG

cystometrogram

CMGN

chronic membranous glomerulonephritis

C-mount adapter

CMSE

cow's milk-sensitive enteropathy

CMV

cisplatin, methotrexate, Velban

cisplatin, methotrexate, vinblastine

cytomegalovirus

CMV colitis

CMV esophagitis

CMV inclusion body

CMV inclusion cyst

CMV infection

CMV ulcerative disease

CMV-associated ulceration

CMV-induced esophageal ulceration

CMV-related ulcer

c-myc

c-myc oncogene

c-myc protooncogene

CNDI

congenital nephrogenic diabetes insipidus

CNNA

culture-negative neutrocytic ascites

CNP

chronic nonbacterial prostatitis

C-type natriuretic peptide

CNS

central nervous system

congenital nephrotic syndrome

CO_2

CO_2 breath test

CO_2 electrolyte

CO_2 laser

CO_2 laser probe

Co

coenzyme

CoA

coenzyme A

coagulase

c. waveform

c. waveform desiccation

coagulase-negative Staphylococcus

coagulating

c. current

c. electrode

c. forceps

coagulation

argon beam plasma c.

argon ion plasma c.

argon plasma c. (APC)

BICAP c.

bipolar c.

Bipolar Circumactive Probe c.

blood c.

Bovie c.

coaptive c.

disseminated intravascular c. (DIC)

EHT c.

electrohydrothermal c.

endoscopic microwave c.

free-beam c.

heater probe c.

c. and hemostatic resection of the prostate (CHRP)

infrared c.

interstitial laser c. (ILC)

laser c.

microwave c.

NOTES

145

coagulation *(continued)*
　　monopolar c.
　　multipolar c.
　　c. necrosis
　　c. probe
　　semen c.
　　c. time
　　tissue c.
coagulative
　　c. laser therapy
　　c. necrosis
coagulator
　　argon beam c.
　　argon plasma c. (APC)
　　Erbe Unit argon plasma c.
　　infrared c.
　　Redfield infrared c.
Coaguloop resection electrode
coagulopathy
　　iatrogenic c.
　　c. pancreatitis
coagulum pyelolithotomy
coalesce
coalescence
coalescent ulcer
coalition
　　Digestive Disease National C.
　　　(DDNC)
coaptive coagulation
coarctation
coarse
　　c. granular cast
　　c. gravel
　　c. material
　　c. nodularity
coarsely granular kidney
coat
　　fibromuscular c.
　　muscular c.
coated biopsy forceps
coaxial
　　c. catheter
　　c. snare
cobalamin deficiency
cobalophilin
cobalt-60
Coban
　　C. dressing
　　C. tape
Cobb collar
cobbler's stitch
cobblestone
　　c. appearance
　　c. appearance of gastric body
　　c. filling defect
　　c. mucosa
　　c. pattern
　　c. pattern of hepatocyte

cobblestone-like monolayer
cobblestoning
　　c. of colon
　　c. of mucosa
　　mucosal c.
　　c. sign
Cobe
　　C. Centrysystem dialyzer 400 HG
　　C. staple gun
　　C. stapler
^{57}**Co B$_{12}$ excretion**
cobra
　　c. catheter
　　c. venom factor (CVF)
cobra-head
　　c.-h. deformity
　　c.-h. sign
cocaine
　　c. hepatotoxicity
　　c. package ingestion
cocarcinogen
cocarcinogenic
　　c. FBA
　　c. fecal bile acid
coccidian
　　c. body
　　c. *Cyclospora*
　　c. sporulation
　　unsporulated c.
coccidian-like
coccidioidal
　　c. cystitis
　　c. endometritis
　　c. peritonitis
Coccidioides immitis **peritonitis**
coccidioidomycosis
coccidiosis
coccidium
coccoides
　　Clostridium c.
coccoid form of *Helicobacter pylori*
coccygeal
　　c. fistula
　　c. pelvis
coccygeus muscle
Cochin China diarrhea
Cochran-Mantel-Haenszel test
CO/CI
　　cardiac output/cardiac index
Cockcroft-Gault
　　C.-G. equation
　　C.-G. formula
Cock operation
Cockroft method
cocktail
　　GI c.
　　lytic c.
CO$_2$-CO$_2$ abundance ratio

^{13}C-octanoic acid gastric emptying breath test
coculture system
CODAS software
code
    genetic c.
Coding Symbols for a Thesaurus of Adverse Reaction Terms (COSTART)
codon
    premature stop c.
coefficient
    glomerular ultrafiltration c.
    mass transfer area c. (MTAC)
    prostatic pressure c. (PPC)
    sieving c. (SC)
    ultrafiltration c.
    c. of variation
coeliac disease
coelioscopy
coenzyme (Co)
coenzyme A (CoA)
coeundi
    impotentia c.
coffee-ground
    c.-g. emesis
    c.-g. material (CGM)
    c.-g. vomitus
Coffey
    C. technique
    C. ureterointestinal anastomosis
Cogentin
cognition
cognitive function
Cohen
    C. antireflux procedure
    C. cross-trigonal reimplantation
    C. cross-trigonal technique
    C. syndrome
    C. test
    C. ureteroneocystostomy
coherent
    c. bundle
    C. model 90-K laser
cohosh
    black c.
coil
    c. catheter
    coiled c.
    endoanal c.
    endoesophageal MRI c.
    endoprostatic c.
    endorectal-pelvic phased-array c.

Gianturco c.
helical c.
Helmholtz double-surface c.
interlocking detachable c.'s
intraurethral c.
MRCP using HASTE with a phased array c.
pelvic phased-array c. (PPA)
secretory c.
spring-wire c.
c. stent
Stylet internal esophageal MRI c.
Coil-Cath catheter
coiled
    c. coil
    c. coil motif
    c. spring sign
coiled-spring appearance
coincubation
    sperm immunobead c.
coinfection
coit
COL4A3 **gene**
COL4A4 **gene**
COL4A5 **gene**
Colace
Colapinto needle
Colaris molecular diagnostic test
Colax-C
Colazal
Colazide
colchicine
cold
    c. biopsy forceps
    c. cup biopsy
    c. cup resection
    c. defect
    c. flushing
    c. forceps ablation
    c. ischemia time (CIT)
    c. knife
    c. knife endoureterotomy
    c. knife hook
    c. knife incision
    c. scissors
    c. snare ablation
    c. snare excision
    C. Spor disinfectant
    c. spot
    c. storage
    c. stress test

C

NOTES

Cole
    C. duodenal retractor
    C. sign
colectasia
colectomy
    abdominal c.
    blind subtotal c.
    laparoscopic c.
    segmental c.
    subtotal c.
    total abdominal c. (TAC)
    transverse c.
    c. ulcerative colitis
coleoptosis
Colestid
colestipol hydrochloride
Coley toxin
coli
    adenomatous polyposis c. (APC)
    aquatosis c.
    attenuated adenomatous polyposis c.
    Campylobacter c.
    enteroadherent *Escherichia c.*
      (EAEC)
    enteroaggregative *Escherichia c.*
      (EaggEC)
    enterohemorrhagic *Escherichia c.*
      (EHEC)
    enteroinvasive *Escherichia c.*
      (EIEC)
    enteropathogenic *Escherichia c.*
      (EPEC)
    enterotoxigenic *Escherichia c.*
      (ETEC)
    Escherichia c.
    familial adenomatous polyposis c.
    familial polyposis c. (FPC)
    flexura lienalis c.
    haustra c.
    juvenile polyposis c.
    labium inferius valvulae c.
    labium superius valvulae c.
    melanosis c.
    nonpathogenic *Escherichia c.*
    pneumatosis c.
    pneumatosis cystoides c. (PCC)
    polyposis c.
    Shiga toxin-producing
      Escherichia c. (STEC)
    tenia c.
colibacillosis
colic
    acute ureteric c.
    appendicular c.
    c. artery
    biliary c. (BC)
    bilious c.

    copper c.
    crapulent c.
    Devonshire c.
    endemic c.
    episodic c.
    esophageal c.
    flatulent c.
    gallstone c.
    gastric c.
    hepatic c.
    c. impression
    c. impression on the liver
    infantile c.
    intestinal c.
    lead c.
    mucous c.
    multiple recurrent renal c.
    c. myoneurosis
    c. omentum
    painter's c.
    pancreatic c.
    c. patch
    c. patch esophagoplasty
    pseudoesophageal c.
    pseudomembranous c.
    renal c.
    saburral c.
    c. sacculation
    saturnine c.
    stercoral c.
    ureteral c.
    uterine c.
    vermicular c.
    verminous c.
    wind c.
    worm c.
    zinc c.
colica
colicky abdominal pain
colicoplegia
colicystopyelitis
coliform
    c. bacillus
    c. bacterium
    c. urinary infection
colipase
colipase-dependent lipase
coliplication
colipuncture
Colirest
colistimethate
colistin
colitic
    c. arthritis
    c. mucosa
colitis, pl. **colitides**
    acute infectious c.

acute self-limited c. (ASLC)
adaptic c.
adenovirus c.
allergic c.
amebic c.
antibiotic-associated c. (AAC)
antibiotic-associated
    pseudomembranous c. (AAPC,
    AAPMC)
bacterial c.
balantidial c.
Balantidium coli c.
Behçet c.
Campylobacter fetus c.
cathartic c.
caustic c.
chronic ulcerative c. (CUC)
CMV c.
    cytomegalovirus colitis
colectomy ulcerative c.
collagenous c.
Crohn c.
c. cystica profunda (CCP)
c. cystica superficialis
cytomegalovirus c. (CMV colitis)
diabetic c.
distal c.
diversion c.
drug-induced c.
eosinophilic c.
familial ulcerative c.
focal c.
fulminant toxic c.
fulminating ulcerative c.
gangrenous ischemic c.
granulomatous transmural c.
c. gravis
hemorrhagic c.
iatrogenic c.
idiopathic c.
indeterminate c. (IC)
infectious c.
inflammatory c.
intractable ulcerative c.
ischemic c.
left-sided c.
lymphocytic c.
microscopic c.
milk-sensitive c.
mucosal ulcerative c. (MUC)
mucous c.
myxomembranous c.

necrotic hemorrhagic c.
neutropenic c.
nonantibiotic c.
nonspecific c.
pantothenic acid deficiency-
    induced c.
patchy c.
c. perineal complication
peroxynitrite-induced c.
c. polyposa
progesterone-associated c.
pseudomembranous c. (PMC)
radiation-induced c.
regional c.
Salmonella c.
segmental ischemic c.
sexually transmitted c.
Shigella c.
single-stripe c. (SSC)
toxic c.
transmural c.
tuberculous c.
ulcerative c. (UC)
uremic c.
viral c.
Yersinia enterocolitica c.
colla (*pl. of* collum)
Collaborative Transplant Study (CTS)
collagen
    alpha-2-beta-1 integrin cell-
        surface c.
    bovine dermal c.
    Contigen glutaraldehyde cross-
        linked c.
    c. deposition
    glutaraldehyde cross-linked c.
        (GAX)
    c. injection
    c. maturation
    c. synthesis
    c. synthesis inhibitor
    c. types I–XIII
    c. vascular disease
collagenase
    interstitial c.
collagenofibrotic glomerulopathy
collagenous
    c. colitis
    c. sprue
collapse
    parenchymal c.
collapsed ileum

NOTES

collapsible tube hydrodynamics
collapsing
    c. FSGS
    c. glomerulopathy
collar
    Cobb c.
    polyglycolic acid c.
    preputial c.
    ulcer c.
collar-button
    c.-b. appearance in colon
    c.-b. ulceration
collar-button-like ulcer
collateral
    c. abdominal circulation
    portal azygous c.
    vasodilation of portasystemic c.
collecting
    c. duct (CD)
    c. duct carcinoma
    c. system
    c. tube
    c. tubule
    c. venule
collection
    American type culture c.
    blood c.
    duodenal fluid c.
    encysted intraabdominal c.
    fluid c.
    24-hour urine c.
    pancreatic fluid c. (PFC)
    perinephric fluid c.
    peripancreatic fluid c.
    pus c.
    quantitative stool c.
    semen c.
collector
    Grass force displacement fluid c.
    Misstique female external
      urinary c.
Colles fascia
colli
    cystitis c.
colliculectomy
colliculitis
colliculus, pl. **colliculi**
    bulbar c.
    seminal c.
    c. seminalis
collimator
    high-sensitivity c.
Collin
    C. abdominal retractor
    C. intestinal forceps
    C. intestinal retractor
    C. knife
    C. mesher

    C. tissue forceps
    C. tongue forceps
Collin-Duval intestinal thumb forceps
Collings
    C. electrode
    C. electrosurgery knife
Collins
    C. indigo carmine solution
    C. intracellular electrolyte solution
    C. umbilical clamp
colliquative
    c. diarrhea
    c. necrosis
    c. proteinuria
Collis
    C. antireflux operation
    C. gastroplasty
    C. repair
collision block
Collis-Nissen
    C.-N. fundoplication
    C.-N. gastroplasty
colloid
    c. osmotic pressure
    c. shift on liver-spleen scan
    c. solution
    sulfur c. (SC)
    ^{99m}Tc albumin c.
    Tc-sulfur c.
    ^{99m}Tc tin c.
    technetium-99m sulfur c. (^{99m}Tc-SC)
    technetium-99m tin c.
colloidal
    c. bismuth subcitrate (CBS)
    c. bismuth suspension
    c. oatmeal
    c. thorium
colloid-producing adenocarcinoma
collum, pl. **colla**
    c. glandis
    c. glandis penis
    c. vesicae biliaris
    c. vesicae felleae
Colly-Seal wafer-type skin barrier
coloanal anastomosis (CAA)
coloboma, heart disease, atresia
    choanae, retarded growth, genital
    hypoplasia, and ear abnormalities
    (CHARGE)
colobronchial fistula
colocalization
colocalized
ColoCARE fecal occult blood test
colocecostomy
colocentesis
colocholecystic fistula
colocholecystostomy
coloclysis

colocolic intussusception
COLO 320 colon cancer cell
colocolonic
    c. anastomosis
    c. fistula
colocolostomy
colocolponeopoiesis
Colocort
colocutaneous fistula
colocystoplasty
    seromuscular c.
colodyspepsia
coloenteric fistula
coloenteritis
colofixation
cologastrocutaneous fistula
Cologel
colography
    computed tomography c.
    CT c.
    magnetic resonance c.
colohepatopexy
coloileal fistula
cololysis
colometrometer
colon
    aganglionic segment of c.
    anterior band of c.
    antral diverticulum of the c.
      (ADC)
    c. ascendens
    ascending c.
    c. cancer
    c. cancer resection
    c. cancer screening
    c. carcinoma
    cathartic c.
    c. cauterization
    closed c.
    cobblestoning of c.
    collar-button appearance in c.
    coned-down appearance of c.
    Crohn disease of c. (CDC)
    c. cutoff sign
    c. descendens
    descending c. (DC)
    distal c.
    diverticula of c.
    endometriosis of c.
    fascia of c.
    foreshortening of the c.
    frenum of valve of c.

gangrenous c.
giant c.
haustra of c.
hepatic flexure of c.
hypoganglionosis of c.
iliac c.
c. impression
c. incarceration
institutional c.
inverted diverticulum of the c.
irritable c. (IC)
knuckle of c.
lateral reflection of c.
c. lavage cytology
lead-pipe c.
left c.
longitudinal band of c.
longitudinal fasciculi of c.
loop of redundant c.
c. medial reflection
mesenteric attachments of c.
mesosigmoid c.
midsigmoid c.
c. motility catheter
pelvic c.
perforation of c.
perisigmoid c.
c. procedure
rectosigmoid c.
right c.
saccular c.
sacculation of c.
c. schistosomiasis
sigmoid c.
c. sigmoideum
c. single-stripe sign
spastic c.
spiculation on c.
spike burst on electromyogram
  of c.
c. splenic flexure
thrifty c.
toxic dilation of c.
c. transit marker study
transverse c.
c. transversum
c. tumor cell lysis
unstable c.
c. urinary conduit
valve of c.
varix of c.
volvulus of c.

C

NOTES

colonalgia
colonic
c. adenocarcinoma
c. adenoma
c. arterial spider
c. bacterium
c. biopsy
c. circular muscle
40-kDa c. antigen
c. dilation
c. distention
c. diverticulosis
c. diverticulum
c. duplication
c. electromyogram
c. epithelial proliferation
c. explosion
c. fistula
c. flora
c. food
c. foreign body
c. gas
c. hamartoma
c. hemorrhage
c. hyperalgesia
c. ileus
c. inertia
c. infiltration
c. insufflation
c. interposition
c. ischemia
c. J-pouch
c. J-pouch reservoir
c. lavage
c. lavage solution
c. leiomyoma
c. lesion identification
c. lipoma
c. loop
c. lymphoid nodule
c. mass
c. metastasis
c. microflora
c. motility
c. mucosal line
c. mucosal pattern
c. mucosal surface
c. myenteric plexus
c. necrosis
c. neoplasia
c. nodular lymphoid hyperplasia
c. obstruction
c. obstruction technique
c. patch
c. perforation
c. permeability
c. pit
c. pitting

c. polyp
c. polyposis
c. polyposis syndrome
c. pouch
c. propulsion
c. prostaglandin
c. pseudoobstruction
c. pseudo-obstruction syndrome
c. purge preparation
c. schistosomiasis
c. solitary ulcer syndrome
c. stent
c. tattoo
c. transabdominal sonography (CTAS)
c. transit study
c. transit test
c. transit time
c. trauma
c. tuberculosis
c. ulcer
c. varix
c. vascular lesion
c. villus
c. volvulus
c. wall
colonization
gut c.
intestinal c.
jejunal c.
stool c.
Colonlite bowel preparation
colonofiberscope
Olympus CG-P-series c.
colonography
CT c.
endoluminal CT c.
magnetic resonance c. (MRC)
colonopathy
colonorrhagia
colonorrhea
colonoscope
ACMI fiberoptic c.
CF-HM magnifying c.
CF-LB3R c.
CF-UHM c.
CF-200Z Olympus c.
double-channel c.
FCS-ML II c.
fiberoptic c.
forward-viewing video c.
Fujinon EC7-CM2 video c.
Fujinon EC-130LT c.
Fujinon EC-200LT c.
Fujinon EC-410MP c.
Fujinon EC-300MS c.
Fujinon EVC-M video c.
Fujinon FE-100LR c.

Innoflex variable stiffness c.
Machida FCS-ML II magnifying c.
magnifying c.
Olympus CF-HM-series
  magnifying c.
Olympus CF-MB/LB c.
Olympus CF-MB-M c.
Olympus CF-MB-series c.
Olympus CF-PL-series c.
Olympus CF-P20S fiberoptic c.
Olympus CF-TL-series forward-
  viewing video c.
Olympus CF-1T100L video c.
Olympus CF-T-series c.
Olympus CF-TVL-series c.
Olympus CF-UHM-series c.
Olympus CF-UM3 c.
Olympus CF-VL-series c.
Olympus CF-200Z c.
Olympus CV-series c.
Olympus EVIS video c.
Olympus PCF-series pediatric c.
Olympus SIF-M magnifying c.
PCF-140L pediatric c.
pediatric c.
Pentax FC-series c.
Pentax VSB-P2900 pediatric c.
single-channel c.
standard c.
Toshiba TCE-M-series c.
video c.
Welch Allyn video c. 8451
colonoscopic
  c. appendectomy
  c. biopsy
  c. decompression
  c. diagnosis
  c. disimpaction
  c. endoluminal ultrasound
  c. polypectomy
  c. removal
  c. sclerotherapy
  c. tattoo
colonoscopist
colonoscopy
  cecal c.
  c. complication
  diagnostic c.
  emergency c.
  high-magnification c.
  magnifying c.
  pediatric c.

c. screening
splenic flexure c.
surveillance c.
tandem c. (TC)
c. technique with an external
  straightener
therapeutic c.
total c.
upper endoscopy and c.
Virtual Vision audiovisual system
  for EGD and c.
colonoscopy-induced hyponatremic
  encephalopathy
colonoscopy-related
  c.-r. emphysema
  c.-r. incarceration
colonostomy
colony count
colony-forming unit (CFU)
colony-stimulating
  c.-s. factor (CSF)
  c.-s. factor-1 (CSF-1)
colopathy
coloperineal fistula
colopexia
colopexostomy
colopexotomy
colopexy
Coloplast
  C. bag
  C. closed pouch
  C. conseal plug
  C. drainable pouch
  C. flange mini cap
  C. flange pouch
  C. irrigation faceplate
  C. irrigation kit
  C. mini pouch
  C. ostomy belt
  C. ostomy irrigation set
  C. skin barrier
  C. skin barrier paste
  C. skin barrier ring
  C. stoma cap
  C. stoma cone
  C. transparent irrigation sleeve
coloplasty pouch
coloplication
coloproctectomy
coloproctia
coloproctitis
coloproctology

C

NOTES

153

coloproctostomy
coloptosis, coloptosia
colopuncture
color
    c. Doppler imaging of ureteral jet into bladder
    c. Doppler ultrasonography
    c. flow Doppler
    c. flow Doppler imaging
    c. flow imaging
    stool c.
    urinalysis c.
    urine c.
color-coded
    c.-c. Doppler sonography
    c.-c. duplex sonography
colorectal
    c. adenocarcinoma
    c. anastomosis
    c. biopsy
    c. cancer (CRC)
    c. cancer screening
    c. cancer syndrome
    c. carcinogenesis
    c. carcinoma (CRC)
    c. disease
    c. endoluminal ultrasound
    c. endometriosis
    c. lymphoma
    c. mass
    c. motility
    c. mucosa
    c. neoplasm
    c. physiologic dysfunction
    c. physiologic study
    c. polyp
    c. resection
    c. snare
    c. stricture
    c. surgery (CRS)
    c. trauma
    c. tumor
    c. tumorigenesis
    c. ulcer
    c. variceal bleeding
    c. villous adenoma
colorectostomy
colorectum
colorimetric detection
Colormate TLc BiliTest System
colorrhagia
colorrhaphy
colorrhea
coloscope
    fiberoptic c.
coloscopy

Coloscreen
    C. Self-test
    C. VPI
Coloshield
colosigmoidostomy
colosigmoid resection
colostomy
    c. bag
    c. bridge
    continent c.
    decompression c.
    descending loop c.
    Devine c.
    diverting loop c.
    divided-stoma c.
    double-barrel c.
    dry c.
    end c.
    end-loop c.
    end-sigmoid c.
    end-to-side ileotransverse c.
    exteriorization c.
    Hartmann c.
    ileoascending c.
    ileosigmoid c.
    ileotransverse c.
    irrigation of c.
    longitudinal c.
    loop transverse c.
    Mikulicz c.
    nonirrigating descending c.
    permanent end c.
    c. pyloric autotransplantation
    resective c.
    c. rod
    sigmoid-end c.
    sigmoid-loop rod c.
    c. soiling
    takedown of c.
    temporary end c.
    terminal c.
    transverse c.
    transverse-loop rod c.
    Turnbull c.
    Wangensteen c.
    wet c.
colosuspension
    Stamey c.
colotomy
    Allingham c.
coloureteral fistula
Colour-Quad-System imaging system
colouterine fistula
colovaginal fistula
colovenous fistula
colovesical fistula
colpocleisis
    Latzko partial c.

colpocystocele
colpocystotomy
colpocystoureterotomy
colpocystourethropexy (CCUP)
colpogram
colpoperineoplasty
colporectopexy
colporrhaphy
colposuspension
    Burch retropubic c.
    laparoscopic needle c.
    laparoscopic retropubic c.
colpoureterotomy
column
    anal c.
    butyl-silane extraction c.
    c. chromatography
    C18 Sep-Pack c.
    hemicrypt c.
    c. of Morgagni
    rectal c.
    Sepharose 4B-coupled-protein-A c.
    variceal c.
columna, pl. columnae
    columnae anales
    columnae rectales
    columnae renales
columnar
    c. cuff
    c. cuff cancer
    c. epithelium
    c. metaplasia
    c. mucosa
columnar-cuboidal adenocarcinoma cell
columnar-lined esophagus (CLE)
Coly-Mycin M, S
colypeptic
CoLyte bowel preparation
coma
    acute hepatic c.
    ammoniagenic c.
    electrolyte imbalance c.
    hepatic c.
comatose
CombiDERM non-adhesive absorbant
  dressing
Combidex
combination
    c. biliary brush catheter
    c. calculus
    prednisone-colchicine c.

combined
    c. androgen blockade (CAB)
    c. chemoradiation therapy
    c. fat- and carbohydrate-induced
      hyperlipidemia
    c. hemorrhoids
    c. hiatal hernia
    c. intracavernous injection and
      stimulation test
    c. kidney and pancreas transplant
      (CKPT)
    c. ureterolysis
comblike redness sign
Combo Cath wire-guided cytology
  brush
comet sign
Comfeel
    C. Purilon
    C. skin adhesive
    C. skin barrier
Comfort Cath I, II catheter
comfrey
Comhaire grading system
co-mitogen
commensal flora
commercial dialysis solution (CDS)
comminution
    stone c.
common
    c. bile duct (CBD)
    c. bile duct compression
    c. bile duct exploration (CBDE)
    c. bile duct microlithiasis (CBDM)
    c. bile duct obstruction
    c. bile duct stent
    c. bile duct stone
    c. bile duct varix
    c. cavity phenomenon
    c. channel
    c. duct (CD)
    c. duct calculus
    c. duct cholangiogram
    c. duct exploration (CDE)
    c. duct sound
    c. duct stone
    c. hepatic artery (CHA)
    c. hepatic duct
    c. iliac artery
    c. iliac vein
    c. penile artery
    c. pH electrode
    c. variable immunodeficiency (CVI)

C

NOTES

communicating hydrocele
communication
    anomalous pancreaticobiliary c.
    cholangiovenous c.
    horseshoe c.
    pseudocyst c.
communis
    arteria hepatica c.
    ductus hepaticus c.
community
    Ashkenazi Jewish c.
comorbid condition
comorbidity
Companion
    C. 2
    C. feeding pump
comparison
    prospective c.
compartment
    infracolic c.
    inframesocolic c.
    posterior pararenal c.
    supracolic c.
Compat
    C. 199205 enteral feeding pump
    C. feeding tube
compatibility
    in vitro c.
Compazine
Compeed Skinprotector dressing
compendium
    urologic drug c.
compensated
    c. cirrhosis
    c. dysphagia for solid food
compensatory testicular hypertrophy
competent
    c. bowel
    c. ileocecal valve
competition
competition-binding assay
competitive protein binding assay
Compleat-B liquid feeding
complement
    c. activation
    C3a c.
    c. fixation test
    c. hemolytic activity
    c. level
    plasma-activated c. 3 (C3a)
    plasma-activated c. 4 (C4a)
    plasma-activated c. 5 (C5a)
    prostate gland C3 c.
    c. receptor type 1 (CR1)
    c. regulatory protein
    total hemolytic c.
complementary
    c. and alternative medicine (CAM)

    c. deoxyribonucleic acid (cDNA)
    c. DNA
complementary, single-stranded, antisense riboprobe
complement-dependent cytotoxicity (CDC)
complement-independent autologous phase
complement-mediated
    c.-m. experimental
      glomerulonephritis
    c.-m. immune glomerular disease
complete
    c. blood count (CBC)
    c. blood count test
    c. bowel obstruction
    c. duplication
    c. hormonal blockage
    c. male epispadias
    c. PEG pull
    c. PEG push
    Pepcid C.
    c. replacement PEG
    c. Savary
    c. surgical exploration (CSE)
    c. ureteral stricture
completion gastrectomy
complex
    adenylate cyclase c.
    AIDS-related c. (ARC)
    anisoylated plasminogen
      streptokinase activator c.
    c. anorectal fistula
    antimajor histocompatibility c.
    avidin-biotin c. (ABC)
    avidin-biotin-peroxidase c.
    calcium-calmodulin c.
    Carman-Kirklin meniscus c.
    Carney c.
    CD3-T cell receptor c.
    c. class II expression
    dorsal vagal c.
    dorsal vein c. (DVC)
    c. enterocele
    epispadias-exstrophy c.
    Eshmun c.
    exstrophy-epispadias c.
    gastroduodenal artery c.
    Golgi c.
    Heymann nephritis antigenic c.
      (HNAC)
    histocompatibility c.
    c. hypospadias
    IGF-BP3 c.
    interdigestive migrating motor c.
    interdigestive myoelectric c.
    lactase-ceramidase c.
    major histocompatibility c. (MHC)

membrane-attack c.
Meyenburg c.
migrating motor c. (MMC)
migrating myoelectric c.
mitochondrial c.
muscle-alginate c.
Mycobacterium avium c.
nephroblastomatosis c. (NBC)
OEIS c.
oligohydramnios c.
oligometric c.
c. papillary infolding
penoscrotal transposition c.
polysaccharide-iron c.
rectal motor c.
refined carbohydrate c.
sling-ring c.
c. stone
streptavidin-biotin peroxidase c.
  (SAB reagent)
T-cell antigen receptor/CD3 c.
thrombin-antithrombin III c.
tuberous sclerosis c. (TSC)
urobilin c.
von Meyenburg c. (VMC)

compliance
bladder c.
c. of bladder
detrusor c.
rectal c.
vesical c.

complication
anastomotic c.
bacterial c.
benign pneumatic colonoscopy c.
bowel preparation c.
cardiopulmonary c.
cardiorespiratory c.
cardiovascular c.
cerebrovascular c.
circumcision c.
colitis perineal c.
colonoscopy c.
endoscopy c.
extraintestinal c.
feeding c.
gastrointestinal c.
hematologic c.
infectious c.
laparoscopy c.
metabolic c.
metastatic c.

neurologic c.
opportunistic c.
postbiopsy vascular c.
postoperative c.
pulmonary c.
renal c.
sclerotherapy c.
significant reported c.
urethral reconstruction c.
vascular access c.

component
Knodell c.
lymphoid c.
secretory c. (SC)
serum amyloid P c.
shock wave lithotripsy cavitation c.
tachykinin c.

composition
adrenal gland c.
urinary c.

Compound-65
Darvon C.-65

compound
bismuth c.
c. cyst
gold c.
guanidino c.
NGD-95-1 antiobesity c.
nitroso c.
tetrapyrrol c.

compressible cavernous body

compression
abdominal c. (AC)
c. anuria
c. button
c. button gastrojejunostomy
celiac axis c.
common bile duct c.
duodenal c.
esophageal c.
extramural common bile duct c.
extrinsic biliary c.
extrinsic pancreatic c.
gastric c.
mechanical variceal c.
renal venous outflow c.
spinal cord c.
c. syndrome
c. ultrasound (CUS)

compressor urethra

compromise
vascular c.

NOTES

Compro suppository
computed
  c. tomographic angiography (CTA)
  c. tomography (CT)
  c. tomography arterial portography
    (CTAP)
  c. tomography colography
  c. tomography during arterial
    portography (CT-AP)
computer-aided
  c.-a. ambulatory gastrojejunal
    manometry
  c.-a. diagnostic system
**computer-controlled sedation infusion
  system**
computer graphic simulation (CGS)
computerization
computerized
  c. dynamic posturography (CDP)
  c. electronic endoscopy
  c. image analysis system
  c. phonoenterography
  c. tomographic hepatic angiography
    (CTHA)
  c. tomography (CT)
Compu-void
comutagenic
Comvax
ConA, con A
  concanavalin A
ConA-anti-con A perfusion
concanavalin A (ConA, con A)
concealed
  c. hemorrhage
  c. hypospadias
  c. penis
  c. umbilical stoma
  c. vomiting
Concentraid Nasal
concentrate
  bile salt c. (BSC)
  Maalox Therapeutic C.
  therapeutic c. (TC)
concentrated urine
concentration
  albumin plasma c.
  aminothiol c.
  amylase c.
  bile phospholipid c. (BPC)
  blood urea c.
  calcium c.
  chloride c.
  dialysate glucose c.
  endothelin-1 c.
  endothelin-3 c.
  c. epidermal growth factor (cEGF)
  expiratory breath ethanol c.
  extrapolated plasma caffeine c.

  fasting plasma caffeine c.
  fluoroquinolone seminal plasma c.
  hyaluronic acid c.
  mean corpuscular hemoglobin c.
    (MCHC)
  millimolar c.
  minimal inhibitory c. (MIC)
  phospholipid-bound choline c.
  plasma caffeine c.
  plasma-free choline c.
  plasma gastrin c.
  plasma norepinephrine c.
  plasma renin c.
  plasma urea c.
  predialysis plasma phosphate c.
  renal vein renin c. (RVRC)
  retinol c.
  semen sperm c.
  serum calcium c.
  sodium butyrate c.
  spermatozoon c.
  testosterone plasma c.
  thyroid hormone serum c.
  timed average urea c. (TACurea)
  total homocysteine plasma c.
  total protein c.
  urine c.
concentric
  c. hyaline inclusion
  c. needle
concentric-needle electrode
concept
  exudate-transudate c.
  Valsalva leak point pressure c.
conceptus dose
concomitant
  c. antireflux surgery
  c. disease
  c. medication effect
concrement
concretion
  bile c.
  fecal c.
  intestinal c.
concurrent hepatic laceration
concussion
  hydraulic abdominal c.
condition
  comorbid c.
  intersex c.
  pathological hypersecretory c.
  physiological c.
  urologic c.
conditioning
  c. film
  interceptive c.
  semantic c.
  c. therapy

condom
    c. catheter
    c. catheter endoscopic ultrasound
    female c.
    c. urinal
conductance
    potassium c.
    urethral electrical c.
conducted current
conduction defect
conductivity
    electrical c.
conduit
    antirefluxing colonic c.
    Bricker ileal c.
    colon urinary c.
    cutaneous appendiceal c.
    ileal urinary c.
    jejunal urinary c.
    Mitrofanoff c.
    nonrefluxing colon c.
    sigmoid c.
    urinary c.
condyloma, pl. **condylomata**
    c. acuminatum
    anal c.
    flat c.
    c. latum
    perianal c.
    pointed c.
condylomatosis
Condylox
cone
    c. biopsy
    Coloplast stoma c.
    hard sonolucent plastic c.
    vaginal c.
coned cecum
coned-down appearance of colon
cone-shaped cecum
cone-tip catheter
confidence
    c. interval (CI)
    c. ring
configuration
    bird-beak c.
    cartwheel c.
    golf-hole c.
    horseshoe c.
    laparoscopy trocar c.
    pouch c.

    rat-tail c.
    W-pouch c.
confluence
confluent
conformal radiation therapy
congenital
    c. adrenal hyperplasia (CAH)
    c. bifid bladder
    c. bilateral absence of the vas deferens (CBAVD)
    c. biliary atresia
    c. biliary cyst
    c. bladder diverticulum
    c. chloride diarrhea
    c. chordee
    c. cloaca
    c. cystic disease
    c. cystosis
    c. diaphragm
    c. diaphragmatic hernia
    c. diverticulosis
    c. double kidney
    c. duodenal atresia
    c. enterocele
    c. enterocyte heparan sulphate deficiency
    c. epispadias
    c. esophageal stenosis
    c. hepatic fibrosis (CHF)
    c. hydrocele
    c. hyperbilirubinemia
    c. hypertrophic pyloric stenosis
    c. hypertrophy of the retinal pigment epithelium (CHRPE)
    c. hypoplasia
    c. intestinal aganglionosis (CIA)
    c. lactic acidosis
    c. malrotation of the gut
    c. megacolon
    c. nephrogenic diabetes insipidus (CNDI)
    c. nephrosis
    c. nephrotic syndrome (CNS)
    c. penile curvature
    c. penile deviation (CPD)
    c. polycystic disease (CPD)
    c. portacaval shunt
    c. pyloric membrane
    c. pylorospasm
    c. renal artery aneurysm
    c. renal mass
    c. sodium diarrhea (CSD)

C

NOTES

congenital *(continued)*
    c. splenic cyst
    c. splenomegaly
    c. ureteral stricture
    c. ureteropelvic junction obstruction
    c. urethral stricture
    c. urethroperineal fistula
    c. urethrorectal fistula
    c. urologic abnormality
    c. uropathy
congenitally altered anatomy
congenitum
    megacolon c.
congested
    c. kidney
    c. mucosa
congestion
    active c.
    hepatic c.
    passive c.
    renal c.
congestive
    c. cirrhosis
    c. heart failure
    c. hepatomegaly
    c. hypertensive gastropathy
    c. splenomegaly
Congo
    C. red dye
    C. red stain
congolense
    Trypanosoma c.
congophilic material
conical
    c. catheter
    c. cecum
    c. centrifuge tube
    c. glans
    c. trocar
conical-tip electrode
conjoined
    c. fiber bundle
    c. tendon
conjugate
    bilirubin ester c.
    bilirubin protein c.
    goat antirabbit HRP c.
    xenobiotic glutathione c.
conjugated
    c. bile acid
    c. bilirubin
    c. estrogen (CE)
    c. hyperbilirubinemia
conjunctival
    c. erythema
    c. icterus
connecting tubule

connective
    c. tissue
    c. tissue disease
    c. tissue disorder
connector
    Luer-Lok c.
    T c.
    Tuohy-Borst c.
    wire loop c.
    Y-port c.
Connell
    C. incision
    C. stitch
    C. suture
connexin 43
conniventes
    valvulae c.
Conn syndrome
conorii
    Rickettsia c.
Conradi line
Conray
    C. 60, 70 contrast material
    C. 280 contrast medium
conscious sedation
Conseal
    C. one-piece continent colostomy system
    C. ostomy irrigation set
consensual reflex
consensus interferon (CIFN)
conserved helix-loop-helix ubiquitous kinase (CHUK)
consistency
    doughy c.
consortial approach
consortium
    Pediatric Peritoneal Dialysis Study c.
constant
    c. infusion excretory urogram (CIXU)
    Michaelis c. (Km)
Constene
constipation
    antepartum c.
    atonic c.
    chronic functional c.
    chronic idiopathic c.
    drug-induced c.
    functional c.
    gastrojejunal c.
    geriatric c.
    idiopathic c.
    intractable c.
    outlet obstruction c.
    postpartum c.

c. predominant irritable bowel
    syndrome
psychogenic c.
slow transit c. (STC)
spastic c.

constipation-predominant irritable bowel syndrome
constitutional
c. hepatic dysfunction
c. hyperbilirubinemia

constricting pain
constriction
mesenteric artery c.
c. ring

constrictive pericarditis
construction
ileal reservoir c.
Lich ureteral implantation for
    neobladder c.
neovagina c.
pelvic ileal reservoir c.
phallic c.
sphincteric c.
U-pouch c.
vaginal c.

constructional apraxia
consumption
alcohol c.
EtOH c.
salt c.
whole-cell oxygen c.

contact
c. bleeding
cell-cell c.
c. dermatitis
c. dissolution
C. Laser vaporization
c. laser vaporization of the
    prostate (CLVP)
c. laxative
c. lithotripsy
c. probe

contact-tip laser system
contagiosum
giant molluscum c.
molluscum c.

container
Safe-T-Flex enteral feeding c.

contamination
fecal c.
c. of food

postautoclave c.
c. of water

content
abdominal c.
bowel c.
gastric c.
hepatic malondialdehyde c.
intestinal c.
luminal c.
mucosal hexosamine c.
renal cortical malondialdehyde c.
reticulocyte hemoglobin c.
total glutathione c.

contexture analysis
Contigen
C. Bard collagen implant
C. glutaraldehyde cross-linked
    collagen

contiguity
appendicitis by c.

contiguous loop
Contimed II pelvic floor muscle monitor
continence
diurnal c.
fecal c.
c. nipple
c. ring
urinary c.

continence-preserving resection
continent
c. abdominal wall stoma
c. anal cap (CAP)
c. catheterizable urinary diversion
c. colostomy
c. cutaneous appendicocystostomy
c. cutaneous diversion
c. cutaneous reservoir
c. ileal reservoir
c. ileal reservoir catheterization
    pouch
c. ileostomy
c. of stool
c. supravesical bowel urinary
    diversion
c. valve

continuity
bowel c.
small bowel c.
urinary c.

continuous
c. ambulatory infusion

NOTES

continuous *(continued)*
    c. ambulatory peritoneal
    c. ambulatory peritoneal dialysis (CAPD)
    c. arteriovenous hemodiafiltration (CAVHDF)
    c. arteriovenous hemodialysis (CAVHD)
    c. arteriovenous hemofiltration (CAVH)
    c. arteriovenous hemofiltration with dialysis
    c. arteriovenous ultrafiltration (CAVU)
    c. bladder drainage
    c. bladder irrigation (CBI)
    c. catheter drainage
    c. cycler-assisted peritoneal dialysis
    c. cycling peritoneal dialysis (CCPD)
    c. drip feeding
    c. hypothermic pulsatile perfusion
    c. incontinence
    c. infusion chemotherapy
    c. murmur
    c. NG suction
    c. prophylaxis
    c. pull-through technique
    c. renal replacement therapy (CRRT)
    c. suction drainage
    c. suture
    c. venovenous hemodiafiltration (CVVHDF)
    c. venovenous hemodialysis (CVVHD)
    c. venovenous hemofiltration (CVVH)
continuous-flow resectoscope
continuously perfused probe
ContiRing
contour
    c. ERCP cannula
    isodose c.
    sawtooth irregularity of bowel c.
contraception
contraceptive
    c. device
    c. pill-induced cholestasia
contractile
    c. apparatus
    c. ring dysphagia
    c. stricture
contractility
    normal detrusor c.
    ureter c.

contraction
    alcohol-induced extracellular volume c.
    anal sphincter c.
    bladder involuntary c.
    clonic c.
    crural c.
    detrusor c.
    fat-induced gallbladder c.
    gallbladder c.
    giant migrating c. (GMC)
    high-amplitude c. (HAPC)
    isotonic c.
    paradoxical puborectalis c.
    peristaltic c.
    phase II c.
    phasic c.
    primary c.
    propagated antroduodenal c.
    propagation of c.
    reflex detrusor c.
    ringlike c.
    secondary c.
    sliding filament model of c.
    slow phasic c.
    tertiary c.
    tonic c.
    voluntary sphincter c.
contraction-relaxation cycle
Contractubex gel
contracture
    bladder neck c.
    Dupuytren c.
    postinflammatory c.
contraindication
    c. to circumcision
    laparoscopy c.
Contrajet ERCP contrast delivery system
contralateral
    c. reflux
    c. testicular biopsy
contrast
    c. agent
    barium enema with air c.
    c. chromoscopy using indigo carmine (CCIC)
    Cysto Conray c.
    dilute iodinated c.
    double c.
    c. enema
    c. enhancement
    c. esophagography
    c. esophagram
    c. filling
    c. fluid
    c. medium
    c. selective cholangiogram

Solutrast 300 c.
water-soluble c.
contrast-associated renal failure
contrast-enhanced
  c.-e. computed tomography
  c.-e. endoscopic ultrasonography
    (CE-EUS)
  c.-e. fast sequence (CE-FAST)
contrast-induced renal failure
control
  androgen gonadotropin feedback c.
  beta-2 microglobulin c.
  bleeding c.
  c. bridle
  endoscopic c.
  EPC pain c.
  fluoroscopic c.
  foot pedal suction c.
  hemorrhage c.
  neural c.
  pain c.
  symptom c.
controlled
  c. expansion (CX)
  c. radial expansion (CRE)
controller
  Actis venous flow c. (VFC)
conus medullaris
ConvaTec
  C. Active Life stoma cap
  C. colostomy pouch
  C. Durahesive Wafer ostomy
  C. Little One Sur-Fit pouch
  C. Sur-Fit two-piece pouch
convection
convective transport
conventional
  c. concentric electromyography
  c. hemodialysis
  c. static scanner
  c. stent
Converspaz
convertase
  C3 c.
converter
  sequential video c.
Converzyme
convexity
convex margin
ConXn
COOH-terminal SH2 domain

Cook
  C. biopsy gun
  18F C. Enforcer
  3.2F C. N-Circle tipless stone
    basket
  C. plastic Luer lock adapter
  C. rectal speculum
  C. stent
  C. tissue morcellator
  C. TPN catheter
  C. urological trocar
Cooke-Apert-Gallais syndrome
coolant
cooled
  c. antenna zone
  c. catheter transurethral microwave
    thermotherapy
  c. catheter TUMT
cooler
  Eissner prostatic c.
cooling
  external c.
  homogenous c.
  ice c.
  immersion c.
  nerve c.
  perfusion c.
  surface c.
  transarterial perfusion c.
  urethral c.
  whole-body c.
cool temperature hemodialysis
Coomassie brilliant blue technique
Coombs test
Coons/Carey endoprosthesis
Coons guide
Cooper
  C. hernia
  C. herniotome
  C. irritable testis
  C. ligament
  C. ligament hernioplasty
  C. ligament sling
cooperi
  fascia propria c.
coordination
  R-wave c.
COPD
  chronic obstructive pulmonary disease
cope
  C. crushing clamp
  C. loop nephrostomy catheter

NOTES

cope *(continued)*
 C. loop nephrostomy tube
 C. modification of a Martel
  intestinal clamp
 C. sign
 C. viscerotomy anchor
 C. wire
copious irrigation
copolymerized substrate
copper
 c. colic
 c. deficiency
 c. nephropathy
copper-binding
 c.-b. protein (CBP)
 c.-b. protein test
copper-deficiency anemia
copracrasia
copremesis
coprolith
coproma
coproplanesia
coproporphyria
 erythropoietic c.
 hereditary c. (HCP)
 variegate c.
coproporphyrin
coprostasis
coracidium
coral calculus
Corbus disease
cord
 Billroth c.
 c. bladder
 genital c.
 gubernacular c.
 hepatic c.
 hepatocytic c.
 c. hydrocele
 inguinal c.
 lipoma of c.
 microsurgical denervation of the
  spermatic c.
 nephrogenic c.
 palpable c.
 spermatic c.
 c. structure
 tethered spinal c.
 tunic of spermatic c.
 umbilical c.
 vocal c.
Cordis-Hakim shunt
corditis
Cordonnier
 C. technique ureterocolonic
  anastomosis
 C. ureteroileal loop

cordotomy
core
 chylomicron c.
 c. needle biopsy
 c. temperature
 c. of tumor
core-cut system
core-through optical urethrotomy
Corgard
Cori
 C. cycle
 C. disease
coring
 c. out
 uterine c.
coring-out procedure
corkscrew
 c. appearance
 c. esophagus
Corlopam
corneae
 Vittaforma c.
corneal
 c. foreign body
 c. reflex
 c. ulcer
Cornelia de Lange syndrome
corner
 c. suture
 C. tampon
cornflake esophageal motility test
cornstarch-rich diet
cornucopia
 sinusoidal endothelium c.
corona, pl. **coronae**
 c. glandis penis
 papillomatosis coronae
coronal
 c. adhesion
 c. epispadias
 c. hypospadias
 c. radiata
 c. sulcus
coronary
 c. artery disease
 c. azygos
 cafe c.
 c. ligament
 c. sinus
Coronavirus **gastroenteritis**
Corpak
 C. feeding tube
 C. weighted-tip, self-lubricating
  tube
corpora (*pl. of* corpus)
corpora cavernosa, sing. **corpus**
 cavernosum

corporal
 c. biopsy
 c. plication procedure
corporeal
 c. aspiration
 c. fibrosis
 Nesbit c.
 c. reconstruction
 c. rotation procedure
 c. sinusoid
 c. venous occlusive dysfunction
corporoplasty
 incisional c.
 modified Essed-Schroeder c.
corporotomy
corpus, pl. **corpora**
 corpora amylacea
 c. callosum agenesis
 c. cavernosum biopsy
 corpora cavernosum dilation
 c. cavernosum muscarinic receptor
 c. cavernosum papaverine injection
 c. cavernosum penile
  electromyography
 c. cavernosum tunica covering
 c. epididymidis
 c. epididymis
 c. gastric mucosa
 c. gastricum
 c. gastritis
 c. Highmore
 Highmore c.
 c. pancreatis
 c. spongiosum
 c. spongiosum fibrosis
 c. spongiosum hypoplasia
 c. spongiosum penis
 c. ventriculare
 c. ventriculi
 c. vesicae biliaris
 c. vesicae felleae
 c. wolffi
corpus cavernosum (*sing. of* corpora
 cavernosa)
corpuscle
 Jaworski c.
 juxtamedullary renal c.
 malpighian c.
 pacinian c.
 renal c.
Correa classification

correction
 chordee c.
 Yates c.
Correctol
correlation
 Pearson-product c.
 Spearman rank c.
Corrigan pulse
corrosive
 c. esophageal stricture
 c. esophagitis
 c. gastritis
Corson
 C. needle
 C. needle electrosurgical probe
Cortef
Cortenema retention enema
cortex, pl. **cortices**
 aberrant suprarenal c.
 adrenal c.
 fetal adrenal c.
 c. glandulae suprarenalis
 kidney c.
 renal c.
cortiadrenal
Corticaine
cortical
 c. abscess
 c. adenoma
 c. arch
 c. collecting duct (CCD)
 c. collecting tubule
 c. interstitial volume fraction
 c. labyrinth
 c. loss
cortices (*pl. of* cortex)
corticoadenoma
 adrenal c.
corticoadrenal
 renal c.
corticomedullary
 c. demarcation
 c. differentiation
corticosteroid
 c. therapy
 c. treatment
corticotropin
corticotropin-releasing hormone (CRH)
Cortifoam
cortisol
 c. hypersecretion
 c. metabolism

C

NOTES

cortisol (*continued*)
    plasma c.
    urinary c.
cortisone acetate
Cortisporin
Cortrophin-Zinc
Cortrosyn stimulation test
corymbifera
    Absidia c.
    Mucor c.
Corynebacterium
    C. minutissimum
    C. parvum
    C. tenuis
cosine curve
cosinor analysis
Cosmegen
cosmesis
costal margin
COSTART
    Coding Symbols for a Thesaurus of
    Adverse Reaction Terms
    COSTART system
cost-effectiveness analysis
Costello
    C. laser ablation of prostate
    C. protocol
costive
costiveness
costochondral
    c. junction
    c. tenderness
costocolic fold
costophrenic blunting
costovertebral
    c. angle tenderness (CVAT)
    c. ligament
    c. sulcus
cosyntropin stimulation test
Cotazym
    C.-S
cotransporter
    c. mRNA
    NA+-glucose c.
    taurine c. (TCT)
Cotrim
co-trimoxazole
cotton
    C. cannulatome
    C. classification
    Oxycel c.
    C. sphincterotome
    c. suture
    c. swab test
Cotton-Huibregtse double pigtail stent
Cotton-Leung biliary stent
cottonseed oil

cotton-tipped applier
cotton-wool spot (CWS)
coudé catheter
cough stress test
Couinaud classification
Coumadin
coumarin
    c. dye laser
    c. green tunable dye laser
    lithotripsy
coumarin-flashlamp-pumped pulsed dye laser
coumestrol
Councill catheter
Councilman
    C. body
    C. lesion
Council tip tube
count
    CD4 lymphocyte c.
    CD8 lymphocyte c.
    CD4+ T-cell c.
    cell c.
    colony c.
    complete blood c. (CBC)
    granulocyte c.
    hemolysis, elevated liver enzymes,
    and low platelet c. (HELLP)
    instrument c.
    lymphocyte c.
    mitosis c.
    needle c.
    peripheral leukocyte c.
    c. per minute (cpm, CPM)
    platelet c.
    red blood cell c.
    sponge c.
    too numerous to c. (TNTC)
    white blood cell c.
    whole crypt mitotic c.
counter
    LKB-Wallac scintillation c.
    RackBeta scintillation c.
countercurrent
    c. exchange
    c. mechanism
    c. multiplication
    c. multiplier
    c. multiplier principle
counterirritation
countertransporter
    sodium-lithium c. (SLC)
coup de sabre
coupling
    capacitive c.
    electromechanical c.
    excitation-contraction c.

pharmacomechanical c.
c. stoichiometry
Courtney
deep postanal space of C.
C. space
Courvoisier
C. gallbladder
C. gastroenterostomy
C. law
C. sign
Courvoisier-Terrier syndrome
couvade syndrome
Couvelaire ileourethral anastomosis
cover
Foxy Pouch c.
laparotomy pad c.
Nu-Hope pouch c.
pad c.
Sur-Fit Pouch c.
covered
c. biliary metal stent
c. self-expanding prosthesis
covering
Camwrap plastic c.
corpus cavernosum tunica c.
Permalume c.
Cowan 1 strain
Cowden
C. disease
C. syndrome
Cowdry type A inclusion body
Cowen
C. disease
C. syndrome
Cowper
C. cyst
C. gland
C. syringocele
cow's
c. milk allergy (CMA)
c. milk protein allergy
c. milk-sensitive enteropathy
(CMSE)
COX
cyclooxygenase
COX enzyme system
COX mRNA
COX-1
cyclooxygenase-1
COX-1 enzyme
COX-1 inhibition

COX-2
cyclooxygenase-2
COX-2 enzyme
COX-2 inhibition
COX-2 inhibitor
COX-2-selective nonsteroidal antiinflammatory drug
Coxiella burnetii
Cox-Mantel test
Cox regression model
coxsackievirus infection (A, B)
CP
chronic pancreatitis
chronic pyelonephritis
CP test
CPA
cyproterone acetate
CPC
choroid plexus cyst
CPD
congenital penile deviation
congenital polycystic disease
CP-EUS
catheter probe-assisted endoluminal
ultrasonography
CPH
chronic persistent hepatitis
CPH-CAH cirrhosis
CPK
creatine phosphokinase
C-plasty
cpm, CPM
count per minute
CPN
celiac plexus neurolysis
chronic pyelonephritis
cisplatin nephropathy
EUS CPN
CPP
cerebral perfusion pressure
CPPS
chronic pelvic pain syndrome
chronic prostate pain syndrome
chronic prostatitis/pelvic pain syndrome
CR1
complement receptor type 1
CR103
OncoScint CR103
cracker test
cradle
acoustically transparent c.
Crafoord thoracic scissors

NOTES

Cragg
  C. Endopro System I stent
  C. thrombolytic brush
cramp
crampy abdominal pain
cranial
  c. mesonephros
  c. pole
craniocaudal
Cranley phleborrheograph
crapulent colic
crapulous diarrhea
crater
  ulcer c.
Crawford clamp
CR Bard Urolase
CR-BSI
  catheter-related bloodstream infection
CRC
  colorectal cancer
  colorectal carcinoma
CRCC
  cystic renal cell carcinoma
Crcl
  creatinine clearance
CRE
  controlled radial expansion
  CRE balloon catheter
C-reactive protein (CRP)
cream
  Analpram-HC anorectal c.
  Ca-Rezz moisture barrier c.
  Dermovate c.
  lidocaine-prilocaine c.
  Prudoxin c.
  rectal c.
  Sween C.
  Topicort C.
  triamcinolone c.
crease
  inguinal c.
  midline abdominal c.
  skin c.
  torso c.
creatine phosphokinase (CPK)
creatinine
  c. clearance (CC, Crcl)
  c. height index (CHI)
  plasma c.
  c. production
  serum c. (SCr)
  c. test
  urinary albumin to c. (UA/C)
creation
  diverting stoma c.
  Politano-Leadbetter tunnel c.
  tunnel c.
creatorrhea

Credé maneuver
^{51}Cr-EDTA
  51-chromium-labeled ethylenediaminetetraacetate
  ^{51}Cr-EDTA excretion
creep
  ureter c.
creeping
  c. of mesenteric fat
Creevy evacuator
CREG
  cross-reactive group
cremaster
  Henle internal c.
  c. muscle
cremasteric
  c. artery
  c. fascia
  c. fiber
  c. muscle
  c. reflex
  c. vessel
Cremer-Ikeda papillotome
crenate margin
Creon 10, 20
crepitus
crescendo decrescendo
crescendoing bowel sound
crescent
  c. fold
  c. gastric cardia
  glomerular c.
  c. snare
crescentic
  c. body
  c. fold disease
  c. glomerulonephritis
  c. nephritis
C-resistance
Crespo operation
CREST
  calcinosis cutis, Raynaud phenomenon, esophageal motility disorder, sclerodactyly, and telangiectasia
  CREST syndrome
crest
  cupula of ampullary c.
  c. factor
  haustral c.
  iliac c.
  jejunal c.
  urethral c.
Creutzfeldt-Jakob disease
crevicular fluid
CRF
  chronic renal failure
CRH
  corticotropin-releasing hormone

CRI
    chronic renal insufficiency
CRIB
    Clinical Risk Index for Babies
cricoid
    c. aneurysm
    c. myotomy
cricomyotomy
cricopharyngeal
    c. achalasia
    c. bar
    c. diverticulum
    c. myotomy
    c. spasm
    c. sphincter
cricopharyngeus muscle
cri du chat syndrome
Crigler-Najjar
    C.-N. disease
    C.-N. jaundice
    C.-N. syndrome (type I, II)
Crile
    C. angle retractor
    C. appendix clamp
    C. bile duct forceps
    C. gall duct forceps
    C. hemostat
    C. hemostatic clamp
    C. malleable retractor
    C. nerve hook
Crile-Wood needle holder
criminal nerve
crinogenic
crisis, pl. **crises**
    abdominal c.
    Addison c.
    adrenal c.
    Dietl c.
    gastric c.
    scleroderma renal c.
crista
    c. urethralis
    c. urethralis masculinae
    c. urethralis virilis
cristate margin
criteria
    Amsterdam c.
    Bosniak c.
    Child liver c.
    Child-Pugh c.
    clinicobiological c.
    DeMeester c.

    Foley c.
    Forrest c.
    Ganau c.
    Hogan/Geenen c.
    King's College ALF c.
    Lown c.
    Manning c.
    manometric c.
    morphometric c.
    Munich inclusion c.
    O'Duffy c.
    Pugh modification of Child c.
    Ranson c.
    Rome c. (I, II)
    Savary-Miller c.
    variceal size inclusion c.
    well-defined anatomical entry c.
critical diarrhea
Criticare
    C. HN elemental liquid feeding
    C. HN-Isocal tube feeding set
CRIT-LINE instrument
Crixivan lithiasis
^{51}Cr-labeled
    ^{51}Cr-l. albumin clearance
    ^{51}Cr-l. EDTA
crochet knot
Crohn
    C. colitis
    C. and Colitis Foundation of
    America (CCFA)
    C. and Colitis Knowledge
    (CCKNOW)
    C. disease (CD)
    C. Disease Activity Index (CDAI)
    C. disease of colon (CDC)
    C. Disease Endoscopic Index of
    Severity (CDEIS)
    C. duodenal ulcer
    C. duodenitis
    C. ileitis
    C. ileocolitis
    C. regional enteritis
    C. small intestine
cromakalim
cromoglycate
    disodium c.
    sodium c.
cromolyn sodium
Cronkhite-Canada syndrome
Crosby capsule
Crosby-Kugler capsule for biopsy

C

NOTES

cross
    gastrointestinal c.
    Maltese c.
    c. vasovasotomy
crossbar
    c. deformity
    inner c.
    outer c.
    c. symptom of Frankel
crossbridge
    c. cycle
    dephosphorylated myosin c.
    myosin c.
cross-clamped, crossclamped
crossed
    c. renal ectopia
    c. testicular ectopia
cross-folding
crosshatch mark
crossmatch
    T-cell c.
crossmatched blood
crossover
    c. design
    c. vasectomy
cross-phosphorylation
cross-reactive group (CREG)
cross-sectional
    8-channel c.-s. anal sphincter probe
cross-trigonal repair
Crotalaria
Croton
    C. lechleri
    C. lechleri tree
croupous
    c. cystitis
    c. membrane
    c. nephritis
CR/OV
    OncoScint CR/OV
        OncoScint colorectal/ovarian
          carcinoma localization
          scintigraphy
crowding
    variable nuclear c.
crow's foot pattern
CRP
    C-reactive protein
CRRT
    continuous renal replacement therapy
CRS
    Cell Recovery System
    cherry red spot
    Chinese restaurant syndrome
    colorectal surgery

CRST
    calcinosis cutis, Raynaud phenomenon,
      sclerodactyly, and telangiectasia
      CRST syndrome
CRT
    chemoradiation therapy
cruciate incision
cruciferous vegetable
crude
    c. drug
    c. urine
crunch
    mediastinal c.
    c. stick anastomosis
crural
    c. contraction
    c. fold
    c. fossa
    c. vein
    c. venous leakage
crus, pl. **crura, cruris**
    c. of diaphragm
    penile c.
    c. penis
    tinea cruris
crush
    c. kidney
    c. syndrome
crusher
    Warthen spur c.
crutched
    c. stick-type biliary duct stent
    c. stick-type polyurethane
      endoprosthesis
Cruveilhier
    C. disease
    C. sign
    C. ulcer
Cruveilhier-Baumgarten
    C.-B. anomaly
    C.-B. cirrhosis
    C.-B. syndrome
Cruz-Chagas disease
cruzi
    Trypanosoma c.
cryoablation
    c. for prostate cancer
    renal c.
    salvage c.
    salvage c. of the prostate
cryofibrinogenemia
cryogenic ablation
cryoglobulinemia
    mixed essential c.
    type II c.
cryoprecipitate
cryoprecipitated plasma

cryopreservation
    sperm c.
    spermatozoon c.
Cryoprobe
cryoprostatectomy
cryospray
cryostat
    c. tissue
    Tissue Tek-II c.
cryosurgery
cryosurgical
    c. ablation
    c. ablation of the prostate (CSAP)
cryotherapy
    endoscopic spray c.
crypt
    c. abscess
    anal c.
    c. architectural distortion
    c. architecture
    c. atrophy
    c. base
    branched c.
    c. cell
    c. cell apoptosis
    c. defensin
    c. epithelium
    forked c.
    c. of Haller
    c. hook
    c. hyperplasia
    c. hypertrophy
    ileal c.
    c. intraepithelial lymphocyte (cIEL)
    Lieberkühn c.
    c. of Littré
    Luschka c.
    Morgagni c.
    mucous c.
    multilocular c.
crypta, pl. **cryptae**
    cryptae mucosae duodeni
Cryptaz
cryptdin
cryptectomy
cryptitis
    neutrophilic c.
cryptococcal pyelonephritis
cryptococcosis
    adrenal c.
    genital c.

    prostatic c.
    renal c.
Cryptococcus neoformans
cryptogenic
    c. chronic hepatitis
    c. cirrhosis
    c. hypertransaminasemia
    c. liver disease
cryptoglandular
cryptolith
cryptorchidectomy
cryptorchidism
    abdominal c.
    bilateral c.
    canalicular c.
    ectopic c.
    femoral c.
    inguinal c.
    nonpalpable c.
    c. torsion
cryptorchidopexy
cryptorchism
cryptosporidia
***Cryptosporidia*-induced diarrhea**
cryptosporidial infection
cryptosporidiosis
    biliary c.
Cryptosporidium
    C. muris
    C. oocyst
    C. parvum
    C. species
crypt-villus
    c.-v. axis
    c.-v. site
    c.-v. unit
crystal
    Boettcher c.
    CaC3 c.
    calcium oxalate monohydrate c.
    Charcot-Leyden c.
    cholesterol monohydrate c.
    cystine c.
    oxalate c.
    phosphate c.
    piezoelectric c.
    Reinke c.
    c. retention
    thymol c.
    triple-phosphate c.
    urate c.
    uric acid c.

C

NOTES

crystal (continued)
  urinalysis sediment microscopy c.
  urinary c.
crystallization
  c. abnormality
  calcium oxalate c.
crystallography
  optical c.
  x-ray c.
crystalloid
  hypertonic c.
  c. solution
crystalluria
crystalluridrosis
crystal-phospholipid interaction
C&S
  culture and sensitivity
  C&S test
CS-5 cryosurgical system
CS-9000 densitometer
CSAP
  cryosurgical ablation of the prostate
CSD
  congenital sodium diarrhea
CSE
  complete surgical exploration
CSF
  cerebrospinal fluid
  colony-stimulating factor
    CSF glucose
    CSF glutamine
    CSF glutamine test
    CSF protein
CSF-1
  colony-stimulating factor-1
CSG
  chronic superficial gastritis
CSI
  cholesterol saturation index
CSM Stretta system
CT
  computed tomography
  computerized tomography
    CT colography
    CT colonography
    CT during arterial portography
      (CTAP)
    helical CT
    CT PEG
    renal helical CT (RHCT)
    CT scan
    CT scan with contrast enhancement
    spiral CT
    unenhanced helical CT
CTA
  computed tomographic angiography

CTAP
  computed tomography arterial
    portography
  CT during arterial portography
CT-AP
  computed tomography during arterial
    portography
CTAS
  colonic transabdominal sonography
CTC
  Child-Turcotte classification
**C-terminal propeptide of type I
  procollagen**
CT-guided
  CT-g. abscess drainage
  CT-g. celiac plexus neurolysis
  CT-g. fine-needle aspiration
  CT-g. liver biopsy
  CT-g. needle-aspiration biopsy
  CT-g. percutaneous endoscopic
    gastrostomy
  CT-g. pseudocyst drainage
CTHA
  computerized tomographic hepatic
    angiography
CTL
  cytolytic T lymphocyte
  cytotoxic T lymphocyte
CTL-mediated lysis
CTPV
  cavernous transformation of the portal
    vein
C-Trak
  C-T. analyzer
  C-T. handheld gamma detector
  C-T. probe
  C-T. surgical guidance system
^{14}C-triolein breath test
CTS
  Collaborative Transplant Study
C-type
  C-t. atrial natriuretic peptide (C-
    ANP)
  C-t. natriuretic peptide (CNP)
cube
  Gelfoam c.
cubilin
cuboidal epithelia
Cub R-200 enteral feeding pump
^{13}C-UBT
  carbon-13 urea breath test
CUC
  chronic ulcerative colitis
Cucurbita pepo
cuff
  c. abscess
  AS-800 c.
  bladder c.

columnar c.
c. electrode
rectal muscle c.
suprahepatic caval c.
cuffed
c. endotracheal tube
c. esophageal endoprosthesis
cuffitis
cul-de-sac
c.-d.-s. of Douglas
c.-d.-s. fluid
c.-d.-s. mass
culdocentesis
culdoplasty
McCall c.
culdoscope
culdoscopy
Cullen sign
Culp
C. spiral flap pyeloplasty
C. ureteropelvioplasty
Culp-DeWeerd
C.-D. spiral flap pyeloplasty
C.-D. ureteropelvioplasty
culture
aerobic c.
allogeneic mixed leukocyte c.
anaerobic c.
bacterial c.
blood c.
calculus c.
glomerular cell c.
c. medium
mixed growth on c.
mixed leukocyte c. (MLC)
semiquantitative c.
c. and sensitivity (C&S)
c. and sensitivity test
shell vial c.
stool c.
tissue c.
urine c.
viral c.
Culturelle
culture-negative neutrocytic ascites (CNNA)
cumulus
Cunningham-Cotton sleeve coaxial dilator
Cunninghamella
Cunningham urinary incontinence clamp

CUOG
Canadian Urology Oncology Group
cup
Bard alligator c.
Bard oval c.
ileostomy c.
stone c.
vaginal fistula c.
cup-and-spill stomach
cup-patch technique
Cuprimine
cuprophane membrane
cupula, pl. **cupulae**
c. of ampullary crest
gas c.
CUR
chronic urinary retention
curative resection
curd
alum c.
cure
krebiozen false cancer c.
C-urea
C-u. breath excretion
C-u. breath test
^{13}**C-urea**
synthetic ^{13}C-u.
C-urea breath test
curette
Spratt c.
C-urinary excretion
Curl Cath catheter
curling
esophageal c.
C. ulcer
Curran syndrome
currant jelly stool
Currarino triad
current
c. algorithm
coagulating c.
conducted c.
cutting c.
c. density
direct c.
electrocoagulating c.
membrane c.
Olympus PSD-10 electrosurgical blend c.
pure cutting c.
Curschmann disease

NOTES

curtsy
- Vincent c.

curvatura
- c. gastrica major
- c. gastrica minor
- c. ventriculi major
- c. ventriculi minor

curvature
- congenital penile c.
- penile c.
- c. of stomach

curve
- angulus on the lesser c.
- cosine c.
- disease-free survival c.
- gallbladder emptying-refilling c.
- Kaplan-Meier c.
- learning c.
- loss of sigmoid c.
- sigmoid c.
- c. of stream
- time-activity c.
- time-concentration c.
- triphasic cystometric c.

curved
- c. bacillus
- c. dissecting forceps
- c. end-to-end anastomosis (CEEA)
- c. flank position
- c. hemostat
- c. Maryland forceps
- c. Mayo clamp
- c. Mayo scissors
- 3.5–10 MHz c. array transducer
- c. transjugular needle

curved-needle surgeon's knot
curvilinear scanning echoendoscope
Curvularia
CUS
- compression ultrasound

CUSA
- Cavitron Ultrasonic Surgical Aspirator
- CUSA dissector

Cushieri maneuver
Cushing
- C. disease
- C. forceps
- C. medicamentosus syndrome
- C. suture
- C. ulcer
- C. vein retractor

cushingoid facies
Cushing-Rokitansky ulcer
cushion
- air c.
- hemorrhoidal c.
- partial water bath and water c.
- Positron Plus c.

- c. sign
- tissue c.

Custom Ultrasonic automatic reprocessor
cut
- blended c.
- electrosurgical c.
- field c.
- c. surface of liver
- c. waveform
- c. waveform desiccation

cutaneobiliary fistula
cutaneous
- c. advancement flap
- c. appendiceal conduit
- c. collateral circulation
- c. dropsy
- c. EGG
- c. electrical field stimulation
- c. electrogastrogram
- c. hemangioma
- c. horn of penis
- c. hyperesthesia
- c. ileocystostomy
- c. lesion
- c. lichen amyloidosis
- c. loop ureterostomy
- c. metastasis
- c. pyelostomy
- c. reflex
- c. T-cell lymphoma
- c. urinary diversion
- c. vesicostomy

cutback
- c. anoplasty
- c. type vaginoplasty
- vaginal c.

cutdown liver
cuticular flap
Cutinova
- C. cavity
- C. foam
- C. hydro
- C. hydro thin

cutis laxa
cutter
- Endopath endoscopic linear c.
- linear staple c.
- Nu-Hope hole c.
- Proximate linear c.
- rib c.
- suture c.

cutting
- c. current
- c. electrode
- c. endoscopic mucosal resection (C-EMR)

c. LR needle
c. wire
CVAT
costovertebral angle tenderness
CVF
cobra venom factor
CVI
common variable immunodeficiency
CVM
childhood visceral myopathy
circular vesicomyotomy
CVP
central venous pressure
CVS
clean-voided specimen
cyclic vomiting syndrome
CVVH
continuous venovenous hemofiltration
CVVHD
continuous venovenous hemodialysis
CVVHDF
continuous venovenous hemodiafiltration
CW
clustered waves
CWS
cotton-wool spot
CX
controlled expansion
CX Plus prosthesis
CXM prosthesis
C282Y
C282Y hemochromatosis
C282Y mutation
cyanate
urea-derived c.
cyanide
potassium c.
cyanoacrylate
c. glue
c. injection
N-butyl c.
2-cyanoacrylate
isobutyl 2-c.
Cyanobacterium-like body
cyanocobalamin
c. injection
c. radioactive agent
cyanosis
enterogenous c.
cyanotic kidney
cybernetic regulation of blood pressure
cyclamate

cyclase
adenylate c. (AC)
guanylate c.
guanylyl c.
ligand-triggered membrane
guanylate c.
cycle
biliary c.
contraction-relaxation c.
Cori c.
crossbridge c.
cyclin/PCNA during cell c.
diurnal c.
gastric c.
glutathione redox c.
Krebs c.
liver-adipose tissue c.
Schiff biliary c.
tricarboxylic acid c.
urea c.
cyclic
c. adenosine monophosphate
(cAMP)
c. guanosine monophosphate
(cGMP)
c. proteinuria
c. urinary disinfectant
c. vomiting
c. vomiting syndrome (CVS)
5′-cyclic
5′-c. adenosine monophosphate
(cAMP)
5′-c. guanosine monophosphate
(cGMP)
cyclical vomiting
cyclin
cyclin-dependent
c.-d. kinase
c.-d. kinase inhibitor
cycling dialysis
cyclin/PCNA during cell cycle
cyclizine
cyclobenzaprine
cyclocytidine
Cyclogyl
cycloheximide
cyclooxygenase (COX)
c. inhibition
c. inhibitor
c. messenger ribonucleoprotein acid
(COX mRNA)
c. metabolite

C

NOTES

cyclooxygenase *(continued)*
   c. pathway
   c. 2-selective nonsteroidal
     antiinflammatory drug
cyclooxygenase-1 (COX-1)
cyclooxygenase-2 (COX-2)
   c. inhibitor
cyclooxygenase-dependent mechanism
cyclopentamine
cyclophosphamide
   cisplatin, doxorubicin, c.
   escalated methotrexate, vinblastine,
     Adriamycin, cisplatin or c. (E-
     MVAC)
   5-fluorouracil, Adriamycin, c.
     (FAC)
   c., Velban, actinomycin-D,
     bleomycin, platinum (VAB-VI)
   vincristine, Adriamycin, c. (VAC)
cycloserine
Cyclospora
   C. cayetanensis
   coccidian *C.*
cyclosporine
   c. arteriolopathy
   c. for microemulsion
   c. nephrotoxicity
   c. toxicity
   c. tubulopathy
cyclosporine-induced optic neuropathy
Cyclotrac-SP radioimmunoassay
cycrimine
cylinder
   AMA inflatable c.
   AMS controlled expansion penile
     prosthesis c.
   AMS 700CX penile prosthesis c.
   banding c.
   Bence Jones c.
   high-pressure inflatable prosthesis c.
   Hostaform plastic c.
   inflated rubber c.
   Mentor Bioflex c.
   suction c.
   Ultrex c.
cylindrical
   c. balloon
   c. confronting cisterna (CCC)
   c. diffuser
   c. mucosal resection
cylindruria
Cymed Micro Skin one-piece drainage
  pouch
CYP3A4
CyPat treatment
cypionate
   c. ester
   testosterone c.

CYP isozyme
cyproheptadine
cyproterone acetate (CPA)
cyst
   adrenal gland c.
   adventitious c.
   air c.
   allantoic c.
   alveolar hydatid c.
   Bartholin c.
   bile duct c.
   biliary c.
   Bowman space c.
   branchiogenous c.
   choledochal c. (grades I, II, III,
     IV, IVa)
   choroid plexus c. (CPC)
   chyle c.
   cluster of grapelike c.'s
   CMV inclusion c.
   compound c.
   congenital biliary c.
   congenital splenic c.
   Cowper c.
   daughter c.
   dermoid c.
   duplication c.
   Echinococcus liver c.
   Entamoeba coli c.
   enteric c.
   enterogenous c.
   epidermal c.
   epidermoid c.
   epididymal c.
   esophageal duplication c.
   extramucosal c.
   extraparenchymal renal c.
   false c.
   fatty c.
   c. fenestration
   Gartner duct c.
   gas c.
   gastric duplication c.
   glomerular c.
   granddaughter c.
   grapelike c.
   hepatic echinococcal c.
   hydatid c.
   ileal duplication c.
   inclusion c.
   intraluminal c.
   intratesticular c.
   isolated c.
   junctional c.
   kidney c.
   lucent c.
   macroscopic liver c.
   median raphe c.

mesenteric c.
mother c.
müllerian duct c.
multilocular c.
multiloculated c.
neoplastic c.
noncommunicating biliary c.
nonepithelial c.
nonparasitic splenic c.
omental c.
ovarian dermoid c.
pancreatic c.
parapelvic c.
parasitic c.
paraurethral c.
parovarian c.
penile c.
peripelvic c.
pilonidal c.
presacral c.
prosthetic utricle c.
c. puncture device
pyelogenic renal c.
renal sinus c.
retention c.
retrorectal c.
Rosen c.
sacrococcygeal pilonidal c.
scrotum c.
sebaceous c.
secondary c.
seminal vesicle hydatid c.
simple renal c.
solitary hepatic c.
sterile c.
tailgut c. (TGC)
Tarlov c.
testicular c.
tunic c.
tunica albuginea c.
unicameral c.
unilocular ovarian c.
urachal c.
urethral c.
urinary c.
vitellointestinal c.

cystadenocarcinoma
biliary c.
pancreatic mucinous c.
stage III papillary serous c.

cystadenoma
biliary c.

ductal c.
ductectatic mucinous c.
glycogen-rich c.
hepatic c.
mucinous c.
ruptured appendiceal c.

Cystagon
cystalgia
cystamine
Cysta-Q
cystathionine gamma-lyase
cystatin C
cystatrophia
cystauchenitis
cystauchenotomy
cystauxe
cysteamine bitartrate
cysteamine-induced duodenal ulcer
cystectasia, cystectasy
cystectomy
palliative c.
partial c.
pilonidal c.
radical c.
salvage c.
simple c.
subtrigonal c.
supratrigonal c.
total c.
cysteine
c. *Brucella* broth
c. calculus
cysteinesulfinic acid
cysteinyl leukotriene
cystelcosis
cystendesis
cystenterostome
cystenterostomy
direct c.
endoscopic c.
cysterethism
cystgastrostomy
surgical c.
cysthypersarcosis
cystic
c. artery
c. bile
c. cystitis
c. degeneration
c. dilation
c. duct (CD)
c. duct angiogram

C

NOTES

cystic *(continued)*
  c. duct catheterization
  c. duct cholangiocatheter
  c. duct cholangiogram
  c. duct cholangiography
  c. duct choledochoscopy
  c. duct leakage
  c. duct lumen
  c. duct stenosis
  c. duct stone
  c. echinococcosis
  c. epithelial proliferation
  c. fibrosis (CF)
  c. fibrosis gene probe
  c. fibrosis transductance regulator
  c. fibrosis transmembrane
    conductance regulator (CFTR)
  c. hamartoma
  c. liver disease
  c. mass
  c. nephroma
  c. plexus
  c. puncture
  c. renal cell carcinoma (CRCC)
  c. Wilms tumor
cystica
  cholecystitis c.
  cystitis c.
  pyelitis c.
  pyeloureteritis c.
  ureteritis c.
  urethritis c.
cystic-choledochal junction
cysticercosis
Cysticercus
  C. bovis
  C. cellulosae
cysticercus disease
cysticohepatic junction
cysticolithectomy
cysticolithotripsy
cysticorrhaphy
cysticotomy
cysticus
  ductus c.
  polypus c.
cystidoceliotomy
cystidolaparotomy
cystidotrachelotomy
cystine
  c. calculus
  c. crystal
  c. dimethylester (CDE)
  c. metabolism
  c. stone
  c. supersaturation
  c. urinary lithiasis

cystinosis
  neuropathic c.
cystinuria
cystis fellea
Cystistat
cystistaxis
cystitis
  acute c.
  acute hemorrhagic c. (AHC)
  allergic c.
  amicrobic c.
  bacterial c.
  candidal c.
  catarrhal c.
  chemical c.
  coccidioidal c.
  c. colli
  croupous c.
  cystic c.
  c. cystica
  dimethyl sulfate c.
  diphtheritic c.
  DMSO c.
  c. emphysematosa
  emphysematous c.
  eosinophilic c.
  exfoliative c.
  follicular c.
  c. follicularis
  gangrenous c.
  glandular c.
  c. glandularis
  hemorrhagic c.
  honeymoon c.
  Hunner interstitial c.
  incrusted c.
  interstitial c.
  mechanical c.
  nonbacterial c. (NBC)
  panmural c.
  papillary c.
  radiation c.
  recurrent c.
  c. senilis feminarum
  subacute c.
  submucous c.
  sympathetic c.
  uncomplicated c.
  viral c.
  xanthogranulomatous c.
Cysto
  C. Conray contrast
  C. Flex stent
  Urovist C.
Cystocath
cystocele
  central c.

grade 4 c.
lateral c.
cystochrome
cystochromoscopy
cystocolostomy
cystocolpoproctography
cystodiaphanoscopy
cystodiathermy
flexible c.
cystodistention
cystodiverticulum
cystoduodenostomy (CDY)
endoscopic c.
cystodynia
cystoenterocele
cystoenterostomy
cystoepiplocele
cystoepithelioma
cystofiberscope
Olympus CYF-3 OES c.
cystofibroma
Cystogam
cystogastric fistula
cystogastrostomy (CGY)
endoscopic c.
endoscopic ultrasound-guided c.
cystogastrotome
cystogenic chemical
cystogram
air c.
chain c.
excretory c. (XC)
gravity c.
micturating c.
postvoiding c. (PVC)
retrograde c. (RC)
static c.
stress c.
surveillance c.
voiding c. (VCG)
cystography
antegrade c.
bead chain c.
radionuclide c.
retrograde c.
suprapubic c.
triple-voiding c.
cystohepatic triangle
Cysto-Hypaque
cystojejunostomy
Roux-en-Y c.
cystolateral pancreatojejunostomy

cystolith
cystolithectomy
cystolithiasis
cystolithic
cystolitholapaxy
cystolithotomy
cystolysis
cystometer
Lewis c.
cystometric
c. biofeedback
c. bladder capacity
cystometrogram (CMG)
filling c.
cystometrographic monitoring
cystometrography
voiding c.
cystometry
filling c.
gas c.
multichannel c.
provoked c.
saline c.
screening c.
simultaneous urethral c.
spontaneous c.
transballoon c.
voiding c.
water c.
cystonephrosis
cystoneuralgia
cystopancreatography
cystopanendoscopy
cystoparalysis
cystopericystectomy
cystoperitoneal shunt
cystopexy
cystophotography
cystophthisis
cystoplasty
augmentation c.
autoaugmentation c.
cecal c.
flap valve c.
Gil-Vernet ileocecal c.
human lyophilized dura c.
laparoscopic c.
nonsecretory sigmoid c.
sigmoid c.
cystoplegia
cystoplelography
cystoproctostomy

NOTES

cystoprostatectomy
    salvage c.
cystoprostatourethrectomy
cystoprostatovesiculectomy
cystoptosis, cystoptosia
cystopyelitis
cystopyelogram
cystopyelonephritis
cystoradiography
cystoradium insertion
cystorectocele
cystorectostomy
cystoresectoscope
    ALR c.
    anterior-posterior c.
    Damon-Julian c.
    Julian c.
cystorrhagia
cystorrhaphy
cystorrhea
cystosarcoma phyllodes
cystoschisis
cystoscope
    Albarran laser c.
    balloon c.
    Braasch direct catheterization c.
    Braasch-Kaplan direct vision c.
    Brown-Buerger c.
    Broyle retrograde c.
    Butterfield c.
    French c.
    InjecTx c.
    Judd c.
    Kelly c.
    Kidd c.
    Laidley double-catheterizing c.
    Lowsley-Peterson c.
    McCarthy-Campbell miniature c.
    McCarthy Foroblique
      panendoscope c.
    McCrea c.
    Miller c.
    Morganstern continuous-flow
      operating c.
    National general purpose c.
    Nesbit c.
    Olympus fiberoptic c.
    Storz c.
    Surgitek graduated c.
    Young c.
cystoscopic
    c. electrohydraulic lithotripsy
    c. urography
cystoscopy
    c. and dilation (C&D)
    percutaneous fetal c.
    steerable c.
    virtual c.

cystosis
    congenital c.
cystospasm
Cystospaz
Cystospaz-M
cystospermitis
cystostaxis
cystostomy
    suprapubic c.
    trocar c.
    c. tube
cystotome
    Kelman air c.
    Kelman double-bladed c.
    Kelman knife c.
    Kelman knife-cannula c.
    McIntyre reverse c.
    Mendez ultrasonic c.
    reverse c.
cystotomy
    open c.
    suprapubic c.
cystotrachelotomy
cystoureteritis
cystoureterogram
cystoureterography
cystoureteropyelitis
cystoureteropyelonephritis
cystourethrectomy
    total c.
cystourethritis
cystourethrocele
cystourethrogram
    micturating c.
    micturition c.
    retrograde c.
    voiding c. (VCUG)
cystourethrography
    chain c.
    expression c.
    isotope voiding c. (IVCU)
    micturating c. (MCU)
    radionuclide voiding c.
    voiding c.
cystourethropexy
    laparoscopic c.
    Marshall-Marchetti-Krantz c.
    obturator shelf c.
    Pereyra-Raz c.
cystourethroplasty
    Kropp c.
    Leadbetter c.
cystourethroscope
    ACMI c.
    microlens c.
    O'Donoghue c.
    Wappler microlens c.

cystourethroscopy
> dynamic c.

cystous

CYT-356 radiolabeled with 111 indium chloride

Cytadren

cytarabine

cytoaggression

Cytocare Prolase II

cytocentrifuge
> c. preparation
> c. set

cytochalasin B

cytochrome
> b558 membrane-bound c.
> c. P450 enzyme
> c. P450 enzyme system
> c. P450 metabolite

cytochrome-c-oxidase deficiency

cytochrome P-450

cytodiagnosis

CytoGam

cytogenetic analysis

cytokeratin
> bile duct type c.
> hepatocyte-type c.
> c. staining

cytokine
> c. antagonist
> antiinflammatory c.
> fibrogenic c.
> fibrosis-promoting c.
> c. gene expression
> GM-CSF c.
> proinflammatory c.
> c. therapy
> c. tumor necrosis factor-α

cytologic
> c. biopsy
> c. brushing
> c. diagnosis
> C. software
> c. specimen

cytology
> aspiration biopsy c.
> balloon c.
> brush c.
> c. brush
> colon lavage c.
> endoscopic brush c.
> endoscopic retrograde c.

> endoscopic transesophageal fine-needle aspiration c.
> c. examination
> exfoliative c.
> fine-needle aspiration c. (FNAC)
> gastric brush c.
> guided-needle aspiration c.
> lavage c.
> needle aspiration c.
> salvage c.
> touch c.
> urine c.
> voiding urine c. (VUC)
> wire-guided c.

cytolysis inhibitor

cytolytic
> c. action
> c. therapy
> c. T lymphocyte (CTL)

cytoma

cytomegalovirus (CMV)
> c. colitis (CMV colitis)
> c. enterocolitis
> c. esophagitis
> c. hepatitis
> c. immune globulin
> c. infection

cytometer
> CAS 200 image c.
> Cell Analysis System 200 image c.
> Dickinson FACS 400-series flow c.
> EPICS C-flow flow c.
> EPICS Elite flow c.
> EPICS 700-series flow c.
> EPICS V-flow c.
> FACScan flow c.

cytometric
> c. analysis
> c. pattern

cytometry
> deoxyribonucleic acid flow c.
> DNA flow c.
> flow c.
> fluorescence-activated flow c.
> image c.
> static image DNA c.

cytopenia

cytophilic antibody

cytophotometry
> static c.

NOTES

cytoplasm
 eosinophilic c.
cytoplasmic
 c. adaptor protein
 c. argyrophilia
 perinuclear antineutrophil c. (p-
   ANC)
 c. staining
 c. urease
cytoprotective prostaglandin
cytoreduction
 ultrasonic c.
cytoreductive surgery
Cytosar
cytosine
 5-methyl c.
cytoskeletal link
cytoskeleton
 prostate gland c.
cytosolic
 c. calcium
 c. face
cytospin collection fluid
CytoTAb
Cytotec
cytotoxic
 c. agent
 c. antibody

 c. chemotherapy
 c. liver disease
 c. T cell
 c. T-cell response
 c. T lymphocyte (CTL)
cytotoxicity
 antibody-dependent cell-mediated c.
   (ADCC)
 antibody-dependent cellular c.
   (ADCC)
 Bartel c.
 cell-mediated c.
 complement-dependent c. (CDC)
 lymphocyte c.
cytotoxin
 c. assay
 c. necrotizing factor
 VacA c.
 vacuolating toxin gene A c.
cytotoxin-associated
 c.-a. gene A (cagA)
 c.-a. gene A protein
Cytoxan
Czerny
 C. rectal speculum
 C. suture
Czerny-Kocher-Perthes incision
Czerny-Lembert suture

D
> daunorubicin
>> D cell

3-D
> 3-D computer reconstruction
> 3-D gadolinium-enhanced MR
>> angiography
> 3-D sonography

D3
> dihydroxyvitamin D3
> 1,25-dihydroxyvitamin D3
>> (1,25(OH)2 D3)
> 25-hydroxyvitamin D3 (25(OH)D3)
> I-alpha-hydroxyvitamin D3
> 1,25(OH)2 D3
>> 1,25-dihydroxyvitamin D3

D-600

D₄
> leukotriene D.

D4S231 marker
D4S414 marker
D16S291 marker
D16S84 marker
DAB
> diaminobenzidine

dacarbazine
> doxorubicin, bleomycin sulfate,
>> vinblastine, d. (ABVD)

dacliximab
Daclizumab
Dacomed
> D. Catalyst VCD
> D. snap gauge

Dacron
> D. interposition graft
> D. mesh
> D. prosthesis
> D. suture

Dacron-impregnated Silastic sheet
DACT
> dactinomycin

dactinomycin (DACT)
DAF
> decay-accelerating factor

DAG
> diacylglycerol
> diffuse antral gastritis
> dimeric acidic glycoprotein

Dagradi esophageal variceal
> **classification**

DAH
> diffuse alveolar hemorrhage

daidzein
daidzin

daily
> d. dialysis
> d. hemodialysis
> d. intermittent peritoneal dialysis
>> (DIPD)
> d. protein intake (DPI)

Daines-Hodgson anastomosis
Dairy-Ease chewable tablet
d-ALA
> delta-aminolevulinic acid

Dale
> D. abdominal binder
> D. Foley catheter holder

DALM
> dysplasia-associated lesion or mass

Dalmane
dalteparin sodium
dam
> rubber d.

damage
> chloroquine-induced d.
> chronic tubular d.
> drug-induced d.
> drug-induced esophageal d. (DIED)
> flucloxacillin-associated liver d.
> gastric mucosal d.
> Graham scale for drug-induced
>> gastric d.
> histologic d.
> hypertensive end-organ d.
> indomethacin-induced mucosal d.
> ischemic tubular d.
> microsomal d.
> oropharyngeal d.
> renal structural d.
> tubular d.

Damon-Julian cystoresectoscope
Danazol
Danbolt-Closs syndrome
Dance sign
dandy
> d. fever
> D. nerve hook

Dane particle
Daniel colostomy clamp
Danish Prostate Symptom Score (DAN-
> **PSS)**
DAN-PSS
> Danish Prostate Symptom Score

Dansac
> D. Karaya Seal one-piece drainage
>> pouch
> D. ostomy irrigation set
> D. skin barrier
> D. Standard Ileo pouch

D

183

dansylcadaverine
Dantec
    D. 12-channel Urocolor Video
      system
    D. Etude system
    D. Menuet system
    D. rotating disk flowmeter
    D. Urodyn 1000 flowmeter
    D. Urodyn 1000 uroflowmeter
danthron
Dantrium
dantrolene sodium
Danubian
    D. endemic familial
    D. endemic familial nephropathy
dapsone
daptomycin for injection
Darbid
Dardik clamp
D-arginine
    enantiomer D.-a.
Daricon
    D. PB
Darier disease
dark
    d. adaptation study
    d. burgundy blood
    d. concentrated urine
    d. spot
    d. stool
darting incision
dartoic
dartoid
dartos
    d. fascia
    d. muscle
    d. pedicled flap
    d. pouch procedure
Darvocet
Darvocet-N 100
Darvon Compound-65
Daseler zone
DASH
    dietary approach to stop hypertension
DAT
    diet as tolerated
data
    long-term followup d.
    perioperative d.
    randomized clinical trial d.
database
    institutional main demographic d.
date fever
Datta procedure
daughter
    d. cyst

    d. endoscopic retrograde
      cholangiopancreatoscopy system
    d. nodule
daunorubicin (D)
DaunoXome
Davat operation
Davidoff cell
David rectal speculum
DaVinci handle instrument
Davis
    D. interlocking sound
    D. intubated ureterostomy
    D. intubated ureterotomy
    D. loop
    D. spatula
    D. technique
Davol
    D. colon tube
    D. feeding bag
    D. feeding tube
    D. sump drain
    D. tunneler
DAWG
    demucosalized augmentation with gastric
      segment
    DAWG procedure
day-care diarrhea
daytime incontinence
DAZ **gene**
DBCP
    dibromochloropropane
DBP
    vitamin-D-binding protein
DBW
    desirable body weight
DC
    descending colon
    dilation catheter
    duodenal cap
    DC locus allelic
DCBE
    double-contrast barium enema
DCC
    deleted in colorectal carcinoma
    DCC gene
D-cell
    antral D-c.
    D-c. density
DCGI
    double-contrast barium examination of
      the upper gastrointestinal tract
DCP
    des-gamma-carboxy prothrombin
3-DCRT
    three-dimensional conformal therapy
DCT
    distal convoluted tubule

3D-CTP
  three-dimensional CT pancreatography
DD
  digestive disease
DD23
    antigen DD23
    DD23 antigen
DDAVP
  deamino D-arginine-vasopressin
  desmopressin
    DDAVP nasal spray
ddC
D-dimer
DDNC
  Digestive Disease National Coalition
DDS
  Denys-Drash syndrome
DDS-Acidophilus
DDV ligator
DE
  duodenal exclusion
de
    d. novo
    d. novo autoimmune hepatitis
    d. novo liver cancer
    d. novo malignancy
    d. novo needle knife technique
    d. novo renal disease
    d. Pezzer catheter
    d. Toni-Debré-Fanconi syndrome
    d. Toni-Fanconi-Debré syndrome
dead
    d. bowel
    d. space
DEAE
  diethylaminoethyl
deafferentation
deafness
    lentigines, electrocardiographic
    conduction abnormalities, ocular
    hypertelorism, pulmonary stenosis,
    abnormal genitalia, retardation of
    growth, and d. (LEOPARD)
de-air
deaminase
    adenosine d.
    porphobilinogen d. (PBG-D)
1-deamino-8-d-arginine vasopressin
deamino D-arginine-vasopressin
  (DDAVP)

Dean
    D. stage
    D. stage I, II radiation proctitis
Dean-MacDonald gastric resection clamp
death
    hepatocellular d.
    ischemic tubular cell d.
    liver d.
Deaver
    D. incision
    D. operating scissors
    D. retractor
    window of D.
Deaver-type blade
deazaaminopterin
DeBakey
    D. clamp
    D. forceps
DeBakey-Cooley retractor
Debove membrane
debrancher
    d. deficiency
    d. enzyme
    d. glycogen storage disease
Debré-de Toni-Fanconi syndrome
debridement
debris
    clots and d.
    degenerating cellular d.
    purulent d.
    stonelike d.
debrisoquin
debulking
    percutaneous d.
    d. therapy
    d. of tumor
    tumor d.
DEC
  diethylcarbamazine
Decadron
decanoate
    nandrolone d.
decapacitation factor
Decapeptyl
decapsulation of kidney
decarboxylase
    histidine d. (HDC)
    ornithine d. (ODC)
    uroporphyrinogen d. (UROD)

D

NOTES

decarboxylation
    amine precursor uptake and d.
    (APUD)
decay-accelerating factor (DAF)
decerebrate posturing
Decholin
decidualis
    periappendicitis d.
Declomycin
decompensated
    d. alcoholic cirrhosis
    d. liver cirrhosis
    d. neobladder
decompensation
    bladder d.
    detrusor muscle d.
decompression
    abdominal d.
    balloon d.
    biliary d.
    bladder d.
    cardiac d.
    d. catheter
    colonoscopic d.
    d. colostomy
    ductal d.
    endoscopic biliary d.
    gastric d.
    hydrostatic d.
    intestinal d.
    long intestinal tube d.
    nasogastric d.
    operative d.
    palliative d.
    PEG-assisted d.
    percutaneous transhepatic d.
    pericardial d.
    portal d.
    surgical d.
    transduodenal endoscopic d.
    d. tube
    tube d.
    variceal d.
decongestant
decontamination
    selective intestinal d. (SID)
decorin
    proteoglycan d.
decorticate posturing
decortication
    renal cyst d.
decrease
    rapid d.
decreased peristalsis
decrescendo
    crescendo d.
decubitus
    d. calculus

    lateral d.
    d. position
    d. ulcer
Deddish-Potts intestinal forceps
dedifferentiate
deep
    d. artery
    d. breathing
    d. cannulation
    d. cervical fascia
    d. dorsal vein
    d. interloop abscess
    d. jaundice
    d. muscular plexus
    d. pain
    d. perineal space
    d. postanal anorectal space
    d. postanal space of Courtney
    d. tendon reflex
    d. trigone
    d. venous thrombosis
de-epithelialization
de-epithelialized flap
deep-seated fungal infection
defecate
    urge to d.
defecating proctogram
defecation
    balloon d.
    fragmentary d.
    infrequent d.
    obstructive d.
    painful d.
    d. syncope
defecatory
    d. difficulty
    d. dyschezia
    d. straining
    d. urgency
defecogram
defecography
    FECOM artificial stool for d.
defecometry
defect
    acidification d.
    acinar d.
    acquired neutrophil chemotaxis d.
    amorphous filling d.
    bony d.
    chain-of-lakes filling d.
    cobblestone filling d.
    cold d.
    conduction d.
    fascial d.
    fetal alcohol syndrome ureter d.
    filling d.
    frondlike filling d.
    hernial d.

hot d.
interventricular d.
intraluminal filling d.
intrapelvic filling d.
isolation d.
lobulated filling d.
mesenteric d.
plaquelike linear d.
polypoid filling d.
portal perfusion d.
renal concentrating d.
tailing d.
uterine lateral fusion d.

defensin
crypt d.

deferens
ampulla of vas d.
congenital bilateral absence of the
vas d. (CBAVD)
ductus d.
ectopic vas d.
vas d.

deferentectomy
deferential artery
deferentis
ampulla ductus d.
diverticulum ampullae ductus d.

deferentitis
deferoxamine mesylate infusion test
defervescence
deficiency
acquired lactose d.
adenine phosphoribosyltransferase d.
adult lactase d.
aldosterone d.
alpha-1-antitrypsin d.
17-alpha-hydroxylase d.
amylo-1,6-glucosidase d.
androgen d.
d. anemia
antithrombin III d.
APRT d.
arginase d.
11-beta-hydroxylase d.
3-beta-hydroxysteroid
dehydrogenase d.
bile salt d.
biotin d.
brancher d.
calcium d.
carbamoyl phosphate synthetase d.
ceramidase d.

chromium d.
cobalamin d.
congenital enterocyte heparan
sulphate d.
copper d.
cytochrome-c-oxidase d.
debrancher d.
20,22-desmolase d.
dietary d.
disaccharidase d.
d. disease
enteropeptidase d.
essential fatty acid d. (EFAD)
estrogen d.
folate d.
follicle-stimulating hormone d.
fructose aldolase d.
fructose diphosphatase d.
fumarylacetoacetate hydrolase d.
glucose-6-phosphatase d.
glucuronyl transferase d.
gonadotropin-releasing hormone d.
growth hormone d.
hepatic phosphorylase d.
hypoxanthine guanine
phosphoribosyltransferase d.
IgA d.
immune d.
intestinal lactase d.
intrinsic sphincter d. (ISD)
iron d.
lactase d.
long-chain acyl-CoA
dehydrogenase d.
magnesium d.
medium-chain acyl-CoA
dehydrogenase d.
niacin d.
nutritional d.
ornithine carbamoyl transferase d.
pancreatic lipase d.
PiZZ alpha-1-antitrypsin d.
potassium d.
protein C d.
protein S d.
pyridoxal 5′-phosphate d.
riboflavin d.
S-adenosylmethionine d.
sodium d.
sucrose-isomaltase d.
testosterone d.
thiamine d.

D

NOTES

deficiency *(continued)*
    triglyceride enzyme d.
    UDPGT d.
    uridine diphosphate
      glucuronosyltransferase d.
    vitamin A d.
    vitamin D d.
    zinc d.
deficiens
    ejaculatio d.
deficit
    lateralizing sensory d.
    neurologic d.
defined-formula diet
defloration pyelitis
Deflux
    D. injectable implant
    D. system implant
deformability
    hepatic d.
deformans
    peritonitis d.
deformity
    Akerlund d.
    bell clapper d.
    bulb d.
    chain-of-lakes d.
    cloverleaf d.
    cobra-head d.
    crossbar d.
    duodenal bulb d.
    gross d.
    hourglass d.
    keyhole d.
    limb d.
    nasal d.
    penile d.
    phrygian cap d.
    swan-neck d.
    trefoil d.
    ureterocele cobra-head d.
    Whitehead d.
    Z-type d.
defunctionalization
defunctionalized bladder
defunctioning efficiency
Defyne urethral assist device
degassed water
degenerating cellular debris
degeneration
    acute hepatocellular d.
    Armanni-Ehrlich d.
    ballooning d.
    cystic d.
    feathery d.
    fistulous d.
    hepatocerebral d.

    hepatolenticular d.
    macular d.
degenerative
    d. change
    d. nephritis
degloving
    penile shaft d.
deglutible
deglutition
    d. disorder
    d. mechanism
    d. reflex
deglutitive
    d. inhibition
    d. pharyngeal chamber
deglutitory
Degos
    D. disease
    D. syndrome
degradation
    gastric mucosal d.
    haptocorrin d.
    proteolytic d.
degradative enzyme
degranulation
    mast cell d.
dehisced
dehiscence
    abdominal incision d.
    d. of cystic stump
    Killian d.
    staple line d.
    suture line d.
    wound d.
DEHOP
    diethylhomospermine
dehydrated ethanol
dehydration
    d. fever
    hyperosmotic nonketotic d.
dehydrocholaneresis
dehydroemetine
dehydroepiandrosterone (DHA)
    d. sulfate (DHAS)
dehydrogenase
    alcohol d. (ADH)
    aldehyde d. (ALDH)
    alpha-ketoacid d.
    benzaldehyde d.
    beta-hydroxyacyl-coenzyme A d.
    3-beta-hydroxysteroid d.
    branched-chain alpha-ketoacid d.
    glutamate d. (GLDH)
    glyceraldehyde phosphate d.
      (GAPD)
    glyceraldehyde-3-phosphate d.
      (GAPDH)
    ketoglutarate d. (KGDH)

lactate d. (LDH)
lactic acid d. (LDH)
long-chain 3-hydroxyacyl coenzyme
  A d. (LCHAD)
medium-chain acyl-CoA d.
  (MCAD)
pyruvate d. (PDH)
sorbitol d. (SDH)
deiodinized formamide
Deisting technique
dejecta
dejection
Dejerine-Sottas syndrome
Delatestryl
delavirdine
delay
  excretory d.
  gastric emptying d.
  outlet d.
delayed
  d. anastomosis
  d. blush
  d. capillary refill
  d. colonic transit
  d. gallbladder emptying
  d. graft function (DGF)
  d. hyperacute transplant rejection
  d. liquid gastric emptying
  d. nephrogram
  d. operative cholangiography
  d. primary closure (DPC)
  d. primary intention
  d. primary intention healing
  d. upstroke
  d. ureteral anastomotic stenosis
  d. vesicoureteral reflux
delayed-release tablet
delayed-type hypersensitivity (DTH)
del Castillo syndrome
deleted
  d. in colon carcinoma gene
  d. in colorectal carcinoma (DCC)
deletion
  chromosome d.
  clonal d.
  d. mutation
  d. and mutation detection
    enhancement gel
  d. polymorphism
  somatic allelic d.
Delflex peritoneal dialysis solution

delivery
  PlasmaKinetic radiofrequency
    energy d.
  vectorial d.
delomorphous cell
Delorme
  D. procedure
  D. rectal prolapse operation
  D. transrectal excision
delta
  d. agent hepatitis
  d. antigen
  d. bilirubin
  d. hepatitis superinfection
  d. over baseline (DOB)
  d. per mil
  d. virus
delta-aminolevulinic acid (d-ALA)
Delta-Cortef
delta-5-pregnenolone
Deltasone
delusional
Demadex
demarcate
demarcation
  corticomedullary d.
DeMartel
  D. appendix clamp
  D. appendix forceps
DeMartel-Wolfson
  D.-W. anastomosis clamp
  D.-W. clamp holder
demasculinization
demeclocycline-induced ascites
DeMeester
  D. acid score
  D. criteria
dementia
  dialysis d.
Demerol
Demethylchlortetracycline
demeure
Deming operation
Demling-Classen sphincterotome
demucosalized
  d. augmentation
  d. augmentation with gastric
    segment (DAWG)
**demucosalized augmentation with gastric
  segment (DAWG)**
denaturation
Denck esophagoscope

D

NOTES

dendritic
> d. calculus
> d. cell therapy
> d. reticular cell

denervated sphincter of Oddi

denervation
> bladder d.
> detrusor d.
> partial bladder d.
> peripheral bladder d.
> sinoaortic d. (SAD)

dengue
> hemorrhagic d.
> d. hemorrhagic fever
> d. hemorrhagic fever infection
> d. virus

Denhardt solution

Denis
> D. Browne abdominal retractor
> D. Browne operation
> D. Browne pouch
> D. Browne urethroplasty technique

Dennis
> D. clamp
> D. intestinal forceps
> D. intestinal tube

Dennis-Brooke ileostomy

Dennis-Varco pancreaticoduodenostomy

Denonvilliers fascia

densa
> lamina d.
> macula d.
> nascent macula d.

dense
> d. adhesion
> d. polyposis

densitometer
> CS-9000 d.
> Hoefer GS 300 laser d.
> Hologic d.

densitometric unit

densitometry
> bone d.
> bone mineral d. (BMD)
> calcaneal ultrasound bone d.
> double x-ray d.
> video d.

density
> bone mineral d. (BMD)
> current d.
> D-cell d.
> fat d.
> filtration slit length d.
> gastrin mRNA:G-cell d.
> d. gradient centrifugation
> intramural microvessel d. (MMD)
> lumbar spine bone mineral d.
>   (LSMB)

> prostate-specific antigen d. (PSAD)
> radiopaque d.
> slit pore length d.

dent
> D. disease
> D. sleeve
> D. sleeve catheter
> D. sleeve device
> D. supplement

dentate
> d. line
> d. margin

denticulatum
> pentastomum d.

denuded mucosa

denutrition

Denver
> D. peritoneovenous shunt
> D. pleuroperitoneal shunt

Denys-Drash syndrome (DDS)

deodorized tincture of opium (DTO)

deoxycholate
> sodium d.

deoxycholic acid

deoxycorticosterone

deoxydoxorubicin

deoxyepinephrine

5′-deoxy-5-fluorouridine (5′-DFUR)

1-deoxy-galactonojirimicin (DGJ)

deoxyribonucleic
> d. acid (DNA)
> d. acid flow cytometry
> d. acid synthesizer

deoxyspergualin (DSP)

15-deoxyspergualin

DePage-Janeway gastrostomy

Depakene

deparaffinization

Depen

dependent rubor

dephosphorylated myosin crossbridge

depletion
> mucous d.
> nephropathy of potassium d.
> plasma volume d.
> potassium d.
> protein d.
> syndrome of chloride d.

deployment
> stent d.

depolarization

Depo-Predate

Depo-Provera

deposit
> C3 d.
> electron-dense mesangial d.
> fatty d.
> hematooxyphilic d.

hemosiderin d.
liver d.
mesangial d.
peritoneal d.
seminal vesicle amyloid d.
subendothelial d.
subepithelial d.
deposition
collagen d.
encrustation d.
heavy-chain d.
ion beam-assisted d.
matrix d.
microdroplet fat d.
perisinusoidal fibrin d.
Depostat
depot
d. injection
Lupron D.
Sandostatin LAR D.
Trelstar d.
Depo-Testosterone
depressed
d. adenoma
d. cancer
d. tumor
depressed-type colorectal cancer
depression
orbital d.
pterygoid d.
respiratory d.
spermatogenesis d.
d. surface
deprivation
androgen d.
neoadjuvant hormonal d.
deranged hemostatic mechanism
derangement
metabolic d.
derivative
atropine d.
ergot d.
fibrate d.
hematoporphyrin d. (HpD)
isoxazole d.
Photofrin d.
photosensitizing hemoporphyrin d.
pivalate d.
sialylated d.
sphingolipid d.
derma

dermal
d. island-flap anoplasty
d. suture
Dermalene suture
Dermalon suture
dermatan sulfate
dermatitidis
Blastomyces d.
dermatitis, pl. **dermatitides**
allergic d.
d. artefacta
atopic d.
contact d.
factitial d.
d. herpetiformis (DH)
irritant d.
seborrheic d.
Toxicodendron d.
dermatofibroma
dermatolymphatic invasion
dermatomyositis
paraneoplastic d.
dermatopathic enteropathy
dermatophyte infection
dermatosis, pl. **dermatoses**
acute febrile neutrophilic d.
d. of hemodialysis
neutrophilic d.
reactive inflammatory vascular d.
dermoid cyst
Dermovate cream
DeRoyal Surgical grab bag
DES
diethylstilbestrol
diffuse esophageal spasm
desaturation
arterial oxygen d.
oxygen d.
des-carboxy-prothrombin
descendens
colon d.
descending
d. colon (DC)
d. diaphragm
d. duodenum
d. inhibitory reflex
d. loop colostomy
d. perineum syndrome
d. urography
descensus
d. aberrans testis
bladder d.

D

NOTES

descensus *(continued)*
    d. paradoxus testis
    rectal d.
    renal d.
    d. uteri
descent
    open renal d.
    pelvic floor d.
    perineal d.
    testicular d.
    total d.
    vaginal d.
Deschamps ligature carrier
DESD
    detrusor external sphincter dyssynergia
deserpidine
**Desferal Mesylate challenge for
  hemochromatosis**
desferrioxamine
des-gamma-carboxy
    d.-g.-c. prothrombin (DCP)
    d.-g.-c. prothrombin level
Desican test
desiccation
    blend waveform d.
    coagulase waveform d.
    cut waveform d.
    electrosurgical d.
design
    crossover d.
    microwave antenna d.
desipramine hydrochloride
desirable body weight (DBW)
Desjardins
    D. gallbladder forceps
    D. gallbladder probe
    D. gallbladder scoop
    D. gall duct probe
    D. gallstone forceps
    D. gallstone probe
    D. gallstone scoop
    D. point
Desmarres paracentesis knife
desmin
desmoid tumor
20,22-desmolase deficiency
desmoplastic
    d. reaction
    d. response
desmopressin (DDAVP)
    d. acetate
    d. response
Desmoreaux lamp
desmosomal junction
desmosome
desoximetasone
desquamated epithelium

desquamation
    tubular cell d.
dessusception
destruction
    fibroproliferative d.
destructive
    d. cholangiopathy
    d. cholangitis
destruens
    adenoma d.
Desyrel
detachment
    mucosal d.
Detachol adhesive remover
detection
    antiliver microsomal antibody d.
    breath isotope bacterial urease d.
    colorimetric d.
    fluorescent d.
    gastroenteropathy d.
    hepatitis B DNA d.
    hepatitis C virus RNA d.
    immunohistochemical d.
    radioactive d.
    RIGScan CR49 test for colorectal
      cancer d.
detection-system
detector
    C-Trak handheld gamma d.
    The Early D.
determinant
    antigenic d.
    clinical d.
    MAb IOT2-recognizing
      monomorphic DR d.
determination
    IHA d.
    indirect hemagglutination d.
detorsion
Detrol LA capsule
detrusodetrusor facilitative reflex
detrusor
    acontractile d.
    d. acontractility
    d. activity index
    d. areflexia
    d. compliance
    d. contraction
    d. contraction strength
    d. denervation
    d. external sphincter dyssynergia
      (DESD)
    d. hyperactivity
    d. hyperreflexia
    hypocontractile d.
    d. hypocontractility
    d. instability (DI)
    d. muscle decompensation

d. muscle flap
d. muscle inhibition
d. muscle instability
d. muscle leak-point pressure
d. muscle myosin
d. muscle overactivity
d. muscle potassium channel
d. muscle pressure-flow micturition study
d. muscle protrusion junction
d. muscle stability
d. muscle trabeculation
d. muscle underactivity
d. myectomy
d. sphincter dyssynergia (DSD)
d. stability
d. urethral dyssynergia
d. urinae

detrusorectomy
detrusorrhaphy
detrusosphincteric inhibitory reflex
detrusourethral inhibitory reflex
detubularization
detubularized
d. right colon reservoir
d. small bowel

detumescence
Deucher abdominal retractor
deuterium oxide
devascularization
paraesophagogastric d.
Sugiura paraesophagogastric d.

devastated urethra
devazepide
developer
Hemoccult SENSA d.

development
embryologic d.

deviated septum
deviation
axis d.
congenital penile d. (CPD)
tongue d.
tracheal d.
ulnar d.
uvular d.

device
Accutorr oscillometric d.
ACMI ulcer measuring d.
Acucise balloon cutting d.
AcuSnare polypectomy d.
AcuTrainer hand-held electronic d.

Aerochamber pediatric spacer d.
angled delivery d. (ADD)
Argon Beamer 2 d.
autostapling d.
band-ligator d.
BAS-300 transurethral thermotherapy d.
bioartificial liver support d.
BladderManager portable ultrasonic d.
broken stent retrieval d.
BSD-300 d.
Button One-Step gastrostomy d.
Carter-Thomason port closure d.
CaverMap surgical d.
charge-coupled d. (CCD)
Circe d.
circular stapling d.
contraceptive d.
cyst puncture d.
Defyne urethral assist d.
Dent sleeve d.
Digiflator digital inflation d.
Dilamezinsert d.
double-headed P190 stapling d.
EEA stapling d.
endoscopically deliverable tissue-transfixing d.
endoscopic hemoclip d.
endoscopic mucosal resection with a ligating d.
ErecAid vacuum erection d.
Erlangen magnetic colostomy d.
external urethral barrier d.
extracorporeal assist d.
extracorporeal liver assist d. (ELAD)
extracorporeal organ bioartificial liver d.
fingerstick d.
flexible delivery d.
flexible Olympus GF-eUM3 d.
fog reduction elimination d. (FRED)
Gastro-Port II feeding d.
GIA autosuture d.
Gould polygraph gastric motility measuring d.
hemoclipping application d.
Hepatix d.
implantable penile venous compression d.

D

NOTES

device *(continued)*
    indwelling stomal d.
    Insuflon insulin delivery d.
    InterStim d.
    IntraSonix TULIP laser d.
    ISOBAR barostat distension d.
    ligation d.
    linear stapling d.
    Macroplastique implantation d.
    Makler insemination d.
    Makler sperm counting d.
    Menuet Compact urodynamic
      testing d.
    Microgyn II urinary incontinence d.
    Microvasive Gold probe bipolar
      electrocautery d.
    miniature ultrasound suction d.
    Mission vacuum constriction d.
    Mission vacuum erection d.
    multiband ligating d.
    Multifire Endo GIA stapling d.
    Nachlas-Linton esophagogastric
      balloon tamponade d.
    needlescope d.
    Nottingham Key-Med introducing d.
    NovolinPen d.
    Olympus clip-fixing d.
    Olympus UES-series snare
      cautery d.
    OraSure salivary collection d.
    OSB gastrostomy d.
    PC Polygraf HR d.
    pneumatic compression d. (PCD)
    PortSaver PercLoop d.
    Pos-T-Vac vacuum erection d.
    prophylactic d.
    Prostathermer d.
    Prostatron transurethral
      thermotherapy d.
    ProTack tacking d.
    pyxigraphic d.
    Q-Maxx side-firing laser d.
    Quantum inflation d. (QID)
    Rigiflator hand-held
      inflation/deflation d.
    RigiScan d.
    ring-type rigidity measuring d.
    robotic-automated assist d.
    roticulator stapling d.
    silicone pressure sensor d.
    Soehendra stent retrieval d.
    SofTouch vacuum erection d.
    Sonoblate ablation d.
    Sony Promavica still capture d.
    Synergist vacuum erection d.
    targeted cryoablation d.
    TA stapling d.
    temporary endoprosthetic d.

    testicular hypothermia d.
    TherMatrx TMx-2000 d.
    Thermex-II transurethral prostate
      heating d.
    thread-locking d.
    transparent elastic band ligating d.
    Trimedyne Optilase 1000 d.
    Turapy d.
    UV-Flash ultraviolet germicidal
      exchange d.
    vacuum constriction d. (VCD)
    vacuum entrapment d.
    vacuum erection d. (VED)
    vacuum extraction d.
    vacuum tumescence d.
    Visiport d.
    VTU-1 vacuum erection d.
    Wallstent delivery d.
    Wedge electrosurgical resection d.
    wire-guided metal spiral retrieval d.
    Wolf Piezolith 2300 lithotripsy d.
device-related urinary tract infection
Devine
    D. colostomy
    D. exclusion
    D. hypospadias repair
Devine-Devine procedure
**Devine-Horton flip flap for hypospadias
repair**
devitalization
devolvulization
    endoscopic d.
Devonshire colic
Dew sign
DEXA
    dual-energy x-ray absorptiometry
dexamethasone
    d. sodium phosphate
    d. suppression test
    vincristine, doxorubicin, d. (VAD)
Dexatrim
dexbrompheniramine
Dexedrine
dexfenfluramine
Dexol 300
Dexon
    D. polyglycolic acid mesh
    D. suture
dexpanthenol
dexter
    ductus hepaticus d.
    ductus lobi caudati d.
dextra
    arteria colica d.
    arteria gastrica d.
    arteria gastroomentalis d.
    flexura coli d.

dextran
    d. 40, 70, 75
    d. clearance
    iron d.
    d. sieving
    d. sodium sulfate (DSS)
dextrin
dextrinizing time
dextrinosis
    limit d.
dextroamphetamine
dextrogastria
dextropropoxyphene
dextrose
DF
    discriminant function
DFT
    Doppler flow test
5′-DFUR
    5′-deoxy-5-fluorouridine
d-galactosamine
DGER
    duodenogastroesophageal reflux
DGF
    delayed graft function
DGJ
    1-deoxy-galactonojirimicin
DGR
    duodenogastric reflux
DH
    dermatitis herpetiformis
    diaphragmatic hernia
DHA
    dehydroepiandrosterone
DHAS
    dehydroepiandrosterone sulfate
DHD
    donor hepatic duct
DHFK
    Dow Hollow Fiber kidney
DHPG
    dihydroxypropoxymethyl guanine
DHT
    dihydrotestosterone
DI
    detrusor instability
    distal intestine
DiaBeta
diabetes
    alimentary d.
    fibrocalculous pancreatic d. (FCPD)
    gestational d.

    d. home screening test
    d. insipidus
    insulin-dependent d.
    d. mellitus
    pancreatic d.
diabetic
    d. autonomic neuropathy
    d. cholecystoparesis
    d. colitis
    d. diarrhea
    d. diet
    d. enteropathy
    d. gastroparesis
    d. gastropathy
    d. impotence
    insulin-treated d.
    d. ketoacidosis
    d. microangiopathy
    d. nephropathy
    d. patient
    d. urine
diabetica
    balanitis d.
diabeticorum
    gastroparesis d.
Diabinese
diabrosis
diacetate
    2′,7′-dichlorofluoresin d.
diachorema
diachoresis
Diacol
diacylglycerol (DAG)
Diacyte DNA ploidy analysis
Diagnex
    D. Blue test
    D. Blue test for gastric acid
diagnosis, pl. **diagnoses**
    colonoscopic d.
    cytologic d.
    differential d.
    endoscopic ultrasonographic d.
    endoscopic ultrasound d.
    enteroscopy d.
    histologic d.
    needle biopsy d.
    noninvasive d.
    pancreatic tumor d.
    pathological d.
    photodynamic d. (PPD)
    prenatal d.
    scintigraphic d.

D

NOTES

diagnosis *(continued)*
    serologic d.
    ultrasonic d.
    wastebasket d.
diagnostic
    d. angiography
    d. aspiration
    d. colonoscopy
    d. duodenoscope
    d. fiberoptic stomatoscopy
    d. imaging evaluation
    d. laparoscope
    d. paracentesis
    d. surgery
    d. uroradiology
diagraph
    Dianon d.
Dialose
Dialume
Dialyflex dialysis fluid
dialysance
dialysate
    bicarbonate d.
    calcium-free d.
    ethanol and phosphate enriched d.
    d. glucose concentration
    high-calcium d.
    low-calcium d.
    peritoneal d.
dialysate-to-plasma ratio
dialysis
    d. access infection
    d. access surgery
    d. adequacy
    automated peritoneal d. (APD)
    chronic ambulatory peritoneal d. (CAPD)
    continuous ambulatory peritoneal d. (CAPD)
    continuous arteriovenous hemofiltration with d.
    continuous cycler-assisted peritoneal d.
    continuous cycling peritoneal d. (CCPD)
    cycling d.
    daily d.
    daily intermittent peritoneal d. (DIPD)
    d. dementia
    d. disequilibrium syndrome
    d. encephalopathy syndrome
    d. equilibrium syndrome
    extended daily d. (EDD)
    extracorporeal d.
    high-efficiency d.
    high-flux d.
    home d.

    d. modality
    nightly intermittent peritoneal d. (NIPD)
    d. osteomalacia
    D. Outcomes Quality Initiative (DOQI)
    peritoneal d. (PD)
    d. to plasma
    profiled d.
    renal d.
    short daily d.
    d. shunt
    slow low-efficiency d. (SLED)
    sustained low-efficiency d. (SLED)
    terminal anuria vesical d.
    title peritoneal d. (TPD)
dialysis-associated hypotension
dialysis-related ascites
dialysis-to-plasma (D-P)
    d.-t.-p. urea ratio
dialysis-to-plasma urea ratio
dialytic
    d. treatment
    d. ultrafiltration (DU)
dialyzer
    AN69 membrane d.
    CA110 d.
    CA cellulose acetate membrane hollow-fiber d.
    Clirans T-series d.
    double d.
    Fresenius AG d.
    Gambro d.
    high-flux d.
    hollow-fiber d.
    d. membrane
    parallel plate d.
    760 polysulfone d.
    Renaflo hollow-fiber d.
    Renalin d.
    Renatron d.
    Terumo d.
diameter
    distal bile duct d.
    inner d. (ID)
    luminal d.
    maximum d.
    outer d. (OD)
    renal artery d.
    unequal calf d.
diaminedichloroplatinum
diamine oxidase
diaminobenzidine (DAB)
    3′,3-d. tetrahydrochloride
diamond
    d. flap
    d. jaw needle holder

D. stent
D. tube
diamorphine
Dianeal K-141
Dianon diagraph
diaphoresis
diaphoretic
diaphragm
congenital d.
crus of d.
descending d.
d. disease
duodenal d.
endoscopic ablation of antral d.
leaves of d.
mucosal ileal d.
pelvic d.
prepyloric antral d.
slit d.
urogenital d.
diaphragmatic
d. abscess
d. breathing
d. hernia (DH)
d. hernial trauma
d. hiatus
d. hump
d. muscle
d. pinch
d. pinchcock
d. surface of liver
diaphragmatocele
diaphragm-like
d.-l. stenosis
d.-l. stricture
diarrhea
acute infectious d.
Aeromonas d.
alcoholic d.
antibiotic-associated d. (AAD)
antibiotic-induced d.
anxiety-related d.
bacterial toxigenic d.
beta-lactam-associated d.
bile acid d. (type 1,2)
bile salt d.
bilious d.
bloody d.
Brainerd d.
cachectic d.
chewing gum d.
choleraic d.

cholera toxin-induced d.
chronic d.
d. chylosa
Clostridium difficile-associated d.
    (CDAD)
Cochin China d.
colliquative d.
congenital chloride d.
congenital sodium d. (CSD)
crapulous d.
critical d.
Cryptosporidia-induced d.
day-care d.
diabetic d.
dientamoeba d.
dysenteric d.
elixir d.
endemic d.
enteral d.
enterotoxin d.
explosive d.
factitious d.
familial chloride d.
fatty acid d.
fermentative d.
flagellate d.
fructose d.
functional d.
gastrogenic d.
gastrogenous d.
gluten-sensitive d.
hemorrhagic d.
hill d.
ileostomy d.
infantile d.
infectious nosocomial d.
infectious viral d.
inflammatory d.
intermittent d.
intractable d.
irritative d.
lactose-associated d.
lienteric d.
liquid d.
magnesium-induced d.
malabsorptive d.
maldigestive d.
mechanical d.
morning d.
mucous d.
nausea, vomiting, d. (NVD)
neurogenic secretory d.

NOTES

D

diarrhea *(continued)*
    nocturnal d.
    osmotic d.
    d. pancreatica
    pancreatogenic d.
    paradoxical d.
    parenteral d.
    postvagotomy d.
    putrefactive d.
    raw milk-associated d.
    rotavirus d.
    rotavirus-associated d.
    runner's d.
    secretory d.
    serous d.
    severe secretory d.
    sodium anion d.
    sorbitol d.
    stercoral d.
    d. stool
    summer d.
    toddler's d.
    toxic d.
    toxigenic d.
    traveler's d.
    tropical d.
    tubercular d.
    unrelenting d.
    viral d.
    virulent d.
    d. and vomiting (D&V)
    watery d.
    white d.
diarrheal, diarrheic
diarrhea-predominant irritable bowel syndrome
diarrheogenic
diary
    voiding d.
Diasonics
    D. DRF ultrasound unit
    D. Therasonic lithotriptor
Diasorb
diastase
    d. digestion
    pancreatic d.
    d. predigestion
diastasis
    palpable rib d.
    pubic d.
    rectus d.
    d. rectus abdominis
    wide pubic d.
diastatic serosal tear
Diastat vascular access graft
diastematomyelia
diastolic murmur
diathermal snare

diathermic
    d. cleaning
    d. fistulotomy
    d. loop
    d. loop biopsy
    d. precut needle
    d. puncture
    d. resection
diathermocoagulation
diathermy
    BICAP bipolar d.
    d. hemorrhoidectomy
    d. scissors
    d. technique
    d. wire
diathesis, pl. **diatheses**
diatrizoate
    meglumine d.
    postdilation meglumine d.
    d. sodium enema
    sodium methylglucamine d.
diatrizoic acid
diazepam emulsified injection
diaziquone
diazo reaction
diazoxide
DIB
    duodenoileal bypass
dibasic
    d. aminoacidopathy
    d. amino acid residue
Dibent Injection
Dibenzyline
dibromochloropropane (DBCP)
dibucaine
DIC
    disseminated intravascular coagulation
    drip infusion cholangiography
    DIC parameter
dichlorofluorescein
dichlorofluoresin
    $2',7'$-d. diacetate
dichotomization
dichroism
    circular d.
Dickinson FACS 400-series flow cytometer
Dickson osteotomy
diclofenac
    d. analgesic therapy
    d. sodium
dicloxacillin
dicyclomine
didanosine
didelphys
    uterus d.
Didrex
Didronel

didymalgia
didymitis
DIED
    drug-induced esophageal damage
diencephalic syndrome
dientamoeba diarrhea
diet

    absolute d.
    acid-ash d.
    ADA d.
    advance to regular d.
    alkaline-ash d.
    Andresen d.
    d. as tolerated (DAT)
    Atkins d.
    baby soft d. (BSD)
    balanced d.
    basal d.
    basic d.
    bland d.
    blenderized d.
    BRAT d.
    BRATT d.
    calcium-rich gluten-free d.
    CAPS-free d.
    challenge d.
    chemically defined d.
    clear liquid d.
    cornstarch-rich d.
    defined-formula d.
    diabetic d.
    disease-specific d.
    Ebstein d.
    elemental d.
    elimination d.
    exclusion d.
    fasting d.
    fen-phen d.
    fiber-deficient d.
    fractionated d.
    fructose-free d.
    full-liquid d.
    galactose-free d.
    gastric d.
    Giordano-Giovannetti d.
    gluten-free d. (GFD)
    gluten-rich d.
    grapefruit d.
    high-bulk, low-fat d.
    high-calorie d.
    high-carbohydrate d.
    high-fat d.
    high-fiber d.
    high-protein d.
    high-roughage d.
    high-starch d.
    hypercaloric d.
    hyperprotidic d.
    immune-enhancing d. (IED)
    Jarotsky d.
    lactose-free d. (LFD)
    liquid d.
    liver d.
    low available carbohydrate d.
    low-calorie d.
    low-fat d. (LFD)
    low-fiber d.
    low-lactose d.
    low-oxalate d.
    low-residue d.
    low-roughage d.
    low-sodium d.
    low-tyrosine, low-phenylalanine d.
    Meulengracht d.
    milk d.
    modified liver d.
    Moro-Heisler d.
    Paleolithic d.
    phen-fen d.
    Portagen d.
    progressive d.
    reducing d.
    regular d.
    rice-fruit d.
    Schmidt d.
    semielemental d.
    Sippy d.
    smooth d.
    soft bland d.
    steroid-dependent d.
    steroid-refractory d.
    d. therapy
    Travasorb Hepatic D.
    Travasorb Renal D.
    vegetarian d.
    very low calorie d. (VLCD)
    Weight Watchers d.
    Western d.

dietary

    d. advice
    d. approach to stop hypertension
    (DASH)
    d. calcium
    d. cholesterol

NOTES

D

dietary *(continued)*
    d. deficiency
    d. energy intake
    d. fat
    d. fiber
    d. gluten
    d. habit
    d. nitrite
    d. oxalate
    d. phosphate
    d. phosphorus
    d. potassium
    d. protein
    d. protein intolerance
    d. protein restriction
    d. purine
    d. sodium
    d. supplementation
dietetic regimen
diethylaminoethyl (DEAE)
diethylcarbamazine (DEC)
diethylenetriamine
    d. pentaacetic acid (DTPA)
    d. pentaacetic acid renal scan
    d. pentaacetic acid renography
diethylenetriamine-pentaacetic acid-
    galactosyl-human serum albumin
    (technetium GSA)
diethylhomospermine (DEHOP)
diethylpropion
diethylstilbestrol (DES)
dieting plateau
dietitian
Dietl crisis
dietogenetics
Dieulafoy
    D. anomaly
    D. cirsoid aneurysm
    D. disease
    D. gastric erosion
    D. gastric lesion
    D. theory
    D. triad
    D. ulcer
    D. vascular malformation
difference
    potential d. (PD)
    transmembrane electrical
      potential d.
    transmucosal potential d. (TMPD)
differential
    d. diagnosis
    d. loading
    d. neuroaxial blockade
    d. renal function test
    d. ureteral catheterization test
    WBC d.
    white blood count d.

differentiated teratoma
differentiation
    cellular d.
    chondrogenic d.
    corticomedullary d.
    endothelial cell d.
    genital d.
    gonadal d.
    impaired cell d.
    osteogenic d.
    rhabdomyoblastic d.
    sexual d.
DiffGAM
difficile
    Clostridium d. (CD)
difficulty
    defecatory d.
Diff-Quik stain
diffractometry
    x-ray d.
Diffu-K
diffuse
    d. alveolar hemorrhage (DAH)
    d. alveolar hemorrhage syndrome
    d. angiodysplasia
    d. angiokeratoma
    d. antral gastritis (DAG)
    d. diabetic glomerulosclerosis
    d. esophageal spasm (DES)
    d. hepatocellular carcinoma
    d. hyperplastic polyposis
    d. liver disease
    d. lobular fibrosis
    d. malignant mesothelioma (DMM)
    d. mesangial proliferation
    d. mesangial sclerosis (DMS)
    d. metastasis
    d. mucosal polyposis
    d. nodular hyperplasia (DNH)
    d. pain
    d. pancreatitis
    d. patchy nephrogram
    d. proliferative glomerulonephritis
    d. redness (DR)
    d. suppurative nephritis
    d. tenderness
    d. varioliform gastritis
    d. vasculitis of polyarteritis nodosa
      type
diffusely tender abdomen
diffuser
    cylindrical d.
diffusion
    disk d.
    interstitial d.
    pericapillary d.
    transcapillary d.
diffusive transport

diffusum
    angiokeratoma corporis d.
Diflucan
diflunisal
difluoromethylornithine
DIF-test
    direct immunofluorescence test
digastric
    d. anterior muscle
    d. impression
    d. posterior muscle
    d. triangle
Di-Gel
DiGeorge
    D. anomaly
    D. syndrome
Digepepsin
digestant
digestion
    brush-border d.
    diastase d.
    proteolytic d.
    RNAse d.
    solid food d.
digestive
    d. apparatus
    d. disease (DD)
    D. Disease National Coalition
        (DDNC)
    d. enzyme
    d. fever
    d. gastrosuccorrhea
    d. glycosuria
    d. system
    d. tract
    d. tube
digestive-respiratory
    d.-r. fistula (DRF)
    d.-r. fistula stent
digestorius
    apparatus d.
    tubus d.
Digibar 190
Digiflator digital inflation device
digit
    sausage d.
digital
    d. manipulation of pubic hair
    d. rectal evacuation
    d. rectal examination (DRE)
    d. subtraction angiography

    d. venous subtraction angiography
        (DSA)
digitalis
digitally guided biopsy
digitonin
Digitrapper
    D. Mark II pH monitoring system
    D. MKIII
    Synthetics dual-channel, solid
        state D.
diglycoaldehyde
Dignity incontinence pants
digoxin
dihydrate
    calcium oxalate d.
    octahedral-shaped d.
dihydroergotoxine
dihydropyridine
dihydrotestosterone (DHT)
    d. gel
    d. synthesis
dihydroxyadenine
    2,8-d. calculus
    d. urinary lithiasis
dihydroxyaluminum
    d. aminoacetate
    d. sodium carbonate
dihydroxyeicosatrienoic acid
dihydroxyphenylalanine (DOPA)
dihydroxypropoxymethyl guanine
    (DHPG)
dihydroxy salt
dihydroxyvitamin D3
    1,25-d. D3 (1,25(OH)2 D3)
    1,25-dihydroxyvitamin D
diiodohydroxyquin
diisopropyliminodiacetic
    d. acid (DISDA, DISIDA)
    d. acid enterogastroesophageal
    reflux study
Dilamezinsert (DMI)
    D. device
    D. penile prosthesis
    D. urologic instrument
Dilantin
dilatation (*var. of* dilation)
dilated
    d. bile duct
    d. gallbladder
    d. loops of bowel
    d. pupil
    d. vein

D

NOTES

dilating
    d. catheter
    d. catheter-gastrostomy tube
      assembly
    d. set
dilation, dilatation
    achalasia balloon d.
    anal d.
    aneurysmal d.
    balloon d.
    biliary d.
    bowel d.
    Brown-McHardy pneumatic mercury
      bougie d.
    capillary d.
    d. catheter (DC)
    cavernous artery d.
    cecal d.
    colonic d.
    corpora cavernosum d.
    cystic d.
    cystoscopy and d. (C&D)
    ductal d.
    Eder-Puestow d.
    endoscopic balloon d. (EBD)
    endoscopic balloon sphincter d.
      (EBSD)
    endoscopic papillary balloon d.
      (EPBD, EPD)
    esophageal d.
    d. of esophagus
    extrahepatic biliary cystic d.
    gastric d.
    Grüntzig balloon d.
    d. of hemorrhoid
    hepatic web d.
    hydrostatic balloon d.
    inadequate d.
    intrahepatic biliary cystic d.
    intrahepatic ductal d.
    Lord d.
    Maloney d.
    mechanical ureteral d.
    medical d.
    mucosal vascular d.
    percutaneous balloon d.
    periportal sinusoidal d.
    peroral esophageal d.
    pneumatic bag esophageal d.
    pneumatic balloon catheter d.
    pneumostatic d.
    prostate gland transurethral
      balloon d.
    pyloric d.
    d. range
    rectal d.
    d. of the stomach
    submucosal vascular d.

    d. therapy
    through-the-scope balloon d.
    tract d.
    transurethral balloon d.
    TTS balloon d.
    upper tract d.
    urethral d.
    Uromat d.
    Wirsung d.
dilator
    achalasia d.
    Achiever balloon d.
    American Dilation System d.
    American Endoscopy d.
    Amplatz fascial d.
    anal d.
    Backhaus d.
    Bakes common duct d.
    balloon d.
    Barnes common duct d.
    biliary balloon d.
    bougie d.
    Brown-McHardy pneumatic d.
    bullet-tip d.
    Celestin graduated d.
    circular anal d.
    Clark common duct d.
    Cunningham-Cotton sleeve
      coaxial d.
    Dotter d.
    Eder-Puestow metal olive d.
    Einhorn d.
    Eliminator PET biliary balloon d.
    ERCP d.
    esophageal balloon d.
    Ferris biliary duct d.
    fluoroscopy-guided balloon d.
    French d.
    Garrett d.
    Grüntzig d.
    Hegar rectal d.
    high-diameter d.
    Hurst bullet-tip d.
    Hurst mercury-filled d.
    Hurst-Tucker pneumatic d.
    KeyMed advanced d.
    Kollmann d.
    Kron bile duct d.
    Kron gall duct d.
    Maloney-Hurst d.
    Maloney mercury-filled
      esophageal d.
    Maloney tapered-tip d.
    mercury-filled d.
    mercury-weighted d.
    metal-olive d.
    Microvasive CRE esophageal d.
    Microvasive Rigiflex balloon d.

modified polyethylene d.
Mosher d.
Murphy common duct d.
Nottingham One-Step tapered d.
Nottingham ureteral d.
Olbert balloon d.
olive-tipped plastic d.
Optilume prostate balloon d.
over-the-endoscope Witzel d.
d. placement
d. placement failure
Plummer d.
pneumatic balloon d.
polyethylene balloon d.
polyvinyl d.
probe d.
prostate balloon d.
Quantum TTC balloon d.
Ramstedt pyloric stenosis d.
rectal d.
Rider-Moeller d.
Rigiflex achalasia d.
Rigiflex TTS balloon d.
Russell peel-away sheath d.
Savary-Gilliard over-the-wire d.
Savary tapered thermoplastic d.
Sippy esophageal d.
Soehendra catheter d.
Starck d.
Stucker bile duct d.
tapered-tip d.
through-the-scope d.
TTS d.
Tucker spindle-shaped d.
vessel d.
Walther d.
Witzel d.
Dilaudid
dilaurate
fluorescein d. (FDL)
dildo, dildoe
dilevalol
dilinoleoylphosphatidylcholine (DLPC)
Dilomine
diltiazem therapy
dilute
d. iodinated contrast
d. Russell viper venom test
(DRVVT)
dilution
agar d.

clonal d.
serial d.
dilutional hyponatremia
dimenhydrinate
dimercaptosuccinic
d. acid (DMSA)
d. acid renal scan
d. acid scintigraphy
dimeric
d. acidic glycoprotein (DAG)
d. IgA
dimerization
dimethyl
d. iminodiacetic acid scan
d. sulfate cystitis
d. sulfoxide (DMSO)
dimethylester
cystine d. (CDE)
1,2-dimethylhydrazine
dimethyl-4-phenylpiperazinium (DMPP)
dimethylpolysiloxane (DMPS)
dimethylsulfoxide
dimethyltriazenoimidazole carboxamide
(DTIC)
diminished
d. bowel sounds
d. branching abnormality
d. gag reflex
diminuta
Hymenolepis d.
diminutive
d. adenomatous polyp
d. colonic polyp
d. hyperplastic polyp
d. polyp (DP)
dimorphic
dimple
celiac d.
dimpling
focal d.
postanal d.
skin d.
Dinamap Plus monitor
dinitrate
isosorbide d.
d. and mononitrate ester
dinitrochlorobenzene (DNCB)
Dinitrophenol
dinner
d. pad
test d.

D

NOTES

dinucleotide
  flavin adenine d.
  nicotinamide adenine d. (NADH)
Diocto
  D.-C
  D.-K
diode
  interstitial d.
  d. laser
Diodrast
Dioeze
Diogenes syndrome
Diomed laser
DIONEX 2000 system
Diosuccin
dioxide
  thorium d.
DiPAS-positive granule
DIPD
  daily intermittent peritoneal dialysis
Dipentum
dipeptidase
  N-acetylated alpha-linked d.
dipeptide
diphallia
diphallus
diphemanil
Diphenatol
diphenhydramine
diphenoxylate
diphenylthiazole
diphosphatase
  adenosine d. (ADPase)
diphosphate
  adenosine d. (ADP)
  d. buffer solution
5′-diphosphate
  uridine 5′-d. (UDP)
diphosphonate
  ^{99m}Tc-labeled stannous methylene d.
diphtheria
diphtheritic
  d. cystitis
  d. enteritis
diphyllobothriasis
Diphyllobothrium
  D. lata
  D. parvum
  D. taenioides
diploid
  d. cell
  d. tumor
diploidy
dipole
dipotassium
  clorazepate d.
dipropionate
  beclomethasone d. (BDP)

Diprospan
dipslide
  Uricult d.
dipstick
  Chemstrip LN d.
  d. protein
  urinalysis d.
  urine d.
Dipylidium caninum
dipyridamole
direct
  d. bilirubin
  d. cautery puncture
  d. current
  d. current electrocoagulation
  d. current electrotherapy trial
  d. cystenterostomy
  d. extension
  d. fragmentation technique
  d. immunobead test
  d. immunofluorescence test (DIF-test)
  d. inguinal hernia
  d. laryngoscopy
  d. manipulation
  d. nerve stimulation graciloplasty
  d. percutaneous jejunostomy (DPJ)
  d. percutaneous jejunostomy tube
  d. percutaneous transhepatic cholangiography
  d. tubular toxicity
  d. vesicoureteral scintigraphy (DVS)
  d. vision
  d. vision internal urethrotomy (DVIU)
  d. vision liver biopsy
direct-beam coupler for TURP
direction
  isoperistaltic d.
director
  grooved d.
  D. Guidewire system
  Larry rectal d.
  probe and groove d.
direct-reading bilirubinometer
Direx Tripter X-1 lithotriptor
dirithromycin
Disa
  D. electromyography
  D. needle electrode
  D. 5500 urograph
disaccharidase
  d. assay
  d. deficiency
  d. enzyme activity
disaccharide
  d. intolerance
  d. lactose

nonabsorbable d.
d. tripeptide
disaggregation
Disalcid Capsules/Tablets
disappearing phenomenon
discharge
    anal d.
    bloody d.
    cervical d.
    chyme d.
    clear d.
    nasal d.
    nipple d.
    purulent d.
    urethral d. (UD)
    vaginal d.
discoid
    d. lupus erythematosus
    d. rash
discoloration
discomfort
    epigastric d.
    postligation d.
    posttreatment d.
    preexisting d.
disconnection
    ureteral endoscopic d.
discontinuation
    transient d.
discontinuity
    pelvic d.
discrete
    d. bleeding source
    d. mass
    d. narrowing
    d. nodule
    d. organ enlargement
discriminant function (DF)
discriminator
    EMI APED amplifier d.
DISDA
    diisopropyliminodiacetic acid
disease
    acalculous gallbladder d.
    acid-peptic d.
    acquired cystic kidney d. (ACKD)
    acquired renal cystic d. (ARCD)
    actinomycotic esophageal d.
    acute abdominal vascular d.
    acute graft-versus-host d.
    acute idiopathic inflammatory
      bowel d.

acute on chronic liver d.
  (AOCLD)
acute polycystic d.
Addison d.
adrenal d.
adult celiac d. (ACD)
adult familial hyaline membrane d.
adult polycystic kidney d. (APKD)
adult polycystic liver d. (APLD)
adynamic bone d. (ABD)
African-American Study of
  Kidney D.
Ajmalin liver d.
Albarran d.
alcoholic liver d. (ALD)
alpha-1-antitrypsin d. (AATD)
alpha-1-antitrypsin deficiency d.
alpha-chain d.
alpha heavy-chain d.
Alstrom d.
alveolar hydatid d.
American Association for the
  Study of Liver D.'s (AASLD)
Andersen d.
anorectal d.
anti-GBM d.
antiglomerular basement
  membrane d.
aplastic bone d.
arteriosclerotic renal artery d.
  (ASO-RAD)
atheroembolic renal d. (AERD)
atherosclerotic renovascular d.
atypical distribution of d.
atypical gallbladder d.
autoimmune thyroid d.
autosomal dominant polycystic
  kidney d. (ADPKD)
autosomally recessively inherited d.
autosomal recessive polycystic
  kidney d. (ARPKD)
Banti d.
Barrett d.
Bassen-Kornzweig d.
Behçet d.
benign anorectal d. (BAD)
Berger d.
Besnier-Boeck-Schaumann d.
Biermer d.
biliary tract d.
black liver d.
bleeding acid-peptic d.

D

NOTES

disease *(continued)*
　Blount d.
　bone d.
　Botkin d.
　Bouchard d.
　Bourneville d.
　bowel d.
　Bowen d.
　Bradley d.
　brancher glycogen storage d.
　branch renal artery d.
　Bright d.
　Brinton d.
　Bruton d.
　Budd d.
　Budd-Chiari d.
　Byler d.
　Cacchi-Ricci d.
　calculous gallbladder d.
　calculus d.
　cardiovascular d.
　Caroli d.
　Castleman d.
　cavernous artery d.
　celiac sprue d.
　cerebrovascular d.
　Chagas d.
　Chagas-Cruz d.
　Cherchevski d.
　Chiari d.
　cholestatic liver d.
　cholesterol ester storage d. (CESD)
　choline deficiency liver d.
　chronic active liver d. (CALD)
　chronic cholestatic liver d.
　chronic glomerular d.
　chronic graft-versus-host d. (c-GVHD)
　chronic granulomatous d.
　chronic inflammatory d.
　chronic inflammatory bowel d. (CIBD)
　chronic liver d.
　chronic obstructive pulmonary d. (COPD)
　chronic parenchymal liver d.
　chronic progressive tubulointerstitial d.
　chylomicron retention d.
　chylopoietic d.
　CMV ulcerative d.
　coeliac d.
　collagen vascular d.
　colorectal d.
　complement-mediated immune glomerular d.
　concomitant d.
　congenital cystic d.

congenital polycystic d. (CPD)
connective tissue d.
Corbus d.
Cori d.
coronary artery d.
Cowden d.
Cowen d.
crescentic fold d.
Creutzfeldt-Jakob d.
Crigler-Najjar d.
Crohn d. (CD)
Cruveilhier d.
Cruz-Chagas d.
cryptogenic liver d.
Curschmann d.
Cushing d.
cysticercus d.
cystic liver d.
cytotoxic liver d.
Darier d.
debrancher glycogen storage d.
deficiency d.
Degos d.
de novo renal d.
Dent d.
diaphragm d.
Dieulafoy d.
diffuse liver d.
digestive d. (DD)
diverticular d.
drug-related liver d.
Dubin-Sprinz d.
Ducrey d.
duodenal ulcer d.
Dupuytren d.
Durand-Nicholas-Favre d.
early-onset graft-versus-host d.
Ebstein d.
echinococcal cyst d.
end-stage liver d. (ESLD)
end-stage renal d. (ESRD)
Epstein d.
estrogen-induced liver d.
extensive pelvic d.
extraabdominal d.
extracapsular d.
extramammary Paget d. (EMPD)
Fabry d.
familial Crohn d.
fatty liver d.
Fenwick d.
fibrocystic d. of the pancreas
fibroobliterative d.
fibropolycystic liver d.
fistulizing Crohn d.
fistulous Crohn d.
Forbes d.
Fournier d.

fulminant Crohn d.
functional bowel d.
gamma heavy-chain d.
Gamna d.
gastric mucosal d.
gastritis-associated peptic ulcer d.
gastroduodenal Crohn d.
gastroesophageal reflux d. (GERD)
Gaucher d.
Gee d.
Gee-Herter d.
Gee-Herter-Heubner d.
Gee-Thaysen d.
Gierke d.
Gilbert d.
Glenard d.
glomerular basement membrane d.
glomerulocystic kidney d.
glycogen storage d.
Goldstein d.
gonococcal perihepatis pelvic
  inflammatory d.
Goodpasture d.
Gordon d.
G protein d.
graft-versus-host d. (GVHD)
granulomatous bowel d.
Graves d.
Grey Turner d.
Gross d.
H d.
Hailey-Hailey d.
halothane-induced d.
Hanot d.
Harley d.
Hartnup d.
HBsAg-negative, anti-HCV-negative
  chronic liver d. (NBNC CLD)
heavy chain deposition d.
Hebra d.
hepatic cystic d.
hepatic Hodgkin d.
hepatic metastatic d.
hepatic venoocclusive d.
hepatic venous web d.
hepatitis C virus-associated
  venoocclusive d.
hepatobiliary fibropolycystic d.
hepatobiliary tract d.
hepatocellular d.
hepatolenticular d.
herring-worm d.

Hers d.
Herter d.
Herter-Heubner d.
Heubner-Herter d.
Hirschsprung d.
Hodgkin d.
homologous protein-overload d.
hookworm d.
Hutinel d.
hydatid cyst d.
hyperacute graft-versus-host d.
hypertensive autosomal dominant
  polycystic kidney d.
hypoplastic glomerulocystic d.
idiopathic inflammatory bowel d.
  (IIBD)
ileocolic d.
ileocolonic Crohn d.
immunodeficiency d.
immunoproliferative small
  intestinal d. (IPSID)
inactive Crohn d.
infantile celiac d.
infantile polycystic d. (IPCD)
infiltrative d.
inflammatory bowel d. (IBD)
intramural atheromatous d.
iron storage d.
ischemic bowel d.
Johne d.
juvenile nephronophthisis-medullary
  cystic d.
Kashin-Beck d.
Katayama d.
Kennedy d.
Keshan d.
kidney glomerulocystic d.
Kimmelstiel-Wilson d.
Kimura d.
Kinnier Wilson d.
Klebs d.
Klemperer d.
Kohlmeier-Degos d.
Kyasanur Forest d.
Kyrle d.
Lane d.
Larrey-Weil d.
Leigh d.
Leiner d.
Leyden d.
Lhermitte-Duclos d.
Liddle d.

D

NOTES

disease *(continued)*
    light chain deposition d. (LCDD)
    Lignac d.
    Lignac-Fanconi d.
    liver d.
    liver hydatid d.
    Löwe d.
    luminal Crohn d.
    lung d.
    Lyell d.
    Lyme d.
    Mackenzie d.
    macrovascular d.
    malabsorption d.
    malignant biliary obstructive d.
    Manson d.
    maple-syrup urine d. (MSUD)
    Marchiafava-Micheli d.
    Marie-Strumpell d.
    Marion d.
    medullary cystic d.
    Ménétrier d.
    Ménière d.
    Menkes d.
    mesenteric inflammatory
      venoocclusive d. (MIVOD)
    mesenteric vascular d.
    metabolic liver d.
    metabolic stone d.
    metastatic Crohn d. (MCD)
    microcystic d. of renal medulla
    microvillus inclusion d.
    Milroy d.
    minimal change d.
    mixed connective tissue d.
      (MCTD)
    Modification of Diet in Renal D.
      (MDRD)
    mucosal d.
    multicystic kidney d.
    Munk d.
    muscle layer d.
    Mya d.
    mycobacterial d.
    myeloproliferative d.
    National Institute of Diabetes,
      Digestive and Kidney D.
      (NIDDK)
    neoplastic d.
    neurohumoral d.
    Niemann-Pick d.
    nil d.
    Nisbet d.
    non-A–G chronic liver d.
    nonalcoholic fatty liver d.
      (NAFLD)
    non-B, non-C chronic liver d.
      (NBNC CLD)

    noncalculous d.
    noncommunicating polycystic d.
    nondiabetic proteinuric renal d.
    nonerosive gastroesophageal
      reflux d.
    nonerosive reflux d. (NERD)
    nonobstructive hepatic
      parenchymal d.
    nonorgan confined d.
    oasthouse urine d.
    obstructive gastroduodenal Crohn d.
    Ohara d.
    oral d.
    organic neurologic d.
    Ormond d.
    Osler-Weber-Rendu d.
    ovarian d.
    Paget extramammary d.
    Paget perianal d.
    panacinar d.
    pancreatic d.
    pancreaticobiliary d.
    parasitic liver d.
    parathyroid d.
    parenchymal liver d.
    Parkinson d.
    paroxysmal motor d.
    patella d.
    Payr d.
    pelvic inflammatory d. (PID)
    peptic reflux d.
    peptic ulcer d. (PUD)
    perforated ulcer d.
    perianal Crohn d.
    perineal Crohn d.
    Peyronie d.
    pilonidal sinus d.
    polycystic kidney d.
    polycystic liver d. (PCLD, PLD)
    Pompe d.
    post jejunoileal bypass hepatic d.
    Potter d.
    predominant hyperparathyroid
      bone d. (PHBD)
    preeclamptic liver d.
    preexisting d.
    primary glomerular d.
    protozoal d.
    pseudoalcoholic liver d.
    pseudo-Whipple d.
    radiation-induced d.
    Rayer d.
    reactive airway d. (RAD)
    recessive polycystic kidney d.
    Recklinghausen d.
    rectal d.
    reflux d.
    Reichmann d.

Reiter d.
renal arterial occlusive d.
renal bone d.
renal cystic d.
renal fibromuscular d.
renal hydatid d.
Rendu-Osler-Weber d.
renovascular d.
rheumatic d.
Rokitansky d.
Rossbach d.
Ruysch d.
Saunders d.
Schilder d.
Schindler d.
schistosomal liver d.
Schönlein-Henoch d.
Schultz d.
scleroderma bowel d.
sexually related intestinal d.
sexually transmitted d. (STD)
sickle cell d.
sigmoid d.
skeletal muscle d.
skin d.
small intestinal Crohn d.
space-occupying d.
Spencer d.
steely-hair d.
Steinert d.
steroid-dependent Crohn d.
steroid-refractory Crohn d.
Stokvis d.
stone d.
Strachan d.
Stühmer d.
subacute liver d.
subserosal d.
suprahilar d.
systemic mast cell d.
Takayasu d.
Tangier d.
terminal ileal d.
testicular Hodgkin d.
Thaysen d.
thin basement membrane d.
  (TBMD)
thin glomerular basement
  membrane d.
thromboembolic d.
thyroid d.
Tis d.

transfusion-related chronic liver d.
tubulointerstitial d.
tufting d.
tunnel d.
unilocular hydatid d.
upper tract d.
uremic medullary cystic d.
urinary tract d.
urologic d.
valvular heart d.
Van Bogaert d.
van Buren d.
van den Bergh d.
vascular d.
venereal d.
venoocclusive liver d.
venous outflow obstructive d.
venous web d.
von Gierke d.
von Hippel-Lindau d.
von Recklinghausen d.
von Rokitansky d.
von Willebrand d.
Wassilieff d.
Weber-Christian d.
Weil d.
Werdnig-Hoffman d.
Westphal-Strümpell d.
Whipple d. (WD)
Wilkie d.
Wilson d. (WD)
Wolman d.
disease-free survival curve
disease-specific
    d.-s. diet
    d.-s. isolation
dish
    Side-Fire reflecting d.
disialosyl Lea
DISIDA
    diisopropyliminodiacetic acid
    DISIDA enterogastroesophageal
      reflux study
    DISIDA scan
disimpaction
    colonoscopic d.
disinfectant
    Abocide d.
    Actril d.
    Asepti-steryl d.
    Burnishine d.
    Calgocide d.

D

NOTES

disinfectant *(continued)*
    Cold Spor d.
    cyclic urinary d.
    Endospore d.
    Enzol d.
    Metricide d.
    Omnicide d.
    ProCide d.
    Sporacidin d.
    Vespore d.
    Wavicide d.
disinfection
    high-level d. (HLD)
disintegration
    endoscopic stone d.
DisIntek reagent strip
disjoined pyeloplasty
disk
    anal d.
    bilaminar embryonic d.
    d. diffusion
    d. kidney
    laser d.
    d. margin
    Marlen double-faced adhesive d.
    Molnar d.
dislodgement
dislodger
    stone d.
dismembered
    d. anastomosis
    d. pyeloplasty
    d. reimplanted appendicocystostomy
dismutase
    superoxide d. (SOD)
disobliteration
disodium
    balsalazide d.
    cefotetan d.
    d. cromoglycate
    d. edetate
Disolan
Disonate
disopyramide phosphate
disorder
    acid-base d.
    acid-related d. (ARD)
    acid secretory d.
    anorexia nervosa and associated d. (ANAD)
    appetite d.
    autoimmune connective tissue d.
    autosomal dominant d.
    blood coagulation d.
    cardiovascular d.
    connective tissue d.
    deglutition d.
    esophageal motility d. (EMD)
    esophageal motor d.
    evacuation d.
    fat storage d.
    feeding d.
    functional bowel d. (FBD)
    functional gastrointestinal d. (FGID)
    gastric motility d.
    Hartnup d.
    humoral immunodeficiency d.
    intestinal motility d.
    iron overload d.
    lower motor neuron bladder d.
    lymphoproliferative d.
    metabolic d.
    mixed connective tissue d.
    motility d.
    myeloproliferative d.
    National Association of Anorexia Nervosa and Associated D.'s
    neurodegenerative d.
    neurologic d.
    nonspecific esophageal motility d. (NEMD)
    papulosquamous d.
    pelvic floor d.
    posttransplant lymphoproliferative d. (PTLD)
    psychological d.
    psychosomatic d.
    pulmonary d.
    rectal evacuatory d. (RED)
    seizure d.
    spastic motor d.
    urachal d.
    vasomotor d.
    vesiculobullous d.
    wound healing d.
disordered
    d. acrosome reaction of spermatozoa
    d. motility
Di-Sosul
dispar
    Entamoeba d.
Di-Spaz
Dispenstirs
displacement
    bowel d.
    fiber lock d.
    fish-hook d.
    gallbladder d.
display
    high-definition video d. (HDVD)
disposable
    d. forceps
    d. pudendal nerve electrode
    d. sheathed flexible sigmoidoscope
    d. trocar

disposable-sheath flexible gastroscope
disruption
    pancreatic duct d.
disruptor
    endocrine d.
Disse
    space of D.
    D. space
dissecting
    d. abdominal aneurysm
    d. balloon
    d. renal artery aneurysm
dissection
    aortic d.
    autonomic nerve-preserving three-space d.
    blunt and sharp d.
    circumferential mucosal d.
    electrosurgical d.
    en bloc d.
    extended obturator node and iliopsoas node d.
    extraperitoneal endoscopic pelvic lymph node d. (EEPLND)
    finger fracture d.
    flap d.
    intersphincteric rectal d.
    intracapsular d.
    intramural air d.
    laparoscopic pelvic lymph node d. (LPLND)
    lateral node d.
    limited obturator node d.
    lymph node d.
    d. margin
    meticulous d.
    minilaparotomy pelvic lymph node d.
    nerve-sparing lymph node d.
    node d.
    partial zonal d. (PZD)
    pelvic d.
    per anum intersphincteric rectal d.
    plane of d.
    rectal d.
    renal hilar d.
    retroperitoneal lymph node d. (RPLD)
    scissors d.
    d. scissors
    sharp d.
    spontaneous d.

    submucosal d.
    suprahilar lymph node d.
    three-field d.
    three-space d.
    ultrasonic d.
    ureteral d.
dissector
    Beaver d.
    CUSA d.
    Kittner d.
    McDonald stone d.
    Mixter d.
    Niblitt d.
    peanut d.
    Spacemaker balloon d.
    sponge d.
    ultrasonic aspirator and d.
disseminated
    d. cancer
    d. CMV infection
    d. histoplasmosis
    d. intravascular coagulation (DIC)
    d. lupus erythematosus (DLE)
    d. metastasis
    d. peritoneal adenomucinosis
dissemination
    metastatic d.
dissimilatory sulfate reduction
dissociated medium
dissolution
    contact d.
    d. of gallstone
    methyl tertbutyl ether stone d.
    MTBE gallstone d.
distal
    d. bile duct
    d. bile duct diameter
    d. blind stomach
    d. colitis
    d. colon
    d. convoluted tubule (DCT)
    d. duodenum
    d. esophageal ring
    d. esophageal stenosis
    d. esophageal stricture
    d. esophagus
    d. gastrectomy
    d. ileitis
    d. intestine (DI)
    d. pancreatectomy
    d. pouch leak
    d. renal tubular acidosis (dRTA)

D

NOTES

distal *(continued)*
    d. renal tubular necrosis
    d. shave section
    d. splenorenal shunt (DSRS)
    d. tubular acting agent
    d. tubule (DT)
    d. ureterectomy
    d. venous plexus
distance
    peritoneal-anal d.
distant
    d. abscess
    d. heart sound
    d. metastasis
distasonis
    Bacteroides d.
distended
    d. abdomen
    d. bladder
distensibility
distensible hydrodynamics
distention, distension
    abdominal d.
    colonic d.
    esophageal balloon d.
    gaseous d.
    gastric d.
    intestinal d.
    intraesophageal balloon d. (IEBD)
    intraluminal d.
    isobaric gastric d.
    postprandial d.
    rectal d.
    d. ulcer
    visible abdominal d.
distomiasis
    intestinal d.
distorted crypt architecture
distortion
    crypt architectural d.
distress
    epigastric d.
    functional bowel d. (FBD)
    mild d.
    moderate d.
    respiratory d.
distribution
    folate d.
    geographic d.
    liver d.
    node d.
    vasoactive intestinal peptide d.
    volume of d. (Vd)
disturbance
    acid-base d.
    gait d.
    phytoestrogen-induced menstrual
      cycle d.

disulfide cross-linked fibril
disulfiram
disulfiram-like effect
dithiothreitol (DTT)
Ditropan
    D. XL
Dittel
    D. operation
    D. sound
Diucardin
Diupres
diuresis
    alcohol d.
    osmotic d.
    postobstructive d.
    tubular d.
    water d.
diuretic
    high-ceiling d.
    hydragogue d.
    kaliuretic d.
    loop d.
    d. nuclear renography
    osmotic d.
    potassium-sparing d.
    refrigerant d.
    d. renal quantitative camera study
    d. renal scintigraphy
    thiazide d.
diuretic-induced hypokalemia
diuria
Diurigen
diurnal
    d. continence
    d. cycle
    d. enuresis
    d. incontinence
    d. urine osmolality
    d. variation
Diutensen-R
diutinum
    erythema elevatum d.
divalent mineral
diversion
    acidosis after urinary intestinal d.
    biliopancreatic d.
    Bricker urinary d.
    Camey enterocystoplasty urinary d.
    Camey I orthotopic urinary d.
    d. colitis
    continent catheterizable urinary d.
    continent cutaneous d.
    continent supravesical bowel
      urinary d.
    cutaneous urinary d.
    Duke pouch cutaneous urinary d.
    external biliary d.
    fecal d.

Gil-Vernet ileocecal cystoplasty
  urinary d.
Gil-Vernet orthotopic urinary d.
Hammock technique urinary d.
hemi-Kock urinary d.
heterotopic d.
ileal conduit urinary d.
ileal neobladder urinary d.
ileocecal cutaneous d.
ileocolic urinary d.
ileocolonic pouch urinary d.
Indiana continent reservoir
  urinary d.
initial proximal d.
jejunal cutaneous urinary d.
Khafagy modified ileocecal
  cystoplasty urinary d.
Kock pouch cutaneous urinary d.
Leadbetter ileal loop d.
Le Bag urinary d.
LeDuc technique urinary d.
Mainz pouch cutaneous urinary d.
orthotopic urinary d.
partial external biliary d.
primary urinary d.
d. proctitis
rectal bladder urinary d.
split-nipple technique urinary d.
Studer reservoir urinary d.
subcutaneous urinary d.
supravesical urinary d.
transductal cystodigestive d.
tunneled technique urinary d.
urinary d.
Wallace technique urinary d.
diversionary ileostomy
diversus
  Citrobacter d.
diverticula (*pl. of* diverticulum)
diverticular
  d. abscess
  d. bleeding
  d. disease
  d. hemorrhage
  d. phlegmon
diverticulectomy
  bladder d.
  endocavitary bladder d.
  Harrington esophageal d.
  pharyngoesophageal d.
  urethral d.
  vesical d.

diverticulitis
  acute d.
  cecal d.
  chronic d.
  duodenal d.
  d. evaluation
  Meckel d.
  perforating d.
  sigmoid d.
diverticulogram
diverticuloma
diverticulopexy
diverticulosis
  acquired d.
  bleeding d.
  colonic d.
  congenital d.
  esophageal intramural d.
  gastric d.
  giant d.
  jejunal d.
diverticulostomy
  endoscopic stapling d.
diverticulotomy
  endoscopic d.
diverticulum, pl. **diverticula**
  d. of Akerlund
  d. ampullae ductus deferentis
  biliary d.
  bladder congenital d.
  bleeding d.
  caliceal d.
  cecal d.
  diverticula of colon
  colonic d.
  congenital bladder d.
  cricopharyngeal d.
  duodenal d.
  epiphrenic d.
  esophageal d.
  false d.
  fluid-filled d.
  d. fulguration
  Ganser d.
  giant d.
  giant colonic d. (GCD)
  Graser d.
  Heister d.
  hepatic d.
  Hutch d.
  hypopharyngeal d.
  d. ilei verum

D

NOTES

diverticulum *(continued)*
    inflamed d.
    intestinal d.
    intraluminal duodenal d. (IDD)
    intramural d.
    inverted sigmoid d.
    juxtapapillary d. (JPD)
    juxtapapillary duodenal d.
    Kirchner d.
    long-neck d.
    Meckel d.
    midesophageal d.
    mucosal d.
    noncommunicating d.
    d. of Nuck
    pancreatic d.
    perforated d.
    periampullary duodenal d.
    peripapillary d.
    Pertik d.
    pharyngeal d.
    pharyngoesophageal d.
    pressure d.
    Rokitansky d.
    ruptured sigmoid d.
    sigmoid d.
    solitary d.
    supradiaphragmatic d.
    traction d.
    unroofing of d.
    urachal d.
    ureteric d.
    urethral d.
    vesical d.
    vesicourachal d.
    volvulated Meckel d.
    Zenker d.
diverting
    d. loop colostomy
    d. loop ileostomy
    d. stoma
    d. stoma creation
divided pancreas
divided-stoma colostomy
division
    urethral plate d.
divisum
    incomplete pancreas d. (IPD)
    pancreas d. (PD)
Dixon-Thomas-Smith clamp
Dizac
DJJ
    duodenojejunal junction
DLC
    dual-lumen catheter
DLE
    disseminated lupus erythematosus

DLPC
    dilinoleoylphosphatidylcholine
DM
    duodenal mucosa
DMEM
    Dulbecco modified Eagle medium
DMI
    Dilamezinsert
        DMI urologic instrument
DMM
    diffuse malignant mesothelioma
DMPP
    dimethyl-4-phenylpiperazinium
DMPS
    dimethylpolysiloxane
DMS
    diffuse mesangial sclerosis
DMSA
    dimercaptosuccinic acid
        DMSA scan
        DMSA scintigraphy
        ^{99m}Tc DMSA
DMSO
    dimethyl sulfoxide
        DMSO cystitis
DNA
    deoxyribonucleic acid
        DNA aneuploidy
        DNA array
        branched chain DNA (bDNA)
        complementary DNA
        DNA flow cytometry
        genomic DNA
        DNA haploid cell
        HBV DNA
        HBV genomic DNA
        hepatitis B-like DNA
        DNA hypomethylation
        DNA immunization
        DNA labeling kit
        DNA laddering
        DNA microarray technology
        DNA ploidy analysis
        DNA ploidy pattern
        DNA polymerase
        DNA polymorphism
        DNA proliferation
        DNA Sequencing System
        single-parameter DNA
        DNA stemline
        DNA synthesis
DNCB
    dinitrochlorobenzene
        DNCB immunological study
DNH
    diffuse nodular hyperplasia
DOB
    delta over baseline

Dobbhoff
    D. biofeedback monitor
    D. bipolar coagulation probe
    D. enteral feeding bag
    D. gastrectomy feeding tube
    D. gastric decompression tube
    D. PEG tube
dobutamine
docetaxel
Dock test meal
Docucal-P
docusate sodium
dodecadactylitis
dodecadactylon
dog-ear of anastomosis
Dogiel type I, II morphology
DO2-haplotype
Dohlman esophagoscope
dolantin
dolasetron
dolichocolon with pseudoobstruction
DoLi S extracorporeal shock wave lithotriptor
Dolobid
dolorimeter
    Chatillon d.
dolorosa
    nephritis d.
dolphin grasping forceps
dolphin-type atraumatic forceps
domain
    alternative cell attachment d.
    carboxyterminal noncollagenous d.
    cleaved extracellular d.
    COOH-terminal SH2 d.
    effector d.
    Kringle d.
    membrane-spanning d. (MDS)
    NH2-terminal SH2 d.
    nucleotide-binding d. (NBD)
    SH2-binding d.
    src-homology 2 d.
dome
    d. of bladder
    gallbladder d.
    d. of liver
    trabeculation of bladder d.
Domeboro solution
dome-shaped internal bumper
dome-tip electrode
domiciliary urinary tract infection
Domino transplant

domperidone
donation
    live renal d.
    organ d.
Donnagel
Donnagel-PG
Donnamar
Donna-Sed
Donnatal
    D. No. 2
Donnazyme
donor
    artificial insemination d. (AID)
    d. dendritic cell
    four antigen-matched d.
    d. hematopoietic cell microchimerism
    d. hepatectomy
    d. hepatic duct (DHD)
    kidney d.
    d. kidney
    living d. (LD)
    living related d.
    living unrelated d. (LURD)
    nitric oxide d.
    d. of nitric oxide
    related living d. (RLD)
    sulphydryl d.
donor/recipient race matching
donor-specific transfusion (DST)
donor-type microchimerism
Donovan body
donovani
    Leishmania d.
    Leishmania donovani d.
donovanosis
Donphen
donut
    circular stapler d.
doom
    triangle of d.
DOPA
    dihydroxyphenylalanine
dopamine
    d. agonist
    d. antagonist
    d. beta hydroxylase
dopaminergic
    d. agonist
    d. medication
Dopar
dopexamine

D

NOTES

Doppler
color flow D.
D. color flow imaging
D. effect
endoscopic color D.
D. flow test (DFT)
D. operation
penile D.
D. perfusion index (DPI)
D. probe
pulsed D.
D. QAD-1
D. Quantum color flow system
D. sonography of the SMA
D. ultrasonography
D. ultrasonography angiography
D. ultrasound intestinal blood flow measurement
DOQI
Dialysis Outcomes Quality Initiative
d'orange
peau d.
Dormia
D. noose
D. stone basket
D. stone basket catheter
Dornier
D. compact lithotriptor
D. electrohydraulic watertank lithotriptor (HM3, HM4)
D. extracorporeal shock wave lithotripsy
D. gallstone lithotriptor
D. HM4 lithotriptor
D. HM3 waterbath lithotriptor
D. MFL 5000 urological workstation
D. MPL 9000 electrohydraulic lithotriptor ultrasound focusing system
D. MPL 9000 gallstone lithotripsy
D. MPL 5000 lithotriptor
D. Urotract cystoscopy table
dorsal
d. bud
d. curve plication
d. lithotomy
d. lithotomy position
d. lumbotomy
d. lumbotomy incision
d. mesogastrium
d. nerve conduction velocity
d. nerve of penis
d. pancreatic artery
d. pancreatic duct
d. penile artery
d. point
d. rhizotomy
d. root ganglia
d. slit
d. tunical tuck
d. vagal complex
d. vein
d. vein complex (DVC)
d. vein patch graft
dorsalis
arteria pancreatica d.
tabes d.
dorsocranial
dorsosacral position
dorsum
d. of penis
d. of testis
dosage
radiation d.
sclerosant d.
dose
breakthrough d.
conceptus d.
dosepak
Hytrin D.
dose-response
dosimeter
single-channel in vivo light d.
dot-blot hybridization
dot-plotted probe
Dotter
D. catheter
D. dilator
Doubilet
D. sphincterotome
D. sphincterotomy
double
d. balloon enteroscopy
d. bite biopsy
d. bladder
d. channel esophagogram
d. contrast
d. dialyzer
d. duct sign
d. enterostomy
d. gallbladder
d. gracilis wrap
d. incontinence
d. J-shaped reservoir
d. loop pouch
d. loop tourniquet
d. penis
d. pyloroplasty
d. pylorus
d. reverse alpha-sigmoid loop
d. stapling technique (DST)
d. tracking of barium
d. uterus
d. x-ray densitometry

**double-accessory channel therapeutic
   endoscope**
double-antibody sandwich system
double-balloon technique
double-barrel
    d.-b. colostomy
    d.-b. ileostomy
    d.-b. reservoir
double-blind randomized study
double-bubble duodenal sign
double-chamber hemodiafiltration
double-channel
    d.-c. colonoscope
    d.-c. endoscope
    d.-c. fistulotome
    d.-c. sphincterotome
    d.-c. videoendoscope
double-contrast
    d.-c. barium enema (DCBE)
    d.-c. barium enema examination
    d.-c. barium examination of the
       upper gastrointestinal tract (DCGI)
    d.-c. barium meal
    d.-c. esophagram
    d.-c. radiography
    d.-c. roentgenography
double-cuff urinary sphincter
double-dose I.V. Timentin
**double-faced island flap for hypospadias
   repair**
double-folded cup-patch technique
double-headed
    d.-h. P190 stapler
    d.-h. P190 stapling device
double-head spermatozoon
double-J
    d.-J. catheter
    d.-J. indwelling catheter stent
    d.-J. silicone stent
    d.-J. Surgitek catheter stent
    d.-J. ureteral stent
double-lumen
    d.-l. balloon catheter
    d.-l. endoprosthesis
    d.-l. gastric laryngeal mask airway
    d.-l. injection catheter
    d.-l. irrigation cannula
    d.-l. tapered-tip papillotome
    d.-l. tube
double-peaked wave
double-pigtail
    d.-p. endoprosthesis

    d.-p. prosthesis
    d.-p. stent
double-puncture laparoscopy
double-spoon forceps
double-stapled
    d.-s. ileal pouch-anal anastomosis
    d.-s. ileal reservoir
double-staple technique
DoubleStent
    D. biliary endoprosthesis
    D. biliary endoprosthesis stent
double-tail spermatozoon
doubling time
doubly ligated
doughnut
    d. lesion
    stapler d.
doughnut-shaped balloon
doughy
    d. abdomen
    d. consistency
Douglas
    D. abscess
    cul-de-sac of D.
    D. fold
    line of D.
    D. pouch
    D. rectal snare
    rectouterine pouch of D.
    semicircular line of D.
doula
Dow-Corning ileal pouch catheter
**Dowd II prostatic balloon dilatation
   catheter**
Dow Hollow Fiber kidney (DHFK)
down
    tacked d.
downhill esophageal varix
downregulation
downscatter
downstage
downstaging
    hormonal d.
downstream
    d. signaling protein
    d. signal transduction
Down syndrome
doxacurium
doxazosin mesylate
doxepin
doxercalciferol injection
Doxinate

D

NOTES

doxorubicin
    d., bleomycin sulfate, vinblastine (ABV)
    d., bleomycin sulfate, vinblastine, dacarbazine (ABVD)
doxycycline-metronidazole-bismuth subcitrate triple therapy
doxycycline monohydrate
Doyen
    D. abdominal retractor
    D. abdominal scissors
    D. gallbladder forceps
    D. intestinal clamp
    D. intestinal forceps
    D. operation
    D. raspatory
    D. rib elevator
DP
    diminutive polyp
D-P
    dialysis-to-plasma
    D-P urea ratio
DP-1 lithotriptor
DPC
    delayed primary closure
DPEG
    dual percutaneous endoscopic gastrostomy
D-penicillamine
DPI
    daily protein intake
    Doppler perfusion index
DPJ
    direct percutaneous jejunostomy
    DPJ tube
DQ2 haplotype
DR
    diffuse redness
    HLA DR
DR2
    DR2 HLA-DRB tissue type
    DR2 1501 HLA-DRB tissue type
    DR2 1502 HLA-DRB tissue type
    DR2 1601 HLA-DRB tissue type
    DR2 1602 HLA-DRB tissue type
DR3
    HLA DR3
    DR3 HLA-DRB tissue type
DR4
    HLA DR4
    DR4 HLA-DRB tissue type
DR5
    heterozygous DR5
DR7
    D. haplotype
    D. HLA-DRB tissue type
DR9 HLA-DRB tissue type

drag
    solvent d.
dragon pyelogram
drain
    Blair silicone d.
    Chaffin-Pratt d.
    cigarette d.
    closed suction d.
    Davol sump d.
    ERCP nasobiliary d.
    fluted J-Vac d.
    four-wing Malecot d.
    Hemovac Suction Standard d.
    Hollister irrigator d.
    Jackson-Pratt d.
    J-Vac d.
    Mikulicz d.
    nasobiliary d. (NBD)
    nasocystic d.
    Nélaton rubber tube d.
    Penrose sump d.
    perineal d.
    Pezzer d.
    Quad-Lumen d.
    Redivac suction d.
    Redon d.
    Relia-Vac d.
    stab-wound d.
    suction d.
    sump d.
    surgical d.
    Synder d.
    Teflon nasobiliary d.
    transnasal pancreatico-biliary d.
    transpapillary d.
    T-tube d.
    two-wing Malecot d.
    van Sonnenberg sump d.
    d. volume
    Wangensteen d.
drainable ostomy pouch
drainage
    antegrade ureteral d.
    bedside d. (BSD)
    biliary d.
    button d.
    caliceal d.
    d. catheter
    closed d.
    continuous bladder d.
    continuous catheter d.
    continuous suction d.
    CT-guided abscess d.
    CT-guided pseudocyst d.
    duodenal d.
    endoscopic biliary d.
    endoscopic nasobiliary d. (ENBD)
    endoscopic nasobiliary catheter d.

endoscopic nasogallbladder d. (ENGBD)
endoscopic pancreatic d.
endoscopic retrograde biliary d. (ERBD)
endoscopic transgastric d.
endoscopic transpapillary cyst d. (ETCD)
external d.
gravity-dependent d.
guided percutaneous d.
incision and d. (I&D)
internal biliary d.
J-Vac closed wound d.
lymphocele internal d.
lymphocele percutaneous d.
nasobiliary d.
nasogastric d.
nasopancreatic d.
open d.
pancreaticoduodenal venous d.
passive chest d.
percutaneous abscess d.
percutaneous antegrade biliary d.
percutaneous biliary d. (PBD)
percutaneous transhepatic d. (PTD)
percutaneous transhepatic biliary d. (PTBD)
postoperative irrigation-suction d.
Pyridium test of vaginal d.
sanguineous d.
serosanguineous d.
suction d.
tidal d.
transduodenal d.
transgastric d.
transhepatic biliary d.
transluminal pseudocyst d.
transmural d. (TMD)
transpapillary d.
T-tube d.
d. tube
Wangensteen d.
wound d.
drainage-resistant pseudocyst
draining sinus
Drake uroflowmeter
Drake-Willock
D.-W. delivery system
D.-W. peritoneal dialysis system
Dramamine
Drapanas shunt

drape
barrier d.
fenestrated d.
Lingeman 3-in-1 procedure d.
Lingeman TUR d.
O'Connor d.
surgical d.
Drash syndrome
DRB gene
DRE
digital rectal examination
Dreiling tube
Dremel Moto-Tool
dressing
Acticoat composite d.
Acticoat foam d.
Adaptic d.
adhesive d.
anorectal d. (ARD)
antiseptic d.
bio-occlusive d.
bolus d.
bulky d.
CarboFlex odor control d.
Coban d.
CombiDERM non-adhesive absorbant d.
Compeed Skinprotector d.
dry sterile d.
Elastoplast d.
d. forceps
gauze d.
Kling d.
LYOfoam d.
Montgomery strap d.
nonadhesive d.
occlusive collodion d.
Op-Site d.
pressure d.
SaliCept freeze-dried d.
Signa Dress Hydrocolloid d.
sterile d.
Tegaderm d.
Telfa d.
Tielle Plus hydropolymer d.
tie-over d.
DRF
digestive-respiratory fistula
DR1 HLA-DRB tissue type
dribble
postmicturition d.
postvoid d.

NOTES

dribbling
    urinary d.
drift
    pronator d.
drilling tract
drink
    Boost Nutritional Energy D.
drinking
    d. habit
    psychogenic water d.
    voluntarily stopping eating and d.
      (VSED)
drip
    alkaline milk d.
    d. infusion cholangiography (DIC)
    d. infusion cholecystography
    intragastric d.
    intravenous d.
    Murphy d.
    postnasal d.
driver
    automatic needle d.
    Haney needle d.
    laparoscopic needle d.
    long vascular needle d.
    needle d.
dromedary hump
dronabinol
drooling
droop
    flank d.
drooping lily sign
droperidol
dropped bladder
dropsical
    d. nephritis
    d. nephropathy
dropsy
    abdominal d.
    cutaneous d.
    nutritional d.
    peritoneal d.
Drosophila melanogaster
dRTA
    distal renal tubular acidosis
drug
    aminobiphosphonate gastrotoxic d.
    anorectic d.
    antagonistic d.
    anticholinergic d.
    antiemetic d.
    antilipemic d.
    antimotility d.
    antimuscarinic d.
    antimycobacterial d.
    antisecretory d.
    antispasmodic d.
    d. carrier system

COX-2-selective nonsteroidal
    antiinflammatory d.
crude d.
cyclooxygenase 2-selective
    nonsteroidal antiinflammatory d.
d. hepatotoxicity
H2 receptor-blocking d.
hydrocholeretic d.
immunoregulatory d.
immunosuppressive d.
d. intoxification
lipid-lowering d.
d. metabolism
neurolytic d.
neuropsychotropic d.
nonnephrotoxic d.
nonsteroidal antiinflammatory d.
    (NSAID)
parasympatholytic d.
parasympathomimetic d.
prokinetic d.
psychotropic d.
d. reaction
recreational d.
d. resistance
second-line d.
serotonergic d.
d. therapy
vasoactive d.
drug-induced
    d.-i. acute hepatic injury
    d.-i. acute pancreatitis
    d.-i. acute tubular necrosis
    d.-i. cholestasia
    d.-i. cirrhosis
    d.-i. colitis
    d.-i. constipation
    d.-i. damage
    d.-i. erection
    d.-i. esophageal damage (DIED)
    d.-i. esophagitis
    d.-i. gastritis
    d.-i. hepatitis
    d.-i. pain
    d.-i. priapism
    d.-i. renal failure
    d.-i. steatosis
    d.-i. ulcer
drug-related liver disease
Drummond
    artery of D.
    marginal artery of D.
DRVVT
    dilute Russell viper venom test
DRw8 HLA-DRB tissue type
DRw10 HLA-DRB tissue type
DRw11 HLA-DRB tissue type
DRw12 HLA-DRB tissue type

DRw13 HLA-DRB tissue type
DRw14 HLA-DRB tissue type
dry
- d. colostomy
- d. ejaculation
- d. heaves
- d. mucous membrane
- d. skin
- d. sterile dressing
- d. swallow
- d. swallow on esophageal manometry
- d. vomiting
- d. weight

DS
- Bactrim DS
- Septra DS
- Sulfatrim DS
- trimethoprim-sulfamethoxazole DS

DSA
- digital venous subtraction angiography

DSD
- detrusor sphincter dyssynergia

D16S283 marker

DSP
- deoxyspergualin

DSRS
- distal splenorenal shunt

DSS
- dextran sodium sulfate

DST
- donor-specific transfusion
- double stapling technique
- duodenal secretin test

DT
- distal tubule

DTH
- delayed-type hypersensitivity

DTIC
- dimethyltriazenoimidazole carboxamide

DTO
- deodorized tincture of opium

DTPA
- diethylenetriamine pentaacetic acid
  - indium-111 DTPA
  - DTPA renal scan
  - DTPA renography

DTT
- dithiothreitol

DU
- dialytic ultrafiltration
- duodenal ulcer

dual
- d. percutaneous endoscopic gastrostomy (DPEG)
- d. percutaneous gastrostomy tube

dual-energy
- d.-e. CT scan
- d.-e. x-ray absorptiometry (DEXA, DXA)

dual-lumen
- d.-l. catheter (DLC)
- d.-l. papillotome

DualMesh hernia repair
dual-photon absorptiometry
Dual-Port system
Dubin-Amelar varicocele classification
Dubin-Johnson syndrome
Dubin-Sprinz
- D.-S. disease
- D.-S. syndrome

Dubowitz syndrome
Duchenne-type muscular dystrophy
duck-bill forceps
Duckett
- D. meatal advancement
- D. procedure

Ducrey disease
ducreyi
- *Haemophilus d.*

duct
- accessory pancreatic d.
- anomalous junction of pancreaticobiliary d.'s (AJPBD)
- anomalous pancreaticobiliary d. (APBD)
- arborization of d.'s
- beaded hepatic d.
- Bellini d.
- Bernard d.
- bifurcation of common bile d.
- bile d.
- branch pancreatic d.
- d. cannulation
- clubbed common bile d.
- collecting d. (CD)
- common d. (CD)
- common bile d. (CBD)
- common hepatic d.
- cortical collecting d. (CCD)
- cystic d. (CD)
- dilated bile d.
- distal bile d.
- donor hepatic d. (DHD)

D

NOTES

duct *(continued)*
  dorsal pancreatic d.
  ductal d.
  ejaculatory d.
  epididymis lymphatic d.
  excretory d.
  extrahepatic bile d.
  fusiform widening of d.
  gall d.
  Gartner d.
  genu of pancreatic d.
  hepatic d.
  horseshoe anomaly of the
    pancreatic d.
  impacted cystic d.
  infected bile d.
  infundibulum of bile d.
  inner medullary collecting d.
    (IMCD)
  interlobular bile d.
  intrahepatic bile d.
  intrapancreatic bile d.
  irregular d.
  left hepatic d. (LHD)
  Leydig d.
  d. lumen
  Luschka d.
  main pancreatic d. (MPD)
  medullary collecting d.
  mesonephric d.
  middle extrahepatic bile d.
  müllerian d.
  narrow-caliber d.
  nontransected pancreatic d.
  normal-caliber d.
  outer medullary collecting d.
  pancreatic d.
  papillomatosis of intrahepatic
    bile d.
  perilobular d.
  peripheral bile d.
  preampullary portion of bile d.
  prepapillary bile d.
  proximal bile d.
  Rathke d.
  right hepatic d.
  d. of Santorini
  serpiginous microcystic d.
  Skene d.
  spiral fold of cystic d.
  Stensen d.
  subvesical d.
  tapered common bile d.
  tear d.
  terminal bile d.
  terminal inner medullary
    collecting d.
  thoracic d.

  upstream pancreatic d.
  vitelline d.
  vitellointestinal d. (VID)
  Wharton d.
  d. of Wirsung
  d. of Wolff
  wolffian d.
ductal
  d. change
  d. cystadenoma
  d. decompression
  d. dilation
  d. duct
  d. epithelial hyperplasia
  d. epithelium
  d. hypertension
  d. obstruction
  d. stricture
  d. system
  d. system perforation
ductectatic
  d. mucinous cystadenoma
  d. tumor
ductogram
  pancreatic d.
ductography
  peroral retrograde
    pancreaticobiliary d.
  postsphincterotomy d.
ductopenia
  idiopathic adulthood d.
ductopenic rejection
ductular structure
ductule
ductuli
  d. aberrantes
  d. biliferi
  d. efferentes
  d. interlobulares
  d. prostatica
ductulus aberrans superior
ductus
  d. biliaris
  d. biliferi
  d. choledochus
  d. cysticus
  d. deferens
  d. ejaculatorius
  d. epididymidis
  d. excretorius glandulae
    bulbourethralis
  d. excretorius vesiculae seminalis
  d. hepaticus communis
  d. hepaticus dexter
  d. hepaticus sinister
  d. lobi caudati dexter
  d. lobi caudati sinister
  d. mesonephricus

d. muelleri
d. pancreaticus
d. pancreaticus accessorius
d. paraurethrales
d. prostatici
d. wolffi

Duecollement
    D. hemicolectomy
    D. maneuver

Duette double-lumen ERCP instrument
Duffield deep surgery scissors
Dufourmentel technique
DUG
    dynamic urinary graciloplasty

Duhamel
    D. operation
    D. pull-through

Duke
    D. pouch
    D. pouch cutaneous urinary
      diversion

Dukes
    D. B-1
    D. classification of carcinoma
    D. signet cell (A, B, C)
    D. stage
    D. staging system

Dul45 cell line
Dulbecco modified Eagle medium
  (DMEM)
Dulcolax bowel preparation
dullness
    hepatic d.
    liver d.
    d. to percussion
    shifting d.
    splenic d.
    tympanitic d.

dull pain
dumbbell-shaped
    d.-s. caliceal extension
    d.-s. shadow

dumdum fever
Dumon-Gilliard
    D.-G. endoprosthesis system
    D.-G. prosthesis introducer
    D.-G. prosthesis pushing tube

dumping
    late d.
    d. stomach
    d. syndrome

dump kidney

duocrinin
duodenal
    d. acidification
    d. adenocarcinoma
    d. adenoma
    d. antrum
    d. atresia
    d. biopsy
    d. bleeding
    d. brake
    d. bulb
    d. bulb deformity
    d. cancer
    d. cap (DC)
    d. carcinoid
    d. C-loop
    d. cluster unit
    d. compression
    d. diaphragm
    d. diverticulitis
    d. diverticulum
    d. drainage
    d. effect
    d. endoscopic polypectomy
    d. erosion
    d. exclusion (DE)
    d. fistula
    d. fluid collection
    d. foreign body
    d. fossa
    d. gastrinoma
    d. hemangiomatosis
    d. hematoma
    d. histoplasmosis
    d. impression
    d. impression on liver
    d. injury
    d. juice
    d. leiomyoma
    d. lesion
    d. loop
    d. lumen
    d. lymphoma
    d. lymphonodular hyperplasia
    d. mass
    d. metastasis
    d. mucosa (DM)
    d. neurofibroma
    d. obstruction
    d. orifice
    d. papilla
    d. perforation

D

NOTES

duodenal *(continued)*
  d. polyp
  d. polyposis
  d. pressure wave
  d. reflux
  d. secretin test (DST)
  d. seromyectomy
  d. stenosis
  d. stump
  d. sweep
  d. switch
  d. telangiectasia
  d. terminus
  d. trauma
  d. tube
  d. tuberculosis
  d. tumor
  d. ulcer (DU)
  d. ulceration
  d. ulcer disease
  d. ulceroinflammatory ulcer
  d. ulcer perforation (DUP)
  d. varix
  d. villus
  d. wall hamartoma
  d. web
duodenale
  Ancylostoma d.
duodenalis, pl. **duodenales**
  Giardia d.
  plica d.
duodenectomy
duodeni
  cryptae mucosae d.
duodenitis
  chronic atrophic d.
  Crohn d.
  erosive d.
duodenobiliary
  d. pressure gradient
  d. reflux
duodenocaval fistula
duodenocholangeitis
duodenocholecystostomy
duodenocholedochotomy
duodenocolic fistula
duodenocystostomy
duodenoduodenostomy
duodenoenterocutaneous fistula
duodenoenterostomy
duodenogastric reflux (DGR)
duodenogastroesophageal reflux (DGER)
duodenogastroscopy
  retrograde d. (RDG)
duodenogastrostomy
  end-to-side d.
duodenogram

duodenography
  hypotonic d.
duodenohepatic
duodenoileal bypass (DIB)
duodenoileostomy
duodenojejunal
  d. angle
  d. flexure
  d. fold
  d. hernia
  d. junction (DJJ)
duodenojejunalis
  flexura d.
duodenojejunostomy
  suprapapillary Roux-en-Y d.
duodenolysis
duodenomesocolic fold
duodenopancreaticocholedochal rupture
duodenopancreatic reflux
duodenorrhaphy
duodenoscope
  diagnostic d.
  Fujinon DUO-XT d.
  Fujinon ED7-XT d.
  Fujinon ED-200XU d.
  Fujinon ED-310XU d.
  Fujinon ED-410XU d.
  Fujinon ED7-XU2 video d.
  Fujinon EVD-XL video d.
  Fujinon EVD-XT d.
  Fujinon FD-100XU d.
  Fujinon 310XU video d.
  JF-200 d.
  JF-IT20 d.
  large-channel therapeutic d.
  master d.
  Olympus EW-series fiberoptic d.
  Olympus JF-series video d.
  Olympus JF1T10 fiberoptic d.
  Olympus JF-V-series video d.
  Olympus JT-series video d.
  Olympus PJF-series pediatric d.
  Olympus TJF-10, -100, -200 d.
  side-viewing fiberoptic d.
  side-viewing video d.
  standard d.
  therapeutic side-viewing d.
  TJF-100,-130 large channel d.
  TJF-10,-20 video d.
  video d.
duodenoscopy
duodenostomy
  Witzel d.
duodenotomy
  transverse d.
duodenum
  Brunner gland of d.
  brunneroma of d.

button of d.
C-loop of d.
closed d.
d. deformed by scarring
descending d.
distal d.
gastric metaplasia of d.
mucous crypt of d.
obstruction d.
scarified d.
ulcer d.
duodenum-preserving pancreatic head resection
Duodopa
Duo-Flow catheter
Duosol
Duo-Tube feeding tube
DUP
duodenal ulcer perforation
DUPAN 2 tumor marker
Duphalac
Duplay operation
duplex
d. Doppler endosonography
d. ileum
d. sonography
duplicated gallbladder
duplicate uterus
duplication
alimentary tract d.
d. anomaly
biliary tree d.
bladder d.
colonic d.
complete d.
d. cyst
gastric d.
incomplete d.
renal d.
tubular colonic d.
urethra d.
Dupuytren
D. contracture
D. disease
D. hydrocele
D. suture
D. tourniquet
durable healing
Duracep biopsy forceps
DURAglide 3 stone balloon catheter
Dura-II positionable penile prosthesis
Duralone

dural patch reconstruction
Duramorph
Durand-Nicholas-Favre disease
Duraphase inflatable penile prosthesis
Durasphere injectable bulking agent
duration
esophageal body contraction d.
mean treatment d.
phasic wave d.
d. time
Duricef
Duroziez sign
Durrani dorsal vein complex ligation needle
duskiness
stomal d.
dusky stoma
Duval
D. distal pancreaticojejunostomy
D. procedure
Duverney foramen
Duvoid
D&V
diarrhea and vomiting
DVC
dorsal vein complex
DVIU
direct vision internal urethrotomy
DVS
direct vesicoureteral scintigraphy
dwarf kidney
dwell period
DXA
dual-energy x-ray absorptiometry
D-xylose
D-x. absorption test
D-x. malabsorption
dyad
mother-infant d.
dyadic relationship
Dyazide
Dyclone
dye
Alcian blue d.
basic d.
cationic d.
Congo red d.
Evans blue d.
indigo carmine d.
indocyanine green d. (ICG)
iodine d.
Kiton red d.

D

NOTES

dye *(continued)*
    d. laser
    metachromatic d.
    methylene blue d.
    orthochromatic d.
    radiopaque d.
    rapid emptying of d.
    rhodamine 6G d.
    d. scattering method
    d. sham intrarenal lesion
    d. spraying
dye-exclusion test
DynaCirc
Dynaflex
    D. penile implant
    D. penile prosthesis
DYNAFLUVE
    dynamic fluorescence video endoscopy
dynamic
    d. closure pressure
    d. cystourethroscopy
    d. fluorescein angiography
    d. fluorescence video endoscopy
    (DYNAFLUVE)
    d. ileus
    d. infusion cavernosometry
    d. infusion cavernosometry and
    cavernosonography
    d. proctography
    d. urethral profile study
    d. urinary graciloplasty (DUG)
dynamoscopy
dynograph
dynorphin
dyphylline
dysarthric
dysautonomia
    Riley-Day syndrome of familial d.
dysautonomy
dyschezia
    defecatory d.
dyscoordinate hyoid movement
dysdiadochokinesia
dysenteriae
    Shigella d.
dysenteric
    d. algid malaria
    d. arthritis
    d. diarrhea
dysentery
    amebic d.
    bacillary d.
    d. bacillus
    balantidial d.
    bilharzial d.
    catarrhal d.
    ciliary d.
    ciliate d.

    epidemic d.
    flagellate d.
    Flexner d.
    fulminant d.
    fulminating d.
    giardiasis d.
    helminthic d.
    institutional d.
    Japanese d.
    malarial d.
    malignant d.
    protozoal d.
    schistosomal d.
    scorbutic d.
    Shiga d.
    Shigella d.
    Sonne d.
    spirillar d.
    spirochetal d.
    sporadic d.
    viral d.
dysesthesia
dysfunction
    anal sphincter d.
    anorectal sensorimotor d.
    autonomic d.
    balanced voiding d.
    bladder neck d.
    Bradley classification of voiding d.
    cardiopulmonary baroreflex d.
    cavernous autonomic nerve d.
    colorectal physiologic d.
    constitutional hepatic d.
    corporeal venous occlusive d.
    ejaculatory d.
    erectile d.
    esophageal body motor d.
    gastric d.
    geriatric voiding d.
    hereditary spastic paraplegia
    voiding d.
    hindgut d.
    human erectile d.
    International Continence Society
    classification of voiding d.
    intrinsic sphincter d. (ISD)
    Lapides classification of voiding d.
    late graft d.
    lower urinary tract d. (LUTD)
    low pressure-low flow voiding d.
    mechanoreceptor d.
    multiple organ system d. (MOSD)
    neurogenic erectile d.
    neuroimmune d.
    neuropathic voiding d.
    neutrophil d.
    nondiabetic neurogenic erectile d.
    nonneurogenic voiding d.

outlet d.
pancreatic exocrine d.
pediatric voiding d.
pelvic floor d.
platelet d.
postgastrectomy d.
postparacentesis circulatory d.
  (PCD)
posttransplant renal d.
progressive renal d.
psychogenic erectile d.
psychologic d.
puborectalis d.
reflex voiding d.
sensory voiding d.
sphincter d.
sphincter of Oddi d. (SOD)
transfer d.
traumatic corporeal veno-
  occlusive d.
tubular cell d.
urodynamic d.
venoocclusive d.
visceral d.

dysfunctional
d. bleeding
d. voiding

dysgenesis
anorectal d.
gonadal d.
mixed gonadal d.

dysgenetic
d. fibrous band
d. gonad

dysgenitalism
dysgerminoma
dysgeusia
dysgonesis
dyskeratosis follicularis
dyskinesia
bile duct d.
biliary d.
primary ciliary d.

dyskinetic
d. cilia syndrome
d. puborectalis

dyslipidemia
dyslipidosis
dysmetabolic syndrome
dysmorphic
d. erythrocyte

d. red blood cell
d. vessel

dysmorphy
extrarenal d.

dysmotility
chronic intestinal d. (CID)
d. dyspepsia
esophageal d.
gallbladder d.

dysmotility-like dyspepsia
dysorexia
dyspareunia
dyspepsia
acid d.
adhesion d.
appendicular d.
appendix d.
atonic d.
biliary d.
catarrhal d.
cholelithic d.
dysmotility d.
dysmotility-like d.
fermentative d.
flatulent d.
functional d.
gastric d.
gastroduodenal d.
mononuclear d.
nervous d.
nonorganic d.
nonulcer d. (NUD)
Optimal Regimen Cures
  Helicobacter-Induced D.
  (ORCHID)
postcholecystectomy flatulent d.
reflex d.
reflux d.
refluxlike d.
ulcer d.
ulcerlike d.

dyspeptica
angina d.

dyspeptic urine
dysperistalsis
dysphagia
d. aortica
Atkinson scoring system for d.
contractile ring d.
esophageal d.
d. inflammatoria
liquid food d.

NOTES

D

dysphagia *(continued)*
    d. lusoria
    malignant d.
    d. nervosa
    neurogenic d.
    oropharyngeal d.
    d. paralytica
    postvagotomy d.
    preesophageal d.
    progressive d.
    sideropenic d.
    soft food d.
    solid food d.
    d. spastica
    transfer d.
    vallecular d.
    d. valsalviana
dysphagic
dysphagy
dysphonia
dysphoria
dysplasia
    acrocephalopolydactylous d.
    anal squamous d.
    anal transitional zone d.
    arteriohepatic d.
    Barrett d.
    bladder d.
    bronchopulmonary d.
    epithelial d.
    fibromuscular d. (FMD)
    fibrous d.
    flat d.
    genital d.
    high-grade d. (HGD)
    kidney d.
    liver cell d.
    low-grade d. (LGD)
    lung d.
    malignant d.
    mucosal d.
    multicystic renal d.
    neuroectodermal d.
    nonulcer d.
    polypoid d.
    renal segmental renal d.
    urothelial d.
dysplasia-associated lesion or mass (DALM)
dysplasia-to-carcinoma sequence
dysplastic
    d. cell
    d. focus
    d. kidney
    d. mucosa
dyspnea
Dysport

dyspragia
    d. angiosclerotica
    d. intermittens
    d. intermittens angiosclerotica intestinalis
    d. intestinalis
dysraphic malformation
dysraphism
    bony d.
    neurospinal d.
    occult spinal d.
    spinal d.
    spine d.
dysreflexia
    autonomic d.
dysrhythmia
    ESWL related d.
    gastric electrical d.
    glucagon-evoked gastric d.
dysspermatogenic sterility
dyssynergia
    biliary d.
    detrusor external sphincter d. (DESD)
    detrusor sphincter d. (DSD)
    detrusor urethral d.
    pelvic floor d.
    rectoanal d.
    rectosphincteric d.
    vesical external sphincter d. (VSD)
    vesicosphincteric d.
dystonia
dystonic phenomenon
dystopia
    d. transversa externa testis
    d. transversa interna testis
dystopic kidney
dystrophic
    d. calcification
    d. penis
dystrophica
    epidermolysis bullosa d.
dystrophy
    adiposogenital d.
    asphyxiating thoracic d.
    Duchenne-type muscular d.
    hyperplastic d.
    Jeune asphyxiating thoracic d.
    muscular d.
    myotonic muscular d.
    oculocerebrorenal d.
    oculopharyngeal muscular d.
    reflex sympathetic d.
    Steinert myotonic d.
dystrypsia
dysuresia
dysuria
    psychic d.

dysuria-pyuria syndrome
dysuric

dyszoospermia

NOTES

D

E
erythrocyte
E sign
E1
E1, E2, E6 protein
prostaglandin E1
E2
prostaglandin E. (PGE2)
E-1023
enzyme immunoassay E.
e10 electrosurgery system
E1b protein
E2F protein
EABV
effective arterial blood volume
Eadie-Hofstee
E.-H. plot
E.-H. transformation
EAEC
enteroadherent *Escherichia coli*
EaggEC
enteroaggregative *Escherichia coli*
Eagle-Barrett syndrome
Eagle minimal essential medium (EMEM)
EAL
endoscopic aspiration lumpectomy
EAM
endoscopic aspiration mucosectomy
EAP
etoposide, Adriamycin, Platinol
ear
bladder e.
Earle
E. hemorrhoid clamp
E. medium
E. rectal probe
E. solution
early
e. gastric cancer (EGC)
e. growth response factor-α
e. satiety
The E. Detector
early-onset graft-versus-host disease
earth-eating
EAS
external anal sphincter
EASIE
Easi-Lav lavage
easily reducible hernia
Easprin

EAST1
enteroaggregative *Escherichia coli* heat-stable enterotoxin 1
Eastern Cooperative Oncology Group (ECOG)
Eastman cystic duct forceps
easy bruisability
easy-to-perform intraprostatic
EATCL
enteropathy-associated T-cell lymphoma
eater
liver e.
EAUS
endoanal ultrasound
EB
epidermolysis bullosa
EBA
extrahepatic biliary atresia
Ebbehoj procedure
EBCT
electron-beam computerized tomography
EBD
endoscopic balloon dilation
EBL
endoscopic band ligation
estimated blood loss
Ebola hemorrhagic fever
ebrotidine
EBRT
external-beam radiation therapy
EBS
estrogen binding site
EBSD
endoscopic balloon sphincter dilation
Ebstein
E. diet
E. disease
E. lesion
EBV
Epstein-Barr virus
EC
epithelial cell
esophageal candidiasis
thymic EC
ECA
enterobacterial common antigen
E-cadherin
EC-cell
antral EC-c.
ECF
extracellular fluid
ECGF
endothelial cell growth factor
Echinacea purpura

E

echinococcal
    e. cyst disease
    e. liver abscess
echinococcosis, echinocacciasis
    biliary e.
    cystic e.
    hepatic e.
    hepatic-alveolar e.
Echinococcus
    E. granulosus
    life cycle of *E.*
    E. liver cyst
    E. multilocularis
echo
    gradient e.
    magnetization prepared-rapid
      gradient e. (MP-RAGE)
    e. pattern
    e. sign
echocolonoscope
    CF-UM3 e.
    Olympus CF-UM3 flexible e.
echo-Doppler
echoduodenoscope
echoduodenoscopy
echoendoscope
    CLA e.
    curvilinear scanning e.
    electronic e.
    GF-UM30P linear-oriented radial
      scanning e.
    linear array e.
    oblique-viewing e.
    Olympus CF-UM-series e.
    Olympus GF-UC30P e.
    Olympus GF-UCT30P linear
      array e.
    Olympus GF-UM30P e.
    Olympus GF-UM29 radial
      scanner e.
    Olympus GIF20 e.
    Olympus GIF-EUM2 e.
    Olympus GIF-series e.
    Olympus GIF-1T10 e.
    Olympus JF-UM20 e.
    Olympus linear array e.
    Olympus UM-20 radial e.
    Olympus VU-M2 e.
    Olympus XIF-UM3 e.
    Pentax FG-36-UX linear array e.
    Pentax linear array e.
    radial sector scanning e.
echoendoscopy (EUS)
echogastroscope
echogenic
    e. cardiac focus
    e. duct margin

    e. foci
    e. liver
echogenicity
    central e.
echographic
    homogeneous e.
echolucent
echomorphologic
echo-poor
    e.-p. layer
    e.-p. lesion
echoprobe
    Olympus XMP-U2 catheter e.
echorich
echotexture
echovirus infection
ECI automatic reprocessor
Eck fistula
Eckhout vertical gastroplasty
ECL
    enhanced chemiluminescence
    enterochromaffin-like
      ECL cell
      ECL cell hyperplasia
      ECL hypertrophy and hyperplasia
      ECL Western blotting
ECLoma
ECLP
    extracorporeal liver perfusion
ECM
    extracellular matrix
    extracolonic malignancy
ECOG
    Eastern Cooperative Oncology Group
      ECOG performance status scale
ecology
    microbial e.
Ecotrin
ECP
    eosinophil cationic protein
ECPL
    endocavitary pelvic lymphadenectomy
ectacolia
ectasia
    antral vascular e.
    Boley vascular e.
    cecal vascular e.
    gastric antral vascular e. (GAVE)
    gastric vascular e. (GVE)
    mucinous ductal e. (MDE)
    precaliceal canalicular e.
    tortuous venous e.
    vascular e.
    venous e.
ectatic
    e. vascular lesion
    e. vessel
ecthyma gangrenosum

ectocolon
ectoderm
ectodermal
ectoperitoneal
ectoperitonitis
ectopia
> crossed renal e.
> crossed testicular e.
> intraabdominal transverse
>   testicular e.
> renal e.
> e. testis
> testis e.
> transverse testicular e.
> ureteral e.
> e. vesica

ectopic
> e. adrenal rest
> e. anus
> e. cryptorchidism
> e. gastric mucosa
> e. gestation
> e. kidney
> e. pancreas
> e. pheochromocytoma
> e. schistosomiasis
> e. scrotum
> e. sigmoid pregnancy
> e. testis
> e. ureter
> e. ureterocele
> e. varix
> e. vas deferens

ectopy
> acquired gastric e.
> gastric mucosal e.

ectoscopy
ECU
> extracorporeal ultrafiltration

ECV
> esophageal collateral vein
> extracellular fluid volume

eczema
> atopic e.

ED1
> monoclonal antibody ED1

EDA+
> extradomain A positive
EDAP LT.01 lithotriptor
EDD
> extended daily dialysis

Edebohls
> E. operation
> E. position

edema
> alimentary e.
> angioneurotic e.
> antral e.
> bullous e.
> cerebral e.
> focal e.
> idiopathic e.
> laryngeal e.
> nephritic e.
> nephrotic e.
> pedal e.
> penile e.
> perianal e.
> pericholecystic e.
> peripheral extremity e.
> pitting e.
> pulmonary e.
> sacral e.

edematous
> e. gallbladder
> e. hyperemic mucosa
> e. pancreatitis
> e. tag

edentulous
Eder-Bernstein gastroscope
Eder-Chamberlin gastroscope
Eder gastroscope
Eder-Hufford
> E.-H. gastroscope
> E.-H. rigid esophagoscope

Eder-Palmer
> E.-P. semiflexible fiberoptic
>   endoscope
> E.-P. semiflexible gastroscope

Eder-Puestow
> E.-P. dilation
> E.-P. dilator shaft
> E.-P. guidewire
> E.-P. metal olive dilator
> E.-P. olive

edetate
> disodium e.

Edex
edge
> e. enhancement
> heaped-up e.
> hepatic e.
> ligament reflecting e.

E

NOTES

edge *(continued)*
    liver e.
    Poupart ligament shelving e.
    ulcer with heaped-up e.
EdGr
    Edmondson grade
    EdGr system
edible vaccine
Edlich gastric lavage tube
Edmondson
    E. grade (EdGr)
    E. grading system
    E. grading system for
      hepatocellular carcinoma
Edna towel clamp
EDNO
    endothelium-derived nitric oxide
EDP
    endoscopic digital pancreatography
EDRF
    endothelium-derived relaxing factor
edrophonium
    e. provocation
    e. test
ED-Spaz
EDTA
    ethylenediamine tetraacetic acid
    ^{51}Cr-labeled EDTA
Edwardsiella tarda
Edwards syndrome
ED7-XU2
    Fujinon ED7-XU2
EEA
    end-to-end anastomosis
    EEA AutoSuture stapler
    EEA stapler gun
    EEA stapling device
    EEA stapling of varices
EEG
    electroencephalography
EEGF
    esophageal epidermal growth factor
EEJ
    electroejaculation
EEPLND
    extraperitoneal endoscopic pelvic lymph
    node dissection
EES
    expandable esophageal stent
E.E.S.
EET
    epoxyeicosatrienoic acid
EFA
    essential fatty acid
EFAD
    essential fatty acid deficiency
effacement
    villous e.

effect
    antinociceptive e.
    antiproteinuric e.
    banana peel e.
    blooming e.
    Bohr e.
    choleretic e.
    concomitant medication e.
    disulfiram-like e.
    Doppler e.
    duodenal e.
    esophageal e.
    first-pass e.
    gastric e.
    gender e.
    Haldane e.
    halo e.
    hypothermic e.
    intracellular flush e.
    irradiation e.
    J-curve e.
    kidney shock wave e.
    local alcohol instillation e.
    membrane e.
    metabolic e.
    mitogenic e.
    mutagenic e.
    normothermic e.
    octreotide e.
    physiological trophic e.
    pinchcock e.
    placebo e.
    preservation times e.
    prokinetic e.
    sieving e.
    snowstorm e.
    soar-crash e.
    systemic e.
    topic e.
    tubulotoxic e.
effective
    e. arterial blood volume (EABV)
    e. dose equivalent radiation
    e. renal plasma flow (ERPF)
effector
    e. cell
    e. domain
    locally acting paracrine e.
    e. response
EFFERdose
    Zantac E.
efferent
    e. glomerular arteriole
    e. limb
    e. loop
    e. loop syndrome
    e. renal sympathetic nerve activity
    (ERSNA)

efferentes
> ductuli e.

Effer-Syllium

efficacy
> poor long-term e.

efficiency
> defunctioning e.

effluent
> anal e.
> ileal e.
> ileostomy e.
> peritoneal dialysis e. (PDE)
> transverse colostomy e.

efflux

effort rupture of esophagus

EG
> eosinophilic gastroenteritis
> esophagogastrectomy
> esophagogastric

EGBT
> esophagogastric balloon tamponade

EGC
> early gastric cancer

EGD
> esophagogastroduodenoscopy

EGE
> eosinophilic gastroenteritis

egesta

EGF
> epidermal growth factor
> ^{125}I-h-EGF
> intragastric EGF
> luminal EGF
> subcutaneous EGF

EGFR
> epidermal growth factor receptor

EGG
> electrogastrography
> cutaneous EGG

eggerthii
> *Bacteroides* e.

egg yolk-cobalamin absorption test (EYCAT)

EGM
> extraglomerular mesangium

egophony

EGS
> electrogalvanic stimulation
> EGS Model 100 electrogalvanic stimulator

EGTA
> esophageal gastric tube airway
> ethylene glycol tetraacetic acid

Egyptian splenomegaly

EHBDA
> extrahepatic bile duct atresia

EHC
> enterohepatic circulation

EHEC
> enterohemorrhagic *Escherichia coli*

EHL
> electrohydraulic lithotripsy
> endoscopic hemorrhoid ligation
> EHL probe

Ehlers-Danlos syndrome

EHM
> extrahepatic metastasis

EHPVO
> extrahepatic portal vein obstruction

Ehrlich
> E. abdominoplasty
> E. reagent

Ehrmann alcohol test meal

EHT
> electrohydrothermal
> EHT coagulation
> EHT electrode

EIA
> enzyme immunoassay
> HCV EIA II
> *Helicobacter pylori* stool antigen EIA
> EIA kit

EIA-2
> second-generation enzyme immunoassay

eicosanoid synthesis

eicosapentaenoic acid (EPA)

EIEC
> enteroinvasive *Escherichia coli*

eight-lumen esophageal manometry catheter

Einhorn
> E. dilator
> E. string test

EIS
> endoscopic injection sclerotherapy

Eisenberger technique

Eissner prostatic cooler

Eitest MONO P-II test

ejaculatio
> e. deficiens

E

NOTES

ejaculatio *(continued)*
    e. praecox
    e. retardata
ejaculation
    antegrade e.
    dry e.
    electrostimulation-induced e.
    e. failure
    premature e.
    retrograde e.
ejaculatorius
    ductus e.
ejaculatory
    e. duct
    e. duct obstruction
    e. duct reflux
    e. duct transurethral resection
    e. duct ultrasonography '
    e. dysfunction
    e. impotence
ejaculum
ejecta
ejection
EJP
    excitatory junction potential
ekiri
eKru
    equivalent residual renal urea clearance
Ektachem slide test
EL2-LS2 flexible video laparoscope
ELAD
    extracorporeal liver assist device
ELAM-1
    endothelial leukocyte adhesion molecule-1
        ligand for ELAM-1
Elastalloy
    E. esophageal endoprosthesis
    E. esophageal stent
elastase
    neutrophil e.
    serum e. 1
elastic
    e. band ligation
    e. bougie
    e. ligature
    e. O ring
    e. scattering spectroscopy
    e. silicone membrane
elastica interna
elasticum
    pseudoxanthoma e.
elastin stain
elastolysis
    generalized e.
Elastoplast dressing
Elavil

ELBF
    estimated liver blood flow
ELBNS
    extraperitoneal laparoscopic bladder neck suspension
elbowed
    e. bougie
    e. catheter
elective resection
electric
    e. tissue morcellator
    e. zone
electrical
    e. blocking
    e. conductivity
    single potential analysis of cavernous e. (SPACE)
    e. waveform
electroblotting
electrocautery
    bipolar e.
    blended e.
    Bovie e.
    Bugbee e.
    e. knife
    light e.
    monopolar e.
    multipolar e.
    needle-knife e. (NKE)
    Neomed e.
    e. pencil
    e. resection
electrocholecystectomy
electrocholecystocausis
electrocoagulating
    e. biopsy forceps
    e. current
electrocoagulation
    bipolar e. (BPEC)
    direct current e.
    endoscopic e.
    Gold probe e.
    monopolar e.
    multipolar e. (MPEC)
    e. necrosis
    snare e.
    transendoscopic e.
electrocystography
electrode
    abdominal patch e.
    ACMI monopolar e.
    antimony monocrystalline e.
    antimony pH e.
    ASSI laparoscopic e.
    ball e.
    bayonet-tip e.
    bipolar glass e.
    Bugbee e.

Buie fulguration e.
button e.
Cameron-Miller e.
coagulating e.
Coaguloop resection e.
Collings e.
common pH e.
concentric-needle e.
conical-tip e.
cuff e.
cutting e.
Disa needle e.
disposable pudendal nerve e.
dome-tip e.
EHT e.
electrohydrothermal e.
e. electrolyte
Eppendorf needle e.
flat spatula e.
foramen e.
glass pH e.
Greenwald Control Tip
  cystoscopic e.
Gyrus bipolar e.
Hamm e.
hook-tip laparoscopic e.
Hulbert e.
indifferent e.
intraluminal reference e.
ion-specific e.
e. jelly
J-hook tip laparoscopic e.
knife e.
loop-tipped e.
McCarthy e.
Microelectrode MI-506 small-caliber
  pH e.
Microglass pH e.
midgastric e.
e. migration
model 440 M1.5, M4 e.
needle e.
needle-tip laparoscopic e.
Neil-Moore e.
Nortech SLED e.
pencil-tipped e.
e. placement
e. probe
renal sympathetic nerve activity
  recording e.
reusable laparoscopic e.
right-angle e.

rollerball e.
single-fiber EMG e.
Smith e.
spatula-tip laparoscopic e.
spoon-tip laparoscopic e.
St. Mark pudendal e.
surface e.
three-quarter circle e.
unipolar glass e.
VaporTrode e.
wire e.
electrodiathermy
electroejaculation (EEJ)
  rectal probe e.
electroejaculator
  G&S E.
electroencephalography (EEG)
electroendosmosis
electroevaporation
electrofulguration
electrogalvanic
  e. stimulation (EGS)
  e. stimulator
electrogastrogram
  cutaneous e.
electrogastrograph
electrogastrography (EGG)
electrohemostasis
electrohydraulic
  e. generator
  e. lithotripsy (EHL)
  e. lithotripsy probe
  e. lithotriptor
  percutaneous transhepatic
    choledochoscopic e.
  e. shock wave lithotripsy (ESWL)
electrohydrothermal (EHT)
  e. coagulation
  e. electrode
electroimmunodiffusion assay
electroincision
electrolithotrity
electrolyte
  e. abnormality
  e. balance
  bicarbonate e.
  calcium e.
  chloride e.
  CO_2 e.
  electrode e.
  e. excretion
  e. flush solution

NOTES

E

electrolyte *(continued)*
 e. imbalance coma
 e. loss
 potassium e.
 e. preparation
 sodium e.
 stool e.
electrolyte-polyethylene glycol lavage solution
electromagnetic
 e. flow transducer
 e. lithotriptor
electromechanical
 e. coupling
 epinephrine-induced
  gastroduodenal e.
 e. impactor (EMI)
electromicroscopy
electromyogram (EMG)
 colonic e.
electromyography
 conventional concentric e.
 corpus cavernosum penile e.
 Disa e.
 intraanal e.
 needle electrode e.
 noninvasive intra-anal e.
 pelvic floor e.
 e. of penile corpus cavernosum muscle
 rhabdosphincter e.
 single-fiber needle e.
 surface pelvic floor e.
 ureteral e.
 video pressure flow e.
electron
 e. immunoperoxidase observation
 e. microscopy
electron-beam computerized tomography (EBCT)
electron-dense mesangial deposit
electronic
 e. barostat
 e. echoendoscope
 e. endoscope
 e. recording nappy
electrophoresis
 agarose gel e.
 horizontal e.
 e. immunoblot analysis
 immunofixation e. (IFE)
 polyacrylamide gel e. (PAGE)
 pulsed field gel e. (PFGE)
 serum e.
 serum protein e. (SPEP)
 urine e.
 urine protein e. (UPEP)

electrophoretic mobility
electrophysiology
 cellular e.
 e. of the gastric musculature
 GI e.
electropneumatic endoscopic lithotriptor
electroresection
electrosensitivity
 mucosal e. (MES)
electrostimulation
electrostimulation-induced ejaculation
electrosurgery
 EUS probe-guided e.
electrosurgical
 e. curved scissors
 e. cut
 e. cutting knife
 e. desiccation
 e. dissection
 e. fulguration
 e. generator
 e. monopolar spatula probe
 e. needle
 e. snare
 e. snare polypectomy
 e. spatula
 e. unit (ESU)
electrotherapy
electrovaporization
 prostate gland e.
 transurethral e.
Elema-Siemens AB pressure transducer
element
 acute-phase response e. (APRE)
 androgen receptor e.
 estrogen response e. (ERE)
 glucocorticoid response e. (GRE)
 hepatic subcellular e.
 thyroid hormone response e. (TRE)
elemental
 e. diet
 e. phosphate
elephantiasis
 genital e.
 e. scroti
elevated WBC
elevation
 mucosal e.
elevator
 Alexander e.
 Doyen rib e.
 Ellik kidney stone e.
 Freer e.
 Stille e.
eleventh
 e. rib flank incision
 e. rib transperitoneal incision

ELF
  etoposide, leucovorin, 5-fluorouracil
  ELF chemotherapy protocol
elimination
  e. diet
  pyelography by e.
  spontaneous partial e.
  stool e.
eliminator
  E. balloon catheter
  E. biliary stent
  Fecal Odor E. (FOE)
  E. nasal biliary catheter set
  E. pancreatic stent
  E. PET biliary balloon dilator
  E. stone extraction basket
ELISA
  enzyme-linked immunosorbent assay
  first-generation ELISA
  gliadin ELISA
  sensitive and specific ELISA
  TG ELISA
  tissue transglutaminase ELISA (TG ELISA)
  ELISA titer
ELISA-I
  enzyme-linked immunosorbent assay I
ELISA-I, -II, -III test
ELISA-II
  enzyme-linked immunosorbent assay II
ELISA-like assay
elixir
  e. diarrhea
  Susano E.
Ellik
  E. evacuator
  E. kidney stone basket
  E. kidney stone elevator
Elliot position
Elliott gallbladder forceps
ellipsoid method
elliptical incision
Ellis types 1, 2 glomerulonephritis
Ellis-van Creveld syndrome
Ellsner gastroscope
Elmiron
ELMISKOP 101 electron microscope
elongated, pseudostratified nucleus
elongation
  calix e.
Eloxatin
Elspar

ELT
  endoscopic laser therapy
eltor
  Vibrio e.
  Vibrio cholerae biotype e.
eluate
  acetonitrile e.
elucidation
ELUS
  endoluminal rectal ultrasonography
elusive
  e. polyp
  e. ulcer
eluted antibody
elutriation
  T-cell depletion by e.
EM
  erythema multiforme
  esophageal manometry
EMA
  endomysial antibody
    antibody to EMA
    IgA EMA
emaciation
EMAG
  environmental metaplastic atrophic gastritis
emasculation
EMB
  eosin-methylene blue
    EMB agar
embarrassment
  circulatory e.
  respiratory e.
embolectomy
  renal artery embolism e.
emboli (*pl. of* embolus)
embolic
  e. agent
  e. nephritis
embolism
  air e.
  bile pulmonary e.
  cholesterol e.
  hemodialysis air e.
  mesenteric arterial e.
  postoperative cholesterol e.
  pulmonary e.
  renal artery e.
embolization
  e. of aneurysm

E

NOTES

embolization *(continued)*
    angiographic variceal e.
    arterial e.
    arteriographic e.
    bilateral pudendal artery e.
    cholesterol crystal e. (CCE)
    Gelfoam e.
    iliac artery e.
    percutaneous transhepatic liver
      biopsy with tract e. (PBTE)
    portal e. (PE)
    renal artery cholesterol e.
    splenic arterial e.
    superselective transcatheter e.
    transarterial catheter e. (TACE)
    transcatheter arterial e. (TAE)
    transcatheter hepatic arterial e.
    transcatheter splenic arterial e.
      (TSAE)
    transcatheter variceal e.
    transhepatic e. (THE)
    varicocele e.
embolization
embolotherapy
    transcatheter e.
embolus, pl. **emboli**
    cholesterol e.
    metallic e.
    pulmonary e.
    renal cholesterol e.
    talc e.
EMBP
    estramustine binding protein
embryoid body
embryologic development
embryology
embryoma
    e. of the kidney
embryonal
    e. adenoma
    e. adenosarcoma
    e. cell carcinoma
    e. nephroma
    e. testicular carcinoma
    e. transitory bladder
    e. tumor
embryonic cleavage
Emcyt
EMD
    esophageal motility disorder
EMDA
    intravesical electromotive drug
    administration
EMEM
    Eagle minimal essential medium
emepronium bromide
emergency
    e. appendectomy

    e. colonoscopy
    e. laparotomy
emergency-to-elective workload
emergent appendectomy
emesis
    bilious e.
    chemotherapy-induced nausea and e.
      (CINE)
    coffee-ground e.
emetatrophia
Emete-Con
emetic reflex
emetine
emetocathartic
emetogenic injury
Emetrol
EMG
    electromyogram
      sphincter EMG
EMI
    electromechanical impactor
      EMI APED amplifier discriminator
      EMI 9813B photomultiplier
eminence
    hypothenar e.
    thenar e.
emissary vein of penis
emission
    gamma e.
    nocturnal e.
Emitasol nasal therapy
Emitrip
emitter
    light e.
EMLA
    eutectic mixture of local anesthetics
      EMLA anesthetic
emollient laxative
EMPD
    extramammary Paget disease
emphysema
    AATD-related e.
    alpha-1-antitrypsin disease-related e.
    colonoscopy-related e.
    endoscopy-related e.
    intestinal e.
    panacinar e.
    panlobular e.
    subcutaneous e.
    unilateral periorbital e.
emphysematosa
    cholecystitis e.
    cystitis e.
emphysematous
    e. cholecystitis
    e. cystitis
    e. gastritis
    e. pyelonephritis

empty
    e. intestine
    e. sella syndrome
emptying
    bladder e.
    delayed gallbladder e.
    delayed liquid gastric e.
    e. delta volume
    gastric e. (GE)
    liquid e.
    neorectal e.
    rapid gastric e.
    rectal e.
    Roux limb e.
    solid e.
    t1/2 time of gastric e.
empyema of gallbladder
empyocele
EMR
    endoscopic magnetic resonance
    endoscopic mucosal resection
EMRC
    endoscopic mucosal resection, cap
      method
EMRL
    endoscopic mucosal resection with
      ligation
EMRT
    endoscopic mucosal resection, tube
      method
EMS
    esophageal manometric sequence
emulsion
    Biafine wound dressing e.
    Calogen LCT e.
    intralipid fat e.
    intravenous lipid e.
    lipid e.
    e. proteinuria
Emulsoil bowel preparation
E-MVAC
    escalated methotrexate, vinblastine,
      Adriamycin, cisplatin or
      cyclophosphamide
E-Mycin
EN
    enema
    enteral nutrition
en
    en bloc dissection
    en bloc distal pancreatectomy
    en bloc kidney transplantation

    en bloc technique
    en bloc ureter
    en bloc vein resection
    en coup de sabre
    en face
    en face view
ENA
    extracted nuclear antigen
    ENA screen
ENaC
    epithelial sodium channel
enalapril
enalkiren
enamel pellicle formation
ENANB
    enterically transmitted non-A, non-B
      ENANB hepatitis
enanthate
    e. ester
    testosterone e.
enantiomer D-arginine
ENBD
    endoscopic nasobiliary drainage
encapsulated
    e. carcinoid tumor
    e. plasmodium
    e. renal cell carcinoma
encapsulation
    peritoneal e.
    tumor e.
Encare tube feeding formula
encasement
    pancreatic duct e.
    ureteral e.
encelialgia
encelitis
Encephalitozoon intestinalis
encephaloid gastric carcinoma
encephalomyopathy
    mitochondrial
      neurogastrointestinal e. (MNGIE)
encephalopathy
    bilirubin e.
    colonoscopy-induced
      hyponatremic e.
    hepatic e. (HE)
    myoclonic e.
    portosystemic e. (PSE)
    postshunt e.
    subclinical hepatic e. (SHE)
    uremic e.
    Wernicke e.

E

NOTES

encephalotrigeminal syndrome
encircle
encirclement
    anal e.
encopresis
encroachment
    scrotal e.
encrustation
    e. analysis
    biofilm related e.
    e. of biomaterial
    e. deposition
    e. of stent
encrusted pyelitis
encysted
    e. bladder
    e. calculus
    e. hydrocele
    e. intraabdominal collection
end
    advanced glycation e. (AGE)
    e. colostomy
    e. expiratory
    e. ileostomy
    e. stoma
endarterectomy
    e. knife
    renal e.
    transaortic e.
endeavor
    Cancer of the Prostate Strategic
    Urologic Research E.
endemic
    e. colic
    e. deep mycosis
    e. diarrhea
    e. hematuria
    e. nonbacterial infantile
    gastroenteritis
end-end stapler
Endep
end-expiratory intragastric pressure
end-filling pressure
end-fire transrectal probe
end-hole ureteral catheter
end-loop
    e.-l. colostomy
    e.-l. ileocolostomy
    e.-l. ileostomy
    e.-l. stoma
endo
    e. catch bag
    E. GIA 30, 60 stapler
    E. GIA suture stapler
    E. Hernia stapler
    E. pants
endoabdominal fascia

endoanal
    e. coil
    e. magnetic resonance imaging
    e. mucosectomy
    e. probe
    e. ultrasound (EAUS)
    e. ultrasound scan
endoappendicitis
Endo-Assist
    E.-A. disposable atraumatic
    grasping forceps
    E.-A. disposable hemostat
    E.-A. disposable ligature carrier
    E.-A. disposable needle holder
    E.-A. reusable knot pusher
endoauscultation
Endo-Avitene
    E.-A. MCH
    E.-A. microfibrillar collagen
    hemostat
Endo-Babcock stapler
Endobag
endobiliary ascariasis
EndoBlade
endobrachyesophagus
endobronchial
    e. fistula
    e. stent
Endocam
endocamera
    Polaroid e. EC-3
endocarditis
    enterococcal e.
    infective e.
    marantic e.
    native valve bacterial e.
    Streptococcus bovis e.
endocavitary
    e. bladder diverticulectomy
    e. pelvic lymphadenectomy (ECPL)
    e. radiation
endocholedochal
Endoclip applier
EndoCoil
    E. biliary stent
    E. esophageal stent
endocolitis
endocrine
    e. cancer
    e. cell
    e. disruptor
    e. mimic
    e. screening
    e. system
    e. therapy
endocrinopathy
Endocut
endocystitis

endocytosis
    fluid-phase e.
endocytotic vesicle
endodermal
endodermic cell
Endodynamics suction polyp trap
endoenteritis
endoesophageal MRI coil
endoesophagitis
endogastric
endogastritis
Endo-Gauge
endogenous
    e. biotin
    e. lipophilic antioxidant
    e. mutation
    e. obesity
    e. opioid
    e. peroxidase
    e. peroxidase activity
    e. pyrogen
    e. renal antigen
endograsper
endoherniorrhaphy
Endolav
    E. lavage pump
    Mcditron EL-100 E.
endoligature
Endoloop suture
EndoLumina bougie
endoluminal
    e. clipping
    e. CT colonography
    e. endoscopy
    e. rectal ultrasonography (ELUS)
    e. ultrasonography-guided fine-
        needle aspiration biopsy
    e. ureteral ultrasound
EndoMate grab bag
endometrial carcinoma
endometrioid
endometrioma
    ovarian e.
endometriosis
    e. of colon
    colorectal e.
    e. vesica
endometritis
    coccidioidal e.
endometrium
endomorph
endomorphic

endomorphy
endomysial
    e. antibody (EMA)
    e. antibody test
    e. IgA
endomysium
    e. antibody
    e. antigen
EndoNet
    Pentax E.
endonuclease
    restriction e.
Endopath
    E. EMS hernia stapler
    E. endoscopic linear cutter
    E. Optiview laparoscopic obturator
    E. 30, 60 stapler
endopeptidase
    neutral e.
    pancreatic e.
endoperitoneal
endoperitonitis
endoperoxide
    PGG2 e.
    PGH2 e.
endophlebitis hepatica obliterans
endophotography
endophytic
endoplasmic
    e. reticulum
    e. reticulum-bound polysome
Endo-P-Probe
endoprobe
    rotating e.
endoprostatic coil
endoprosthesis
    biliary e.
    Celestin e.
    Coons/Carey e.
    crutched stick-type polyurethane e.
    cuffed esophageal e.
    double-lumen e.
    double-pigtail e.
    DoubleStent biliary e.
    Elastalloy esophageal e.
    endoscopic biliary e.
    esophageal e.
    exchange of e.
    expandable biliary e.
    expandable metal mesh e.
    IntraStent DoubleStrut biliary e.
    KeyMed Atkinson e.

E

NOTES

endoprosthesis *(continued)*
    large-bore biliary e.
    Medoc-Celestin e.
    pancreatic e.
    peroral e.
    pigtail e.
    3/4-pigtail plastic e.
    plastic e.
    polyethylene e.
    Proctor-Livingston e.
    self-expandable stainless steel
      braided e.
    straight e.
    Titan e.
    transpapillary endoscopic e.
    UroLume e.
    Wallstent e.
    Wilson-Cook e.
endopyelotomy
    Acucise e.
    antegrade e.
    e. failure
    e. incision
    retrograde e.
    e. stent
    ureteroscopic e.
endopyeloureterotomy
    percutaneous e.
endoradiosonde
endorectal
    e. advancement flap
    e. coil magnetic resonance imaging
    e. ileal pouch
    e. ileal pull-through
    e. probe
    e. surface coil MRI
    e. ultrasound (ERUS)
endorectal-pelvic phased-array coil
endosac
endo-scissors
    rotating e.-s.
endoscope
    AccuSharp e.
    ACMI e.
    battery-powered e.
    cap-fitted e.
    CCD e.
    CF-HM e.
    charge-coupled device e.
    Cho/Dyonics two-portal e.
    double-accessory channel
      therapeutic e.
    double-channel e.
    Eder-Palmer semiflexible
      fiberoptic e.
    electronic e.
    end-viewing e.
    EVIS 140 Q series e.

EVIS 140 S wide-screen e.
FCS two-channel ultra high-
  magnification e.
FG-series two-channel e.
FGS-ML-series two-channel e.
FGS-series two-channel e.
FGS-SML-series two-channel e.
fiberoptic e.
flexible fiberoptic e.
forward-viewing e.
Fujinon EG-FP-series e.
Fujinon EVE-series e.
Fujinon EVG-CT e.
Fujinon EVG-FP-series e.
Fujinon EVG-F-series e.
Fujinon FP-series e.
Fujinon UGI-FP-series video e.
GIF N30 fiberoptic pediatric e.
GIF XP20 e.
GIF XQ10 upper e.
Hirschowitz e.
e. impaction
intraductal e.
JFB III e.
JF-20 side-viewing fiberoptic e.
J-shaped e.
Karl Storz e.
Kussmaul e.
large-channel e.
lateral-viewing e.
LoPresti e.
magnifying e.
Messerklinger e.
mother-daughter e.
Navigator flexible e.
near-infrared electronic e.
oblique-viewing e.
Olympus Aloka GF-EU-series e.
Olympus CF-UM20 ultrasound e.
Olympus CF-200Z e.
Olympus CV-series e.
Olympus DES-series e.
Olympus EUM-20 e.
Olympus EUS-series e.
Olympus EVIS Q-series e.
Olympus EVIS 140 Q video e.
Olympus GF-series video e.
Olympus GF-UM30P e.
Olympus GF-UM20 radial
  scanning e.
Olympus GF-UM20 ultrasound e.
Olympus GIF-D2 e.
Olympus GIF-HM-series e.
Olympus GIF-J-series e.
Olympus GIF-P e.
Olympus GIF-Q200 e.
Olympus GIF-2T200 e.
Olympus GIF-T-series e.

Olympus GIF-XP-series e.
Olympus GIF-XV-series e.
Olympus JF-series video e.
Olympus JF1T e.
Olympus JF-T-series e.
Olympus JF-TV-series e.
Olympus JF-V-series e.
Olympus PJF e.
Olympus PJF-series pediatric e.
Olympus P-series e.
Olympus Q200 video e.
Olympus SIF-SW fiberoptic e.
Olympus SIF-100 video push e.
Olympus SSIF-VI KAI
  fiberoptic e.
Olympus 2T100 e.
Olympus UM-series e.
Olympus V-series e.
Olympus XCF-XK-series e.
Olympus XGF-UCT30 e.
Olympus XP-series e.
Olympus XQ-200, XQ-230
  video e.
pediatric e.
Pentax EC-series video e.
Pentax EG-2901,-2940,-3800 e.
Pentax ESI-2000 fiberoptic e.
Pentax FD-series video e.
Pentax FG-38X e.
Pentax VSB-2000 fiberoptic e.
rigid e.
semiflexible e.
semirigid e.
side-viewing e.
Simpson e.
Surgenomic e.
therapeutic e.
Toshiba video e.
transcutaneous sonogram e.
two-channel e.
UGI e.
ultrasound e.
ultrathin e.
upper GI e.
video e.
Visicath e.
Weerda e.
Welch Allyn video e.
endoscope-body position relationship
endoscopic
  e. ablation of antral diaphragm
  e. adrenalectomy

e. alligator forceps
e. aspiration lumpectomy (EAL)
e. aspiration mucosectomy (EAM)
e. atrophic gastritis
e. balloon dilation (EBD)
e. balloon sphincter dilation
  (EBSD)
e. band ligation (EBL)
e. band ligation of varix
e. band ligator
e. BICAP probe
e. biliary decompression
e. biliary drainage
e. biliary endoprosthesis
e. biliary sphincterotomy
e. biliary stent
e. biliary stent placement
e. biopsy forceps
e. biopsy site
e. botulinum toxin injection
e. brush cytology
e. camera
e. clipping
e. color Doppler
e. color Doppler assessment
e. color Doppler ultrasonography
e. control
e. cystenterostomy
e. cystoduodenostomy
e. cystogastrostomy
e. devolvulization
e. digital pancreatography (EDP)
e. diverticulotomy
e. Doppler probe
e. electrocoagulation
e. electrohydraulic lithotripsy
e. enterogastric reflux gastritis
e. epinephrine injection
e. erythematous/exudative gastritis
e. esophagitis
e. esophagogastric variceal ligation
e. examination
e. extirpation cicatricial obliteration
e. extraction pancreatic duct stone
e. finding
e. fine-needle puncture
e. fistulotomy
e. flowprobe
e. four-quadrant tattoo
e. fulguration
e. gastrostomy
e. gastrostomy tube

NOTES

E

endoscopic *(continued)*
- e. grasping forceps
- e. guidance
- e. heat probe
- e. hemoclip device
- e. hemoclipping
- e. hemoclip therapy
- e. hemorrhagic gastritis
- e. hemorrhoid ligation (EHL)
- e. hemostasis
- e. hemostatic therapy
- e. Ho:YAG lithotripsy
- e. incision
- e. India ink injection
- e. injection sclerosis
- e. injection sclerotherapy (EIS)
- e. injection therapy
- e. jejunostomy
- e. laser cautery
- e. laser cholecystectomy
- e. laser recanalization
- e. laser therapy (ELT)
- e. light source
- e. magnetic extractor
- e. magnetic resonance (EMR)
- e. magnetic resonance scanning
- e. management
- e. manometry
- 20-MHz e. ultrasound probe
- e. microwave
- e. microwave coagulation
- e. monitoring
- e. mucosal resection (EMR)
- e. mucosal resection, cap method (EMRC)
- e. mucosal resection, tube method (EMRT)
- e. mucosal resection with a ligating device
- e. mucosal resection with ligation (EMRL)
- e. mucosectomy
- e. nasobiliary catheter drainage
- e. nasobiliary drainage (ENBD)
- e. nasogallbladder drainage (ENGBD)
- e. optical urethrotomy
- e. pancreatic drainage
- e. pancreatic duct sphincterotomy
- e. pancreatic sphincterotomy (EPS)
- e. pancreatic stenting (EPS)
- e. pancreatic therapy
- e. papillary balloon dilation (EPBD, EPD)
- e. papillotomy (EPT)
- e. papillotomy and stenting
- e. patchiness
- e. photography
- e. pulsed dye laser
- e. pulsed dye laser lithotripsy
- e. raised erosive gastritis
- e. reflectance
- e. reflectance spectrophotometry
- e. resection of antral web
- e. retroflexion
- e. retrograde biliary drainage (ERBD)
- e. retrograde biliary stenting
- e. retrograde cannulation
- e. retrograde cholangiogram
- e. retrograde cholangiography (ERC)
- e. retrograde cholangiopancreatography (ERCP)
- e. retrograde cholangiopancreatography catheter
- e. retrograde cholecystoendoprosthesis (ERCCE)
- e. retrograde cytology
- e. retrograde ileography
- e. retrograde pancreatography (ERP)
- e. retrograde parenchymography (ERP)
- e. retrograde parenchymography of pancreas (ERPP)
- e. retrograde sclerotherapy
- e. rugal hyperplastic gastritis
- e. scissors
- e. sclerotherapy (ES)
- e. sessile
- e. sessile polypectomy
- e. sewing machine
- e. sigmoidopexy
- e. small bowel biopsy
- e. snare
- e. snare ampullectomy
- e. snare resection
- e. sphincterectomy
- e. sphincter of Oddi manometry
- e. sphincterotomy (ES, EST)
- e. sphincterotomy-induced duodenal perforation
- e. sphincterotomy-induced pancreatitis
- e. spray cryotherapy
- e. stapling diverticulostomy
- e. stent exchange
- e. stigma
- e. stigmata of hemorrhage
- e. stone disintegration
- e. stone manipulation
- e. stone removal
- e. stricturoplasty
- e. stricturotomy
- e. strip biopsy
- e. surveillance

e. suture-cutting forceps
e. system
e. technology
e. thermal ablation
e. thermo-disinfector
e. transesophageal fine-needle
  aspiration
e. transesophageal fine-needle
  aspiration cytology
e. transgastric drainage
e. transpapillary biopsy
e. transpapillary cannulation
e. transpapillary catheterization of
  the gallbladder (ETCG)
e. transpapillary cyst drainage
  (ETCD)
e. transpapillary drainage of
  pancreatic abscess
e. treatment
e. ultrasonographic diagnosis
e. ultrasonographic imaging
e. ultrasonography (EUS)
e. ultrasound (EUS)
e. ultrasound-assisted band ligation
e. ultrasound diagnosis
e. ultrasound evaluation
e. ultrasound-guided celiac plexus
  block
e. ultrasound-guided
  cystogastrostomy
e. ultrasound-guided fine-needle
  aspiration (EUS-FNA)
e. ultrasound-guided fine-needle
  injection
e. variceal band ligation
e. variceal ligation (EVL)
e. variceal sclerotherapy
e. washing pipe
e. Waterpik
endoscopically
e. deliverable tissue-transfixing
  device
e. normal patient
endoscopic-controlled lithotripsy
endoscopist
endoscopy
advanced therapeutic e.
American Society for
  Gastrointestinal E. (ASGE)
5-aminolevulinic acid-induced
  fluorescence e.
anal e.

CE-AD gastric lesion staging by e.
CE-M gastric lesion staging by e.
CE-SM gastric lesion staging by e.
e. complication
computerized electronic e.
dynamic fluorescence video e.
  (DYNAFLUVE)
endoluminal e.
enhanced magnification e.
Erlanger active stimulator for
  interventional e.
fiberoptic e.
flexible e.
fluorescent electronic e.
gastrointestinal e.
high-altitude e.
high-magnification e.
high-resolution e.
infrared e.
intestinal e.
intraoperative e. (IOE)
intraoperative biliary e.
open access e. (OAE)
outpatient e.
pancreaticobiliary e.
pediatric e.
peripartum e.
peroral e.
postsurgical e.
primary diagnostic e.
e. procedure
rapid exchange technique for
  therapeutic e.
screening e.
e. suite
surveillance e.
TEM transanal e.
therapeutic pancreaticobiliary e.
therapeutic upper e.
transcolonic e.
transesophageal e.
transmural e.
transnasal e.
UGI e.
ultra-high-magnification e.
ultrathin e.
upper alimentary e.
upper gastrointestinal e. (UGIE)
video e.
virtual e.
wireless capsule e.
e. with iodine staining

E

NOTES

endoscopy-related emphysema
Endoshears
EndoSheath
    Vision System E.
endosnare
endosonographically targeted injection
endosonographic staging
endosonography
    anal e. (AES)
    anorectal e.
    duplex Doppler e.
    high-frequency e.
    e. instrument
    rectal e.
endosonography-guided
    e.-g. celiac plexus neurolysis
    e.-g. drainage of pancreatic
      pseudocyst
EndoSound
    E. endoscopic ultrasound catheter
    E. ultrasound probe
Endospore disinfectant
Endostapler
Endostat II bipolar/monopolar
  electrosurgical generator
endostethoscope
Endotek machine
endothelia (*pl. of* endothelium)
endothelial
    e. cell
    e. cell differentiation
    e. cell growth factor (ECGF)
    e. leukocyte adhesion molecule-1
      (ELAM-1)
    e. tube
endothelial-dependent relaxation
endothelialis
    hepatic e.
endothelin (ET)
    e. A (EtA)
    e. antagonist
    e. A receptor
    e. B (EtB)
    e. receptor
    renal e.
    selective e. A
endothelin-1 (ET-1)
    e.-1 concentration
endothelin-3 (ET-3)
    e. concentration
endothelioma
endotheliosis
    glomerular e.
endothelium, pl. **endothelia**
    gastrointestinal e.
    sinusoidal e.

endothelium-dependent
    e.-d. fibrinolysis
    e.-d. vasodilation
endothelium-derived
    e.-d. nitric oxide (EDNO)
    e.-d. relaxing factor (EDRF)
    e.-d. relaxing hormone
endotherapy
Endotorque
    Greenen E.
endotoxemia
    systemic e.
endotoxin
    e. antibody
    bacterial e.
endotracheal
    e. intubation
    e. tube (ET)
    e. tube placement
ENDO-Tube nasal jejunal feeding tube
endoureteral ultrasound sonography
endoureterotomy
    cold knife e.
endourologic
    e. biopsy
    e. management
endourological cold-knife incision
endourology
    reconstructive e.
    therapeutic e.
endovascular
    e. stent grafting
    e. stenting
    e. treatment
Endovations disposable cytology brush
endovenous
endowment
    original e.
Endozime
    E. AW bacteriostatic enzyme
      cleaner
    E. sponge
endplate
    motor e.
end-point dilution titer
Endrate
end-sigmoid colostomy
end-stage
    e.-s. cirrhosis
    e.-s. liver disease (ESLD)
    e.-s. renal disease (ESRD)
    e.-s. renal failure
end-to-end
    e.-t.-e. anastomosis (EEA)
    e.-t.-e. branch reanastomosis
    e.-t.-e. enterostomy
end-to-side
    e.-t.-s. anastomosis

e.-t.-s. arteriotomy
e.-t.-s. choledochojejunostomy
e.-t.-s. duodenogastrostomy
e.-t.-s. ileotransverse colostomy
e.-t.-s. portacaval shunt
e.-t.-s. reimplantation
e.-t.-s. vasoepididymostomy
   technique

Enduron
Enduronyl
end-viewing

e.-v. endoscope
e.-v. gastroscope

enema (EN)

air-contrast barium e. (ACBE)
5-aminosalicylic acid e.
analeptic e.
antegrade colonic e. (ACE)
antegrade continence e. (ACE)
5-ASA e.
barium e. (BE)
blind e.
cleansing hypertonic phosphate e.
contrast e.
Cortenema retention e.
diatrizoate sodium e.
double-contrast barium e. (DCBE)
flatus e.
Fleet Babylax e.
flexible barium e.
flocculation on barium e.
full-column barium e.
Gastrografin e.
glycerin e.
high e.
hydrocortisone e.
hydrogen peroxide e.
Hypaque e.
Kayexalate e.
lactulose e.
Malone antegrade continence e.
meglumine diatrizoate e.
mesalamine e.
methylene blue e.
nuclear e.
NuLytely e.
nutrient e.
oil retention e.
pancreatic e.
phosphate e.
Phospho-Soda e.
povidone-iodine e.

prednisolone e.
puddling on barium e.
retention e.
retrograde flow on barium e.
Rowasa e.
saline cleansing e.
single-contrast barium e.
small bowel e.
soapsuds e. (SSE)
sorbitol e.
steroid foam e.
sucralfate retention e.
sulfasalazine e.
tap water e.
theophylline olamine e.
tranexamic acid e.
turpentine e.
e.'s until clear
water-soluble contrast e.

enemator
enemiasis
energy

apparent digestive e. (ADE)
e. dispersive x-ray analysis
mean e.

Enfamil with iron formula
enflurane
enforcer

18F Cook E.

ENGBD

endoscopic nasogallbladder drainage

Engerix-B

HBV E.-B

engorgement

liver e.
venous e.

engraftment
enhanced

e. chemiluminescence (ECL)
e. chemiluminescence Western
  blotting
e. magnification endoscopy
e. reverse transcriptase polymerase
  chain reaction assay

enhancement

contrast e.
CT scan with contrast e.
edge e.
hybrid rapid acquisition with
  relaxation e. (HRARE)

ENK

enkephalin

NOTES

E

1-ENK
  leucine-enkephalin
enkephalin (ENK)
enlarged
  e. prostate
  e. uterus
enlargement
  benign prostatic e. (BPE)
  bladder e.
  calix e.
  discrete organ e.
  ovarian e.
  parotid gland e.
  salivary gland e.
  tonsillar e.
  tube e.
  uterine e.
enolase
  neuron-specific e. (NSE)
enorchia
Enovil
enoxacin
enoxaparin
  e. sodium
  e. sodium injection
enrich
  E. feeding
  E. protein and calorie supplement
ENS
  enteric nervous system
ensheathing trocar
ensnarement
Ensure
  E. HIN tube feeding formula
  E. Plus
  E. Plus formula
  E. Plus liquid feeding
  E. pudding
entactin
entamebiasis
entamebic abscess
Entamoeba
  E. coli cyst
  E. dispar
  E. histolytica
  E. histolytica abscess
enteradenitis
Entera-Flo
enteral
  e. alimentation
  e. diarrhea
  e. feeding
  e. nutrition (EN)
enteralgia
enterectasis
enterectomy
enterelcosis

enteric
  e. adenovirus
  e. cyst
  e. excitatory motoneuron
  e. fever
  e. fistula
  e. ganglia
  e. ganglion cell
  e. hormone
  e. hyperoxaluria
  e. immunogen
  e. infection
  e. inhibitory motoneuron
  e. interneuron
  e. nervous system (ENS)
  e. neuronal circuit
  e. neuronal reflex
  e. oxaluria
  e. pathogen
  e. secretomotor circuit
  e. vasodilator neuron
enterically
  e. transmitted non-A, non-B
    (ENANB)
  e. transmitted non-A, non-B
    hepatitis (ET-NANBH)
enteric-coated
  e.-c. aspirin
  e.-c. capsule
entericus
  liquor e.
  succus e.
enteritidis
  Salmonella e.
enteritis
  Campylobacter fetus e.
  choleriform e.
  chronic cicatrizing e.
  Clostridium difficile e.
  Crohn regional e.
  e. cystica chronica
  diphtheritic e.
  eosinophilic e.
  granulomatous e.
  e. gravis
  hemorrhagic e.
  idiopathic diffuse ulcerative
    nongranulomatous e.
  leishmanial e.
  mucomembranous e.
  mucous e.
  myxomembranous e.
  e. necroticans
  pellicular e.
  phlegmonous e.
  e. polyposa
  protozoan e.
  pseudomembranous e.

radiation e.
regional e. (RE)
segmental e.
Streptococcus e.
tuberculous e.
ulcerative e.
viral e.
Yersinia e.
enteroadherent *Escherichia coli* (EAEC)
enteroaggregative
　　e. *Escherichia coli* (EaggEC)
　　e. *Escherichia coli* heat-stable
　　enterotoxin 1 (EAST1)
enteroanastomosis
enteroanthelone
enteroapocleisis
Enterobacter
　　E. aerogenes
　　E. cloacae
　　E. hafniae
　　E. liquefaciens
Enterobacteriaceae
enterobacterial common antigen (ECA)
enterobiliary
Enterobius vermicularis
enterobrosis, enterobrosia
enterocele
　　complex e.
　　congenital e.
　　iatrogenic e.
　　partial e.
　　e. pulsion
　　e. sac
　　secondary e.
　　simple e.
　　e. traction
enterocentesis
enteroceptive
enterocholecystostomy
enterocholecystotomy
enterochromaffin cell
enterochromaffin-like (ECL)
　　e.-l. cell
enterocinesia
enterocinetic
enterocleisis
　　omental e.
enteroclysis
　　small bowel e.
　　e. tube

enterococcal
　　e. endocarditis
　　e. sepsis
Enterococcus
　　E. faecalis
enterococcus, pl. enterococci
　　vancomycin-resistant e. (VRE)
enterocolectomy
enterocolic fistula
enterocolitica
　　Yersinia e.
enterocolitis
　　Aeromonas-associated e.
　　antibiotic-induced e.
　　bacterial e.
　　cytomegalovirus e.
　　gangrenous ischemic e.
　　granulomatous e.
　　hemorrhagic e.
　　Hirschsprung-associated e. (HAEC)
　　necrotizing e. (NEC)
　　nontuberculous mycobacteria-
　　　associated e.
　　pericrypt eosinophilic e.
　　pseudomembranous e.
　　radiation e.
　　regional e.
　　Salmonella typhimurium e.
enterocolostomy
enterocutaneous
　　e. fistula
　　e. intubation
enterocyst
enterocystocele
enterocystoma
enterocystoplasty
　　Camey e.
　　clam e.
　　sigmoid e.
enterocyte
　　e. apoptosis
　　CD23 e.
　　intestinal e.
　　small intestinal e.
Enterocytozoon bieneusi
enterodiol
enterodynia
enteroendocrine cell
enteroenteral fistula
enteroenteric
　　e. anastomosis
　　e. fistula

E

NOTES

enteroenterostomy
    Braun e.
    Parker-Kerr closed method of end-
      to-end e.
    two-layer e.
enterogastric reflex
enterogastritis
enterogastrone
enterogenic proteinuria
enterogenous
    e. cyanosis
    e. cyst
enteroglucagon
enterogram
enterograph
enterography
enterohemorrhagic *Escherichia coli*
  (EHEC)
enterohepatic circulation (EHC)
enterohepatitis
enterohepatocele
enteroidea
enteroinsular axis
enterointestinal
enteroinvasive *Escherichia coli* **(EIEC)**
enterokinase
enterokinesia
enterokinetic
enterolactone
enterolith
    calcified e.
enterolithiasis
enterolithotomy
enterology
enterolysis
enteromegalia
enteromegaly
enteromenia
enteromesenteric occlusion
enterometer
enteromycodermitis
enteromycosis
enteromyiasis
enteron
enteronitis
    polytropous e.
enteroparesis
enteropathic
    e. organism
    e. reactive arthritis
enteropathica
    acrodermatitis e.
enteropathogen
enteropathogenic *Escherichia coli*
  (EPEC)
enteropathy
    allergic e.
    bile salt-losing e.

    choleretic e.
    chronic bacterial e.
    cow's milk-sensitive e. (CMSE)
    dermatopathic e.
    diabetic e.
    food-sensitive e.
    gluten-sensitive e. (GSE)
    HIV-1 e.
    idiopathic e.
    protein-losing e.
    radiation e.
    soya-induced e.
enteropathy-associated T-cell lymphoma
  (EATCL)
enteropeptidase deficiency
enteroperitoneal abscess
enteropexy
enteroplasty
enteroplegia
enteroplex
enteroplexy
Enteroport feeding pump
enteroproctia
enteroptosis
enteroptychia
enteroptychy
enterorrhagia
enterorrhaphy
enterorrhea
enterorrhexis
enteroscope
    magnifying e.
    Olympus SIF-10 e.
    Olympus SIF-M-series video e.
    Olympus SIF-Q240 e.
    Olympus SIF-SW-series video e.
    Olympus SIF-100 video push e.
    Olympus SSIF-series video e.
    Olympus XSIF-series video e.
    Pentax VSB-P-series e.
    push e.
    Sonde e.
    temporary e.
    tube e.
    video push e.
enteroscopy
    e. diagnosis
    double balloon e.
    intraoperative e. (IOE)
    push e.
    push-type e.
    Roux-en-Y limb e.
    small bowel e. (SBE)
    Sonde e.
    total peroral intraoperative e.
    transgastrostomic e. (TGE)
    video small bowel e.
    virtual e.

enterosepsis
enterosorption
enterospasm
enterostasis
enterostaxis
enterostenosis
enterostomal therapy (ET)
enterostomy
 double e.
 end-to-end e.
 gun-barrel e.
 tube e.
 Witzel e.
Entero-Test
enterotome
enterotomy
 antimesenteric e.
 inadvertent e.
 e. incision
 longitudinal e.
enterotoxemia
enterotoxication
enterotoxigenic *Escherichia coli* (ETEC)
enterotoxin
 Clostridium difficile e.
 e. diarrhea
 enteroaggregative *Escherichia coli*
  heat-stable e. 1 (EAST1)
 heat-labile e.
 heat-stable e. (ST)
enterotoxism
enterotropic
enterourethral fistula
enterourethrostomy
enterourinary fistula
enterovaginal fistula
enterovenous
enterovesical fistula
enterovirus
enterozoon, pl. enterozoa
Enterra
 E. gastrointestinal pacemaker
 E. therapy
enthesis
enthetic
entocele
entoderm
Entolase
Entozyme
Entract
 E. catheter

E. stent
 E. stone retriever
Entralife HN tube feeding formula
entrapment
 e. of bowel
 e. sack
 e. sack introducer
Entri-Pak
 E.-P. enteral feeding bag
 E.-P. tube feeding formula
EntriStar
 E. feeding tube
 E. polyurethane PEG tube
Entrition
 E. Entri-Pak feeding
 E. tube feeding formula
entropion
 eversion e.
entry site
ENtube-Pedi feeding tube
enucleation
enucleator
 Young e.
Enulose
enuresis
 adult-onset e.
 e. alarm
 e. alarm technique
 diurnal e.
 learned e.
 monosymptomatic nocturnal e.
  (MNE)
 nocturnal e.
 psychologic e.
 sleep e.
enuretic absence
envelope 2 antigen (anti-E2)
environment
 acidic e.
 bactericidal stomach e.
environmental metaplastic atrophic
 gastritis (EMAG)
enzimoimmunoassay MEIA Abbott
Enzol disinfectant
Enzygnost antiHIV 1+2 test
enzymatic
 e. fat necrosis
 e. spectrophotometric analysis
enzyme
 angiotensin-converting e. (ACE)
 AP marker e.
 brancher e.

E

NOTES

enzyme *(continued)*
    brush-border marker e.
    carboxypeptidase B-like e.
    catecholamine synthetic e.
    cellular e.
    e. change
    circulating e.
    COX-1 e.
    COX-2 e.
    cytochrome P450 e.
    debrancher e.
    degradative e.
    digestive e.
    gluconeogenesis-associated e.
    glycolytic e.
    glycosaminoglycan-degrading e.
    HK e.
    e. immunoassay (EIA)
    e. immunoassay E-1023
    insulin-degrading e. (IDE)
    Ku-Zyme HP pancreatic e.
    lactase e.
    LDH e.
    lipase e.
    lipolytic e.
    liver e.
    lysosomal e.
    NAG lysosomal marker e.
    pancreatic e.
    plasma e.
    proteinase e.
    proteolytic e.
    e. replacement therapy
    restriction e.
    SDH e.
    zinc-requiring e.
enzyme-conjugated anti-IgA antibody
enzyme-linked
    e.-l. immunosorbent assay (ELISA)
    e.-l. immunosorbent assay I
      (ELISA-I)
    e.-l. immunosorbent assay II
      (ELISA-II)
enzymic protein
enzymology
Enzymun test
EOA
    esophageal obturator airway
EOB-DTPA
    gadolinium EOB-DTPA (Gd-EOB-
      DTPA)
EOG
    eosinophilic gastroenteritis
EORTC
    European Organization for Research and
    Treatment of Cancer

eosin
    hematoxylin and e. (H&E)
    e. stain
eosin-methylene
    e.-m. blue (EMB)
    e.-m. blue agar
eosinophil
    e. cationic protein (ECP)
    e. protein X (EPX)
eosinophilia
eosinophilic
    e. ascites
    e. ballooning
    e. cholangiopathy
    e. colitis
    e. cystitis
    e. cytoplasm
    e. enteritis
    e. esophagitis
    e. gastritis
    e. gastroenteritis (EG, EGE, EOG)
    e. gastroenteritis syndrome
    e. gastroenteropathy
    e. granuloma
    e. ileal perforation
    e. major basic protein
eosinophiluria
Eovist
EP2-EP3 protein
EPA
    eicosapentaenoic acid
EPBD
    endoscopic papillary balloon dilation
EPC pain control
EPD
    endoscopic papillary balloon dilation
EPEC
    enteropathogenic *Escherichia coli*
ephedrine sulfate
EpHM
    intraesophageal pH monitoring
EPI
    exocrine pancreatic insufficiency
epicardia
epicardial
epicritic pain
EPICS
    EPICS C-flow flow cytometer
    EPICS Elite flow cytometer
    EPICS 700-series flow cytometer
    EPICS V-flow cytometer
epicystitis
epicystotomy
epidemic
    e. dysentery
    e. gangrenous proctitis
    e. hemorrhagic fever
    e. hepatitis

e. hypochlorhydria
e. nausea
e. nephritis
e. nephropathy
e. nonbacterial gastroenteritis
e. vomiting
epidemica
nephropathia e.
epidemiologic
epidemiological
epidemiology
epidermal
e. cyst
e. growth factor (EGF)
e. growth factor receptor (EGFR)
e. stria
epidermidis
Staphylococcus e.
epidermoid
e. carcinoma
e. cyst
epidermolysis
e. bullosa (EB)
e. bullosa acquisita
e. bullosa dystrophica
Epidermophyton floccosum
epididymal
e. abscess
e. cyst
e. infection
e. sarcoidosis
e. sperm aspiration (ESA)
e. tubule
e. tunic
epididymectomy
epididymidectomy
epididymidis
cauda e.
corpus e.
ductus e.
globus major e.
globus minor e.
vas e.
epididymis, pl. **epididymides**
appendix e.
body of e.
caput e.
cauda e.
corpus e.
e. epithelium
e. filariasis
e. lymphatic duct

e. marsupialization
e. micropuncture
microsurgical extraction of sperm
from e. (MASE)
e. obstruction
e. percutaneous puncture
e. secretion
epididymisoplasty
epididymitis
acute e.
mumps e.
spermatogenic e.
epididymodeferentectomy
epididymodeferential
epididymography
epididymoorchitis
pediatric cryptococcal e.
epididymoplasty
epididymotomy
epididymovasectomy
epididymovasostomy
microsurgical e. (MSEV)
epididymovesiculography
epidural
e. catheter
e. space
epifluorescence microscopy
epigastralgia
epigastric
e. angle
e. artery
e. discomfort
e. distress
e. fold
e. fossa
e. hernia
e. incision
e. pain
e. puncture
e. spot
e. zone
epigastrica
plica e.
epigastrium
epigastrocele
epigastrography
impedance e.
epigenetic
epiglottis
epi-illumination
7-beta-epimer of chenodeoxycholic acid
Epimorph

E

NOTES

epinephrectomy
epinephrine
epinephrine-induced gastroduodenal
  electromechanical
epinephritis
epinephroma
epinephros
epiphenomenon
epiphrenic diverticulum
epiplocele
epiploectomy
epiploenterocele
epiploic
    e. abscess
    e. appendage
    e. appendix
    e. foramen
epiploicum
    foramen e.
epiploitis
epiploon
    great e.
    lesser e.
epiplopexy
epiploplasty
epiplorrhaphy
epipodophyllotoxin
epirubicin
episcleritis
episiotomy scar
episode
    multiple acute rejection e.
episodic
    e. colic
    e. vomiting
epispadia (*var. of* epispadias)
epispadiac
    e. opening
    e. orifice
epispadial
epispadias, epispadia
    balanitic e.
    complete male e.
    congenital e.
    coronal e.
    female e.
    incontinent e.
    male e.
    penile e.
    penopubic e.
    e. repair
    subsymphyseal e.
epispadias-exstrophy complex
epistaxis
    Gull renal e.
    renal e.
epitaxial nucleation

epithelia
    CF e.
    cuboidal e.
    nontumorous e.
    oviduct e.
    tumorous e.
epithelial
    e. cell (EC)
    e. dysplasia
    e. endocrine cell
    e. growth factor
    e. inclusion body
    e. membrane antigen
    e. restitution and renewal
    e. sodium channel (ENaC)
    e. tumor
epitheliitis
epithelioid
    e. granuloma
    e. leiomyoma
epithelium
    adenomatous e.
    airway e.
    Barrett e.
    bladder e.
    celomic e.
    columnar e.
    congenital hypertrophy of the
      retinal pigment e. (CHRPE)
    crypt e.
    desquamated e.
    ductal e.
    epididymis e.
    flattening of ileal e.
    follicle-associated e.
    gastric foveolar e.
    gastric-type surface e.
    germinal e.
    heterotopic cylindric ciliated e.
    hyperplastic foveolar e.
    metaplastic e.
    nonkeratinizing squamous e.
    parietal e.
    proliferation of the gastric e.
    seminiferous tubule e.
    short-segment Barrett e.
    specialized columnar e. (SCE)
    squamous e.
    surface e.
    transitional e.
    villous e.
epithelium-lined tubule
epitope
    antibody to GOR e.
    B-cell e.
    Goodpasture e.
    HLA class II-restricted T-cell e.
    immunodominant T-cell e.

Lewis Y carbohydrate e.
nephritogenic e.
T-cell e.
epitrochlear
epityphlitis
epityphlon
Epivir-HBV
EPL
extracorporeal piezoelectric lithotripsy
Piezolith EPL
E.P. Mycin
EPO
erythropoietin
glycosylation of EPO
Epo
Epodyl
epoetin
e. alfa
e. beta
Epogen
Epon 812 resin
epoophoron
epoprostenol sodium
epoxyeicosatrienoic acid (EET)
EPP
erythropoietic proporphyria
Eppendorf
E. needle electrode
E. tube
Epping jaundice
EPS
endoscopic pancreatic sphincterotomy
endoscopic pancreatic stenting
expressed prostatic secretions
epsilon-aminocaproic acid
EPSP
excitatory postsynaptic potential
Epstein
E. disease
E. nephrosis
E. syndrome
Epstein-Barr
E.-B. viral infection
E.-B. virus (EBV)
EPT
endoscopic papillotomy
EPX
eosinophil protein X
Equagesic
Equalactin
equal fluid balance

equation
Cockcroft-Gault e.
Harris-Benedict energy
requirement e.
Henderson-Hasselbalch e.
Nernst e.
Portsmouth predictor e.
Equilet
equilibrium
acid-base e.
Gibbs-Donnan e.
solute e.
equina
cauda e.
equivalent
meconium ileus e. (MIE)
e. residual renal urea clearance
(eKru)
equivocal
equol
ER
estrogen receptor
ERA
estrogen receptor assay
eradication therapy
ER alpha
estrogen receptor alpha
ERBD
endoscopic retrograde biliary drainage
ER beta
estrogen receptor beta
Erbe Unit argon plasma coagulator
Erbotom F2 electrocoagulation unit
ERC
endoscopic retrograde cholangiography
ERCCE
endoscopic retrograde
cholecystoendoprosthesis
ERCP
endoscopic retrograde
cholangiopancreatography
ERCP balloon extractor
ERCP cannula
ERCP cannulation
ERCP catheter
ERCP conventional prosthesis
ERCP dilator
ERCP guidewire
ERCP manometry
ERCP nasobiliary drain
ERCP sphincterotome
ERCP-guided biopsy

E

NOTES

ERCP-induced splenic rupture
ERE
  estrogen response element
ErecAid
  E. vacuum erection device
  E. vacuum system
erectile
  e. dysfunction
  e. potency
  e. sinusoid
erection
  artificial e.
  artificial e. test
  drug-induced e.
  e. hemodynamics
  intraoperative penile e.
  Medicated Urethral System for E.
    (MUSE)
  medication-associated e.
  nocturnal e.
  nonbuckling e.
  penile e.
  pharmacologically induced e.
  psychogenic e.
  reflex e.
  reflexogenic e.
  vacuum constriction e.
ERF
  esophagorespiratory fistula
Ergamisol
ergonovine test
ergot
  e. alkaloid
  e. derivative
ergotamine
erigendi
  impotentia e.
erigentes
  nervi e.
ERK
  extracellular signal-regulated protein
    kinase
Erlangen
  E. magnetic colostomy device
  E. papillotome
  E. pull-type precut papillotomy
  E. pull-type sphincterotomy
Erlanger active stimulator for
  interventional endoscopy
eroded polyp
E-rosetted
erosion
  aphthous e.
  Cameron e.
  cancerous e.
  cervical e.
  chronic e.

Dieulafoy gastric e.
duodenal e.
gastric antral e.
gastric mucosal e.
gravity-induced e.
idiopathic chronic e.
implant e.
limiting plate e.
linear e.
mucosal e.
salt and pepper duodenal e.
stress e.
erosive
  e. duodenitis
  e. esophagitis
  e. gastritis
  e. gastropathy
  e. prepyloric change
erosive-hemorrhagic gastritis
erotic vomiting
ERP
  endoscopic retrograde pancreatography
  endoscopic retrograde parenchymography
ERPF
  effective renal plasma flow
ERPP
  endoscopic retrograde parenchymography
    of pancreas
ERSNA
  efferent renal sympathetic nerve activity
ERT
  estrogen replacement therapy
eructation
  nervous e.
ERUS
  endorectal ultrasound
Eryc
EryPed
erysipelas
Ery-Tab
erythema
  conjunctival e.
  e. elevatum diutinum
  joint e.
  e. multiforme (EM)
  necrolytic migratory e.
  e. nodosum
  palmar e.
  e. toxicum
  urethral meatal e.
erythematosus
  discoid lupus e.
  disseminated lupus e. (DLE)
  lupus e.
  procainamide-induced systemic
    lupus e.
  systemic lupus e. (SLE)

erythematous
 e. gastropathy
 e. streak
erythrasma
Erythrocin
erythrocyte (E)
 e. aggregation
 e. cast
 dysmorphic e.
 eumorphic e.
 e. lysis assay
 neuraminidase-treated sheep e.
 e. sedimentation rate (ESR)
 e. sedimentation rate test
 e. sickling
erythrocytosis
 absolute e.
 stress e.
erythrocyturia
erythroid
 e. colony formation
 e. hypoplasia
erythromycin
 e. base
 e. estolate hepatotoxicity
 e. ethylsuccinate
 e. lactobionate
erythromycin-induced cholecystitis
erythroplasia
 Queyrat e.
 Zoon e.
erythropoiesis
 ineffective e.
erythropoietic
 e. coproporphyria
 e. proporphyria (EPP)
 e. protoporphyria
erythropoietin (EPO)
 human recombinant e.
 e. hyporesponsiveness
 recombinant e.
 recombinant human e. (rh-EPO)
 e. therapy
ES
 endoscopic sclerotherapy
 endoscopic sphincterotomy
ESA
 epididymal sperm aspiration
Esbach method
Esca Buess + fistula funnel

escalated methotrexate, vinblastine, Adriamycin, cisplatin or cyclophosphamide (E-MVAC)
Escherichia
 E. coli
 E. faecalis
escutcheon
 female e.
 male e.
E-selectin expression
Eshmun complex
Esidrix
ESI fiberoptic sigmoidoscope
Esimil
ESKA-Buess esophageal tube
ESLD
 end-stage liver disease
esmolol
esogastritis
esomeprazole magnesium
EsophaCoil
 E. prosthesis
 E. self-expanding esophageal stent
esophagalgia
esophageal
 e. A, B ring
 e. achalasia
 e. acid clearance
 e. acid infusion test
 e. adenocarcinoma
 e. atresia
 e. balloon dilator
 e. balloon distention
 e. balloon tamponade
 e. banding
 e. banding technique
 e. band ligation
 e. biopsy
 e. body contraction amplitude
 e. body contraction duration
 e. body motor dysfunction
 e. bougienage
 e. cancer
 e. candidiasis (EC)
 e. cast
 e. clearing
 e. colic
 e. collateral vein (ECV)
 e. compression
 e. condyloma acuminatum
 e. condyloma virus
 e. contractile ring

E

NOTES

esophageal *(continued)*
   e. curling
   e. dilation
   e. dilation treatment
   e. diverticulum
   e. duplication cyst
   e. dysmotility
   e. dysphagia
   e. ectopic sebaceous gland
   e. effect
   e. endoprosthesis
   e. epidermal growth factor (EEGF)
   e. extirpation
   e. fistula
   e. foreign body
   e. function test
   e. fungal infection
   e. gastric tube airway (EGTA)
   e. globus
   e. globus sensation
   e. groove
   e. hyperkeratosis
   e. hyperkinesia
   e. hypomotility
   e. impression
   e. inlet
   e. intramural diverticulosis
   e. intramural hematoma
   e. intramural pseudodiverticulosis
   e. intubation
   e. I stent
   e. leiomyoma
   e. Lewy body
   e. lumen
   e. malignancy
   e. manometric sequence (EMS)
   e. manometry (EM)
   e. mass
   e. motility
   e. motility disorder (EMD)
   e. motility perfused catheter
   e. motor disorder
   e. mucosa
   e. mucosal ring
   e. muscular ring
   e. myotomy
   e. obstruction
   e. obturator airway (EOA)
   e. osteophyte
   e. paralysis
   e. perforation
   e. perfusate
   e. perfusion catheter
   e. peristalsis
   e. peristaltic pressure
   e. pH monitoring
   e. photodynamic therapy
   e. plexus

   e. polyp
   e. prosthesis
   e. reflux
   e. resection
   e. rupture
   e. scleroderma
   e. shunt
   e. single balloon
   e. sling procedure
   e. sound
   e. spasm
   e. sphincter
   e. sphincter relaxation
   e. squamous cell carcinoma
   e. squamous papilloma
   e. stenosis
   e. stethoscope
   e. Strecker stent
   e. stricture
   e. tear
   e. transection
   e. transit scan
   e. transit time
   e. trauma
   e. tube
   e. tuberculosis
   e. tumor
   e. ulcer
   e. ulceration
   e. valve (ESV)
   e. variceal bleeding
   e. variceal hemorrhage (EVH)
   e. variceal sclerosant
   e. variceal sclerosis
   e. variceal sclerotherapy (EVS)
   e. varix
   e. wall
   e. wall thickness (EWT)
   e. web
   e. Z stent with anchor

esophagectasia
esophagectasis, esophagectasia
esophagectomy
   Ivor Lewis two-stage subtotal e.
   transhiatal blunt e.
   transhiatal radical e.
   transhiatal simple e.
   transthoracic e.
   e. with thoracotomy
esophagi (*pl. of* esophagus)
esophagism
   hiatal e.
esophagismus
esophagitis
   acid-pepsin reflux e.
   acid-peptic e.
   acute corrosive e.
   acute necrotizing e.

alkaline reflux e.
aspergillosis e.
bacterial e.
Barrett e.
Candida e.
candidal e.
caustic e.
chemical-induced e.
chronic peptic e.
CMV e.
corrosive e.
cytomegalovirus e.
e. dissecans superficialis
drug-induced e.
endoscopic e.
eosinophilic e.
erosive e.
herpes simplex e.
herpetic e.
herpetiform e.
histological e.
infectious e.
Leishmania e.
Los Angeles Classification (grade A, B, C, D) e.
Monilia e.
monilial e.
mucormycosis e.
nonerosive e.
nonreflux e.
nonspecific e.
peptic e.
pill e.
pill-induced e.
polycystic chronic e.
radiation e.
reflux e. (RE)
refractory e.
retention e.
Savary-Gilliard e. (grade I, II)
severe erosive e.
severe reflux e.
stasis e.
streptococcal e.
thrush e.
tuberculous e.
tuberculous infectious e.
ulcerative reflux e.
esophagobronchial fistula
esophagocardial malignancy
esophagocardiomyotomy
esophagocardioplasty

esophagocele
esophagocolic anastomosis
esophagocologastrostomy
esophagocoloplasty
esophagoduodenostomy
esophagodynia
esophagoenterostomy
esophagoesophagostomy
esophagofiberscope
esophagofundopexy
esophagogastrectomy (EG)
    Ivor Lewis e.
    thoracoabdominal e.
esophagogastric (EG)
    e. balloon tamponade (EGBT)
    e. fat pad
    e. intubation
    e. junction
    e. junction cancer
    e. pH-metry
    e. tamponade
    e. variceal bleeding
    e. varix
esophagogastroanastomosis
esophagogastroduodenoscopy (EGD)
    pediatric e.
    small-caliber e.
esophagogastromyotomy
esophagogastropexy
    intercostal pedicle e.
esophagogastroplasty
    Grondahl-Finney e.
esophagogastroscopy
    Abbott e.
    Clagett-Barrett e.
    intrathoracic e.
    Johnson e.
    Thal e.
    Woodward e.
esophagogastrostomy
    Abbott e.
    Barrett-Clagett e.
    Clagett e.
    Clagett-Barrett e.
    intrathoracic e.
    Johnson e.
    Thal e.
    Woodward e.
esophagogram
    double channel e.
    solid-column e.
    tube e.

E

NOTES

esophagography
    contrast e.
esophagojejunal anastomosis
esophagojejunoplasty
esophagojejunostomy
    loop e.
    Roux-en-Y e.
esophagolaryngectomy
esophagology
esophagomalacia
esophagomediastinal fistula
esophagometer
esophagomycosis
esophagomyotomy
    Heller e.
esophagopharynx
esophagoplasty
    colic patch e.
esophagopleural fistula
esophagoplication
esophagoprobe
    Olympus ultrasonic e.
esophagoproximal gastrectomy
esophagoptosis
esophagopulmonary fistula
esophagorespiratory fistula (ERF)
esophagosalivary reflex
esophagosalivation
esophagoscope
    ACMI fiberoptic e.
    ballooning e.
    Blom-Singer e.
    Boros e.
    Broyle e.
    Bruening e.
    Brunings e.
    Chevalier Jackson e.
    child e.
    Denck e.
    Dohlman e.
    Eder-Hufford rigid e.
    Eutaw-Hoffman e.
    fiberoptic e.
    Foregger rigid e.
    Foroblique fiberoptic e.
    full-lumen e.
    Haslinger e.
    Holinger e.
    Hufford e.
    infant e.
    Jackson e.
    Jasbee e.
    Jesberg e.
    J-scope e.
    Kalk e.
    large-bore rigid e.
    Lell e.
    LoPresti fiberoptic e.

    Moersch e.
    Mosher e.
    Moure e.
    Negus rigid e.
    Olympus EF-series e.
    optical e.
    oval e.
    oval-open e.
    Roberts folding e.
    Roberts-Jesberg e.
    Roberts oval e.
    Sam Roberts e.
    Schindler e.
    Storz e.
    Tesberg e.
    Tucker e.
    Universal e.
    Yankauer e.
esophagoscopy
    flexible e.
    rigid e.
    video e.
esophagospasm
esophagostenosis
esophagostoma
esophagostomy
esophagotome
esophagotomy
esophagotracheal fistula
esophagram
    barium e.
    contrast e.
    double-contrast e.
esophagraphy
esophagus, pl. esophagi
    abdominal e.
    achalasia-like e.
    aperistaltic e.
    A ring of e.
    atonic e.
    Barrett e. (BE)
    black e.
    B ring of e.
    cervical e.
    closed e.
    columnar-lined e. (CLE)
    corkscrew e.
    dilation of e.
    distal e.
    effort rupture of e.
    external coat of e.
    Heller-Belsey correction of
      achalasia of e.
    Heller-Nissen correction of
      achalasia of e.
    hypersensitive e.
    introitus esophagi
    long-segment Barrett e. (LSBE)

nutcracker e.
pneumatic bag dilation of e.
primary malignant melanoma of
the e. (PMME)
pseudowatermelon e.
scleroderma of e.
short-segment Barrett e. (SSBE)
spastic e.
strictured e.
thoracic e.
tortuous e.
variceal sclerotherapy in e.

esorubicin
esprolol plus Viagra
ESR
erythrocyte sedimentation rate
ESR immunological study
immunological study
ESRD
end-stage renal disease
Essed
E. plication method
E. surgical procedure
essential
e. amino acid
e. fatty acid (EFA)
e. fatty acid deficiency (EFAD)
e. hematuria
EST
endoscopic sphincterotomy
estazolam
**Esteem advanced vacuum therapy for
impotence**
ester
cholesterol e.
cholesteryl e.
cypionate e.
dinitrate and mononitrate e.
enanthate e.
injectable e.
N^G-nitro-L-arginine methyl e. (L-
NAME)
esterase
leukocyte e.
e. stain
urinary leukocyte e.
esterification
esterified fecal acid
esthesioneuroblastoma
estimate
ultrasonography e.

estimated
e. blood loss (EBL)
e. liver blood flow (ELBF)
Estracyt
estradiol
e. releasing silicone vaginal ring
e. transderm patch
estramustine
e. binding protein (EMBP)
e. phosphate
e. phosphate sodium
Estring estradiol vaginal ring
estrogen
e. binding site (EBS)
conjugated e. (CE)
e. deficiency
e. receptor (ER)
e. receptor alpha (ER alpha)
e. receptor assay (ERA)
e. receptor beta (ER beta)
e. replacement therapy (ERT)
e. response element (ERE)
e. testicular secretion
estrogen binding site (EBS)
estrogen-induced
e.-i. cholestasia
e.-i. liver disease
estrone
ESU
electrosurgical unit
ESV
esophageal valve
ESWL
electrohydraulic shock wave lithotripsy
extracorporeal shock wave lithotripsy
Modulith SL 20 device for ESWL
ESWL related dysrhythmia
ET
endothelin
endotracheal tube
enterostomal therapy
ET-1
endothelin-1
ET-3
endothelin-3
EtA
endothelin A
EtA, EtB antagonist
EtA, EtB receptor
EtB
endothelin B

E

NOTES

ETCD
  endoscopic transpapillary cyst drainage
ETCG
  endoscopic transpapillary catheterization
  of the gallbladder
ETEC
  enterotoxigenic *Escherichia coli*
E-test
ethacrynic acid
ethambutol
Ethamolin
ethanol (EtOH, ETOH)
  e. abuse
  dehydrated e.
  gastric first-pass metabolism of e.
    (GFPM)
  e. injection
  e. injection therapy
  e. and phosphate enriched dialysate
  e. sclerotherapy
ethanolamine
  e. oleate
  e. oleate sclerosant
ethanolamine oleate
ethanol-enriched
ethanol-induced tumor necrosis (ETN)
ethanolism
ethanol-specific impairment
Ethaquin
ethaverine
ethchlorvynol
ether
    methyl tert-butyl e., methyl tertiary
      butyl ether (MTBE)
    methyl tertiary butyl e. (MTBE)
    trimethylsilyl e.
Ethezyme debriding ointment
Ethibond suture
Ethicon
    E. CDH29 stapler
    E. TLH30 stapler
    E. trocar
ethidium
  e. bromide
  e. bromide staining
Ethiflex suture
Ethilon suture
ethinylestradiol
ethiofos
ethionamide
ethmoid
ethoglucid
ethopropazine
ethosuximide
Ethox feeding tube
ethoxysclerol
Ethril
ethyl alcohol

ethylcellulose
ethylchlorformate polymerized antigen
ethylene
  e. glycol
  e. glycol tetraacetic acid (EGTA)
  e. oxide
  e. oxide gas (ETO)
ethylenediamine
  e. tetraacetic acid (EDTA)
  theophylline e.
ethylenediaminetetraacetate
  51-chromium-labeled e. (^{51}Cr-EDTA)
ethylene oxide gas (ETO)
ethylsuccinate
  erythromycin e.
5-ethynyluracil
Ethyol
etidronate
etiology
etiopathogenesis
ETN
  ethanol-induced tumor necrosis
ET-NANBH
  enterically transmitted non-A, non-B
    hepatitis
ETO
  ethylene oxide gas
  ETO sterilization
etodolac
EtOH, ETOH
  ethanol
  EtOH consumption
etomidate
etoposide
  e., Adriamycin, Platinol (EAP)
  e., ifosfamide, cisplatin
  e. injection
  e., leucovorin, 5-fluorouracil (ELF)
  platinum, e. (PE)
Etude cystometer uroflowmeter
EU
  excretory urography
eubacterial strain
Eubacterium
    E. lentum
    E. limosum
Eucestoda
euchlorhydria
eucholia
euchylia
euglycemic hyperinsulinemia
Eulexin plus LHRH-A
  chemotherapy/radiation therapy
  protocol
eumorphic
  e. erythrocyte
  e. red blood cell
eupancreatism

eupepsia
eupepsy
eupeptic
euperistalsis
Euphorbia resinifera
Euro-Collins
    E.-C. fluid
    E.-C. solution
European Organization for Research and Treatment of Cancer (EORTC)
Eurotransplant kidney allocation
EUS
    echoendoscopy
    endoscopic ultrasonography
    endoscopic ultrasound
        EUS CPN
        EUS probe-guided electrosurgery
EUS-AD gastric lesion staging by endoscopic ultrasonography
EUS-FNA
    endoscopic ultrasound-guided fine-needle aspiration
EUS-guided
    EUS-g. fine-needle aspiration
    EUS-g. FNA
EUS-M gastric lesion staging by endoscopic ultrasonography
EUS-SM gastric lesion staging by endoscopic ultrasonography
Eutaw-Hoffman esophagoscope
eutectic
    e. mixture
    e. mixture of local anesthetics (EMLA)
Eutonyl
euvolemic
Evac-Q-Kit
    E.-Q.-K. bowel preparation
, **Evac-Q-Kwik**
    E.-Q.-K. bowel preparation
evacuation
    digital rectal e.
    e. disorder
    hematobilia e.
    ileal reservoir e.
    e. pouchography
    e. proctography
    rectal e.
    stool e.
evacuator
    Creevy e.
    Ellik e.

    McCarthy e.
    Toomey e.
    Urovac bladder e.
Evac-U-Gen
Evac-U-Lac
Evac-U-Lax
evagination
Evalose
evaluation
    acute physiology, age and chronic health e. (APACHE)
    adolescent urologic e.
    diagnostic imaging e.
    diverticulitis e.
    endoscopic ultrasound e.
    followup e.
    geriatric incontinence e.
    Heart Outcomes Prevention E. (HOPE)
    manometric e.
    medical e.
    metabolic e.
    peripheral nerve e. (PNE)
    presurgical medical e.
    pretransplant e.
    risk e.
    serum metabolic e.
    sexual e.
    status e.
    urinary tract four-glass e.
    urodynamic e.
    videourodynamic e.
evanescent
Evans
    E. blue
    E. blue dye
EVE Fujinon videocolonoscope
event
    thromboembolic e.
eventration
Everett pile forceps
Everett-TeLinde operation
eversion
    e. entropion
    e. normal
    e. operation
    e. orchiopexy
    vaginal e.
evert
everted umbilicus
everting suture

E

NOTES

EVH
> esophageal variceal hemorrhage

evidence
> solid e.

eviration

EVIS
> EVIS Exera
> EVIS EXERA Video System
> EVIS 140 Q series endoscope
> EVIS 140 S wide-screen endoscope

evisceration
> pelvic e.
> total abdominal e. (TAE)

EVL
> endoscopic variceal ligation

evoked potential

EVS
> esophageal variceal sclerotherapy

Ewald
> E. breakfast
> E. gastroscope
> E. node
> E. test meal
> E. tube

Ewing sarcoma

EWT
> esophageal wall thickness

ex
> ex vivo
> ex vivo cannulation
> ex vivo liver-directed gene therapy
> ex vivo perfusion

exacerbation of pain

examination
> abdominal tomodensitometric e.
> adolescent genitourinary e.
> anorectal e.
> arterioportographical e.
> bidigital rectal e.
> bladder e.
> cytology e.
> digital rectal e. (DRE)
> double-contrast barium enema e.
> endoscopic e.
> fistula in ano endoscopic e.
> followup e.
> merthiolate fresh stool e.
> microscopic urine e.
> motor e.
> nonrehydrated guaiac e.
> parasite e.
> peroral pneumocolon e.
> prostate gland color flow
>   Doppler e.
> rectal e.
> reflux small bowel e.
> retrograde small bowel e.

> tomodensitometric e.
> vertical strip pattern breast e.

exanthematicus
> ichthyismus e.

exanthesis arthrosia

excavated gastric carcinoma

excavatio, pl. **excavationes**
> e. rectouterina
> e. rectovesicalis
> e. vesicouterina

excavation
> ischiorectal e.
> rectoischiadic e.

excavatum
> pectus e.

excel
> E. disposable biopsy forceps

excess
> base e.
> e. mucus

excessive
> e. bleeding
> e. straining

exchange
> cation e.
> countercurrent e.
> e. of endoprosthesis
> endoscopic stent e.
> guidewire e.
> plasma e.
> short-dwell hypertonic e.
> sodium e.
> stent e.
> wire-guided balloon-assisted
>   endoscopic biliary stent e.

exchanger
> cation e.
> heat e.
> thymocyte NA+/H+ e.

excision
> abdominoperineal e.
> adrenal gland laparoscopic e.
> Allingham rectum e.
> bladder e.
> cold snare e.
> Delorme transrectal e.
> full-thickness local e. (FTLE)
> Gibson e.
> laparoscopic abdominoperineal e.
> laser hemorrhoid e.
> mesorectal e.
> pouch e.
> sinus e.
> total mesorectal e. (TME)
> transanal e.

excitation-contraction coupling

excitatory
    e. junction potential (EJP)
    e. postsynaptic potential (EPSP)
excitotoxic food poisoning
exclusion
    Devine e.
    e. diet
    duodenal e. (DE)
    subtotal gastric e.
excoriation
excrement
excrementitious
excrescence
    polypoid e.
excreta
excrete
excretion
    basal renal e.
    biliary e.
    calcium e.
    calculation of renal ammonium e.
    ^{57}Co B$_{12}$ e.
    ^{51}Cr-EDTA e.
    C-urea breath e.
    C-urinary e.
    electrolyte e.
    fecal fat e. (FFE)
    glucose e.
    24-hour fecal fat e.
    net acid e. (NAE)
    pulmonary methane e.
    e. pyelography
    quantified protein e.
    renal acid e.
    renal ammonium e.
    renal phosphate e.
    renal sodium e.
    urate renal e.
    urinary chloride e.
    urinary kallikrein e.
    urinary protein e.
    urinary sodium e. (UNaV)
    urinary urea nitrogen e. (UUN)
    waste nitrogen e.
    water e.
    whole-kidney fractional e.
excretor
    methane (CH4) e.
    non-CH4 e.
excretory
    e. azoospermia
    e. cystogram (XC)

    e. delay
    e. duct
    e. function
    e. urogram (XU)
    e. urography (EU, EXU)
excursion
    respiratory e.
excystation
exdwelling ureteral occlusion balloon catheter
exendin
exenteration
    anterior pelvic e.
    pelvic e.
    posterior pelvic e.
    supralevator pelvic e.
    total pelvic e.
exenterative surgery for pelvic cancer
exenteritis
Exera
    EVIS E.
exercise
    Kegel pelvic muscle e.
    pelvic floor e. (PFE)
    vaginal cone for pelvic floor e.'s
exercise-associated acute renal failure
exercise-induced hematuria
exeresis
    palliative e.
exertional rhabdomyolysis
exertion-induced pain
exfoliative
    e. cystitis
    e. cytology
    e. epithelial colonic cell
    e. gastritis
exisulind
exit
    e. site
    e. site of catheter
    e. site infection
Ex-Lax
Exna
exocolitis
exocrine
    e. function
    e. pancreas
    e. pancreatic hypoplasia
    e. pancreatic insufficiency (EPI)
exocytosis
    granulocyte e.
exoenzyme-S

E

NOTES

exogastric
exogastritis
exogenous
    e. androgen
    e. calcium
    e. cholecystokinin or cerulein
    e. IGF-1
    e. obesity
    e. PGE2
    e. thiol
exomphalos
exon (1–5)
exon skipping
exopeptidase
    pancreatic e.
exophytic
    e. adenocarcinoma
    e. lesion
    e. mass
    e. wart
exotoxin
    Pseudomonas e. A
expandable
    e. biliary endoprosthesis
    e. esophageal stent (EES)
    e. intrahepatic portacaval shunt
      stent
    e. metallic stent
    e. metal mesh endoprosthesis
    e. olive
expander
    rectal e.
expanding retroperitoneal hematoma
expansile abdominal mass
expansion
    controlled e. (CX)
    controlled radial e. (CRE)
    intravascular volume e.
    mesangial matrix e.
    plasma volume e.
    volume e.
expenditure
    resting energy e. (REE)
experience
    initial clinical e.
experienced rectal spasm
experiment
    Nussbaum e.
experimental background
expiratory
    e. breath ethanol concentration
    end e.
explant
exploration
    common bile duct e. (CBDE)
    common duct e. (CDE)
    complete surgical e. (CSE)

    laparoscopically guided
      transcystic e.
    laparoscopic transcystic duct e.
    renal e.
    transcystic duct/common bile
      duct e. (TCD/CBDE)
exploratory
    e. celiotomy
    e. laparotomy
explosion
    colonic e.
explosive
    e. diarrhea
    e. doubling time
    e. vomiting
exponential rate
exposure
    occupational toxin e.
    postural quantitative analysis of
      acid e.
    radiation e.
    toxin e.
expressed prostatic secretions (EPS)
expression
    breast cancer-associated protein
      pS2 e.
    carbohydrate antigen 19-9
      immunohistochemical e.
    complex class II e.
    e. cystourethrography
    cytokine gene e.
    E-selectin e.
    fibronectin e.
    p53 e.
    renal tissue kallikrein e.
    tissue-specific gene e.
exquisite
    e. pain
    e. tenderness
exquisitely tender abdomen
exsanguinating hemorrhage
exsanguination
exsiccation fever
exstrophic bladder plate
exstrophy
    bladder e.
    cloacal e.
    e. closure
    vesical e.
exstrophy-epispadias
    e.-e. complex
extended
    e. daily dialysis (EDD)
    e. left subcostal incision
    e. obturator node and iliopsoas
      node dissection
    e. pelvic lymphadenectomy
    e. pyelolithotomy

e. pyelotomy
e. right hepatectomy

extensibility

penile e.

extension

caliceal e.
direct e.
dumbbell-shaped caliceal e.
e. fiber
full e.

extensive pelvic disease
exteriorization colostomy
externa

fascia spermatica e.
lamina rara e. (LRE)
muscularis e.

external

e. anal sphincter (EAS)
e. anal sphincter muscle
e. anorectal mucosal prolapse
e. biliary diversion
e. biliary fistula
e. biliary lavage
e. coat of esophagus
e. cooling
e. cooling appliance
e. drainage
e. hemorrhoid
e. iliac artery
e. inguinal ring
e. ligament
e. oblique
e. oblique aponeurosis
e. oblique fascia
e. oblique muscle
e. proctotomy
e. rectal sphincter
e. rotation
e. shock wave lithotripsy
e. skin tag
e. spermatic fascia
e. spermatic vein
e. sphincter ani profundus muscle
e. sphincterotomy
e. stimulus
e. straightener
e. striated urinary sphincter
e. swelling
e. trauma
e. ureteral catheter
e. urethral barrier device
e. urethral sphincter

e. urethrotomy
e. vacuum therapy

external-beam

e.-b. irradiation
e.-b. radiation therapy (EBRT)

externally releasable knot
externi

urethritis orificii e.

extirpation

esophageal e.
surgical e.

extra

e. heart sound
E. Stiff Amplatz wire

extraabdominal disease
extraanatomical renal revascularization technique
extracapillary crescent formation
extracapsular

e. disease
e. tumor

extracellular

e. calcium
e. fluid (ECF)
e. fluid volume (ECV)
e. hyperosmolarity
e. lipid
e. matrix (ECM)
e. potassium
e. signal-regulated protein kinase (ERK)
e. superoxide

extracolonic malignancy (ECM)
extracorporeal

e. anastomosis
e. assist device
e. cardiopulmonary circuit
e. dialysis
e. lithotripsy
e. liver assist device (ELAD)
e. liver perfusion (ECLP)
e. organ bioartificial liver device
e. partial nephrectomy
e. piezoelectric lithotripsy (EPL)
e. piezoelectric lithotriptor
e. piezoelectric shock wave lithotripsy
e. renal preservation
e. repair
e. shock wave
e. shock wave lithotripsy (ESWL)
e. shock wave lithotriptor

E

NOTES

extracorporeal *(continued)*
  e. surgery
  e. ultrafiltration (ECU)
  e. whole organ perfusion
extract
  pollen e.
  pygeum e.
  Serenoa repens e.
extracted
  e. ductal sperm
  e. nuclear antigen (ENA)
extraction
  e. balloon
  e. balloon technique
  basket e.
  e. bile duct stone
  bolus e.
  foreign body e.
  harpoon e.
  e. pancreatic stone
  stone e.
  testicular sperm e. (TESE)
extractor
  Applied Biosystems 340A nucleic
    acid e.
  endoscopic magnetic e.
  ERCP balloon e.
  Glassman stone e.
  Soehendra stent e.
  E. three-lumen retrieval balloon
    catheter
  E. XL triple-lumen retrieval
    balloon
eXtract specimen bag
extractum senna
extradomain A positive (EDA+)
extradural electrical stimulation
extraesophageal symptom
**extraglandular endocrine cell
  proliferation**
extraglomerular mesangium (EGM)
extragonadal
  e. germ cell cancer
  e. germ cell neoplasm
extrahepatic
  e. bile duct
  e. bile duct atresia (EHBDA)
  e. bile duct cancer
  e. bile duct obstruction
  e. biliary atresia (EBA)
  e. biliary cystic dilation
  e. biliary obstruction
  e. biliary stricture
  e. cholestasia
  e. metastasis (EHM)
  e. portal vein
  e. portal vein obstruction (EHPVO)

  e. portal venous hypertension
  e. shunt
extraintestinal complication
extralymphatic metastasis
extramammary Paget disease (EMPD)
extramedullary
  e. hematopoiesis
  e. plasmacytoma
extramucosal
  e. cyst
  e. mass
extramural
  e. common bile duct compression
  e. lesion
  e. pseudocyst
**extraordinary urinary frequency
  syndrome of childhood**
extrapancreatic
  e. nerve plexus
  e. pseudocyst
extraparenchymal renal cyst
extraperitoneal
  e. endoscopic pelvic lymph node
    dissection (EEPLND)
  e. excision of lower one-third of
    ureter
  e. fascia
  e. laparoscopic bladder neck
    suspension (ELBNS)
  e. laparoscopic nephrectomy
  e. laparoscopy
  e. supracostal live donor
    nephrectomy
  e. tissue
  totally e. (TEP)
**extrapolated plasma caffeine
  concentration**
extraprostatitis
extrapudendal pelvic nerve
extrapulmonary *Pneumocystis carinii*
  infection
extrapyramidal function assessment
extrarenal
  e. antigen
  e. azotemia
  e. calix
  e. dysmorphy
  e. mass
  e. renal pelvis
  e. uremia
  e. vasculitis
extrasphincteric
  e. anal fistula
  e. approach
extraurethral incontinence
extravaginal torsion
extravasate

extravasated
    e. bile
    e. iodinated contrast material
extravasation
    e. of contrast medium
    peripelvic e.
    pyelosinus e.
    red blood cell e.
    urinary e.
    urine e.
extravascular space
extraversion
    urinary e.
extravesical
    e. anastomosis
    e. reimplantation
    e. seromuscular tunnel
    e. ureteral reimplantation technique
    e. ureterolysis
extravisceral aneurysm
extremitas, pl. **extremitates**
extremity
    anterior e.
    inferior e.
    posterior e.
    superior e.
    c. weakness
extrinsic
    e. biliary compression

    e. mass
    e. pancreatic compression
    e. ureteral obstruction
    e. ureteropelvic junction obstruction
extrude
extruding mucus
extubate
extussusception
EXU
    excretory urography
exuberant granulation tissue
exudate
    fibrinopurulent e.
    mucopurulent e.
    pharyngeal e.
    whitish e.
exudate-transudate concept
exudative
    e. ascites
    e. nephritis
    e. peritonitis
exulceratio simplex
EYCAT
    egg yolk-cobalamin absorption test
eyelet
Ez-HBT
E-Z Paque
EZ vascular 35 linear stapler

NOTES

E

F-18, ^{18}**F**
    fluorine-18
F9 cell
F2 focal point
Faber
    F. anemia
    F. syndrome
fabianii
    Hansenula f.
FABP
    fatty acid binding protein
Fabricius
    bursa of F.
Fabry disease
FAC
    5-fluorouracil, Adriamycin,
      cyclophosphamide
face
    cytosolic f.
    en f.
    linear streaks en f.
    stable f.
faceplate
    Coloplast irrigation f.
    Marlen Neoprene All-Flexible f.
    Torbot f.
    United Surgical Hypalon f.
faceted gallstone
facial tenderness
facies
    f. abdominalis
    f. anterior pancreatis
    cushingoid f.
    f. diaphragmatica hepatis
    f. hepatica
    f. inferior hepatis
    f. inferior pancreatis
    moon f.
    f. posterior hepatis
    f. posterior pancreatis
    Potter f.
    f. superior hepatis
    f. visceralis hepatis
faciodigital syndrome
FACS
    fluorescence-activated cell sorter
FACScan
    fluorescence-activated cell sorter scan
FACScan flow cytometer
factitial
    f. dermatitis
    f. proctitis
factitious diarrhea
Factive

factor
    f. VIII
    acidic fibroblast growth f.
    acid-inhibitory f.
    adverse prognostic f.
    alcoholic prognostic f.
    angiogenic f.
    f. VIII antigen
    atrial natriuretic f. (ANF)
    autocrine motility f. (AMF)
    bacterial virulence f.
    basic fibroblast growth f. (bFGF)
    basic fibroblastic growth f.
    B-cell differentiation f.
    beta-fibroblastic growth f.
    beta-HCG autocrine motility f.
    binary f.
    bladder cancer angiogenic f.
    brain-derived neurotrophic f.
      (BDNF)
    chemotactic f.
    clotting f.
    cobra venom f. (CVF)
    colony-stimulating f. (CSF)
    concentration epidermal growth f.
      (cEGF)
    crest f.
    cytotoxin necrotizing f.
    decapacitation f.
    decay-accelerating f. (DAF)
    endothelial cell growth f. (ECGF)
    endothelium-derived relaxing f.
      (EDRF)
    epidermal growth f. (EGF)
    epithelial growth f.
    esophageal epidermal growth f.
      (EEGF)
    fibroblast-derived f.
    fibroblast growth f. (FGF)
    gastric inhibitor f.
    glial cell line-derived
      neurotrophic f. (GDNF)
    glial-derived neurotrophic f.
      (GDNF)
    glycyrrhetinic acid like f. (GALF)
    granulocyte-macrophage colony-
      stimulating f. (GM-CSF)
    growth f.
    guanine nucleotide-releasing f.
      (GNRF)
    f. H
    heat-labile f. (HLF)
    heparin-binding epidermal growth f.
      (HB-EGF)
    hepatocyte growth f. (HGF)

F

factor *(continued)*
    histamine-releasing f. (HRF)
    host f.
    human epidermal growth f. (h-EGF)
    human growth f. (HGF)
    insulinlike growth f. (IGF)
    insulinlike growth f.-2 (IGF-2)
    intrinsic f. (IF)
    keratinocyte growth f.
    luminal CCK-releasing f.
    luteinizing hormone-follicle-stimulating hormone releasing f.
    macrophage colony-stimulating f. (M-CSF)
    migration inhibition f. (MIF)
    mineralocorticoid-independent f.
    müllerian inhibiting f.
    nerve growth f. (NGF)
    neurohumoral f.
    new differentiation f. (NDF)
    nuclear roundness f.
    osteoclast-activating f.
    oxidase cytosolic f.
    paracrine f.
    pathogenetic f.
    platelet f. 4
    platelet-activating f. (PAF)
    platelet-derived growth f. (PDGF)
    P-Mod-S f.
    polypeptide growth f.
    prognostic f.
    progression f.
    prostatic antibacterial f.
    psychological f.
    salivary epidermal growth f. (sEGF)
    scatter f.
    serum blocking f.
    somatotropin release-inhibiting f. (SRIF)
    sperm motility-inhibiting f.
    sperm survival f.
    testis-determining f.
    transcription f.
    transfer f.
    transforming growth f. (TGF)
    transforming growth f. beta-1 (TGF-beta-1)
    transforming growth f. beta-2 (TGF-beta-2)
    transforming growth f. beta-3 (TGF-beta-3)
    tumor necrosis f. (TNF)
    urethral resistance f. (URA)
    vascular endothelial growth f. (VEGF)
    vascular permeability f. (VPF)
    von Willebrand f.
    f. Xa
    f. XIa
    f. XIIa
    washout f.
    Wyanoids Relief F.

factor-1
    colony-stimulating f. (CSF-1)
    heparin-binding growth f.
    insulinlike growth f. (IGF-1)
    salivary epidermal growth f.

factor-alpha
    cytokine tumor necrosis f.-a.
    early growth response f.-a.

factor-beta-1,-2,-3
Fader Tip ureteral stent
faecalis
    Enterococcus f.
    Escherichia f.
    Streptococcus f.

FAG
    fundic atrophic gastritis
Fahrenheit thermometer
failed
    f. adaptation
    f. nipple valve
    f. transplant

failure
    acute hepatic f.
    acute intrinsic renal f.
    acute liver f. (ALF)
    acute renal f. (ARF)
    anemia of chronic renal f.
    bile secretory f.
    chronic renal f. (CRF)
    congestive heart f.
    contrast-associated renal f.
    contrast-induced renal f.
    dilator placement f.
    drug-induced renal f.
    ejaculation f.
    endopyelotomy f.
    end-stage renal f.
    exercise-associated acute renal f.
    fulminant hepatic f. (FHF)
    fulminant hepatocellular f.
    fulminant liver f.
    hyperacute liver f. (HALF)
    intubation f.
    irradiation f.
    kidney f.
    late-onset hepatic f.
    liver f.
    multiorgan system f.
    multiple organ f. (MOF)
    multiple organ system f. (MOSF)
    multiple system organ f. (MSOF)

multisystem organ f. (MSOF)
nephrotoxic acute renal f.
nonoliguric acute renal f.
oliguric renal f.
parenchymatous acute renal f.
postischemic acute renal f.
pouch f.
radiocontrast-induced acute renal f.
renal f.
respiratory f.
shock wave lithotripsy f.
subacute liver f. (SALF)
subfulminant liver f.
f. to thrive
treatment f.
vascular access f.

Fairley
F. bladder washout localization technique
F. bladder washout test

falciform
f. body
f. ligament

falciparum
f. malaria
Plasmodium f.

Falk appendectomy spoon

fallax
Clostridium f.

fallopian
f. arch
f. tube

Fallot tetralogy

F2-alpha
prostaglandin F2-alpha (PGF2-alpha)

false
f. aneurysm
f. channel formation
f. colonic obstruction
f. cyst
f. diverticulum
f. membrane
f. tympanites

false-negative (FN)
false-positive (FP)
f.-p. scintiscan

FAM
5-fluorouracil, Adriamycin, mitomycin C

famciclovir

FAMe
fluorouracil, Adriamycin, mitomycin C

familial
f. adenomatous polyposis (FAP)
f. adenomatous polyposis coli
f. aggregation
f. amyloid polyneuropathy (FAP)
f. atypical multiple mole melanoma (FAMM)
f. atypical multiple mole melanoma syndrome
f. chloride diarrhea
f. chloridorrhea
f. cholemia
f. cholestasia
f. chronic idiopathic jaundice
f. colon cancer
f. colonic varix
f. colorectal polyposis
f. Crohn disease
Danubian endemic f.
f. fat-induced hyperlipidemia
f. gastrointestinal polyposis
f. hamartomatous polyposis
f. hepatitis
f. hyperaldosteronism
f. hyperbetalipoproteinemia
f. hypercholesteremic xanthomatosis
f. hypercholesterolemia
f. hyperchylomicronemia
f. hyperlipoproteinemia (type I–V)
f. hyperprebetalipoproteinemia
f. hypertriglyceridemia
f. hypocalciuric hypercalcemia (FHH)
f. hypocalciuric hypocalcemia
f. intestinal neurofibromatosis
f. intestinal polyposis
f. intestinal pseudoobstruction
f. juvenile nephronophthisis
f. juvenile nephrophthisis
f. juvenile polyposis (FJP)
f. Mediterranean fever (FMF)
f. microvillus atrophy
f. nephritis serum
f. nephrosis
f. nonhemolytic jaundice
f. pancreatitis
f. paroxysmal polyserositis (FPP)
f. pheochromocytoma
f. polyposis coli (FPC)
f. polyposis syndrome
f. predisposition
f. recurrent polyserositis

F

NOTES

familial *(continued)*
    f. ulcerative colitis
    f. unconjugated hyperbilirubinemia
    f. visceral myopathy (FVM)
    f. visceral neuropathy (FVN)
family
    Caliciviridae virus f.
    inter-alpha inhibitor f.
    secretin-glucagon-vasoactive intestinal peptide f.
    S100 super f.
    tachykinin-bombesin f.
FAMM
    familial atypical multiple mole melanoma
    FAMM syndrome
famotidine
    f. maintenance treatment
    f. pharmacokinetics
FAMTX
    fluorouracil, Adriamycin, methotrexate with leucovorin rescue
FANA
    fluorescent antinuclear antibody
Fanconi-de Toni-Debre syndrome
Fanconi syndrome
fan elevator retractor
fan-shaped biopsy technique
fan-type laparoscopic retractor
FAP
    familial adenomatous polyposis
    familial amyloid polyneuropathy
    5-fluorouracil, Adriamycin, Platinol
Farabeuf retractor
farmer's lung
fascia, pl. **fasciae, fascias**
    anal f.
    anterior rectus f.
    anterior renal f.
    Buck f.
    Camper f.
    f. of Camper
    Colles f.
    f. of colon
    cremasteric f.
    dartos f.
    deep cervical f.
    Denonvilliers f.
    f. diaphragmatis pelvis inferior
    f. diaphragmatis pelvis superior
    endoabdominal f.
    external oblique f.
    external spermatic f.
    extraperitoneal f.
    fusion f.
    Gerota f.
    inferior f.
    internal abdominal f.
    internal oblique f.

    internal spermatic f.
    investing f.
    ischiorectal f.
    kidney Gerota f.
    f. lata buttress
    f. lata suburethral sling
    lateral oblique f.
    f. latum
    levator f.
    lumbodorsal f.
    lumbosacral f.
    paraconal f.
    pelvic f.
    f. pelvis
    f. pelvis visceralis
    f. penis profunda
    f. penis superficialis
    perineal f.
    perirenal f.
    posterior renal f.
    prevertebral f.
    f. propria cooperi
    prostatic f.
    psoas f.
    pubocervical f.
    pubovesicocervical f.
    rectal f.
    rectosacral f.
    rectovesical f.
    rectus f.
    renal f.
    f. renalis
    rim of f.
    Scarpa f.
    spermatic f.
    f. spermatica externa
    f. spermatica interna
    subperitoneal f.
    subserous f.
    superficial f.
    transversalis f.
    umbilicovesical f.
    f. of urogenital trigone
    vesicopelvic f.
    Waldeyer f.
fascial
    f. capsule
    f. defect
    f. layer
    f. sling approach
    f. stranding
fasciculata
    zona f.
fasciculate bladder
fasciculated bladder
fasciculation
fasciitis
    necrotizing f.

fasciocutaneous flap
Fasciola
    F. gigantica
    F. hepatica
    F. hepatica infestation
fascioliasis
    hepatic f.
Fascioloides magna
fasciolopsiasis
Fasciolopsis buski
Fas **gene**
fashion
    Heineke-Mikulicz f.
    helical f.
    LeDuc f.
    retrograde f.
fast
    f. cholinergic input
    f. spin-echo acquisition MRI
    f. twitch striated muscle fiber
fasted-to-fed pattern
fastener
    Brown-Mueller T-bar f.
    ROC XS suture f.
fastidium cibi
fasting
    f. diet
    intermediate f.
    f. motor pattern
    partial f.
    f. plasma caffeine concentration
    f. serum gastrin
    f. serum gastrin level
    total f.
FastPack system
FasTrac hydrophilic coated guidewire
fat
    abdominal f.
    autologous f.
    f. cast
    f. cell
    creeping of mesenteric f.
    f. density
    dietary f.
    fecal f.
    f. free (FF)
    herniated preperitoneal f.
    f. indigestion
    f. infiltration
    ischiorectal f.
    macrovesicular f.
    microvesicular f.

    f. pad
    paratesticular f.
    pericolonic f.
    perinephric f.
    peripelvic f.
    perirectal f.
    perirenal f.
    perivesical f.
    preperitoneal f.
    properitoneal f.
    protruding f.
    retroperitoneal f.
    serosal creeping f.
    f. storage disorder
    subcutaneous f.
    submucosal f.
    f. wrapping
fat-free supper (FFS)
fatigue
    structural f.
    suture f.
fat-induced gallbladder contraction
fat-soluble
    f.-s. bilirubin
    f.-s. vitamin
fat-storing liver cell
fat-suppressed spin-echo (FSSE)
fatty
    f. acid
    f. acid binding protein (FABP)
    f. acid diarrhea
    f. acid-free bovine serum albumin
    f. ascites
    f. cast
    f. cirrhosis
    f. cyst
    f. deposit
    f. food
    f. food intolerance
    f. infiltration of liver
    f. kidney
    f. liver (FL)
    f. liver cell (FLC)
    f. liver disease
    f. liver hepatitis
    f. liver and kidney syndrome
     (FLKS)
    f. liver of pregnancy
    f. meal
    f. meal sonogram (FMS)
    f. metamorphosis
    f. necrosis

NOTES

fatty (*continued*)
    f. omental apron
    f. stool
    f. tissue
favored gait
FB-25K jumbo biopsy forceps
FBA
    fecal bile acid
        cocarcinogenic FBA
FBD
    functional bowel disorder
    functional bowel distress
FBDSI
    Functional Bowel Disorder Severity
      Index
FBI
    food-borne illness
FBV
    fiber bundle volume
***FCC-COCA1* gene**
F-circle
FCIS
    Flint Colon Injury Scale
FCPD
    fibrocalculous pancreatic diabetes
FCS-ML
        FCS-ML II colonoscope
        FCS-ML II fiberscope
        FCS-ML II gastroscope
FCS two-channel ultra high-
  magnification endoscope
FDI
    frequency-duration index
FDL
    fluorescein dilaurate
        FDL test
FDP
    fibrin/fibrinogen degradation product
Fe
    Slow Fe
feathery degeneration
feature
    AESOP ReView f.
    manometric f.
    pathognomonic f.
febrile
    f. morbidity
    f. pleomorphic anemia
    f. proteinuria
    f. urine
fecal
    f. abscess
    f. alpha-1-antitrypsin test
    f. analysis
    f. bile acid (FBA)
    f. calprotectin
    f. concretion
    f. contamination

    f. contamination of food
    f. contamination of water
    f. continence
    f. diversion
    f. fat
    f. fat excretion (FFE)
    f. fat test
    f. fistula
    f. flora
    f. fluid
    f. frequency (FF)
    f. homogenate
    72-hour f. fat test
    f. impaction
    f. incontinence
    f. leukocyte
    f. leukocyte count test
    f. marker
    f. material
    f. obstruction
    f. occult blood test (FEOT, FOBT)
    f. occult blood testing
    F. Odor Eliminator (FOE)
    f. paradoxical puborectalis spasm
    f. peritonitis
    f. PMN-elastase
    f. reservoir
    f. residue
    f. seepage
    f. soiling
    f. spillage
    f. stasis
    f. tagging
    f. transmission
    f. tumor
    f. urobilinogen
    f. vomiting
fecalith
fecaloid
fecaloma
fecal-oral
    f.-o. route
    f.-o. transmission
fecaluria
Fecatest
feces
    impacted f.
    inspissated f.
    retained f.
Fechtner syndrome
FECOM artificial stool for
  defecography
feculence
feculent vomitus
fecundity
fed
    f. motor pattern
    f. response

Federici sign
fedotozine
feedback
    tubuloglomerular f. (TGF)
feeding
    Amin-Aid powdered f.
    bolus f.
    Build Up enteral f.
    Citrotein liquid f.
    Clinifeed Iso enteral f.
    Compleat-B liquid f.
    f. complication
    continuous drip f.
    Criticare HN elemental liquid f.
    f. disorder
    Enrich f.
    Ensure Plus liquid f.
    enteral f.
    Entrition Entri-Pak f.
    Finkelstein f.
    Flexical enteral f.
    forced f., forcible f.
    Fortison enteral f.
    gastric f.
    gastrostomy f.
    f. gastrostomy
    f. gastrostomy tube
    gavage f.
    half-strength f.
    Hepatic-Aid powdered f.
    HN f.
    hyperosmotic f.
    intermittent drip f.
    intravenous f.
    Isocal HCN liquid f.
    Isotein HN f.
    isotonic f.
    jejunostomy elemental diet f.
    jejunostomy tube f.
    lactose-free f.
    Lonalac f.
    low-residue f.
    Magnacal liquid f.
    Meritene liquid f.
    modified sham f.
    nasal f.
    nasoenteric f.
    nasojejunal f.
    Osmolite HN enteral f.
    parenteral f.
    Portagen f.
    postoperative regimen for oral
      early f. (PROEF)
    Precision Isotein HN powdered f.
    Precision Isotonic powdered f.
    Precision LR powdered f.
    Renu enteral f.
    Resource enteral f.
    semielemental enteral f.
    sham f.
    Stresstein liquid f.
    Sustacal HC liquid f.
    Sustagen liquid f.
    thermic effect of f. (TEF)
    transitional f.
    transpyloric f.
    TraumaCal enteral f.
    Traum-Aid HBC enteral f.
    Travasorb HN powdered f.
    Travasorb MCT liquid f.
    Travasorb STD liquid f.
    tube f.
    f. tube placement
    f. vessel
    Vital f.
    Vitaneed f.
    Vivonex HN powdered f.
    Vivonex TEN f.
Feen-a-Mint
FEFEK
    fractional excretion of potassium
Fehland intestinal clamp
Feldene
Feleki instrument
FELI
    fractional excretion of lithium
felineus
    Opisthorchis f.
fellea
    cystis f.
    vesica f.
    vesicula f.
felleae
    collum vesicae f.
    corpus vesicae f.
    fossa cystidis f.
    fundus vesicae f.
felodipine
Felty syndrome
female
    f. catheter
    f. condom
    f. epispadias

F

NOTES

female *(continued)*
    f. escutcheon
    f. hypospadias
    f. pelvis
    f. perineum
    f. urethral syndrome
feminae
    hydrocele f.
    ostium urethrae externum f.
    tunica spongiosa urethrae f.
feminarum
    cystitis senilis f.
Femina vaginal weight
feminina
    urethra f.
feminizing
    f. genitoplasty
    f. surgery
femoral
    f. artery
    f. bruit
    f. canal
    f. cryptorchidism
    f. hemodialysis catheter
    f. hernia
    f. ligament
    f. nerve
    f. testis
    f. triangle
FemSoft insert
FENa
    fractional excretion of sodium
fenbufen
fencing reflex
fenestrated
    f. catheter
    f. cup biopsy forceps
    f. drape
    f. ellipsoid spiked open span
      biopsy forceps
    f. spiked open-span jumbo biopsy
      forceps
fenestration
    cyst f.
fenfluramine
Fenger gallbladder probe
fenofibrate
fenoldopam
fenoprofen
fen-phen diet
fentanyl
Fenwick disease
Fenwick-Hunner ulcer
Feosol
FEOT
    fecal occult blood test
Ferguson
    F. abdominal scissors

    F. anal retractor
    F. anoscope
    F. gallstone scoop
    F. hemorrhoidectomy
    F. needle
    F. technique
    F. tenaculum forceps
Ferguson-Moon rectal retractor
Feridex IV
fermentative
    f. diarrhea
    f. dyspepsia
Ferrein
    F. tube
    F. tubule
ferricytochrome-C
Ferris
    F. biliary duct dilator
    F. common duct scoop
ferritin
    anionic f.
    cationized f.
    serum f.
ferrofluid
ferromagnetic tamponade
ferrous
    f. salt poisoning
    f. sulfate
fertile eunuch syndrome
fertility status
fertilization
    in vitro f.
ferumoxides injectable solution
ferumoxsil
ferumoxsil
Festal
    F. II
Festalan
fetal
    f. adrenal cortex
    f. adrenal gland hemorrhage
    f. alcohol syndrome ureter defect
    f. arginine vasopressin
    f. bladder aspiration
    f. calf serum
    f. liver-derived B cell
    f. macrosomia
    f. sulfoglycoprotein antigen (FSA)
fetalis
    nonimmune hydrops f. (NIHF)
fetid
fetoprotein
    alpha f. (AFP)
    alpha-1-f.
    beta f.
    fucosylated alpha f.
    fucosylation index of alpha f.
    gamma f.

fetor
　　fetor f.
fetus
　　Campylobacter f.
Feulgen
　　F. reaction
　　F. staining
fever
　　Aden f.
　　Assam f.
　　beaver f.
　　bilious remittent f.
　　bouquet f.
　　breakbone f.
　　Burdwan f.
　　cachectic f.
　　Charcot intermittent f.
　　dandy f.
　　date f.
　　dehydration f.
　　dengue hemorrhagic f.
　　digestive f.
　　dumdum f.
　　Ebola hemorrhagic f.
　　enteric f.
　　epidemic hemorrhagic f.
　　exsiccation f.
　　familial Mediterranean f. (FMF)
　　filarial f.
　　food f.
　　hemorrhagic f.
　　hemorrhagic f. with renal syndrome
　　hepatic intermittent f.
　　inanition f.
　　intermittent hepatic f.
　　Katayama f.
　　Kinkiang f.
　　Korean hemorrhagic f.
　　Lassa hemorrhagic f.
　　low-grade f.
　　Manchurian hemorrhagic f.
　　Mediterranean f.
　　polka f.
　　Q f.
　　solar f.
　　spiking f.
　　thirst f.
　　typhoid f.
　　urticarial f.
　　viral hemorrhagic f.
　　Yangtze Valley f.
fexofenadine

FF
　　fat free
　　fecal frequency
　　follicular fluid
FFE
　　fecal fat excretion
^{18}**F-fluorodeoxyglucose**
FFP
　　fresh frozen plasma
FFS
　　fat-free supper
FGF
　　fibroblast growth factor
FGID
　　functional gastrointestinal disorder
FG-series two-channel endoscope
FGS-ML II gastroscope
FGS-ML-series two-channel endoscope
FGS-series two-channel endoscope
FGS-SML-series two-channel endoscope
FG-32UA
　　　　Pentax FG-32UA
　　　　Pentax/Hitachi FG-32UA
FHF
　　fulminant hepatic failure
FHH
　　familial hypocalciuric hypercalcemia
FHVP
　　free hepatic venous pressure
fialuridine (FIAU)
FIAU
　　fialuridine
fiber
　　　　afferent f.
　　　　autonomic nerve f.
　　　　f. bundle
　　　　f. bundle volume (FBV)
　　　　circular muscle f.
　　　　cremasteric f.
　　　　dietary f.
　　　　extension f.
　　　　fast twitch striated muscle f.
　　　　GBM collagen f.
　　　　hypogastric f.
　　　　intrapelvic somatic f.
　　　　f. lock displacement
　　　　oblique gastric f.
　　　　optical f.
　　　　oxidative-glycolytic f.
　　　　pain f.
　　　　psyllium husk f.
　　　　ragged-red f.

F

NOTES

fiber *(continued)*
  sacral afferent f.
  sling muscle f.
  slow twitch striated muscle f.
  SLT 7 laser f.
  splanchnic afferent f.
  UltraLine f.
  Urolase neodymium:YAG laser f.
  viscoelastic collagen f.
Fiberall
fibercolonoscope
  Olympus CF-20 f.
FiberCon
fiber-deficient diet
fiberduodenoscope
fiberendoscope
fibergastroscope
  fluorescence f.
fiberoptic
  f. bundle
  f. catheter
  f. colonoscope
  f. coloscope
  f. endoscope
  f. endoscopy
  f. esophagoscope
  f. gastroscope
  f. injection sclerotherapy (FIS)
  f. instrument technology
  f. light cable
  f. panendoscopy
  f. sensor
  f. sigmoidoscope
  f. sigmoidoscopy
fiberoptics
fiberscope
  CF-HM f.
  FCS-ML II f.
  gastrointestinal f.
  GIF-HM f.
  Hirschowitz gastroduodenal f.
  Olympus Aloka EU-MI ultrasound gastrointestinal f.
  Olympus GF-EU1 gastrointestinal f.
  Olympus GIF-Q30 f.
  Olympus OES f.
  Olympus XK-series oblique-viewing flexible f.
  pediatric f.
  Pentax f.
  side-viewing f.
  ultrasound gastrointestinal f.
fiberTome system
fibrae
  f. oblique gastricae
  f. oblique ventriculi
fibrate derivative

fibril
  disulfide cross-linked f.
  twisted beta-pleated sheet f.
fibrillary glomerulonephritis
fibrin
  f. calculus
  f. glue
  f. injection
  f. score
  f. seal
  f. sealant
  f. split product (FSP)
  f. sponge
  f. spraying
  f. strand
  f. tissue adhesive
fibrin/fibrinogen degradation product (FDP)
fibrinogen degradation product
fibrinoid necrosis
fibrinolysis
  endothelium-dependent f.
fibrinolytic activity
fibrinopeptide-A
fibrinopurulent exudate
fibroadenoma
fibroadenomatosis
  biliary f.
fibroadipose tissue
fibroblast
  f. ECM adhesion assay
  f. growth factor (FGF)
  HE9 f.
  interstitial f.
  perivascular f.
  f. PMN adhesion assay
  quiescent human f.
  3T3 murine f.
fibroblast-derived factor
fibrocalculous pancreatic diabetes (FCPD)
fibrocongestive splenomegaly
fibrocystic
  f. change
  f. disease of the pancreas
fibrodysplastic
fibroelastic
  f. connective tissue stroma
  f. tissue
fibroelastosis
fibrofatty
  f. adventitia
  f. infiltration of the pancreas
fibrogastroscopy
fibrogenesis
fibrogenic
  f. cascade
  f. cytokine

fibroid
f. induration
f. polyp
uterine f.
fibrolamellar
f. hepatocarcinoma
f. hepatocellular carcinoma (FL-HCC)
f. hepatoma
fibrolipomatous nephritis
fibroma
kidney f.
ovarian f.
renal f.
testicular f.
f. of testis
fibromatogenic
fibromatoid
fibromatosis
aggressive f.
mesenteric f.
penile f.
f. ventriculi
fibromatous
fibromectomy
fibromuscular
f. coat
f. dysplasia (FMD)
f. hyperplasia
fibromyalgia
fibromyoma
fibromyxoma
fibronectin
f. expression
f. monoclonal antibody
plasma f.
urinary f.
fibronectin-binding protein
fibroobliterative disease
fibroplasia
adventitial f.
intimal f.
medial f.
perimedial f.
string-of-beads appearance of renal medial f.
subadventitial f.
fibroplastica
gastritis granulomatosa f.
fibropolycystic liver disease
fibroproliferative destruction
fibropurulent perisplenitis

fibrosa
appendix f.
capsula f.
tunica f.
fibrosarcoma
kidney f.
fibrosing
f. cholestatic hepatitis B
f. piecemeal necrosis
fibrosis
acholangic biliary f.
alcoholic f.
anal f.
arachnoid f.
biliary f.
cavernous f.
chronic sclerosing hyaline f.
congenital hepatic f. (CHF)
corporeal f.
corpus spongiosum f.
cystic f. (CF)
diffuse lobular f.
hepatic f.
idiopathic retroperitoneal f.
interlobular f.
interstitial f.
intralobular f.
liver f.
mixed intralobular f.
noncirrhotic portal f. (NCPF)
pancreatic f.
paravariceal f.
penile f.
pericentral f.
periductal f.
perilobular f.
peripancreatic f.
periportal f.
periportal-perisinusoidal f.
perisinusoidal f.
periureteral f.
perivenular f.
portal-to-portal f.
portal tract f.
postoperative retroperitoneal f.
progressive perivenular alcoholic f. (PPAF)
retroperitoneal f.
f. score
secondary biliary f.
segmental bile duct f.
sinusoidal f.

F

NOTES

fibrosis *(continued)*
>   stripe interstitial f.
>   transmural f.
>   tubulointerstitial f.
>   vesical f.

fibrosis-promoting cytokine
fibrotic corpus cavernosum
fibrous
>   f. appendage of liver
>   f. capsule of liver
>   f. cavernitis
>   f. chordee
>   f. dysplasia
>   f. histiocytoma
>   f. nephritis
>   f. obliterative cholangitis
>   f. sheath
>   f. stroma
>   f. tissue
>   f. tunic
>   f. tunic of liver

fibrovascular polyp
Ficoll-Hypaque
>   F.-H. density gradient centrifuge
>   F.-H. gradient centrifugation
>   F.-H. gradient sedimentation

FIDUS probe
field cut
field-of-view camera
Fiessinger-Leroy-Reiter syndrome
figure-of-eight suture
filament
>   actin f.
>   Charcot-Boettcher crystals and f.'s

filamentous morphology
filarial
>   f. abscess
>   f. fever
>   f. funiculoepididymitis
>   f. hydrocele
>   f. lymphedema
>   f. orchitis

filariasis
>   amicrofilaremic f.
>   epididymis f.
>   late period f.
>   occult f.
>   prepatent period f.

filiform
>   f. bougie
>   f. and follower
>   f. polyp
>   f. polyposis
>   f. stricture
>   f. tip

filling
>   bladder f.
>   contrast f.

>   f. cystometrogram
>   f. cystometry
>   f. defect
>   gallbladder f.
>   muscle f.
>   rectal f.

film
>   Bard protective barrier f.
>   conditioning f.
>   high abdominal plain f.
>   organic conditioning f.
>   plain f.
>   postevacuation f.
>   soft x-ray f.

filmy adhesion
filter
>   Amicon D-20 f.
>   Baermann stool f.
>   Baxter CA-210 f.
>   charcoal f.
>   fluorescence excitation f.
>   Fresenius F-40 f.
>   Gambro FH88H f.
>   Gene Screen nylon membrane f.
>   Greenfield f.
>   Hospal Biospal f.
>   interference barrier f.
>   Millex-GS 0.22-mm pore-size f.
>   Millex-GV 0.22-mm f.
>   Millipore f.
>   Percoll f.
>   Renal System HF250 f.
>   suprarenal Greenfield f.
>   Sur-Fit auto lock closed-end pouch
>   with f.
>   Sur-Fit Natura opaque closed-end
>   pouch with f.
>   Zeta probe nylon f.

filtered
>   f. fraction
>   f. glucose

filtering
>   high-pass f.

filtrate
>   Folin f.

filtration
>   f. barrier
>   f. fraction
>   glomerular f.
>   kidney magnesium f.
>   f. slit length density
>   spontaneous ascites f.

filtration-slit membrane
fimbriae
final
>   f. motor neuron
>   f. position

finasteride

finding
cholangiographic f.
endoscopic f.
focal f.
manometric f.
RNA-based f.
roentgen f.
sensory f.
spinal fluid f.
ultrasonographic f.
fine
f. gastric mucosal pattern
f. granular cast
f. needle
f. needle vasography
f. reticular pattern
f. tissue forceps
finely
f. fatty foamy liver
f. granular kidney
fine-needle
f.-n. aspiration (FNA)
f.-n. aspiration biopsy (FNAB)
f.-n. aspiration cytology (FNAC)
f.-n. capillary biopsy
f.-n. percutaneous cholangiogram
f.-n. transhepatic cholangiogram
f.-n. transhepatic cholangiography
(FNTC, FNTHC)
fine-toothed forceps
finger
clubbed f.
f. clubbing
f. fracture dissection
f. fracture technique
f. intrinsic
f. ring
zinc f.
fingerbreadth
fingerlike
f. epithelial process
f. villus
fingerprick latex agglutination test
fingerprinting
peptide mass f.
fingerstick device
fingertip lesion
Finkelstein feeding
Finney
F. Flexirod penile prosthesis
F. gastroenterostomy
F. operation

F. pyloroplasty
F. strictureplasty
Finochietto retractor
FIO₂
fractional percentage of inspired oxygen
Fioricet
Fiorinal
Firlit-Kluge stent
First-Choice drainable pouch
first-degree relative
first-generation ELISA
first-line screening technique
first-order kinetics
first-pass
f.-p. effect
f.-p. metabolism (FPM)
first-set phenomenon
first-stage repair
FIS
fiberoptic injection sclerotherapy
Fischer test meal
FISH
fluorescence in situ hybridization
fish
f. bone ingestion
f. oil
f. oil supplementation
f. tapeworm
Fishberg method
Fisher
F. Accumet pH meter
F. Capillary System
F. exact probability test
F. two-tailed exact test
fish-hook displacement
Fishman-Doubilet test
fishmouth
f. anastomosis
f. incision
fish-scale gallbladder
fissura, pl. **fissurae**
f. ligamenti teretis
f. ligamenti venosi
fissural
fissure
Allingham f.
anal f.
f. in ano
anterior f.
cecal f.
f. for ligamentum teres
f. for ligamentum venosum

NOTES

F

285

fissure *(continued)*
    longitudinal f.
    portal f.
    posterior f.
    f. of round ligament
    transverse f.
    umbilical f.
fissurectomy
fissured tongue
fissure-like ulceration
fist fornication
fistula, pl. **fistulae, fistulas**
    abdominal f.
    airway-arterial f.
    amphibolic f., amphibolous f.
    anal f.
    f. in ano
    f. in ano endoscopic examination
    anorectal f.
    anovaginal f.
    antecubital arteriovenous f.
    anterior f.
    aortoduodenal f. (ADF)
    aortoenteric f.
    aortoesophageal f.
    aortogastric f.
    aortograft duodenal f.
    aortosigmoid f.
    arterial-enteric f.
    arterioportal f.
    arteriovenous f. (AVF)
    AV f.
    benign duodenocolic f.
    biliary f.
    biliary-bronchial f.
    biliary-cutaneous f.
    biliary-duodenal f.
    biliary-enteric f.
    bilioenteric f.
    f. bimucosa
    bladder f.
    blind f.
    Blom-Singer tracheoesophageal f.
    brachioaxillary bridge graft f. (BAGF)
    brachiosubclavian bridge graft f. (BSGF)
    Brescia-Cimino f.
    bronchobiliary f.
    bronchoesophageal f. (BEF)
    bronchopancreatic f.
    caliceal f.
    cholecystenteric f.
    cholecystobiliary f.
    cholecystocholedochal f.
    cholecystocolonic f.
    cholecystoduodenal f.
    cholecystoduodenocolic f.

    choledochocolonic f.
    choledochoduodenal f.
    choledochoenteric f.
    chylous f.
    f. cibalis
    coccygeal f.
    colobronchial f.
    colocholecystic f.
    colocolonic f.
    colocutaneous f.
    coloenteric f.
    cologastrocutaneous f.
    coloileal f.
    colonic f.
    coloperineal f.
    coloureteral f.
    colouterine f.
    colovaginal f.
    colovenous f.
    colovesical f.
    complex anorectal f.
    congenital urethroperineal f.
    congenital urethrorectal f.
    cutaneobiliary f.
    cystogastric f.
    digestive-respiratory f. (DRF)
    duodenal f.
    duodenocaval f.
    duodenocolic f.
    duodenoenterocutaneous f.
    Eck f.
    endobronchial f.
    enteric f.
    enterocolic f.
    enterocutaneous f.
    enteroenteral f.
    enteroenteric f.
    enterourethral f.
    enterourinary f.
    enterovaginal f.
    enterovesical f.
    esophageal f.
    esophagobronchial f.
    esophagomediastinal f.
    esophagopleural f.
    esophagopulmonary f.
    esophagorespiratory f. (ERF)
    esophagotracheal f.
    external biliary f.
    extrasphincteric anal f.
    fecal f.
    forearm graft arteriovenous f.
    f. formation
    gastric f.
    gastrocolic f.
    gastrocutaneous f.
    gastroduodenal f.
    gastroenteric f.

gastrointestinal f.
gastrojejunocolic f.
genitourinary f.
graft-enteric f.
hepatic f.
hepaticopulmonary f.
hepatopleural f.
horseshoe f.
H-type f.
iatrogenic prostatourethral-rectal f.
iatrogenic rectourethral f.
ileosigmoid f.
ileovesical f.
intersphincteric anal f.
intestinal f.
intrahepatic AV f.
intrahepatic spontaneous
  arterioportal f.
ischiorectal f.
jejunocolic f.
kidney arteriovenous f.
low intersphincteric anal f.
malignant esophagopericardial f.
Mann-Bollman f.
mesenteric arteriovenous f.
mucous f.
pancreatic cutaneous f.
pancreaticopleural f.
pancreatic-portal vein f.
pararectal f.
parietal f.
pelvirectal f.
perianal f.
perineal urinary f.
perirectal f.
pleurobiliary f.
postbiopsy f.
postoperative pleurobiliary f.
posttraumatic pancreatic-cutaneous f.
pouch f.
primary arteriovenous f.
f. probe
prostatourethral f.
prostatourethral-rectal f.
pseudocystobiliary f.
radiocephalic f.
rectal f.
rectolabial f.
rectoneovaginal f.
rectourethral f.
rectourinary f.
rectovaginal f.

rectovesical f.
rectovestibular f.
rectovulvar f.
renal arteriovenous f.
renogastric f.
residual rectoperineal f.
respiratory-esophageal f.
retroperitoneal f.
seton treatment of high anal f.
sigmoidovesical f.
spermatic f.
splanchnic AV f.
splenic AV f.
splenobronchial f.
stercoral f.
suprapapillary f.
suprasphincteric f.
sylvian f.
thigh graft arteriovenous f.
Thiry f.
Thiry-Vella f. (TVF)
thoracic f.
tracheoesophageal f. (TEF)
transsphincteric anal f.
ulcerogenic f.
umbilical f.
urachal f.
ureterocolic f.
urctcrocutancous f.
ureterouterine f.
ureterovaginal f.
urethral f.
urethrocavernous f.
urethrocutaneous f.
urethrorectal f.
urethrovaginal f.
urinary umbilical f.
urogenital f.
vaginal f.
vasocutaneous f.
Vella f.
vesical f.
vesicocolic f.
vesicocolonic f.
vesicocutaneous f.
vesicoenteric f.
vesicointestinal f.
vesicorectal f.
vesicosalpingovaginal f.
vesicoumbilical f.
vesicouterine f.
vesicovaginal f. (VVF)

F

NOTES

fistula *(continued)*
    vesicovaginorectal f.
    vulvorectal f.
fistulation
    spreading f.
fistulectomy
fistulization
fistulizing Crohn disease
fistuloenterostomy
fistulogram
fistulography
fistulotome
    double-channel f.
    needle-knife f.
fistulotomy
    choledochoduodenal f.
    diathermic f.
    endoscopic f.
    laying-open f.
    needle-knife f. (NKF)
    Parks method of anal f.
    Parks staged f.
    primary f.
fistulous
    f. Crohn disease
    f. degeneration
    f. orifice
    f. tract
FITC
    fluorescein isothiocyanate
Fite stain
Fitz
    F. law
    F. syndrome
Fitz-Hugh and Curtis syndrome
five-port fan placement
fixation
    f. anomaly
    intestinal f.
    pubic f.
    sacrospinalis ligament vaginal f.
    sacrospinous ligament vaginal f.
    tissue f.
fixative
    Saccomanno f.
    Zamboni f.
fixed
    f. drain pipe urethra
    f. drug reaction
    f. ring retractor
    f. segment of bowel
Fix and Perm permeabilizing kit
FJP
    familial juvenile polyposis
FK506
FL
    fatty liver
    full liquid

flabby abdomen
flaccid penis
flagella
    polar sheathed f.
flagellate
    f. diarrhea
    f. dysentery
Flagyl
flail chest
flame photometry
flammeus
    nevus f.
flange
    Assura pediatric skin barrier f.
flank
    f. approach
    f. approach adrenalectomy
    bulging f.
    f. droop
    f. incision
    f. mass
    f. nephrectomy
    f. pain
    f. position
    f. roll positioning
    f. surgery
flanking sequence
FLAP
    fluorouracil, leucovorin rescue,
      Adriamycin, Platinol
flap
    abdominal fasciocutaneous f.
    advancement of rectal f.
    advancement sleeve f.
    axial f.
    Bakamjian f.
    Boari bladder f.
    Boari-Ockerblad f.
    Byars f.
    circumferential transanal sleeve
      advancement f.
    cutaneous advancement f.
    cuticular f.
    dartos pedicled f.
    de-epithelialized f.
    detrusor muscle f.
    diamond f.
    f. dissection
    endorectal advancement f.
    fasciocutaneous f.
    forearm f.
    foreskin f.
    Fortunoff f.
    gracilis muscle f.
    House f.
    ischemia or soughing of the f.
    island groin f.
    island pedicle f.

latissimus dorsi free f.
liver f.
Martius labial fat pad f.
Mathieu island onlay f.
microvascular f.
musculocutaneous f.
myocutaneous f.
Ockerblad-Boari f.
omental pedicle f.
onlay island f.
paraexstrophy skin f.
parameatal-based f.
pedicle island f.
pedicle muscle f.
penile island f.
random f.
rectus abdominis
  musculocutaneous f.
rectus femoris f.
renal capsular f.
Scardino f.
surgical f.
f. technique
tensor fasciae latae f.
tubed groin f.
tubularized cecal f.
upper arm f.
U-shaped skin f.
vaginal f.
f. valve
f. valve antireflux procedure
f. valve cystoplasty
vastus lateralis muscle f.
ventrum penis f.
flapping tremor sign
flap-valve mechanism
flare
f. cell
pancreatic f.
flare-up
FLASH
flat low-angle shot
FLASH pulse sequence
flashlamp pumped dye laser
flash pulmonary edema with anuria
flat
f. abdomen
f. adenoma
f. carcinoma
f. condyloma
f. depressed lesion
f. dysplasia

f. elevated lesion
f. hyperplasia
f. low-angle shot (FLASH)
f. plate of abdomen
f. polycyclic ulceration
f. rectal adenocarcinoma
f. spatula electrode
f. ulcer
flattened
f. duodenal fold
f. epithelial microfold cell
flattening
histogram f.
f. of ileal epithelium
flat-type carcinoma
flatulence
flatulent
f. colic
f. dyspepsia
Flatulex
flatus
f. enema
f. incontinence
f. tube insertion
Flavimonas
flavin
f. adenine dinucleotide
f. mononucleotide
flavivirus
Flavobacterium meningosepticum
flavoxate hydrochloride
flavus
Aspergillus f.
FLC
fatty liver cell
flea-bitten kidney
flecainide
Fleet
F. Babylax enema
F. Bisacodyl
F. bowel preparation
F. Enema Mineral Oil
F. Flavored Castor Oil
F. Phospho-Soda
F. Phospho-Soda buffered saline
  laxative
fleroxacin
Fletcher's Castoria
flexed
Flexeril
flexible
f. aspiration needle

NOTES

F

flexible *(continued)*
   f. barium enema
   f. bronchocopy simulator
   f. cystodiathermy
   f. delivery device
   f. dental suction
   f. endoscopic overtube
   f. endoscopy
   f. esophagoscopy
   f. fiberoptic choledochoscope
   f. fiberoptic endoscope
   f. forward-viewing panendoscope
   f. gastroscope
   f. laparoscopy
   f. nephroscope
   f. nephroscopy
   f. Olympus GF-eUM3 device
   f. sigmoidoscope
   f. sigmoidoscopy
   f. ureteropyeloscopy
   f. ureterorenoscopy
   f. ureteroscope
   f. video laparoscope (FVL)
flexible-tip guidewire
Flexical enteral feeding
Flexicath silicone subclavian cannula
Flexi-Flate
   F.-F. I, II penile prosthesis
   F.-F. penile implant
Flexiflo
   F. Companion enteral feeding pump
   F. II enteral feeding pump
   F. Inverta-PEG gastrostomy kit
   F. Inverta-PEG tube
   F. Lap G laparoscopic gastrostomy kit
   F. Lap J laparoscopic jejunostomy kit
   F. over-the-guidewire gastrostomy kit
   F. stoma creator tube
   F. Stomate low-profile gastrostomy tube
   F. Top-Fill Enteral Nutrition System
   F. tungsten-weighted feeding tube
   F. Versa-PEG tube
Flexima biliary stent
Flexirod penile prosthesis
Flexner dysentery
flexneri
   Shigella f.
FlexSure
   F. HP test
   F. whole-blood test
flexura, pl. **flexurae**
   f. coli dextra
   f. coli sinistra
   f. duodeni inferior
   f. duodeni superior
   f. duodenojejunalis
   f. hepatica cell
   f. lienalis coli
   f. perinealis recti
   f. sacralis recti
flexure
   anorectal f.
   colon splenic f.
   duodenojejunal f.
   hepatic f.
   left colonic f.
   perineal f.
   right colonic f.
   sigmoid f.
   splenic f.
Flexxicon
   F. Blue dialysis catheter
   F. II PC internal jugular catheter
FLH
   focal lymphoid hyperplasia
FL-HCC
   fibrolamellar hepatocellular carcinoma
FLI
   fluorescent light intensity
Flint Colon Injury Scale (FCIS)
flip-flap
   Mathieu-Horton-Devine f.-f.
   f.-f. procedure
   f.-f. technique
flipped T wave
FLKS
   fatty liver and kidney syndrome
floating
   f. gallbladder
   f. gallstone
   f. stent
   f. stool
   f. table
Flocare 500 feeding pump
floccosum
   Epidermophyton f.
flocculate
   calcific f.
flocculation on barium enema
flocculus
   calcific f.
Flo-Gard pump
Flolan
Flomax
Flood syndrome
floor
   inguinal f.
   f. of inguinal region
   pelvic f.

floppy
    f. Nissen fundic wrap
    f. Nissen fundoplication
floppy-tipped guidewire
flora
    bacterial f.
    colonic f.
    commensal f.
    fecal f.
    GI tract f.
    gut f.
    intestinal f.
    normal f.
    protective probiotic f.
    proximal human colonic f.
florid
    f. bile duct lesion
    f. polyposis
Florida
    F. pouch urinary reservoir
    F. urinary pouch
Floropryl
flosulide
flow
    azygos blood f.
    bile f. (BF)
    blood f.
    cavernous artery blood f.
    f. cytometric analysis
    f. cytometric study
    f. cytometry
    effective renal plasma f. (ERPF)
    estimated liver blood f. (ELBF)
    forearm blood f.
    gastric mucosal blood f.
    hepatic blood f.
    hepatofugal f.
    hepatopetal f.
    high-velocity f.
    light f.
    f. microsphere fluorescent
      immunoassay technique
    mucosal blood f.
    nephron plasma f.
    noninvasive assessment of
      urinary f.
    obstruction of bile f.
    outer cortical blood f. (OCBF)
    pancreatic blood f.
    peak f.
    petal-fugal f.
    plasma f.

    f. rate
    renal blood f. (RBF)
    renal plasma f. (RPF)
    splanchnic blood f.
    splenic venous blood f.
    turbulent f.
    urinary f.
    f. volume
flower
    passion f.
flowmeter
    Dantec rotating disk f.
    Dantec Urodyn 1000 f.
    laser Doppler f.
    Life-Tech f.
    Model 500F electromagnetic f.
    Transonics laser-Doppler f.
flowprobe
    endoscopic f.
Flow-Thru feeding tube
Floxin
floxuridine
flucloxacillin
flucloxacillin-associated liver damage
flucloxacillin-induced delayed cholestatic
    hepatitis
fluconazole
fluctuant mass
fluctuation
    GB vol+ f.
flucytosine
fludarabine phosphate
Fluhrer rectal probe
fluid
    f. absorptive capacity
    f. analysis
    ascitic f.
    ascitic tumor f. (ATF)
    BiCart dialysis f.
    bile-stained f.
    bile-tinged f.
    bloody peritoneal f.
    cerebrospinal f. (CSF)
    f. challenge
    chylous ascitic f.
    citrate replacement f.
    cloudy f.
    f. collection
    contrast f.
    crevicular f.
    cul-de-sac f.
    cytospin collection f.

F

NOTES

fluid *(continued)*
    Dialyflex dialysis f.
    Euro-Collins f.
    extracellular f. (ECF)
    fecal f.
    follicular f. (FF)
    forward motility protein of
      epididymal f.
    free f.
    intracellular f. (ICF)
    intraglandular f.
    irrigating f.
    IV f.
    LDH level of ascitic f.
    LKB Optiphase 2 scintillation f.
    f. loss
    malodorous f.
    milky f.
    motor oil peritoneal f.
    nonmalodorous f.
    oviductal f.
    peripancreatic f.
    peritoneal f.
    peritubular f.
    f. phase marker
    prune juice peritoneal f.
    renal tubular f.
    f. replacement therapy
    f. restriction
    f. resuscitation
    sanguineous f.
    seminal f.
    f. sequestration
    serosanguineous f.
    f. shift
    straw-colored f.
    synovial f.
    testicular interstitial f. (TIF)
    f. transport
    turbid peritoneal f.
    University of Wisconsin f.
    f. wave
fluid-air interface
fluid-debris level
fluid-filled
    f.-f. balloon
    f.-f. diverticulum
    f.-f. sac
    f.-f. small bowel
fluidity
    hepatocellular basolateral plasma
      membrane f.
fluid-phase
    f.-p. endocytosis
    f.-p. pinocytosis
fluke
    giant intestinal f.
    liver f.

flulike syndrome
flumazenil
flumecinol
flunarizine
flunisolide
fluocinolone
fluorescein
    f. dilaurate (FDL)
    f. dilaurate test
    f. isothiocyanate (FITC)
    f. isothiocyanate-conjugated antibody
    f. isothiocyanate-labeled monoclonal
      antibody
    linear f.
    scattered f.
    sodium f. (NaF)
    f. string test
    superficial f.
fluoresceinuria
fluorescence
    f. angiography
    f. excitation filter
    f. fibergastroscope
    pericentral pyridine nucleotide f.
    periportal pyridine nucleotide f.
    f. in situ hybridization (FISH)
fluorescence-activated
    f.-a. cell sorter (FACS)
    f.-a. cell sorter scan (FACScan)
    f.-a. flow cytometry
fluorescent
    f. antinuclear antibody (FANA)
    f. detection
    f. electronic endoscopy
    f. gene scanning
    f. image analysis
    f. light intensity (FLI)
    f. treponemal antibody absorption
      (FTA-ABS)
    f. treponemal antibody absorption
      test
fluoride
    phenyl-methane-sulfonyl f.
fluorine-18 (F-18, ^{18}F)
5-fluorocytosine
fluorodeoxyuridine (FUDR)
fluorodopan
fluorometholone
FluoroPlus Roadmapper
fluoroquinolone
    f. seminal plasma concentration
    f. therapy
fluoroscope
    C-arm f.
fluoroscopic
    f. control
    f. guidance
    f. monitoring

fluoroscopy
    C-arm f.
    oblique f.
fluoroscopy-guided balloon dilator
Fluoro Tip ERCP cannula
Fluorotome double-lumen sphincterotome
fluorouracil
    f., Adriamycin, methotrexate with leucovorin rescue (FAMTX)
    f., Adriamycin, mitomycin C (FAMe)
    etoposide, leucovorin, 5-f. (ELF)
    f., leucovorin rescue, Adriamycin, Platinol (FLAP)
    MeCCNU, Oncovin, f. (MOF)
5-fluorouracil (5-FU)
    5-f., Adriamycin, cyclophosphamide (FAC)
    5-f., Adriamycin, mitomycin C (FAM)
    5-f., Adriamycin, Platinol (FAP)
    5-f., mitomycin C radiation (FUMIR)
fluorourodynamics
fluoxetine hydrochloride
fluoxymesterone
FLUP
    front-loading ultrasound probe
fluphenazine
flurbiprofen
flush
    carcinoid f.
    saline f.
    f. stoma
flushing
    cold f.
    f. syndrome
flush-tank sign
flutamide therapy
fluted J-Vac drain
fluvastatin
fluvialis
    Vibrio f.
fluvoxamine
flux
    bilious f.
    celiac f.
    lumen-to-bath sodium f.
    proton f.
    sodium f.
FMD
    fibromuscular dysplasia

FMF
    familial Mediterranean fever
fMLP
    N-formyl-methyonyl-leucyl-phenylalanine
    fMLP chemoattractant receptor
fMLP-stimulated O_2
fMRI
    functional magnetic resonance imaging
FMS
    fatty meal sonogram
FN
    false-negative
FNA
    fine-needle aspiration
    EUS-guided FNA
FNAB
    fine-needle aspiration biopsy
FNAC
    fine-needle aspiration cytology
FNH
    focal nodular hyperplasia
FNTC
    fine-needle transhepatic cholangiography
FNTHC
    fine-needle transhepatic cholangiography
foam
    f. cell
    Cutinova f.
    hydrocortisone f.
foamy
    f. liver
    f. stool
Fobi pouch
FOBT
    fecal occult blood test
    FOBT-positive
focal
    f. accumulation of tracer
    f. bacterial nephritis
    f. biliary cirrhosis
    f. carcinoma
    f. colitis
    f. collagen synthesis
    f. colonic mucosal ulcer
    f. dimpling
    f. edema
    f. fatty infiltration
    f. fatty infiltration of liver
    f. finding
    f. ileus
    f. lymphoid hyperplasia (FLH)

F

NOTES

focal *(continued)*
    f. necrotizing glomerulonephritis
    f. nodular hyperplasia (FNH)
    f. nonfatty infiltration of liver
    f. pancreatitis
    f. proliferative glomerulonephritis
    f. sclerosis
    f. segmental glomerulosclerosis
      (FSGS)
    f. stricture
    f. tenderness
    f. tumor
focus, pl. **foci**
    aberrant crypt f. (ACF)
    dysplastic f.
    echogenic foci
    echogenic cardiac f.
    f. of tumor
    tumor f.
focused shock wave
FOE
    Fecal Odor Eliminator
Foerster
    F. abdominal ring retractor
    F. sponge forceps
Fogarty
    F. balloon
    F. balloon biliary catheter
    F. biliary probe
    F. clamp
    F. irrigation catheter
fog reduction elimination device
   (FRED)
folate
    f. anemia
    f. deficiency
    f. distribution
    f. malabsorption
    polyglutamate f.
    red blood cell f.
    serum f.
fold
    aryepiglottic f.
    cecal f.
    cholecystoduodenocolic f.
    costocolic f.
    crescent f.
    crural f.
    Douglas f.
    duodenojejunal f.
    duodenomesocolic f.
    epigastric f.
    flattened duodenal f.
    gastric f.
    gastropancreatic f.
    giant gastric f.
    gluteal f.
    haustral f.

    Heister f.
    Hensing f.
    hepatopancreatic f.
    ileocolic f.
    inferior duodenal f.
    inguinal f.
    interhaustral f.
    Jonnesco f.
    Kerckring f.
    left pancreaticogastric f.
    middle rectal f.
    mucosal f.
    Nélaton f.
    palatopharyngeal f.
    paraduodenal f.
    parietocolic f.
    f. pattern
    peritoneum lateral umbilical f.
    peritoneum medial f.
    peritoneum median f.
    rectal f.
    rugal f.
    semilunar-shaped f.
    sentinel f.
    sigmoid f.
    spiral f.
    superior duodenal f.
    thickness of skin f. (TSF)
    Tourneux f.
    Treves f.
    triradiate cecal f.
    vascular cecal f.
    vertical f.
folded fundus
Foley
    F. catheter
    F. criteria
    F. operation
    F. Y-plasty
    F. Y-plasty pyeloplasty
    F. Y-type ureteropelvioplasty
    F. Y-V plasty
    F. Y-V pyeloplasty
    F. Y-V ureteropelvioplasty
foliaceus
    pemphigus f.
foliate papilla
folic
    f. acid
    f. acid malabsorption
Folin
    F. filtrate
    F. gravimetric method
    F. phenol reagent
Folin-Benedict-Myers method
Folin-Denis method
folinic acid

follicle
- ileal f.
- Lieberkühn f.
- lymphoid f.
- mucosal lymphoid f.

follicle-associated epithelium

follicle-stimulating
- f.-s. hormone (FSH)
- f.-s. hormone deficiency
- f.-s. hormone inhibin regulation
- f.-s. hormone secretion

follicular
- f. atresia
- f. cholecystitis
- f. cystitis
- f. fluid (FF)
- f. gastritis
- f. lymphoid hyperplasia

follicularis
- cystitis f.
- dyskeratosis f.
- keratosis f.

folliculitis

folliculus, pl. **folliculi**
- f. lymphatica
- folliculi lymphatici aggregati
- folliculi lymphatici gastrici
- folliculi lymphatici recti
- folliculi lymphatici solitarius
- folliculi lymphatici splenici

follitropin alfa for injection

Follmann balanitis

follower
- filiform and f.

following bougie

followthrough
- small bowel f. (SBFT)

followup
- f. evaluation
- f. examination

fomepizole

Fontana-Masson stain

food
- f. allergen
- f. allergy
- f. ball
- bland f.
- f. bolus
- f. bolus impaction
- f. bolus obstruction
- caffeine, alcohol, pepper, spicy f.'s (CAPS)
- f. chain
- f. challenge
- cholecystokinetic f.
- colonic f.
- compensated dysphagia for solid f.
- contamination of f.
- fatty f.
- fecal contamination of f.
- f. fever
- gas-producing f.
- *Lactobacillus plantarum*-fermented f.
- f. particle
- f. poisoning
- f. residue
- sieving of solid f.
- solid f.
- f. supplement

food-borne illness (FBI)

food-sensitive enteropathy

foot
- f. pedal suction control
- f. process (FP)

footprint

foramen
- f. of Bochdalek
- Duverney f.
- f. electrode
- epiploic f.
- f. epiploicum
- greater sciatic f.
- f. of Morgagni
- omental f.
- f. omentale
- pleuroperitoneal f.
- f. of Winslow

Forbes disease

force
- isometric f.

forced
- f. alimentation
- f. feeding

forceps
- ACMI Martin endoscopy f.
- Adair-Allis f.
- Adson-Brown tissue f.
- Adson tissue f.
- Allen intestinal f.
- alligator jaws Olympus FG 6L grasping f.
- alligator-type grasping f.
- Allis f.
- atraumatic locking/grasping f.

F

NOTES

forceps *(continued)*

Babcock intestinal f.
Backhaus towel f.
Bainbridge intestinal f.
Ballenger f.
Bard Precisor direct bite f.
Barracuda flexible cystoscopic hot
  biopsy f.
Barrett intestinal f.
Barrett-Murphy intestinal thumb f.
basket f.
basket-type crushing f.
bayonet-type f.
Beardsley intestinal f.
Beasley-Babcock f.
Beck aorta f.
Beebe hemostatic f.
Behrend cystic duct f.
Best gallstone f.
Bevan gallbladder f.
Billroth f.
biopsy f.
bipolar coagulating f.
bite biopsy f.
Blake gallstone f.
Blalock pulmonary artery f.
Blanchard hemorrhoid f.
bowel f.
Bozeman f.
Bridge deep-surgery f.
Brunner intestinal f.
Brunner tissue f.
Buie biopsy f.
Buie pile f.
bulldog f.
Carmalt f.
Child intestinal f.
Children's Hospital intestinal f.
claw f.
coagulating f.
coated biopsy f.
cold biopsy f.
Collin-Duval intestinal thumb f.
Collin intestinal f.
Collin tissue f.
Collin tongue f.
Crile bile duct f.
Crile gall duct f.
curved dissecting f.
curved Maryland f.
Cushing f.
DeBakey f.
Deddish-Potts intestinal f.
DeMartel appendix f.
Dennis intestinal f.
Desjardins gallbladder f.
Desjardins gallstone f.
disposable f.

dolphin grasping f.
dolphin-type atraumatic f.
double-spoon f.
Doyen gallbladder f.
Doyen intestinal f.
dressing f.
duck-bill f.
Duracep biopsy f.
Eastman cystic duct f.
electrocoagulating biopsy f.
Elliott gallbladder f.
Endo-Assist disposable atraumatic
  grasping f.
endoscopic alligator f.
endoscopic biopsy f.
endoscopic grasping f.
endoscopic suture-cutting f.
Everett pile f.
Excel disposable biopsy f.
FB-25K jumbo biopsy f.
fenestrated cup biopsy f.
fenestrated ellipsoid spiked open
  span biopsy f.
fenestrated spiked open-span jumbo
  biopsy f.
Ferguson tenaculum f.
fine tissue f.
fine-toothed f.
Foerster sponge f.
foreign body-retrieving f.
Foss intestinal clamp f.
Fujinon biopsy f.
gallstone f.
Gavin-Miller intestinal f.
Gemini gall duct f.
Gerald f.
Gilbert cystic duct f.
Glassman-Allis intestinal f.
Glenn diverticulum f.
Gold deep surgery f.
grasping f.
grasp tripod f.
Gray cystic duct f.
Green cystic duct f.
Haberer intestinal f.
Halsted f.
Hamilton deep surgery f.
Harrington f.
Hasson bullet-tip f.
Hasson needle-nose f.
Hasson ring f.
Hasson spike-tooth f.
Healy intestinal f.
hook f.
Hosemann f.
hot biopsy f.
hot flexible f.
Jarvis hemorrhoid f.

jeweler's f.
Johns Hopkins gallbladder f.
Judd-Allis intestinal f.
Judd-DeMartel gallbladder f.
Julian splenorenal f.
jumbo biopsy f.
Keen Edge disposable biopsy f.
Kelly f.
Kelly-Murphy f.
Kent deep surgery f.
Kleppinger f.
Kocher f.
Koerte gallstone f.
Lahey-Babcock f.
Lahey gall duct f.
Lalonde hook f.
lancet-shaped biopsy f.
Lane intestinal f.
Laplace f.
Lawrence deep surgery f.
Leonard deep surgery f.
Lillie intestinal f.
Lockwood-Allis intestinal f.
long-jaw disposable f.
loop-type snare f.
loop-type stone-crushing f.
Lovelace f.
Lower gall duct f.
Luer hemorrhoid f.
Maxum reusable f.
Mayo-Blake gallstone f.
Mayo-Pean f.
Mayo-Robson intestinal f.
Mazzariello-Caprini f.
McGill f.
McGivney hemorrhoid f.
McNealey-Glassman-Mixter f.
Medicon-Jackson rectal f.
Michigan intestinal f.
Microvasive disposable alligator-
  shaped f.
Microvasive radial jaw 3 biopsy f.
Mikulicz peritoneal f.
Miller rectal f.
Millin f.
Mill-Rose RiteBite biopsy f.
Mixter gallstone f.
mosquito f.
Moynihan artery f.
Moynihan gall duct f.
Muir hemorrhoid f.
Nelson f.

Nissen gall duct f.
Nussbaum intestinal f.
Ochsner f.
O'Hara f.
Olympus alligator-jaw endoscopic f.
Olympus basket-type endoscopic f.
Olympus Endo-Therapy disposable
  biopsy f.
Olympus FB 20C endoscopic f.
Olympus FBK 13 f.
Olympus FB 25K endoscopic f.
Olympus FG-12U wide mouth f.
Olympus FK-13-1 biopsy f.
Olympus FS-K-series endoscopic
  suture-cutting f.
Olympus grasping rat-tooth f.
Olympus hot biopsy f.
Olympus magnetic extractor f.
Olympus mini-snare f.
Olympus pelican-type endoscopic f.
Olympus rat-tooth endoscopic f.
Olympus reusable oval cup f.
Olympus rubber-tip endoscopic f.
Olympus shark-tooth endoscopic f.
Olympus tripod-type endoscopic f.
Olympus W-shaped endoscopic f.
Ombrédanne f.
Orr gall duct f.
packing f.
Payr pyloric f.
Péan f.
pelican biopsy f.
Pennington f.
Percy intestinal f.
perforating f.
pinch f.
Porter duodenal f.
Positrap three prong non-retracting
  grasping f.
Potts f.
Potts-Smith f.
Precisor Direct Bite biopsy f.
Precisor disposable biopsy f.
radial jaw bladder biopsy f.
radial jaw hot biopsy f.
radial jaw 3 Max Capacity with
  needle biopsy f.
radial jaw 3 single-use biopsy f.
Rampley sponge-holding f.
Randall stone f.
Ratliff-Blake gallstone f.
Ratliff-Mayo f.

F

NOTES

forceps *(continued)*
    rat-tooth Olympus FG 8L
      grasping f.
    Reich-Nechtow f.
    f. removal
    ring f.
    RiteBite biopsy f.
    Robbers f.
    Robson intestinal f.
    Rochester-Carmalt f.
    Rochester gallstone f.
    Rochester-Mixter f.
    Rochester-Ochsner f.
    Rochester-Péan f.
    Rudd Clinic hemorrhoidal f.
    Russian tissue f.
    Schindler peritoneal f.
    Schnidt gall duct f.
    Schnidt thoracic f.
    Schoenberg intestinal f.
    Scudder intestinal f.
    Seitzinger tripolar cutting f.
    Semken tissue f.
    shark tooth f.
    Singley intestinal f.
    smooth tissue f.
    spiral gallstone f.
    sponge f.
    sponge-holding f.
    spoon f.
    Steinmann intestinal f.
    Stille-Barraya intestinal f.
    Stille gallstone f.
    stone-grasping f.
    stone-holding basket f.
    straight Maryland f.
    SureBite biopsy f.
    Therma Jaw disposable hot
      biopsy f.
    The Shark disposable biopsy f.
    Thorek gallbladder f.
    Thorek-Mixter gallbladder f.
    three-armed basket f.
    three-pronged grasping f.
    tissue f.
    tonsil f.
    toothed tissue f.
    traumatic grasping f.
    tripod grasping f.
    Troutman rectus f.
    Turner-Warwick stone f.
    Turrell-Wittner rectal f.
    Varco gallbladder f.
    Westphal gall duct f.
    Williams intestinal f.
    W-shaped f.
    Yeoman rectal biopsy f.
    Yeoman-Wittner rectal f.
    Young intestinal f.
forcible feeding
Forder retractor
Fordyce
    angiokeratoma of F.
    F. granule
    F. spot
forearm
    f. blood flow
    f. flap
    f. graft arteriovenous fistula
Foregger rigid esophagoscope
foregut
foreign
    f. body
    f. body extraction
    f. body ingestion
    f. body management
    f. body reaction
    f. body removal
    f. body-retrieving forceps
    f. body sensation
    f. body trauma
    f. object
foreign-body appendicitis
foreshortening of the colon
foreskin
    f. flap
    f. manual retraction
    f. restoration
Forest I, II lesion
forestomach
forgotten stent
fork
    stimulation f.
forked crypt
form
    band f.
    trophozoite f.
    wax-matrix slow-release f.
    WBC immature f.'s
Formad kidney
formaldehyde
    gelatin resorcinol and f. (GRF)
    f. solution
formalin
    intravesical f.
formalin-fixed tissue
formamide
    deiodinized f.
formate
formation
    abscess f.
    adhesion f.
    bacterial biofilm f.
    beta-pleated sheet f.

bile acid-independent bile f.
  (BAIBF)
bone f.
branching tubule f.
calculous f.
enamel pellicle f.
erythroid colony f.
extracapillary crescent f.
false channel f.
fistula f.
gallstone f.
germinal center f.
Gothic arch f.
idiopathic calcium (renal) stone f.
  (ICSF)
kerion f.
median bar f.
micelle f.
physicochemical basis of
  gallstone f.
pseudoaneurysm f.
recurrent calcium stone f.
scar tissue f.
stone granuloma f.
struvite crystal f.

formatio reticularis
forme
  f. fruste
  f. tardive
formed stool
former
  calcium oxalate stone f.
  pouch f.
  stone f.
formigenes
  Oxalobacter f.
formin
formononctin
formula, pl. **formulas, formulae**
  Advance f.
  Attain tube feeding f.
  Callaway f.
  Cockcroft-Gault f.
  Encare tube feeding f.
  Enfamil with iron f.
  Ensure HIN tube feeding f.
  Ensure Plus f.
  Entralife HN tube feeding f.
  Entri-Pak tube feeding f.
  Entrition tube feeding f.
  Formula 2 tube feeding f.
  heartburn relief f. (Maalox HRF)

hydrolyzed whey f.
Isomil SF f.
I-Soyalac f.
Jevity tube feeding f.
Lofenalac f.
Lonalac f.
Natural stool f.
Nursoy f.
Nutramigen f.
Portagen f.
predigested protein f.
Pregestimil f.
ProSobee liquid f.
RCF f.
Reabilan HN tube feeding f.
Similac PM 60/40 low-iron f.
SMA f.
Soyalac f.
soy-based f.
van Slyke f.
Vitaneed tube feeding f.

Formulex
formyl peptide receptor
fornication
  fist f.
fornix, pl. **fornices**
  caliceal f.
  gastric f.
Foroblique
  50-degree F. optic laparoscope
  F. fiberoptic esophagoscope
  F. lens
  F. resectoscope
Forrest
  F. classification
  F. criteria
Forssell sinus
Fortaz
Forte
  Robinul F.
Fortison enteral feeding
fortuitum
  Mycobacterium f.
Fortuna syringe
Fortunoff flap
forward
  0-degree f. optic laparoscope
  f. motility protein of epididymal
    fluid
forward-viewing
  f.-v. endoscope

F

NOTES

forward-viewing *(continued)*
    f.-v. telescope
    f.-v. video colonoscope
foscarnet
    f. therapy
    f. treatment
fosfomycin tromethamine
fosinopril
Foss
    F. anterior resection clamp
    F. bifid gallbladder retractor
    F. biliary duct retractor
    F. intestinal clamp
    F. intestinal clamp forceps
fossa, pl. **fossae**
    Biesiadecki f.
    Broesike f.
    f. caecalis
    crural f.
    f. cystidis felleae
    duodenal f.
    epigastric f.
    Gruber-Landzert f.
    Hartmann f.
    hypochondriac f.
    iliac f.
    inferior digital f.
    intrabulbar f.
    ischiorectal f.
    Jonnesco f.
    Landzert f.
    lateral f.
    f. of male urethra
    f. of Morgagni navicular
    f. navicularis
    f. navicularis urethra
    f. ovalis
    paravesical f.
    piriform f.
    prostatic f.
    rectal f.
    retrocolic f.
    f. subinguinalis
    subsigmoid f.
    Treitz f.
    f. vesicae biliaris
fotemustine
Fothergill sign
Fouchet test
foul-smelling
    f.-s. odor
    f.-s. stool
foundation
    American Digestive Health F.
      (ADHF)
    American Liver F. (ALF)
four
    f. antigen-matched donor

    f. lines sign
    f. phases of swallowing
four-glass test
Fourier
    F. transform analysis
    F. transform infrared spectroscopy
      (FTIR)
four-lumen
    f.-l. polyvinyl manometric catheter
    f.-l. tube
Fournier
    F. disease
    F. gangrene
    F. sign
    F. syphiloma
four-port diamond placement
four-pronged polyp grasper
four-quadrant
    f.-q. incision
    f.-q. jumbo biopsy
    f.-q. tattooing
four-wing Malecot drain
fovea
    Morgagni f.
foveola, pl. **foveolae**
    gastric f.
    f. gastricae
foveola-gland ratio
foveolar
    f. gastric mucosa
    f. hyperplasia
foveolate
Fowler position
Fowler-Stephens
    F.-S. maneuver
    F.-S. orchidopexy
    F.-S. orchiopexy
    F.-S. procedure
    F.-S. test
Foxy Pouch cover
FP
    false-positive
    foot process
FPC
    familial polyposis coli
FPM
    first-pass metabolism
FPP
    familial paroxysmal polyserositis
FQ
    orphanin F.
fraction
    alpha-gliadin f.
    anionic IgG 4 f.
    cortical interstitial volume f.
    filtered f.
    filtration f.
    gallbladder ejection f. (GBEF)

globulin f.
mesangial volume f.
micronized flavonidic f.
non-T-cell f.
packing f.
plasma protein f.
recombination f.

fractional
f. clearance
f. excretion of lithium (FELI)
f. excretion of potassium (FEFEK)
f. excretion of sodium (FENa)
f. percentage of inspired oxygen (FIO$_2$)
f. proximal reabsorption
f. weight change

fractionated
f. diet
f. voiding

fractionation of bilirubin

fracture
micronized purified flavonoid f. (MPFF)
pelvis f.
penis f.
trabecular bone f.

fragilis
Bacteroides f.

fragment
anucleate f.
autotransplantation of splenic f.
N-terminal f.
nuclear f.
residual f.

fragmentary defecation

fragmentation
laser-induced f.
stone f.
ultrasonic f.

Fragmin

Fraley
F. sign
F. syndrome

frame
nitinol mesh-covered f.
Stryker f.

frameshift

Framingham risk-factor approach

Francis test

Franco operation

frank
f. blood

f. blood in stool
f. cirrhosis
F. operation
f. pus

Frankel
crossbar symptom of F.

Frankfeldt rectal snare

Franklin-Silverman biopsy cannula

Franz abdominal retractor

Fraser syndrome

Frazier
F. suction tip
F. suction tube

FreAmine amino acid solution

FRED
fog reduction elimination device

FREDDY Nd:YAG laser

Frederick-Miller tube

frederiksenii
Yersinia f.

Fredet-Ramstedt
F.-R. operation
F.-R. pyloromyotomy

Fredrickson classification

free
f. acetate
f. air
f. band of colon
fat f. (FF)
f. fatty acid
f. fecal bile acid
f. fluid
f. hepatic venous pressure (FHVP)
f. jejunal graft
f. prostate-specific antigen
f. radical
f. radical scavenger
f. reflux
f. resection
f. ribosome
f. subphrenic gas
f. testosterone
f. thyroxine (FT4)
f. tie
f. to total prostate-specific antigen (F:T PSA, FTPSA, F:T PSA)
f. to total PSA

free-beam
f.-b. coagulation
f.-b. laser system

F

NOTES

freedom
  F. Clear long seal male external
    catheter line
  F. Clear LS male external catheter
    line
  F. Clear sport sheath male external
    catheter line
  F. Clear SS male external catheter
    line
freehand
  f. biopsy
  f. cannulation
freeing up of adhesion
Freer elevator
free-standing ambulatory surgical center
free-to-total PSA ratio
freezing
  gastric f.
Freiburg biopsy set
fremitus
frena (*pl. of* frenum)
frenal
French
  F. bougie
  F. Cope loop nephrostomy catheter
  F. cystoscope
  F. dilator
  F. double-J ureteral stent
  F. eye needle
  F. introducer set
  F. mushroom tip catheter
  F. Pharmacovigilance system
  F. pigtail nephrostomy catheter
  F. scale
  F. Swan-Ganz balloon
  F. Teflon pyeloureteral catheter
  F. T-tube
frenectomy
frenoplasty
Frenta
  F. Mat feeding pump
  F. System II feeding pump
frenulum, pl. **frenula**
  f. of duodenal papilla
  f. of ileocolic valve
  f. of Morgagni
  f. of prepuce
  f. preputii penis
  f. valvae ilealis
  f. valvae ileocaecalis
frenum, pl. **frena**
  f. of valve of colon
frequency
  fecal f. (FF)
  operating f.
  pulse repetition f. (PRF)
  f. of stool
  urinary f.

**frequency-doubled-double pulse ND:YAG
  laser**
frequency-duration index (FDI)
frequency-urgency-pain syndrome
frequent hemodialysis
Fresenius
  F. AG dialyzer
  F. F-40 filter
  F. 2008H hemodialysis machine
  F. volumetric dialysate balancing
    system
fresh
  f. clot
  f. frozen plasma (FFP)
Freund adjuvant
freundii
  Citrobacter f.
Frey
  F. gastric pit
  F. hair
Freyer operation
friability
  cervical f.
friable mucosa
friction
  f. knot
  f. rub
friction-fit adapter
Friderichsen-Waterhouse syndrome
Friedländer bacillus
Friedman perineal retractor
**Frimberger-Karpiel 12 o'clock
  papillotome**
Fritsch retractor
Froehlich (*var. of* Fröhlich)
frog leg position
frog-spawn-like mucosa
Fröhlich, Froehlich
  F. syndrome
frondlike filling defect
frontal tenderness
front-loading ultrasound probe (FLUP)
Frostberg reversed 3 sign
frothy
frozen section
fructose
  f. aldolase
  f. aldolase deficiency
  f. diarrhea
  f. diphosphatase deficiency
  f. intolerance
  seminal plasma f.
fructose-1,6-bisphosphatase
fructose-free diet
fruity odor
fruste
  forme f.
Frykman-Goldberg procedure

FSA
　fetal sulfoglycoprotein antigen
FSGS
　focal segmental glomerulosclerosis
　　collapsing FSGS
FSH
　follicle-stimulating hormone
FSP
　fibrin split product
F60S polysulfone
FSSE
　fat-suppressed spin-echo
FT4
　free thyroxine
FTA-ABS
　flouuescent treponemal antibody
　　absorption
　fluorescent treponemal antibody
　　absorption
　　FTA-ABS test
FTIR
　Fourier transform infrared spectroscopy
FTLE
　full-thickness local excision
FTPSA, F:T PSA
　frcc to total prostate specific antigen
5-FU
　5-fluorouracil
fucosidosis
fucosylated alpha fetoprotein
fucosylation index of alpha fetoprotein
fucosyltransferase gene
FUDR
　fluorodeoxyuridine
fugax
　　proctalgia f.
Fujinon
　　F. biopsy forceps
　　F. CEG-FP-series videoelectroscope
　　F. DUO-XT duodenoscope
　　F. EB-410S bronchoscope
　　F. EC7-CM2 video colonoscope
　　F. EC-130LT colonoscope
　　F. EC-200LT colonoscope
　　F. EC-410MP colonoscope
　　F. EC-300MS colonoscope
　　F. ED7-XT duodenoscope
　　F. ED7-XU2
　　F. ED-200XU duodenoscope
　　F. ED-310XU duodenoscope
　　F. ED-410XU duodenoscope
　　F. ED7-XU2 video duodenoscope

　　F. EG-310D gastroscope
　　F. EG-200FP gastroscope
　　F. EG-FP-series endoscope
　　F. EG-410HR gastroscope
　　F. ES-200ER sigmoidoscope
　　F. EVC-M video colonoscope
　　F. EVD-XL video duodenoscope
　　F. EVD-XT duodenoscope
　　F. EVE-series endoscope
　　F. EVG-CT endoscope
　　F. EVG-FP-series endoscope
　　F. EVG-F-series endoscope
　　F. FD-100XU duodenoscope
　　F. FE-100LR colonoscope
　　F. FG-series endoscopic camera
　　F. FP-series endoscope
　　F. FS-100ER sigmoidoscope
　　F. GF-100PE gastroscope
　　F. PRO-PC flexible fiberoptic
　　sigmoidoscope
　　F. 400 series super image video
　　gastroscope
　　F. SIG-E2 fiberoptic sigmoidoscope
　　F. SIG-EK-series flexible fiberoptic
　　sigmoidoscope
　　F. SIG-E-series flexible fiberoptic
　　sigmoidoscope
　　F. SIG-ET-series flexible fiberoptic
　　sigmoidoscope
　　F. SP-501 sonoprobe system
　　F. UGI-FP-series video endoscope
　　F. video endoscopy cart
　　F. video endoscopy system
　　F. 310XU video duodenoscope
FUL
　functional urethral length
fulguration
　　diverticulum f.
　　electrosurgical f.
　　endoscopic f.
full
　　f. extension
　　f. liquid (FL)
　　f. range of motion
full-bladder technique
full-column barium enema
Fuller
　　F. operation
　　F. rectal shield
full-length viral genome
full-liquid diet
full-lumen esophagoscope

F

NOTES

fullness
 abdominal f.
 adnexal f.
 postprandial f.
 pyloric f.
full-surface micro mesh teeth
full-thickness
 f.-t. biopsy
 f.-t. graft
 f.-t. local excision (FTLE)
fulminant
 f. Crohn disease
 f. dysentery
 f. hepatic failure (FHF)
 f. hepatitis (A–E)
 f. hepatocellular failure
 f. liver failure
 f. toxic colitis
 f. viral hepatitis (FVH)
fulminating
 f. appendicitis
 f. dysentery
 f. pancreatitis
 f. ulcerative colitis
fumagillin
fumarylacetoacetate hydrolase deficiency
fumigatus
 Aspergillus f.
FUMIR
 5-fluorouracil, mitomycin C radiation
function
 anal sphincter f.
 bladder neck sphincteric f.
 bladder storage f.
 bowel f.
 cardiopulmonary baroreflex f.
 Carnot f.
 cine-loop memory f.
 cognitive f.
 delayed graft f. (DGF)
 discriminant f. (DF)
 excretory f.
 exocrine f.
 gallbladder f.
 gastrin cell f.
 graft f.
 impaired colonic motor f.
 International Index of Erectile F. (IIEF)
 kidney f.
 Leydig cell secretory f.
 Maddrey discriminant f.
 native kidney f.
 neoanal f.
 P450 f.
 pharyngoesophageal f.
 proximal tubule f.
 puborectalis muscle f.

 pudendal nerve f.
 rectoanal f.
 rectosigmoid f.
 renal f.
 Sertoli cell secretory f.
 sexual f.
 sieving f.
 sphincter f.
 splenic f.
 split renal f.
functional
 f. bladder capacity
 f. bleeding
 f. bowel disease
 f. bowel disorder (FBD)
 F. Bowel Disorder Severity Index (FBDSI)
 f. bowel distress (FBD)
 f. bowel syndrome
 f. castration
 f. constipation
 f. cystic duct obstruction
 f. diarrhea
 f. disorder stomach
 f. dyspepsia
 f. gastrointestinal disorder (FGID)
 f. hepatic volume
 f. impotence
 f. incontinence
 f. magnetic resonance imaging (fMRI)
 f. pain
 f. plasminogen
 f. profile length
 f. urethral length (FUL)
fundal
 f. gastritis
 f. plication
 f. pouch
 f. varix
fundectomy
fundi (*pl. of* fundus)
fundic
 f. atrophic gastritis (FAG)
 f. biopsy
 f. clot
 f. gland atrophy
 f. gland gastritis
 f. gland heterotopia
 f. gland polyp
 f. mucosa
 f. plexus
 f. varix
fundic-antral junction
fundiform ligament
fundoplasty
 Gomez f.
 Thal f.

fundoplication
Belsey 270-degree f.
Belsey Mark IV 240-degree f.
Belsey partial f.
Belsey two-thirds wrap f.
circumferential f.
Collis-Nissen f.
floppy Nissen f.
Hill esophageal f.
intrathoracic Nissen f.
laparoscopic Nissen f. (lap Nissen)
laparoscopic Nissen and Toupet f.
Nissen 360-degree wrap f.
Nissen laparoscopic f.
partial f.
Rossetti modification of Nissen f.
slipped Nissen f.
supraphysiological f.
Toupet partial posterior f.
fundopyloric mucosal border
fundus, pl. **fundi**
bald gastric f.
folded f.
gallbladder f.
gastric f.
f. gastricus
f. rotation gastroplasty
f. of stomach
f. ventricularis
f. ventriculi
f. vesicae biliaris
f. vesicae felleae
f. vesicae urinaria
fundusectomy
fungal
f. ball
f. bezoar
f. infection
f. liver abscess
f. peritonitis
f. pyelonephritis
f. spore
fungating growth
fungemia
fungi (*pl. of* fungus)
Fungi-Fluor
F.-F. chitin stain
F.-F. procedure
fungiform papilla
Fungizone
fungoides
mycosis f.

fungosa
gastrosia f.
gastroxynsis f.
funguria
fungus, pl. **fungi**
ovoid f.
f. testis
funicular
f. hydrocele
f. inguinal hernia
f. stump
funiculate
funiculi (*pl. of* funiculus)
funiculitis
funiculoepididymitis
filarial f.
funiculoepididymitus
funiculopexy
funiculus, pl. **funiculi**
hepatic f.
f. spermaticus
funis
funisitis
funnel
Esca Buess + fistula f.
stent f.
funnel-neck prostate
fura-2, pentapotassium salt
Furacin
Furadantin
furazolidone
Furlow
F. cylinder inserter
F. introducer
**Furlow-Fisher modification of Virag 1
operation**
Furniss
F. anastomosis clamp
F. ureterointestinal anastomosis
Furniss-Clute duodenal clamp
furnissii
Vibrio f.
furor medicus
furosemide washout renogram
Furoxone
furrier suture
furrow
Liebermeister f.
furuncle
furunculosis
Fusarium solani
fused kidney

F

NOTES

fusible calculus
fusiform
    f. renal artery aneurysm
    f. widening of duct
fusion
    f. fascia
    tissue f.
    urethrohymenal f.
    viral membrane f.
Fusobacterium
Futura resectoscope sheath

F value
FVH
    fulminant viral hepatitis
FVL
    flexible video laparoscope
FVM
    familial visceral myopathy
FVN
    familial visceral neuropathy
Fx1A antibody
fyn protein

G

G cell
G protein
G protein disease
G syndrome
gabapentin
gabexate mesylate
Gabriel proctoscope
gadolinium
g. chelate
g. EOB-DTPA (Gd-EOB-DTPA)
Gadolite oral suspension
GAG
glycosaminoglycan
gag
Millard mouth g.
mouth g.
g. reflex
g. response
GAGUA
glycosaminoglycan uronate
gain
interdialytic weight g. (IDWG)
symptomatic fluid g.
weight g.
gait
antalgic g.
ataxic g.
broad-based g.
g. disturbance
favored g.
parkinsonian g.
spastic g.
steppage g.
Trendelenburg g.
unsteady g.
galactitol
galactodes
urina g.
Galacto-Light assay
galactoma
galactopexy
galactose-1-phosphate uridyltransferase
galactose elimination capacity (GEC)
galactose-free diet
galactosemia
Indiana variant g.
Rennes variant g.
galactosidase
beta g.
galactosyltransferase isoenzyme II
galacturia
galanin antiserum
Galant reflex
Galeati gland

galeni
porus g.
galenic preparation
GALF
glycyrrhetinic acid like factor
gall
g. duct
g. duct spoon
gallamine
gallbladder (GB)
adenomyoma of g.
g. adenomyomatosis
g. bag positioner
g. bed
bilobed g.
g. calculus
g. carcinoma
cholesterolosis of g.
chronically inflamed g.
g. contraction
Courvoisier g.
dilated g.
g. displacement
g. dome
double g.
duplicated g.
g. dysmotility
edematous g.
g. ejection fraction (GBEF)
g. ejection rate (GBER)
g. emptying-refilling curve
empyema of g.
endoscopic transpapillary
catheterization of the g. (ETCG)
g. filling
fish-scale g.
floating g.
g. function
g. function test
g. fundus
gangrene of g.
hourglass constriction of g.
g. hydrops
g. ileus
inflamed g.
infundibulum of g.
g. lift
mobile g.
mucocele of g.
multiseptate g.
nonfunctioning g.
nonvisualization of g.
notch of g.
palpable g.
perforation of g.

G

gallbladder *(continued)*
    porcelain g.
    robin's egg-blue g.
    g. scan
    g. scoop
    g. series (GBS)
    g. sludge
    stasis g.
    g. stasis
    g. stone
    strawberry g.
    thick-walled g.
    thin-walled g.
    g. torsion
    torsion of g.
    trauma of g.
    g. trauma
    g. trocar
    g. varix
    g. volume
    g. wall
    g. wall abscess
    wandering g.
Gallie transplant
gallinaginis
    caput g.
gallium
    g. imaging
    g. nitrate
    g. scan
gallium-67
gallop rhythm
Galloway-Mowat syndrome (GMS)
gallows-type retractor
gallstone
    asymptomatic g.
    bilirubin pigment g.
    black pigment g.
    brown pigment g.
    calcified g.
    cholesterol-containing g.
    g. colic
    dissolution of g.
    faceted g.
    floating g.
    g. forceps
    g. formation
    g. ileus
    g. incidence
    innocent g.
    intragastric g.
    g. migration
    mixed-cholesterol g.
    mulberry g.
    g. pancreatitis
    g. pattern
    pigment g.
    pigmented g.

    g. probe
    radiolucent g.
    retained g.
    silent g.
    symptomatic g.
    unextractable g.
gallstone-solubilizing agent
Gal 4 protein
GALT
    gastrointestinal-associated lymphoid
      tissue
    gut-associated lymphoid tissue
galvanic probe
Gambee
    G. anastomosis
    G. stitch
    G. suture
Gambian sleeping sickness
Gambro
    G. AK10 machine
    G. dialyzer
    G. FH88H filter
    G. Lundia Minor artificial kidney
gamete
    g. intrafallopian transfer (GIFT)
    g. micromanipulation
gametic
gametocidal
gametocide
gametocyst
gamma
    g. aminobutyric acidergic neuron
    g. emission
    g. fetoprotein
    g. globulin
    g. globulin therapy
    g. heavy-chain disease
    g. interferon
    g. light chain
    g. scintillation camera
    g. seminoprotein
    g. split-sling wrap
    g. transverse colon loop
gamma-aminobutyric
    g.-a. acid
    g.-a. acid accumulation
gammaglobulin
    antithymocyte g. (ATGAM)
gamma-glutamyl
    g.-g. transferase (GGT)
    g.-g. transferase level
    g.-g. transpeptidase (GGTP)
gamma glutamyltransferase
    serum g. g.
gamma-lyase
    cystathionine g.-l.
Gammatone II gamma camera

gammopathy
  monoclonal g.
Gamna
  G. disease
  G. nodule
GAN-19 needle
Ganau criteria
ganciclovir
Gandy-Gamna nodule
ganglial
ganglion, pl. **ganglia**
  basal ganglia
  celiac-superior mesenteric ganglia
  g. cell loss
  dorsal root ganglia
  enteric ganglia
  intramural ganglia
  nodose ganglia
  subserous ganglia
  Troisier g.
ganglionated plexus
ganglioneuroblastoma
ganglioneuroma
  adrenal cortex g.
ganglioneuromatosis
ganglion-free muscle strip
ganglioside
  GM3 g.
gangliosides
gangraenosa
  balanitis g.
gangrene
  cecal g.
  Fournier g.
  g. of gallbladder
  gas g.
  ischemic penile g.
gangrenosum
  ecthyma g.
  pyoderma g. (PG)
gangrenous
  g. appendicitis
  g. appendix
  g. balanitis
  g. bowel
  g. cholecystitis
  g. colon
  g. cystitis
  g. ischemic colitis
  g. ischemic enterocolitis
  g. necrosis

Gans
  incisura dextra of G.
Ganser diverticulum
Gantanol
  Azo G.
Gant clamp
Gantrisin
  Azo G.
gantry
GAP
  glans approximation procedure
  GAP test
gap
  anion g.
  glottic g.
  g. junction
  osmolarity g.
  stool osmotic g.
  underwater spark g.
  urinary anion g.
GAPD
  glyceraldehyde phosphate dehydrogenase
GAPDH
  glyceraldehyde-3-phosphate
  dehydrogenase
Garamycin
garbled speech
Garden prognostic system
Gardner-Diamond syndrome
Gardnerella vaginalis
Gardner syndrome (GS)
gargle
  viscous Xylocaine g.
garnet
  holmium:yttrium aluminum g.
   (Ho:YAG)
Garren
  G. balloon
  G. gastric bubble
Garren-Edwards
  G.-E. balloon
  G.-E. gastric (GEG)
  G.-E. gastric bubble
Garrett dilator
Gartner
  G. duct
  G. duct cyst
gas
  g. abscess
  arterial blood g. (ABG)
  bowel g.
  g. chromatography

G

NOTES

gas *(continued)*
    g. chromatography/mass
      spectroscopy (GC/MS)
    colonic g.
    g. cupula
    g. cyst
    g. cystometry
    g. density line
    ethylene oxide g. (ETO)
    free subphrenic g.
    g. gangrene
    hydrogen g.
    g. isotope ratio mass spectrometry
    g. pattern
    g. sterilization
    g. thermometer
gas-bloat syndrome
gaseous
    g. cholecystitis
    g. distention
    g. pericholecystitis
gas-forming
    g.-f. liver abscess
    g.-f. organism in bowel wall
    g.-f. pyogenic liver infection
gasket
    Seal-tight adhesive g.
    United Surgical Seal Tite g.
gasless
    g. laparoscopic approach
    g. laparoscopy
GASP
    gastric augment and single pedicle tube
gas-producing food
gasserian syndrome
Gasser syndrome
gassiness
gassy
gaster
gastralgia
gastrectasis, gastrectasia
gastrectomized patient
gastrectomy
    antecolic g.
    Billroth I, II g.
    completion g.
    distal g.
    esophagoproximal g.
    high subtotal g.
    Horsley g.
    partial g.
    physiologic g.
    Pólya g.
    proximal g.
    subtotal g.
    total g.
    von Haberer-Aguirre g.

gastric
    g. accommodation test
    g. achlorhydria
    g. acid
    g. acidity
    g. acidity reduction
    g. acid pump inhibitor
    g. acid rebound
    g. acid secretion
    g. actinomycosis
    g. adenocarcinoma
    g. adenopapillomatosis
    g. air bubble
    g. analysis
    g. aneurysm
    g. angioma
    g. angiomyolipoma
    g. anisakiasis
    g. anoxia
    g. antral erosion
    g. antral sessile polyp
    g. antral vascular ectasia (GAVE)
    g. antrum
    g. arteriography
    g. arteriovenous malformation
    g. artery
    g. aspirate
    g. aspiration
    g. aspiration tube
    g. atony
    g. atresia
    g. augment and single pedicle tube
      (GASP)
    g. bacterial overgrowth (GBO)
    g. balloon
    g. balloon implantation
    g. bezoar
    g. bladder
    g. bladder replacement
    g. bleeding time (GBT)
    g. brush cytology
    g. bypass (GBP)
    g. bypass surgery
    g. calculus
    g. cancer
    g. capacity
    g. carcinoid
    g. carcinoid tumor
    g. carcinoma
    g. carcinosarcoma
    g. cardia
    g. carditis
    g. cell kinetics
    g. channel
    g. chloroma
    g. chromoscopy
    g. coin removal
    g. colic

g. compression
g. content
g. crisis
g. cycle
g. decompression
g. diet
g. dilation
g. distention
g. diverticulosis
g. duplication
g. duplication cyst
g. dysfunction
g. dyspepsia
g. effect
g. electrical dysrhythmia
g. electrical stimulation
g. emptying (GE)
g. emptying delay
g. emptying half-time (GET1/2)
g. emptying scan
g. emptying scintigraphy
g. emptying test
g. emptying time (GET)
g. epithelial cell infiltration
g. epithelial cell replication
g. feeding
g. first-pass metabolism of ethanol (GFPM)
g. fistula
g. fold
g. foreign body
g. fornix
g. foveola
g. foveolar epithelium
g. freezing
g. function test
g. fundus
g. fundus wrap
Garren-Edwards g. (GEG)
g. gland
g. hemorrhage
g. heterotopia
g. hyperacidity
g. hyperemia
g. hyperplastic polyp
g. hypersecretion
g. hypochlorhydria
g. hypomotility
g. hypothermia
g. hypothermia machine
g. ileus
g. impression

g. impression on liver
g. indigestion
g. inflammatory fibroid polyp
g. inhibitor factor
g. inhibitory peptide (GIP)
g. inhibitory polypeptide (GIP)
g. insufficiency
g. juice
g. Kaposi sarcoma
g. laryngeal mask airway (GLMA)
g. lavage
g. lavage tube
g. leiomyoma
g. leiomyosarcoma
g. lesion
g. lipoma
g. luminal pH
g. lymphoma
g. malaria
g. mass
g. mechanosensory threshold
g. metaplasia
g. metaplasia of duodenum
g. microenvironment
g. motility disorder
g. mucormycosis
g. mucosal atrophy
g. mucosal barrier
g. mucosal blood flow
g. mucosal damage
g. mucosal degradation
g. mucosal disease
g. mucosal ectopia in rectum (GMER)
g. mucosal ectopy
g. mucosal erosion
g. mucosal injury
g. mucosal laminin receptor
g. mucosal pattern classification
g. mucosal prolapse
g. mucus
g. muscularis mucosa
g. mycosis
g. myoelectrical activity
g. neobladder
g. neobladder procedure
g. neurasthenia
g. neurectomy
g. notch
g. omentum
g. outlet
g. outlet obstruction (GOO)

NOTES

G

gastric *(continued)*
   g. outline
   g. oxyntic cell receptor
   g. pacemaker cell
   g. pacemaker region
   g. parietography
   g. partition
   g. perforation
   g. petechia
   g. pH monitor
   g. pigment
   g. pit
   g. pitting
   g. plasma
   g. plasmacytoma
   g. plexus
   g. pneumocystosis
   g. polyp
   g. polypectomy
   g. polyposis
   g. pool
   g. pouch
   g. pseudolymphoma
   g. red spot
   g. remnant
   g. resection (GR)
   g. residuum
   g. retention
   g. rupture
   g. sclerosis
   g. secretory test
   g. sedative
   g. serosa
   g. stapling
   g. stasis
   g. stump
   g. syphilis
   g. tear
   g. teratoma
   g. tetany
   g. tone
   g. transit time
   g. transposition
   g. trauma
   g. tuberculosis
   g. ulcer
   g. ulceration
   g. urease activity
   g. variceal ligation
   g. varix
   g. varix bleeding
   g. vascular ectasia (GVE)
   g. vein
   g. venacaval shunt
   g. vertigo
   g. volume
   g. volvulus

   g. window
   g. xanthoma
gastrica
   achylia g.
   adenasthenia g.
   adenohypersthenia g.
   area g.
   myasthenia g.
   zymosis g.
gastricae
   areae g.
   fibrae oblique g.
   foveola g.
   rugae g.
   sordes g.
gastrici
   folliculi lymphatici g.
gastric-juice ammonia assay
gastric-type surface epithelium
gastricum
   corpus g.
gastricus
   fundus g.
   liquor g.
   status g.
   succus g.
Gastrimmune
^{125}I-gastrin
gastrin
   antral g.
   basic g. (BG)
   g. cell
   g. cell function
   g. cell hyperfunction
   fasting serum g.
   ^{125}I-g.
   g. gene
   g. mRNA
   g. mRNA:G-cell density
   g. mRNA level
   g. mRNA species
   g. receptor
   G. RIA kit II
   serum g.
   g. stain
   g. stimulation test
gastrin-17
gastrinoma
   duodenal g.
gastrin-releasing
   g.-r. peptide (GRP)
   g.-r. peptide/bombesin
gastrin-secreting
   g.-s. cell
   g.-s. non-beta islet cell tumor
gastritis
   acute erosive g. (AEG)
   acute hemorrhagic g.

alcoholic hemorrhagic g.
alkaline reflux g.
antral atrophic g. (AAG)
antral-predominant g.
antrum g.
aspirin-induced g.
atrophic g.
autoimmune metaplastic atrophic g.
  (AMAG)
bile reflux g.
bleeding g.
Campylobacter pyloridis g.
catarrhal g.
chemical g.
chronic active g.
chronic atrophic g. (CAG)
chronic cystic g.
chronic erosive g.
chronic follicular g.
chronic interstitial g.
chronic nonimmune g.
chronic superficial g. (CSG)
cirrhotic g.
corpus g.
corrosive g.
g. cystica polyposa
g. cystic profunda
diffuse antral g. (DAG)
diffuse varioliform g.
drug-induced g.
emphysematous g.
endoscopic atrophic g.
endoscopic enterogastric reflux g.
endoscopic
  erythematous/exudative g.
endoscopic hemorrhagic g.
endoscopic raised erosive g.
endoscopic rugal hyperplastic g.
environmental metaplastic
  atrophic g. (EMAG)
eosinophilic g.
erosive g.
erosive-hemorrhagic g.
exfoliative g.
follicular g.
fundal g.
fundic atrophic g. (FAG)
fundic gland g.
giant hypertrophic g.
g. granulomatosa fibroplastica
granulomatous g.
Helicobacter pylori-induced g.

hemorrhagic g.
histological chronic active g.
hyperpeptic g.
hypertrophic lymphocytic g. (HLG)
idiopathic chronic erosive g.
interstitial g.
isolated granulomatous g.
lymphocytic g. (LG)
metaplastic atrophic g.
multifocal atrophic g. (MAG)
mycotic g.
nonautoimmune fundic atrophic g.
nonerosive nonspecific g.
nonspecific erosive g.
oxyntic mucosal g.
phlegmonous g.
polypous g.
postgastrectomy g.
postoperative g.
proliferative hypertrophic g.
pseudomembranous g.
purulent g.
radiation g.
reflux bile g.
severe g.
specific g.
stress g.
superficial g.
suppurative g.
Sydney classification of g.
syphilitic g.
toxic g.
tuberculous g.
type A, B g.
type B antral g.
ulcerative g.
uremic g.
varioliform g.
g. varioliformis
verrucous g.
viral g.
zonal g.
gastritis-associated peptic ulcer disease
gastroadenitis
gastroadynamic
gastroalbumorrhea
gastroanastomosis
gastroatonia
gastroblennorrhea
gastrocamera
  Olympus GTF-A g.
gastrocardiac syndrome

NOTES

G

Gastroccult test
gastrocele
gastrochronorrhea
gastrocolic
    g. fistula
    g. ligament
    g. omentum
    g. reflex
gastrocolitis
gastrocolostomy
gastrocutaneous
    g. fistula
    g. fistulous tract
gastrocystoplasty
gastrodiaphanoscopy
gastrodiaphany
gastroduodenal
    g. artery (GDA)
    g. artery complex
    g. carcinoid
    g. Crohn disease
    g. double ulcer
    g. dyspepsia
    g. fistula
    g. hypertrophy
    g. lumen
    g. misperfusion
    g. mucosa
    g. mucosal injury
    g. mucosal protection
gastroduodenal-to-renal
    g.-t.-r. artery bypass
    g.-t.-r. artery bypass graft
gastroduodenectomy
gastroduodenitis
    neutrophilic g.
gastroduodenoenterostomy
gastroduodenopancreatectomy
gastroduodenoscopy
    Billroth g.
gastroduodenostomy
    Billroth I g.
    Jaboulay g.
gastrodynia
gastroenteralgia
gastroenteric fistula
gastroenteritis
    acute g. (AGE)
    acute infectious nonbacterial g.
    astrovirus g.
    Calicivirus g.
    Coronavirus g.
    endemic nonbacterial infantile g.
    eosinophilic g. (EG, EGE, EOG)
    epidemic nonbacterial g.
    infantile g.
    infectious g.
    nonbacterial g.

    Norwalk g.
    rotavirus g.
    viral g.
    winter g.
gastroenteroanastomosis
gastroenterocolitis
gastroenterocolostomy
gastroenterologic
gastroenterologist
gastroenterology
    American College of G. (ACG)
gastroenteropancreatic (GEP)
    g. tumor
gastroenteropathy
    g. detection
    eosinophilic g.
    protein-losing g.
gastroenteroplasty
gastroenteroptosis
gastroenterostomy (GE)
    Balfour g.
    Billroth g. (type I, II)
    Braun-Jaboulay g.
    Courvoisier g.
    Finney g.
    Heineke-Mikulicz g.
    Hill esophageal g.
    Hofmeister g.
    percutaneous g. (PGE)
    Pólya g.
    Roux-en-Y g.
    Schoemaker g.
    truncal vagotomy and g.
gastroenterotomy
gastroepiploic
    g. arcade
    g. artery (GEA)
    g. blood vessel
gastroesophageal (GE)
    g. hernia
    g. incompetence
    g. junction
    g. reflux (GER)
    g. reflux disease (GERD)
    g. reflux scan
    g. scintigraphy
    g. scintiscan
    g. sphincter
    g. variceal plexus
    g. varix (type 1, 2)
gastroesophagitis
gastroesophagostomy
    cervical g.
gastrogalvanization
gastrogastrostomy
gastrogavage
gastrogenic diarrhea
gastrogenous diarrhea

Gastrografin
- G. contrast medium
- G. enema
- G. GI series
- G. swallow

GastrograpH
- G. ambulatory pH monitoring system
- G. Mark III pH analyzer

gastrohepatic
- g. bare area
- g. ligament
- g. omentum

gastrohydrorrhea

gastroileac augmentation

gastroileal reflex

gastroileitis

gastroileostomy

gastroiliac reflex

gastrointestinal (GI)
- g. absorption
- g. allergy
- g. assistant
- g. autonomic nerve tumor
- g. biota
- g. bleed
- g. bleeding (GIB)
- g. blood loss test
- g. cancer
- g. cancer-associated antigen (GICA)
- g. complication
- g. cross
- g. endoscopy
- g. endothelium
- g. eosinophilic granuloma
- g. fiberscope
- g. fistula
- g. fungal ball
- g. hamartomatous polyp
- g. histoplasmosis
- g. immunodeficiency syndrome
- g. intubation
- g. Kaposi sarcoma
- g. lavage
- g. lesion
- g. lipoma
- g. motility
- g. myenteric plexus
- g. needle
- g. neuroendocrinology
- g. neurofibroma
- g. peptide hormone

- g. polyposis (GIP)
- g. reflux
- g. regularity peptide
- g. smooth muscle
- g. stoma
- g. stromal tumor
- G. Symptom Rating Scale (GSRS)
- g. system (GIS)
- g. telangiectasia
- g. therapeutic system (GITS)
- g. tract (GIT)
- g. tract hemorrhage
- g. transit
- G. Tumor Study Group (GITSG, GTSG)
- upper g. (UGI)

gastrointestinal-associated lymphoid tissue (GALT)

gastrointestinalis
- pseudoleukemia g.

gastrojejunal
- g. constipation
- g. loop obstruction syndrome

gastrojejunocolic fistula

gastrojejunostomy
- antecolic long-loop isoperistaltic g.
- Billroth g. (type I, II)
- compression button g.
- Hofmeister-Shoemaker g.
- loop g.
- percutaneous endoscopic g. (PEG-J)

gastrokinesograph

gastrokinetic agent

gastrolavage

gastrolienal ligament

gastrolith

gastrolithiasis

gastrologist

gastrology

gastrolysis

Gastrolyte oral solution

gastromalacia

GastroMark

gastromegaly

gastromotor insufficiency

gastromycosis

gastromyotomy

gastromyxorrhea

gastronesteostomy

gastropancreatic
- g. fold

G

NOTES

gastropancreatic *(continued)*
 g. ligament
 g. reflex
gastropancreatitis
gastroparalysis
gastroparesis
 diabetic g.
 g. diabeticorum
 idiopathic g.
 nondiabetic g.
 postvagotomy g.
 transient g.
gastroparietal
gastropathic
gastropathology
gastropathy
 aphthous g.
 benign hyperplastic g.
 cardiofundic g.
 chemical g.
 congestive hypertensive g.
 diabetic g.
 erosive g.
 erythematous g.
 hemorrhagic g.
 hypertensive g.
 hypertrophic g.
 idiopathic hypertrophic g.
 nonsteroidal antiinflammatory
  drug g.
 NSAID g.
 papulous g.
 portal hypertensive g. (PHG)
 prolapse g.
 protein-losing g.
 varioliform g.
gastroperiodynia
gastroperitonitis
gastropexy
 Boerema anterior g.
 Hill posterior g.
 Horsley g.
gastrophotography
gastrophrenic ligament
gastrophthisis
gastroplasty (GP)
 Collis g.
 Collis-Nissen g.
 Eckhout vertical g.
 fundus rotation g.
 Gomez horizontal g.
 greater curvature banded g.
 horizontal g.
 Laws g.
 Mason vertical banded g.
 Silastic ring vertical g.
 silicone elastomer ring vertical g.
  (SRVG)

 Stamm g.
 tubular vertical g.
 unbanded g.
 vertical banded g. (VBG)
 vertical ring g. (VRG)
 vertical Silastic ring g.
gastroplegia
gastroplication
Gastro-Port II feeding device
gastroprokinetic
gastroprotection
 adaptive g.
gastroprotective
gastroptosis
gastroptyxis
gastropylorectomy
gastropyloric
Gastroreflex ambulatory pH
 monitor/recorder
gastrorenal shunt
gastrorrhagia
gastrorrhaphy
gastrorrhea continua chronica
gastrorrhexis
gastroschisis
 Silastic silo reduction of g.
gastroscope
 ACMI g.
 Benedict g.
 Bernstein g.
 Cameron omniangle g.
 Chevalier Jackson g.
 disposable-sheath flexible g.
 Eder g.
 Eder-Bernstein g.
 Eder-Chamberlin g.
 Eder-Hufford g.
 Eder-Palmer semiflexible g.
 Ellsner g.
 end-viewing g.
 Ewald g.
 FCS-ML II g.
 FGS-ML II g.
 fiberoptic g.
 flexible g.
 Fujinon EG-310D g.
 Fujinon EG-200FP g.
 Fujinon EG-410HR g.
 Fujinon GF-100PE g.
 Fujinon 400 series super image
  video g.
 GFC g.
 GFT Olympus g.
 Herman-Taylor g.
 Hirschowitz g.
 Housset-Debray g.
 Janeway g.
 Jenning-Streifeneder g.

Kelling g.
Krentz g.
Mancke flex-rigid g.
Mikulicz g.
Olympus GIF-K-series g.
Olympus GIF-XQ30 flexible g.
Olympus 2T-2000 twin-channel
  therapeutic g.
pediatric g.
Pentax EUP-EC124 ultrasound g.
peroral g.
Schindler semiflexible g.
Sielaff g.
Taylor g.
Tomenius g.
Universal g.
Wolf-Henning g.
Wolf-Knittlingen g.
Wolf-Schindler semiflexible g.
XQ230 Olympus g.
gastroscopic
gastroscopy
  cap-fitted g.
  high-magnification g.
  infrared transillumination g.
Gastrosed
gastrosia fungosa
gastrosis
gastrospasm
Gastrospirillum hominis
gastrosplenic
  g. ligament
  g. omentum
gastrostaxis
gastrostenosis
gastrostogavage
gastrostolavage
gastrostomy
  Beck g.
  Beck-Jianu g.
  g. bumper
  button g.
  g. button
  CT-guided percutaneous
    endoscopic g.
  DePage-Janeway g.
  dual percutaneous endoscopic g.
    (DPEG)
  endoscopic g.
  g. feeding
  feeding g.
  Glassman g.

Janeway g.
jejunal tube through percutaneous
  endoscopic g. (JETPEG)
Kader g.
Martin g.
Marwedel g.
Olympus g.
percutaneous g. (PG)
percutaneous endoscopic g. (PEG)
plug g.
Russell percutaneous endoscopic g.
g. scarring
Ssabanejew-Frank g.
Stamm g.
Surgitek One-Step percutaneous
  endoscopic g.
g. tube
g. tube migration
ultrasound-assisted percutaneous
  endoscopic g.
venting percutaneous g. (VPG)
Witzel g.
gastrosuccorrhea
  digestive g.
  g. mucosa
gastrotome
gastrotomy
gastrotonometer
gastrotonometry
gastrotoxic
gastrotoxin
gastrotropic
Gastrovist contrast medium
gastroxia
gastroxynsis fungosa
Gastrozepine
Gas-X
gate
  sampling g.
gatekeeper gene
Gates
  method of G.
Gatta prognostic system
Gaucher
  G. cell
  G. disease
  G. splenomegaly
Gauderer-Ponsky PEG operation
Gauder Silicon PEG catheter
Gau gastric balloon
gauge
  Chatillon Digital Force g.

G

NOTES

gauge *(continued)*
    Dacomed snap g.
    intraabdominal pressure g.
    LeVeen inflator with pressure g.
    snap g.
    Statham P23 strain g.
Gaur balloon distension technique
Gauthier classification for extrahepatic bile duct atresia
Gautier ureteroscope
gauze
    g. dressing
    Iodoform g.
    g. pack
    g. sponge
    Surgicel g.
    Vaseline g.
    Xeroform g.
gavage
    1090 G. Bag
    g. feeding
Gavard muscle
GAVE
    gastric antral vascular ectasia
    GAVE syndrome
Gavin-Miller intestinal forceps
Gaviscon
Gaviscon-2
GAX
    glutaraldehyde cross-linked collagen
GAX-collagen
gay bowel syndrome
Gaymar water-circulating blanket
Gazayerli
    G. endoscopic retractor
    G. knot pusher
GB
    gallbladder
    GB virus C/hepatitis G virus (GBV-C/HGV)
    GB vol+ fluctuation
GBC-590
GBEF
    gallbladder ejection fraction
GBER
    gallbladder ejection rate
GBM
    glomerular basement membrane
    GBM collagen fiber
    perimesangial GBM
    GBM polyanion
GBO
    gastric bacterial overgrowth
GBP
    gastric bypass
GBS
    gallbladder series
    group B streptococcus

GBT
    gastric bleeding time
GBV-C/HGV
    GB virus C/hepatitis G virus
GBV-C/HGV-RNA
    hepatitis G-RNA
GC
    gonococcus
    granular cast
GC-16
    Surgitek graduated cystocope G.
GCD
    giant colonic diverticulum
G-cell
    G.-c. gastrin release
    G.-c. hyperplasia
GC/MS
    gas chromatography/mass spectroscopy
G-CSF
GCT
    giant cell transformation
    granular cell tumor
GCW
    glomerular capillary wall
GDA
    gastroduodenal artery
    GDA aneurysm
G:D-cell ratio
Gd-EOB-DTPA
    gadolinium EOB-DTPA
GDNF
    glial cell line-derived neurotrophic factor
    glial-derived neurotrophic factor
GDSS
    Glasgow Dyspepsia Severity Score
GE
    gastric emptying
    gastroenterostomy
    gastroesophageal
    GE junction
    GE reflux
    GE RT 3200 Advantage II
GEA
    gastroepiploic artery
    GEA graft
GEC
    galactose elimination capacity
Gee disease
Gee-Herter disease
Gee-Herter-Heubner
    G.-H.-H. disease
    G.-H.-H. syndrome
Gee-Thaysen disease
GEG
    Garren-Edwards gastric
    GEG bubble
gel
    agar g.

agarose g.
Betadine g.
chondrocyte-alginate g.
Contractubex g.
deletion and mutation detection
  enhancement g.
dihydrotestosterone g.
g. filtration chromatography
ILE-SORB absorbent g.
IntraDose g.
percutaneous testosterone g.
polyacrylamide g.
Sephacryl S-300 HR g.
Simaal G.
Simaal G. 2
viscoelastic g.

Gelamal
gelatin
g. Hank buffered salt solution
  (GHBSS)
g. resorcinol and formaldehyde
  (GRF)
g. sponge
g. sponge packing

gelatinous
g. ascites
g. nodule

gelatin-subbed slide
GELdose
Zantac G.

Gelfoam
G. cube
G. embolization
G. particles transarterial
  embolization treatment

Gellhorn pessary
Gelpi self-retaining retractor
gelsolin
recombinant human g.

Gelusil
open-label G.

Gelusil-II
Gelusil-M
gemcitabine HCl
Gemella
gemfibrozil
gemifloxacin
Gemini
G. gall duct forceps
G. paired wire helical basket

Gemzar

gender
g. effect
g. reassignment

gene
g. A
adenomatous polyposis coli g.
ADPKD1 g.
alpha g.
angiotensin-converting enzyme g.
APC tumor suppressor g.
APOB g.
apolipoprotein B g.
ATP7A g.
break cluster homology g.
cagA g.
caretaker g.
g. carrier
C-beta g.
c-Ha-ras g.
G. Clean II kit
COL4A3 g.
COL4A4 g.
COL4A5 g.
DAZ g.
DCC g.
deleted in colon carcinoma g.
DRB g.
Fas g.
FCC-COCA1 g.
fucosyltransferase g.
gastrin g.
gatekeeper g.
HDA-DR3 g.
HFE g.
HLA class II g.
HLA-DQw2 g.
HLA-DR3 g.
hMLH1 g.
human kidney chloride channel g.
immunogenic g.
KAL1 g.
kallikrein-like g.
K-*ras* g.
Ki-*ras* g.
g. linkage
LMP g.
MCC g.
MCH g.
MDM2 g.
MDR1 g.
Menkes disease g.
metastasis g.

NOTES

gene *(continued)*
    MLH1 g.
    MSH2 g.
    MTS1 g.
    MTS2 g.
    MUC-1 g.
    multidrug-resistance g.
    MutL g.
    MutS g.
    NM23 g.
    OB g.
    p53 g.
    p15 g.
    P15/INK4B g.
    p16 g.
    p18 g.
    P21/WAF1 g.
    P27Kip1 g.
    PAX2 g.
    PAX8 g.
    PKD1, PKD2 g.
    polymorphic g.
    prodynorphin g.
    proenkephalin g.
    proopiomelanocortin g.
    Rb g.
    G. Screen nylon membrane filter
    serine threonine kinase g. 11
      (*STK11*)
    SRY g.
    STK11 g.
    suppressor g.
    TAP g.
    TAP2 peptide transporter g.
    TGF-beta-1 g.
    g. therapy
    TNF-alpha g.
    TP40 g.
    TP53 g.
    tumor suppressor g.
    uromodulin g.
    V-alpha g.
    V-beta g.
    VHL g.
    von Hippel Lindau g.
    WTI g.
gene-blotting study
gene-linkage analysis (GLA)
general
    g. anesthesia
    g. endotracheal anesthesia (GETA)
    g. peptic ulcer
generalized
    g. elastolysis
    g. glycogenosis
    g. nephrographic (GNG)
    g. peritonitis

generation
    anti-HCV antibody 3rd g.
    Chiron RIBA HCV test system
      second g.
    interdialytic urea g.
    Ortho HCV ELISA test system
      second g.
generator
    banana plug dipolar g.
    electrohydraulic g.
    electrosurgical g.
    Endostat II bipolar/monopolar
      electrosurgical g.
    implantable pulse g. (IPG)
    isolated g.
    Itrel pulse g.
    Medstone STS shock-wave g.
    microexplosive g.
    Northgate SD-100 EHL g.
    piezoelectric g.
    spark-gap shock wave g.
    Symmetry endo-bipolar g.
    Valleylab SSE2L g.
genetic
    g. alteration
    g. code
    g. hemochromatosis (GH)
    g. heterogeneity
    g. marker
    g. predisposition
    g. susceptibility
    G.'s Systems microplate reader
      spectrophotometer
gene-transfer therapy
geniohyoid muscle
genistein
genital
    g. burn
    g. cord
    g. cryptococcosis
    g. differentiation
    g. dysplasia
    g. elephantiasis
    g. end bulb
    g. human papillomavirus
    g. mesonephros
    g. rash
    g. reconstruction
    g. scabies
    g. swelling
    g. tract
    g. tuberculosis
    g. ulcer
    g. wart
genitalia
    adolescent g.
    ambiguous external g.
    anomalous g.

genitocerebral evoked potential study
genitocrural
genitofemoral nerve
genitography
    retrograde g.
genitoinfectious
genitomesenteric band
genitoplasty
    fcminizing g.
    masculinizing g.
genitourinary
    g. carcinoma
    g. fistula
    g. neoplasm
    g. prolapse
    g. region
    g. surgeon
    g. tract
    g. tuberculosis
genodermatosis
genome
    full-length viral g.
    retroviral g.
genome/ml
genomic
    g. deoxyribonucleic acid
    g. DNA
    g. DNA probe
    g. imprinting
    g. instability
    g. sequence
    g. site
genotoxic
genotype
    ADPKD1 g.
    ADPKD2 g.
    hepatitis C virus g.
    g. III 2a
    g. II, III
    g. IV 2b
    g. V 3
Genta
    G. method
    G. stain
Gentafair
Gentamar
gentamicin sulfate
gentian violet
gentle
    G. Nature
    G. Touch colostomy appliance

genuine
    g. stress incontinence (GSI)
    g. stress urinary incontinence
    (GSUI)
genu of pancreatic duct
Geocillin
geographic
    g. distribution
    g. tongue
    g. variance
Geopen
geophagia, geophagism, geophagy
geotrichosis
Geotrichum candidum
GEP
    gastroenteropancreatic
GER
    gastroesophageal reflux
Gerald forceps
GERD
    gastroesophageal reflux disease
    Los Angeles classification of
    GERD
    RS associated with GERD
Gerhardt
    G. table
    G. test
geriatric
    g. constipation
    g. incontinence
    g. incontinence evaluation
    g. urinary tract infection
    g. urology
    g. voiding dysfunction
geriatrics
Geridium
Geriplex-FS
Gerlach valve
germ
    g. cell carcinoma
    g. cell hypoplasia
    g. cell neoplasm
    g. cell tumor
    g. layer
germander
germicide
    liquid chemical g. (LCG)
germinal
    g. center formation
    g. epithelium
germinomatous
germline mutation

G

NOTES

Gerota
　　G. capsule
　　G. fascia
gestation
　　ectopic g.
gestational
　　g. diabetes
　　g. thyrotoxicosis
　　g. trophoblastic tumor (GTT)
GET
　　gastric emptying time
GET1/2
　　gastric emptying half-time
GETA
　　general endotracheal anesthesia
GFC gastroscope
GFD
　　gluten-free diet
GFPM
　　gastric first-pass metabolism of ethanol
GFR
　　glomerular filtration rate
　　　　AmB-induced reduction GFR
　　　　amphotericin B-induced reduction
　　　　　　glomerular filtration rate
　　　　single-nephron GFR
GFS Mark II inflatable penile prosthesis
GFT Olympus gastroscope
GF-UM20
GF-UM30P linear-oriented radial scanning echoendoscope
GG
　　Lactobacillus GG (LGG)
GGT
　　gamma-glutamyl transferase
　　GGT test
GGTP
　　gamma-glutamyl transpeptidase
　　GGTP liver function test
GGU
　　giant gastric ulcer
GH
　　genetic hemochromatosis
GHBSS
　　gelatin Hank buffered salt solution
Ghedini-Weinberg serologic test
GHP
　　^{99m}Tc GHP
GI
　　gastrointestinal
　　Gingival Index
　　GI bleeding scan
　　GI cancer
　　GI cocktail
　　GI electrophysiology
　　Imagent GI

GI tract
GI tract flora
GIA
　　GIA autosuture apparatus
　　GIA autosuture device
　　GIA instrument
　　GIA stapler
Gianotti-Crosti syndrome
giant
　　g. anorectal condyloma acuminatum
　　g. cell
　　g. cell adenocarcinoma
　　g. cell hepatitis
　　g. cell transformation (GCT)
　　g. colon
　　g. colonic diverticulum (GCD)
　　g. diverticulosis
　　g. diverticulum
　　g. fibrous mesothelioma
　　g. gastric fold
　　g. gastric ulcer (GGU)
　　g. hypertrophic gastritis
　　g. intestinal fluke
　　g. migrating contraction (GMC)
　　g. mitochondria
　　g. molluscum contagiosum
　　g. peptic ulcer
Gianturco
　　G. coil
　　G. expandable (self-expanding) metallic biliary prosthesis
　　G. expandable (self-expanding) metallic biliary stent
　　G. metal urethral stent
　　G. Z-stent
Gianturco-Rosch
　　G.-R. biliary Z-stent
　　G.-R. self-expandable Z-stent stent
Gianturco-Roubin flexible coil stent
Gianturco-Z stent
Giardia
　　G. *duodenalis*
　　G. *intestinalis*
　　G. *lamblia*
giardiasis dysentery
GIB
　　gastrointestinal bleeding
Gibbon
　　G. hernia
　　G. hydrocele
　　G. indwelling ureteral stent
Gibbs-Donnan equilibrium
Gibson
　　G. excision
　　G. incision
Gibson-Balfour abdominal retractor
GICA
　　gastrointestinal cancer-associated antigen

Giemsa
- G. method
- G. stain

Giemsa-stained section

Gierke disease

GIF
- GIF N30 fiberoptic pediatric endoscope
- GIF XP20 endoscope
- GIF XQ10 upper endoscope

GIF-HM fiberscope

GIFT
- gamete intrafallopian transfer

GIF1T130
- Olympus large-channel endoscope GIF1T130

gigantica
- *Fasciola g.*

Gigasept

Gilbert
- G. cholemia
- G. cystic duct forceps
- G. disease
- G. sign
- G. syndrome

Gilbert-Behçet syndrome

Gilbert-Dreyfus syndrome

Gilchrist
- G. ileocecal bladder
- G. procedure

Gill renal tourniquet

Gilman-Abrams gastric tube

Gil-Vernet
- G.-V. dorsal lumbotomy incision
- G.-V. extended pyelolithotomy
- G.-V. ileocecal cystoplasty
- G.-V. ileocecal cystoplasty urinary diversion
- G.-V. operation
- G.-V. orthotopic urinary diversion
- G.-V. position
- G.-V. procedure
- G.-V. retractor
- G.-V. technique

ginger root

gingival
- G. Index (GI)
- g. papilloma

gingivostomatitis
- herpetic g.

ginkgo

ginseng

Giordano-Giovannetti diet

Giordano sphincter

GIP
- gastric inhibitory peptide
- gastric inhibitory polypeptide
- gastrointestinal polyposis
- 10-cm needle GIP

GIP/Med-Globe needle

Giraldes
- organ of G.

girdle
- Neptune g.
- shoulder g.

Gironcoli hernia

girth
- abdominal g.

GIS
- gastrointestinal system

GIT
- gastrointestinal tract

Gitelman syndrome

GITS
- gastrointestinal therapeutic system

GITSG
- Gastrointestinal Tumor Study Group

Gittes
- G. bladder neck suspension
- G. needle
- G. technique
- G. urethral suspension procedure
- G. urethropexy

Gittes-Loughlin
- G.-L. bladder neck suspension
- G.-L. procedure

GL
- glucagon

GLA
- gene-linkage analysis

glabella reflex

glabrata
- *Candida g.*
- *Torulopsis g.*

glabrous cirrhosis

Glahn test

gland
- accessory sex g.
- adrenal g.
- Albarran g.
- anal intramuscular g.
- Bartholin g.
- Brunner g.
- bulbourethral g.

NOTES

G

gland *(continued)*
    cardiac-type g.
    Cowper g.
    esophageal ectopic sebaceous g.
    Galeati g.
    gastric g.
    hilum of suprarenal g.
    Home g.
    Lieberkühn g.
    Littré g.
    Luschka cystic g.
    medulla of suprarenal g.
    metaplastic gastric fundic g.
    middle g.
    misplaced g.
    mucous g.
    mucus-secreting g.
    oxyntic g.
    paraurethral g.
    periductal g.
    periurethral g.
    preputial g.
    pyloric g.
    Skene g.
    suprarenal g.
    trapped prostate g.
    urethral g.
    vestibular g.
    Von Ebner g.
glandis
    collum g.
glandula, pl. **glandulae**
glandular
    g. cystitis
    g. metaplasia
    g. structure
glandularis
    cystitis g.
    pyelitis g.
    ureteritis g.
    urethritis g.
glandule
glandulectomy
glandulopexy
glandulous
glans
    g. approximation procedure (GAP)
    conical g.
    g. hyperemia
    g. penis
    g. penis papilla
glansplasty
    meatal advancement and g.
    (MAGPI)
glanular hypospadias
glanuloplasty
Glasgow
    G. coma scale

    G. criteria for severity of
    pancreatitis
    G. Dyspepsia Severity Score
    (GDSS)
glass
    g. penile prosthesis
    g. pH electrode
    g. pH-electrodes - MIC
Glasser gastrostomy tube
Glassman
    G. basket
    G. brush
    G. gastrostomy
    G. noncrushing gastrointestinal
    clamp
    G. stone extractor
Glassman-Allis intestinal forceps
Glaxo stain
Glazyme APF-EIA-TEST test
GLDH
    glutamate dehydrogenase
Gleason
    G. cancer grade
    G. grading system
    G. score
gleet
gleety
Glenard
    G. disease
    G. syndrome
Glenn
    G. diverticulum forceps
    G. technique
Glenn-Anderson
    G.-A. advancement
    G.-A. technique
    G.-A. ureteroneocystostomy
gliadin
    g. ELISA
    g. IgA
gliadin-specific T-cell clone
glial cell line-derived neurotrophic factor (GDNF)
glial-derived neurotrophic factor (GDNF)
glibornuride
gliclazide
Glidewire
    angle-tip G.
    G. Gold surgical guidewire
    Terumo G.
glide wire
Glidex coated Percuflex catheter
glimepiride
glioblastoma multiforme
glioma-polyposis syndrome
glipizide
glischruria

Glisson
    G. capsule
    G. cirrhosis
    G. sphincter
glissonitis
glitter cell
GLMA
    gastric laryngeal mask airway
global sclerosis
globi (*pl. of* globus)
globoside
globular
    g. albuminuria
    g. hyalin
    g. proteinuria
globulin
    alpha-2 g.
    alpha-1-antitrypsin g.
    antilymphocyte g.
    antithymocyte g. (ATG)
    Bence Jones g.
    cytomegalovirus immune g.
    g. fraction
    gamma g.
    hepatitis B hyperimmune g.
    human hepatitis B immune g.
    immune serum g.
    Minnesota antilymphocyte g.
    prophylactic gamma g.
    sex hormone binding g. (SHBG)
    testosterone-binding g.
    testosterone-estrogen-binding g.
    tetanus g.
    thyroxine-binding g.
globulinuria
globus, pl. **globi**
    esophageal g.
    g. hystericus
    g. major
    g. major epididymidis
    g. minor
    g. minor epididymidis
glomerular
    g. arteriole
    g. basement membrane (GBM)
    g. basement membrane disease
    g. capillary
    g. capillary hypertension
    g. capillary pressure
    g. capillary wall (GCW)
    g. cell culture
    g. cell proliferation

    g. contractile cell
    g. crescent
    g. cyst
    g. endothelial myxovirus-like microtubular inclusion
    g. endotheliosis
    g. epithelial cell
    g. epithelial cell toxin puromycin aminonucleoside
    g. extracellular matrix
    g. fibronectin mRNA
    g. filtration
    g. filtration rate (GFR)
    g. hematuria
    g. hypercellularity
    g. hyperfiltration
    g. hypertrophy
    g. injury
    g. ischemia
    g. macrophage infiltration
    g. mesangium
    g. metabolism
    g. microvascular thrombosis
    g. morphology
    g. necrosis
    g. neutrophil infiltration
    g. podocyte
    g. proteinuria
    g. sclerosis
    g. tip lesion (GTL)
    g. tuft
    g. ultrafiltrate
    g. ultrafiltration
    g. ultrafiltration coefficient
glomerulation
glomeruli (*pl. of* glomerulus)
glomerulitis
glomerulocapillary
glomerulocapsular nephritis
glomerulocystic kidney disease
glomerulonephritis,
    pl. **glomerulonephritides (GN)**
        acute g. (AGN)
        acute mesangial proliferative g.
        acute poststreptococcal g. (APSGN)
        anti-GBM g.
        antiglomerular basement membrane g.
        antithymocyte antibody-induced g.
        biopsy-verified chronic g.
        chronic g. (CG, CGN)
        chronic membranous g. (CMGN)

G

NOTES

glomerulonephritis *(continued)*
    chronic renal failure g.
    complement-mediated
      experimental g.
    crescentic g.
    diffuse proliferative g.
    Ellis types 1, 2 g.
    fibrillary g.
    focal necrotizing g.
    focal proliferative g.
    idiopathic crescentic g.
    idiopathic membranous g.
    idiopathic rapidly progressive g.
      (IRPGN)
    IgA g.
    immune complex g. (IC-GN)
    immunotactoid g.
    membranoproliferative g. (type I,
      II) (MPGN)
    membranous g. (MGN)
    mesangiocapillary g.
    mesangioproliferative g.
    necrotizing crescentic g. (NCGN)
    pauciimmune antineutrophil
      cytoplasmic antibody-associated g.
    pauciimmune crescentic g.
    postinfectious g.
    poststreptococcal g. (PSGN)
    poststreptococcal acute g.
    proliferative g.
    rapidly progressive g. (RPGN)
    recurrent focal sclerosing g.
    tropical mesangiocapillary g.
    type I mesangiocapillary g.
glomerulopathy
    Adriamycin g.
    amyloid-like g.
    collagenofibrotic g.
    collapsing g.
    immunotactoid g. (ITGP)
    inflammatory g.
    lipoprotein g.
    nonamyloid g.
    proteinuric g.
    toxic g.
glomerulosa
    zona g.
glomerulosclerosis
    diffuse diabetic g.
    focal segmental g. (FSGS)
    segmental g.
glomerulose
glomerulotubular balance
glomerulus, pl. **glomeruli**
    amyloidotic g.
    atubular g.
    capsula g.
    human g.

    kidney g.
    malpighian g.
    obsolescent g.
    renal g.
    Ruysch g.
    vas afferens glomeruli
    vas efferens glomeruli
glomus tumor
glossitis
    Rider-Moeller g.
glossodynia
Glo-tip biliary catheter
glottic
    g. gap
    g. spasm
glove
    SensiCare synthetic powder-free
      surgical g.
    Tactyl 1 g.
GLPT
    glutamate pyruvate transaminase
glucagon (GL)
    g. precipitation
    g. stain
glucagon-evoked gastric dysrhythmia
glucagonoma syndrome
glucocerebrosidase
glucocorticoid
    g. response element (GRE)
    g. treatment
glucocorticoid-induced
    g.-i. hypercalcemia
    g.-i. hypercalcemic nephrolithiasis
gluconate
    calcium g.
    iron g.
    quinidine g.
gluconeogenesis
gluconeogenesis-associated enzyme
**gluconeogenic-competent human
    proximal tubule cell**
gluconeogenic pathway
glucoreceptor
glucose
    G. analyzer II test
    CSF g.
    g. excretion
    filtered g.
    g. intolerance
    luminal g.
    g. test
    g. tolerance
    g. transport
    g. transporter
    g. uptake
    urinary g.
glucose-6-phosphatase deficiency
glucose-6-phosphate isomerase

glucose-dependent insulinotropic peptide
glucose-galactose malabsorption
glucosuria
  renal g.
Glucotrol
glucuronate
  trimetrexate g.
glucuronidase
glucuronidation
glucuronide
glucuronosyltransferase
  uridine diphosphate g. (UDPGT)
glucuronyl
  g. transferase
  g. transferase deficiency
glue
  cyanoacrylate g.
  fibrin g.
  hemostatic surgical g.
  tissue g.
glutamate
  g. dehydrogenase (GLDH)
  g. pyruvate transaminase (GLPT)
glutamic
  g. acid
  g. acid hydrochloride
glutamic-oxaloacetic transaminase (GOT)
glutamic-pyruvic transaminase (GPT)
glutaminase
  mitochondrial phosphate-
    dependent g.
  phosphate-dependent g. (PDG)
  phosphate-independent g. (PIG)
glutamine
  g. aminotransferase pathway
  CSF g.
  g. nitrogen
  g. test
glutamyl transpeptidase (GTP)
glutaral
glutaraldehyde
  activated alkaline g.
  g. alarm
  g. cross-linked collagen (GAX)
  g. cross-linked collagen injection
glutaraldehyde-induced proctitis
glutathione (GSH)
  g. metabolism
  g. peroxidase
  g. redox cycle
  g. S-transferase (GST)
  g. S-transferase M1

  g. S-transferase pi
  g. transferase
gluteal
  g. artery
  g. fold
  g. nerve
gluten
  g. challenge
  dietary g.
  g. sensitivity
  g. solution
  wheat g.
gluten-dependent population
gluten-free diet (GFD)
gluten-rich diet
gluten-sensitive
  g.-s. diarrhea
  g.-s. enteropathy (GSE)
gluteus
  g. maximus
  g. maximus transposition
Gluzinski test
glyburide
glycated albumin
glyceraldehyde-3-phosphate
  dehydrogenase (GAPDH)
glyceraldehyde phosphate dehydrogenase
  (GAPD)
glycerin
  g. enema
  g. suppository
glycerol
Glycerol-T
glycerylphosphorylcholine
  alpha g.
glyceryl trinitrate (GTN)
glycine
glycocalyx
  podocyte g.
glycochenodeoxycholate
glycogen
  g. inclusion
  g. nephrosis
  g. phosphorylase
  g. storage disease
glycogenic acanthosis
glycogenosis
  brancher deficiency g.
  generalized g.
  hepatophosphorylase deficiency g.
  hepatorenal g.
  type III g.

G

NOTES

glycogen-rich cystadenoma
glycol
    ethylene g.
    polyethylene g. (PEG)
    polyethylene g. 600
glycolate
glycolipid
    mucin-type g.
glycolysis
    aerobic g.
    anaerobic g.
glycolytic
    g. enzyme
    g. inhibition
glycoprotein
    g. accumulation
    acidic epididymal g.
    alpha-1-acid g.
    dimeric acidic g. (DAG)
    heterodimeric g.
    microfil-associated g. (MAGP)
    N-linked g.
    TAG-72 g.
glycoprotein-2
    sulfated g. (SGP-2)
glycoprotein-producing tumor
glycopyrrolate test
glycosaminoglycan (GAG)
    g. heparin
    g. layer
    g. uronate (GAGUA)
glycosaminoglycan-degrading enzyme
glycosidase
glycoside
    anthracene g.
    cardiac g.
glycosphingolipid
glycosuria
    alimentary g.
    digestive g.
glycosylation
    g. of EPO
    nonenzymatic g.
    g. process
glycosyltransferase
glycyl prolinuria
glycyltryptophan test
glycyrrhetinic acid like factor (GALF)
glycyrrhiza
    syrup of g.
Glynazan
glyoxylate
Glypressin
GM3 ganglioside
GMC
    giant migrating contraction

GM-CSF
    granulocyte-macrophage colony-
      stimulating factor
      GM-CSF cytokine
Gmelin test
GMER
    gastric mucosal ectopia in rectum
GMP
    guanosine 5′-monophosphate
GMS
    Galloway-Mowat syndrome
GN
    glomerulonephritis
gnawing pain
GNG
    generalized nephrographic
      GNG phase imaging
GNRF
    guanine nucleotide-releasing factor
GnRH
    gonadotropin-releasing hormone
goat antirabbit HRP conjugate
goblet
    g. cell
    g. cell hyperplasia
    g. cell metaplasia
Goelet retractor
goiter
    nontoxic g.
gold
    cationic colloidal g. (CCG)
    g. compound
    7C G. urine test
    G. deep surgery forceps
    g. nephropathy
    G. probe
    G. Probe Direct bipolar hemostasis
      catheter
    G. probe electrocoagulation
    G. Probe electrohemostasis catheter
    g. salt
    g. seed implant
    g. seed implantation technique
gold-198 (^{198}Au)
Goldberg Anorectic Attitude scale
Goldblatt
    G. clamp
    G. hypertension
    G. kidney
    G. phenomenon
Goldenhar syndrome
Goldman classification of operative risk
Goldschmiedt technique
Goldstein
    G. disease
    G. hematemesis
    G. Microspike approximator clamp
Goldston syndrome

Goldwasser suture carrier
golf-hole configuration
Golgi
    G. apparatus
    G. complex
Goligher
    G. extraperitoneal ileostomy
    G. modification
    G. retractor
GoLYTELY
    G. bowel preparation
    G. solution
Gomco
    G. suction
    G. suction tube
    G. umbilical clamp
Gomez
    G. fundoplasty
    G. horizontal gastroplasty
    G. horizontal gastroplasty with
      reinforced stoma
Gompertzian tumor kinetics
gonad
    dysgenetic g.
    intersex g.
    streak g.
    vanishing g.
gonadal
    g. artery
    g. differentiation
    g. dysgenesis
    g. ligament
    g. vein
    g. vein valve
    g. vessel
gonadectomize
gonadectomy
gonadial
gonadoblastoma
gonadoblastoma
gonadocytoma
gonadoliberin
gonadopathy
gonadotherapy
gonadotoxic
gonadotoxicity
    chemotherapy g.
gonadotroph
gonadotrophin
gonadotropin
    human chorionic g. (HCG)
    human menopausal g.

gonadotropin-releasing
    g.-r. hormone (GnRH)
    g.-r. hormone deficiency
    g.-r. hormone pulsatile secretion
    g.-r. hormone test
gonaduct
Gonal-F
gonangiectomy
gondii
    Toxoplasma g.
gonecyst
gonecystic calculus
gonecystis
gonecystitis
gonecystolith
gonecystopyosis
gonococcal
    g. perihepatis pelvic inflammatory
      disease
    g. proctitis
    g. urethritis (GU)
gonococcus (GC)
gonocyte
    seminiferous tubule g.
gononephrotome
gonophore
gonorrhea
    rectal g.
gonorrheal
    g. bubo
    g. proctitis
    g. urethritis
gonorrhoeae
    Neisseria g.
GOO
    gastric outlet obstruction
goodness-of-fit testing
Goodpasture
    G. disease
    G. epitope
    G. reactivity
    G. syndrome
good performance unit
Goodsall rule
Goodwin
    G. cup-patch principle
    G. technique
    G. technique ureterocolonic
      anastomosis
Goodwin-Hohenfellner technique
Goodwin-Scott technique
Gopalan syndrome

G

NOTES

GOR
 antibody to G. (anti-GOR)
Gordon
 G. disease
 G. syndrome
gordonae
 Mycobacterium g.
Gore-Tex
 G.-T. catheter
 G.-T. graft
 G.-T. sling reinforcement
 G.-T. soft tissue patch
 G.-T. strip
gorge
gorget
 probe g.
 Teale g.
Gorlin
 G. basal cell nevus syndrome
Gorlin-Chaudhry-Moss syndrome
goserelin acetate
Gosset appendectomy retractor
GOT
 glutamic-oxaloacetic transaminase
Gothic arch formation
Gott
 G. shunt
 G. tube
Gottron sign
gouge
 Capener g.
Gould
 G. inverted mattress suture
 G. polygraph gastric motility
  measuring device
 G. pressure monitor
 G. pressure transducer
Goulding procedure
Gouley catheter
gout
gouty
 g. kidney
 g. proteinuria
 g. urethritis
 g. urine
Gowers
 G. attack
 G. sign
 G. syndrome
Goyrand hernia
GP
 gastroplasty
gp330 receptor
G3PDH
 G3PDH CDNA probe
 G3PDH mRNA species
GPL unit

GPT
 glutamic-pyruvic transaminase
GR
 gastric resection
Grabstald (Memorial) staging system
gracilis
 g. muscle
 g. muscle flap
 g. musculocutaneous unit
 g. myocutaneous neovagina
 g. neosphincter
graciloplasty
 direct nerve stimulation g.
 dynamic urinary g. (DUG)
 intramuscular perineural
  stimulation g.
 stimulated g.
grade
 g. 4 cystocele
 Edmondson g. (EdGr)
 Gleason cancer g.
 hemorrhoid g.
 Hetzel-Dent esophagitis g.
 Matts g. (1–4)
 M.D. Anderson g.
 mucosal PMN g.
 Roenigk g.
 Savary-Miller II g.
 tumor g.
graded
 g. alcohol
 g. esophageal balloon distention
  test
gradient
 A-a g.
 acinar g.
 albumin g.
 biliary-duodenal pressure g.
 duodenobiliary pressure g.
 g. echo
 hepatic venous pressure g. (HVPG)
 serum-ascites albumin g. (SAAG)
 transcapillary hydrostatic pressure g.
 transmural hydrostatic pressure g.
gradient-recalled acquisition in a steady state (GRASS)
grading
 histologic g.
 tumor g.
graft
 aortic g.
 aortoenteric g.
 aortohepatic arterial g.
 aortorenal bypass g.
 g. atherosclerosis
 autogenous tunica vaginalis g.
 g. bed

biologic collagen-based tissue-matrix g.
bladder mucosal g.
bovine g.
branched vascular g.
buccal mucosal patch g.
bypass g.
C g.
cadaveric segmental g.
Dacron interposition g.
Diastat vascular access g.
dorsal vein patch g.
free jejunal g.
full-thickness g.
g. function
gastroduodenal-to-renal artery bypass g.
GEA g.
Gore-Tex g.
hepatic-to-renal artery saphenous vein bypass g.
HLA identical kidney g.
Horton-Devine dermal g.
iliac-to-renal artery bypass g.
Impra g.
interposition Dacron g.
live-donor segmental g.
loop forearm g.
g. loss
Marlex g.
Martius g.
meshed g.
mucosal g.
omental pedicle flap g.
patch g.
pedicle g.
pedicled omental g.
g. placement
portacaval H g.
postauricular Wolfe g.
prosthetic arterial g.
reduced-size g.
renal artery g.
segmental liver g.
seromuscular intestinal patch g.
skin g.
g. spatulation
splenorenal bypass g.
split-thickness skin g.
superior mesenteric-to renal artery saphenous vein bypass g.
sural nerve g.

g. survival
synthetic vascular g.
Thiersch g.
Thiersch-Duplay tube g.
tube g.
tubed free skin g.
vascular access g. (VAG)
Vectra hemodialysis access g.
V-Y sliding skin g.
Y-V sliding skin g.

graft-enteric fistula
grafting
  endovascular stent g.
graft-versus-host disease (GVHD)
Graham
  G. catheter
  G. closure
  G. closure with omental pouch
  G. deep surgery scissors
  G. plication
  G. scale for drug-induced gastric damage
  G. test
Gram
  G. stain
  G. stain of stool
  G. stain of stool test
gram-negative
  g.-n. bacterium
  g.-n. rod
  g.-n. sepsis
gram-positive
  g.-p. bacterium
  g.-p. organism
  g.-p. sepsis
Gram-stain morphology
granddaughter cyst
granisetron
granny knot
Grant gallbladder retractor
granular
  g. cast (GC)
  g. cell myoblastoma
  g. cell tumor (GCT)
  g. induration
  g. kidney
granularity
granulation
  healing by g.
granule
  acidophilic PAS-positive g.
  carcinoid secretory g.

G

NOTES

granule *(continued)*
    DiPAS-positive g.
    Fordyce g.
    hemosiderin g.
    Kretz g.
    perichromatin g.
    Weibel-Palade g.
    zymogen g.
granulocyte
    g. count
    g. exocytosis
granulocyte-macrophage colony-stimulating factor (GM-CSF)
granulocytic
    g. sarcoma
    g. sarcoma of stomach
granulocytopenia
granuloma
    amebic g.
    barium g.
    caseating g.
    eosinophilic g.
    epithelioid g.
    gastrointestinal eosinophilic g.
    hepatic g.
    g. inguinale
    noncaseating tubercle-like g.
    nonnecrotizing g.
    plasma cell g.
    portal zone g.
    pulmonary g.
    pyogenic g.
    sperm g.
    stone g.
    suture g.
    umbilical g.
granulomatis
    Calymmatobacterium g.
granulomatosa
    Miescher cheilitis g.
granulomatosis
    lipophagia g.
    lipophagic intestinal g.
    Wegener g.
granulomatous
    g. bowel disease
    g. cheilitis
    g. cholangitis
    g. enteritis
    g. enterocolitis
    g. gastritis
    g. hepatitis
    g. ileitis
    g. peritonitis
    g. prostatitis
    g. transmural colitis
granulosa
    appendicitis g.

    g. cell tumor
    urethritis g.
granulosa-theca cell tumor
granulosus
    Echinococcus g.
granzyme B
grapefruit diet
grapelike cyst
Graser diverticulum
grasp
    g. biopsy
    palmar g.
    plantar g.
    g. tripod forceps
grasper
    Allis tooth g.
    atraumatic g.
    bowel g.
    four-pronged polyp g.
    laparoscopic g.
    Polaris g.
    polyp g.
    three-pronged g.
    traumatic locking g.
    tripod g.
    umbilical port g.
grasping forceps
GRASS
    gradient-recalled acquisition in a steady state
grass
    G. force displacement fluid collector
    G. Model SIU5A stimulation isolation unit
    G. Model S9 stimulator
Grassi
    G. nerve
    G. test
gravel
    coarse g.
Graves
    G. disease
    G. technique
gravidarum
    hyperemesis g.
    icterus g.
    nephritis g.
gravid uterus
gravimetric
    g. technique
    g. weighing
gravis
    colitis g.
    enteritis g.
    icterus g.
    myasthenia g.

gravity
    g. cavernosometry
    g. cystogram
    urinalysis specific g.
    g. urinary incontinence
    urinary specific g.
    urine specific g.
gravity-dependent drainage
gravity-induced erosion
Grawitz
    G. cachexia
    G. tumor
gray
    G. cystic duct forceps
    g. scale
    g. scale imaging
    g. scale sonography
    g. scale ultrasonography
    g. scale ultrasound
GRE
    glucocorticoid response element
great
    g. epiploon
    g. lacuna
    g. pancreatic artery
greater
    g. celandine
    g. curvature banded gastroplasty
    g. curvature of stomach
    g. curvature ulcer
    g. curve position
    g. omentum
    g. peritoneal sac
    g. sciatic foramen
greedy bowel
green
    G. cystic duct forceps
    indocyanine g.
    g. Mersilene suture
    g. sputum
    g. stool
Greenen
    G. Endotorque
    G. pancreatic stent
Greene retractor
Greenfield
    G. caval catheter
    G. filter
Greenville gastric bypass
Greenwald
    G. Control Tip cystoscopic
    electrode

    G. needle
    G. Roth Grip-Tip suture guide
    G. sound
Greer EZ Access drainage pouch
Gregoir-Lich procedure
Greishaber self-retaining retractor
Grey
    G. Turner disease
    G. Turner sign
    G. Turner sign of retroperitoneal
    hemorrhage
GRF
    gelatin resorcinol and formaldehyde
GRFoma
Grice suture needle
gridiron incision
Griess test
Griffen Roux-en-Y bypass
Griffith point
Grimelius
    G. silver stain
    G. staining
    G. technique
Grimelius-positive cell
grip
    hook g.
    power g.
    precision g.
    three-finger g.
    two-finger g.
Grip-Tip suture guide
griseofulvin
gritty tumor
G-RNA
    hepatitis G-RNA (GBV-C/HGV-RNA)
Grocco sign
Grocott methenamine silver stain
groin incision
Grondahl-Finney esophagogastroplasty
groove
    anal intersphincteric g.
    esophageal g.
    innominate g.
    intersphincteric g.
    Liebermeister g.
    oval-form colonic g.
    g. pancreatitis
    paracolic g.
    radial g.
    spindle colonic g.
grooved director

NOTES

G

grooving
transurethral g. of prostate
gross
g. deformity
G. disease
g. hematuria
G. test
ground-glass
g.-g. appearance
g.-g. body of Hadziyannis
g.-g. cell
group
ABH blood g.
ABO blood g.
Astra/Merck G.
Benelux Multicentre Trial Study G.
g. B streptococcus (GBS)
Canadian Urology Oncology G.
(CUOG)
cross-reactive g. (CREG)
g. C rotavirus
Eastern Cooperative Oncology G.
(ECOG)
Gastrointestinal Tumor Study G.
(GITSG, GTSG)
hydroxyl g.
International Germ Cell Cancer
Collaborative G. (IGCCCG)
Laparoscopic Colorectal Surgery G.
(LCSSG)
Leuprolide Depot Neoadjuvant
Prostate Cancer Study G.
Lewis blood g.
National Prostatic Cancer
Treatment G. (NPCTG)
National Wilms Tumor Study G.
(NWTSG)
phytyl g.
radical resection g.
growth
cancer cell g.
g. factor
g. factor beta
g. factor isoform
fungating g.
g. hormone deficiency
g. regulation
somatic g.
GRP
gastrin-releasing peptide
Gruber-Landzert fossa
Grüntzig, Gruentzig
G. balloon
G. balloon catheter
G. balloon dilation
G. dilator

Grynfeltt
G. hernia
G. triangle
GS
Gardner syndrome
GSA
technetium GSA
diethylenetriamine-pentaacetic
acid-galactosyl-human serum
albumin
GSE
gluten-sensitive enteropathy
G&S Electroejaculator
GSH
glutathione
GSH prodrug
GSI
genuine stress incontinence
GSRS
Gastrointestinal Symptom Rating Scale
GST
glutathione S-transferase
GSUI
genuine stress urinary incontinence
GTL
glomerular tip lesion
GTL-16 gastric carcinoma cell
GTN
glyceryl trinitrate
GTP
glutamyl transpeptidase
guanosine triphosphate
GTPase activating protein
GTP-dependent signaling protein
GTP-regulatory protein
GTSG
Gastrointestinal Tumor Study Group
GTT
gestational trophoblastic tumor
G-tube
button-type G-t.
Moss G-t.
GU
gonococcal urethritis
guaiac
bicolor g. (BG)
g. gum
g. test
guaiac-impregnated slide
guaiac-negative stool
guaiac-positive stool
guanabenz
guanadrel
guanethidine
parenteral g.
guanfacine
guanidine thiocyanate
guanidinium thiocyanate buffer

guanidino compound
guanine
    dihydroxypropoxymethyl g. (DHPG)
    g. nucleotide
    g. nucleotide-regulatory protein
    g. nucleotide-releasing factor
      (GNRF)
guanoclor
guanosine
    g. monophosphate
    g. 5'-monophosphate (GMP)
    g. monophosphate pathway
    g. triphosphate (GTP)
guanoxan
guanylate cyclase
guanylyl cyclase
guard
    mouth g.
guarding
    abdominal g.
    involuntary g.
    muscle g.
    g. reflex
    g. sign
    voluntary g.
guard-ring tocodynamometer
guar gum
gubernacular
    g. cord
    g. vein
gubernaculum
    chorda g.
Guenzberg test
Guerin
    valve of G.
guidance
    choledochoscopic g.
    endoscopic g.
    fluoroscopic g.
guide
    catheter g.
    Coons g.
    Greenwald Roth Grip-Tip suture g.
    Grip-Tip suture g.
    image g. (IG)
    J-wire g.
    light g. (LG)
    Lunderquist-Ring torque g.
    master image g.
    Roth Grip-Tip suture g.
    soft-tipped wire g.
    suture g.

    TFE-coated wire g.
    tracer Hybrid wire g.
guided
    g. percutaneous drainage
    g. transcutaneous biopsy
guided-needle aspiration cytology
guide-eye instrument
guideline
    Appropriate Use of Gastrointestinal
      Endoscopy g.
    string g.
guidewire (*See also* wire)
    Amplatz Super Stiff g.
    Bard Director g.
    Bentson floppy-tipped g.
    Bentson-type Glidewire g.
    cannula with preloaded 0.35-
      inch g.
    Eder-Puestow g.
    ERCP g.
    g. exchange
    FasTrac hydrophilic coated g.
    flexible-tip g.
    floppy-tipped g.
    Glidewire Gold surgical g.
    HPC g.
    hydrophilic-coated g.
    hydrophilic polymer-coated
      steerable g.
    Hydro Plus coated g.
    Jagwire g.
    Lumenator injectable g.
    Lumina g.
    Lunderquist g.
    Microvasive angled hydrophilic g.
    Microvasive Geenen Endotorque g.
    Microvasive Glidewire g.
    g. and mini-snare technique
    nonconductive g.
    olive over g.
    g. passage
    Pathfinder exchange g.
    Placer g.
    slipper-tipped g.
    g. sphincterotomy
    Teflon-coated g.
    Terumo hydrophilic g.
    Terumo/Meditech g.
    Terumo-Radiofocus hydrophilic
      polymer-coated g.
    Wilson-Cook Protector g.
    Wilson-Cook THSF-series g.

NOTES

G

guidewire *(continued)*
    Wilson-Cook Tracer g.
    Zebra exchange g.
guidewire/basket lasso
guiding catheter
Guillain-Barré syndrome
guillotine
    g. incision
    g. needle biopsy
gullet
Gull renal epistaxis
gum
    guaiac g.
    guar g.
    Karaya g.
gumma
gummatous necrosis
gummosa
    periarteritis g.
gun
    Bard Biopty g.
    biopsy g.
    Biopty g.
    Cobe staple g.
    Cook biopsy g.
    EEA stapler g.
    introducer g.
    Mentor g.
    modified caulking g.
    Moss T-anchor introducer g.
    spring-loaded biopsy g.
gun-barrel enterostomy
gunpowder lesion
gurgle
gurgling bowel sounds
Gussenbauer suture
gustatory
    g. hyperesthesia

    g. hypoesthesia
    g. sweating
gustatory-salivary reflex
gut
    artificial g.
    caffeine g.
    g. colonization
    congenital malrotation of the g.
    g. flora
    g. hormone
    nervous g.
    plain g.
    g. rest
gut-associated lymphoid tissue (GALT)
gut-hormone profile
gutter
    lateral g.
    left g.
    paracolic g.
    right g.
guttered T tube
Guyon
    G. sign
    G. sound
GVE
    gastric vascular ectasia
GVHD
    graft-versus-host disease
gynandroblastoma
gynecologic laparoscopy
gynecomastia
gynecomastia-aspermatogenesis syndrome
gynoblastoma
Gyrus
    G. bipolar electrode
    G. endourology system

H2
    histamine-2
        H2 blocker
        H2 breath test
        H2 receptor
        H2 receptor antagonist (H2RA)
        H2 receptor-blocker
        H2 receptor-blocking drug
H2-antagonist therapy
H2-receptor antagonist therapy
H3 histone
H-600 normothermic irrigation
H63D mutation
HA
    hyaluronan
HAA
    hepatitis-associated antigen
HAART
    highly active antiretroviral therapy
Haberer
        H. abdominal spatula
        H. intestinal clamp
        H. intestinal forceps
        vena marginalis epididymis of H.
habit
        bowel h.
        dietary h.
        drinking h.
habitus
        body h.
        marfanoid h.
Hadefield-Clarke syndrome
Hadju-Cheney acroosteolysis syndrome
Hadziyannis
        ground-glass body of H.
HAE
    hereditary angioedema
HAEC
    Hirschsprung-associated enterocolitis
haeckelii
        Psorospermium h.
haematobium
        Schistosoma h.
haemolyticus
        Haemophilus h.
Haemophilus
        H. ducreyi
        H. haemolyticus
        H. influenzae
haemorrhagica
        achylia gastrica h.
Hafnia alvei
hafniae
        Enterobacter h.
Hafter diet trick

Hagner operation
HAI
    hepatic arterial infusion
    histological activity index
Hailey-Hailey disease
hair
        h. ball
        digital manipulation of pubic h.
        Frey h.
hairy
        h. leukoplakia
        h. tongue
HAL
    hand-assisted laparoscopy
Halban procedure
Halcion
Haldane effect
Haldane-Priestly tube
Hald-Bradley classification
Haldol
Hale
        H. colloidal iron stain
        H. colloidal iron technique
Haley's M-O
HALF
    hyperacute liver failure
half-body irradiation
**half-Fourier acquisition single-shot turbo
    spin-echo (HASTE)**
half-hitch knot
half-life
half-normal saline
half-strength feeding
half-time
        gastric emptying h.-t. (GET1/2)
haliphagia
halitosis
Hallberg biliointestinal bypass
Halle point
Haller
        crypt of H.
HALNU
    hand-assisted laparoscopic
        nephroureterectomy
halo effect
haloperidol
halothane hepatotoxicity
halothane-induced
        h.-i. disease
        h.-i. hepatitis
HALS
    hand-assisted laparoscopic surgery
Halsted
        H. anastomosis
        H. forceps

H

Halsted (*continued*)
  H. hemostat
  H. hernioplasty
  H. inguinal herniorrhaphy
  H. interrupted mattress suture
  H. interrupted quilt suture
  H. method
  H. operation
Halsted-Bassini
  H.-B. hernia repair
  H.-B. herniorrhaphy
HALT-C
  hepatitis C antiviral long-term treatment
  to prevent cirrhosis
  HALT-C study
Haltran
Ham
  H. F12 medium
  H. test
hamartoma
  ampullary h.
  angiomatous lymphoid h.
  Brunner gland h.
  colonic h.
  cystic h.
  duodenal wall h.
  mesenchymal h.
  pancreatic h.
  Peutz-Jeghers h.
  renal h.
hamartomatous
  h. gastric polyp
  h. lesion
  h. polyposis
Hamel test
Hamilton deep surgery forceps
Hamilton-Thorn motility analyzer
Hamm electrode
hammock
  omental h.
  H. technique
  H. technique urinary diversion
Hampton
  H. line
  H. sign
hand-assisted
  h.-a. laparoscopic
    nephroureterectomy (HALNU)
  h.-a. laparoscopic surgery (HALS)
  h.-a. laparoscopy (HAL)
hand-held retractor
Handi-Cath catheter kit
handling
  renal tubular sodium h.
  tubular sodium h.
HandPort system
handsewn anastomosis
hand temperature

Haney
  H. needle driver
  H. retractor
Hanger test
hanging panniculus
Hank
  H. balanced salt solution (HBSS)
  H. buffer solution
Hanley
  H. method
  H. rectal bladder procedure
Hanot
  H. cirrhosis
  H. disease
  H. syndrome
Hanot-Chauffard syndrome
Hanot-Rössle syndrome
Hansel stain
Hansenula fabianii
Hanta virus
HAP
  hepatic arterial-dominant phase
  high-amplitude peristalsis
  HAP image
hapatotoxic range
HAPC
  high-amplitude contraction
HA-PI
  hepatic arterial pulsatility index
haploid cell
haplotype
  DQ2 h.
  DR7 h.
  histocompatibility h.
  HLA DQ2 h.
  HLA DR17 h.
haptocorrin degradation
haptoglobin
  serum h.
**Hara classification of gallbladder
  inflammation**
hard
  h. adhesion
  h. sonolucent plastic cone
  h. stool
harderoporphyria
harderoporphyrinogen
Har-el pharyngeal tube
Harewood suspension procedure
Harley disease
harmonic
  h. scalpel
  h. scalpel coagulating shears
harpoon extraction
Harrington
  H. Deaver retractor
  H. esophageal diverticulectomy

H. forceps
H. splanchnic retractor
Harrington-Mayo scissors
Harris
H. band
H. hematoxylin
H. segregator
H. tube
H. tube suction
Harris-Benedict energy requirement equation
Harrison spot test
hartford
Salmonella h.
Hartmann
H. closure of rectum
H. colostomy
H. fossa
H. operation
H. point
H. pouch
H. procedure
H. reconstruction technique
H. solution
Hartnup
H. disease
H. disorder
H. syndrome
Harvard pump
harvest
harvester
Arandel cell h
Brandel cell h
harvesting en bloc
Harvey-Bradshaw index
Harvey Stone clamp
Hashimoto
H. struma
H. thyroiditis
Hashizume endoscopic ligator kit
Hashmat shunt
Hashmat-Waterhouse shunt
Haslinger esophagoscope
Hasson
H. bullet-tip forceps
H. method
H. needle-nose forceps
H. open laparoscopy cannula
H. ring forceps
H. spike-tooth forceps
H. trocar

HASTE
half-Fourier acquisition single-shot turbo spin-echo
HASTE sequence
HAT
hepatic artery thrombosis
hatching
blastocyst h.
h. test
H+-ATPase
vacuolar H+-ATPase
Haudek sign
Hauri technique
Hausted all-purpose chair
haustra (*pl. of* haustrum)
haustral
h. blunting
h. crest
h. fold
h. indentation
h. marking
h. pattern
h. pouch
haustration
haustrum, pl. **haustra**
cecal h.
haustra coli
haustra of colon
Hautmann ileal neobladder
HAV
hepatitis A virus
Havrix
Hawaii
H. agent
H. virus
Hawes-Pallister-Landor syndrome
Hayem
H. icterus
H. jaundice
Hayes
H. anterior resection clamp
H. colon clamp
Hayflick phenomenon
Haymann nephrosis
Hay test
HB
Tagamet HB
HBAg
hepatitis B antigen
HBcAb
hepatitis B core antibody

NOTES

H

HBcAg
    hepatitis B core antigen
      HBcAg immunostaining
      recombinant HBcAg (rHBcAg)
HBeAb, HbeAb
    hepatitis Be antibody
      HBeAb antibody
HBeAg, HbeAg
    hepatitis B early antigen
      HBeAg antigen
      HBeAg immunological study
      purified HBeAg
HBeAg-positive
HBe antibody
HB-EGF
    heparin-binding epidermal growth factor
HBIG
    hepatitis B immunoglobulin
HBIg
    hepatitis B immunoglobulin
HBOT
    hyperbaric oxygen therapy
HBsAb
    hepatitis B surface antibody
HBsAg
    hepatitis B surface antigen
      HBsAg immunological study
      HBsAg subtype
HBsAg-negative, anti-HCV-negative
chronic liver disease (NBNC CLD)
HBSS
    Hank balanced salt solution
HBV
    hepatitis B virus
      HBV DNA
      HBV Engerix-B
      HBV genomic DNA
HBV-associated DNA polymerase
HBV-specific T cell
HBVV
    hepatitis B virus vaccine
HC-1
    Anusol HC-1
HCA
    hepatocellular adenoma
HCC
    hepatocellular carcinoma
HCG
    human chorionic gonadotropin
HCl
    hydrochloric acid
    hydrochloride
      alprostadil/prazosin HCl
      benazepril HCl
      gemcitabine HCl
      liposomal daunorubicin HCl
      lomefloxacin HCl
      1% pramoxine HCl

      sibutramine HCl
      tamsulosin HCl
      Tris HCl
      Vancocin HCl
HCN
    high calorie and nitrogen
      Isocal HCN
HCO^{3-}
    luminal HCO^{3-}
    peritubular HCO^{3-}
    HCO^{3-} reabsorption
HCP
    hereditary coproporphyria
HCS
    hematocystic spot
HCTZ
    hydrochlorothiazide
HCTZ-TA
    hydrochlorothiazide-triamterene
HCV
    hepatitis C virus
      HCV antibody
      HCV DupliType test
      HCV EIA II
      HCV ELISA test
      HCV genotype 1b
      HCV protein
      HCV RNA
HD
    hemodialysis
HDA-DR3 gene
HDAg
    hepatitis D antigen
HDC
    high-dose chemotherapy
    histidine decarboxylase
H disease
HDL
    high-density lipoprotein
HDL-C
    high-density lipoprotein cholesterol
HDV
    hepatitis delta virus
    hepatitis D virus
HDVD
    high-definition video display
HE
    hepatic encephalopathy
H&E
    hematoxylin and eosin
      H&E stain
HE9 fibroblast
head
    Medusa h.
    h. of pancreas
    h. symptom
headlamp
    Keeler Magnalite h.

healed
    h. ulcer
    h. yellow atrophy
healing
    delayed primary intention h.
    durable h.
    h. by first intention
    h. by granulation
    h. per primam intentionem
    h. per secundam intentionem
    h. by primary intention
    h. by secondary intention
    h. by second intention
    wound h.
health
    National Institutes of H. (NIH)
    h. outcome
health-related quality of life (HRQOL)
Healy intestinal forceps
Heaney
    H. clamp
    H. retractor
heaped-up edge
heart
    H. Outcomes Prevention Evaluation (HOPE)
    h. rate monitoring
    h. transplant
    h. transplantation
heartburn
    nocturnal h.
    h. of pregnancy
    h. relief formula (Maalox HRF)
heart-kidney transplant
heart-lung machine
heat
    h. exchanger
    h. probe
    h. probe thermocoagulation
    h. shock protein (HSP)
    h. therapy
heater
    h. probe (HP)
    h. probe coagulation
    h. probe therapy
    h. probe thermocoagulation
    telescope h.
heat-inactivated fetal calf serum
heating
    preferential h.
heat-labile
    h.-l. enterotoxin

    h.-l. factor (HLF)
    h.-l. toxin (LT)
heat-stable enterotoxin (ST)
heat-sterilized by autoclave
heave
    dry h.'s
heavy
    h. chain deposition disease
    h. silk suture
heavy-chain deposition
Hebra disease
Hectorol injection
Heelift smooth boot
Hegar
    H. intrarectal bougie
    H. rectal dilator
h-EGF
    human epidermal growth factor
heidelberg
    Salmonella h.
Heidenhain
    H. cell
    H. pouch
Heifitz clip
heilmanii
    Helicobacter h.
Heimlich maneuver
Heineke-Mikulicz
    H.-M. fashion
    H.-M. gastroenterostomy
    H.-M. incision
    H.-M. operation
    H.-M. principle
    H.-M. pyloroplasty
    H.-M. strictureplasty
Heiss loop
Heister
    H. diverticulum
    H. fold
    spiral valve of H.
    H. valve
Heitz-Boyer procedure
HeLa cell
helical
    H. basket
    h. coil
    h. computed tomography
    h. CT
    h. fashion
helical-ridged ureteral stent
Helicide
helicine artery

NOTES

H

Helicobacter
  H. heilmanii
  H. hepaticus
  H. pylori (HP)
  H. pylori breath excretion test
  H. pylori-induced gastritis
  H. pylori-like organism (HPLO)
  H. pylori stool antigen EIA
Helicobacter-**induced gastric injury**
Helicoblot 2.1 test
Helicosol
Helidac therapy
heliotrope sign
Heliotropium
Helisal
  H. Rapid Blood diagnostic kit
  H. rapid blood test
helium insufflation
helium-neon laser
Helivax
helix-loop-helix protein
helix-turn-helix protein
Heller
  H. cardiomyotomy
  H. esophagomyotomy
  H. myotomy
  H. operation
Heller-Belsey correction of achalasia of esophagus
Heller-Dor procedure
Heller-Nelson syndrome
Heller-Nissen correction of achalasia of esophagus
HELLP
  hemolysis, elevated liver enzymes, and low platelet count
    HELLP syndrome
Helmholtz double-surface coil
helminth
helminthemesis
helminthiasis
helminthic
  h. abscess
  h. appendicitis
  h. dysentery
  h. infection
  h. pseudotumor
helminthism
Helmstein balloon
helper T cell
Helvetius ligament
Hemaccel
hemagglutination
  indirect h. (IHA)
hemangioblastoma
  cerebral h.
  spinal h.

hemangioblastomatosis
  cerebelloretinal h.
  von Hippel-Lindau cerebellar h.
hemangioendothelial sarcoma
hemangioepithelioma
hemangioma
  capillary h.
  cavernous h.
  cutaneous h.
  hepatic h.
  h. laser treatment
  polypoid colorectal cavernous h.
  renal h.
  scrotal h.
  strawberry h.
  urethral h.
  vascular h.
hemangiomatosis
  duodenal h.
  splenic capillary h.
hemangiopericytoma
hemangiosarcoma
Hemaseel APR kit fibrin sealant
hematemesis
  Goldstein h.
Hematest test
hematin cast
hematobilia evacuation
hematocele
hematocelia
hematochezia
hematochyluria
hematocolpos
hematocrit
  hemoglobin and h. (H&H)
hematocystic spot (HCS)
hematocystis
hematocyturia
hematogenic metastasis
hematogenous
  h. micrometastasis
  h. proteinuria
  h. pyelitis
  h. pyelonephritis
  h. spread of infection
hematologic
  h. abnormality
  h. complication
  h. study
hematological stain
hematoma
  butterfly h.
  duodenal h.
  esophageal intramural h.
  expanding retroperitoneal h.
  intrahepatic h.
  intramural duodenal h. (IDH)
  kidney h.

mesenteric h.
parenchymal h.
perianal h.
perinephric h.
perirenal h.
pulsatile h.
rectus abdominis h.
rectus sheath h. (RSH)
renal h.
retroperitoneal h.
septal h.
subcapsular h.
warfarin-associated subcapsular h.
wound h.
hematometrocolpos
hematomphalocele
hematonephrosis
hematooxyphilic deposit
hematopathology
hematopoiesis
extramedullary h.
hepatic extramedullary h.
hematopoietic
h. cell
h. cell transplantation
h. lineage
hematoporphyrin
h. derivative (IIpD)
h. derivative therapy
hematoscheocele
hematospermatocele
hematospermia
hematoxylin
h. and eosin (H&E)
h. and eosin stain
Harris h.
hematuresis
hematuria
adolescent stress h.
angioneurotic h.
anticoagulant-induced h.
benign familial h.
endemic h.
essential h.
exercise-induced h.
glomerular h.
gross h.
idiopathic h.
initial h.
macroscopic h.
microscopic h.
nonglomerular h.

painful h.
painless h.
renal h.
stress h.
terminal h.
total h.
urethral h.
vesical h.
h. with clots
hematuria-dysuria syndrome
hemaurochrome
HemaWipe test
heme
h. pigment-induced acute tubular
necrosis
h. test
heme-albumin
intravenous h.-a.
heme-negative stool
heme-porphyrin assay
heme-positive
h.-p. NG aspirate
h.-p. stool
HemeSelect
hemiacidrin irrigation
hemianopsia
hemiballismus
hemiblock
anterior h.
hemibody irradiation
hemicolectomy
Duecollement h.
laparoscopic-assisted h.
hemicolon
hemicrypt column
hemifundoplication
Toupet h.
hemigastrectomy and vagotomy (H&V)
hemihepatectomy
hemihypertrophy
hemi-Kock
h.-K. neobladder
h.-K. pouch
h.-K. procedure
h.-K. system
urethral h.-K.
h.-K. urinary diversion
heminephrectomy
heminephroureterectomy
hemiorchiectomy
hemiparesis
hemiplegia

NOTES

H

hemipylorectomy
hemipyonephrosis
hemiscrotectomy
hemiscrotum
hemispherium, pl. **hemispheria**
    h. bulbi urethra
hemizona assay
hemobilia
Hemoccult
    H. II
    H. II card
    H. II test
    H. SENSA
    H. SENSA developer
    H. SENSA slide
    H. SENSA test
hemocholecyst
hemochromatosis
    African h.
    C282Y h.
    Desferal Mesylate challenge for h.
    genetic h. (GH)
    hereditary human leukocyte antigen-linked h.
    idiopathic h.
    perinatal h.
    precirrhotic h.
hemochromatotic cirrhosis
Hemoclip
hemoclipping
    h. application device
    endoscopic h.
hemoconcentration
hemoculture
hemocyanin
    keyhole limpet h. (KLH)
hemocytometer
hemodiafiltration
    continuous arteriovenous h.
     (CAVHDF)
    continuous venovenous h.
     (CVVHDF)
    double-chamber h.
    online h.
hemodialysis (HD)
    h. air embolism
    h. associated anemia
    continuous arteriovenous h.
     (CAVHD)
    continuous venovenous h.
     (CVVHD)
    conventional h.
    cool temperature h.
    daily h.
    dermatosis of h.
    frequent h.
    intermittent h. (IHD)

    nocturnal h.
    h. patient
    h. population
    sequential ultrafiltration h.
    simplified nocturnal home h.
     (SNHHD)
    single-pass h.
    sorbent h.
    standard h.
    venovenous continuous h.
hemodialysis-associated ascites
hemodialyzer
    ALTRA-FLUX h.
    1550 Baxter h.
    2008E h.
    ultrafiltration h.
hemoductal pancreatitis
hemodynamics
    erection h.
    hepatic arterial h.
    intraglomerular h.
    intrarenal h.
    renal h.
hemofilter
hemofiltration
    arteriovenous h.
    continuous arteriovenous h.
     (CAVH)
    continuous venovenous h. (CVVH)
    simultaneous hemodialysis and h.
    h. therapy (HFT)
    venovenous h.
hemoflagellate parasite
hemoglobin
    h. content index (IHb)
    h. and hematocrit (H&H)
    mean corpuscular h. (MCH)
    mucosal blood h.
hemoglobinemia
    paroxysmal nocturnal h.
hemoglobin and hematocrit (H&H)
hemoglobinopathy
    sickle h.
hemoglobinuria
    intermittent h.
    paroxysmal nocturnal h. (PNH)
Hemoject
    H. injection catheter
    H. needle
hemolysin
hemolysis
    h., elevated liver enzymes, and
     low platelet count (HELLP)
    sulfasalazine-induced oxidative h.
hemolytic
    h. anemia
    h. jaundice

h. splenomegaly
h. streptococcus
hemolytic-uremic syndrome (HUS)
hemonephrosis
hemoperfusion
    albumin-coated resin h.
    charcoal h.
    hepatic venous isolation by
      direct h. (HVI-DHP)
    h. with charcoal
hemopericardium
hemoperitoneum
Hemophan membrane
hemophilia
    renal h.
hemophiliac
hemoptysis
hemopyelectasis, hemopyelectasia
HemoQuant
    H. assay
    H. fecal blood test
hemorrhage
    acute nonvariceal upper
      gastrointestinal h.
    adrenal h.
    bland pulmonary h.
    colonic h.
    concealed h.
    h. control
    diffuse alveolar h. (DAH)
    diverticular h.
    endoscopic stigmata of h.
    esophageal variceal h. (EVH)
    exsanguinating h.
    fetal adrenal gland h.
    gastric h.
    gastrointestinal tract h.
    Grey Turner sign of
      retroperitoneal h.
    hepatic h.
    internal h.
    intestinal h.
    intraabdominal h.
    intracranial h.
    intramural intestinal h.
    intraperitoneal h.
    kidney h.
    lower gastrointestinal h.
    neonatal adrenal gland h.
    nonvariceal upper GI h.
    pancreatitis-related h.
    postgastrectomy h.

    postpolypectomy h.
    refractory variceal h.
    renal cyst h.
    retroperitoneal h.
    stigmata of recent h. (SRH)
    stress ulcer h.
    subcapsular h.
    subconjunctival h.
    subepithelial h.
    submucosal gastric h.
    torrential h.
    upper GI h.
    variceal h.
hemorrhagic
    h. ascites
    h. colitis
    h. cystitis
    h. dengue
    h. diarrhea
    h. enteritis
    h. enterocolitis
    h. fever
    h. fever with renal syndrome
    h. gastritis
    h. gastropathy
    h. hypotension
    h. necrotizing pancreatitis
    h. nephritis
    h. nephrosonephritis
    h. radiation injury
    h. speck
    h. telangiectasia
hemorrhoid
    bleeding h.
    cloverleaf excision of h.
    combined h.'s
    dilation of h.
    external h.
    h. grade
    internal h.
    ligation of h.
    Lord dilation of h.
    mixed h.'s
    mucocutaneous h.'s
    necrotic h.
    prolapsed internal h.
    prolapsing fourth-degree h.
    h. reduction
    rubber band ligation of h.
    strangulated h.
    thrombosed internal and external h.

NOTES

H

hemorrhoidal
 h. banding
 h. clamp
 h. cushion
 h. plexus
 h. prolapse
 h. sclerotherapy
 h. tag
 h. zone
hemorrhoidectomy
 ambulatory h.
 closed h.
 diathermy h.
 Ferguson h.
 laser h.
 Lord method h.
 Milligan-Morgan h.
 modified Whitehead h.
 open h.
 radical h.
 semiopen h.
 stapled h.
 sutured h.
HemoSelect test
hemosiderin
 h. deposit
 h. granule
hemosiderin-laden macrophage
hemosiderosis
hemospermia
 h. spuria
 h. vera
hemostasis
 endoscopic h.
hemostasis
hemostat
 Carmalt h.
 Crile h.
 curved h.
 Endo-Assist disposable h.
 Endo-Avitene microfibrillar
   collagen h.
 Halsted h.
 Kelly h.
 Kocher h.
 microfibrillar collagen h. (MCH)
 Mixter h.
 mosquito h.
 Ochsner h.
 Rochester-Péan h.
 Westphal h.
hemostatic
 h. agent
 h. bond strength
 h. clamp
 h. surgical glue
 h. suture
 h. therapy

hemosuccus pancreaticus
HemoTherapies liver dialysis unit
hemothorax
hemotympanum
Hemovac Suction Standard drain
hemp seed calculus
hemuresis
Henderson-Hasselbalch equation
Hendren
 H. clamp
 H. technique
Hendrickson lithotrite
Henke triangle
Henle
 H. ampulla
 H. band
 H. internal cremaster
 internal cremaster of H.
 loop of H. (LH)
 H. loop
 H. sphincter
 H. tubule
Henning sign
Henoch-Schönlein purpura
Henry approach
henselae
 Bartonella h.
Hensing fold
Hepa
 Amino Mel H.
hepadnavirus
Hepahydrin
Hepaplastin test
hepar
 h. adiposum
 h. lobatum
heparan sulfate proteoglycan (HSPG)
heparin
 h. bolus
 glycosaminoglycan h.
 intravesical h.
 low molecular weight h. (LMWH)
heparinase
heparin-binding
 h.-b. epidermal growth factor (HB-
   EGF)
 h.-b. growth factor-1
heparin-induced
 h.-i. lipolysis
 h.-i. thrombocytopenia (HIT)
heparinization
 regional h.
heparinized saline
hepatalgia
HepatAmine amino acid solution
HepatAssist Liver Support System
hepatectomy
 donor h.

extended right h.
partial h.
recipient h.
triple lobe h.

hepatic
  h. abnormality
  h. abscess
  h. adenoma
  h. adhesion
  h. allograft
  h. amebiasis
  h. amyloidosis
  h. angiomatosis
  h. angiosarcoma
  h. architecture
  h. arterial-dominant phase (HAP)
  h. arterial hemodynamics
  h. arterial infusion (HAI)
  h. arterial infusion chemotherapy
  h. arterial pulsatility index (HA-PI)
  h. arterial vascular resistance
  h. arteriogram
  h. arteriography
  h. artery
  h. artery aneurysm
  h. artery infusion pump
  h. artery ligation
  h. artery thrombosis (HAT)
  h. bed
  h. bifurcation
  h. blood flow
  h. blood pool scan
  h. calculus
  h. candidal infection
  h. capsule
  h. capsulitis
  h. circulation
  h. cirrhosis
  h. clearance
  h. colic
  h. coma
  h. congestion
  h. copper overload
  h. cord
  h. cystadenoma
  h. cystic disease
  h. deformability
  h. diverticulum
  h. duct
  h. duct stone
  h. dullness
  h. echinococcal cyst

  h. echinococcosis
  h. edge
  h. encephalopathy (HE)
  h. endothelialis
  h. extramedullary hematopoiesis
  h. fascioliasis
  h. fibrosis
  h. fistula
  h. flexure
  h. flexure of colon
  h. funiculus
  h. funiculus of Rauber
  h. glycogen store
  h. granuloma
  h. hemangioma
  h. hemorrhage
  h. hilar region
  h. hilum
  h. Hodgkin disease
  h. hydrothorax
  h. hypoxia
  h. insufficiency
  h. intermittent fever
  h. iron index (HII)
  h. lectin
  h. leiomyosarcoma
  h. ligament
  h. lipase (HL)
  h. lobectomy
  h. malignancy
  h. malondialdehyde content
  h. mass lesion
  h. metabolism
  h. metastatic disease
  h. 3-methylglutaryl coenzyme A reductase (HMG-CoA)
  h. osteodystrophy
  h. outflow tract
  h. parenchyma
  h. peliosis
  h. perfusion index (HPI)
  h. phosphorylase deficiency
  h. porphyria
  h. resection
  h. rudiment
  h. rupture
  h. sarcoidosis
  h. schistosomiasis
  h. sclerosis
  h. segmentectomy
  h. sinusoid
  h. span

NOTES

H

hepatic *(continued)*
   h. steatosis
   h. stellate cell (HSC)
   h. stimulatory substance (HSS)
   h. subcellular element
   h. subsegmentectomy
   h. telangiectasia
   h. toxemia
   h. trauma
   h. triad
   h. triglyceride lipase (HTGL)
   h. tumor
   h. tumor index (HTI)
   h. uptake
   h. urea
   h. uroporphyrinogen decarboxylase
    activity
   h. vein (HV)
   h. vein catheterization
   h. vein injury
   h. vein occlusion
   h. vein thrombosis
   h. vein wedge pressure
   h. venogram
   h. venography
   h. venoocclusive disease
   h. venous isolation by direct
    hemoperfusion (HVI-DHP)
   h. venous outflow
   h. venous outflow obstruction
    (HVOO)
   h. venous pressure
   h. venous pressure gradient
    (HVPG)
   h. venous pressure gradient
    reduction
   h. venous web disease
   h. venule
   h. web
   h. web dilation
   h. wedge pressure
hepatica
   adiposis h.
   facies h.
   Fasciola h.
Hepatic-Aid powdered feeding
hepatic-alveolar echinococcosis
hepaticocholedochostomy
hepaticocystic junction
hepaticodochotomy
hepaticoduodenostomy
hepaticoenterostomy
hepaticogastrostomy
hepaticojejunal anastomosis
hepaticojejunostomy
   Roux-en-Y h.
hepaticoliasis
hepaticolithotomy

hepaticolithotripsy
hepaticopulmonary fistula
hepaticostomy
hepaticotomy
hepatic-to-renal
   h.-t.-r. artery saphenous vein
    bypass
   h.-t.-r. artery saphenous vein
    bypass graft
hepaticus
   fetor h.
   Helicobacter h.
   peliosis h.
hepatis
   area nuda h.
   facies diaphragmatica h.
   facies inferior h.
   facies posterior h.
   facies superior h.
   facies visceralis h.
   impressio esophagealis h.
   incisura vesicae felleae h.
   ligamentum teres h.
   peliosis h.
   pons h.
   ponticulus h.
   porta h.
hepatitic
hepatitis, pl. **hepatitides**
   h. A
   active chronic h.
   acute h. (AH)
   acute alcoholic h.
   acute mononucleosis-like h.
   acute parenchymatous h.
   acute self-limited h.
   acute viral h. (AVH)
   h. A inactivated and hepatitis B
    (recombinant) vaccine
   alcoholic h. (AH)
   amebic h.
   anesthetic h.
   anicteric viral h.
   autoimmune h. (AIH)
   h. A vaccine
   h. A virus (HAV)
   h. B
   h. B antigen (HBAg)
   h. B core antibody (HBcAb)
   h. B core antigen (HBcAg)
   h. B DNA detection
   h. Be antibody (HBeAb, HbeAb)
   h. Be antigen
   h. B early antigen (HBeAg,
    HbeAg)
   h. B hyperimmune globulin
   h. B immunoglobulin (HBIG,
    HBIg)

h. B-like DNA
h. B-like DNA virus
blood-borne non-A, non-B h.
h. B surface antibody (HBsAb)
h. B surface antigen (HBsAg)
h. B surface antigen
  subdeterminant
h. B vaccine
h. B virus (HBV)
h. B virus-encoded antigen
h. B virus vaccine (HBVV)
h. C
h. C antiviral long-term treatment
  to prevent cirrhosis (HALT-C)
capsula fibrosa h.
h. carrier
cholangiolitic h.
cholestatic viral h.
chronic h. (CH)
chronic active h. (CAH)
chronic active viral h. (CAVH)
chronic active viral h., non-A,
  non-B (CAVH-NAB)
chronic active viral h., type B
  (CAVH-B)
chronic aggressive h. (CAH)
chronic autoimmune h.
chronic h. B, C
chronic benign h. (CBH)
chronic fibrosing h.
chronic interstitial h.
chronic lobular h. (CLH)
chronic persistent h. (CPH)
chronic progressive h.
chronic type B h.
chronic viral h.
cryptogenic chronic h.
h. C viremia
h. C virus (HCV)
h. C virus-associated venoocclusive
  disease
h. C virus DupliType test
h. C virus enzyme immunoassay
h. C virus genotype
h. C virus RNA
h. C virus RNA detection
cytomegalovirus h.
h. D
h. D antigen (HDAg)
delta agent h.
h. delta virus (HDV)
de novo autoimmune h.

drug-induced h.
h. D superinfection
h. D virus (HDV)
h. E
ENANB h.
enterically transmitted non-A, non-
  B h. (ET-NANBH)
epidemic h.
h. E virus (HEV)
h. F
familial h.
fatty liver h.
fibrosing cholestatic h. B
flucloxacillin-induced delayed
  cholestatic h.
fulminant h. (A–E)
fulminant viral h. (FVH)
giant cell h.
granulomatous h.
h. G-RNA (GBV-C/HGV-RNA)
h. G virus (HGV)
halothane-induced h.
herpetic h.
hyperglobulinemic h.
idiopathic autoimmune chronic h.
h. infection (A–E)
infectious h.
intrahepatic h.
ischemic h.
isoniazid-induced h.
lobular h.
long incubation h.
lupoid h.
malarial h.
MS-1, -2 h.
murine h.
NANB h.
neonatal h.
newborn h.
non-A–E h.
non-A–G fulminant h.
non-A, non-B h.
non-A, non-B, non-C h.
non-A, non-B posttransfusion h.
nonspecific reactive h.
normal carrier h.
occult h.
oxacillin-associated anicteric h.
persistent chronic h.
persistent viral h. (PVII)
persistent viral h., non-A, non-B
  (PVH-NANB)

NOTES

H

349

hepatitis *(continued)*
    persistent viral h., type B (PVH-B)
    plasma cell h.
    posttransfusion h.
    quiescent h.
    h. serologic marker
    serum h.
    short incubation h.
    spontaneous reactivation of h.
    subacute h.
    subclinical h.
    superimposed alcoholic h.
    syphilitic h.
    terbutaline h.
    toxic h.
    transfusion-associated h.
    h. type 1
    type 1, 2 autoimmune h.
    viral h.
    viral h. type A, B
hepatitis-associated antigen (HAA)
Hepatix device
hepatization
hepatobiliary
    h. capsule
    h. cholescintigraphy
    h. fibropolycystic disease
    h. malignancy
    h. manifestation
    h. scan
    h. scintigraphy
    h. tract disease
    h. tree
hepatoblastoma
hepatocanalicular
    h. cholestasia
    h. jaundice
hepatocarcinogenesis
hepatocarcinogenic
hepatocarcinoma
    fibrolamellar h.
hepatocele
hepatocellular
    h. adenoma (HCA)
    h. atypia
    h. ballooning
    h. basolateral plasma membrane
     fluidity
    h. carcinoma (HCC)
    h. cholestasia
    h. death
    h. disease
    h. injury
    h. jaundice
    h. necrosis
    h. protein
hepatocerebral degeneration
hepatocholangeitis

hepatocholangiocarcinoma
hepatocholangiocystoduodenostomy
hepatocholangioduodenostomy
hepatocholangioenterostomy
hepatocholangiogastrostomy
hepatocholangiojejunostomy
hepatocholangiostomy
hepatocholangitis
hepatocirrhosis
hepatocolic ligament
hepatocystic
hepatocystis
hepatocystocolic ligament
hepatocyte
    ballooning degeneration of h.
    cobblestone pattern of h.
    h. growth factor (HGF)
    lipid-laden h.
    h. lysosome
    h. necrosis
    periportal h.
    polygonal h.
    porcine h.
    h. proliferation inhibitor (HPI)
    h. protein synthesis
    pseudoductular transformation of h.
    h. transplantation
hepatocyte-type cytokeratin
hepatocytic cord
hepatoduodenal
    h. ligament
    h. reflection
hepatoduodenal-peritoneal reflection
hepatoduodenostomy
hepatodynia
hepatodysentery
hepatoenterostomy
hepatofugal
    h. arterioportal shunt
    h. flow
    h. portosystemic venous shunt
hepatogastric ligament
hepatogastroduodenal ligament
hepatogastroenterology
hepatogenic, hepatogenous
    h. jaundice
hepatography
hepatohemia
hepatoid adenocarcinoma
hepatoiminodiacetic acid (HIDA)
hepatojugular reflux
hepatolenticular
    h. degeneration
    h. disease
hepatolith
hepatolithectomy
hepatolithiasis
hepatologist

hepatology
hepatoma
    fibrolamellar h.
hepatomegaly
    congestive h.
hepatomphalocele
hepatomphalos
hepatonephoric syndrome
hepatonephromegaly
hepatopancreatica
    ampulla h.
hepatopancreatic fold
hepatopancreatoduodenectomy
hepatopathic
hepatopathy
    radiation h.
hepatopetal flow
hepatopexy
hepatophosphorylase deficiency
  glycogenosis
hepatophrenic ligament
hepatopleural fistula
hepatoportal sclerosis
hepatoportoenterostomy
    Kasai-type h.
hepatoptosis
hepatopulmonary syndrome (HPS)
hepatorenal
    h. angle
    h. bypass
    h. glycogenosis
    h. ligament
    h. space of Morison
    h. syndrome (HRS)
hepatorrhagia
hepatorrhaphy
hepatorrhea
hepatorrhexis
hepatoscopy
hepatosplenic T-cell lymphoma
hepatosplenomegaly
hepatosplenopathy
hepatostomy
hepatotherapy
hepatotomy
hepatotoxemia
hepatotoxic
hepatotoxicity
    acetaminophen h.
    Amanita mushroom h.
    anesthetic h.
    anticonvulsant agent h.

antidepressant drug h.
antidiabetic agent h.
antineoplastic drug h.
antipsychotic drug h.
antithyroid drug h.
carbamazepine h.
cardiovascular drug h.
chemotherapeutic agent h.
cocaine h.
drug h.
erythromycin estolate h.
halothane h.
hydrazide h.
nitrofurantoin h.
2-nitropropane h.
phenylbutazone h.
potentiation of drug h.
valproic acid h.
yellow phosphorus h.
hepatotoxin
hepatoumbilical ligament
Hep-B-Gammagee
HepBzyme
HEPES
    HEPES buffer
    HEPES solution
hepG2 cell
Heprofile ELISA test
heptahelical receptor protein
Heptalac
Heptavax-B
Heptazyme
Her-2/neu oncogene
heracleifolia
    Cimicifuga h.
herald
    h. bleed
    h. patch
Herbgels
    BioFIT H.
Herculink
    H. Plus biliary stent
hereditary
    h. angioedema (HAE)
    h. coproporphyria (HCP)
    h. flat adenoma syndrome (HFAS)
    h. fructose intolerance
    h. hemorrhagic telangiectasia (HHT)
    h. human leukocyte antigen-linked
      hemochromatosis
    h. internal anal sphincter myopathy
    h. nephritis

NOTES

H

hereditary *(continued)*
    h. nonpolyposis colon cancer (HNPCC)
    h. nonpolyposis colorectal cancer
    h. nonpolyposis colorectal cancer syndrome
    h. nonpolyposis colorectal carcinoma
    h. osteoonychodysplasia
    h. pancreatitis (HP)
    h. papillary renal cancer (HPRC)
    h. prostate cancer 1 locus (HPC-1)
    h. spastic paraplegia voiding dysfunction
    h. tyrosinemia
Hering
    canal of H.
Herlitz junctional epidermolysis bullosa
Hermansky-Pudlak syndrome
Herman-Taylor gastroscope
hermaphroditism
hermaphroditismus
hermetically
hernia, pl. **herniae**
    abdominal wall h.
    antevesical h.
    axial hiatal h.
    Barth h.
    Béclard h.
    bladder h.
    Bochdalek h.
    cecal h.
    Cheatle-Henry h.
    Cloquet h.
    combined hiatal h.
    congenital diaphragmatic h.
    Cooper h.
    diaphragmatic h. (DH)
    direct inguinal h.
    duodenojejunal h.
    easily reducible h.
    epigastric h.
    femoral h.
    funicular inguinal h.
    gastroesophageal h.
    Gibbon h.
    Gironcoli h.
    Goyrand h.
    Grynfeltt h.
    Hesselbach h.
    Hey h.
    hiatal h., hiatus h.
    Holthouse h.
    h. hydrocele
    incarcerated intrathoracic h.
    h. incarceration
    incisional h.
    incomplete h.

    indirect inguinal h.
    inguinal h. (IH)
    inguinofemoral h.
    inguinoscrotal h.
    inguinosuperficial h.
    interstitial h.
    intraepiploic h.
    intrailiac h.
    irreducible h.
    h. knife
    Krönlein h.
    lateral ventral h.
    Laugier h.
    Lesgaft h.
    levator ani h.
    Littré h.
    Madden repair of incisional h.
    Maydl h.
    mesenteric h.
    mesentericoparietal h.
    mesocolic h.
    metachronous contralateral hernias
    Morgagni h.
    multiorgan h.
    obturator h.
    occult levator ani h.
    pantaloon h.
    paracolostomy h.
    paraduodenal h.
    paraesophageal diaphragmatic h.
    paraesophageal hiatal h.
    paraesophageal h. (type I, II)
    parahiatal h.
    paraileostomal h.
    parapubic h.
    parastomal h.
    parietal h.
    h. pouch
    properitoneal h.
    reducible h.
    h. repair
    retrograde h.
    retroperitoneal h.
    retrosternal h.
    Richter h.
    Rieux h.
    right inguinal h. (RIH)
    Rokitansky h.
    rolling hiatal h.
    h. sac
    sciatic h.
    scrotal h.
    sliding esophageal hiatal h.
    spigelian h.
    h. stapler
    strangulated h.
    traumatic diaphragmatic h.
    Treitz h.

umbilical h.
ureteral h.
h. uteri inguinale
Velpeau h.
ventral h.
vesicle h.
voluminous hiatus h.

hernial
h. defect
h. repair

herniated preperitoneal fat
herniation
paracolostomy h.
ureteroneocystostomy h.

hernioenterotomy
herniolaparotomy
hernioplasty
Cooper ligament h.
Halsted h.
mesh plug h.
open mesh-plug h.

herniorrhaphy
Anson-McVay femoral h.
Bassini inguinal h.
Halsted-Bassini h.
Halsted inguinal h.
Hill hiatus h.
Lichtenstein h.
Macewen h.
Madden incisional h.
McVay h.
pants-over-vest h.
Ponka h.
Shouldice inguinal h.
ventral h.
vest-over-pants h.

herniotome
Cooper h.

herniotomy
herpangina
herpes
anorectal h.
h. labialis
h. pharyngitis
h. progenitalis
h. simplex
h. simplex esophagitis
h. simplex infection
h. simplex virus (HSV)
h. simplex virus thymidine kinase
(HSK-tk)

h. zoster
h. zoster virus

herpesvirus
Kaposi sarcoma-associated h.
h. simplex (HVS)

herpetic
h. esophagitis
h. gingivostomatitis
h. hepatitis
h. stomatitis
h. ulcer

herpetiform esophagitis
herpetiformis
dermatitis h. (DH)

Herrick kidney clamp
herring worm
herring-worm disease
Hers disease
Herter
H. disease
H. infantilism

Herter-Heubner disease
Herzberg test
hesitancy
urinary h.

Hesselbach
H. hernia
H. ligament
H. triangle

Hess operation
HETE
hydroxyeicosatetraenoic acid

heterochromatin
heteroconjugate
antilymphocyte h.

heterodimer
heterodimeric
h. glycoprotein
h. protein

heteroduplex analysis
heterogeneity
cancer cell h.
genetic h.
intratumoral h.

heterogeneous texture
heterogenous pseudocyst
heterologous
h. anti-GBM antibody
h. liver perfusion

heterotopia
fundic gland h.
gastric h.

NOTES

H

heterotopic
    h. cylindric ciliated epithelium
    h. diversion
    h. gastric mucosa
    h. pancreas
heterotrimer
heterotrimeric G protein
heterozygosity
heterozygote
heterozygous
    h. DR5
    h. ornithine transcarbamylase (HOTC)
HE-TUMT
    high-energy transurethral microwave thermotherapy
Hetzel-Dent
    H.-D. esophagitis grade
    H.-D. scale
Hetzel score
Heubner-Herter disease
HEV
    hepatitis E virus
Hewlett-Packard IVUS imaging system
Hexabrix
hexagon snare
hexamethonium bromide
hexobarbital
hexocyclium
hexokinase (HK)
Hey
    H. hernia
    H. ligament
Heyde syndrome
Heyer-Schulte
    H.-S. Small-Carrion sizing set
    H.-S. stent
Heymann
    H. antibody
    H. nephritis
    H. nephritis antigenic complex (HNAC)
HFAS
    hereditary flat adenoma syndrome
HFE **gene**
HFT
    hemofiltration therapy
HFU
    high-intensity focused ultrasound
HFUPS
    high-frequency ultrasound probe sonography
HG
    Cobe Centrysystem dialyzer 400 HG
HgCl2
    mercury chloride

HGD
    high-grade dysplasia
HGF
    hepatocyte growth factor
    human growth factor
      recombinant HGF
HGF-stimulated renal epithelial cell
HGV
    hepatitis G virus
H&H
    hemoglobin and hematocrit
HHM
    humoral hypercalcemia of malignancy
HHT
    hereditary hemorrhagic telangiectasia
HIAA
    hydroxyindoleacetic acid
5-HIAA
    5-hydroxyindoleacetic acid
hiatal
    h. esophagism
    h. hernia
hiatus
    aortic h.
    diaphragmatic h.
    h. hernia
    patulous h.
    vena cava h.
Hibiclens
Hibidil solution
Hibistat
Hibond N+ nylon membrane
hiccup, hiccough, pl. **hiccups**
Hickman
    H. catheter
    H. percutaneous introducer
HIDA
    hepatoiminodiacetic acid
      HIDA scan
      ^{99m}Tc HIDA
hidden antigen
hidradenitis suppurativa
hiemis
    hyperemesis h.
HIFU
    high-intensity focused ultrasound
Higgins
    H. India ink
    H. technique
    H. ureterointestinal anastomosis
high
    h. abdominal plain film
    h. anion gap metabolic acidosis
    h. calorie
    h. calorie and nitrogen (HCN)
    h. enema
    h. fundal lesion
    h. intermuscular abscess

h. intraluminal pressure
h. ligation
h. ligation of hernia sac
h. lithotomy
h. neurological lesion
h. nitrogen (HN)
h. rectal washout
h.-resolution endoluminal
  sonography (HRES)
h. resting anal pressure
h. small bowel obstruction
h. subtotal gastrectomy
h. testis
h. transection
h. transection of the inferior
  mesenteric artery
high-affinity
  h.-a. low-capacity system
  h.-a. receptor
  h.-a. sodium-dependent phosphate
    transport system
high-altitude endoscopy
high-amplitude
  h.-a. contraction (HAPC)
  h.-a. peristalsis (HAP)
high-bulk, low-fat diet
high-calcium dialysate
high-calorie diet
high-carbohydrate diet
high-ceiling diuretic
high-compliance latex balloon
high-definition video display (HDVD)
high-density
  h.-d. lipoprotein (HDL)
  h.-d. lipoprotein cholesterol (HDL-
    C)
high-diameter dilator
high-dose
  h.-d. chemotherapy (HDC)
  h.-d. consensus interferon
  h.-d. intravenous urography
  h.-d. IVU
  h.-d. pulse steroid
high-echoic area
high-efficiency dialysis
high-ending vagina
high-energy
  h.-e. modification
  h.-e. protocol
  h.-e. transurethral microwave
    thermotherapy (HE-TUMT)
  h.-e. TUMT

higher host susceptibility
high-fat diet
high-fiber diet
high-flow priapism
high-flux
  h.-f. dialysis
  h.-f. dialysis membrane
  h.-f. dialyzer
  h.-f. polysulfone
  h.-f. polysulfone membrane
high-frequency
  h.-f. endosonography
  h.-f. intraluminal ultrasound
  h.-f. miniprobe
  h.-f. sonography
  h.-f. ultrasound probe sonography
    (HFUPS)
high-grade
  h.-g. cholestasia
  h.-g. dysplasia (HGD)
  h.-g. obstruction
  h.-g. synchronous colon cancer
  h.-g. tumor
high-intensity
  h.-i. focused ultrasonography
  h.-i. focused ultrasound (HFU,
    HIFU)
high-level disinfection (HLD)
highlight
  human genome h.
high-loop cutaneous ureterostomy
highly
  h. active antiretroviral therapy
    (HAART)
  h. selective vagotomy
high-lying side
high-magnification
  h.-m. colonoscopy
  h.-m. endoscopy
  h.-m. gastroscopy
Highmore
  H. body
  corpus H.
  H. corpus
high-pass filtering
high-performance liquid chromatography
  (HPLC)
high-pitched bowel sounds
high-power
  h.-p. field (hpf)
  h.-p. photomicrograph

NOTES

H

high-pressure
  h.-p. antireflux barrier
  h.-p. arterial baroreceptor
  h.-p. inflatable prosthesis cylinder
  h.-p. liquid chromatography (HPLC)
  h.-p. zone (HPZ)
high-protein diet
high-resolution
  h.-r. endoluminal sonography
    (HRES)
  h.-r. endoscopy
  h.-r. 25-megahertz ultrasonography
  h.-r. real-time scanner
high-riding bladder
high-roughage diet
high-sensitivity collimator
high-speed electrical tissue morcellator
high-starch diet
high-velocity flow
HII
  hepatic iron index
hila (*pl. of* hilum)
hilar
  h. bile duct stenting
  h. carcinoma
  h. cholangiocarcinoma
  h. clamp
  h. mass
  h. plate
  h. retractor
  h. structure scar tissue
hill
  H. antireflux operation
  h. diarrhea
  H. esophageal antireflux repair
  H. esophageal fundoplication
  H. esophageal gastroenterostomy
  H. hiatus hernia repair
  H. hiatus herniorrhaphy
  H. median arcuate repair
  H. posterior gastropexy
  H. rectal retractor
Hill-Ferguson rectal retractor
Hilton white line
hilum, pl. **hila**
  hepatic h.
  renal h.
  h. renale
  h. renalis
  splenic h.
  h. stimulation
  h. of suprarenal gland
hilus
  liver h.
  renal h.
hindgut
  h. carcinoid

  h. dysfunction
  h. pattern
hind kidney
Hind-SITE 20/20 system
Hinkle-James rectal speculum
Hinman
  H. procedure
  H. reflux
  H. syndrome
Hinman-Allen syndrome
Hippel-Lindau syndrome
hippocratic succussion
Hippuran clearance technique
hippurate
  methenamine h.
hippuric acid
Hiprex
hirschfeldii
  Salmonella h.
Hirschmann
  H. anoscope
  H. pile clamp
  H. speculum
Hirschowitz
  H. endoscope
  H. gastroduodenal fiberscope
  H. gastroscope
Hirschsprung-associated enterocolitis (HAEC)
Hirschsprung disease
hirsute papilloma of penis
hirsutism
  adrenal h.
hirsutoid papilloma
His
  angle of H.
  bundle of H.
Hismanal
Histalog stimulation test
histamine
  h. H2 antagonist
  h. H2-receptor antagonist
  h. test
histamine-2 (H2)
  h. 2 receptor antagonist (H2RA)
histamine-producing mast cell
histamine-releasing factor (HRF)
histamine-resistant achlorhydria
histaminergic type 2 receptor
histatin
histidine decarboxylase (HDC)
histiocyte
  pigmented h.
histiocytic lymphoma
histiocytoma
  fibrous h.
  kidney malignant fibrous h.

histiocytosis
    Langerhans cell h.
    malignant h.
Histoacryl injection
histochemical pattern
histochemical-ultrastructural analysis
histochemistry
histocompatibility
    h. antigen
    h. complex
    h. haplotype
    h. testing
histocytochemical technique
Histofine
    H. SAB kit
    H. SAB-PO kit
histogram flattening
histologic
    h. anal canal
    h. cirrhosis
    h. damage
    h. diagnosis
    h. grading
    h. patchiness
    h. sign
histological
    h. activity index (HAI)
    h. chronic active gastritis
    h. esophagitis
histology
    bladder h.
histolytica
    Entamoeba h.
histometry
histomorphometric
histone
    H3 h.
histopathology
    renal h.
Histoplasma capsulatum
histoplasmosis
    disseminated h.
    duodenal h.
    gastrointestinal h.
    intestinal h.
    mediastinal h.
    recurrent colonic h.
history
    positive family h.
    psychosexual h.
histrionic personality

HIT
    heparin-induced thrombocytopenia
Hitachi
    H. 717 analyzer
    H. 737 autoanalyzer
    H. F-2000 fluorescence
      spectrophotometer
hitch
    psoas h.
HIV
    human immunodeficiency virus
    HIV infection
    HIV P24 antigen
HIV-1 enteropathy
HIVAN
    HIV-associated nephropathy
    human immunodeficiency virus-
      associated nephropathy
HIV-associated nephropathy (HIVAN)
hive
Hi-Vegi-Lip
HK
    hexokinase
    HK enzyme
hK3
H+/K+-ATPase
    H+/K+-ATPase acid pump inhibitor
    H+/K+-ATPase enzyme system
H-K-ATPase proton pump
HL
    hepatic lipase
HLA
    human leukocyte antigen
    HLA class II gene
    HLA class II phenotype
    HLA class II restricted
    HLA class II-restricted interferon-
      gamma
    HLA class II-restricted T-cell
      epitope
    HLA DQ2 haplotype
    HLA DR
    HLA DR3
    HLA DR4
    HLA DR17 haplotype
    HLA identical kidney graft
    HLA mismatch
    solubilized HLA
      solubilized human leukocyte
      antigen
    HLA typing
    HLA typing immunological study

NOTES

H

HLA-A
HLA-B
HLA-B8
HLA-DP allele
HLA-DQ2 molecule
HLA-DQ typing
HLA-DQw2 gene
HLA-DR
    H.-D. antigen
    H.-D. DNA typing
    H.-D. matching
    H.-D. typing
HLA-DR+
HLA-DR2 subtyping
HLA-DR3 gene
HLA-identical sibling
HLA-matched kidney
HLD
    high-level disinfection
HLF
    heat-labile factor
    HLF cell
HLG
    hypertrophic lymphocytic gastritis
HM4
    Dornier electrohydraulic watertank lithotriptor (HM3, HM4)
    HM4 lithotriptor
^{1}H magnetic resonance spectroscopy
HMB-45
    HMB-45 monoclonal antibody
    HMB-45 monoclonal antibody marker
HM-CAP serological test
HMG-CoA
    hepatic 3-methylglutaryl coenzyme A reductase
hMLH1 gene
HN
    high nitrogen
    hypertensive nephrosclerosis
    HN feeding
HNAC
    Heymann nephritis antigenic complex
HNPCC
    hereditary nonpolyposis colon cancer
hobnailed cell
hobnail liver
Hochenegg operation
hockey-stick incision
Hodge intestinal decompression tube
Hodgkin disease
Hodgson
    H. technique of modified Lich procedure
    H. XX procedure
hoe
    Joe h.

Hoefer GS 300 laser densitometer
Hoehn and Yahr stage
Hoesch test
Hoffmann-Steinberg gastric reservoir
Hofmeister
    H. anastomosis
    H. gastroenterostomy
    H. operation
    H. procedure
    H. technique
Hofmeister-Shoemaker gastrojejunostomy
Hogan/Geenen criteria
Hoguet maneuver
H_2O_2-induced injury
holder
    Adson needle h.
    Bihrle dorsal clamp-T-C needle h.
    Bookler swivel-ball laparoscope h.
    Bovie h.
    Capillary System slide h.
    Cath-Secure catheter h.
    Crile-Wood needle h.
    Dale Foley catheter h.
    DeMartel-Wolfson clamp h.
    diamond jaw needle h.
    Endo-Assist disposable needle h.
    Jacobson needle h.
    Kilner needle h.
    Lloyd-Davis knee and leg h.
    Mason needle h.
    Mayo-Hegar needle h.
    microneedle h.
    microvascular needle h.
    needle h.
    Sarot needle h.
    Stratte needle h.
    T-C needle h.
    Young needle h.
hold-up
    bolus h.-u.
Holinger esophagoscope
Hollander test
Hollande solution
Hollenhorst plaque
hollisae
    Vibrio h.
Hollister
    H. Convex insert
    H. First Choice pouch
    H. Guardian F skin barrier
    H. Holligard pouch
    H. irrigator drain
    H. Karaya 5 ostomy pouch
    H. Karaya Seal pouch
    H. Premium paste
    H. Premium pouch
    H. urostomy bag
hollow-fiber dialyzer

hollow viscus
holmium laser resection of the prostate
    (HoLRP)
holmium:YAG laser
holmium:yttrium aluminum garnet
    (Ho:YAG)
holodiastolic
Hologic densitometer
holosystolic
HoLRP
    holmium laser resection of the prostate
Holter
    H. Pediatric Pump 903, 907
    H. valve
    vesicovaginal H.
Holthouse hernia
Holt-Oram syndrome
Holyoke
    H. brief
    H. pants
homatropine methylbromide
home
    H. Care Simplimatt Plus zoned
      foam mattress
    h. dialysis
    H. gland
    12-hour h. pad test
    H. lobe
    h. parenteral nutrition (HPN)
    h. screening test
    short daily at h.
    h. uroflowmetry
homeostasis
    calcium h.
    calcium-phosphate h.
    sodium h.
homeostatic therapy
Homer Wright rosette
HomeSelect test
homing
    lymphoblast h.
hominis
    Blastocystis h.
    Gastrospirillum h.
    Mycoplasma h.
    Trichomonas h.
homocladic anastomosis
homocysteine
    h. level
    plasma h.
    protein-bound h.
    total h. (tHcy)

homocystinuria
homodimer
homodimerization
    ligand-dependent receptor h.
homogenate
    cecal h.
    fecal h.
    mucosal h.
    sphincter of Oddi h.
homogeneity
homogeneous
    h. ablation
    h. echographic
    h. texture
homogenous
    h. cooling
    h. nucleation
    h. radioimmunoassay
homologous
    h. protein-overload disease
    h. serum jaundice
homosexual rectal trauma
homotransplant
homotransplantation
    renal h.
homovanillic acid (HVA)
homozygote
homozygous sickle cell anemia
honeycomb pattern
honeymoon cystitis
hood
    latex h.
hooded prepuce
hook
    Adson dissecting h.
    Barr fistula h.
    cold knife h.
    Crile nerve h.
    crypt h.
    Dandy nerve h.
    h. forceps
    h. grip
    Joseph h.
    h. knife
    Neivert polyp h.
    nerve h.
    Pratt crypt h.
    Pratt rectal h.
    Pucci-Seed h.
    Rosser crypt h.
    h. scissors
    Shambaugh fistula h.

NOTES

H

hook (*continued*)
    Stewart crypt h.
    Whitaker h.
hooked catheter
hooklet
    hydatid h.
hook-tip laparoscopic electrode
hookworm disease
Hooper deep surgery scissors
HOPE
    Heart Outcomes Prevention Evaluation
    HOPE study
Hopkins
    H. II rod lens
    H. rod-lens system for rigid
        choledochoscope
    H. symptom checklist
    H. telescope
hordein
hordeolum
Horizon prostatic stent
horizontal
    h. electrophoresis
    h. folds of rectum
    h. gastroplasty
    h. mattress suture
    h. transmission
hormonal
    h. downstaging
    h. therapy
hormone
    adrenocorticotropic h. (ACTH)
    h. antagonist
    antidiuretic h. (ADH)
    corticotropin-releasing h. (CRH)
    endothelium-derived relaxing h.
    enteric h.
    follicle-stimulating h. (FSH)
    gastrointestinal peptide h.
    gonadotropin-releasing h. (GnRH)
    gut h.
    human menopausal h.
    international unit of male h.
    luteinizing h. (LH)
    luteinizing hormone-follicle-
        stimulating h. (LH-FSH)
    luteinizing hormone-releasing h.
        (LHRH)
    parathyroid h. (PTH)
    peptide h.
    plasma parathyroid h. (PTH)
    h. receptor
    secosteroid h.
    thyroid h.
    thyrotropin-releasing h.
hormone-secreting tumor syndrome
hormone-stimulated cAMP synthesis

horn
    anterior h.
    H. sign
Horner syndrome
horseradish peroxidase-conjugated anti-
    rabbit IgG
horseshoe
    h. abscess
    h. anomaly of the pancreatic duct
    h. communication
    h. configuration
    h. fistula
    h. kidney
    h. track
Horsley
    H. anastomosis
    H. gastrectomy
    H. gastropexy
    H. pyloroplasty
    H. suture
hortobezoar
Horton-Devine
    H.-D. dermal graft
    H.-D. flip-flap hypospadias repair
    H.-D. operation
Hosemann forceps
hose-pipe appearance of terminal ileum
Hospal Biospal filter
The Hospital Anxiety and Depression
    Inventory
host
    h. factor
    immunocompetent h.
    immunocompromised h.
Hostaform plastic cylinder
hostility score
HOT
    Hypertension Optimal Treatment
    HOT trial
hot
    h. appendix
    h. biopsy
    h. biopsy forceps
    h. biopsy technique
    h. defect
    h. flexible forceps
    h. spot
    h. squeeze
    h. wire balloon
HOTC
    heterozygous ornithine transcarbamylase
Hounsfield unit (HU)
24-hour
    24-h. ambulatory esophageal pH
        monitoring
    24-h. ambulatory gastric pH
        monitor
    24-h. ambulatory manometry study

24-h. ambulatory pH-metry
24-h. ambulatory pH test
24-h. creatinine clearance
24-h. esophageal pH probe
24-h. fecal fat excretion
24-h. gastric acidity test
24-h. home pH-metry
24-h. intraesophageal pH study
24-h. urine collection

hourglass
h. constriction of gallbladder
h. deformity
h. narrowing
h. stomach
h. stricture

house
H. advancement anoplasty
H. flap

Housset-Debray gastroscope
Houston
H. muscle
valve of H.
H. valve

Howard test
Howel-Evans syndrome
Howell
H. needle
H. Rotatable BII papillotome

Howell-Jolly body
Howmedica slit catheter
Howship-Romberg sign
Ho:YAG
holmium:yttrium aluminum garnet

HP
heater probe
Helicobacter pylori
hereditary pancreatitis
hyperplastic polyp
Ku-Zyme HP
HP thermocoagulation

HPA
hypothalamic-pituitary-adrenal
hypothalamic-pituitary axis

HPC
hydrophilic-coated
HPC guidewire

HPC-1
hereditary prostate cancer 1 locus

Hp Chek screening system
HpD
hematoporphyrin derivative

HpD dye
low-dose HpD

hpf
high-power field

Hpfast rapid urease test
HPI
hepatic perfusion index
hepatocyte proliferation inhibitor

HPLC
high-performance liquid chromatography
high-pressure liquid chromatography

HPLO
Helicobacter pylori-like organism

HPN
home parenteral nutrition

HP-NAP
neutrophil-activating protein of
Helicobacter pylori

HPRC
hereditary papillary renal cancer
HPRC syndrome

HPS
hepatopulmonary syndrome
hypertrophic pyloric stenosis

HpSA
Premier Platinum HpSA
HpSA test

HPT
human proximal tubule
hyperparathyroidism

Hp-test
Jatrox Hp-t.

HPUS
hydrogen peroxide ultrasound

HPV
human papillomavirus

HPV 16
human papillomavirus 16

HPZ
high-pressure zone

H2RA
histamine-2 receptor antagonist
H2 receptor antagonist

HRARE
hybrid rapid acquisition with relaxation
enhancement

H-related protein
HRES
high-resolution endoluminal sonography

HRF
histamine-releasing factor

NOTES

H

HRF *(continued)*
    Maalox HRF
        heartburn relief formula
HRQOL
    health-related quality of life
HRS
    hepatorenal syndrome
HSC
    hepatic stellate cell
HSE
    hypertonic saline-epinephrine
        HSE solution
H-shaped
        H-s. ileal pouch-anal anastomosis
        H-s. tilt tag
HSK-tk
    herpes simplex virus thymidine kinase
HSP
    heat shock protein
HSP-70
        HSP-70 cDNA
        HSP-70 messenger ribonucleoprotein
        acid level
        HSP-70 mRNA
HSPG
    heparan sulfate proteoglycan
HSS
    hepatic stimulatory substance
HSV
    herpes simplex virus
5-HT
    5-hydroxytryptamine
    serotonin
        5-HT test
HT-29 cell
HTGL
    hepatic triglyceride lipase
H-thymidine
3H-thymidine
HTI
    hepatic tumor index
HTLV-I
    human T-cell leukemia virus of type I
        antibody to HTLV-I (anti-HTLV-I)
HTLV-I-associated myelopathy
H-type fistula
HU
    Hounsfield unit
Huan
    Jin Bu H.
Hueter maneuver
Hufford esophagoscope
Huggins operation
Huibregtse biliary stent
Huibregtse-Katon papillotome
Hulbert
    H. electrode

H. electrosurgical knife
H. endo-electrode set
Hulka clip
hum
    venous h.
human
    h. adenovirus 12
    h. albumin
    h. apo A-I DNA probe
    h. chorionic gonadotropin (HCG)
    h. chromosome 6
    h. cytochrome P-450 enzyme
    system
    h. cytotoxic T cell
    h. epidermal growth factor (h-EGF)
    h. erectile dysfunction
    h. fibronectin cDNA probe
    h. gastrin probe
    h. genome highlight
    h. glandular kallikrein 3
    h. glomerulus
    h. growth factor (HGF)
    h. gut bacterium
    h. hepatitis B immune globulin
    h. immunodeficiency virus (HIV)
    h. immunodeficiency virus-
    associated nephropathy (HIVAN)
    h. insulin
    h. intestinal epithelial Coco-2 cell
    h. kidney chloride channel gene
    h. leukocyte antigen (HLA)
    h. leukocyte antigen renal allograft
    h. lymphoblastoid interferon (L-
    IFN)
    h. lymphocyte chromosomal
    aberration test
    h. lyophilized dura cystoplasty
    h. menopausal gonadotropin
    h. menopausal hormone
    h. motilin receptor
    h. papillomavirus (HPV)
    h. papillomavirus 16 (HPV 16)
    h. PDGF receptor
    h. proximal tubule (HPT)
    h. recombinant erythropoietin
    h. recombinant TGF
    h. serum albumin
    h. serum I-FABP
    h. T-cell leukemia virus of type I
    (HTLV-I)
    h. T-cell lymphotrophic virus (type
    I, II)
    h. umbilical vein endothelial cell
    (HUVEC)
humanized monoclonal antibody
humeral neck
Humicade

humoral
    h. arm
    h. hypercalcemia of malignancy
        (HHM)
    h. immunity
    h. immunodeficiency disorder
hump
    diaphragmatic h.
    dromedary h.
hunger pain
hungry bone syndrome
Hunner
    H. interstitial cystitis
    H. stricture
    H. ulcer
hunt
    H. colostomy clamp
    H. test
hunterian chancre
Hunter line
Hunt-Lawrence pouch
Hunt-Limo-Basto gastric reservoir
Huppert-Cole test
Huppert test
Hurst
    H. bougienage
    H. bullet-tip dilator
    H. mercury bougie
    H. mercury-filled dilator
Hurst-Tucker pneumatic dilator
Hurst-type bougie
Hurwitz
    H. dialysis catheter
    H. esophageal clamp
    H. intestinal clamp
HUS
    hemolytic-uremic syndrome
husband
    artificial insemination h. (AIH)
Huschke ligament
husk
    ispaghula h.
Hutch diverticulum
Hutinel disease
HUVEC
    human umbilical vein endothelial cell
HV
    hepatic vein
H&V
    hemigastrectomy and vagotomy
HVA
    homovanillic acid

HVI-DHP
    hepatic venous isolation by direct
        hemoperfusion
HVOO
    hepatic venous outflow obstruction
HVPG
    hepatic venous pressure gradient
HVR1
    hypervariable region 1
HVS
    herpesvirus simplex
HWA 486
Hyalgan
hyalin
    alcoholic h.
    globular h.
hyaline
    h. arteriolar nephrosclerosis
    h. cast
    Mallory h.
hyalinized stroma
hyalinosis
    arteriolar h.
hyaluronan (HA)
hyaluronate
    sodium h.
hyaluronic
    h. acid
    h. acid concentration
hyaluronidase activity
hybridization
    dot-blot h.
    fluorescence in situ h. (FISH)
    nucleic acid h.
    quantitative liquid h.
    reverse dot h.
    sequence-sequence oligonucleotide h.
    in situ h.
    Southern blot h.
hybridoma-derived monoclonal antibody
**hybrid rapid acquisition with relaxation
    enhancement (HRARE)**
Hybritech
    H. method
    H. PSA scan
    H. Tandem prostate specific
        antigen assay
    H. Tandem PSA ratio test
    H. Tandem-R assay kit
    H. Tandem-R PSA assay
Hy-Cal calorie supplement
Hycamtin

NOTES

H

363

hycanthone mesylate
hydatid
   h. cyst
   h. cyst disease
   h. cyst intrahepatic rupture
   h. hooklet
   Morgagni h.
   h. resonance
   h. sand
hydatidiform mole
hydatidocele
hydatidosis
   renal h.
hydatidosus
   polypus h.
hydatiduria
Hydergine
Hyde shunt
Hydra
   H. Vision Es urological imaging
     system
   H. Vision IV urology system
   H. Vision Plus urological system
hydraeroperitoneum
hydragogue diuretic
hydralazine
hydramnios
   acute h.
hydrargyria, hydrargyrism
hydrate
   chloral h.
hydrated pyelogram
hydration
   intravenous h.
hydraulic
   h. abdominal concussion
   h. capillary infusion system
   h. hinge penile prosthesis
hydrazide hepatotoxicity
hydrazine sulfate
Hydrea
hydremic
   h. ascites
   h. nephritis
hydrepigastrium
hydrindantin
hydro
   Cutinova h.
   H. Plus coated guidewire
   H. Plus stent
hydroappendix
hydrobilirubin
hydrobromide
hydrocalix, hydrocalyx
hydrocalycosis
hydrocele
   abdominoscrotal h.
   communicating h.

   congenital h.
   cord h.
   Dupuytren h.
   encysted h.
   h. feminae
   filarial h.
   funicular h.
   Gibbon h.
   hernia h.
   Maunoir h.
   meconium h.
   h. muliebris
   noncommunicating h.
   Nuck h.
   postoperative h.
   h. repair
   simple h.
   h. wall
hydrocelectomy
   h. bottle procedure
   h. dartos pouch procedure
   h. plication technique
   h. scleral therapy
hydrocephalus
   normal-pressure h.
hydrochloric
   h. acid (HCl)
   h. acid secretion
   h. acid test
hydrochloride (HCl)
   alosetron h.
   amiloride h.
   amitriptyline h.
   bethanechol h.
   bupivacaine h.
   buspirone h.
   ciprofloxacin h.
   colestipol h.
   desipramine h.
   flavoxate h.
   fluoxetine h.
   glutamic acid h.
   hydroxyzine h.
   imipramine h.
   irinotecan h.
   lomefloxacin h.
   meperidine h.
   midazolam h.
   nefazodone h.
   oxyphencyclimine h.
   papaverine h.
   phenazopyridine h.
   phenoxybenzamine h.
   pramoxine h.
   prazosin h.
   procaine h.
   propoxyphene h.
   pseudoephedrine h.

quinine urea h.
ranitidine h.
sevelamer h.
tetracycline h.
thioridazine h.
tocainide h.
tolazoline h.
vancomycin h.
yohimbine h.
hydrochlorothiazide (HCTZ)
h. and reserpine
h. and spironolactone
h. and triamterene
hydrochlorothiazide-triamterene (HCTZ-TA)
hydrocholecystis
hydrocholeretic drug
Hydrocil Instant
hydrocirsocele
hydrocodone
hydrocolpos
hydrocortisone
1% h.
h. acetate
h. acetate rectal aerosol
h. enema
h. foam
Hydrocortone Acetate
hydrodilation
hydrodistention
bladder h.
HydroDIURIL
hydrodynamics
collapsible tube h.
distensible h.
Hydroflex
H. penile implant
H. penile prosthesis
H. sphincter
hydroflumethiazide
hydrogen
h. adenosine triphosphatase
h. breath test
h. gas
h. gas clearance
h. gas clearance technique
h. ion
h. ion production
h. peroxide
h. peroxide enema
h. peroxide ultrasound (HPUS)

hydrography
MR h.
hydrohematonephrosis
hydrohepatosis
hydrolase
carboxylic ester h. (CEH)
lactase-phlorizin h. (LPH)
hydrolysis
intragastric h.
urea h.
hydrolyze
hydrolyzed whey formula
Hydromer
H. coated polyurethane stent
H. grafted catheter
hydrometrocolpos
hydromorphone
Hydromox
Hydromox-R
hydronephrosis
bilateral h.
prenatal fetal h.
h. in utero
hydronephrotic
hydropancreatosis
Hydro-Par
hydroperinephrosis
hydroperitoneum, hydroperitonia
hydroperoxide
lipid h.
hydrophila
Aeromonas h.
hydrophilic
h. polymer-coated steerable guidewire
h. wire
hydrophilic-coated (HPC)
h.-c. guidewire
hydrophilicity
hydrophobic binding region
hydrophone
Imotec needle h.
needle h.
hydropic nephrosis
hydropigenous nephritis
hydropneumoperitoneum
hydropneumothorax
Hydropres
Hydropres-25
Hydropres-50
hydrops
h. abdominis

NOTES

H

hydrops *(continued)*
    gallbladder h.
    nonimmune h.
hydropyonephrosis
hydrorchis
hydrosarcocele
hydroscheocele
Hydro-Serp
Hydroserpine
hydrostatic
    h. balloon
    h. balloon catheter
    h. balloon dilation
    h. decompression
    h. pressure
    h. pressure therapy
hydrothorax
    cirrhotic h.
    hepatic h.
Hydro-T Tabs
hydroureter
hydroureteronephrosis
hydroureterosis
hydrouria
Hydroxacen
hydroxide
    aluminum h.
    ammonium h.
    magnesium h.
hydroxyapatite
6-hydroxybenzoate
hydroxychloroquine
18-hydroxycorticosterone
18-hydroxycortisol
hydroxyeicosatetraenoic
    h. acid (HETE)
    20-h. acid
5-hydroxyindoleacetic acid (5-HIAA)
hydroxyindoleacetic acid (HIAA)
hydroxyl
    h. group
    h. radical
    h. radical scavenger
hydroxylamine
hydroxylase
    17-alpha-h. deficiency
    11-beta-h. deficiency
hydroxylated vitamin D
hydroxyl-free radical
3-hydroxy 3-methylglutaric aciduria
hydroxyquinoline
hydroxystilbamidine
5-hydroxytryptamine (5-HT)
hydroxyurea
25-hydroxyvitamin
    25-h. D
    25-h. D3 (25(OH)D3)
    25-h. D level

hydroxyzine hydrochloride
hydruria
hydruric
hygiene
    perianal h.
Hygroton
hymen
    imperforate h.
hymenal band
hymenolepiasis
Hymenolepis
    H. diminuta
    H. nana
hymenotomy
hyodeoxycholate
hyodysenteriae
    Serpulina h.
hyointestinalis
    Campylobacter h.
hyoscine butylbromide
Hyoscine-N-Butylbromide
hyoscyamine
    sublingual h.
    h. sulfate
Hyosophen
hypanakinesia, hypanakinesis
Hypaque
    H. contrast medium
    H. enema
    H. swallow
hypazoturic nephropathy
hyperabduction
hyperabsorption
hyperacid
hyperacidity
    gastric h.
hyperactive
    h. bowel sounds
    h. rectosigmoid junction
hyperactivity
    detrusor h.
hyperacute
    h. graft-versus-host disease
    h. liver failure (HALF)
    h. rejection
hyperadiposis
hyperaldosteronism
    familial h.
    primary h.
    secondary h.
hyperalgesia
    colonic h.
    selective jejunal h.
    visceral h.
hyperalimentation
    central h.
    intravenous h. (IVH)

parenteral h.
peripheral h.
hyperalimentosis
hyperalkalinity
hyperaminoaciduria
hyperammonemia
hyperammonemic syndrome
hyperamylasemia
hyperandrogenism
hyperbaric
h. oxygen
h. oxygen chamber
h. oxygen therapy (HBOT)
h. oxygen toxicity
hyperbetalipoproteinemia
familial h.
hyperbilirubinemia
congenital h.
conjugated h.
constitutional h.
familial unconjugated h.
idiopathic unconjugated h.
neonatal conjugated h.
unconjugated h.
hypercalcemia
familial hypocalciuric h. (FHH)
glucocorticoid-induced h.
iatrogenic h.
h. of malignancy
hypercalcemic
h. nephrolithiasis
h. nephropathy
hypercalciuria
absorptive h.
idiopathic h. (IH)
renal h.
resorptive h.
hypercaloric diet
hypercarbia
hypercatabolic
hypercatharsis
hypercathartic
hypercellularity
glomerular h.
interstitial h.
mesangial h.
hyperchloremia
hyperchloremic metabolic acidosis
hyperchlorhydria
hypercholecystokininemia
hypercholesterolemia
familial h.

hypercholesterolemic cadaveric renal transplant
hypercholia
hyperchromatic nucleus
hyperchylia
hyperchylomicronemia
familial h.
hypercoagulability
hypercoagulable state
hypercontinence
hypercontinent
hypercontractile external sphincter response
hyperdense
hyperdibasic aminoaciduria
hyperdiploidy
hyperdistention
hyperdiuresis
hyperdopaminemia
hyperdynamic
h. circulation
h. ileus
h. precordium
h. syndrome
hypereccrisia
hypereccritic
hyperechoic
h. shadowing
h. spot
h. stranding
hyperemesis
h. gravidarum
h. hiemis
hyperemetic
hyperemia
gastric h.
glans h.
postprandial portal h.
reactive h.
splanchnic h.
hyperemic
h. border zone
h. mucosa
hypereosinophilia syndrome
hyperesthesia
cutaneous h.
gustatory h.
hyperesthetic
hyperfibrinogenemia
hyperfiltration
capillary h.
glomerular h.

NOTES

H

hyperfiltration *(continued)*
 h. injury
 renal h.
 h. theory
hyperfractionated radiation therapy
hyperfunction
 adrenal cortex h.
 antral gastrin cell h.
 gastrin cell h.
hyperganglionosis
hypergastrinemia
 clinical h.
 h. with acid hypersecretion
hypergenitalism
hyperglobulinemic hepatitis
hyperglycemia
hyperglycemic clamping
hypergonadotropic hypogonadism
HyperHep
hyperhepatia
hyperhidrosis
hyperhomocystinemia
hyperhydrochloria
hyperinfection
hyperingestion
hyperinsulinemia
 euglycemic h.
hyperinsulinism
 alimentary h.
hyperkalemia
hyperkaluria
hyperkeratosis
 esophageal h.
 h. palmaris et plantaris
hyperkinesia
 esophageal h.
hyperkinesis
 paroxysmal anal h.
hyperleydigism
hyperlipidemia
 carbohydrate-induced h.
 combined fat- and carbohydrate-
  induced h.
 familial fat-induced h.
 idiopathic h.
 mixed h.
hyperlipoproteinemia
 acquired h.
 familial h. (type I–V)
hyperlithic
hyperlithuria
hypermagnesemia
hypermetabolic state
hypermobile kidney
hypermobility
 bladder neck h.
 urethral h.
hypermotility

hypernatremia
 hypervolemic h.
hypernephritis
hypernephroid
hypernephroma
hypernephronia
hypernutrition
hyperorchidism
hyperorexia
hyperosmolar
 h. liquid
 h. perfusate
hyperosmolarity
 extracellular h.
hyperosmotic
 h. feeding
 h. laxative
 h. nonketotic dehydration
 h. urine
hyperoxaluria
 absorptive h.
 acquired h.
 enteric h.
 idiopathic h.
 mild h.
 primary h. type I (PH-I)
 primary h. type II
hyperoxaluric stone
hyperpancreaorrhea
hyperpancreatism
hyperpancreorrhea
hyperparathyroidism (HPT)
 primary h. (PrHPT)
 secondary h.
 tertiary h.
hyperpepsia
hyperpepsinemia
hyperpepsinia
hyperpepsinogenemia
hyperpeptic gastritis
hyperperfusion
hyperperistalsis
hyperphagia
 weight loss with h.
hyperphagic
hyperphosphate ion-urea
hyperphosphatemia
hyperpipecolatemia
hyperplasia
 adenomatous h. (AH)
 adrenal zona glomerulosa h.
 antral G-cell h.
 atypical adenomatous h. (AAH)
 benign prostatic h. (BPH)
 biliary epithelia h.
 bilobar h.
 Brunner gland h.
 colonic nodular lymphoid h.

congenital adrenal h. (CAH)
crypt h.
diffuse nodular h. (DNH)
ductal epithelial h.
duodenal lymphonodular h.
ECL cell h.
ECL hypertrophy and h.
fibromuscular h.
flat h.
focal lymphoid h. (FLH)
focal nodular h. (FNH)
follicular lymphoid h.
foveolar h.
G-cell h.
goblet cell h.
incomplete basal cell h.
insulin h.
intimal h.
islet cell h.
lymphoid nodular h.
lymphonodular h.
median lobe h.
mesonephric h.
mesothelial h. (MH)
myointimal h.
neointimal h.
nodular h.
nodular lymphoid h. (NLH)
nodular h. of prostate
nodular regenerative h. (NRH)
nonantral endocrine cell h.
papillary h.
parathyroid h.
polypoid gastric rugal h.
polypoid lymphoid h.
polypoid lymphomatous h.
postatrophic h.
prostate gland benign h.
prostatic h.
Rokitansky-Aschoff sinus h.
symptomatic benign prostatic h.
trilobar h.
hyperplasiogenic polyp
hyperplasmic obesity
hyperplastic
h. adenomatous polyp
h. arteriolar nephrosclerosis
h. cholecystosis
h. dystrophy
h. epithelial gastric polyp
h. foveolar epithelium
h. gastric polyp

h. nodule
h. obesity
h. polyp (HP)
h. polyposis
hyperplasticity
hyperpolarization
membrane h.
hyperprebetalipoproteinemia
familial h.
hyperprochoresis
hyperprolactinemia
hyperproliferation
hyperproteinemia
hyperproteosis
hyperprotidic diet
hyperpyrexia
hyperreflexia
autonomic h.
detrusor h.
neurogenic h.
hyperreflexic
h. bladder
h. motor urge incontinence
hyperreninemia
hyperreninemic
hyperresonance
hyperresonant abdomen
hyperresponsiveness
hyperrugosity
hypersalivation
hypersecreting tumor
hypersecretion
acid h.
cortisol h.
gastric h.
hypergastrinemia with acid h.
h. obstruction hypothesis
salivary h.
hypersensitive esophagus
hypersensitivity
h. angiitis
antiepileptic drug h. (AHS)
cholestatic h.
delayed-type h. (DTH)
paraaminosalicylate h.
phenindione h.
h. reaction
visceral h.
hypersplenism
hypersthenuria
hyperstimulation
hypersuprarenalism

NOTES

H

369

hypertension
    accelerated h.
    African-American Study of Kidney Disease and H. (AASK)
    allograft-mediated h.
    angiotensin-dependent h.
    dietary approach to stop h. (DASH)
    ductal h.
    extrahepatic portal venous h.
    glomerular capillary h.
    Goldblatt h.
    idiopathic portal h. (IPH)
    intraglomerular h.
    intrahepatic portal h.
    isolated systolic h. (ISH)
    lithotripsy-induced h.
    noncirrhotic portal h.
    H. Optimal Treatment (HOT)
    H. Optimal Treatment trial
    pancreatic ductal h.
    portal h. (PHT)
    presinusoidal intrahepatic portal h.
    refractory h.
    renal h.
    renin-mediated renovascular h.
    renovascular h.
    h. resistance axis
    salt-sensitive h.
    secondary h.
    splenoportal h.
    systemic h.
hypertensive
    h. autosomal dominant polycystic kidney disease
    h. end-organ damage
    h. gastropathy
    h. lower esophageal sphincter
    h. lower esophageal sphincter syndrome
    h. nephrosclerosis (HN)
    h. renal injury
hypertestosteronism
hyperthermia
    malignant h.
    microwave h.
    transrectal prostatic h. (TPH)
hyperthyroidism
hyperthyroxinemia
hypertonia
    anal canal h.
hypertonic
    h. bladder
    h. crystalloid
    h. infusion
    h. saline
    h. saline-epinephrine (HSE)
    h. saline-epinephrine solution

hypertonicity
hypertransaminasemia
    cryptogenic h.
hypertrichosis lanuginosa acquisita
hypertriglyceridemia
    familial h.
hypertrophic
    h. cirrhosis
    h. gastropathy
    h. lymphocytic gastritis (HLG)
    h. obesity
    h. osteoarthropathy
    h. pyloric stenosis (HPS)
    h. pylorus
hypertrophy
    benign prostatic h. (BPH)
    Billroth h.
    bilobar h.
    h. of column of Bertin
    compensatory testicular h.
    crypt h.
    gastroduodenal h.
    glomerular h.
    muscle h.
    prostatic h.
    renal h.
    renovascular h.
    rugal h.
    symptomatic benign prostatic h.
    trilobar h.
hypertyrosinemia
hyperuricemia
hyperuricosuria
hyperuricuria
hypervariable
    h. deoxyribonucleic acid
    h. region 1 (HVR1)
hypervolemia
hypervolemic hypernatremia
hyphema
hyphemia
    intertropical h.
    tropical h.
Hypnovel
%HYPO
    percentage of hypochromic red cell
hypoacidity
    luminal h.
hypoactive bowel sounds
hypoactivity
hypoalbuminemia
hypoalbuminemic patient
hypoaldosteronism
    hyporeninemic h.
    isolated h.
hypoalimentation
hypoandrogenism
hypobetalipoproteinemia

hypobicarbonatemia
hypocalcemia
    asymptomatic h.
    familial hypocalciuric h.
hypocapnia
hypochloremia
hypochloremic hypokalemic metabolic alkalosis
hypochlorhydria
    epidemic h.
    gastric h.
hypochlorhydric cirrhosis
hypochloruric nephropathy
hypocholia
hypochondria (*pl. of* hypochondrium)
hypochondriac
    h. fossa
    h. region
hypochondriacal patient
hypochondriasis
hypochondrium, pl. **hypochondria**
hypochromic
    h. microcytic anemia
    h. red cell
hypochylia
hypocitraturia
hypocomplementemia
hypocontractile detrusor
hypocontractility
    detrusor h.
hypocystotomy
hypodiaphragmatic
hypodiploidy
hypoeccrisis
hypoeccritic
hypoechoic
    h. cancer
    h. lesion
    h. periphery
    h. ringed layer
    h. thickening
hypoesthesia
    gustatory h.
hypoestrogenic urethritis
hypoestrogenism
hypofibrinogenemia
hypofunction
hypogammaglobulinemia
hypogammaglobulinemic
hypoganglionosis of colon
hypogastric
    h. artery

    h. artery aneurysm
    h. fiber
    h. nerve
    h. node
    h. papillary zone
    h. plexus
    h. region
    h. vessel
hypogastrium
hypogastrocele
hypogastroschisis
hypogenetic nephritis
hypogenitalism
hypogeusia
hypoglycemia
    alcohol-induced h.
    postprandial h.
hypoglycin
    acetyl coenzyme h. A
hypogonadal state
hypogonadism
    hypergonadotropic h.
    hypogonadotropic h.
hypogonadotropic hypogonadism
hypohepatia
hypohydrochloria
hypokalemia
    diuretic-induced h.
hypokalemic
    h. metabolic alkalosis
    h. nephropathy
    h. nephrosis
    h. renal tubular acidosis
hypokaluria
hypolactasia
    adult h.
hypoleydigism
hypomagnesemia
hypomagnesuria
hypometabolic
hypometabolism
hypomethylation
    DNA h.
hypomotility
    esophageal h.
    gastric h.
hypomyxia
hyponatremia
    dilutional h.
    thiazide-induced h.
hypoorchidism
hypoosmotic urine

NOTES

hypopancreatism
hypopancreorrhea
hypoparathyroidism
hypopepsia
hypopepsinia
hypoperfusion
    renal h.
hypoperistalsis syndrome
hypoperistaltic
hypopharyngeal
    h. cancer
    h. diverticulum
hypopharynx
hypophosphatasia
hypophosphatemia
    X-linked h. (XLH)
hypophosphatemic rickets
hypophosphaturia
hypophrenic
hypophysectomy
hypoplasia
    bile duct h.
    bladder h.
    congenital h.
    corpus spongiosum h.
    erythroid h.
    exocrine pancreatic h.
    germ cell h.
    intrahepatic biliary duct h.
    oligonephronic h.
    prostate gland h.
    thymic h.
    unilateral renal h.
hypoplastic
    h. blind-ending spermatic vessel
    h. glomerulocystic disease
    h. kidney
hypoposia
hypoproteinemia
hypoproteinosis
hypoprothrombinemia
hypopyon
hyporeninemic hypoaldosteronism
hyporesponsiveness
    cardiac beta-adrenoreceptor h.
    erythropoietin h.
hypospadiac
hypospadias
    anterior h.
    balanic h.
    complex h.
    concealed h.
    coronal h.
    female h.
    glanular h.
    middle h.
    penile h.
    penoscrotal h.

    perineal h.
    posterior h.
    pseudovaginal perineoscrotal h.
    scrotal h.
    subcoronal h.
hypospermatogenesis
hyposplenism
hypostasis
hypostatic
hyposthenuria
    renal h.
hyposuprarenalism
hypotension
    dialysis-associated h.
    hemorrhagic h.
    intradialytic h. (IDH)
    systemic h.
hypotestosteronism
hypothalamic-pituitary-adrenal (HPA)
hypothalamic-pituitary axis (HPA)
hypothalamic-pituitary-testicular-penile
    axis
hypothalamic suppression
hypothalamus
hypothenar eminence
hypothermia
    gastric h.
    intraoperative kidney h.
    renal h.
hypothermic
    h. effect
    h. pulsatile perfusion
    h. storage
hypothesis
    affinity-avidity h.
    hypersecretion obstruction h.
    Keller h.
hypothyroidism
hypotonia
    rectal h.
hypotonic
    h. bladder
    h. duodenography
hypouremia
hypouresis
hypouricemia
hypouricuria
hypourocrinia
hypoventilation
    benzodiazepine-induced h.
    sedation-induced h.
hypovolemia
    nephrosis with h.
    nephrosis without h.
    watery diarrhea, hypokalemia,
      and h. (WDHH)
hypovolemic
    h. anemia

h. shock
h. variance
hypoxanthine guanine phosphoribosyltransferase deficiency
hypoxemia
hypoxia
hepatic h.
pericentral h.
hypoxia-induced rhabdomyolysis
Hypoxis rooperi
Hyrtl sphincter
hysterectomy
hysteresis
hysterical vomiting

hystericus
globus h.
hysterocele
hysterocystopexy
hysterosacropexy
Ivalon sponge h.
polyvinyl alcohol sponge h.
hysterosalpingectomy
laparoscopic h.
hysteroscopy
Hy-Tape
Hytrin Dosepak
Hyzine-50

NOTES

H

I-125, ¹²⁵**I**
    iodine-125
        I-125 iothalamate clearance
        ProstaSeed I-125
I-131
    iodine-131
I1307K allele
IA
    intraarterial
I-alpha-hydroxyvitamin D3
IAS
    internal anal sphincter
    intraabdominal sepsis
iatrogenic
    i. chymobilia
    i. coagulopathy
    i. colitis
    i. enterocele
    i. hypercalcemia
    i. hypercalcemic nephrolithiasis
    i. immunodeficiency syndrome
    i. malabsorption
    i. pancreatic trauma
    i. pneumothorax
    i. prostatourethral-rectal fistula
    i. rectourethral fistula
    i. tumor perforation
    i. urinary lithiasis
IBB
    intestinal brush border
IBC
    iron-binding capacity
IBD
    inflammatory bowel disease
IBDQ
    Inflammatory Bowel Disease
      Questionnaire
IBS
    inflammatory bowel syndrome
    irritable bowel syndrome
ibuprofen
IBW
    ideal body weight
IC
    indeterminate colitis
    intracisternal
    irritable colon
IC351
ICA
    ileocolic anastomosis
      ICA test
ICAM-1
    intercellular adhesion molecule-1
ICC
    interstitial cells of Cajal

ice
    i. cooling
    i. slush
    i. water test
iced
    i. intestine
    i. lactated Ringer solution
    i. saline
    i. saline lavage
IceSeeds
ice-water swallow
ICF
    intracellular fluid
ICG
    indocyanine green dye
      ICG clearance
      ICG test
IC-GN
    immune complex glomerulonephritis
ICGN
    ICR strain-derived glomerular nephritis
ichthyismus exanthematicus
ICIT
    intracavernosal injection therapy
ICL
    intracorporeal laser lithotripsy
ICP
    intrahepatic cholestasia of pregnancy
ICR strain-derived glomerular nephritis (ICGN)
ICS
    International Continence Society
ICSF
    idiopathic calcium (renal) stone
      formation
ICSI
    intracytoplasmic sperm injection
ICT
    isolated cortical tubule
ictal
icteric
    i. necrosis
    i. sclerae
    i. skin
icterogenic
icterohepatitis
icteroid
icterus
    benign familial i.
    conjunctival i.
    i. gravidarum
    i. gravis
    Hayem i.
    i. melas
    i. neonatorum

icterus *(continued)*
    i. praecox
    scleral i.
ictometer
ictus
ID
    inner diameter
    intraduodenal
I&D
    incision and drainage
IDA
    iminodiacetic acid
idarubicin
IDD
    intraluminal duodenal diverticulum
IDDM
    insulin-dependent diabetes mellitus
IDE
    insulin-degrading enzyme
ideal body weight (IBW)
identification
    colonic lesion i.
    lesion i.
IDH
    intradialytic hypotension
    intramural duodenal hematoma
idiopathic
    i. achalasia
    i. adulthood ductopenia
    i. ascites
    i. autoimmune cholangitis
    i. autoimmune chronic hepatitis
    i. bile acid malabsorption
    i. calcium (renal) stone formation (ICSF)
    i. chronic erosion
    i. chronic erosive gastritis
    i. colitis
    i. constipation
    i. crescentic glomerulonephritis
    i. diffuse ulcerative nongranulomatous enteritis
    i. edema
    i. enteropathy
    i. esophageal ulcer (IEU)
    i. fibrosing pancreatitis
    i. fibrous retroperitonitis
    i. gastric acid secretion
    i. gastroparesis
    i. hematuria
    i. hemochromatosis
    i. hypercalciuria (IH)
    i. hypereosinophilic syndrome (IHES)
    i. hyperlipidemia
    i. hyperoxaluria
    i. hypertrophic gastropathy
    i. hypertrophic pyloric stenosis

    i. hypocomplementemic interstitial nephritis
    i. infertility
    i. inflammatory bowel disease (IIBD)
    i. intestinal pseudoobstruction
    i. megacolon
    i. megarectum
    i. membranous glomerulonephritis
    i. nephralgia
    i. nephrotic syndrome
    i. obstruction
    i. portal hypertension (IPH)
    i. proctitis
    i. proctocolitis
    i. rapidly progressive glomerulonephritis (IRPGN)
    i. recurrent pancreatitis (IRP)
    i. retroperitoneal fibrosis
    i. steatorrhea
    i. thrombocytopenic purpura
    i. unconjugated hyperbilirubinemia
    i. varix
    i. volvulus
idiotype-anti-idiotype interaction
idioventricular
IDL
    intermediate-density lipoprotein
IDPN
    intradialytic parenteral nutrition
IDST
    intraductal secretin test
IDUS
    intraductal ultrasonography
    intraductal ultrasound
IDWG
    interdialytic weight gain
IEBD
    intraesophageal balloon distention
IEC-6 cell
IED
    immune-enhancing diet
IEHL
    intracorporeal electrohydraulic lithotripsy
IEL
    intestinal epithelial cell
    intraepithelial leukocyte
    intraepithelial lymphocyte
        IEL T cell
IEM
    ineffective esophageal motility
IEU
    idiopathic esophageal ulcer
IF
    intrinsic factor
I-FABP
    intestinal fatty acid-binding protein
        human serum I-FABP

I

IFE
    immunofixation electrophoresis
Ifex, Taxol, Platinol (ITP)
IFN-alpha
    interferon-alfa
        IFN-alpha therapy
IFN-alpha-2b therapy
IFN-gamma
    interferon-gamma
IFOBT
    immunological fecal occult blood test
IFP
    inflammatory fibroid polyp
IG
    image guide
    intragastric
        IG bundle
Ig
    immunoglobulin
IgA
    immunoglobulin A
        IgA deficiency
        dimeric IgA
        IgA EMA
        endomysial IgA
        gliadin IgA
        IgA glomerulonephritis
        IgA immunological study
        jejunal IgA
        IgA kappa chain myeloma
        IgA nephropathy
        IgA neuropathy
        IgA polymerization
        secretory IgA (sIgA)
        IgA tTG
        IgA tTG assay
IgA1
    immunoglobulin A1
IgA2
    immunoglobulin A2
IgA-antigliadin
IgA-producing cell
IGCCCG
    International Germ Cell Cancer
      Collaborative Group
        IGCCCG classification
IgD
    immunoglobulin D
IgE
    immunoglobulin E
IGF
    insulinlike growth factor

IGF-1
    insulinlike growth factor-1
        exogenous IGF-1
IGF-2
    insulinlike growth factor-2
IGF-binding protein-1 mRNA
IGFBP-1
    insulinlike growth factor-binding protein-
      1
IGF-BP3 complex
IGF-1R
        IGF-1R mRNA
        IGF-1R RNA
IgG
    immunoglobulin G
        IgG AGA
        IgG alpha-gliadin antibody
        IgG anti-HAV-positive
        horseradish peroxidase-conjugated
          anti-rabbit IgG
        IgG immunological study
        polyclonal IgG
        IgG reticulin antibody
        IgG serology
IgG1
    immunoglobulin G1
IgG2a
    immunoglobulin G2a
        IgG2a antibody
IgG-producing cell
Iglesias
        I. fiberoptic resectoscope
        I. method of aspiration
IgM
    immunoglobulin M
        IgM anti-HAV
        IgM anti-HAV antibody
        IgM anti-HBc antibody
        anti-*Helicobacter pylori* IgM
        IgM immunological study
        monoclonal IgM
        IgM nephropathy
IgM-antigliadin
IgM-HA antibody
IgM-HEV antibody titer
IGP
    injection gold probe
IGV
    isolated gastric varices (type 1, 2)
IH
    idiopathic hypercalciuria
    inguinal hernia

NOTES

IHA
  indirect hemagglutination
  intrahepatic atresia
    IHA determination
IHb
  hemoglobin content index
IHD
  intermittent hemodialysis
IHES
  idiopathic hypereosinophilic syndrome
IHPS
  infantile hypertrophic pyloric stenosis
IIBD
  idiopathic inflammatory bowel disease
IIEF
  International Index of Erectile Function
[^{123}I]IMP
  iodoamphetamine
[^{123}I]iodoamphetamine radionuclide
IJ
  intrajejunal
IkBa protein
IL
  ileum
  interleukin
IL-1
  interleukin-1
IL-2
  interleukin-2
    IL-2 receptor
IL-6
  interleukin-6
    IL-6 receptor
IL-8
  interleukin-8
    IL-8 receptor
IL-10
  interleukin-10
    recombinant IL-10
IL-3 receptor
IL-4 receptor
ILA surgical stapler
ILC
  interstitial laser coagulation
ILDL
  intermediate low-density lipoprotein
ileac
ileal
  i. artery
  i. artery stent
  i. atresia
  i. biopsy
  i. bladder
  i. blood vessel
  i. brake
  i. conduit urinary diversion
  i. crypt
  i. duplication cyst
  i. effluent
  i. follicle
  i. ileoscopy
  i. inflow tract
  i. interposition
  i. intestinal antireflux valve
  i. J-pouch
  i. loop
  i. loopography
  i. low-pressure bladder substitute pouch
  i. Malone cecostomy
  i. neobladder
  i. neobladder urinary diversion
  i. neobladder urinary pouch
  i. nipple valve
  i. orthotopic bladder substitute
  i. outflow tract
  i. papilla
  i. patch ureteroplasty
  i. pouch-anal anastomosis (IPAA)
  i. pouch-distal rectal anastomosis
  i. pull-through
  i. reflux
  i. resection (IR)
  i. reservoir
  i. reservoir construction
  i. reservoir evacuation
  i. segment (IS)
  i. sleeve
  i. S-pouch
  i. spout
  i. stasis
  i. ureter
  i. ureteral substitution
  i. urinary conduit
  i. varix
  i. W-pouch
ilealis
  frenulum valvae i.
  ostium valvae i.
  papilla i.
  valva i.
ileectomy
ilei
  arteriae i.
ileitis
  backwash i.
  Crohn i.
  distal i.
  granulomatous i.
  Meckel i.
  obstructive dysfunctional i.
  pouch i.
  prestomal i.
  regional i. (RI)
  terminal i.

ileoanal
   i. anastomosis
   i. endorectal pull-through
   i. pouch
   i. pull-through procedure
   i. reservoir
ileoascending colostomy
ileocaecalis
   frenulum valvae i.
   papilla i.
   valva i.
ileocecal
   i. bladder
   i. continent urinary reservoir
   i. cutaneous diversion
   i. fat pad
   i. insufficiency
   i. intestinal antireflux valve
   i. intussusception
   i. junction
   i. papilla
   i. pouch
   i. region
   i. resection
   i. segment
   i. segment transposition
   i. sphincter
   i. syndrome
   i. tuberculosis
   i. ureterosigmoidostomy
ileocecale
   ostium i.
ileocecalis
   plica i.
ileocecocystoplasty bladder augmentation
ileocecostomy
ileococcygeus muscle
ileocolectomy
ileocolic
   i. anastomosis (ICA)
   i. artery
   i. disease
   i. fold
   i. intussusception
   i. plexus
   i. resection
   i. urinary diversion
   i. vessel
ileocolica
   arteria i.
ileocolitis
   Crohn i.

   transmural i.
   tuberculous i.
   i. ulcerosa chronica
ileocolonic
   i. bladder
   i. Crohn disease
   i. neobladder
   i. pouch
   i. pouch urinary diversion
   i. transit
ileocolonoscopy
ileocolostomy
   end-loop i.
   LeDuc-Camey i.
ilcocolotomy
ileoconduit
ileocystoplasty
   Camey i.
   clam i.
   LeDuc-Camey i.
ileocystostomy
   cutaneous i.
ileoentectropy
ileogastric reflex
ileogastrostomy
ileogram
ileography
   endoscopic retrograde i.
ileoileal intussusception
ileoileostomy
ileojejunitis
ileopexy
ileoproctostomy (IP)
ileorectal anastomosis (IRA)
ileorectostomy
ileorenal bypass
ileorrhaphy
ileoscopy
   ileal i.
ileosigmoid
   i. anastomosis
   i. colostomy
   i. fistula
   i. knot
ileosigmoidostomy
ileostogram
ileostomate
ileostomist
ileostomy
   i. bag
   Bishop-Koop i.
   blow-hole i.

NOTES

ileostomy *(continued)*
> Brooke i.
> i. closure
> continent i.
> i. cup
> Dennis-Brooke i.
> i. diarrhea
> diversionary i.
> diverting loop i.
> double-barrel i.
> i. effluent
> end i.
> end-loop i.
> Goligher extraperitoneal i.
> incontinent i.
> J-loop i.
> Kock continent i.
> Kock reservoir i.
> loop i. (LI)
> loop end i.
> mucosal i.
> permanent loop i.
> pouched i.
> i. rod
> split i.
> i. stoma
> temporary loop i.
> terminal i.
> Turnbull end-loop i.

ileotomy
ileotransverse
> i. colon anastomosis
> i. colostomy

ileotransversostomy
ileoureteric stenosis
ileovesical
> i. anastomosis
> i. fistula

ileovesicostomy
> incontinent i.
> traverse retubularized i.
> Yang-Monti i.

ILE-SORB absorbent gel
ileum (IL)
> antimesenteric border of distal i.
> collapsed i.
> duplex i.
> hose-pipe appearance of terminal i.
> neoterminal i.
> i. nipple
> terminal i.

ileus
> adhesive i.
> adynamic i.
> colonic i.
> dynamic i.
> focal i.
> gallbladder i.

> gallstone i.
> gastric i.
> hyperdynamic i.
> mechanical i.
> meconium i.
> occlusive i.
> paralytic i.
> i. paralyticus
> postoperative i.
> spastic i.
> i. subparta
> terminal i.
> verminous i.

iLEX skin protectant paste
ilia (*pl. of* ilium)
iliac
> i. artery
> i. artery aneurysm
> i. artery embolization
> i. bend
> i. colon
> i. crest
> i. fossa
> i. roll
> i. spine
> i. vein

iliac-to-renal artery bypass graft
iliacus muscle
iliococcygeus muscle
iliocolotomy
iliofemoral triangle
iliohypogastric nerve
ilioinguinal
> i. nerve
> i. ring

iliopectineal line
iliopsoas
> i. ring
> i. sign
> i. test

^{131}I-lipiodol isotope
ilium, pl. **ilia**
ILL
> intracorporeal laser lithotripsy

illness
> food-borne i. (FBI)

illuminated St. Mark's retractor
illumination system
Ilopan
iloprost
Ilosone
Ilozyme
ILS
> intraluminal stapler

ILUS
> intraluminal ultrasound
>> ILUS catheter

IM
 Rocephin IM
IMA
 inferior mesenteric artery
image
 i. analysis
 axial i.
 B-mode ultrasound i.
 i. cytometry
 i. guide (IG)
 i. guide bundle
 HAP i.
 longitudinal i.
 point-counting i.
 i. processing
 sagittal i.
 transverse i.
 T1-weighted i.
 T2-weighted i.
Imagent GI
image-processing unit
imager
 Tesla Signa MR i.
imaging
 anorectal i.
 bladder i.
 B-mode i.
 color flow i.
 color flow Doppler i.
 Doppler color flow i.
 endoanal magnetic resonance i.
 endorectal coil magnetic
  resonance i.
 endoscopic ultrasonographic i.
 functional magnetic resonance i.
  (fMRI)
 gallium i.
 GNG phase i.
 gray scale i.
 LaparoScan laparoscopic
  ultrasonic i.
 magnetic resonance i. (MRI)
 nuclear hepatobiliary i.
 parathyroid i.
 planar i.
 radiolabeled i.
 radionuclide renal i.
 renal helical CT i.
 RHCT i.
 sonoelasticity i.
 technetium i.
 thallium i.

 thermal i.
 transcutaneous ultrasound i.
 uniplanar i.
imbalance
 acid base i.
imbedded microtransducer
imbricate
IMCD
 inner medullary collecting duct
IMED 430 enteral feeding pump
Imerslund syndrome
imidazole aminoaciduria
imidazolecarboxamide
imidoacetic acid radioactive agent
imiglucerase
iminodiacetic acid (IDA)
iminoglycinuria
imipenem
imipenem-cilastatin
imipramine hydrochloride
imiquimod
immature teratoma
immediate blush
immersion
 i. cooling
 water i.
immitis
 Candida i.
immotile cilia syndrome
ImmTher
Immu-4
Immudia-HemSp
immune
 i. complex glomerulonephritis (IC-
  GN)
 i. deficiency
 i. electron microscopy
 i. response
 i. serum (IS)
 i. serum globulin
 i. suppression
 i. system
immune-enhancing diet (IED)
immune-mediated
 i.-m. infertility
 i.-m. interstitial nephritis
 i.-m. reaction
immunity
 acquired i.
 adaptive i.
 cell-mediated i.
 cellular i.

NOTES

immunity *(continued)*
    humoral i.
    immunologic i.
    innate i.
    natural i.
    nonimmunologic i.
immunization
    DNA i.
    parenteral i.
immunoadsorption
immunoassay
    Abbott TDx monoclonal
      fluorescence polarization i.
    enzyme i. (EIA)
    hepatitis C virus enzyme i.
    Magic Lite chemiluminometric i.
    microparticle enzyme i. (MEIA)
    rapid enzyme i.
    second-generation enzyme i. (EIA-2)
    TDX fluorescent polarization i.
immunobead assay
immunobead-reacting antigen
immunobiology
immunoblot test
ImmunoCard
    I. STAT!
    I. STAT! Rotavirus test
immunocompetency
immunocompetent host
immunocompromised host
immunocyte
immunocytochemical stain
immunocytochemistry
    vacuolar type proton pump i.
immunocytology
ImmunoCyt test
immunodeficiency
    acquired i.
    common variable i. (CVI)
    i. disease
    severe combined i. (SCID)
immunodepression
immunodiffusion
    radial i.
    i. test
immunodominant T-cell epitope
immunoelectrophoresis
immunoenhancing
immunofixation electrophoresis (IFE)
immunofluorescence
    indirect i.
    i. microscopy
    negative i.
immunofluorescent antibody test
immunogen
    enteric i.

immunogenic gene
immunoglobulin (Ig)
    i. A (IgA)
    i. A1 (IgA1)
    i. A2 (IgA2)
    i. A endomysial antibody
    i. A nephropathy
    i. A transglutaminase antibody
      (IgA tTG)
    biliary i.
    i. D (IgD)
    i. E (IgE)
    i. G (IgG)
    i. G1 (IgG1)
    i. G2a (IgG2a)
    i. G2a antibody
    i. G antigliadin antibody (IgG
      AGA)
    i. G clearance
    hepatitis B i. (HBIG, HBIg)
    intravenous i. (IVIg)
    i. M (IgM)
    i. neuropathy
    secretory i. A
    i. superfamily adhesion molecule
immunohistochemical
    i. detection
    i. method
    i. stain
    i. staining
immunohistochemistry
    p53 i.
immunohistology
immunologic
    i. abnormality
    i. immunity
immunological
    i. fecal occult blood test (IFOBT)
    i. rapid urease test
    i. study
immunology
    intestinal i.
immunomodulatory
    i. action
    i. gene therapy
    i. therapy
immunonephelometry
immunoneutralization
immunoperoxidase
    light and electron i.
    i. stain
    i. staining
    i. staining technique
immunopositivity
immunoprecipitation

immunoproliferative small intestinal disease (IPSID)
immunoradiometric assay (IRMA)
immunoreactive methionine-enkephalin (IRME)
immunoreactivity
    cholecystokinin-like i. (CCK-LI)
    PYY-like i.
    vasoactive intestinal polypeptide i. (VIP-IR)
immunoregulatory drug
immunoscintigraphy
    ^{111}In-CYT-103 i.
immunosorbent
immunostain
immunostaining
    HBcAg i.
    in situ i.
    i. technique
immunosuppressed patient
immunosuppression
    posttransplant i.
immunosuppressive
    i. drug
    i. regimen
    i. therapy
immunosurveillance
immunotactoid
    i. glomerulonephritis
    i. glomerulopathy (ITGP)
immunotherapy
    adoptive i.
    BCG i.
    intravesical i.
    Pacis BCG bladder cancer i.
    specific i.
immunotyping
Imodium
    I. A-D
Imotec needle hydrophone
impact
    I. lithotriptor system
    I. nutritional supplement
impacted
    i. ampullary stone
    i. calculus
    i. cystic duct
    i. feces
    i. stool
impaction
    acute esophageal food i. (AEFI)
    endoscope i.

fecal i.
food bolus i.
meat i.
rectal i.
stone and basket i.
impactor
    electromechanical i. (EMI)
    stone i.
impaired
    i. cell differentiation
    i. colonic motor function
    i. gastric absorption
    i. lecithin synthesis
    i. regeneration syndrome (IRS)
    i. urinary concentrating ability
impairment
    anabolic steroid spermatogenesis i.
    ethanol-specific i.
    memory i.
impassable ureter
impedance
    i. epigastrography
    i. planimetry
    i. plethysmography (IPG)
    rectal i.
impedancometry
    intraluminal electrical i.
    multiple intraluminal i.
imperforate
    i. anus
    i. hymen
implant
    Contigen Bard collagen i.
    Deflux injectable i.
    Deflux system i.
    Dynaflex penile i.
    i. erosion
    Flexi-Flate penile i.
    gold seed i.
    Hydroflex penile i.
    iridium-192 wire i.
    islet cell i.
    Jonas i.
    leuprolide acetate i.
    Lifecath peritoneal i.
    Macroplastique i.
    malleable i.
    palladium-103 seed i.
    penile i.
    retropubic i.
    Surgitek Flexi-Flate II penile i.
    testicular i.

NOTES

implant *(continued)*
    transperineal seed i.
    Zoladex i.
implantable
    i. neuromodulation system
    i. penile venous compression
      device
    i. pulse generator (IPG)
implantation
    artificial genitourinary sphincter i.
    artificial urinary sphincter i.
    bulbous urethral cuff i.
    gastric balloon i.
    intracavitary i.
    i. metastasis
    metastatic i.
    percutaneous transperineal seed i.
    radioactive seed i.
    real-time 3-D biplanar transperineal
      prostate i.
    second-cuff i.
    ureter i.
    ureteral intestinal i.
implementation
    strict i.
implication
    clinical i.
impotence
    arteriogenic i.
    diabetic i.
    ejaculatory i.
    Esteem advanced vacuum therapy
      for i.
    functional i.
    organic i.
    orgastic i.
    paretic i.
    psychic i.
    psychogenic i.
    secondary i.
    symptomatic i.
    vasculogenic i.
    venogenic i.
    venous leak i.
impotentia
    i. coeundi
    i. erigendi
Impra graft
impressio, pl. **impressiones**
    i. esophagealis hepatis
impression
    cardiac i. on the liver
    colic i.
    colon i.
    digastric i.
    duodenal i.
    esophageal i.
    gastric i.

    liver i.
    renal i.
    suprarenal i.
Impress Softpatch
imprinting
    genomic i.
improved graft survival
IMPT
    intensity-modulated proton therapy
IMRT
    intensity-modulated radiation therapy
Imuran
IMV
    inferior mesenteric vein
IMX
    IMX Hg assay
IMx PSA system
In
    indium
in
    i. situ
    i. situ end labeling (ISEL)
    i. situ hybridization
    i. situ immunostaining
    i. utero programming
    i. vitro
    i. vitro clearance
    i. vitro compatibility
    i. vitro fertilization
    i. vitro incubation
    i. vitro synergism
    i. vivo
    i. vivo clearance
    i. vivo microscopy
    i. vivo veritas
In-111 pentretreotide
Inactin
inactivated pepsin (IP)
inactivation
    oncogene i.
inactive
    i. Crohn disease
    i. schistosomiasis
inactivity
    physical i.
inadequate
    i. bowel preparation
    i. dilation
inadvertent enterotomy
in-and-out catheterization
inanition fever
Inapsine
inborn error of metabolism
incarcerated
    i. bowel
    i. intrathoracic hernia
    i. omentum

i. prolapse
i. snare
incarceration
colon i.
colonoscopy-related i.
hernia i.
penile i.
i. symptom
InCare PRES 9300 system
in-center
short daily i.-c.
incentive spirometry
incidence
angle of i.
gallstone i.
incidental
i. adenoma
i. appendectomy
i. splenectomy
incidentaloma
adrenal gland i.
incipient
i. nephropathy
i. proteinuria
incision
Amussat i.
anterolateral thoracotomy i.
apron skin i.
Battle i.
Battle-Jalaguier-Kammerer i.
Bevan abdominal i.
bilateral subcostal i.
bilateral transabdominal i.
bucket-handle i.
burrowing i.
buttonhole i.
celiotomy i.
Cheatle-Henry i.
Cherney i.
chevron i.
choledochotomy i.
circumumbilical i.
cold knife i.
Connell i.
cruciate i.
Czerny-Kocher-Perthes i.
darting i.
Deaver i.
dorsal lumbotomy i.
i. and drainage (I&D)
eleventh rib flank i.
eleventh rib transperitoneal i.

elliptical i.
endopyelotomy i.
endoscopic i.
endourological cold-knife i.
enterotomy i.
epigastric i.
extended left subcostal i.
fishmouth i.
flank i.
four-quadrant i.
Gibson i.
Gil-Vernet dorsal lumbotomy i.
gridiron i.
groin i.
guillotine i.
Heineke-Mikulicz i.
hockey-stick i.
infraumbilical i.
inguinal i.
inverted-U abdominal i.
Joel-Cohen i.
Kammerer-Battle i.
Kehr i.
Kocher i.
LaRoque herniorrhaphy i.
i. line
lower abdominal transverse i.
low transverse i.
lumbodorsal i.
lumbotomy i.
Mallard i.
McBurney i.
median i.
midabdominal transverse i.
midline lower abdominal i.
midline upper abdominal i.
minilaparotomy i.
mini-Pfannenstiel i.
modified Gibson i.
muscle-cutting i.
muscle-splitting i.
oblique i.
omega-shaped i.
paramedian i.
pararectus i.
perineal i.
Pfannenstiel i.
plaque i.
posterior transthoracic i.
precut i.
pyelotomy i.
radial i.

NOTES

incision *(continued)*
    relaxing i.
    Rockey-Davis i.
    Salmon backcut i.
    Sanders i.
    Schuchardt relaxing i.
    smiling i.
    stab i.
    stepladder i. technique
    steri-stripped i.
    subcostal flank i.
    subcostal transperitoneal i.
    supracostal i.
    surgical i.
    teardrop i.
    thoracoabdominal i.
    transperitoneal anterior subcostal i.
      (TASI)
    transpubic i.
    transurethral i. (TUI)
    transverse semilunar skin i.
    Turner-Warwick i.
    unilateral subcostal i.
    vertical midline i.
    Wangensteen i.
    xiphoid-to-pubis midline
      abdominal i.
    xiphoid-to-umbilicus i.
    Y-shaped i.
incisional
    i. biopsy
    i. corporoplasty
    i. hernia
incisor
incisura
    i. angularis
    i. dextra of Gans
    i. vesicae felleae hepatis
inclusion
    i. body
    concentric hyaline i.
    i. cyst
    glomerular endothelial myxovirus-
      like microtubular i.
    glycogen i.
    intracytoplasmic tuboreticular i.
      (TRI)
    tubuloreticular i. (TRI)
incompetence
    gastroesophageal i.
    LES i.
    neurogenic sphincteric i.
incompetent
    i. ileocecal valve
    i. sphincter
incomplete
    i. basal cell hyperplasia
    i. cirrhosis

    i. duplication
    i. hernia
    i. pancreas divisum (IPD)
    i. passage
    i. polypectomy
    i. rectal prolapse
    i. relaxation
    i. voiding
inconspicuous penis
incontinence
    adolescent i.
    anal i.
    anatomic stress i.
    anterior fecal i.
    bladder i.
    bowel i.
    continuous i.
    daytime i.
    diurnal i.
    double i.
    extraurethral i.
    fecal i.
    flatus i.
    functional i.
    genuine stress i. (GSI)
    genuine stress urinary i. (GSUI)
    geriatric i.
    gravity urinary i.
    hyperreflexic motor urge i.
    ischemic fecal i.
    mixed i.
    Miyazaki-Bonney test for stress i.
    neurogenic refractory urge i.
    nocturnal i.
    overflow fecal i.
    pad test for urinary i.
    paradoxical i.
    paralytic i.
    passive i.
    postprostatectomy i.
    posttraumatic i.
    postvoid i.
    rectal i.
    recurrent stress i.
    reflex i.
    Resident Assessment Protocol for i.
    i. score
    secondary i.
    sphincteric i.
    stool i.
    stress i. (type 0, I, II, III)
    stress urinary i. (SUI)
    Teflon paste injection for i.
    type 0–3 stress urinary i.
    unconscious i.
    urge i.
    urgency i.

urinary exertional i.
urinary stress i.
incontinent
i. epispadias
i. ileostomy
i. ileovesicostomy
incontinentia
i. alvi
i. urinae
incoordination
pharyngeal-UES i.
incretin
incrustation
stent i.
incrusted cystitis
incubation
in vitro i.
incurable cancer
Incystene
¹¹¹In-CYT-103 immunoscintigraphy
indapamide
indentation
haustral i.
independent predictor
Inderal
Indermil adhesive
indeterminate colitis (IC)
index, pl. **indices**
American Urological Association
symptom i.
apoptotic i.
AUA Symptom I.
biliary saturation i.
body mass i. (BMI)
Bouchard i.
BPH impact i. (BII)
brachial pressure i.
Broder i.
cardiac output/cardiac i. (CO/CI)
CD activity i.
i. of cell proliferation
cholesterol saturation i. (CSI)
clitoral i.
creatinine height i. (CHI)
Crohn Disease Activity I. (CDAI)
detrusor activity i.
Doppler perfusion i. (DPI)
frequency-duration i. (FDI)
Functional Bowel Disorder
Severity I. (FBDSI)
Gingival I. (GI)
Harvey-Bradshaw i.

hemoglobin content i. (IHb)
hepatic arterial pulsatility i. (HA-PI)
hepatic iron i. (HII)
hepatic perfusion i. (HPI)
hepatic tumor i. (HTI)
histological activity i. (HAI)
insulin sensitivity i.
Karnofsky i.
Knodell i.
Kruger i.
Maine Medical Assessment
Program i.
i. of malnutrition
mean shunt i.
mitosis-karyorrhexis i. (MKI)
mitotic i.
MMAP i.
modified Barthel degree of
disability i.
National Institutes of Health
Chronic Prostatitis Symptom I.
(NIH-CPSI)
Nepean Dyspepsia I. (NDI)
nutritional i.
obesity i.
obstruction i.
oxygen saturation i. (ISO_2)
parietal cell i.
PCNA-labeling i. (PCNA-LI)
Pediatric Crohn Disease Activity I.
(PCDAI)
Penetrating Abdominal Trauma I.
(PATI)
penile-brachial i. (PBI)
penile-brachial pressure i. (PBPI)
Perianal Crohn Disease Activity I.
(PDAI)
portal shunt i. (PSI)
portal vein congestive i. (PVCI)
postthaw sperm motility i.
p_2 penile brachial i.
prognostic nutritional i. (PNI)
PSA free/total i.
Psychological General Well
Being I. (PGWBI)
pulsatility i.
Quetelet BMI i.
renal failure i.
renal resistive i.
renal vascular resistance i. (RVRI)
resistive i. (RI)

NOTES

i. colic
i. diarrhea
i. gastroenteritis
i. hypertrophic pyloric stenosis (IHPS)
i. leishmaniasis
i. nephrotic syndrome
i. pellagra
i. polycystic disease (IPCD)
infantilism
Herter i.
sexual i.
infantis
Bifidobacterium i.
Salmonella i.
infantum
Leishmania i.
Leishmania donovani i.
infarct
bile i.
bilirubin i.
Brewer i.
small bowel i.
uric acid i.
Zahn i.
infarcted bowel
infarction
acute nonocclusive bowel i.
intestinal i.
mesenteric i.
myocardial i.
nonocclusive intestinal i.
occlusive i.
omental i.
segmental ileal i.
segmental testicular i.
small intestinal i.
total i.
infected
i. bile duct
i. necrosis
i. pancreatic necrosis (IPN)
i. pseudocyst
i. tract
infection
active systemic bacterial i.
adenovirus i.
antifungal esophageal i.
antifungal-resistant opportunistic i.
Aspergillus i.
asymptomatic urinary tract i. (AUTI)

bacterial i.
biomaterial-associated i.
bladder *Candida* i.
blood stream i. (BSI)
i. calculus
Candida i.
candidal i.
catheter-related bloodstream i. (CR-BSI)
catheter tunnel i.
Chlamydia trachomatis i.
CMV i.
coliform urinary i.
coxsackievirus i. (A, B)
cryptosporidial i.
cytomegalovirus i.
deep-seated fungal i.
dengue hemorrhagic fever i.
dermatophyte i.
device-related urinary tract i.
dialysis access i.
disseminated CMV i.
domiciliary urinary tract i.
echovirus i.
enteric i.
epididymal i.
Epstein-Barr viral i.
esophageal fungal i.
exit site i.
extrapulmonary *Pneumocystis carinii* i.
fungal i.
gas-forming pyogenic liver i.
geriatric urinary tract i.
helminthic i.
hematogenous spread of i.
hepatic candidal i.
hepatitis i. (A–E)
herpes simplex i.
HIV i.
intestinal i.
intraabdominal i.
isolated urinary tract i.
liver cyst i.
metasynchronous bacterial urinary tract i.
monilial i.
multiple hepatitis virus i.
Mycobacterium i.
necrotizing i.
nematode i.
nosocomial fungal i.

NOTES

infection *(continued)*
    nosocomial urinary tract i.
    opportunistic i.
    parasitic i.
    pediatric urinary tract i.
    perianal i.
    perineal i.
    peristomal i.
    peritoneal fungal i.
    pneumococcal i.
    polymicrobial i.
    Polyomavirus i.
    postsplenectomy i.
    recurrent urinary tract i.
    renal allograft i.
    renal cyst i.
    retroperitoneal i.
    retrovirus i.
    rotavirus i.
    seminal vesicle i.
    i. stone
    strongyloid i.
    synchronous urinary tract i.
    torulopsis i.
    tunnel i.
    uncomplicated urinary tract i.
    unresolved urinary tract i.
    urinary tract i. (UTI)
    varicella-zoster i.
    Vibrio fetus i.
    viral i.
    whipworm i.
    wound i.
infection-related interstitial nephritis
infectious
    i. avian nephrosis
    i. colitis
    i. complication
    i. esophagitis
    i. gastroenteritis
    i. hepatitis
    i. jaundice
    i. mononucleosis heterophil
      antibody
    i. nosocomial diarrhea
    i. pancreatic necrosis
    i. splenomegaly
    i. viral diarrhea
infective
    i. endocarditis
    i. jaundice
    i. splenomegaly
INFeD
Infergen
inferior
    i. adrenal vein
    i. anal nerve
    i. anal plexus

    arteria epigastrica i.
    arteria mesenterica i.
    arteria pancreatica i.
    arteria rectalis i.
    i. digital fossa
    i. duodenal fold
    i. extremity
    i. fascia
    fascia diaphragmatis pelvis i.
    flexura duodeni i.
    i. hemorrhoidal artery
    i. hypogastric plexus
    i. mesenteric artery (IMA)
    i. mesenteric vein (IMV)
    i. pancreatic artery
    i. pancreaticoduodenal artery
    i. phrenic artery
    i. pole
    i. rectal nerve
    i. rectal vein
    i. vena cava (IVC)
    i. vena cava thrombosis
inferiores
    arteriae pancreaticoduodenales i.
inferomedial
infertility
    idiopathic i.
    immune-mediated i.
    tubal i.
infestation
    Ascaris i.
    biliary i.
    Fasciola hepatica i.
    parasitic i.
infiltrate
    chronic inflammatory cell i.
    lobular inflammatory i.
    lobular mononuclear cell i.
    MN i.
    mononuclear histiocytic portal i.
    PMN i.
    polymorphonuclear inflammatory i.
    sparse inflammatory i.
infiltrating adenocarcinoma
infiltration
    bacterial mucosal i.
    cellular i.
    colonic i.
    fat i.
    focal fatty i.
    gastric epithelial cell i.
    glomerular macrophage i.
    glomerular neutrophil i.
    lymphohistiocytic i.
    massive malignant i.
    neutrophilic i.
    panmucosal inflammatory cell i.
    perirectal fat i.

plasma cell portal i.
portal plasma cell i.
serosal i.
tumor i.
infiltrative
    i. disease
    i. lymphoma
inflamed
    i. appendix
    i. diverticulum
    i. gallbladder
    i. mucosa
inflammation
    cervical i.
    Hara classification of gallbladder i.
    interstitial i.
    intralobular i.
    kidney i.
    i. marker
    microbiliary i.
    parenchymal i.
    periportal i.
    portal eosinophilic i.
    portal tract i.
    transmural i.
    traumatic i.
    tubulointerstitial i.
    vaginal i.
inflammatoria
    dysphagia i.
inflammatory
    i. bowel disease (IBD)
    I. Bowel Disease Questionnaire (IBDQ)
    i. bowel syndrome (IBS)
    i. colitis
    i. diarrhea
    i. fibroid polyp (IFP)
    i. glomerulopathy
    i. pancreatitis
    i. pseudotumor
    i. renal mass
    i. response
inflatable penile prosthesis (IPP)
inflated rubber cylinder
inflator
    LeVeen i.
InflatoRing
infliximab
    i. IV infusion
    Remicade i.

influenzae
    Haemophilus i.
influenza virus
influx
    Rb i.
infold
infolding
    complex papillary i.
infracolic compartment
infradiaphragmatic radiotherapy
infragastric pancreoscopy
infrahepatic vena cava
inframammary region
inframesocolic compartment
infraorbital
infrapatellar bursa
infrared
    i. coagulation
    i. coagulator
    i. endoscopy
    i. photocoagulation (IRC)
    i. spectroscopy
    i. transillumination gastroscopy
infrarenal template procedure
infraumbilical
    i. incision
    i. mound
infravesical prostatic obstruction
infrequent
    i. defecation
    i. voider-lazy bladder syndrome
Infumorph
infundibular stenosis
infundibuliform
infundibulopelvic
    i. angle
    i. ligament
    i. stenosis
infundibuloplasty
infundibulum
    i. of bile duct
    caliceal i.
    i. of gallbladder
Infusaid
    I. chemotherapy implantable pump
    I. hepatic pump
infuser
    UROS i.
infusion
    acid i.
    atropine i.
    circadian-shaped i.

NOTES

infusion *(continued)*
    citrate i.
    continuous ambulatory i.
    hepatic arterial i. (HAI)
    hypertonic i.
    infliximab IV i.
    insulin/glucagon i.
    intraarterial vasopressin i.
    intraduodenal lipid i.
    intravariceal i.
    intravenous urea i.
    intravenous vasopressin i.
    lipid i.
    monooctanoin i.
    multiple vitamin for i.
    i. nephrotomography
    pentagastrin i.
    i. pump (IP)
    i. pyelography
    Remicade IV i.
    saline i.
    solvent i.
    total dose i.
    transcatheter arterial i.
    vasopressin i.

ingested
    i. foreign body
    i. foreign object

ingestion
    acid i.
    alkali i.
    battery i.
    button battery i.
    caustic i.
    cocaine package i.
    fish bone i.
    foreign body i.
    lye i.
    mercuric oxide battery i.
    razor blade i.
    safety pin i.

Ingold M3, M4 glass electrode pH monitor

ingrowth
    mesodermal i.
    i. of tumor

inguinal
    i. adenopathy
    i. bulge
    i. canal
    i. cord
    i. crease
    i. crease compound nevus
    i. cryptorchidism
    i. floor
    i. fold
    i. hernia (IH)
    i. incision
    i. ligament
    i. ligament of Blumberg
    i. lymphadenopathy
    i. lymph node
    i. reservoir inserter
    i. ring
    i. sphincter
    i. triangle
    i. varicocelectomy

inguinale
    granuloma i.
    hernia uteri i.

inguinoabdominal
inguinocrural
inguinofemoral hernia
inguinoperitoneal
inguinoscrotal hernia
inguinosuperficial hernia
INH
inhalation aerosol
inhaler
    Allis i.
    Vanceril i.

inheritance
    kallikrein i.

inhibin
    beta i.

inhibition
    alcohol dehydrogenase i.
    5-alpha-reductase i.
    antisense DNA i.
    i. assay
    bladder i.
    COX-1 i.
    COX-2 i.
    cyclooxygenase i.
    deglutitive i.
    detrusor muscle i.
    glycolytic i.
    laminin receptor i.
    lipoxygenase i.
    micturition reflex i.
    presynaptic i.
    renin i.
    spinobulbospinal micturition
     reflex i.

inhibitor
    ACE i.
    alpha-glucosidase i.
    5-alpha-reductase i.
    angiotensin-converting enzyme i. (ACEI)
    aromatase i.
    ATPase i.
    azasteroid i.
    calcineurin i.
    carbonic anhydrase i. (CAI)
    C-1 esterase i.

chain-terminating i.
collagen synthesis i.
COX-2 i.
cyclin-dependent kinase i.
cyclooxygenase i.
cyclooxygenase-2 i.
cytolysis i.
gastric acid pump i.
hepatocyte proliferation i. (HPI)
H+/K+-ATPase acid pump i.
inter-alpha-trypsin i. (ITI)
lipoxygenase i.
5-lipoxygenase i.
metalloproteinase i.
monoamine oxidase i.
nitric oxide synthase i.
pancreatic secretory trypsin i.
  (PSTI)
PDE5 i.
  phosphodiesterase type 5 inhibitor
phosphodiesterase i.
phosphodiesterase type 5 i. (PDE5
  inhibitor)
plasminogen activator i. (PAI)
plasminogen activator i. type 1
  (PAI-1)
plasminogen activator i. type 2
  (PAI-2)
protease i.
proteinase i.
proton pump i. (PPI)
purine synthesis i.
rapamycin i.
rectoanal i.
sertraline serotonin reuptake i.
serum alpha$_1$-protease i.
topoisomerase I i.
trypsin i.
tumor-derived angiogenic i.
urinary trypsin i.
wheat amylase i.

inhibitory
i. intestinointestinal reflex
i. postsynaptic potential (IPSP)
i. syndrome
inhomogeneity of parenchyma
inhomogeneous hyperechoic mass
initial
i. clinical experience
i. hematuria
i. proximal diversion

initiation
micturition reflex manual i.
voiding i.
initiative
Dialysis Outcomes Quality I.
  (DOQI)
National Kidney Foundation-Data
  Outcomes Quality I. (NKF-DOQI)
InjecAid system
injectable
i. ester
Macroplastique i.
injection
adrenalin i.
Albunex i.
Antizol for i.
BCG live intravesical i.
Benzacot I.
botulinum toxin i.
BTX i.
Camptosar i.
i. catheter
collagen i.
corpus cavernosum papaverine i.
cyanoacrylate i.
cyanocobalamin i.
daptomycin for i.
depot i.
diazepam emulsified i.
Dibent I.
doxercalciferol i.
endoscopic botulinum toxin i.
endoscopic epinephrine i.
endoscopic India ink i.
endoscopic ultrasound-guided fine-
  needle i.
endosonographically targeted i.
enoxaparin sodium i.
ethanol i.
etoposide i.
fibrin i.
follitropin alfa for i.
glutaraldehyde cross-linked
  collagen i.
i. gold probe (IGP)
Hectorol i.
Histoacryl i.
intracytoplasmic sperm i. (ICSI)
intralesional steroid i.
intraperitoneal i.
intrasphincteric botulinum toxin i.
intravariceal i.

NOTES

injection *(continued)*
    iopamidol i.
    iron sucrose i.
    lipiodol i.
    local depot i.
    moxisylyte i.
    mycophenolate mofetil intravenous
      for i.
    papaverine i.
    paravariceal i.
    PEG-interferon alfa-2b powder
      for i.
    PEG-Intron powder for i.
    percutaneous ethanol i. (PEI)
    periurethral collagen i.
    PGE1 i.
    polidocanol i.
    Polytef i.
    polytetrafluoroethylene paste i.
    polytetrafluoroethylene periurethral i.
    Renovist I.
    sclerosant i.
    i. sclerosis
    i. sclerotherapy
    sham i.
    i. site
    sodium hyaluronate i.
    sodium morrhuate i.
    sodium tetradecyl i.
    somatropin i.
    submucosal saline i.
    submucosal Teflon i.
    subureteric Teflon i. (STING)
    tangential colonic submucosal i.
    ^{99m}Tc-DISIDA contrast i.
    technetium Tc 99m Exametazime i.
    i. therapy
    Tisseel fibrin sealant i.
    transduodenal i.
    trigger point i.
injector
    Olympus i.
    Teflon i.
    Virag i.
InjecTx cystoscope
injury
    acid i.
    Ajmalin liver i.
    alcohol-induced gastric i.
    alkaline i.
    antecedent pancreatic i.
    bile salt i.
    bladder i.
    blast i.
    bowel i.
    cavernous artery i.
    cell-mediated hepatic i.
    closed i.

    drug-induced acute hepatic i.
    duodenal i.
    emetogenic i.
    gastric mucosal i.
    gastroduodenal mucosal i.
    glomerular i.
    Helicobacter-induced gastric i.
    hemorrhagic radiation i.
    hepatic vein i.
    hepatocellular i.
    H_2O_2-induced i.
    hyperfiltration i.
    hypertensive renal i.
    intestinal radiation i.
    ischemia-reperfusion i.
    juxtahepatic venous i.
    liver transplantation preservation i.
    major deceleration i.
    medication-induced i.
    microangiopathic renal i.
    mucosal i.
    NSAID-induced gastric i.
    NSAID-induced intestinal i.
    obstetric i.
    open i.
    oxidant i.
    oxidative cell i.
    pancreatic i.
    paraquat-induced upper
      gastrointestinal i.
    pill-induced esophageal i.
    pinch i.
    PMN-mediated endothelial cell i.
    radiation i.
    rectal i.
    renal vascular i.
    reperfusion i.
    spinal cord i. (SCI)
    splenic i.
    straddle i.
    stress-related mucosal i.
    tubular epithelial cell i.
    tubular morphologic i.
    tubulointerstitial i.
    ureteral i.
    urethra blowout i.
    vascular i.

ink
    autoclaved India i.
    China i.
    Higgins India i.
    India i.
    Koh-I-Noor Universal India i.
    osmolarity of the i.
    Pelikan brand India i.
    solution-diluted India i.

inlay
    Turner-Warwick i.

Inlay-Tabs
> Ursinus I.-T.

inlet
> esophageal i.
> i. patch
> i. patch mucosa
> i. port
> i. pouch (IP)
> thoracic i.

[111]**In-leukocyte technique**

in-line blood gas monitor

Inmed whistle tip urethral catheter

innate immunity

inner
> i. crossbar
> i. diameter (ID)
> i. medulla
> i. medullary collecting duct
> (IMCD)

innervation
> adrenal gland i.
> afferent i.
> bladder i.
> cholinergic i.
> intrinsic excitatory i.
> kidney i.
> pelvis i.
> prostate gland i.
> rectal i.
> seminal vesicle i.
> serosal afferent i.
> striated muscle i.

innocens
> *Serpulina i.*

innocent gallstone

innocuous

Innoflex variable stiffness colonoscope

Inno-LiPA assay

innominate
> i. bone
> i. groove

Innova home incontinence therapy system

inoculated medium

inoculum size

inorganic iodine

iNOS
> induced nitric oxide synthase

inositol
> i. lipid
> i. ring
> i. triphosphate

> i. 1,4,5-triphosphate (IP3)
> i. 1,4,5-triphosphate Ca2+

input
> fast cholinergic i.
> nociceptive sensory i.

insemination
> intrauterine i. (IUI)
> subzonal i. (SUZI)

insensible loss of water

insert
> FemSoft i.
> Hollister Convex i.
> Nu-Hope Convex i.
> Reliance urinary control i.
> Sur-Fit Natura disposable convex i.
> United Surgical Convex i.
> urinary control urethral i.

inserter
> Furlow cylinder i.
> inguinal reservoir i.

insertion
> biliary endoprosthesis i.
> chromosome i.
> cystoradium i.
> flatus tube i.
> jejunal tube i.
> J-tube i.
> i. mutation
> PEG i.
> Sengstaken-Blakemore tube i.
> subclavian catheter i.
> i. tube

InSIGHT
> I. manometry
> I. manometry system

insipidus
> congenital nephrogenic diabetes i.
> (CNDI)
> diabetes i.
> nephrogenic diabetes i. (NDI)
> neurogenic diabetes i.

insorption

inspiration

inspiratory

inspissated
> i. bile
> i. bile syndrome
> i. feces
> i. sump syndrome

instability
> bladder post-cystourethropexy i.
> chromosome i. (CIN)

NOTES

instability (*continued*)
>   detrusor i. (DI)
>   detrusor muscle i.
>   genomic i.
>   microsatellite i. (MSI)

instant
>   i. camera
>   Hydrocil I.
>   i. photography

instantaneous clearance

InStent EsophaCoil stent

instillation
>   intravesical i.
>   i. therapy

institutional
>   i. colon
>   i. dysentery
>   i. main demographic database

instrument
>   Bard Biopty i.
>   Bard BladderScan bladder
>   volume i.
>   biopsy i.
>   BIP biopsy i.
>   i. count
>   CRIT-LINE i.
>   DaVinci handle i.
>   Dilamezinsert urologic i.
>   DMI urologic i.
>   Duette double-lumen ERCP i.
>   endosonography i.
>   Feleki i.
>   GIA i.
>   guide-eye i.
>   mechanical radial-scanning i.
>   oblique forward-viewing i.
>   ProLine endoscopic i.
>   Quinton suction biopsy i.
>   Radiometer 85 i.
>   Roboprep G i.
>   Sharpoint cutting i.
>   slotted i.
>   small-diameter endosonographic i.
>   spring-loaded type biopsy i.
>   standardized i.
>   XQ video i.

instrumentation
>   biliary i.
>   Karl Storz i.
>   Microvasive i.

instrument-track seeding

insufficiency
>   acute renal i. (ARI)
>   adrenal i.
>   Angiotensin-Converting Enzyme
>   Inhibition in Progressive Renal I.
>   (AIPRI)
>   chronic renal i. (CRI)

>   exocrine pancreatic i. (EPI)
>   gastric i.
>   gastromotor i.
>   hepatic i.
>   ileocecal i.
>   pancreatic exocrine i.
>   primary adrenal i.
>   progressive renal i.
>   pyloric i.
>   renal i.
>   vascular i.

insufflation
>   air i.
>   colonic i.
>   helium i.
>   i. of stomach

insufflator
>   carbon dioxide i.
>   nitrous oxide i.

Insuflon insulin delivery device

insular structure

insulated
>   i. curved scissors
>   i. straight scissors

insulation-tipped electrosurgical knife

insulin
>   human i.
>   i. hyperplasia
>   Lente i.
>   NPH i.
>   protamine zinc i.
>   i. reaction
>   i. receptor-related receptor
>   i. resistance
>   i. resistance syndrome
>   Semilente i.
>   i. sensitivity index
>   i. stain
>   Ultralente i.

insulin-degrading enzyme (IDE)

insulin-dependent
>   i.-d. diabetes
>   i.-d. diabetes mellitus (IDDM)

insulin/glucagon
>   i./g. infusion
>   putative hepatotrophic factors i./g.

insulinlike
>   i. growth factor (IGF)
>   i. growth factor-1 (IGF-1)
>   i. growth factor-2 (IGF-2)
>   i. growth factor-binding protein-1
>   (IGFBP-1)

insulinoma

insulinopenia

insulin-transferrin-sodium selenite

insulin-treated diabetic

insult
>   ischemic i.

intact
>   i. hormone assay
>   i. proprioception
>   i. PTH

intake
>   caloric i.
>   clandestine i.
>   daily protein i. (DPI)
>   dietary energy i.
>   i. and output (I&O)

Intal

integrated
>   i. assessment
>   i. automatic stone-tissue detection system
>   i. clearance

integrating spherical power meter

integrin
>   alpha-3-beta-1 i.
>   alpha-5-beta-1 i.
>   B1, B2 i.
>   beta-1 chain i.
>   membrane-spanning i.

integrity
>   mucosal i.

integument

intensified radiographic imaging system (IRIS)

intensity
>   fluorescent light i. (FLI)

intensity-modulated
>   i.-m. proton therapy (IMPT)
>   i.-m. radiation therapy (IMRT)

intention
>   delayed primary i.
>   healing by first i.
>   healing by primary i.
>   healing by second i.
>   healing by secondary i.

intentionem
>   healing per primam i.
>   healing per secundam i.

intention-to-treat (ITT)

interaction
>   bacterial host i.
>   cell-cell i.
>   cervical mucus-sperm i.
>   crystal-phospholipid i.
>   idiotype-anti-idiotype i.
>   vasoactive peptide-cytokine i.

interactive video technology (IVT)

inter-alpha inhibitor family

inter-alpha-trypsin inhibitor (ITI)

intercalated cell

intercalatum
>   *Schistosoma i.*

intercapillary nephrosclerosis

Interceed absorbable adhesion barrier

intercellular
>   i. adhesion molecule-1 (ICAM-1)
>   i. space

interceptive conditioning

Interceptor M3 triple-channel, solid state monitor

intercolonoscopy

interconversion

intercostal
>   i. pedicle esophagogastropexy
>   i. scan
>   i. space

intercourse
>   receptive anal i.

interdialytic
>   i. urea generation
>   i. weight gain (IDWG)

interdigestive
>   i. antroduodenal motility
>   i. migrating motor complex
>   i. myoelectric complex

interdigitate

interdigitating teeth

interest
>   region of i.

interface
>   fluid-air i.

interference barrier filter

interferential electrical stimulation

interferon
>   i. alfa-2a
>   i. alfa-2b
>   i. alfacon-1
>   i. alfa-n1
>   i. alfa-n3
>   alpha i.
>   i. alpha
>   i. alpha-2b
>   i. alpha-2b therapy
>   i. alpha therapy
>   beta i.
>   consensus i. (CIFN)
>   gamma i.
>   high-dose consensus i.
>   human lymphoblastoid i. (L-IFN)

NOTES

interferon *(continued)*
    i. inducer
    low-dose i.
    pegylated i.
    recombinant human alpha i.
    i. treatment
    i. type I
interferon-alpha
    lymphoblastoid i.-a.
alpha-2-a-interferon
interferon-beta
interferon-alfa (IFN-alpha)
    i.-a. 2-beta
    recombinant i.-a. (rIFN-alpha)
interferon-gamma (IFN-gamma)
    basal i.-g.
    HLA class II-restricted i.-g.
    nucleocapsid antigen-stimulated i.-g.
    i.-g. stimulation
interfoveolar muscle
Intergroup Rhabdomyosarcoma Study (IRS)
interhaustral
    i. fold
    i. septum
interlabial
    i. rhabdomyosarcoma
    i. sarcoma botryoid
interleukin (IL)
interleukin-1 (IL-1)
    i. receptor antagonist
interleukin-2 (IL-2)
    i. receptor-blocking agent
    recombinant i.
    serum i.
interleukin-6 (IL-6)
    serum i.
interleukin-8 (IL-8)
interleukin-10 (IL-10)
interleukin-1b urinary marker
interlobar
    i. renal artery
    i. vein
interlobular
    i. bile duct
    i. fibrosis
interlobulares
    ductuli i.
interlocking
    i. detachable coils
    i. ligature
interloop abscess
intermedia
    Yersinia i.
intermediate
    i. biomarker
    i. fasting
    i. junction

    i. low-density lipoprotein (ILDL)
    malignant teratoma, i. (MTI)
    i. mesenteric lymph node
    i. polyposis
    i. space
    thiol i.
intermediate-density lipoprotein (IDL)
intermedius
    Citrobacter i.
intermesenteric abscess
intermicrovillar area
intermittens
    dyspragia i.
intermittent
    i. calcitriol therapy
    i. catheterization
    i. click
    i. diarrhea
    i. drip feeding
    i. hemodialysis (IHD)
    i. hemoglobinuria
    i. hepatic fever
    i. obstruction
    i. pain
    i. positive pressure breathing (IPPB)
    i. proteinuria
    i. pulse
    i. self-catheterization (ISC)
    i. self-obturation
    i. suctioning
interna
    elastica i.
    fascia spermatica i.
    lamina rara i. (LRI)
internal
    i. abdominal fascia
    i. abdominal ring
    i. anal sphincter (IAS)
    i. biliary drainage
    i. biliary lavage
    i. cremaster of Henle
    i. fiberoptic cable
    i. hemorrhage
    i. hemorrhoid
    i. iliac artery
    i. iliac vein
    i. inguinal ring
    i. oblique
    i. oblique fascia
    i. oblique muscle
    I. Ostomy Association (IOA)
    i. procidentia
    i. proctotomy
    i. pudendal artery
    i. pudendal vein
    i. rectal sphincter
    i. ribosome entry site (IRES)

i. rotation
i. septation
i. spermatic fascia
i. spermatic vessel
i. sphincterotomy
i. urethrotomy

international
i. androgen unit
I. Association for Enterostomal Therapy
I. Autoimmune Hepatitis Group score
I. Biomedical Mode 745-100 microcapillary infusion system
I. Continence Society (ICS)
I. Continence Society classification of voiding dysfunction
I. Continence Society voiding function classification
I. Germ Cell Cancer Collaborative Group (IGCCCG)
I. Germ Cell Cancer Collaborative Group classification
I. Index of Erectile Function (IIEF)
I. Prognostic Index score
I. Prostate Symptom Score (IPSS)
i. unit of male hormone
i. unit per liter (IU/L)

interneuron
enteric i.

internist tumor
internodal strand
internuclear ophthalmoplegia
internum
orificium urethrae externum i.
ostium urethrae i.

interosseous
interpersonal sensitivity
interphase PBMC
interpolar region
interposition
colonic i.
i. Dacron graft
i. flap of omentum
ileal i.
omental i.
i. operation

interrogans
Leptospira i.

interrupted
i. manual mucomucosal absorbable suture
i. seromuscular suture
intersex
i. condition
i. gonad
intersexuality
intersphincteric
i. anal fistula
i. anorectal space
i. groove
i. perirectal abscess
i. plane
i. rectal dissection
i. resection
i. sulcus
InterStim device
interstitial
i. brachytherapy
i. cells of Cajal (ICC)
i. cell tumor of testis
i. collagenase
i. cystitis
i. diffusion
i. diode
i. fibroblast
i. fibrosis
i. gastritis
i. hernia
i. hypercellularity
i. immunocompetent cell
i. inflammation
i. irradiation
i. laser coagulation (ILC)
i. mononuclear cell
i. pancreatitis
i. photodynamic therapy
i. rejection
i. scarlatinal nephritis
i. syphilitic nephritis
i. volume
interstitium
medullary i.
renal i.
intersymphyseal
i. bar
i. stitch
intertriginous region
intertrigo
candidal i.
intertropical hyphemia

NOTES

interureteral
interureteric ridge
interval
  i. appendectomy
  confidence i. (CI)
intervention
  angiographic i.
interventional
  i. technique
  i. uroradiology
interventricular defect
interview
  SSIAM i.
intestinal
  i. adaptation
  i. anastomosis
  i. angina
  i. anthrax
  i. antireflux valve
  i. atony
  i. atresia
  i. atrophy
  i. bacterium
  i. bag
  i. biopsy
  i. brush border (IBB)
  i. bypass
  i. calculus
  i. capillariasis
  i. clamp
  i. colic
  i. colonization
  i. concretion
  i. content
  i. decompression
  i. distention
  i. distomiasis
  i. diverticulum
  i. emphysema
  i. endocrine cell
  i. endoscopy
  i. enterocyte
  i. epithelial cell (IEL)
  i. fatty acid-binding protein (I-FABP)
  i. fistula
  i. fixation
  i. flora
  i. hemorrhage
  i. histoplasmosis
  i. immunology
  i. indigestion
  i. infarction
  i. infection
  i. intoxication
  i. intussusception
  i. ischemia
  i. juice

  i. lactase deficiency
  i. lamina propria
  i. lipodystrophy
  i. loop
  i. lumen
  i. lymphangiectasia
  i. malrotation
  i. metaplasia (type I–III)
  i. motility disorder
  i. mucosa
  i. myiasis
  i. myoneurosis
  i. myxoneurosis
  i. necrosis
  i. obstruction (IO)
  i. parasite
  i. peptide
  i. perforation
  i. perfusion
  i. permeability
  i. permeability measurement
  i. pneumatosis
  i. polyposis
  i. polyposis-cutaneous pigmentation syndrome
  i. prolapse
  i. protozoa
  i. pseudoobstruction
  i. radiation injury
  i. schistosomiasis
  i. sedative
  i. sling
  i. sling placement
  i. spirochete
  i. stasis
  i. steatorrhea
  i. stenosis
  i. stricture
  i. surgery
  i. tract
  i. transit study
  i. tuberculosis
  i. ureteral replacement
  i. viability
  i. villous architecture
  i. villus
  i. volvulus
  i. web
intestinalis, pl. **intestinales**
  arteriae intestinales
  dyspragia i.
  dyspragia intermittens angiosclerotica i.
  Encephalitozoon i.
  Giardia i.
  lipodystrophia i.
  mycosis i.
  myxorrhea i.

pneumatosis i.
pneumatosis cystoides i. (PCI)
sepsis i.
Septata i.
trunci intestinales
intestine
bacterial metabolism in i.
blind i.
Crohn small i.
distal i. (DI)
empty i.
iced i.
jejunoileal i.
kink in i.
malrotation of i.
mesenterial i.
milking of i.
segmental i.
small i.
straight i.
villous coat of small i.
intestinofugal neuron
intestinogastric reflex
intestinointestinal
intestinorum
pneumatosis cystoides i.
intimal
i. fibroplasia
i. hyperplasia
intimin
intolerance
dietary protein i.
disaccharide i.
fatty food i.
fructose i.
glucose i.
hereditary fructose i.
lactose i.
intoxication
drug i.
intoxication
acute methanol i.
alcohol i.
intestinal i.
metal i.
methanol i.
quinidine i.
systemic mercury i.
intraabdominal
i. abscess
i. adhesion
i. bile leakage

i. desmoid tumor
i. hemorrhage
i. ileal reservoir
i. infection
i. mass
i. pressure
i. pressure gauge
i. sepsis (IAS)
i. transverse testicular ectopia
i. viscus
intraanal
i. electromyography
i. pressure
i. wart
intraaortic endovascular sonography
intraappendicular
intraarterial (IA)
i. chemotherapy
i. chemotherapy catheter
i. digital subtraction angiography
i. vasopressin infusion
intraassay precision
intraballoon pressure
intrabulbar fossa
intracapillary thrombosis
intracapsular dissection
intracavernosal
i. injection therapy (ICIT)
i. injection treatment
i. pressure
intracavernous
i. injection and stimulation test
i. injection therapy
intracavitary
i. application brachytherapy
i. implantation
i. radiation boost therapy
i. topical therapy
i. transducer
intracellular
i. acidity
i. acification
i. buffering
i. fluid (ICF)
i. flush effect
i. pH
i. potassium
i. signaling system
intracellulare
Mycobacterium i.
intracholedochal
i. manometric catheter

NOTES

intracholedochal *(continued)*
   i. pressure
   i. stent
intracisternal (IC)
IntraCoil nitinol stent
intracolonic Kaposi sarcoma
intracorporeal
   i. anastomosis
   i. electrohydraulic lithotripsy
     (IEHL)
   i. injection therapy
   i. laser lithotripsy (ICL, ILL)
   i. needle breakage
   i. shock wave lithotripsy
intracranial
   i. hemorrhage
   i. pressure monitoring
intractable
   i. constipation
   i. diarrhea
   i. tumor
   i. ulcer
   i. ulcerative colitis
   i. vomiting
intracuticular suture
intracystic epithelial proliferation
intracytoplasmic
   i. calcium
   i. CMV inclusion body
   i. mucin
   i. sperm injection (ICSI)
   i. tuboreticular inclusion (TRI)
intradermal
   i. suture
   i. tattooing technique
intradialytic
   i. hypotension (IDH)
   i. parenteral nutrition (IDPN)
   i. period
   i. symptom
intradiverticular papilla
IntraDose gel
Intraducer peritoneal cannula
intraductal
   i. cholangioscopy
   i. endoscope
   i. imaging catheter
   i. lithiasis
   i. mucin-hypersecreting neoplasm
   i. mucin-producing tumor
   i. oncocytic papillary neoplasm
     (IOPN)
   i. papillary mucinous neoplasm
     (IPMN)
   i. papillary mucinous tumor
     (IPMT)
   i. papillary and mucinous tumors
     of pancreas (IPMY)

   i. papillary tumor (IPT)
   i. pressure
   i. secretin test (IDST)
   i. ultrasonography (IDUS)
   i. ultrasound (IDUS)
   i. ultrasound probe
intraduodenal (ID)
   i. lipid infusion
intraepiploic hernia
intraepithelial
   i. body
   i. cancer
   i. leukocyte (IEL)
   i. lymphocyte (IEL)
   i. lymphocytosis
intraesophageal
   i. acid test
   i. balloon distention (IEBD)
   i. peristaltic pressure
   i. pH
   i. pH monitoring (EpHM)
   i. pH test
   i. stent
   i. variceal pressure
intrafamilial clustering of *Helicobacter pylori*
intragastric (IG)
   i. acidity
   i. balloon
   i. bubble
   i. continuous pH-meter
   i. drip
   i. EGF
   i. gallstone
   i. hydrolysis
   i. pH
   i. pH mapping
   i. pH monitor record
   i. pressure
   i. volume
intraglandular fluid
intraglomerular
   i. hemodynamics
   i. hypertension
   i. mesangial cell
   i. pressure
intragraft
intrahaustral contraction ring
intrahepatic
   i. abscess
   i. antigen-dependent lymphocyte-
     hepatocyte
   i. artery-systemic shunt
   i. ascariasis
   i. atresia (IHA)
   i. AV fistula
   i. bile duct
   i. biliary cystic dilation

i. biliary duct hypoplasia
i. biliary stricture
i. cholangioentcrostomy
i. cholangiojejunostomy
i. cholelithiasis
i. cholestasia
i. cholestasia of pregnancy (ICP)
i. ductal dilation
i. hematoma
i. hepatitis
i. invasion
i. lymphocyte
i. portal hypertension
i. portal obstruction
i. radicle
i. sclerosing cholangitis
i. shunt
i. spontaneous arterioportal fistula
i. stone

intrailiac hernia
intrajejunal (IJ)
intralesional
i. steroid injection
i. treatment
intralipid fat emulsion
intralobar
intralobular
i. fibrosis
i. inflammation
intraluminal
i. clot
i. cyst
i. distention
i. duodenal diverticulum (IDD)
i. electrical impedancometry
i. esophageal pressure
i. filling defect
i. lipolysis
i. manometry
i. pH-pressure relationship
i. pouch
i. pressure recording
i. probe
i. proliferation
i. radiotherapy
i. reference electrode
i. Silastic esophageal stent
i. stapler (ILS)
i. stone
i. ultrasound (ILUS)
i. urethral pressure

intramesenteric
i. abscess
i. desmoid tumor
intramucosal
i. cancer
i. carcinoma
i. metastasis
intramural
i. air dissection
i. aneurysm
i. atheromatous disease
i. colonic air
i. diverticulum
i. duodenal hematoma (IDH)
i. fistulous tract
i. ganglia
i. intestinal hemorrhage
i. lesion
i. microvessel density (MMD)
i. secretory reflex
i. ureter
intramuscular perineural stimulation
graciloplasty
intranuclear CMV inclusion body
intraoperative
i. angiography
i. autologous transfusion
i. biliary endoscopy
i. cavernous nerve stimulation
i. cholangiogram
i. cholangiography (IOC)
i. electron beam radiotherapy
i. endoscopy (IOE)
i. enteroscopy (IOE)
i. kidney hypothermia
i. mortality
i. penile erection
i. phlebography
i. radiation therapy (IORT)
i. radiotherapy (IORT)
i. ultrasonography (IOUS)
intrapancreatic
i. bile duct
i. nerve
intrapapillary terminus
intraparavariceal procedure
intraparenchymal tumor
intrapelvic
i. filling defect
i. somatic fiber
intraperitoneal (IP)
i. abscess

NOTES

intraperitoneal *(continued)*
- i. adhesion
- i. air
- i. cavity
- i. chemotherapy
- i. hemorrhage
- i. hyperthermic chemotherapy (IPHC)
- i. hyperthermic perfusion (IPHP)
- i. injection
- i. mesh repair
- i. onlay mesh hernia repair (IPOM)
- i. perforation
- i. viscus
- i. volume

intraportal endovascular ultrasonography (IPEUS)
intraportally
intraprostatic
- easy-to-perform i.
- i. spiral
- i. stent
- i. temperature
- i. temperature-guided treatment
- i. temperature measurement
- i. vasculature

intrapulmonary shunting
intrarectal
- i. intussusception
- i. retroflexion
- i. ultrasonography

intrarenal (IR)
- i. calculus
- i. chemolysis
- i. collecting system
- i. hemodynamics
- i. matrix-degrading enzyme cascade
- i. reflux
- i. renal artery aneurysm
- i. vascular thrombosis

IntraSonix TULIP laser device
intrasphincteric botulinum toxin injection
intrasplenic pseudocyst
IntraStent DoubleStrut biliary endoprosthesis
intratesticular cyst
intrathecal
- i. catheter
- i. chemotherapy

intrathoracic
- i. esophagogastroscopy
- i. esophagogastrostomy
- i. Nissen fundoplication
- i. stomach

intratubular
- i. germ cell neoplasia (ITGCN)
- i. obstruction

intratumoral
- i. heterogeneity

intraurethral
- i. coil
- i. PGE$_1$
- i. pressure
- i. prostaglandin suppository (IPS)
- i. swab specimen

intrauterine
- i. growth restriction (IUGR)
- i. insemination (IUI)

intravaginal
- i. electrical stimulation
- i. torsion

intravariceal
- i. ethanolamine oleate
- i. infusion
- i. injection
- i. injection sclerotherapy
- i. pressure

intravasation
intravascular
- i. lipolysis
- i. thrombosis
- i. ultrasound (IVUS)
- i. ultrasound catheter
- i. volume
- i. volume expansion

intravenous (IV)
- i. albumin
- i. cholangiogram (IVC)
- i. cholangiography (IVC)
- i. cholecystography
- i. drip
- i. drug abuse
- i. feeding
- i. heme-albumin
- i. H2 receptor antagonist (IVH2RA)
- i. hydration
- i. hyperalimentation (IVH)
- i. immunoglobulin (IVIg)
- i. lipid emulsion
- i. nitroglycerin
- i. nutrition (IVN)
- i. pyelogram (IVP)
- i. pyelography
- i. renal angiography
- i. secretin test
- i. urea infusion
- i. urogram (IVU)
- i. urography (IVU)
- i. vasopressin infusion

intravesical
- i. alum

i. alum irrigation
i. anastomosis
i. bacillus Calmette-Guérin
i. BCG
i. capsaicin
i. chemotherapy
i. electromotive drug administration
  (EMDA)
i. formalin
i. heparin
i. hyaluronic acid
i. immunotherapy
i. instillation
i. migration
i. oxybutynin
i. pressure
i. silver nitrate
i. ureterocele
i. ureterolysis
intrinsic
i. enzymatic activity
i. excitatory innervation
i. factor (IF)
i. factor secretion
finger i.
i. proteinuria
i. reflex
i. sphincter deficiency (ISD)
i. sphincter dysfunction (ISD)
i. striated muscle of the urethra
i. striated sphincter
i. ureteral stricture
i. ureteropelvic junction obstruction
i. urethral sphincter
introducer
Atkinson i.
Dumon-Gilliard prosthesis i.
entrapment sack i.
Furlow i.
i. gun
Hickman percutaneous i.
KeyMed Nottingham i.
LapSac i.
Nottingham Key-Med i.
Nottingham semirigid i.
pull-apart i.
semirigid Nottingham i.
i. set
split sheath i.
Wilson-Cook prosthesis i.
introitus esophagi
Introl bladder neck support prosthesis

intromission
Intromit
Intron
  I. A multidose pen
  Rebetol with I.
Intropin
intubate
intubated ureterotomy
intubation
  catheter-guided endoscopic i.
    (CAGEIN)
  endotracheal i.
  enterocutaneous i.
  esophageal i.
  esophagogastric i.
  i. failure
  gastrointestinal i.
  nasal i.
  nasogastric i.
  nasotracheal i.
  oral i.
  orotracheal i.
  pyloric i.
  terminal ileum i. (TII)
intumescence
intumescent
intussuscepted
  i. ileal triple nipple
  i. nipple valve
intussusception
  agonic i.
  appendiceal i.
  bowel i.
  cecocolic i.
  colocolic i.
  ileocecal i.
  ileocolic i.
  ileoileal i.
  intestinal i.
  intrarectal i.
  jejunogastric i.
  postmortem i.
  rectal i.
  retrograde i.
  sigmoidoanal i.
  triple i.
intussusceptum
intussuscipiens
inulin
  i. clearance
  plasma i.
  i. solution

NOTES

Inutest test
invaginated membrane
invaginating ampulla of Vater
invagination
    i. of the ampulla
    stomal i.
    stump i.
    i. technique
invasion
    capillary-lymphatic i.
    dermatolymphatic i.
    intrahepatic i.
    neural i.
    periportal i.
    stromal i.
    vascular i.
    venous i.
    Wilms tumor capsule i.
invasive
    i. adenocarcinoma
    i. carcinoma
    i. colorectal polyp
    i. diagnostic test
    i. enteric pathogen
    i. procedure
inventory
    Beck Depression I.
    Minnesota Multiphasic
      Personality I.
    Ostomy Assessment I. (OAI)
    The Hospital Anxiety and
      Depression I.
    Urogenital Distress I. (UDI)
invermination
Inversine
inversion
    i. appendectomy
    i. of bladder
    chromosome i.
inversion-ligation appendectomy
inversus
    abdominal situs i.
    situs i.
inverted
    i. diverticulum of the colon
    i. papilloma
    i. sigmoid diverticulum
    i. testis
    i. U-pouch ileal reservoir
    i.-V peritoneotomy
inverted-U
    i.-U abdominal incision
    i.-U pouch
inverted-V
    i.-V peritoneotomy
    i.-V sign
inverter
    Mayo-Kelly appendix i.

inverting suture
investigation
    Lapides cystometric i.
    radiological i.
investing fascia
Invicorp
involuntary
    i. guarding
    i. reflex rigidity
involution
    prostate gland i.
involvement
    multifocal i.
    tubercular i.
IO
    intestinal obstruction
I&O
    intake and output
IOA
    Internal Ostomy Association
IOC
    intraoperative cholangiography
iocetamic
    i. acid
    i. acid contrast medium
Iodamoeba buetschlii
iodide
    isopropamide i.
    Lugol i.
    i. nephropathy
    propidium i.
iodinated
    i. contrast agent
    i. contrast material
iodine
    i. dye
    i. hippurate scanning
    inorganic i.
    Lugol i.
    i. scan
    i. staining
iodine-123 iodoamphetamine
iodine-125 (I-125, ^{125}I)
iodine-131 (I-131)
    radioactive i.
iodine-131-labeled
  metaiodobenzylguanidine
iodipamide
    i. meglumine
    i. meglumine contrast medium
    sodium i.
iodism
iodoamphetamine ([^{123}I]IMP)
    iodine-123 i.
iodoantipyrine clearance
iodochlorhydroxyquin
iodocholesterol scan
Iodoform gauze

Iodohippurate
iodophor
Iodopyracet
iodoquinol
IOE
    intraoperative endoscopy
    intraoperative enteroscopy
iohexol
ion
    i. beam-assisted deposition
    i. channel
    i. chromatography
    hydrogen i.
    i. laser
    phosphate i. (PI)
Ionamin
ionizing radiation
ionomycin
ionophore
ion-sensitive field effect transistor
ion-specific electrode
iontophoresis
ion-urea
    hyperphosphate i.-u.
    phosphate i.-u. (PI-urea)
iopamidol
    i. contrast imaging agent
    i. injection
iopanoic
    i. acid
    i. acid contrast medium
IOPN
    intraductal oncocytic papillary neoplasm
iopromide
IORT
    intraoperative radiation therapy
    intraoperative radiotherapy
IOT29, clone K20 monoclonal antibody
iothalamate
    i. clearance
    i. level
    sodium i.
iothalamate-125
iothalamic acid
iotroxate
    meglumine i.
IOUS
    intraoperative ultrasonography
ioversol
ioxaglate
IP
    ileoproctostomy

    inactivated pepsin
    infusion pump
    inlet pouch
    intraperitoneal
        IP chemotherapy
IP3
    inositol 1,4,5-triphosphate
IPAA
    ileal pouch-anal anastomosis
^{131}I para-aminohippuric acid
IPCD
    infantile polycystic disease
IPD
    incomplete pancreas divisum
ipecac
    i. abuse
    i. syrup
ipecac-induced
    i.-i. cardiotoxicity
    i.-i. myopathy
    i.-i. vomiting
IPEC-J2 cell
IPEUS
    intraportal endovascular ultrasonography
IPG
    impedance plethysmography
    implantable pulse generator
IPH
    idiopathic portal hypertension
IPHC
    intraperitoneal hyperthermic
      chemotherapy
IPHP
    intraperitoneal hyperthermic perfusion
I-Plant brachytherapy seed
IPMN
    intraductal papillary mucinous neoplasm
IPMT
    intraductal papillary mucinous tumor
IPMY
    intraductal papillary and mucinous
      tumors of pancreas
IPN
    infected pancreatic necrosis
ipodate contrast medium
IPOM
    intraperitoneal onlay mesh hernia repair
IPP
    inflatable penile prosthesis
IPPB
    intermittent positive pressure breathing
ipratropium

NOTES

iproniazid
iproniazid-induced jaundice
iproplatin
IPS
> intraurethral prostaglandin suppository

IPSID
> immunoproliferative small intestinal disease

ipsilateral adrenalectomy
IPSP
> inhibitory postsynaptic potential

IPSS
> International Prostate Symptom Score

IPT
> intraductal papillary tumor

IR
> ileal resection
> intrarenal

¹⁹²Ir
> iridium-192
>> ¹⁹²Ir wire

IRA
> ileorectal anastomosis

IRC
> infrared photocoagulation

IRES
> internal ribosome entry site

iridectomy scar
iridium
> i. prosthesis
> i. ribbon
> i. seed

iridium-192 (¹⁹²Ir)
> iridium-192 wire implant

iridium-192-loaded stent
irinotecan hydrochloride
IRIS
> intensified radiographic imaging system

iritis
IRMA
> immunoradiometric assay

IRME
> immunoreactive methionine-enkephalin

iron
> i. deficiency
> i. dextran
> i. gluconate
> i. nephropathy
> oral i.
> i. overload disorder
> i. poisoning
> serum i. (SI)
> i. storage disease
> i. store
> i. sucrose injection

iron-binding capacity (IBC)
iron-deficiency anemia
iron-dependent oxidant

IRP
> idiopathic recurrent pancreatitis

IRPGN
> idiopathic rapidly progressive glomerulonephritis

irradiate
irradiated tumor vaccine
irradiation
> i. effect
> external-beam i.
> i. failure
> half-body i.
> hemibody i.
> interstitial i.
> Nd:YAG laser i.
> total body i. (TBI)
> total lymphoid i. (TLI)
> ultraviolet i.

irreducible hernia
irregular
> i. amputated mucosal pattern
> i. duct
> i. pupil
> i. rhythm

irregularity
> cervical i.

irretrievable object
irrigant
> Neosporin G.U. I.

irrigating
> i. fluid
> i. patient

irrigation
> acetohydroxamic acid i.
> bladder i.
> bowel i.
> catheter i.
> i. of colostomy
> continuous bladder i. (CBI)
> copious i.
> i. fluid absorption syndrome
> hemiacidrin i.
> H-600 normothermic i.
> intravesical alum i.
> pulsed i.
> rectal pulsed i.
> rectum i.
> Renacidin i.
> Sur-Fit Natura Visi-Flow i.
> whole-gut i.

irrigation-suction
> postoperative i.-s.

irrigator/aspirator
> Nezhat-Dorsey i.

irritable
> i. bladder
> i. bowel syndrome (IBS)
> i. colon (IC)

i. colon syndrome
i. gut syndrome
i. stricture
i. testis
irritant dermatitis
irritative
i. diarrhea
i. symptom
IRS
impaired regeneration syndrome
Intergroup Rhabdomyosarcoma Study
IRS-IV trial
IS
ileal segment
immune serum
Isaacs-Ludwig arteriole
ISC
intermittent self-catheterization
ischemia
acute gastric i.
acute occlusive mesenteric i.
atherosclerosis-induced cavernosal i.
AVF-induced renal i.
colonic i.
glomerular i.
intestinal i.
kidney i.
mesenteric i.
midgut i.
mucosal i.
myocardial i.
i. necrosis
nonocclusive mesenteric i.
outer medullary i.
renal i.
i. or soughing of the flap
tubular i.
visceral i.
warm i.
ischemia-reperfusion injury
ischemic
i. bowel
i. bowel disease
i. colitis
i. fecal incontinence
i. hepatitis
i. insult
i. penile gangrene
i. tubular cell death
i. tubular damage
ischial tuberosity
ischioanal

ischiocavernosus muscle
ischiorectal
i. anorectal space
i. aponeurosis
i. excavation
i. fascia
i. fat
i. fistula
i. fossa
i. fossa plane
i. perirectal abscess
i. region
ischochymia
ISD
intrinsic sphincter deficiency
intrinsic sphincter dysfunction
ISEL
in situ end labeling
isethionate
pentamidine i.
ISH
isolated systolic hypertension
island
i. flap procedure
i. groin flap
lipid i.
mucosal i.
i. pedicle flap
islet
i. amyloid polypeptide
i. cell
i. cell adenoma
i. cell antibody (ICA test)
i. cell carcinoma
i. cell hyperplasia
i. cell implant
i. cell of Langerhans
i. cell tumor
Langerhans i.
Isletest-ICA
Ismelin
Is-5-Mn
isosorbide-5-mononitrate
ISO_2
oxygen saturation index
isoamyl alcohol
ISOBAR barostat distension device
isobaric gastric distention
isobutyl 2-cyanoacrylate
Isocal
I. HCN
I. HCN liquid feeding

NOTES

isocarboxazid
isodose contour
isoechoic
isoenzyme
>alkaline phosphatase i.
>Regan i.
>serum pepsinogen i. (I, II)

isoflavone
isoflurane
isoform
>growth factor i.

isoiodide
isolate
isolated
>i. cortical tubule (ICT)
>i. cyst
>i. gastric varices (type 1, 2) (IGV)
>i. generator
>i. granulomatous gastritis
>i. hepatocyte perfusion
>i. hypoaldosteronism
>i. renal mucormycosis
>i. retained antrum syndrome
>i. systolic hypertension (ISH)
>i. urinary tract infection

isolation
>body substance i. (BSI)
>category-specific i.
>i. defect
>disease-specific i.

isoleucine
>peptide histidine i. (PHI)

isomannide
IsoMed constant flow infusion system
isomerase
>glucose-6-phosphate i.

isometric
>i. force
>i. tubular vacuolization

Isomil
>I. SF
>I. SF formula

isomotic lavage
isoniazid
isoniazid-induced hepatitis
isoosmolar liquid
isopentane
isoperistaltic
>i. anastomosis
>i. direction
>i. ileal reservoir

isoprenaline
isoprenologue
isopropamide iodide
isopropanol
isoproterenol
Isoptin

Isordil
isosorbide dinitrate
isosorbide-5-mononitrate (Is-5-Mn)
Isospora belli
isosporan parasite
isosporiasis
Isotein HN
>I. HN feeding

isoterm
>Langmuir adsorption i.

isothiocyanate
>fluorescein i. (FITC)

isotonic
>i. contraction
>i. feeding
>i. saline

isotope
>^{131}I-lipiodol i.
>i. meal
>i. nephrography
>i. renal scan
>i. renogram
>i. renography
>i. study
>^{99m}Tc-MAG-3 i.
>technetium-99m mercaptoacetythiglycine i.
>i. voiding cystourethrography (IVCU)

isotropic
>i. probe 2818
>i. scan

isovaleric
>i. acid
>i. acidemia

isovolemic variance
Isovue
Isovue-300
isoxazole derivative
isoxsuprine
I-Soyalac formula
isozyme
>CYP i.

ispaghula husk
isradipine
Israel
>I. operation
>I. retractor

issue
>adequacy i.

isthmectomy
isthmic
isthmus, pl. **isthmi**
>i. prostatae
>i. urethra

Isuprel
isuria

itch
>jock i.
>swimmer's i.

iterative bifid branching system

ITGCN
>intratubular germ cell neoplasia

ITGP
>immunotactoid glomerulopathy

ITI
>inter-alpha-trypsin inhibitor

Itis
>bundle of I.

Ito
>I. cell
>I. cell sarcoma

ITP
>Ifex, Taxol, Platinol

itraconazole

Itrel pulse generator

ITT
>intention-to-treat

^{125}I-Tyr1-somatostatin

IUGR
>intrauterine growth restriction

IUI
>intrauterine insemination

IU/L
>international unit per liter

IV
>intravenous
>>IV fluid
>>IV fluid therapy
>>piggybacking of IV
>>IV sedation

IVAC needleless IV System

Ivalon
>I. sponge

>I. sponge hysterosacropexy
>I. sponge rectopexy
>I. sponge-wrap operation
>I. suture

Ivanissevitch ligation

IVC
>inferior vena cava
>intravenous cholangiogram
>intravenous cholangiography

IVCU
>isotope voiding cystourethrography

Ivemark syndrome

ivermectin

IVH
>intravenous hyperalimentation

IVH2RA
>intravenous H2 receptor antagonist

IVIg
>intravenous immunoglobulin

IVN
>intravenous nutrition

Ivor
>I. Lewis esophagogastrectomy
>I. Lewis two-stage subtotal esophagectomy

IVP
>intravenous pyelogram

IVT
>interactive video technology

IVU
>intravenous urogram
>intravenous urography
>>high-dose IVU
>>one-shot IVU

IVUS
>intravascular ultrasound
>>IVUS catheter

NOTES

J

J chain
J line
J needle
J pelvic ileal pouch
J reservoir
J wire

Jaboulay
J. button
J. gastroduodenostomy
J. procedure
J. pyloroplasty

Jaboulay-Doyen-Winkleman
J.-D.-W. operation
J.-D.-W. technique

jackknife position

Jackson
J. esophageal bougie
J. esophagoscope
J. membrane
J. staging system
J. veil

Jackson-Pratt
J.-P. catheter
J.-P. drain

Jacobson needle holder

Jacobs-Palmer laparoscope

Jacoby test

Jadassohn syndrome

Jaffe
J. picrate reaction
J. test

Jagwire guidewire

Jaksch test

Jamaican
J. vomiting sickness
J. vomiting syndrome

Jamshidi liver biopsy needle

Janeway
J. gastroscope
J. gastrostomy
J. lesion

Jansen retractor

Jansen-type metaphyseal chondrodysplasia

Janus
J. System III

Japanese
J. cancer classification
J. classification of cancer
J. dysentery
J. schistosomiasis

japonicum
Schistosoma j.

Jarit rotator

Jarotsky diet

Jarvis
J. hemorrhoid clamp
J. hemorrhoid forceps
J. pile clamp

Jasbee esophagoscope

Jass staging for rectal carcinoma

Jatrox
J. *Helicobacter pylori* test
J. Hp-test

jaundice
acholuric j.
benign postoperative j.
black j.
Budd j.
catarrhal j.
cholestatic j.
chronic idiopathic j.
cloxacillin-induced cholestatic j.
Crigler-Najjar j.
deep j.
Epping j.
familial chronic idiopathic j.
familial nonhemolytic j.
Hayem j.
hemolytic j.
hepatocanalicular j.
hepatocellular j.
hepatogenic j.
homologous serum j.
infectious j.
infective j.
iproniazid-induced j.
latent j.
leptospiral j.
malignant obstructive j.
mechanical j.
neonatal j.
newborn j.
nonhemolytic j.
nonobstructive j.
obstructive j.
painless j.
parenchymal j.
physiologic j.
regurgitation j.
retention j.
shrapnel-induced obstructive j.
ticrynafen-induced j.

jaundiced skin

Jaworski
J. body
J. corpuscle
J. test

jaw wiring

413

J/cm
    joule per centimeter
J-curve effect
Jeffrey introducer set
jejunal
    j. bypass
    j. colonization
    j. crest
    j. cutaneous urinary diversion
    j. diverticulosis
    j. drainage and biopsy
    j. feeding tube
    j. gluten challenge
    j. IgA
    j. interposition of Henle loop
    j. limb
    j. pouch
    j. syndrome
    j. tube insertion
    j. tube through percutaneous
      endoscopic gastrostomy (JETPEG)
    j. ulcer
    j. urinary conduit
    j. varix
    j. villus
jejunales
    arteriae j.
jejunectomy
jejuni
    Campylobacter j.
jejunitis
    nongranulomatous j.
    ulcerative j.
jejunocecostomy
    ulcerative jejunitis j.
jejunocolic fistula
jejunocolostomy
jejunogastric intussusception
jejunoileal (JI)
    j. atresia
    j. bypass (JIB)
    j. bypass surgery
    j. fold pattern reversal
    j. intestine
    j. shunt
jejunoileitis
    nongranulomatous ulcerative j.
jejunoileostomy
    Roux-en-Y distal j.
jejunoileum
jejunojejunostomy
jejunoplasty
jejunorrhaphy
jejunostomy
    direct percutaneous j. (DPJ)
    j. elemental diet feeding
    endoscopic j.
    laparoscopic-guided feeding j.

    long Roux-en-Y pouch j.
    loop j.
    needle-catheter j.
    percutaneous endoscopic j. (PEJ)
    Roux-en-Y j.
    j. tract choledochoscopy
    j. tube
    j. tube feeding
    Witzel j.
jejunotomy
jejunum
    j. antigen
    Roux-en-Y loop of j.
Jelco catheter
jelly
    Anestacon 2% lidocaine
      hydrochloride j.
    carboxymethyl cellulose j.
    electrode j.
    lidocaine hydrochloride j.
    Lubraseptic j.
    Snap-It lubricating j.
    spermicidal j.
    Xylocaine j.
JEM-100B and 100S electron
  microscope
Jenamicin
Jenckel
    J. cholecystoduodenostomy
    J. cholecystoduodenostomy method
Jendrassik-Grof method
Jenning-Streifeneder gastroscope
JEOL
    JEOL 100 CX electron microscope
    JEOL JSM 35 CF scanning
      electron microscope
jerk
    absent ankle j.
    ankle j.
Jesberg esophagoscope
jet
    j. nebulizer
    j. stream phenomenon
    ureteral j.
Jetco-spray cannula
jetlike bleeding
JETPEG
    jejunal tube through percutaneous
      endoscopic gastrostomy
Jeune
    J. asphyxiating thoracic dystrophy
    J. syndrome
Jevity
    J. isotonic liquid nutrition
    J. tube feeding formula
jeweler's forceps
Jewett
    J. bladder carcinoma classification

J. classification of bladder
carcinoma
J. sound
J. staging system
Jewett-Strong system
Jewett-Whitmore Cancer Staging System
JF-200
J. duodenoscope
J. side-viewing videoendoscope
JF-20 side-viewing fiberoptic endoscope
JFB III endoscope
JF-IT20 duodenoscope
JG
juxtaglomerular
J-hook tip laparoscopic electrode
JI
jejunoileal
JIB
jejunoileal bypass
Jin Bu Huan
J-loop ileostomy
J-Maxx stent
Jobert de Lamballe suture
Job syndrome
jock itch
Joe hoe
Joel-Cohen incision
Johanson-Blizzard syndrome
Johne disease
Johns
J. Hopkins gallbladder forceps
J. Hopkins gallbladder retractor
J. Hopkins prostate cancer grading
system
Johnson
J. esophagogastroscopy
J. esophagogastrostomy
Johnston buttonhole procedure
joint
j. erythema
sacroiliac j.
Jolles test
Jonas
J. implant
J. penile prosthesis
Jones-Politano technique
Jones silver stain
Jonnesco
J. fold
J. fossa
J. operation

Joseph
J. hook
J. syndrome
Joubert syndrome
joule per centimeter (J/cm)
Joyce-Loebl Magiscan image analysis
system
JP
juvenile polyposis
JPD
juxtapapillary diverticulum
J-pexy
omental J-p.
J-pouch
colonic J-p.
JPS
juvenile polyposis syndrome
JR-St cell
J-scope esophagoscope
J-shaped
J-s. endoscope
J-s. ileal pouch
J-s. ileal pouch-anal anastomosis
J-s. ileal reservoir
JT1001 prostate cancer vaccine
J-tube
J-t. insertion
wire-guided J-t.
J-turn of the scope
J-type maneuver
Judd
J. cystoscope
J. pyloroplasty
J. ventral hernia repair
Judd-Allis intestinal forceps
Judd-DeMartel gallbladder forceps
jugular
juice
acid-peptic j.
duodenal j.
gastric j.
intestinal j.
pancreatic j.
pure pancreatic j. (PPJ)
Julian
J. cystoresectoscope
J. splenorenal forceps
jumbo
j. biopsy
j. biopsy forceps
jumentosa
urina j.

NOTES

junction
anomalous pancreatobiliary duct j. (APBDJ)
anorectal j.
cardioesophageal j. (CE, CEJ)
cardioesophageal mucosal j.
choledochopancreatic ductal j.
costochondral j.
cystic-choledochal j.
cysticohepatic j.
desmosomal j.
detrusor muscle protrusion j.
duodenojejunal j. (DJJ)
esophagogastric j.
fundic-antral j.
gap j.
gastroesophageal j.
hepaticocystic j.
hyperactive rectosigmoid j.
ileocecal j.
intermediate j.
mucosal j.
NS3/NS4 j.
NS4/NS5 j.
pancreaticobiliary ductal j.
pancreaticocholedochoductal j.
patulous gastroesophageal j.
penopubic j.
penoscrotal j.
pharyngoesophageal j.
prostatovesical j.
pyloroduodenal j.
rectosigmoid j.
saphenofemoral j.
squamocolumnar mucosal j.
tracheoesophageal j.
ureteropelvic j. (UPJ)
ureterovesical j. (UVJ)

junctional
j. cyst
j. intestinal metaplasia
juvenile
j. cirrhosis
j. nephronophthisis
j. nephronophthisis-medullary cystic disease
j. polyposis (JP)
j. polyposis coli
j. polyposis syndrome (JPS)
j. retention polyp
j. xanthogranuloma
juxtacapillary process
juxtaglomerular (JG)
j. apparatus
j. apparatus tumor
j. body
juxtahepatic venous injury
juxtamedullary
j. arteriole
j. renal corpuscle
juxtapapillary
j. diverticulum (JPD)
j. duodenal diverticulum
juxtaposed mesenteric lymph node
juxtapyloric ulcer
juxtaregional node
juxtavesical ureter
J-Vac
J-V. closed wound drainage
J-V. drain
J-V. suction reservoir
J-wave phenomenon
J-wire guide

K2

    vitamin K2

K-141

    Dianeal K-141

K+

    Ca^{2+}-activated K+

K562 erythroid line

kabure

Kader

    K. gastrostomy
    K. operation

KAL1 **gene**

kala azar

Kaleorid

kaliopenic nephropathy

Kaliscinski

    K. plication
    K. ureteral folding technique

kaliuretic diuretic

Kalk esophagoscope

kallidin

kallikrein

    human glandular k. 3
    k. inheritance
    plasma k.
    tissue k.
    urinary k.

kallikrein-like gene

Kallmann syndrome

Kammerer-Battle incision

Kanagawa phenomenon

kanamycin nephropathy

Kane umbilical clamp

Kangaroo

    K. Delivery System
    K. 200, 330 enteral feeding pump
    K. 324 feeding pump
    K. gastrostomy tube

kansasii

    Mycobacterium k.

K antigen

Kantor string sign

Kantrex

kanyemba

Kaodene

kaolin

Kaopectate

Kapectolin

Kaplan-Meier

    K.-M. analysis
    K.-M. curve
    K.-M. method

Kaposi

    K. sarcoma (KS)
    K. sarcoma-associated herpesvirus

kappa

    k. light chain
    k. receptor opioid agonist

Kapp-Beck colon clamp

Kapsinow test

KAR

    killer-activating receptor

Karaya

    K. gum
    K. 5 paste
    K. powder
    K. ring ileostomy appliance
    K. 5 seal

Karl

    K. Storz Calcutript
    K. Storz endoscope
    K. Storz flexible ureteropyeloscope
    K. Storz instrumentation
    K. Storz-Lutzeyer lithotriptor

Karmen unit

Karnofsky

    K. index
    K. performance status
    K. performance status scale
    K. score

Karroo syndrome

Kartagener syndrome

karyometry

karyotype

    chromosome k.

Kasai

    K. classification for extrahepatic
      bile duct atresia
    K. operation
    K. peritoneal venous shunt
    K. portoenterostomy
    K. procedure

Kasai-type hepatoportoenterostomy

Kashin-Beck disease

Kashiwado test

Kaslow intestinal tube

Kasugai

    chronic pancreatitis of K.
    K. classification

Katayama

    K. disease
    K. fever
    K. syndrome

KATO-III cell

Kato test

Kaufman syndrome

Kawasaki syndrome

Kaye

    K. nephrostomy tamponade balloon
    K. tamponade balloon catheter

K

Kayexalate enema
Kayser-Fleischer ring
KB
  ketone body
KBR
  ketone body ratio
KC
  Kupffer cell
KCl
  potassium chloride
Kearns-Sayre syndrome (KSS)
Keeler
  K. Magnalite headlamp
  K. panoramic loupe
Keen Edge disposable biopsy forceps
Keflex
Keftab
Kefzol
Kegelcisor
Kegel pelvic muscle exercise
Kehr
  K. incision
  K. sign
  K. T-tube
Keith needle
Kelami classification
Keller
  K. hydrodynamic hypothesis of
    sieving
  K. hypothesis
Kelling
  K. gastroscope
  K. test
Kelling-Madlener procedure
Kellogg's Castor Oil
Kelly
  K. abdominal retractor
  K. clamp
  K. cystoscope
  K. fistula scissors
  K. forceps
  K. hemostat
  K. operation
  K. plication
  K. plication procedure
  K. proctoscope
  K. rectal speculum
  K. sigmoidoscope
  K. sign
  K. sphincteroscope
Kelly-Deming operation
Kelly-Kennedy modification
Kelly-Murphy forceps
Kelly-Stoeckel operation
Kelman
  K. air cystotome
  K. double-bladed cystotome

  K. knife-cannula cystotome
  K. knife cystotome
keloid
kelotomy
Kelsey pile clamp
Kemadrin
Kennedy disease
Kent deep surgery forceps
Keofeed
  K. enteral feeding bag
  K. 500 enteral feeding pump
  K. II enteral feeding pump
  K. II feeding tube
keratin
  antibody to k.
keratinization
  single cell k.
keratinocyte growth factor
keratitis
  seborrheic k.
keratoacanthoma
keratoderma blennorrhagica
keratosis, pl. **keratoses**
  k. blennorrhagica
  k. follicularis
  lace-like k.
keratotic pseudoepitheliomatous balanitis
Kerckring
  circular folds of K.
  K. fold
  valve of K.
kerion formation
Kerlix wrap
kernicterus
Kernig sign
Kerr kink
Keshan disease
Kessler-Kleinert suture
ketamine
ketanserin
keto
  k. acid
  k. acid-amino acid supplement
ketoacidosis
  diabetic k.
7-ketocholesterol
ketoconazole
ketogenesis
ketoglutaramate (KGM)
  alpha k.
ketoglutarate (KG)
  k. dehydrogenase (KGDH)
ketone
  k. body (KB)
  k. body ratio (KBR)
  k. body test
  urinary k.
ketoprofen analgesic therapy

ketorolac tromethamine
ketosteroid
17-ketosteroid
ketotifen
keyhole
    k. deformity
    k. limpet hemocyanin (KLH)
KeyMed
    K. advanced dilator
    K. advanced esophageal dilator set
    K. Atkinson endoprosthesis
    K. automatic reprocessor
    K. disposable variceal injection
      needle
    K. heater probe thermocoagulation
    K. Nottingham introducer
    K. unit
Keystone technique
KG
   ketoglutarate
   alpha-KG
KGDH
   ketoglutarate dehydrogenase
   alpha-KGDH
KGM
   ketoglutaramate
   alpha-KGM
Khafagy modified ileocecal cystoplasty
  urinary diversion
KHB
   Krebs-Henseleit bicarbonate buffer
Ki-67 stain
Kidd cystoscope
kidney
   abdominal k.
   k. abscess
   k. adenoma
   k. adysplasia
   k. agenesis
   allocating cadaveric k.
   k. allograft
   amyloid k.
   k. amyloidosis
   k. angiomyolipoma
   k. aplasia
   k. arteriovenous fistula
   artificial k.
   k. ascent
   Ask-Upmark k.
   k. ballottement
   cadaver k.
   cake k.

k. calcification
k. calix
k. carbuncle
k. carcinoma
k. carcinosarcoma
k. clearance
clear cell carcinoma of k.
k. clear cell sarcoma
coarsely granular k.
congenital double k.
congested k.
k. cortex
crush k.
cyanotic k.
k. cyst
decapsulation of k.
disk k.
k. donor
donor k.
Dow Hollow Fiber k. (DHFK)
dump k.
dwarf k.
k. dysplasia
dysplastic k.
dystopic k.
ectopic k.
k. electrolyte clearance rate
k. electrolyte excretion rate
embryoma of the k.
k. failure
fatty k.
k. fibroma
k. fibrosarcoma
finely granular k.
flea-bitten k.
Formad k.
k. function
fused k.
Gambro Lundia Minor artificial k.
k. Gerota fascia
k. glomerulocystic disease
k. glomerulus
Goldblatt k.
gouty k.
granular k.
k. hematoma
k. hemorrhage
hind k.
HLA-matched k.
horseshoe k.
hypermobile k.
hypoplastic k.

NOTES

kidney *(continued)*
k. inflammation
k. innervation
k. internal splint/stent (KISS)
k. internal splint/stent catheter
k. ischemia
lardaceous k.
k. leiomyosarcoma
k. liposarcoma
k.'s, liver, spleen (KLS)
living donor k.
k. lobe
lumbar k.
lump k.
k. lymphoblastoma
k. magnesium filtration
malacoplakia of k.
k. malacoplakia
k. malignant fibrous histiocytoma
k. mass
maximal tubular excretory capacity
    of k.
k. medulla
medullary sponge k.
mortar k.
multicystic k. (MCK)
multicystic dysplastic k. (MCDK)
multilobar k.
multilobular k.
mural k.
murine k.
myelin k.
myeloma k.
k. nephroma
obstructed k. (OBK)
k. oncocytoma
k. ossifying tumor
k. osteogenic sarcoma
Page k.
palpable k.
pancake k.
k. pedicle clamp
pelvic k.
pole of k.
presacral ectopic k.
primordial k.
k. pseudotumor
k. punch
putty k.
pyramid of k.
k. rhabdomyosarcoma
right k. (RK)
Rokitansky k.
Rose-Bradford k.
sacciform k.
k. scarring
sclerotic k.
k. shock wave effect

sigmoid k.
k. size
soapy k.
solitary k.
k. sparing operation
k. stone
supernumerary k.
k.s, ureters, bladder (KUB)
k.s, ureters, bladder radiography
thoracic k.
k. transillumination
k. transplant
k. transplantation
k. transplant recipient
unilateral fused k.
unipapillary k.
k. variant
k. vascular pedicle
k. vasculature
k. weight (KW)
k. worm
Kiernan space
Kifa skin clip
killer
natural k. (NK)
k. T cell
killer-activating receptor (KAR)
Killian
K. dehiscence
K. rectal speculum
K. suction tube
K. triangle
Kilner needle holder
KilRoid single-handed ligator
Kim Care contour brief
Kimmelstiel-Wilson (KW)
K.-W. disease
K.-W. syndrome
Kimura disease
kinase
conserved helix-loop-helix
    ubiquitous k. (CHUK)
cyclin-dependent k.
extracellular signal-regulated
    protein k. (ERK)
herpes simplex virus thymidine k.
    (HSK-tk)
ligand-triggered protein tyrosine k.
mitogen-activated protein k.
    (MAPK)
muscle-brain isoenzyme of
    creative k. (CK-MB)
myosin light-chain k.
protein k. A
protein k. C (PKC)
protein serine k.
protein threonine k.
protein tyrosine k.

pyruvate k.
tyrosine protein k.
3-kinase
PI 3-k.
Kinberg test
Kinesed
kinetic
bromodeoxyuridine cell k.'s
capacity-limited k.'s
first-order k.'s
k. gallbladder study
gastric cell k.'s
Gompertzian tumor k.'s
Michaelis-Menten k.'s
k. parameter
urea k.'s
Kinevac
King
5-15 K. Armstrong unit
K. technique
King-Armstrong unit
King's College ALF criteria
kinin
kink
k. in bowel
k. in intestine
Kerr k.
Kinkiang fever
kinking
Kinnier Wilson disease
Ki-*ras*
K.-*r.* gene
K.-*r.* gene mutation
Kirchner diverticulum
Kirschner abdominal retractor
Kirsten-*ras*
K.-*r.* oncogene
K.-*r.* oncogen mutation
Kish urethral illuminate catheter
KISS
kidney internal splint/stent
KISS catheter
kissing
k. prostatic lobes
k. ulcers
kit
Abbott HCV EIA 2nd
generation k.
Abbott HCV 2.0 test k.
Bard-Stiegmann-Goff variceal
ligation k.
BIO101 MERmaid k.

Boehringer k.
Carey-Coons biliary
endoprosthesis k.
Cavilon diabetes foot care k.
Coloplast irrigation k.
DNA labeling k.
EIA k.
Fix and Perm permeabilizing k.
Flexiflo Inverta-PEG gastrostomy k.
Flexiflo Lap G laparoscopic
gastrostomy k.
Flexiflo Lap J laparoscopic
jejunostomy k.
Flexiflo over-the-guidewire
gastrostomy k.
Gastrin RIA k. II
Gene Clean II k.
Hashizume endoscopic ligator k.
Helisal Rapid Blood diagnostic k.
Histofine SAB k.
Histofine SAB-PO k.
Hybritech Tandem-R assay k.
MERmaid k.
Moss G-tube PEG k.
Nichols IRMA k.
OctreoScan k.
Ott/Mayo Channel Sampling k.
Percufix catheter cuff k.
Predicta TGF-β1 k.
propHiler urinary pH testing k.
Pros-Check k.
Pulse-Pak infusion k.
PyloriTek *Helicobacter pylori*
test k.
Random Primed DNA Labeling k.
rapid urease testing k.
RIA k.
Russell gastrostomy k.
RUT k.
Sacks-Vine gastrostomy k.
Serodia commercial k.
Steigmann-Goff endoscopic
ligator k.
StoneRisk diagnostic monitoring k.
Tandem-R assay k.
UltraTag RBC k.
Uri-Kit culture k.
UriSite urine collection k.
Uri-Three culture k.
Vectastain ABC k.
Versa-PEG gastrostomy k.

K

NOTES

kit *(continued)*
  Vesica percutaneous bladder neck
    suspension k.
  Wilson-Cook feeding tube k.
Kitano knot
Kiton red dye
Kittner dissector
Klatskin
  K. liver biopsy needle
  K. stenosis
  K. tumor
Klebanoff
  K. common duct bougie
  K. common duct sound
  K. gallstone scoop
Klebs disease
Klebsiella
  K. oxytoca
  K. pneumoniae
Kleinert
  K. pants
  K. Safe and Dry panty and pad
    system
Kleinschmidt appendectomy clamp
Klemm sign
Klemperer disease
Kleppinger forceps
KLH
  keyhole limpet hemocyanin
KLH-ImmuneActivator
Klinefelter syndrome
Kling dressing
Klippel-Trenaunay-Weber syndrome
Klonopin
KLS
  kidneys, liver, spleen
Km
  Michaelis constant
KMI 60 enteral feeding pump
knee-chest position
knee-elbow position
knife, pl. **knives**
  Bard-Parker k.
  k. blade
  cautery k.
  cold k.
  Collin k.
  Collings electrosurgery k.
  Desmarres paracentesis k.
  electrocautery k.
  k. electrode
  electrosurgical cutting k.
  endarterectomy k.
  hernia k.
  hook k.
  Hulbert electrosurgical k.
  insulation-tipped electrosurgical k.
  Lempert paracentesis k.

  Mori k.
  needle k.
  optical laser k.
  optical urethrotome k.
  Orandi k.
  skin k.
  urethrotome k.
knife-like pain
knob
  lateral deflection control k.
knobby process
knock
  pericardial k.
Knodell
  K. component
  K. criteria for histology activity
  K. index
  K. score
knot
  crochet k.
  curved-needle surgeon's k.
  externally releasable k.
  friction k.
  granny k.
  half-hitch k.
  ileosigmoid k.
  Kitano k.
  laparoscopic k.
  one-handed k.
  Roeder loop k.
  self-tightening slip k.
  square k.
  surgeon's k.
  Tim k.
knotting
  stochastic k.
knowledge
  Crohn and Colitis K. (CCKNOW)
knuckle of colon
Ko-Airan maneuver
Kocher
  K. anastomosis
  K. clamp
  K. dilatation ulcer
  K. forceps
  K. gallbladder retractor
  K. hemostat
  K. incision
  K. maneuver
  K. operation
  K. pylorectomy
  K. ureterosigmoidostomy procedure
kocherization
Koch postulate
Kock
  K. continent ileostomy
  K. neobladder
  K. nipple

K

K. nipple valve
K. pouch cutaneous urinary diversion
K. pouch modified procedure
K. reservoir
K. reservoir ileostomy
K. technique
K. urinary pouch
Kockogram
Kodak Ektachem 700 machine
Kodsi scale
Koenig, König
K. syndrome
Koerte gallstone forceps
Koh-I-Noor Universal India ink
Kohlmeier-Degos disease
Kohlrausch valve
KOH smear
koilocytosis
Kollmann dilator
Kolmogorov-Smirnov test
kolypeptic
Kondremul
König (*var. of* Koenig)
Konigsberg
K. catheter
K. 5-channel solid-state catheter assembly
K. microtransducer
Konsyl
Konsyl-D
Kontrast U
Koplik spot
Korean
K. hemorrhagic fever
K. hemorrhagic nephrosonephritis
Koro syndrome
Korsakoff syndrome
Kossa stain
Koyanagi technique for hypospadias repair
K-Pek
K-Phen-50
K-Phos Neutral
K-*ras*
K.-*r.* gene
K.-*r.* oncogene
Kraske
K. operation
K. parasacral approach
K. position
K. roll

kraurosis
penile k.
Krause
K. arm rest
K. ligament
Krazy Glue sclerosant
krebiozen false cancer cure
Krebs
K. cycle
K. solution
Krebs-Henseleit bicarbonate buffer (KHB)
Krebs-Ringer
K.-R. bicarbonate buffer
K.-R. solution
Kreha
polysaccharide K. (PSK)
Krentz gastroscope
Kretz
K. Combison 330 ultrasound scanner
K. granule
K. 311 ultrasound scanner
K. ultrasound system
Kringle domain
Kristalose
kristensenii
Yersinia k.
Krokicwicz test
Kron
K. bile duct dilator
K. gall duct dilator
Krönlein hernia
Kropp
K. bladder neck reconstruction
K. cystourethroplasty
K. operation
K. procedure
K. technique
Kruger index
Krukenberg
K. tumor
K. veins
krusei
Candida k.
Kruskal-Wallis
K.-W. analysis of variance
K.-W. test
krypton laser
KS
Kaposi sarcoma
KSG-504 CCK antagonist

NOTES

423

KSS
Kearns-Sayre syndrome
KTP
potassium-titanyl phosphate
KTP 532 laser
KTP laser probe
KTP laser prostatectomy
KTP 532
Laserscope KTP 532
KTP/Nd:YAG laser treatment
K-tube
Kt/V urea
KUB
kidneys, ureters, bladder
KUB radiography
Kudrox
Kugel hernia patch
Kulchitsky cell
Kumpe catheter
Kunkel syndrome
Kupffer
K. cell (KC)
K. cell sarcoma

Kuracil
Kussmaul
K. breathing
K. endoscope
Ku-Zyme
K.-Z. HP
K.-Z. HP pancreatic enzyme
Kveim test
KW
kidney weight
Kimmelstiel-Wilson
kwashiorkor
Kwell
Kyasanur Forest disease
kymography
balloon k.
kyphoscoliosis
kyphosis
Kyrle disease
Kytril

L-364,781 CCK antagonist
L-365,260 CCK antagonist
LA
    Los Angeles
    lupus anticoagulant
        LA classification
LAAL
    lower anterior axillary line
Labbe
    L. syndrome
    L. triangle
labeled red blood cell scan
labeling
    in situ end l. (ISEL)
    terminal uridine deoxynucleotide
        nick end l. (TUNEL)
labetalol
labialis
    herpes l.
labial ulceration
labile
    acid l.
labium
    l. inferius valvulae coli
    l. majus muscle
    l. minus muscle
    l. superius valvulae coli
    l. urethra
laboratory
    l. abnormality
    Venereal Disease Research L.
        (VDRL)
labyrinth
    cortical l.
    Ludwig l.
    renal l.
    Santorini l.
lab zymogen
lace-like keratosis
laceration
    concurrent hepatic l.
    longitudinal l.
    lower pole l.
    Mallory-Weiss l.
    rectal l.
    splenic l.
    vascular l.
lacrimal duct probe
lactaciduria
LactAid
lactase
    l. deficiency
    l. enzyme
lactase-ceramidase complex
lactase-phlorizin hydrolase (LPH)

lactate
    l. dehydrogenase (LDH)
    Ringer l.
lactated Ringer solution
lacteal
    central l.
    l. vessel
lactic
    l. acid
    l. acid dehydrogenase (LDH)
    l. acidosis
Lactinex
lactobacilli preparation
Lactobacillus
    L. acidophilus
    L. agilis
    L. bifidus
    L. bulgaricus
    L. casei
    L. GG (LGG)
    L. plantarum
    L. plantarum-fermented food
    L. plantarum-fermented oat
    L. plantarum 299v
    L. reuteri
    L. rhamnosus
lactobezoar
lactobionate
    erythromycin l.
lactoferrin
lacto-N-fucopentaose
    sialylated l.-N-f.
lactose
    disaccharide l.
    l. hydrogen breath testing (LHBT)
    l. intolerance
    l. malabsorption (LMA)
    l. maldigestor
    l. tolerance test
lactose-associated diarrhea
lactose-free
    l.-f. diet (LFD)
    l.-f. feeding
lactovegetarian
lactovegetarianism
Lactrase
lactulose
    l. enema
    l. hydrogen breath test (LHBT)
    l. solution
lactulose-mannitol
    l.-m. permeability test
    l.-m. ratio
lacuna, pl. lacunae
    great l.

L

lacuna *(continued)*
    l. magna
    Morgagni lacunae
    l. of muscle
    l. of urethra
    urethral l.
lacunar abscess
lacunula, pl. **lacunulae**
lacunule
Ladd
    L. band
    L. correction of malrotation of
      bowel
    L. operation
    L. procedure
    L. syndrome
laddering
    DNA l.
Laënnec cirrhosis
Lafora body
LAGB
    Lap-Band adjustable gastric banding
      system
    LAGB system
lag phase
Lahey
    L. aneurysm needle
    L. gall duct forceps
    L. liver transplant bag
Lahey-Babcock forceps
Laidley double-catheterizing cystoscope
Laird-McMahon anorectoplasty
LAK cell
lake
    bile l.
Lalonde hook forceps
LAMA
    laser-assisted microanastomosis
L-AmB
    liposomal-amphotericin B
Lambda Plus PDL 1, 2 laser system
Lambert-Eaton myasthenic syndrome
lamblia
    Giardia l.
lambliasis
lamina
    basal l.
    l. densa
    l. muscularis mucosae
    proper l.
    l. propria
    l. propria lymphoid cell
    l. rara externa (LRE)
    l. rara interna (LRI)
    vascular l.
laminar cortical necrosis
laminated calcification
laminectomy

laminin
    32/67-kD l. receptor
    l. receptor
    l. receptor inhibition
lamivudine
lamotrigine
lamp
    Desmoreaux l.
    slit l.
    Wood l.
    xenon l.
Lancereaux nephritis
lancet-shaped biopsy forceps
lancinating pain
Landau
    L. reflex
    L. trocar
landmark
    bony l.
Landzert fossa
Lane
    L. band
    L. disease
    L. gastroenterostomy catheter
    L. gastroenterostomy clamp
    L. intestinal clamp
    L. intestinal forceps
    L. operation
Lange
    L. skin-fold calipers
    L. test
Langerhans
    L. cell
    L. cell histiocytosis
    L. islet
    islet cell of L.
    L. lineage
Langer line
Langhans
    L. cell
    L. line
Langmuir adsorption isoterm
Lanoxin
lanreotide
lansoprazole, amoxicillin, clarithromycin
lanthanum carbonate
Lanza scale
Lanz point
LAP
    leucine aminopeptidase
    leukocyte alkaline phosphatase
    LAP test
lap
    laparotomy
    l. Nissen
    l. pad
    l. sponge
    l. tape

laparator
    Weck high flow l.
laparectomy
laparocele
laparocholecystotomy
laparocolectomy
laparocolostomy
laparocystectomy
laparoendoscopy
laparoenterostomy
Laparofan
laparogastroscopy
Laparolift system
LaparoLith
laparonephrectomy
laparorrhaphy
LaparoSAC
LaparoScan laparoscopic ultrasonic imaging
laparoscope
    50-degree Foroblique optic l.
    0-degree forward optic l.
    10-degree operating l.
    diagnostic l.
    EL2-LS2 flexible video l.
    flexible video l. (FVL)
    Jacobs-Palmer l.
    Olympus A5256 l.
    operative l.
laparoscopic
    l. abdominoperineal excision
    l. abdominoperineal resection
    l. adjustable gastric banding
    l. adrenalectomy
    l. adrenal gland surgery
    l. Allis clamp
    l. antireflux surgery (LARS)
    l. appendectomy
    l. biopsy
    l. biopsy of liver
    l. bladder neck suspension
    l. bladder neck suture suspension procedure
    l. Burch urethropexy
    l. cannula
    l. cholecystectomy (LC)
    l. clip application
    l. colectomy
    l. colorectal cancer surgery
    L. Colorectal Surgery Group (LCSSG)
    l. colposuspension technique

l. contact ultrasonography (LCU)
l. cystoplasty
l. cystourethropexy
l. dismembered pyeloplasty
l. gastric bypass
l. grasper
l. Heller myotomy
l. hysterosalpingectomy
l. intracorporal ultrasound (LICU)
l. knot
l. laser-assisted autoaugmentation
l. laser cholecystectomy (LLC)
l. living donor nephrectomy
l. lymphocelectomy
l. lysis
l. marsupialization
l. needle colposuspension
l. needle driver
l. nephroureterectomy
l. Nissen fundoplication (lap Nissen)
l. Nissen and Toupet fundoplication
l. orchiopexy
l. partial nephrectomy
l. pelvic lymphadenectomy
l. pelvic lymph node dissection (LPLND)
l. photography
l. pyelolithotomy
l. radical nephrectomy (LRN)
l. radical prostatectomy
l. retraction system
l. retropubic colposuspension
l. seromyotomy
l. stapler
l. suture rectopexy
l. tie clip
l. transcystic duct exploration
l. transcystic duct stenting of papilla
l. transcystic papillotomy
l. trocar sleeve
l. ultralow anterior resection
l. ultrasound (LUS)
l. ureteral reanastomosis
l. ureterolithotomy
l. ureterolysis
l. urinary diversion procedure
l. uterolysis
l. vagotomy
l. varicocelectomy
l. varicocele repair
l. varix ligation

L

NOTES

laparoscopically
    l. assisted colorectal resection
    l. assisted panenteroscopy
    l. guided transcystic exploration
laparoscopic-assisted
    l.-a. approach
    l.-a. hemicolectomy
laparoscopic-guided feeding jejunostomy
laparoscopist
laparoscopy
    l. complication
    l. contraindication
    double-puncture l.
    extraperitoneal l.
    flexible l.
    gasless l.
    gynecologic l.
    hand-assisted l. (HAL)
    pulmonary gas embolism during l.
    single-puncture l.
    standard l. (SL)
    therapeutic l.
    l. trocar configuration
    l. trocar placement
laparoscopy-guided subhepatic
    cholecystostomy
Laparoshield laparoscopic smoke
    filtration system
LaparoSonic coagulating shears
laparosplenectomy
laparotomy (lap)
    emergency l.
    exploratory l.
    negative l.
    l. pack
    l. pad
    l. pad cover
    second-look l.
    l. sponge
    l. tape
laparotyphlotomy
Lap-Band adjustable gastric banding
    system (LAGB)
Lapides
    L. classification
    L. classification of voiding
      dysfunction
    L. cystometric investigation
    L. test
    L. vesicostomy
Lapides-Ball urethropexy
Laplace
    L. forceps
    L. law
    law of L.
Lapra-Ty clip
LapSac introducer
Lapwall laparotomy sponge

LAR
    low anterior resection
LAR/CAA
    low anterior resection in combination
      with coloanal anastomosis
lardaceous kidney
large
    l. bowel
    l. bowel cancer
    l. bowel carcinoma
    l. bowel obstruction
    l. cell change (LCC)
    l. common duct stone
    l. needle size
large-bore
    l.-b. biliary endoprosthesis
    l.-b. cannula
    l.-b. catheter
    l.-b. double-pigtail stent
    l.-b. gastric lavage tube
    l.-b. heat probe
    l.-b. rigid esophagoscope
    l.-b. Tygon tubing
large-channel
    l.-c. endoscope
    l.-c. therapeutic duodenoscope
large-diameter bougie
large-droplet fatty liver
large-forceps biopsy
large-particle biopsy
large-volume paracentesis (LVP)
L-arginine
lari
    Campylobacter l.
Larodopa
LaRoque
    L. herniorrhaphy incision
    L. repair
    L. technique
Larrey-Weil disease
Larry
    L. rectal director
    L. rectal probe
LARS
    laparoscopic antireflux surgery
larval nephrosis
larva migrans
    visceral l. m.
larvata
    appendicitis l.
laryngeal
    l. carcinoma
    l. edema
    l. jack-assisted retrograde
      esophageal membranotomy
    l. jack technique
    l. vestibule

laryngitis
    reflux l.
laryngopharyngectomy
laryngoscope
    Olympus ENF-P-series l.
laryngoscopy
    direct l.
laryngospasm
larynx
LAS
  lymphadenopathy syndrome
laser
    l. ablation
    ADD'Stat l.
    l. adjustable silicone gastric
     banding (LASGB)
    alexandrite l.
    argon ion l.
    argon-pumped dye l.
    balloon l.
    Candela Model MDL 2000 l.
    Candela 405-nm pulsed dye l.
    carbon dioxide l.
    L. CHRP rigid fiber scope system
    l. clipping
    CO_2 l.
    l. coagulation
    Coherent model 90-K l.
    coumarin dye l.
    coumarin-flashlamp-pumped pulsed
     dye l.
    l. desorption/ionization mass
     spectrometry
    diode l.
    Diomed l.
    l. disk
    l. Doppler flowmeter
    l. Doppler velocimetry
    dye l.
    endoscopic pulsed dye l.
    flashlamp pumped dye l.
    FREDDY Nd:YAG l.
    frequency-doubled-double pulse
     ND:YAG l.
    helium-neon l.
    l. hemorrhoidectomy
    l. hemorrhoid excision
    holmium:YAG l.
    ion l.
    krypton l.
    KTP 532 l.
    l. laparoscopic vagotomy

Lateralase l.
lateral-firing l.
Lithognost flash-lamp pulsed dye l.
l. lithotripsy (LL)
l. lithotriptor
l. lithotriptor basket
LX-20 l.
medical l.
Medilas fiberTome l.
l. microscope
Molectron Nd:YAG l.
Myriadlase Side-Fire l.
Nd:YAG l.
neodymium:yttrium garnet l.
Olympus Nd:YAG l.
OmniPulse MAX holmium l.
l. partial nephrectomy
l. photoablation
l. photocoagulation
l. photodestruction
l. plume
Prolase II lateral firing Nd:YAG l.
l. prostatectomy
pulsed dye neodymium:YAG l.
pulse dye l.
Pulsolith l.
pumped-dye l.
Q-switched alexandrite l.
Q-switched Nd:YAG l.
rhodamine 6G dye l.
l. sclerosis
Side-Fire l.
SLT contact MTRL l.
l. surgery
l. temperature
l. therapy
l. thermocoagulation
l. tissue weld
l. tissue welding
l. tissue welding solder
Trimedyne holmium l.
tunable pulsed dye l.
Ultraline l.
ultrasound-guided l.
Urolase l.
l. vaporization
VersaPulse Select l.
visual endoscopically controlled l.
l. welding
l. welding technique
l. writer
YAG l.

L

NOTES

laser-assisted
    l.-a. endoscopic myotomy
    l.-a. microanastomosis (LAMA)
    l.-a. tissue welding technique
laser-Doppler Periflux PF-3 probe
laser-guided biopsy
laser-induced
    l.-i. fluorescence spectroscopy
      (LIFS)
    l.-i. fragmentation
    l.-i. intracorporeal shock wave
      lithotripsy (LISL)
LaserMed laser pointer
Laserscope
    L. KTP 532
    L. YAG 1064
Lasersonic ACMI Ultraline
laserthermia
lasertripsy
LaserTripter
    Candela MDA-200 L.
    L. MDL 3000
LASGB
    laser adjustable silicone gastric banding
Lashmet-Newburgh method
Lasix
L-asparaginase
Lassa hemorrhagic fever
lasso
    guidewire/basket l.
    l. snare
    l. technique
last-generation serologic ELISA test
lata (*pl. of* latum)
lata
    Diphyllobothrium l.
latamoxef sodium
Latarjet
    nerve of L.
late
    l. dumping
    l. dumping syndrome
    l. graft dysfunction
    l. period filariasis
latency
    pudendal nerve terminal motor l.
latent
    l. jaundice
    l. nephritis
late-onset
    l.-o. ataxia
    l.-o. hepatic failure
lateral
    l. abdominal region
    l. bending technique
    l. branch
    l. chordee
    l. cutaneous paresthesia

    l. cystocele
    l. decubitus
    l. decubitus position
    l. deflection control knob
    l. fossa
    l. fossa of preputial space
    l. gutter
    l. internal pelvic reservoir
    l. lithotomy
    l. lobe
    l. margin
    l. node dissection
    l. oblique fascia
    l. pancreaticojejunostomy
    l. prostatomy
    l. pyelography
    l. rectal ligament
    l. reflection of colon
    l. sphincterotomy
    l. ventral hernia
    l. window technique
Lateralase laser
lateral-firing laser
lateralizing sensory deficit
lateral-lateral pouch
lateral-viewing endoscope
latex
    l. agglutination assay
    l. allergy
    l. balloon
    l. fixation test
    l. hood
    l. sclerosant
latex-base skin cement
latissimus
    l. dorsi detrusor myoplasty
    l. dorsi free flap
    l. dorsi muscle
latum, pl. lata
    condyloma l.
    fascia l.
Latzko
    L. partial colpocleisis
    L. technique
Laubry-Soulle syndrome
laudanum
Laugier hernia
Launois-Cléret syndrome
Laurence-Moon-Bardet-Biedl syndrome
Laurence-Moon-Biedl syndrome
Lauren gastric carcinoma classification
lavage
    abdominal l.
    l. bowel preparation
    cisapride-assisted l.
    closed continuous l.
    colonic l.
    l. cytology

Easi-Lav l.
external biliary l.
gastric l.
gastrointestinal l.
iced saline l.
internal biliary l.
isomotic l.
Lazarus-Nelson peritoneal l.
nasocystic catheter l.
nasogastric l.
norepinephrine l.
oral l.
PEG l.
peritoneal l.
polyethylene glycol-based l.
rapid colonic l.
l. solution
stomach l.
l. and suction
Waterpik l.

lavage-induced
l.-i. cardiac asystole
l.-i. pill malabsorption

law
Bell l.
Courvoisier l.
Fitz l.
Laplace l.
l. of Laplace
Meyer-Weigert l.
Poiseuille l.
Poiseuille-Hagen l.
Salmon l.
Tait l.
Weigert-Meyer l.

lawn mower technique
Lawrence   .
L. Add-A-Cath
L. deep surgery forceps
L. gastric reservoir

Laws
L. gastroplasty
L. gastroplasty with Silastic collar-reinforced stoma

laxa
cutis l.

laxation
laxative
l. abuse
anthracene-type l.
anthraquinone l.
bulk l.

bulk-producing l.
contact l.
emollient l.
Fleet Phospho-Soda buffered saline l.
hyperosmotic l.
lubricant l.
osmotic l.
saline l.
sodium phosphate-based l.
stimulant l.
stool-softening l.
surfactant l.

LaxCaps
Phillips L.
Laxinate 100
laxity
ligamentous l.
Lax-Senna
Black-Draught L.-S.
layer
Bernard glandular l.
echo-poor l.
fascial l.
germ l.
glycosaminoglycan l.
hypoechoic ringed l.
seromuscular l.
subcutaneous l.
submucosal vaginal smooth musculofascial l.
submucous l.
subserosal l.
laying-open fistulotomy
lay-open method
Lazarus-Nelson
L.-N. peritoneal lavage
L.-N. technique
lazy bladder syndrome
LB 9501 luminometer
LBM
lean body mass
LC
laparoscopic cholecystectomy
liver cirrhosis
LCA
lithocholic acid
liver cell adenoma
LCA-DCA
lithocolic acid-deoxycholic acid ratio
LCA-DCA ratio

L

NOTES

LCAT
lecithin-cholesterol acyltransferase
LCC
large cell change
LCDD
light chain deposition disease
L cell
LC-EMR
lift-and-cut endoscopic mucosal resection
LCFA
long-chain fatty acid
LCG
liquid chemical germicide
LCHAD
long-chain 3-hydroxyacyl coenzyme A
dehydrogenase
L-citrulline
lck protein
LCSSG
Laparoscopic Colorectal Surgery Group
LCT
long-chain triglyceride
LCU
laparoscopic contact ultrasonography
LD
living donor
LDH
lactate dehydrogenase
lactic acid dehydrogenase
LDH enzyme
LDH isoenzyme 5
LDH level of ascitic fluid
LDH test
LDL
low-density lipoprotein
LDL Direct test
oxidized LDL
LDL susceptibility
LDLC
low-density lipoprotein cholesterol
LDLT
living donor liver transplantation
LDP-02 antibody
LDS
ligating and dividing stapler
LDS stapler
Le
Le Bag
Le Bag ileocolonic pouch
Le Bag neobladder
Le Bag pouch reservoir
Le Bag urinary diversion
Le Bag urinary pouch
Le Fort sound
Lea
disialosyl L.
monosialosyl L.
Leach technique

lead
l. citrate
l. citrate stain
l. colic
l. nephropathy
l. poisoning
l. wire
Leadbetter
L. and Clarke technique
L. and Clarke ureteral anastomosis
L. cystourethroplasty
L. ileal loop diversion
L. maneuver
L. modification technique
L. procedure
L. tunneling technique
Leadbetter-Politano
L.-P. reimplantation
L.-P. ureteroneocystostomy
L.-P. ureterovesicoplasty
leading bar
lead-pipe
l.-p. appearance
l.-p. colon
leaf
chaparral l.
l. of mesentery
leafless tree appearance
leaflike villus
leak
anastomotic l.
distal pouch l.
lymphatic l.
l. pressure
proximal pouch l.
renal calcium l.
leakage
anastomotic l.
biliary l.
bilious l.
l. bypass cable
cavernovenous l.
crural venous l.
cystic duct l.
intraabdominal bile l.
postmicturition continuous l.
postoperative biliary l.
precipitant l.
tube l.
venous l.
leaking
leak-point pressure (LPP)
lean body mass (LBM)
learned enuresis
learning curve
leather-bottle stomach
leaves of diaphragm
Leber amaurosis

Lebsche shears
LE cell
lecimibide
lecithin
 polyunsaturated l.
lecithin-cholesterol acyltransferase
 (LCAT)
lectin
 hepatic l.
 l. reactivity
 l. staining
lecturescope
LeDuc
 L. fashion
 L. technique
 L. technique urinary diversion
 L. ureteral anastomosis
LeDuc-Camey
 L.-C. ileocolostomy
 L.-C. ileocystoplasty
leech
 mechanical l.
leflunomide (LFM)
LeFort procedure
left
 l. colon
 l. colonic flexure
 l. decubitus position
 l. gastroomental artery
 l. gutter
 l. hepatic duct (LHD)
 l. hepatic duct stricture
 l. hepatic lobe (LHL)
 l. hepatic vein (LHV)
 l. lateral decubitus position
 l. lobe
 l. lower quadrant (LLQ)
 l. pancreaticogastric fold
 l. upper quadrant (LUQ)
 l. ureter
left-sided
 l.-s. appendicitis
 l.-s. clonus
 l.-s. colitis
left-to-right subtotal pancreatectomy
Legionella pneumophila
Leigh disease
Leiner disease
leiomyoblastoma
leiomyoma, pl. **leiomyomata, leiomyomas**
 bizarre l.
 colonic l.

 duodenal l.
 epithelioid l.
 esophageal l.
 gastric l.
 parasitic l.
 l. of seminal vesicle
 testicular l.
 Zenker l.
leiomyosarcoma
 bladder l.
 gastric l.
 hepatic l.
 kidney l.
 low-grade l.
 paratesticular l.
 prostate gland l.
 rectal l.
 small intestine l.
 spermatic cord l.
Leishmania
 L. donovani
 L. donovani chagasi
 L. donovani donovani
 L. donovani infantum
 L. esophagitis
 L. infantum
leishmanial enteritis
leishmaniasis, leishmaniosis
 infantile l.
 visceral l.
Lell esophagoscope
Lembert inverting seromuscular suture
lemostenosis
Lempert paracentesis knife
Lendrum stain
length
 anal canal l. (ACL)
 functional profile l.
 functional urethral l. (FUL)
 peripheral capillary filtration slit l.
 telomere l.
 total slit pore l.
Lennhoff sign
lens
 30-degree l.
 70-degree l.
 120-degree l.
 Foroblique l.
 Hopkins II rod l.
 narrow l.
 objective l.
 right-angle l.

L

NOTES

lenta
    cholangitis l.
Lente insulin
lentigines, electrocardiographic conduction abnormalities, ocular hypertelorism, pulmonary stenosis, abnormal genitalia, retardation of growth, and deafness (LEOPARD)
lentigo
Lentivirus
lentum
    Eubacterium l.
Leonard
    L. Arm
    L. deep surgery forceps
LEOPARD
    lentigines, electrocardiographic conduction abnormalities, ocular hypertelorism, pulmonary stenosis, abnormal genitalia, retardation of growth, and deafness
        LEOPARD syndrome
Leo test
Lepley-Ernst tube
leprae
    Mycobacterium l.
leprosy
leptin level
Leptospira interrogans
leptospiral
    l. jaundice
    l. nephritis
leptospirosis
leptum
    Clostridium l.
Leriche syndrome
LES
    lesser esophageal sphincter
    lower esophageal sphincter
        LES incompetence
        LES locator
        LES pressure
        LES relaxation
        transient relaxations of the LES
Lesch-Nyhan syndrome
Lescol
Leser-Trélat sign
Lesgaft
    L. hernia
    L. space
    L. triangle
lesion
    acetowhite l.
    acute gastric mucosal l.
    ampullary l.
    anal squamous intraepithelial l.
    angiodysplastic l.
    Antopol-Goldman l.

aortoostial l.
aphthous-type l.
apple-core l.
Armanni-Ebstein l.
Baehr-Lohlein l.
bilobed polypoid l.
blanching of l.
bleeding l.
Bosniak l. (category I–IV)
bull's eye l.
Cameron l.
cauda equina l.
colonic vascular l.
Councilman l.
cutaneous l.
Dieulafoy gastric l.
doughnut l.
duodenal l.
dye sham intrarenal l.
Ebstein l.
echo-poor l.
ectatic vascular l.
exophytic l.
extramural l.
fingertip l.
flat depressed l.
flat elevated l.
florid bile duct l.
Forest I, II l.
gastric l.
gastrointestinal l.
glomerular tip l. (GTL)
gunpowder l.
hamartomatous l.
hepatic mass l.
high fundal l.
high neurological l.
hypoechoic l.
l. identification
intramural l.
Janeway l.
local glomerular l.
localized l.
Lohlein-Baehr l.
lower motor neuron l.
lumbar spinal cord l.
lymphoepithelial l.
macroorchidism l.
macroscopic l.
Mallory-Weiss l.
mesenteric vascular l.
metachronous l.
metastatic l.
minute polypoid l.
mucosal l.
mulberry l.
multicentric l.
napkin-ring annular l.

neoplastic l.
nodular l.
nonerosive gastric mucosal l.
nonneoplastic l.
ocular l.
pancreas l.
pancreatic l.
papillary l.
penile l.
perianal l.
photon-deficient l.
plaquelike l.
pliable l.
polypoid l.
precancerous l.
preoperative l.
primary glomerular l.
right-sided l.
ringlike l.
ruptured peliotic l.
satellite l.
scirrhous l.
semipedunculated l.
sessile l.
short-segment l.
skip l.
space-occupying l.
stenotic l.
stress l.
subglottic l.
submucosal upper gastrointestinal
  tract l.
synchronous l.
target l.
traumatic l.
trophic l.
tubulovillar l.
uremic gastrointestinal l.
vascular l.
vasculitic l.
vegetative l.
wire-loop l.

LESP
lower esophageal sphincter pressure
LESR
lower esophageal sphincter relaxation
lesser
l. curvature of stomach
l. curvature ulcer
l. epiploon
l. esophageal sphincter (LES)
l. omentum

l. pancreas
l. peritoneal sac
**Lester Martin modification of Duhamel
  operation**
lethargic
LE-TUMT
low-energy transurethral microwave
  thermotherapy
Leube test meal
leucine
l. aminopeptidase (LAP)
l. aminopeptidase test
l. metabolism
radiolabeled l.
l. zipper
l. zipper sequence
leucine-enkephalin (1-ENK)
Leucomax
leucovorin rescue
leu-enkephalin
leukemia
acute lymphoblastic l.
acute lymphocytic l.
acute myelomonocytic l.
chylous l.
testicular l.
Leukeran
leukobilin
leukocyte
l. adherence inhibition test
l. alkaline phosphatase (LAP)
l. alkaline phosphatase test
chemotaxis of polymorphonuclear l.
l. common antigen
l. esterase
l. esterase test
fecal l.
intraepithelial l. (IEL)
peritoneal l.
polymorphonuclear l. (PMNL)
l. scintography
tether circulating l.
l. trafficking
WBC l.
leukocytoclastic vasculitis
leukocytosis
leukopenia
acute l.
leukoplakia
bladder l.
hairy l.

L

NOTES

leukoplakia *(continued)*
    oral l.
    l. of penis
leukotriene
    l. A$_4$
    l. C$_4$
    cysteinyl l.
    l. D$_4$
leukourobilin
leu-peptide
leupeptin
leuprolide
    l. acetate
    l. acetate implant
    L. Depot Neoadjuvant Prostate
    Cancer Study Group
Leutrol
Leuvectin
levamfetamine
levamisole
Levaquin
Levarterenol
Levatol
levator
    l. ani
    l. ani hernia
    l. ani muscle
    l. ani syndrome
    l. fascia
    l. plate
    l. span
    l. veli palatini muscle
Levbid
LeVeen
    L. ascites shunt
    L. catheter
    L. inflation syringe
    L. inflator
    L. inflator with pressure gauge
    L. peritoneal shunt
    L. peritoneovenous shunt
    L. valve
level
    air-fluid l.
    Albarran deflecting l.
    alpha-1-antitrypsin l.
    alpha-fetoprotein l.
    ammonia l.
    AMP l.
    anti-M2 antimitochondrial
     antibody l.
    blood alcohol l. (BAL)
    blood lead l. (BLL)
    blood urea l.
    breath ethane l.
    complement l.
    des-gamma-carboxy prothrombin l.
    fasting serum gastrin l.

    fluid-debris l.
    gamma-glutamyl transferase l.
    gastrin mRNA l.
    homocysteine l.
    HSP-70 messenger ribonucleoprotein
     acid l.
    25-hydroxyvitamin D l.
    iothalamate l.
    leptin l.
    lipoprotein X l.
    motilin plasma l.
    pentane excretion l.
    pepsinogen l. (A, B, C)
    pericardial air-fluid l.
    polyamine l.
    protein C, S l.
    red blood cell folate l.
    serum gastrin l.
    serum leptin l.
    serum urate l.
    somatostatin MRNA l.
    stairstep air-fluid l.
    theophylline l.
    thyroid-stimulating hormone l.
    transferrin saturation l.
    uric acid l.
    urinary cGMP l.
    whole-blood trough l.
Levin
    L. tube
    L. tube aspiration
levocarnitine
levodopa/carbidopa
levodopa dopaminergic medication
levofloxacin
levorphanol
levothyroxine
Levovist contrast agent
Levsinex Timecaps
Levsin/SL
levulose test
Lewis
    L. A blood group antigen
    L. acid
    L. blood group
    L. B, X, Y antigen
    L. classification for vascular
     anomalies of the gastrointestinal
     tract
    L. cystometer
    L. Y carbohydrate epitope
Lewis-Tanner esophagectomy procedure
Lewy syringe
Lexipafant
lexipafant
Lexirin
Leyden disease

Leydig
    L. cell
    L. cell adenoma
    L. cell secretion
    L. cell secretory function
    L. cell tumor
    L. duct
leydigarche
LFD
    lactose-free diet
    low-fat diet
LFM
    leflunomide
LFS
    liver function series
LFT
    liver function test
LG
    light guide
    lymphocytic gastritis
        LG bundle
LGD
    low-grade dysplasia
LGG
    Lactobacillus GG
LGIB
    lower gastrointestinal bleeding
L-glutamine
L-glyceric aciduria
LGV
    lymphogranuloma venereum
LH
    loop of Henle
    luteinizing hormone
LHBT
    lactose hydrogen breath testing
    lactulose hydrogen breath test
LHD
    left hepatic duct
Lhermitte-Duclos disease
LH-FSH
    luteinizing hormone-follicle-stimulating
      hormone
LHL
    left hepatic lobe
LHRH
    luteinizing hormone-releasing hormone
LHV
    left hepatic vein
LI
    loop ileostomy

libera
    tenia l.
libidinal
libido
Librax
Libritabs
Lich
    L. extravesical technique
    L. procedure
    L. ureteral implantation for
      neobladder construction
lichen
    l. nitidus
    l. planus
    l. sclerosus
    l. sclerosus et atrophicus
    l. simplex chronicus
lichenoid reaction
Lich-Gregoire
    L.-G. anastomosis
    L.-G. repair
    L.-G. technique
    L.-G. ureterolysis
Lichtenstein
    L. hernial repair
    L. herniorrhaphy
LICU
    laparoscopic intracorporal ultrasound
lidamidine
Liddle
    L. disease
    L. mutation
    L. syndrome
Lidex
lidocaine
    l. hydrochloride jelly
    l. topical anesthetic
    viscous l.
lidocaine-prilocaine cream
lidofenin
    ^{99m}Tc l.
Lidox
Lidoxide
Lieberkühn
    L. ampulla
    L. crypt
    L. follicle
    L. gland
Lieberman
    L. proctoscope
    L. sigmoidoscope

NOTES

L

Liebermeister
    L. furrow
    L. groove
lieenulus (*var. of* lienculus)
lien
    l. accessorius
    l. mobilis
lienal artery
lienalis
    arteria l.
    penicilli arteriae l.
lienculus, lieenulus, lienunculus
lienectomy
lienis
    pulpa l.
    trabeculae l.
lienitis
lienocele
lienomalacia
lienomedullary
lienomyelogenous
lienomyelomalacia
lienopancreatic
lienopathy
lienophrenic ligament
lienorenal ligament
lienteric
    l. diarrhea
    l. stool
lientery
lienunculus
lienunculus (*var. of* lienculus)
lieutaudi
    trigonum vesicae l.
Lieutaud uvula
life
    l. cycle of *Echinococcus*
    health-related quality of l.
      (HRQOL)
    quality of l. (QOL)
Lifecath peritoneal implant
LIFE-GI
    light induced fluorescence endoscopy
      system
lifelong obesity
Lifemed catheter
LifeSite hemodialysis access system
lifestyle
    l. modification (LSM)
    l. therapy
Life-Tech flowmeter
L-IFN
    human lymphoblastoid interferon
Li-Fraumeni syndrome
LIFS
    laser-induced fluorescence spectroscopy
lift
    gallbladder l.

lift-and-cut
    l.-a.-c. biopsy
    l.-a.-c. endoscopic mucosal resection
      (LC-EMR)
    l.-a.-c. method
    l.-a.-c. technique
lifting sign
ligament
    Arantius l.
    Bellini l.
    Camper l.
    Carcassonne perineal l.
    cardinal l.
    cholecystoduodenal l.
    Clado l.
    Cooper l.
    coronary l.
    costovertebral l.
    external l.
    falciform l.
    femoral l.
    fissure of round l.
    fundiform l.
    gastrocolic l.
    gastrohepatic l.
    gastrolienal l.
    gastropancreatic l.
    gastrophrenic l.
    gastrosplenic l.
    gonadal l.
    Helvetius l.
    hepatic l.
    hepatocolic l.
    hepatocystocolic l.
    hepatoduodenal l.
    hepatogastric l.
    hepatogastroduodenal l.
    hepatophrenic l.
    hepatorenal l.
    hepatoumbilical l.
    Hesselbach l.
    Hey l.
    Huschke l.
    infundibulopelvic l.
    inguinal l.
    Krause l.
    lateral rectal l.
    lienophrenic l.
    lienorenal l.
    lumbodorsal l.
    l. of Mackenrodt
    medial umbilical l.
    median arcuate l.
    mucosal suspensory l.
    periurethral l.
    phrenicocolic l.
    phrenicoesophageal l.
    Poupart l.

pubocervical l.
puboprostatic l.
pubourethral l.
pubovesical l.
rectosacral l.
l. reflecting edge
reflecting edge of l.
round l.
sacrospinous l.
sacrotuberous l.
sacrouterine l.
shelving edge of Poupart l.
splenocolic l.
splenopancreatic l.
splenorenal l.
suspensory l.
l. of Treitz
triangular l.
umbilical l.
urethropelvic l.
uterosacral l.
vesical l.

ligamentous laxity
ligamentum
l. teres
l. teres cardiopexy
l. teres hepatis
l. venosum

ligand
l. for ELAM-1
reciprocal l.
l. recognition

ligand-dependent receptor homodimerization
ligand-gated channel
ligandin
ligand-triggered
l.-t. membrane guanylate cyclase
l.-t. protein tyrosine kinase

ligase
Thermus aquaticus DNA l.

ligated
doubly l.
suture l.

ligating and dividing stapler (LDS)
ligation
band l.
Barron l.
bidirectional l.
bile duct l. (BDL)
l. device
elastic band l.

endoscopic band l. (EBL)
endoscopic esophagogastric
variceal l.
endoscopic hemorrhoid l. (EHL)
endoscopic mucosal resection
with l. (EMRL)
endoscopic ultrasound-assisted
band l.
endoscopic variceal l. (EVL)
endoscopic variceal band l.
esophageal band l.
gastric variceal l.
l. of hemorrhoid
hepatic artery l.
high l.
Ivanissevitch l.
laparoscopic varix l.
loop l.
mini-loop l.
open retroperitoneal high l.
penile vein l.
postureteral l.
rubber band l. (RBL)
spermatic vein l.
stump l.
transesophageal l.
transgastric l.
triple rubber band l.
tubal l.
variceal band l.
varix l.

ligator
Bandito single-band l.
Barron rubber band l.
DDV l.
endoscopic band l.
KilRoid single-handed l.
McGivney hemorrhoidal l.
multiple band l.
NAMI DDV l.
O'Regan hemorrhoid l.
RapidFire multiple band l.
rubber band l. (RBL)
Rudd Clinic hemorrhoidal l.
Saeed multiband l.
Saeed multiple l.
Saeed six-shooter l.
Speedband Superview l.
Stiegmann-Goff Clearvue
endoscopic l.
Stiegmann-Goff variceal l.

L

NOTES

ligator *(continued)*
    variceal l.
    Wilson-Cook l. (4, 6, 10 band)
Ligat test
ligature
    elastic l.
    interlocking l.
    purse-string, pursestring l.
    retroperitoneoscopic vein l.
    l. sign
    silk l.
    Surgiwip suture l.
    suture l.
light
    bili l.
    l. cable
    l. chain deposition disease (LCDD)
    l. electrocautery
    l. and electron immunoperoxidase
    l. and electron immunoperoxidase
      observation
    l. emitter
    l. flow
    l. guide (LG)
    l. guide bundle
    l. induced fluorescence endoscopy
      system (LIFE-GI)
    l. micrographic study
    l. microscopy
    l. monitoring probe
    l. reflex
Lightwood syndrome
Lignac
    L. disease
    L. syndrome
Lignac-Fanconi
    L.-F. disease
    L.-F. syndrome
lignan
likelihood ratio
Likert scale
Lillie intestinal forceps
limb
    afferent ileal l.
    ascending l.
    blind l.
    l. deformity
    efferent l.
    jejunal l.
    Roux l.
    Roux-en-Y jejunal l.
    thick ascending l. (TAL)
    vertebral, anal, cardiac,
      tracheoesophageal fistula, renal, l.
      (VACTERL)
limbus, pl. **limbi**
LIM 2537 cell
limerence

limit dextrinosis
limited
    l. obturator node dissection
    l. range of motion
limiting
    l. dilution assay
    l. plate
    l. plate erosion
limosum
    Eubacterium l.
limy bile
Lincoln deep surgery scissors
lincomycin
lindane
line
    Aldrich-Mees l.
    anocutaneous l.
    anorectal l.
    anterior axillary l. (AAL)
    arcuate l.
    arterial l.
    B cell l.
    Beacon surgical l.
    Brödel l.
    Cantlie l.
    CaSki cell l.
    cell l.
    central venous pressure l.
    colonic mucosal l.
    Conradi l.
    dentate l.
    l. of Douglas
    Dul45 cell l.
    Freedom Clear long seal male
      external catheter l.
    Freedom Clear LS male external
      catheter l.
    Freedom Clear sport sheath male
      external catheter l.
    Freedom Clear SS male external
      catheter l.
    gas density l.
    Hampton l.
    Hilton white l.
    Hunter l.
    iliopectineal l.
    incision l.
    J l.
    K562 erythroid l.
    Langer l.
    Langhans l.
    lower anterior axillary l. (LAAL)
    lower midclavicular l. (LMCL)
    lymphoblastoid cell l.
    midaxillary l.
    midclavicular l. (MCL)
    milkman's l.
    mucosal l.

murine mesangial cell l.
myelomonocytic cell l.
neuronal cell l.
pararectal l.
pectinate l.
Poupart l.
pubic hair l.
pubococcygeal l.
pubosacral l.
Rex-Cantli-Serege l.
Richter-Monroe l.
Seraflo blood l.
Sergent white adrenal l.
skin l.
suture l.
T-cell l.
l. of Toldt
total parenteral nutrition l.
TPN l.
transverse umbilical l.
upper midclavicular l. (UMCL)
white anococcygeal l.
Z l.

linea
l. alba
l. nigra

lineage
hematopoietic l.
Langerhans l.

linear
l. analog pain score
l. array echoendoscope
l. array transducer
l. convex array scanner
l. erosion
l. fluorescein
l. 35-Mhz transducer
l. mode
l. probe
l. proctotomy
l. regression
l. staple cutter
l. stapler
l. stapling device
l. streaks en face
l. ulcer
l. ulceration

Lingeman
L. 3-in-1 procedure drape
L. TUR drape

lingua, pl. **linguae**
pityriasis l.

lingual lipase
linguatuliasis
lingula
linitis
l. plastica
l. plastica carcinoma

link
cytoskeletal l.

linkage
gene l.

Linnartz intestinal clamp
linoleic acid
linsidomine chlorohydrate
Linton
L. shunt
L. tourniquet clamp

Linton-Nachlas tube
Lioresal
Lipancreatin
LIP angle
liparocele
lipase
bile salt-stimulated l. (BSSL)
Cherry-Crandall method for testing serum l.
colipase-dependent l.
l. enzyme
hepatic l. (HL)
hepatic triglyceride l. (HTGL)
lingual l.
lipoprotein l. (LPL)
pancreatic l.
serum l.
l. test

lipid
l. bilayer
biliary l.
l. emulsion
extracellular l.
l. hydroperoxide
l. infusion
inositol l.
l. island
l. maldigestion
membrane-based l.
l. metabolism
l. nephrosis
l. oxidation rate
l. peroxidation

lipid-laden
l.-l. clear cell
l.-l. hepatocyte

L

NOTES

lipid-lowering drug
lipidosis
    ceramide lactoside l.
    Schwann cell l.
lipid-to-protein ratio
lipiduria
lipiodol
    l. injection
    l. transarterial embolization
      treatment
lipoblastic sarcoma
lipoblastoma
lipocele
lipodystrophia intestinalis
lipodystrophy
    intestinal l.
    mesenteric l.
lipofection reagent
lipofuscin
lipogranuloma
    mesenteric l.
lipogranulomatosis
lipoidal
lipoid nephrosis (LN)
lipolysis
    heparin-induced l.
    intraluminal l.
    intravascular l.
    LPL-mediated l.
lipolytic enzyme
lipoma
    colonic l.
    l. of cord
    gastric l.
    gastrointestinal l.
    submucosal ileal l.
lipoma-like tissue
lipomatosis
    pelvic l.
lipomatous
    l. ileocecal valve
    l. nephritis
    l. paranephritis
    l. tissue
lipomeningocele
lipomyelocystocele
lipomyelomeningocele
lipophagia granulomatosis
lipophagic intestinal granulomatosis
lipophagy
lipopolysaccharide (LPS)
lipoprotein
    apolipoprotein B-containing l.
    l. glomerulopathy
    high-density l. (HDL)
    intermediate-density l. (IDL)
    intermediate low-density l. (ILDL)
    l. lipase (LPL)

    liver-specific membrane l. (LSP)
    low-density l. (LDL)
    l. metabolism
    oxidized l.
    oxidized low density l. (Ox-LDL)
    very low density l. (VLDL)
    l. X
    l. X level
liposarcoma
    bladder l.
    kidney l.
    spermatic cord l.
liposclerotic mesenteritis
liposomal-amphotericin B (L-AmB)
liposomal daunorubicin HCl
Liposorber LA-15 System lithotriptor
Liposyn II fat emulsion solution
lipothymia
Lipoxide
lipoxin
lipoxygenase
    l. blockade
    l. inhibition
    l. inhibitor
    l. pathway
5-lipoxygenase inhibitor
Lipshultz urology microsurgical set
liquefaciens
    Aeromonas l.
    Enterobacter l.
    Serratia l.
liquefaction
    semen l.
liquefactive necrosis
Liqui-Char
liquid
    l. antacid
    l. chemical germicide (LCG)
    l. chromatographic assay
    l. diarrhea
    l. diet
    l. emptying
    l. food dysphagia
    full l. (FL)
    hyperosmolar l.
    isoosmolar l.
    Peptamen L.
    L. Pred
    l. scintillation spectrometer
    l. stool
Liqui-Doss
Liqui-E
liquor
    l. entericus
    l. gastricus
    l. pancreaticus
    l. seminis
lisinopril

LISL
>   laser-induced intracorporeal shock wave
>   lithotripsy

list
>   Mood Adjective Check L.

Listeria monocytogenes

liter
>   international unit per l. (IU/L)

lithagogue
lithangiuria
lithectasy
lithectomy
lithiasis
>   ammonium acid urate urinary l.
>   asymptomatic urinary l.
>   calcium oxalate urinary l.
>   calcium phosphate urinary l.
>   Crixivan l.
>   cystine urinary l.
>   dihydroxyadenine urinary l.
>   iatrogenic urinary l.
>   intraductal l.
>   magnesium ammonium phosphate
>   urinary l.
>   matrix urinary l.
>   pediatric urinary l.
>   renal l.
>   silicate urinary l.
>   staghorn urinary l.
>   struvite urinary l.
>   triamterene urinary l.
>   uric acid urinary l.
>   urinary l.
>   xanthine urinary l.

lithium
>   l. clearance (CLi)
>   fractional excretion of l. (FELI)

lithocenosis
lithocholate
lithocholic
>   l. acid (LCA)
>   l. acid-deoxycholic acid ratio

lithoclast
>   Swiss L.

Lithoclast endoscopic lithotriptor
lithoclysmia
lithocolic acid-deoxycholic acid ratio
(LCA-DCA)
lithocystotomy
lithodialysis
lithogenesis
>   urinary l.

lithogenic bile
Lithognost flash-lamp pulsed dye laser
lithokonion
litholabe
litholapaxy
>   Bigelow l.

litholysis
>   chemical l.

litholyte
litholytic
lithometer
lithomyl
lithonephritis
lithonephrotomy
lithophone
lithoscope
Lithostar
>   L. nonimmersion lithotriptor
>   L. Plus
>   L. Plus electromagnetic lithotriptor
>   bidimensional x-ray focusing
>   system
>   Siemens L.

Lithostat
lithostathine molecule
lithotome
lithotomist
lithotomy
>   bilateral l.
>   dorsal l.
>   high l.
>   lateral l.
>   Marian l.
>   median l.
>   mediolateral l.
>   perineal l.
>   l. position
>   prerectal l.
>   rectovesical l.
>   suprapubic l.
>   vaginal l.
>   vesical l.
>   vesicovaginal l.

lithotresis
>   ultrasonic l.

lithotripsy
>   alexandrite laser l.
>   biliary l.
>   blind l.
>   contact l.
>   coumarin green tunable dye
>   laser l.

L

NOTES

lithotripsy *(continued)*
    cystoscopic electrohydraulic l.
    Dornier extracorporeal shock
      wave l.
    Dornier MPL 9000 gallstone l.
    electrohydraulic l. (EHL)
    electrohydraulic shock wave l.
      (ESWL)
    endoscopic-controlled l.
    endoscopic electrohydraulic l.
    endoscopic Ho:YAG l.
    endoscopic pulsed dye laser l.
    external shock wave l.
    extracorporeal l.
    extracorporeal piezoelectric l. (EPL)
    extracorporeal piezoelectric shock
      wave l.
    extracorporeal shock wave l.
      (ESWL)
    intracorporeal electrohydraulic l.
      (IEHL)
    intracorporeal laser l. (ICL, ILL)
    intracorporeal shock wave l.
    laser l. (LL)
    laser-induced intracorporeal shock
      wave l. (LISL)
    mechanical l.
    Medstone extracorporeal shock
      wave l.
    pancreatoscopic laser l. (PSLL)
    peroral shock wave l. (PSWL)
    piezoelectric l.
    pneumatic l.
    pressure regulated
      electrohydraulic l.
    l. retreatment
    shock wave l. (SWL)
    l. table
    tunable dye laser l.
    ultrasonic l.
    ureteroscopic intracorporeal
      electrohydraulic l.
    visible-light l.
lithotripsy-induced hypertension
lithotriptic
lithotriptor, lithotripter
    American endoscopy mechanical l.
    Breakstone l.
    Calcutript electrohydraulic l.
    Circon-ACMI l.
    Diasonics Therasonic l.
    Direx Tripter X-1 l.
    DoLi S extracorporeal shock
      wave l.
    Dornier compact l.
    Dornier gallstone l.
    Dornier HM4 l.
    Dornier HM3 waterbath l.

    Dornier MPL 5000 l.
    DP-1 l.
    EDAP LT.01 l.
    electrohydraulic l.
    electromagnetic l.
    electropneumatic endoscopic l.
    extracorporeal piezoelectric l.
    extracorporeal shock wave l.
    HM4 l.
    Karl Storz-Lutzeyer l.
    laser l.
    Liposorber LA-15 System l.
    Lithoclast endoscopic l.
    Lithostar nonimmersion l.
    manual l.
    Medispec Econolith spark plug l.
    Medstone STS l.
    MFL 5000 l.
    Modulith SL 20 l.
    MonoLith single-piece mechanical l.
    Northgate SD-3 dual-purpose l.
    Olympus BML-3Q, -4Q l.
    out-of-scope l.
    percutaneous ultrasonic l.
    piezoelectric shock wave l.
    Piezolith EPL l.
    Piezolith 2300, 2500 model l.
    pneumatic endoscopic l.
    Richard Wolf Piezolith l.
    second-generation l.
    shock wave l.
    Siemens Lithostar Plus System
      C l.
    Sonotrode l.
    Storz Monolith l.
    Swiss lithoclast l.
    Technomed Sonolith 3000 l.
    Therasonics l.
    third-generation l.
    tubeless l.
    ultrasonic l.
    Waltz endoscopic l.
    water cushion l.
    Wilson-Cook mechanical l.
    Wolf Piezolith 2300 l.
    Wolf Sonolith l.
lithotriptoscope
lithotriptoscopy
lithotrite
    Hendrickson l.
    Lowsley l.
    Marmite l.
    Reliquet l.
    Rotolith l.
    Thompson l.
    Wolf l.
lithotrity
lithous

lithoxiduria
lithuresis
lithureteria
litmus milk test
littoral
  l. cell
  l. cell angioma
Littré
  crypt of L.
  L. gland
  L. hernia
Livaditis circular myotomy
live
  l. attenuated virus
  l. donor nephrectomy
  l. renal donation
live-donor segmental graft
liver
  l. abscess
  l. acinus
  acute fatty l.
  l. Ah receptor
  alcoholic fatty l.
  ballottable l.
  bare area of l.
  l. bed
  biliary cirrhotic l.
  l. biopsy
  l. breath
  l. cancer
  l. capsule
  cardiac impression on the l.
  caudate eminence of l.
  caudate lobe of l.
  l. cell adenoma (LCA)
  l. cell carcinoma
  l. cell dysplasia
  l. cell plate
  centrilobular region of l.
  l. cirrhosis (LC)
  cirrhotic l.
  colic impression on the l.
  cutdown l.
  cut surface of l.
  l. cyst infection
  l. death
  l. deposit
  l. dialysis system
  l. dialysis unit
  diaphragmatic surface of l.
  l. diet
  l. disease

  l. distribution
  dome of l.
  l. dullness
  duodenal impression on l.
  l. eater
  echogenic l.
  l. edge
  l. engorgement
  l. enzyme
  l. failure
  fatty l. (FL)
  fatty infiltration of l.
  l. fibrosis
  fibrous appendage of l.
  fibrous capsule of l.
  fibrous tunic of l.
  finely fatty foamy l.
  l. flap
  l. flap sign
  l. fluke
  foamy l.
  focal fatty infiltration of l.
  focal nonfatty infiltration of l.
  l. function profile
  l. function series (LFS)
  l. function test (LFT)
  gastric impression on l.
  l. hilus
  hobnail l.
  l. hydatid disease
  l. impression
  l. iron store
  l., kidneys, spleen (LKS)
  laparoscopic biopsy of l.
  large-droplet fatty l.
  lobe of l.
  lobular architecture of l.
  l. lymphoma
  macrovesicular fatty l.
  l. meal
  l. membrane antigen
  l. metastasis
  nodular l.
  l. nodule
  noncirrhotic l.
  nonparasitic cyst of l.
  nutmeg l.
  l. parenchyma
  phlegmonous alcoholic fatty l.
  polycystic l.
  polycystic disease of l. (PDL)
  polylobar l.

L

NOTES

liver *(continued)*
    potato l.
    l. protein store
    pyogenic l.
    quadrate lobe of l.
    renal impression on l.
    l. resection
    sagittal fissure of l.
    l. scan
    segmentectomy of l.
    shock l.
    shrunken l.
    l. sinusoid
    small-droplet fatty l.
    l. span
    stasis l.
    subacute atrophy of l.
    subchronic atrophy of l.
    suprarenal area of l.
    tender l.
    l. transplant
    l. transplantation
    l. transplantation preservation injury
    l. trauma
    undersurface of l.
    undifferentiated embryonal sarcoma
        of l.
    l. volume
    wandering l.
liver-adipose tissue cycle
liver-deprived epithelial clonic cell
liver-directed autoreactivity
liver-kidney
    l.-k. microsomal antibody
    l.-k. microsome (LKM)
Liver Panel Plus 9
liver-specific
    l.-s. antigen
    l.-s. membrane lipoprotein (LSP)
    l.-s. protein
liver-spleen scan
living
    l. donor (LD)
    l. donor kidney
    l. donor liver transplantation
        (LDLT)
    l. donor transplant
    l. related donor
    l. unrelated donor (LURD)
Livingston triangle
livor mortis
LKB Optiphase 2 scintillation fluid
LKB-Wallac scintillation counter
LKM
    liver-kidney microsome
    LKM specificity
LKS
    liver, kidneys, spleen

LL
    laser lithotripsy
LLC
    laparoscopic laser cholecystectomy
LLC-PK1-FBPase+ cell
LLCPK renal tubular cell
Lloyd
    L. Davies stirrups
    L. Davies Trendelenburg position
    L. Davis position
    L. sign
Lloyd-Davis
    L.-D. knee and leg holder
    L.-D. sigmoidoscope
LLQ
    left lower quadrant
LMA
    lactose malabsorption
LMCL
    lower midclavicular line
LMP **gene**
LMW
    low molecular weight
LMWH
    low molecular weight heparin
LN
    lipoid nephrosis
    lupus nephritis
LNa
    low sodium
LNaCl
    low salt
L-NAME
    N^G-nitro-L-arginine methyl ester
L-NMMA
    N^G-monomethyl-L-arginine
L-N-monomethyl-arginine
load
    osmotic l.
    virus l.
loading
    differential l.
    methionine l.
    peripheral l.
    uniform l.
    water l.
lobar
    l. atrophy
    l. nephronia
lobatum
    hepar l.
lobe
    caudate l.
    Home l.
    kidney l.
    kissing prostatic l.'s
    lateral l.
    left l.

left hepatic l. (LHL)
l. of liver
median l.
predominant median l.
quadrate l.
renal l.
Riedel l.
right l.

lobectomy
hepatic l.

lobi (*pl. of* lobus)
lobucavir
lobular
l. architecture
l. architecture of liver
l. hepatitis
l. inflammatory infiltrate
l. mononuclear cell infiltrate
l. necroinflammation

lobulated
l. border
l. filling defect
l. mass

lobulation
portal l.

lobule
l. of pancreas
portal l.

lobuli (*pl. of* lobulus)
lobulization
lobulose
lobulus, pl. **lobuli**
lobuli testis

lobus, pl. **lobi**
local
l. alcohol instillation effect
l. anesthesia
l. depot injection
l. glomerular lesion
l. recurrence
l. scarring

localization
bleeding site l.
manometric l.
pancreatic tumor l.
target l.

localized
l. amyloidosis
l. lesion
l. pain

localizing tenderness

locally
l. acting paracrine effector
l. made rapid urease test (LRUT)

location
tumor l.

locator
LES l.
lower esophageal sphincter locator
lower esophageal sphincter l. (LES
locator)

LoCholest
loci (*pl. of* locus)
locker room syndrome
locking suture
lock stitch
lock-stitch suture
Lockwood-Allis intestinal forceps
LOCM
low-osmolar contrast medium

locomote
locomotor
locus, pl. **loci**
hereditary prostate cancer 1 l.
(HPC-1)

Loeffler syndrome
Loewe (*var. of* Löwe)
Lofenalac formula
logarithmic rate
Logen
logistic regression analysis
log-rank test
Lohlein-Baehr lesion
Lohlein nephritis
loin
l. pain
l. pain hematuria syndrome (LPHS)

lollipop tree sign
Lomanate
lomefloxacin
l. HCl
l. hydrochloride
l. TMP/SMX

Lomotil
lomustine
Lonalac
L. feeding
L. formula

Lone
L. Star retractor
L. Star self-retractor

long
l. anal sphincter

L

NOTES

447

long *(continued)*
    l. incubation hepatitis
    l. intestinal tube
    l. intestinal tube decompression
    l. Roux-en-Y pouch jejunostomy
    l. seal (LS)
    l. terminal repeat (LTR)
    l. vascular needle driver
long-chain
    l.-c. acyl-CoA dehydrogenase deficiency
    l.-c. fatty acid (LCFA)
    l.-c. 3-hydroxyacyl coenzyme A dehydrogenase (LCHAD)
    l.-c. triglyceride (LCT)
longitudinal
    l. band of colon
    l. choledochotomy
    l. colostomy
    l. enterotomy
    l. esophageal stricture
    l. fasciculi of colon
    l. fissure
    l. image
    l. laceration
    l. myotomy
    l. nephrotomy of Boyce
    l. pancreaticojejunostomy
    l. subepithelial venous plexus
    l. ulcer
    l. view
longitudinalis
    plica l.
long-jaw disposable forceps
long-limb surgical bypass
Longmire operation
long-neck diverticulum
long-nosed
    l.-n. retriever snare
    l.-n. sphincterotome
long-segment
    l.-s. Barrett esophagus (LSBE)
    l.-s. CLE
long-term
    l.-t. antibiotic
    l.-t. catheter use
    l.-t. followup data
    l.-t. indwelling catheter
    l.-t. low-dose maintenance chemoprophylaxis
    l.-t. outcome
longum
    Bifidobacterium l.
Lonox
loop
    afferent l.
    air-filled l.
    alpha sigmoid l.

Biebl l.
bipolar urological l.
blind l.
bowel l.
Bradley l.
brain stem-sacral l.
l. caliber
cerebral-sacral l.
l. choledochojejunostomy
closed afferent l.
closed efferent l.
colonic l.
contiguous l.
Cordonnier ureteroileal l.
Davis l.
diathermic l.
l. diuretic
double reverse alpha-sigmoid l.
duodenal l.
efferent l.
l. end ileostomy
l. esophagojejunostomy
l. forearm graft
gamma transverse colon l.
l. gastrojejunostomy
Heiss l.
l. of Henle (LH)
Henle l.
ileal l.
l. ileostomy (LI)
intestinal l.
jejunal interposition of Henle l.
l. jejunostomy
l. ligation
N l.
N-shaped sigmoid l.
ostomy l.
l. ostomy bridge
polyglactin monofilament l.
polyglyconate monofilament l.
puborectalis l.
l. of redundant colon
resectoscope l.
reverse alpha sigmoid l.
Roeder l.
Roux-en-Y l.
sentinel l.
sigmoid l.
l. stoma
Surgitite ligating l.
l. suture
transverse l.
l. transverse colostomy
Vapor Cut l.
vesical-sacral-sphincter l.
Wedge l.
looped cautery
loopogram

loopography
    ileal l.
    retrograde l.
loop-tipped electrode
loop-type
    l.-t. snare forceps
    l.-t. stone-crushing forceps
Looser-Milkman stria
loose stool
loperamide
Lopez enteral valve
Lopid
Lopressor
LoPresti
    L. endoscope
    L. fiberoptic esophagoscope
Lopurin
Lorabid
loracarbef
Lorad
    L. StereoGuide
    L. StereoGuide prone breast biopsy
      system
lorazepam
Lord
    L. dilation
    L. dilation of hemorrhoid
    L. method hemorrhoidectomy
lordosis
    lumbar l.
Lorenzo oil
Lortat-Jacob hepatic resection
Los Angeles (LA)
    LA classification
    LA classification of GERD
    LA Classification (grade A, B, C,
      D) esophagitis
losartan
Losec
Losotron Plus
losoxantrone
loss
    autoimmune sensorineural hearing l.
    cortical l.
    electrolyte l.
    estimated blood l. (EBL)
    fluid l.
    ganglion cell l.
    graft l.
    negligible blood l.
    nephron l.
    obligatory dialysate protein l.

    psoas l.
    sensory l.
    l. of sigmoid curve
    weight l.
Lotheissen-McVay technique
Lotrel
Lotrimin
Lotrisone
Lotronex
loupe
    Keeler panoramic l.
    surgical l.
    wide-angled l.
lovastatin
Lovelace forceps
Lovenox
low
    l. anterior resection (LAR)
    l. anterior resection in combination
      with coloanal anastomosis
      (LAR/CAA)
    l. available carbohydrate diet
    l. coloanal anastomosis
    l. intermittent suction
    l. intersphincteric anal fistula
    l. molecular weight (LMW)
    l. molecular weight heparin
      (LMWH)
    l. molecular weight protein
    l. molecular weight protein
      ribonuclease
    l. pressure bladder substitute
    l. pressure-low flow voiding
      dysfunction
    l. salt (LNaCl)
    l. small bowel obstruction
    l. sodium (LNa)
    l. transverse incision
    l. turnover osteomalacia (LTOM)
    l. urethral pressure (LUP)
low-affinity, high-capacity system
low-affinity transporter
low-calcium dialysate
low-calorie diet
low-compliance
    l.-c. balloon
    l.-c. bladder
    l.-c. perfusion system
low-density
    l.-d. lipoprotein (LDL)
    l.-d. lipoprotein cholesterol (LDLC)
    l.-d. lipoprotein susceptibility

L

NOTES

low-dose
    l.-d. HpD
    l.-d. interferon
Löwe, Loewe
    L. disease
low-energy
    l.-e. program
    l.-e. protocol
    l.-e. transurethral microwave thermotherapy (LE-TUMT)
    l.-e. TUMT
lower
    l. abdominal transverse incision
    l. anterior axillary line (LAAL)
    l. esophageal B ring
    l. esophageal contraction ring
    l. esophageal mucosal ring
    l. esophageal sphincter (LES)
    l. esophageal sphincter circular muscle
    l. esophageal sphincter locator (LES locator)
    l. esophageal sphincter pressure (LESP)
    l. esophageal sphincter relaxation (LESR)
    l. esophageal sphincter tone
    L. gall duct forceps
    l. gastrointestinal bleeding (LGIB)
    l. gastrointestinal hemorrhage
    l. GI bleeding
    l. GI tract foreign body
    l. infundibulopelvic angle
    l. midclavicular line (LMCL)
    l. motor neuron bladder disorder
    l. motor neuron lesion
    l. nephron nephrosis
    l. panendoscopy
    l. pole laceration
    l. ureter
    l. urinary tract dysfunction (LUTD)
    l. urinary tract symptom (LUTS)
Lowery method
Lowe syndrome
low-fat diet (LFD)
low-fiber diet
low-flow priapism
low-flux
    l.-f. cuprophane membrane
    l.-f. dialysis membrane
    l.-f. polysulfone membrane
low-grade
    l.-g. dysplasia (LGD)
    l.-g. fever
    l.-g. leiomyosarcoma
    l.-g. positive smear
low-lactose diet
low-loop cutaneous ureterostomy

low-lying rectal cancer
low-magnification electron micrograph
low-molecular
Lown criteria
low-osmolar contrast medium (LOCM)
low-oxalate diet
low-pitched bowel sounds
low-power photomicrograph
low-pressure
    l.-p. cardiopulmonary baroreceptor
    l.-p. pouch
    l.-p. venous system
low-pulsatility arterial waveform
low-residue
    l.-r. diet
    l.-r. feeding
low-roughage diet
Lowsium
Lowsley
    L. lithotrite
    L. operation
    L. retractor
    L. tractor
Lowsley-Peterson cystoscope
low-sodium diet
low-tyrosine, low-phenylalanine diet
low-volume sclerotherapy
loxiglumide
lozenge
    tetracaine l.
Lozol
LP
    lymphomatous polyposis
L-PAM
    L-phenylalanine mustard
LPH
    lactase-phlorizin hydrolase
LPHS
    loin pain hematuria syndrome
LPL
    lipoprotein lipase
LPL-mediated lipolysis
LPLND
    laparoscopic pelvic lymph node dissection
LPP
    leak-point pressure
LPS
    lipopolysaccharide
LRE
    lamina rara externa
L-rhamnose
LRI
    lamina rara interna
LRN
    laparoscopic radical nephrectomy
LRUT
    locally made rapid urease test

LS
    long seal
LSBE
    long-segment Barrett esophagus
LSC 7000 curved array transducer
L-selectin
LSM
    lifestyle modification
LSMB
    lumbar spine bone mineral density
LSP
    liver-specific membrane lipoprotein
LT
    heat-labile toxin
LTOM
    low turnover osteomalacia
LTR
    long terminal repeat
Lubb syndrome
Lubraseptic jelly
lubricant
    l. laxative
    Surgilube l.
Lubri-flex ureteral stent
lucent cyst
Lucey-Driscoll syndrome
Luder-Sheldon syndrome
Ludwig labyrinth
Luer
    L. hemorrhoid forceps
    L. syringe
Luer-Lok
    L.-L. connector
    L.-L. syringe
Lugol
    L. chromoendoscopy
    L. iodide
    L. iodine
    L. iodine solution
    L. solution stain
Lugol-combined upper gastrointestinal videoendoscopy
Lukes-Collins classification
lumbar
    l. appendicitis
    l. artery
    l. kidney
    l. lordosis
    l. nephrectomy
    l. nephrotomy
    l. plexus
    l. spinal cord lesion

    l. spine bone mineral density (LSMB)
    l. vein
lumbocolostomy
lumbocolotomy
lumbocostoabdominal triangle
lumbodorsal
    l. fascia
    l. incision
    l. ligament
lumbosacral
    l. fascia
    l. plexus
    l. trunk
lumbotomy
    dorsal l.
    l. incision
lumbricoides
    Ascaris l.
lumen, pl. **lumina**
    bile duct l.
    bowel l.
    cystic duct l.
    duct l.
    duodenal l.
    esophageal l.
    gastroduodenal l.
    intestinal l.
    rectal l.
    scalloped bowel l.
    l. of seminiferous tubule
    single l.
Lumenator injectable guidewire
lumen-seeking catheter
lumen-to-bath sodium flux
lumina (*pl. of* lumen)
Lumina guidewire
Luminal
luminal
    l. acid
    l. acid clearance
    l. amoxicillin
    l. antigliadin
    l. bulge
    l. CCK-releasing factor
    l. content
    l. contrast study
    l. Crohn disease
    l. diameter
    l. EGF
    l. glucose
    l. HCO_3^-

L

NOTES

luminal *(continued)*
    l. hypoacidity
    l. narrowing
    l. nutrition
    l. secretagogue
    l. sodium
    l. stenosis
luminol-enhanced chemiluminescence
luminometer
    LB 9501 l.
Lumi-Phos 530
lumpectomy
    endoscopic aspiration l. (EAL)
lump kidney
Lunar DPX total-body scanner
lunatus
    penis l.
Lunderquist guidewire
Lunderquist-Ring torque guide
Lundh
    L. meal
    L. test
lung
    l. cancer
    l. disease
    l. dysplasia
    farmer's l.
    l. purpura
LUP
    low urethral pressure
lupoid hepatitis
Lupron Depot
lupus
    l. anticoagulant (LA)
    l. erythematosus
    l. nephritis (LN)
LUQ
    left upper quadrant
LURD
    living unrelated donor
LUS
    laparoscopic ultrasound
Luschka
    accessory duct of L.
    L. crypt
    L. cystic gland
    L. duct
lusoria
    arteria l.
    dysphagia l.
lusorian artery
LUTD
    lower urinary tract dysfunction
luteinized granulosa-theca cell tumor
luteinizing
    l. hormone (LH)
    l. hormone-follicle-stimulating
    hormone (LH-FSH)

    l. hormone-follicle-stimulating
    hormone releasing factor
    l. hormone-releasing hormone
    (LHRH)
    l. hormone-releasing hormone
    antagonist
Lütkens sphincter
LUTS
    lower urinary tract symptom
Lutz automatic reprocessor
luxation
Luy segregator
LVP
    large-volume paracentesis
LX-20 laser
Lycopodium serratum
lye ingestion
Lyell
    L. disease
    L. syndrome
Lyme disease
lymph
    l. channel
    l. node
    l. node adenopathy
    l. node dissection
    l. node metastasis
    l. scrotum
lymphadenectomy
    endocavitary pelvic l. (ECPL)
    extended pelvic l.
    laparoscopic pelvic l.
    mediastinal l.
    mesorectal l.
    minilaparotomy staging pelvic l.
    paraaortic l.
    pelvic l.
    prophylactic l.
    retroperitoneal l.
    thoracoabdominal retroperitoneal l.
    three-field l.
    two-field l.
lymphadenitis
lymphadenopathy
    cervical l.
    inguinal l.
    malignant peribiliary l.
    mediastinal l.
    perihepatic l.
    l. syndrome (LAS)
lymphangiectasia, lymphangiectasis
    intestinal l.
    pancreatic l.
    peritoneal l.
    primary intestinal l. (PIL)
lymphangiogram
lymphangiography

lymphangioma
scrotal l.
lymphangitic streak
lymphangitis
penis sclerosing l.
sclerosing l.
lymphapheresis
lymphatic
l. channel
l. leak
l. metastasis
l. microcyst
l. obstruction
l. package
l. transport
l. vessel
lymphatica
folliculus l.
lymphedema
filarial l.
lymphoblast homing
lymphoblastoid
l. cell line
l. interferon-alpha
lymphoblastoma
kidney l.
renal l.
lymphocele
l. aspiration
l. internal drainage
l. percutaneous drainage
l. spontaneous regression
lymphocelectomy
laparoscopic l.
pelvic l.
lymphocyst
lymphocyte
B l.
CD8 l.
CD45RO l.
CD8+ T l.
l. costimulatory molecule
l. count
crypt intraepithelial l. (cIEL)
cytolytic T l. (CTL)
l. cytotoxicity
cytotoxic T l. (CTL)
intraepithelial l. (IEL)
intrahepatic l.
l. migration
naive B and T l.
peripheral blood l. (PBL)

sinusoidal l.
T l.
thymus-derived l.
total l. (TTL)
tumor-infiltrating l. (TIL)
virgin l.
WBC l.
lymphocyte-hepatocyte
intrahepatic antigen-dependent l.-h.
lymphocyte-target cell
lymphocytic
l. colitis
l. gastritis (LG)
l. vasculitis
lymphocytosis
intraepithelial l.
lymphocytotoxic antibody
lymphocyturia
lymphoepithelial lesion
lymphogenic metastasis
lymphogranuloma venereum (LGV)
lymphography
lymphohemangioma
bladder l.
lymphohistiocytic infiltration
lymphoid
l. aggregate
l. cholangitis
l. component
l. follicle
l. interstitial pneumonia
l. nodular hyperplasia
l. nodule
l. polyp
l. tumor
lymphokine-activated killer cell
lymphokine production
lymphoma
benign l.
bladder l.
Burkitt l.
colorectal l.
cutaneous T-cell l.
duodenal l.
enteropathy-associated T-cell l.
(EATCL)
gastric l.
hepatosplenic T-cell l.
histiocytic l.
infiltrative l.
liver l.
MALT l.

L

NOTES

lymphoma *(continued)*
    marginal zone l.
    Mediterranean l.
    mucosa-associated lymphoid
      tissue l.
    nodular l.
    non-Hodgkin l. (NHL)
    penis l.
    polypoid l.
    primary B-cell l.
    primary hepatosplenic l. (PHSL)
    prostate gland l.
    retroperitoneal l.
    seminal vesicle l.
    small intestinal malignant l.
    small non-cleaved-cell l.
    T-cell l.
    testicular l.
    ulcerative l.
lymphomatosis
lymphomatous
    l. nodule
    l. polyposis (LP)
lymphomononuclear cell
lymphonodular hyperplasia
lymphonodulus, pl. **lymphonoduli**
    lymphonoduli splenici
lymphoplasmacytosis
lymphoproliferative
    l. disorder
    l. syndrome
lymphosarcoma

lymphoscintigraphy
lymphovascular permeation
Lynch syndrome (I, II)
LYOfoam dressing
Lyon
    L. ring
    L. ring-constrictive band
**lyophilized dura mater for pubovaginal
   sling**
Lyphocin
lyse
lysine
lysinuria
lysis
    l. of adhesion
    colon tumor cell l.
    CTL-mediated l.
    laparoscopic l.
    mesangial l.
    tumor cell l.
lysolecithin
lysosomal
    l. accumulation
    l. enzyme
    l. membrane
    l. swelling
lysosome
    hepatocyte l.
lysozyme
lysyl-bradykinin
lytic cocktail
Lytren electrolyte solution

μV
microvolt
M
microfold
M antibody
M cell
M1
antibody to Leu M1
glutathione S-transferase M1
M30
Zeiss morphomate M30
M344
M344 antigen
antigen M344
MAA
macroaggregated albumin
^{99m}Tc MAA
Maalox
M. HRF
M. Plus
M. spray
M. Therapeutic Concentrate
MAB
maximal androgen blockade
MAb, mAb
monoclonal antibody
anti-class II MAb
MAb IOT2-recognizing
monomorphic DR determinant
MABP
mean arterial blood pressure
Macalister
valve of M.
Macaluso stent remover
MacConkey agar
Macdonald test
Macewen
M. hernia operation
M. herniorrhaphy
MACH1
metronidazole, amoxicillin,
clarithromycin, *H. pylori*, one-week
therapy
MACH1 study
Machado-Guerreiro test
Machida
M. choledochoscope
M. FCS-ML II magnifying
colonoscope
machine
A2008 ABGII hemodialysis m.
Accuson-128 color flow
Doppler m.
Belzer m.
endoscopic sewing m.

Endotek m.
Fresenius 2008H hemodialysis m.
Gambro AK10 m.
gastric hypothermia m.
heart-lung m.
Kodak Ektachem 700 m.
MOX TM-100 portable renal
preservation m.
Narco esophageal motility m.
Nova II m.
perfusion m.
Phillips ultrasound m.
portable renal preservation m.
Primus Prostate M.
Mackenrodt
ligament of M.
Mackenzie
M. disease
M. point
MacLean test
Maclet magnetic ring
macroaggregated albumin (MAA)
macroamylasemia
macroangiodynamic
macroangiopathic hemolytic anemia
Macrobid
macrocephaly
macrocrystal
macrocyclic triene
macrocyst
adrenocortical m.
Macrodantin
macrogenitosomia
macroglobulinemia
Waldenström m.
macrolide
m. antibiotic
m. antimicrobial
macromolecular
m. secretion
m. uronate (MMUA)
macromolecule
radiolabeled m.
macronidia
macronodular cirrhosis
macroorchidism lesion
macropenis
macrophage
bile-laden m.
ceroid-laden m.
m. colony-stimulating factor (M-
CSF)
hemosiderin-laden m.
parasitizing m.
peritoneal m.

M

macrophage-rich inflammatory response
macrophage-TGF-beta axis
macrophallus
Macroplastique
    M. implant
    M. implantation device
    M. injectable
    M. soft tissue synthetic bulking
      agent
macroprolactinoma
macroproteinuria
macroregenerative nodule
macroscopic
    m. hematuria
    m. lesion
    m. liver cyst
macrosomia
    fetal m.
macrosteatosis
macrothrombocyte
macrovascular disease
macrovesicular
    m. fat
    m. fatty liver
    m. steatosis
macula, pl. **maculae**
    m. densa
macular degeneration
macule
maculopapular
Madayag biopsy needle
Madden
    M. incisional herniorrhaphy
    M. intestinal clamp
    M. repair
    M. repair of incisional hernia
    M. technique
Maddrey discriminant function
Mad Hatter syndrome
Madigan prostatectomy
Madsen-Iversen
    M.-I. scale
    M.-I. scoring system
Madsen symptom score
mafenide acetate
Maffucci syndrome
MAG
    multifocal atrophic gastritis
MAG-3
    mercaptotriglycylglycine
    MAG-3 renal scan
    TechneScan MAG-3
magaldrate
Magic Lite chemiluminometric
  immunoassay
magna
    arteria pancreatica m.

    Fascioloides m.
    lacuna m.
Magnacal liquid feeding
MagnaScanner
    Picker Vista M.
magnesia
    citrate of m.
    milk of m. (MOM)
    Phillips Milk of M.
magnesium
    m. ammonium phosphate
    m. ammonium phosphate urinary
      lithiasis
    m. carbonate
    m. citrate
    m. deficiency
    esomeprazole m.
    m. hydroxide
    m. metabolism
    m. oxide
    m. salt
    m. trisilicate
magnesium-induced diarrhea
magnetic
    m. bore
    m. internal ureteral stent
    m. resonance
    m. resonance angiography (MRA)
    m. resonance cholangiography
      (MRC)
    m. resonance
      cholangiopancreatography (MRCP)
    m. resonance colography
    m. resonance colonography (MRC)
    m. resonance imaging (MRI)
    m. resonance pancreatography
      (MRP)
    m. resonance spectroscopy (MRS)
    m. resonance urography (MRU)
    m. stimulation
    m. susceptibility test
magnetization prepared-rapid gradient
  echo (MP-RAGE)
magnetoencephalography (MEG)
magnetometry
magnification chromoendoscopy
magnifying
    m. colonoscope
    m. colonoscopy
    m. endoscope
    m. enteroscope
Mag-OX 400
MAGP
    microfil-associated glycoprotein
    MAGP microfibrillar protein
MAGPI
    meatal advancement and glansplasty

meatal advancement, glanuloplasty,
penoscrotal junction meatotomy
MAGPI operation

Magsal

mahogany-colored stool

Mahurkar catheter

MAI

Mycobacterium avium-intracellulare

main

m. pancreatic duct (MPD)
m. pancreatic duct stent

Maine

M. Medical Assessment Program
(MMAP)
M. Medical Assessment Program
index

Mainstay urologic soft tissue anchor

maintenance treatment

Mainz

M. pouch augmentation
M. pouch cutaneous urinary
diversion
M. pouch II
M. pouch operation
M. pouch urinary reservoir
M. urinary pouch

Mainz-type ureterosigmoidostomy

maitre

tour de m.

Maixner cirrhosis

major

curvatura gastrica m.
curvatura ventriculi m.
m. deceleration injury
m. GI surgery
globus m.
m. histocompatibility complex
(MHC)
m. papilla
papilla duodeni m.

majus

Chelidonium m.
omentum m.

Makkas operation

Makler

M. cannula
M. counting chamber
M. insemination device
M. sperm counting device

malabsorption

bile acid m. (BAM)
m. disease

D-xylose m.
folate m.
folic acid m.
glucose-galactose m.
iatrogenic m.
idiopathic bile acid m.
lactose m. (LMA)
lavage-induced pill m.
m. syndrome
vitamin B_{12} m.

malabsorptive diarrhea

malacia

tracheobronchial m.

malacoplakia, malakoplakia

bladder m.
kidney m.
m. of kidney
m. vesica

malacotomy

maladaptive response

maladjustment

Structured and Scaled Interview to
Assess M. (SSIAM)

Malakit *Helicobacter pylori* Biolab

malakoplakia (*var. of* malacoplakia)

malaria

algid m.
bilious remittent m.
dysenteric algid m.
falciparum m.
gastric m.
malignant tertian m.
pernicious m.
quartan m.

malariae

Plasmodium m.

malarial

m. dysentery
m. hepatitis
m. nephropathy

malate

malayi

Brugia m.

maldescended testicle

maldescent

maldigestion

lipid m.

maldigestion-absorption syndrome

maldigestive diarrhea

maldigestor

lactose m.

M

NOTES

male
    m. catheter
    m. epispadias
    m. escutcheon
    m. genitalia melanoma
    m. pelvis
    m. perineum
    m. sterility
    m. Turner syndrome
maleate
    methysergide m.
    perhexiline m.
Malecot
    M. gastrostomy tube
    M. nephrostomy tube
    M. reentry catheter
    M. suprapubic catheter
malemission
malformation
    anorectal m.
    anus m.
    arteriovenous m. (AVM)
    bronchopulmonary foregut m.
    Chiari m.
    cloacal m.
    Dieulafoy vascular m.
    dysraphic m.
    gastric arteriovenous m.
    mermaid m.
    polypoid vascular m.
    pulmonary arteriovenous m.
    scrotal arteriovenous m.
    sink-trap m.
    submucosal arterial m.
    submucosal vascular m.
    vascular m.
malignancy
    m. associated cellular marker
    bulky m.
    de novo m.
    esophageal m.
    esophagocardial m.
    extracolonic m. (ECM)
    hepatic m.
    hepatobiliary m.
    humoral hypercalcemia of m.
      (HHM)
    hypercalcemia of m.
    nonskin m.
    pancreaticobiliary m.
    paratesticular m.
    periampullary m.
    peritoneal m.
malignant
    m. acanthosis nigricans
    m. ascites
    m. atrophic papulosis
    m. B-cell syndrome

    m. biliary obstruction
    m. biliary obstructive disease
    m. cachexia
    m. carcinoid syndrome
    m. dysentery
    m. dysphagia
    m. dysplasia
    m. esophagopericardial fistula
    m. histiocytosis
    m. hyperthermia
    m. malnutrition
    m. melanoma
    m. meniscus sign
    m. mesenchymal tumor
    m. mesenchymoma
    m. nephrosclerosis
    m. nuclear structure
    m. obstructive jaundice
    m. peribiliary lymphadenopathy
    m. pheochromocytoma
    m. polyp
    m. potential
    m. pseudoachalasia
    m. rectal stricture
    m. renal mass
    m. seeding
    m. stenosis
    m. teratoma (MT)
    m. teratoma, intermediate (MTI)
    m. teratoma, trophoblastic (MTT)
    m. tertian malaria
    m. ulcer
maljunction
    pancreaticobiliary m.
mall
    space of M.
Mallard incision
malleability
    pelvic m.
malleable
    m. blade
    m. implant
    m. prosthesis
    m. retractor
    m. scoop
Mallinckrodt catheter
Mallory
    M. hyaline
    M. hyaline body
Mallory-Azan stain
Mallory-Weiss
    M.-W. laceration
    M.-W. lesion
    M.-W. mucosal rupture
    M.-W. syndrome
    M.-W. tear
malnourished

malnutrition
    index of m.
    malignant m.
    protein-calorie m. (PCM)
    protein-energy m.
malnutrition-related diabetes mellitus (MRDM)
malodorous
    m. fluid
    m. stool
malondialdehyde
Malone
    M. antegrade colonic enema stoma procedure
    M. antegrade continence enema
    M. antegrade continent enema channel
    M. cecostomy
    M. continent appendicostomy
Maloney
    M. bougie
    M. dilation
    M. mercury-filled esophageal dilator
    M. tapered-tip dilator
Maloney-Hurst dilator
malpighian
    m. body
    m. corpuscle
    m. glomerulus
malpighii
    stratum m.
Malpighi pyramid
malrotation
    intestinal m.
    m. of intestine
    midgut volvulus with m.
MALT
    mucosa-associated lymphoid tissue
    MALT lymphoma
maltase
maltase-glucoamylase
Maltese cross
MALToma
    mucosa-associated lymphoid tissue
maltophilia
    Stenotrophomonas m.
    Xanthomonas m.
maltose tetrapalmitate
Maltsupex
Maly test
mammalgia

mammalian
    m. cell membrane
    m. transgenesis
mammillated
mammillation
mammilliform
mammose
management
    m. algorithm
    American Academy of Wound M. (AAWC)
    antibiotic m.
    endoscopic m.
    endourologic m.
    foreign body m.
    mechanical endoscopic m.
    seton m.
    stone m.
Manchester-Fothergill operation
Manchester virus
Manchurian hemorrhagic fever
Mancke flex-rigid gastroscope
Mandelamine
mandelate
    methenamine m.
mandelic acid
mandible
mandril set
maneuver
    alpha-loop m.
    avoidance m.
    bunching m.
    Credé m.
    Cushieri m.
    Duecollement m.
    Fowler-Stephens m.
    Heimlich m.
    Hoguet m.
    Hueter m.
    J-type m.
    Ko-Airan m.
    Kocher m.
    Leadbetter m.
    Mattox m.
    Mendelsohn m.
    Müller m.
    peroral m.
    Prentiss m.
    Pringle m.
    straightening m.
    suppressive m.

M

NOTES

maneuver *(continued)*
    U-turn m.
    Valsalva m.
mangafodipir trisodium
manifestation
    hepatobiliary m.
    otolaryngologic m.
Manifold II slot-blot apparatus
manipulation
    direct m.
    endoscopic stone m.
    pancreatic duct m.
    postureteroscopic m.
mannan
    yeast strain m.
Mann-Bollman fistula
Manning criteria
mannitol
mannose-specific adhesion
Mann-Whitney rank sum test
Mann-Williamson
    M.-W. operation
    M.-W. ulcer
manofluorography (MFG)
manometer
manometric
    m. criteria
    m. evaluation
    m. feature
    m. finding
    m. localization
    m. pattern
    m. sensor
    m. study
manometry
    ambulatory m.
    anal vector m.
    aneroid m.
    anorectal m.
    antral m.
    antroduodenal m.
    antroduodenojejunal m.
    balloon reflex m.
    biliary m.
    m. catheter
    computer-aided ambulatory
      gastrojejunal m.
    dry swallow on esophageal m.
    endoscopic m.
    endoscopic sphincter of Oddi m.
    ERCP m.
    esophageal m. (EM)
    InSIGHT m.
    intraluminal m.
    papillary m.
    perendoscopic m.
    PIP on esophageal m.

    point of respiratory reversal on
      esophageal m.
    pull-through m.
    rectosigmoid m.
    sphincter of Oddi m. (SOM)
    transileostomy m.
Manson
    M. disease
    M. schistosomiasis
mansonelliasis
mansoni
    Schistosoma m.
Mansson
    M. operation
    M. urinary pouch
Mantel-Haenszel test
manual lithotriptor
MAO
    maximal acid output
MAP
    mean arterial pressure
      MAP kinase signaling cascade
      systemic MAP
map
    acid-base m.
MAPK
    mitogen-activated protein kinase
maple-syrup urine disease (MSUD)
mapping
    anal m.
    bladder m.
    cavernous nerve m.
    intragastric pH m.
maprotiline
Maquet endoscopy table
Maranon syndrome
marantic endocarditis
marasmus
Marblen
Marburg virus
Marcaine block
marcescens
    Serratia m.
Marchand adrenals
Marchiafava-Micheli
    M.-M. disease
    M.-M. syndrome
Marcillin
Mardis soft stent
Mardi test
Marechal-Rosen test
Marezine
Marfan
    M. epigastric puncture
    M. syndrome
marfanoid habitus
margin
    anal m.

cell-positive m.
circumferential m.
convex m.
costal m.
crenate m.
cristate m.
dentate m.
disk m.
dissection m.
echogenic duct m.
lateral m.
medial m.
obtuse m.
subcostal m.
superior m.
marginal
  m. artery of Drummond
  m. ulcer
  m. zone lymphoma
margo, pl. **margines**
Marian
  M. lithotomy
  M. operation
marianum
  Silybum m.
Marie-Strumpell disease
marina
  Anisakis m.
Marinesco-Sjögren syndrome
Marinol
Marion disease
mark
  crosshatch m.
  M. IV Moss decompression-feeding
    catheter
marked tube
marker
  anthropometric m.
  antigen m.
  biochemical m.
  biologic m.
  bone turnover m.
  B5 tumor m.
  CA 1-18 tumor m.
  CA 72-4 tumor m.
  CEAker colorectal cancer m.
  cell cycle m.
  C100-3 hepatitis C m.
  chromosomal m.
  m. chromosome
  chromosome m.
  D4S231 m.

D4S414 m.
D16S84 m.
D16S283 m.
D16S291 m.
DUPAN 2 tumor m.
fecal m.
fluid phase m.
genetic m.
hepatitis serologic m.
HMB-45 monoclonal antibody m.
inflammation m.
interleukin-1b urinary m.
malignancy associated cellular m.
molecular m.
OA-519 prognostic prostate
  carcinoma m.
p-ANC genetic m.
pancreatic cancer m.
plasma membrane m.
polycationic m.
radiopaque m.
serologic m.
serum m.
Spot endoscopic m.
m. stitch
surrogate m.
tape m.
m. transit study
tumor m.
viral hepatitis m.
marking
  haustral m.
  red wale m.
Markov model
Marlen
  M. double-faced adhesive disk
  M. Gas Relief drainage pouch
  M. Neoprene All-Flexible faceplate
  M. Odor-Ban ileostomy pouch
  M. Solo ileostomy pouch
  M. Zip Klosed pouch
Marlex
  M. band
  M. graft
  M. hernial repair
  M. mesh
  M. mesh abdominal rectopexy
  M. plug technique
Marmite lithotrite
marneffei
  Penicillium m.
Marogen

M

NOTES

maroon blood
maroon-colored stool
marrow transplant recipient
MARS
  molecular adsorbents recirculating system
Marseille pancreatitis classification
Marshall
  M. and Tanner pubertal staging
  M. test
  M. U-stitch suture
Marshall-Bonney test
Marshall-Marchetti-Birch operation
Marshall-Marchetti-Krantz (MMK)
  M.-M.-K. cystourethropexy
  M.-M.-K. operation
  M.-M.-K. procedure
  M.-M.-K. urethropexy
Marshall-Marchetti test
marshmallow
  barium-impregnated m.
  m. bolus
marsupialization
  epididymis m.
  laparoscopic m.
  renal cyst m.
marsupium
Martel clamp
Martin
  M. anoplasty
  M. gastrostomy
  M. operation
Martin-Davis rectal speculum
Martius
  M. fascial sling
  M. fat pad
  M. graft
  M. labial fat pad flap
  M. operation
  M. scarlet blue stain
Martius-Harris operation
Martorell hypertensive ulcer
Marwedel gastrostomy
MAS
  mean allograft survival
  multiple anal sphincterotomies
masculinae
  crista urethralis m.
  ostium urethrae externum m.
masculinizing genitoplasty
masculinum
  ovarium m.
masculinus
  uterus m.
  utriculus m.
MASE
  microsurgical extraction of sperm from
    epididymis

mask
  Bili m.
  m. phenomenon
  Prohibit anti-fog face m.
Mason
  M. abdominotranssphincteric
    resection
  M. needle holder
  M. operation
  M. vertical banded gastroplasty
mass
  abdominal wall m.
  adjusted body m. (ABM)
  adnexal m.
  adrenal gland m.
  appendiceal m.
  asymptomatic m.
  body cell m. (BCM)
  colonic m.
  colorectal m.
  congenital renal m.
  cul-de-sac m.
  cystic m.
  discrete m.
  duodenal m.
  dysplasia-associated lesion or m.
    (DALM)
  esophageal m.
  exophytic m.
  expansile abdominal m.
  extramucosal m.
  extrarenal m.
  extrinsic m.
  flank m.
  fluctuant m.
  gastric m.
  hilar m.
  inflammatory renal m.
  inhomogeneous hyperechoic m.
  intraabdominal m.
  kidney m.
  lean body m. (LBM)
  lobulated m.
  malignant renal m.
  mediastinal m.
  mushroom-shaped m.
  neoplastic renal m.
  palpable m.
  parovarian m.
  periampullary m.
  perirectal m.
  m. peristalsis
  phlegmonous m.
  pleural m.
  polypoid m.
  pulsatile m.
  rectal m.
  renal m.

salivary m.
scrotal m.
soft tissue m.
submucosal m.
testicular m.
m. transfer area coefficient (MTAC)
transformary m.
traumatic renal m.
tubular excretory m.
vaginal m.
vascular renal m.

massage
prostatic m.
masseter strength
Masset test
massive
m. bowel resection syndrome
m. hepatic necrosis
m. malignant infiltration
Masson
M. trichrome
M. trichrome stain
M. trichrome staining technique
Masson-Fontana stain
mast
m. cell
m. cell degranulation
master
m. duodenoscope
m. IG bundle
m. image guide
MasterFlex pump
Masters intestinal clamp
Masters-Schwartz liver clamp
masticatory-salivary reflex
Mastisol liquid surgical adhesive
mastocytosis
systemic m.
mastoiditis
masturbation
traumatic m.
Masugi nephritis
matairesinol
matching
donor/recipient race m.
HLA-DR m.
optimizing HLA m.
optimizing human leukocyte antigen m.
material
anastomotic m.

coarse m.
coffee-ground m. (CGM)
congophilic m.
Conray 60, 70 contrast m.
extravasated iodinated contrast m.
fecal m.
iodinated contrast m.
microcrystalline m.
proteinaceous cast m.
purulent m.
suture m.
Triangle gelatin-sealed sling m.
maternal morbidity
Mathews rectal speculum
Mathieu
M. island onlay flap
M. procedure
M. technique
Mathieu-Horton-Devine flip-flap
Matrigel
Matritech NMP22 test for bladder cancer
matrix
m. calculus
m. deposition
extracellular m. (ECM)
glomerular extracellular m.
m. metalloproteinase (MMP)
nuclear m.
pericellular m. (PCM)
prostate gland tissue m.
m. urinary lithiasis
Matson operation
matted node
Mattox maneuver
mattress
Bedge antireflux m.
Home Care Simplimatt Plus zoned foam m.
m. suture
Matts grade (1–4)
maturation
collagen m.
mucosal barrier m.
normal m.
osteoclast m.
stone m.
mature teratoma
maturing the stoma
maturity-onset diabetes of the young (MODY)

M

NOTES

matutinus
> vomitus m.

Mauch double-sheathed plastic wash pipe

Maunoir hydrocele

Maunsell-Weir operation

Mavigraph color video printer

Maxaquin

Max-EPA capsule

Maxeran

MaxForce
> M. TTS balloon
> M. TTS biliary balloon dilatation catheter
> M. TTS high performance balloon dilatation catheter

maximal
> m. acid output (MAO)
> m. androgen blockade (MAB)
> m. toleration (MT)
> m. toleration volume (MTV)
> tubular m. (Tm)
> m. tubular excretory capacity of kidney

maximum
> m. (anal) resting pressure (MRP)
> m. bladder capacity
> m. coagulative necrosis
> m. cystometric capacity
> m. diameter
> m. free flow rate
> m. squeeze pressure (MSP)
> m. tolerable volume (MTV)
> m. urethral closure pressure (MUCP)
> m. urinary flow rate
> m. vasal pressure (MVP)

maximus
> gluteus m.

Maxisorb test plate

Maxolon

Maxon-loop

Maxon suture

Maxum reusable forceps

Maxzide

Maydl
> M. hernia
> M. operation
> M. procedure
> M. ureterosigmoidostomy

Mayer
> M. acid alum hematoxylin stain
> M. hematoxylin solution

Mayer-Rokitansky-Kuster-Hauser syndrome

Mayer-Rokitansky syndrome

May-Grünwald-Giemsa stain

Mayo
> M. abdominal clamp
> M. abdominal retractor
> M. bladder
> M. Clinic system test for primary biliary cirrhosis
> M. common duct probe
> M. common duct scoop
> M. common duct spoon
> M. gallstone scoop
> M. grading system
> M. operation
> M. scissors
> M. stand
> M. trocar-point needle

Mayo-Adams appendectomy retractor

Mayo-Blake gallstone forceps

Mayo-Hegar needle holder

Mayo-Kelly appendix inverter

Mayo-Noble dissecting scissors

Mayo-Ochsner suction trocar cannula

Mayo-Pean forceps

Mayo-Robson
> M.-R. gallstone scoop
> M.-R. intestinal clamp
> M.-R. intestinal forceps
> M.-R. position

Mays operation

Mazicon

mazindol

Mazzariello-Caprini forceps

MBS
> modified barium swallow

MC
> mesangial cell
> methotrexate, cisplatin

MCA
> middle colic artery

MCAD
> medium-chain acyl-CoA dehydrogenase

McArdle syndrome

McBurney
> M. incision
> M. point
> M. retractor
> M. sign

MCC
> mutated colorectal carcinoma
> *MCC* gene

McCall culdoplasty

McCarthy
> M. electrode
> M. evacuator
> M. Foroblique panendoscope cystoscope

McCarthy-Campbell miniature cystoscope

McCleery-Miller intestinal clamp

McCormack gastric mucosal sign
McCort sign
McCrea
    M. cystoscope
    M. sound
McCune-Albright syndrome
MCD
    metastatic Crohn disease
MCDK
    multicystic dysplastic kidney
McDonald
    M. cerclage
    M. stone dissector
McDougal prostatectomy clamp
MCF-7 tumor
MCFA
    medium-chain fatty acid
McGaw
    M. plastic bottle
    M. volumetric pump
McGill
    M. forceps
    M. pain questionnaire
McGivney
    M. hemorrhoidal ligator
    M. hemorrhoid forceps
M-CH
    mitomycin adsorbed onto activated
    charcoal
MCH
    mean corpuscular hemoglobin
    microfibrillar collagen hemostat
    Endo-Avitene MCH
    MCH gene
MCHA
    microsome antibody
MCHC
    mean corpuscular hemoglobin
    concentration
m-chlorophenyl-piperazine
McIndoe procedure
McIntyre reverse cystotome
MCK
    multicystic kidney
MCL
    midclavicular line
    MCL port
McLean pile clamp
McNealey-Glassman-Mixter forceps
McNeer classification
McNemar ascites test

MCP
    membrane cofactor protein
    monocyte chemotactic protein
MCP-1
    monocyte chemoattractant protein-1
M-CSF
    macrophage colony-stimulating factor
MCT
    mean colonic transit
    medium-chain triglyceride
    medullary carcinoma of thyroid
    MCT oil
MCTD
    mixed connective tissue disease
MCU
    micturating cystourethrography
MCV
    mean corpuscular volume
    methotrexate, cisplatin, vinblastine
    molluscum contagiosum virus
McVay
    M. herniorrhaphy
    M. inguinal hernial repair
    M. operation
MD-60 contrast medium
M.D. Anderson grade
MDCA
    mean distal contraction amplitude
MDCK epithelial cell
MDE
    mucinous ductal ectasia
MDLO
    metoclopramide, dexamethasone,
    lorazepam, ondansetron
MDM2 gene
MDP
    ^{99m}Tc MDP
MDR
    minimum daily requirement
MDR1 gene
MDRD
    Modification of Diet in Renal Disease
MDS
    membrane-spanning domain
MDT renogram
Meadox Surgimed Doppler probe
MEA-1
    multiple endocrine adenomatosis type I
MeAIB
    methylaminoisobutyric acid
MEA-II
    multiple endocrine adenomatosis type II

M

NOTES

meal
    barium m.
    Boas test m.
    Boyden test m.
    butter m.
    Dock test m.
    double-contrast barium m.
    Ehrmann alcohol test m.
    Ewald test m.
    fatty m.
    Fischer test m.
    isotope m.
    Leube test m.
    liver m.
    Lundh m.
    motor test m.
    normal saline m.
    opaque m.
    pH standardized m.
    retention m.
    Riegel test m.
    Salzer test m.
    small bowel m.
    solid egg white m.
    standard fatty m.
    test m.

meal-stimulated
    m.-s. acid output (MSAO)
    m.-s. pancreatic secretion

mean
    m. allograft survival (MAS)
    m. arterial blood pressure (MABP)
    m. arterial pressure (MAP)
    m. colonic transit (MCT)
    m. corpuscular hemoglobin (MCH)
    m. corpuscular hemoglobin
      concentration (MCHC)
    m. corpuscular volume (MCV)
    m. distal contraction amplitude
      (MDCA)
    m. energy
    m. input time (MIT)
    m. prostatic volume
    m. renal volume
    m. resistance time (MRT)
    m. shunt index
    m. TIMP-1/GAPDH rate
    m. TIMP-3/GAPDH ratio
    m. transit time (MTT)
    m. treatment duration
    m. venous outflow (MVO)

Meares-Stamey technique
measure
    antiendotoxin m.
    cGy radiation m.
    temporizing m.
measurement
    anorectal m.

    anthropometric m.
    bulbocavernous reflex latency m.
    Doppler ultrasound intestinal blood
      flow m.
    intestinal permeability m.
    intraprostatic temperature m.
    microfluorometric m.
    physiologic m.
    planimetric m.
    plasma bile acid m.
    pressure m.
    rectal compliance m.
    RigiScan m.
    serum bile acid m.
    m. test
    urethral pressure m.
    Vector volume m.
    velocity m.
    voiding urethral pressure m.
      (VUPM)

measuring-mounting (MM)
    m.-m. catheter
meatal
    m. advancement
    m. advancement and glansplasty
      (MAGPI)
    m. advancement, glanuloplasty,
      penoscrotal junction meatotomy
      (MAGPI)
    m. atresia
    m. spreader
    m. stenosis
    m. stenosis after circumcision
meat impaction
meatoplasty
    Stacke m.
    V-flap m.
meatorrhaphy
meatoscope
meatoscopy
    ureteral m.
meatotome
meatotomy
    meatal advancement, glanuloplasty,
      penoscrotal junction m. (MAGPI)
    m. scissors
    ureteral m.
    ventral m.
    Y-V m.
meatus, pl. meatus
    retrusive m.
    urethral m.
    m. urinarius
mebendazole
mebeverine
mebrofenin
mecamylamine

mecasermin
MeCCNU, Oncovin, fluorouracil (MOF)
mechanical
    m. anastomosis
    m. assist system
    m. biliary obstruction
    m. cystitis
    m. diarrhea
    m. duct obstruction
    m. endoscopic management
    m. extrahepatic obstruction
    m. ileus
    m. intestinal obstruction
    m. jaundice
    m. leech
    m. lithotripsy
    m. product
    m. radial-scanning instrument
    m. rotating probe
    m. small bowel obstruction
    m. stress wave
    m. ureteral dilation
    m. variceal compression
    m. ventilation
mechanism
    Albarran m.
    antireflux flap-valve m.
    cell-mediated m.
    countercurrent m.
    cyclooxygenase-dependent m.
    deglutition m.
    deranged hemostatic m.
    flap-valve m.
    Mitrofanoff m.
    neuroparacrine m.
    peptidergic m.
    pinchcock m.
    renal autoregulatory m.
    sphincteric m.
    swallowing m.
    T-cell-dependent m.
    tubuloglomerular feedback m.
    urethral closure m.
mechanoreceptor dysfunction
mechanosensitive afferent
Mecholyl
mecillinam
Meckel
    M. diverticulitis
    M. diverticulum
    M. ileitis
    M. rod

    M. scan
    M. syndrome
Meckel-Gruber syndrome
meclizine
meclofenamate
    sodium m.
meconium
    m. hydrocele
    m. ileus
    m. ileus equivalent (MIE)
    m. peritonitis
    m. plug
    m. plug syndrome
Mectra tissue sample retainer
Medena tube
media (*pl. of* medium)
medial
    m. fibroplasia
    m. margin
    m. preoptic area
    m. umbilical ligament
median
    m. arcuate ligament
    m. bar formation
    m. bar of Mercier
    m. furrow of the prostate
    m. incision
    m. lithotomy
    m. lobe
    m. lobe hyperplasia
    m. operative time
    m. raphe cyst
mediastinal
    m. crunch
    m. histoplasmosis
    m. lymphadenectomy
    m. lymphadenopathy
    m. lymph node sampling
    m. mass
    m. shift
    m. thickening
    m. tube
    m. tumor
    m. widening
mediastinitis
mediastinum
    m. germ cell tumor
    m. testis
mediated
    plasmid m.
mediation
    autoimmune immunoglobulin m.

M

NOTES

mediator
    mesenchymal inductive m.
medical
    m. dilation
    m. evaluation
    m. laser
    m. therapy
    m. vagotomy
medically induced achlorhydria
medicamentosus
    pseudopolyposis m.
Medicare patient
**Medicated Urethral System for Erection
(MUSE)**
medication
    m. allergy
    anticholinergic m.
    m. bezoar
    bromocriptine dopaminergic m.
    carbidopa dopaminergic m.
    dopaminergic m.
    levodopa dopaminergic m.
    pergolide dopaminergic m.
    psychopharmacologic m.
    psychotropic m.
    m. teratogenesis
medication-associated
    m.-a. erection
    m.-a. suppression of gastric
      secretion
medication-induced injury
medicine
    complementary and alternative m.
      (CAM)
    nuclear m. (NM)
    teratogenic m.
**MediClenze hygiene and water therapy
system**
Medicone
Medicon-Jackson rectal forceps
medicus
    furor m.
Medicut
    M. cannula
    M. catheter
Mediflex-Gazayerli retractor
Mediflex MD-7 endoscopic video system
Medi-Ject
Medi-Jector Choice
Medilas fiberTome laser
Medina
    M. ileostomy catheter
    M. tube
mediolateral lithotomy
medisect
Medisense Pen 2 glucose meter
**Medispec Econolith spark plug
lithotriptor**

Medi-Tech
    M.-T. bipolar catheter
    M.-T. bipolar probe
    M.-T. steerable catheter
Mediterranean
    M. fever
    M. lymphoma
Meditron EL-100 Endolav
medium, pl. **media**
    arteria colica media
    arteria rectalis media
    Balch 1 broth m.
    Baricon contrast m.
    Baroflave contrast m.
    Barosperse contrast m.
    Biligrafin contrast m.
    Biliscopin contrast m.
    Bilivist contrast m.
    Bilopaque contrast m.
    Biloptin contrast m.
    Campy-BAP culture m.
    Cary-Blair m.
    chocolate agar m.
    Cholebrine contrast m.
    Cholografin contrast m.
    Conray 280 contrast m.
    contrast m.
    culture m.
    dissociated m.
    Dulbecco modified Eagle m.
      (DMEM)
    Eagle minimal essential m.
      (EMEM)
    Earle m.
    extravasation of contrast m.
    Gastrografin contrast m.
    Gastrovist contrast m.
    Ham F12 m.
    Hypaque contrast m.
    inoculated m.
    iocetamic acid contrast m.
    iodipamide meglumine contrast m.
    iopanoic acid contrast m.
    ipodate contrast m.
    low-osmolar contrast m. (LOCM)
    MD-60 contrast m.
    meglumine diatrizoate contrast m.
    meglumine iotroxate contrast m.
    Niopam contrast m.
    OCT m.
    Oragrafin contrast m.
    Reno-M contrast m.
    RPMI-1640 m.
    Selenite-F enrichment m.
    Skirrow m.
    sodium iodipamide contrast m.
    Solu-Biloptin contrast m.
    sorbitol-MacConkey m.

Telepaque contrast m.
Thorotrast contrast m.
tyropanoate contrast m.
Urografin 290 contrast m.
water-soluble contrast m.
medium-chain
m.-c. acyl-CoA dehydrogenase (MCAD)
m.-c. acyl-CoA dehydrogenase deficiency
m.-c. fatty acid (MCFA)
m.-c. triglyceride (MCT)
medium-power photomicrograph
medium-term result
Medivator automatic reprocessor
Medoc-Celestin
M.-C. endoprosthesis
M.-C. pulsion tube
medorrhea
Medrad Mrinnervu endorectal colon probe
Medralone
Medrol
medronate
^{99m}Tc m.
medroxyprogesterone acetate
MEDS
microsurgical extraction of ductal sperm
Medstone
M. extracorporeal shock wave lithotripsy
M. IRIS system
M. STS lithotripsy system
M. STS lithotriptor
M. STS shock-wave generator
Medtrax
M. urology database
M. urology software
medulla
adrenal m.
m. glandulae suprarenalis
inner m.
kidney m.
outer m.
renal m.
suprarenal m.
m. of suprarenal gland
medullaris
conus m.
medullary
m. carcinoma of thyroid (MCT)
m. collecting duct

m. cystic disease
m. interstitial osmolality
m. interstitium
m. oxygenation
m. pyramid
m. sponge kidney
m. thyroid carcinoma
medullation
medullectomy
medulliadrenal
medulloadrenal
medulloblastoma
medulloid
medullosuprarenoma
medusae
caput m.
Medusa head
Meeker gallbladder clamp
mefenamic acid
mefloquine
Mefoxin
Mefoxin-saline solution
MEG
magnetoencephalography
megabladder
megacalycosis
Megace
megacolon
acquired functional m.
acute m.
aganglionic m.
congenital m.
m. congenitum
idiopathic m.
toxic m.
megacystic
m. mucinous neoplasm
m. syndrome
megacystis
bladder congenital m.
megacystis-megaureter
m.-m. association
m.-m. syndrome
megacystis-microcolon-intestinal hypoperistalsis syndrome
megaduodenum
megaesophagus
Chagasic m.
megakaryocyte
megalin
Megalink biliary stent
megaloblastic anemia

M

NOTES

megalocystis
megaloesophagus
megalogastria
megalopenis
megalophallus
megaloureter
megalourethra
megameatus
megameatus-intact prepuce (MIP)
megamitochondria
megarectum
    idiopathic m.
megasigmoid syndrome
megaureter
    m. classification
    obstructive m.
    primary obstructive m.
    primary refluxing m.
    secondary refluxing m.
    unilateral m.
megaurethra
megavitamin
megestrol acetate
meglumine
    m. diatrizoate
    m. diatrizoate contrast medium
    m. diatrizoate enema
    iodipamide m.
    m. iotroxate
    m. iotroxate contrast medium
    Urovist M.
MEGX
    monoethylglycinexylidide
MEIA
    microparticle enzyme immunoassay
Meigs syndrome
Meissner plexus
melaninogenicus
    Bacteroides m.
melanogaster
    Drosophila m.
melanoma
    adrenal gland m.
    bladder malignant m.
    familial atypical multiple mole m.
    (FAMM)
    m. intratumor pressure
    male genitalia m.
    malignant m.
    metastatic m.
melanorrhagia
melanorrhea
melanosis
    m. coli
    penile m.
melanotic
    m. neuroectodermal tumor of
    infancy (MNTI)

melas
    icterus m.
melasma
    m. addisonii
    m. suprarenale
melatonin
Melchior ileal neobladder
melena
    m. neonatorum
    m. spuria
    m. vera
melenemesis
melenic stool
melitensis
    Brucella m.
melituria
Melkersson-Rosenthal syndrome
mellitus
    diabetes m.
    insulin-dependent diabetes m.
    (IDDM)
    malnutrition-related diabetes m.
    (MRDM)
    non-insulin-dependent diabetes m.
    (NIDDM)
    posttransplant diabetes m. (PTDM)
    streptozotocin-induced diabetes m.
    type 2 diabetes m.
meloxicam
melphalan
Meltzer-Lyon test
Meltzer sign
membranate
membrane
    antiglomerular basement m.
    antitubular basement m.
    antral m.
    basement m.
    basolateral m. (BLM)
    biocompatible m.
    bioincompatible m.
    brush-border m. (BBM)
    m. catheter technique
    cell m.
    cellulose-based m.
    cellulose diacetate m.
    Chwalla m.
    cloacal m.
    m. cofactor protein (MCP)
    congenital pyloric m.
    croupous m.
    cuprophane m.
    m. current
    Debove m.
    dialyzer m.
    dry mucous m.
    m. effect
    elastic silicone m.

false m.
filtration-slit m.
glomerular basement m. (GBM)
Hemophan m.
Hibond N+ nylon m.
high-flux dialysis m.
high-flux polysulfone m.
m. hyperpolarization.
invaginated m.
Jackson m.
low-flux cuprophane m.
low-flux dialysis m.
low-flux polysulfone m.
lysosomal m.
mammalian cell m.
microvillous m.
moist mucous m.
MSI nylon m.
mucous m.
NaK-ATPase m.
nuclear m.
m. oxygenator
m. permeability
m. peroxidation
phrenoesophageal m.
polymethylmethacrylate m.
polysulfone m.
porous filter m.
posttransplant antiglomerular
  basement m.
Preclude peritoneal m.
prostate-specific m. (PSM)
Seprafilm bioresorbable m.
serous m.
small intestinal m.
thin basement m. (TBM)
Toldt m.
m. trafficking
m. transport protein
tubular basement m. (TBM)
urea-impermeable m.
urothelial basement m. (UBM)
membrane-attack complex
membrane-based lipid
membrane-coated SEMS
membrane-covered stent
membrane-spanning
m.-s. domain (MDS)
m.-s. integrin
membranolysis
membranoproliferative glomerulonephritis
(type I, II) (MPGN)

membranotomy
laryngeal jack-assisted retrograde
  esophageal m.
membranous
m. glomerulonephritis (MGN)
m. nephropathy
m. neuropathy
m. urethra
membrum virile
Memokath catheter
memory
m. impairment
m. T cell
m. wire
Memotherm
M. colorectal stent
M. Flexx biliary stent
M. nitinol stent
MEN
multiple endocrine neoplasia
MEN 2A
  multiple endocrine neoplasia 2A
MEN 2B
  multiple endocrine neoplasia 2B
MEN I syndrome
menaquinone (MK)
mendelian pattern
Mendelsohn maneuver
Mendez ultrasonic cystotome
Ménétrier disease
Menghini
M. liver biopsy needle
M. technique
M. technique for percutaneous liver
  biopsy
Menghini-type coring bevel
Ménière disease
meningismus
meningitis
pyogenic m.
meningomyelocele
meningosepticum
Flavobacterium m.
meniscus sign
Menkes
M. disease
M. disease gene
M. syndrome
menouria
MENS
multiple endocrine neoplasia syndrome

M

NOTES

mentagrophytes
> *Trichophyton m.*

Mentor
> M. Alpha 1 inflatable penile prosthesis
> M. Bioflex cylinder
> M. GFS penile prosthesis
> M. gun
> M. IPP penile prosthesis
> M. malleable penile prosthesis
> M. Mark II penile prosthesis
> M. nonhydrophilic PVC catheter
> M. Response VCD
> M. straight catheter

Mentor-Piston VCD
Mentor-Touch VCD
Menuel cavernosometry
Menuet
> M. Compact primary urodynamic analyzer
> M. Compact urodynamic testing device

MEOS
> microsomal ethanol oxidizing system

mepenzolate bromide
meperidine
> m. conscious sedation
> m. hydrochloride

mephentermine
mepiperphenidol
meprobamate
mercaptan
mercaptoethane sulfonate
2-mercaptoethanesulfonic acid (mesna)
6-mercaptopurine (6-MP)
mercaptotriglycylglycine (MAG-3)
Mercedes Benz sign
Mercier
> M. bar
> median bar of M.
> M. operation

mercurialism
mercurial nephrosis
mercuric
> m. chloride-induced ARF
> m. chloride-induced nephritis
> m. chloride nephrotoxicity
> m. oxide
> m. oxide battery ingestion

mercury
> m. bougienage treatment
> m. chloride (HgCl2)
> millimeter of m. (mmHg, mm Hg)
> m. poisoning

mercury-containing balloon
mercury-filled dilator
mercury-weighted
> m.-w. dilator

> m.-w. rubber bougie
> m.-w. tube

Meridia
Merindino operation
Meritene liquid feeding
MERmaid kit
mermaid malformation
meropenem
Merrem
Mersilene
> M. mesh
> M. for pubovaginal sling
> M. strut
> M. suture
> M. tape

merthiolate fresh stool examination
merycism
MES
> mucosal electrosensitivity

MESA
> microepididymal sperm aspiration
> microsurgical epididymal sperm aspiration

mesalamine
> m. enema
> m. rectal suppository
> m. sodium

mesalazine
mesangial
> m. angle
> m. cell (MC)
> m. deposit
> m. hypercellularity
> m. lysis
> m. matrix expansion
> m. nephropathy
> m. pattern
> m. proliferation
> m. volume fraction

mesangiocapillary glomerulonephritis
mesangiolysis
mesangioproliferative glomerulonephritis
mesangium
> extraglomerular m. (EGM)
> glomerular m.

mesaraica
> tabes m.

mesenchyma cell
mesenchymal
> m. change
> m. hamartoma
> m. inductive mediator
> m. protein

mesenchyme
> metanephrogenic m.

mesenchymoma
> benign m.
> malignant m.

mesenterectomy
mesenterial intestine
mesenteric
  m. adenitis
  m. angiogram
  m. apoplexy
  m. arterial embolism
  m. arterial thrombosis
  m. arteriography
  m. arteriovenous fistula
  m. artery
  m. artery constriction
  m. attachment
  m. attachments of colon
  m. circulation
  m. cyst
  m. defect
  m. fibromatosis
  m. hematoma
  m. hernia
  m. infarction
  m. inflammatory venoocclusive
    disease (MIVOD)
  m. ischemia
  m. lipodystrophy
  m. lipogranuloma
  m. lymph node (MLN)
  m. panniculitis (MP)
  m. rupture
  m. sensory receptor
  m. steal syndrome
  m. stranding
  m. tear
  m. triangle
  m. tumefaction
  m. varix
  m. vascular disease
  m. vascular lesion
  m. vascular occlusion
  m. vasculitis
  m. vein
  m. vein thrombosis (MVT)
  m. window
mesenterica
  tabes m.
mesentericoparietal hernia
mesenteriolum
mesenteriopexy
mesenteriorrhaphy
mesenteriplication
mesenteritis
  liposclerotic m.

  retractile m.
  sclerosing m.
mesenterium
mesenteroaxial gastric volvulus
mesenterorenal bypass
mesentery
  leaf of m.
  small intestine m. (SIM)
mesentorrhaphy
mesh
  Dacron m.
  Dexon polyglycolic acid m.
  Marlex m.
  Mersilene m.
  m. plug hernioplasty
  polypropylene m.
  polytetrafluoroethylene m.
  Sperma-Tex preshaped m.
  m. stent
  m. stent prosthesis
  Surgipro m.
  synthetic m.
  Trelex m.
  Vicryl m.
  Visilex m.
meshed graft
mesher
  Collin m.
mesna
  2-mercaptoethanesulfonic acid
Mesnex
mesoappendicitis
mesoappendix
mesoblastic nephroma
mesocaval
  m. anastomosis
  m. H-graft shunt
  m. interposition shunt
mesocecum
mesocolic
  m. band
  m. hernia
  m. shelf
mesocolica
  taenia m.
mesocolon
mesocolonic vessel
mesocolopexy
mesocoloplication
mesodermal ingrowth
mesogastric

M

NOTES

mesogastrium
    dorsal m.
    ventral m.
mesoileum
mesometrium
mesonephric
    m. adenoma
    m. duct
    m. hyperplasia
    m. nephron
    m. remnant
    m. tubule
mesonephricus
    ductus m.
mesonephros, pl. **mesonephroi**
    caudal m.
    cranial m.
    genital m.
mesopexy
mesophilic bacterium
mesor
mesorectal
    m. excision
    m. lymphadenectomy
    m. tissue
mesorectum
mesoridazine
mesorrhaphy
mesosigmoid colon
mesosigmoidopexy
mesothelial
    m. hyperplasia (MH)
    m. metaplasia
mesothelioma
    benign cystic m.
    benign m. of genital tract
    diffuse malignant m. (DMM)
    giant fibrous m.
    peritoneal m.
    well-differentiated papillary m.
      (WDPM)
mesotrypsin
message-2
    testosterone repressed prostate m.-2
      (TRPM-2)
messenger
    m. ribonucleic acid (mRNA)
    m. RNA (mRNA)
    m. RNA molecule
    T-cell second m.
    ureteral peristalsis second m.
Messerklinger endoscope
Mestinon
mesylate
    doxazosin m.
    gabexate m.
    hycanthone m.
    nafamostat m.

metaanalysis
metaanalytic review
metabolic
    m. acidosis
    m. alkalosis
    m. balance
    m. bone survey
    m. calculus
    m. complication
    m. derangement
    m. disorder
    m. effect
    m. evaluation
    m. liver disease
    m. predictor
    m. range
    m. rate
    m. stone
    m. stone disease
    m. therapy
metabolism
    albumin m.
    basal m. (BM)
    bile salt m. (BSM)
    calcium m.
    citrate m.
    cortisol m.
    cystine m.
    drug m.
    first-pass m. (FPM)
    glomerular m.
    glutathione m.
    hepatic m.
    inborn error of m.
    leucine m.
    lipid m.
    lipoprotein m.
    magnesium m.
    oxalate m.
    phosphorus m.
    protein m.
    sulfur amino acid m.
    tryptophan m.
metabolite
    arachidonic acid m.
    cyclooxygenase m.
    cytochrome P450 m.
    reactive oxygen m.
    toxic m.
metachromatic dye
metachronous
    m. adenoma
    m. colon cancer
    m. contralateral hernias
    m. lesion
    m. neoplasia
    m. small bowel adenocarcinoma
    m. tumor

metadysentery
MetaFluor system
Metagonimus yokogawai
Metahydrin
metaicteric
metaiodobenzylguanidine (MIBG)
    iodine-131-labeled m.
metal
    m. ball-tip catheter
    m. bar retractor
    m. clip
    m. intoxication
    m. olive
    m. sound
    m. stent
    m. wing clamp
    M. Z stent
metallic
    m. biliary stent
    m. biliary stent migration
    m. embolus
    m. staple
    m. stent placement
metallic-tip catheter
metalloenzyme
metalloproteinase
    m. inhibitor
    matrix m. (MMP)
    tissue m. (TIMP)
    tissue inhibitor of m.
    tissue inhibitor of m.-2 (TIMP-2)
metallothionein
metal-olive dilator
metal-tipped stent pusher
metal-weighted Silastic feeding tube
metamorphosis
    fatty m.
Metamucil
metanephric
    m. tubule
    m. vesicle
metanephrine
metanephrogenic mesenchyme
metanephros, pl. metanephroi
metaplasia
    Barrett m.
    bladder squamous m.
    cardia intestinal m. (CIM)
    columnar m.
    gastric m.
    glandular m.
    goblet cell m.

    intestinal m. (type I–III)
    junctional intestinal m.
    mesothelial m.
    myeloid m.
    osseous m.
    pancreatic acinar m. (PAM)
    specialized intestinal m. (SIM)
metaplasia-dysplasia-carcinoma sequence
metaplastic
    m. atrophic gastritis
    m. epithelium
    m. gastric fundic gland
    m. ossification
    m. polyp
metaproterenol
metapyrone stimulation test
metaraminol
metastasis, pl. metastases
    brain m.
    colonic m.
    cutaneous m.
    diffuse m.
    disseminated m.
    distant m.
    duodenal m.
    extrahepatic m. (EHM)
    extralymphatic m.
    m. gene
    hematogenic m.
    implantation m.
    intramucosal m.
    liver m.
    lymphatic m.
    lymph node m.
    lymphogenic m.
    neoplasm m.
    percutaneous image-guided thermal
      ablation of hepatic m.
    periesophagogastric lymph node m.
    port site m.
    m. suppression
    tumor, node, m. (TNM)
metastatic
    m. adenocarcinoma
    m. cancer
    m. carcinoid syndrome
    m. cascade
    m. cholangiocarcinoma
    m. complication
    m. Crohn disease (MCD)
    m. dissemination
    m. fat necrosis

M

NOTES

metastatic *(continued)*
    m. implantation
    m. lesion
    m. melanoma
    m. neuroblastoma
    m. orchitis
    m. prostatic carcinoma
    m. renal cell carcinoma (MRCC)
Metastron
metasulfobenzoate
    prednisolone m.
metasynchronous bacterial urinary tract infection
Metatensin
metaxalone
met-enkephalin
    methionine-enkephalin
        met-enkephalin peptide
        plasma met-enkephalin
meteorism
meter
    Aleo m.
    Fisher Accumet pH m.
    integrating spherical power m.
    Medisense Pen 2 glucose m.
    One Touch blood glucose m.
    Synectics 6000 digital pH-meter m.
metformin
methacholine
methacrylate
    methyl m.
methadone
methamphetamine
methane (CH4) excretor
methanethiol
Methanobrevibacter smithii
methanogen
methanogenesis
methanogenic archaea
methanol intoxication
methantheline bromide
methapyrilene
methdilazine
Methedrine
methemalbumin
methemoglobinemia
methenamine
    m. hippurate
    m. mandelate
methicillin
methicillin-resistant *Staphylococcus aureus* **(MRSA)**
methimazole
Methiodal
methionine-enkephalin (met-enkephalin)
    immunoreactive m.-e. (IRME)
methionine loading
methixene

method
    ablate-and-chip m.
    acid guanidine thiocyanate-phenol-chloroform m.
    acid hematin m.
    Addis m.
    anthrone m.
    avidin-biotin-peroxidase complex m.
    barostat m.
    Beck m.
    Bence Jones protein m.
    Benedict and Franke m.
    Benedict-Osterberg m.
    Benedict-Talbot body surface area m.
    Bertrand m.
    Biogenex antigen retrieval m.
    Brown and Wickham pressure profile m.
    cap m.
    cholesterol-cholesteroloxidase-phenol 4-aminophenazone m.
    cinefluoroscopic m.
    Cockroft m.
    dye scattering m.
    ellipsoid m.
    endoscopic mucosal resection, cap m. (EMRC)
    endoscopic mucosal resection, tube m. (EMRT)
    Esbach m.
    Essed plication m.
    Fishberg m.
    Folin-Benedict-Myers m.
    Folin-Denis m.
    Folin gravimetric m.
    m. of Gates
    Genta m.
    Giemsa m.
    Halsted m.
    Hanley m.
    Hasson m.
    Hybritech m.
    immunohistochemical m.
    Jenckel cholecystoduodenostomy m.
    Jendrassik-Grof m.
    Kaplan-Meier m.
    Lashmet-Newburgh m.
    lay-open m.
    lift-and-cut m.
    Lowery m.
    Metzer-Boyce m.
    microwave-assisted streptavidin-biotin peroxidase m.
    Morison m.
    noninvasive m.
    Okamoto m.
    Papanicolaou m.

Parker-Kerr closed m.
partial hood assisted lift-and-cut m.
Patterson-Parker m.
pause-squeeze m.
Payr m.
percutaneous sampling m.
Permutit m.
phosphotungstic acid-magnesium
chloride precipitation m.
pull m.
Quimby m.
radiochromium-labeled
erythrocyte m.
Reddick-Saye m.
Rehfuss m.
Schwartz m.
Sengstaken-Blakemore m.
Shohl-Pedley m.
Sjöqvist m.
standard radioenzymatic m.
suck-and-cut m.
Sumner m.
thermally active m.
thiourea-resorcinol m.
trapezoid m.
triangulation stapling m.
turn-and-suction m.
two-devices-in-one-channel m.
Volhard-Fahr m.
Warthin-Starry m.
Waterston m.
Woolf m.
methotrexate (MTX)
m., cisplatin (MC)
m., cisplatin, vinblastine (MCV)
m., vinblastine, Adriamycin,
cisplatin (MVAC, M-VAC)
m., vinblastine, epirubicin, cisplatin
(M-VEC)
methotrimeprazine
methoxamine
methoxsalen
methoxyflurane anesthesia
methoxyphenamine
methscopolamine
m. bromide
methyclothiazide
methyl
m. CCNU
m. methacrylate
m. red test
m. salicylate

m. tert-butyl ether (MTBE)
m. tertbutyl ether stone dissolution
m. tertiary butyl ether (MTBE)
methylaminoisobutyric acid (MeAIB)
methylate
phentolamine m.
methylatropine nitrate
methylbromide
anisotropine m.
homatropine m.
methylcellulose
2-methylcitric acid
5-methyl cytosine
methyldopa
parenteral m.
methyldopate
methylene
m. blue
m. blue dye
m. blue enema
m. blue stain
5,10-m.-tetrahydrofolate reductase
(MTHFR)
methylhistamine
3-methylhistidine
urinary 3-m.
methylmalonic acid
methylnitrate
atropine m.
methylphenidate
1-methyl-4-phenyl-1,2,3,6-
tetrahydropyridine (MTPT)
6-methylprednisolone
methylprednisolone acetate
methylsulfate
neostigmine m.
methyl-tert-butyl ether therapy
methyltestosterone
methyltestosterone-induced cholestasis
methysergide maleate
Meticorten
meticulous dissection
Metizol
metoclopramide
m., dexamethasone, lorazepam,
ondansetron (MDLO)
m. premedication
metocurine
metolazone
metoprolol tartrate
Metricide disinfectant

M

NOTES

metrifonate
metrizamide
metrizoate
MetroGel
metronidazole
    m., amoxicillin, clarithromycin, *H.*
    pylori, one-week therapy
    (MACH1)
    omeprazole, amoxicillin, m. (OAM)
metronidazole-resistant strain
Metryl 500
metschnikovii
    Vibrio m.
metyrapone stimulation test
metyrosine
Metzenbaum scissors
Metzer-Boyce method
Meulengracht diet
Mevacor
Mewissen infusion catheter
Mexican hat sign
mexiletine
Meyenburg complex
Meyer-Weigert law
mezlocillin
MFG
    manofluorography
MFL 5000 lithotriptor
MGN
    membranous glomerulonephritis
MH
    mesothelial hyperplasia
MHC
    major histocompatibility complex
    MHC class I, II antigen
MHC-bound
MHV
    middle hepatic vein
Mi-Acid
Miami pouch
MIB-1
    monoclonal antibody MIB-1
    MIB-1 staining
MIBG
    metaiodobenzylguanidine
MIC
    minimal inhibitory concentration
    MIC gastroenteric tube
    MIC gastrostomy tube
    glass pH-electrodes - MIC
micaceous growth of penis
mica operation
micellar solubilization
micelle formation
Michaelis constant (Km)
Michaelis-Gutmann body
Michaelis-Menten kinetics

Michal
    M. II technique
    M. procedure (I, II)
Michel clip
Michigan
    M. intestinal forceps
    M. Kidney Registry
Mick
    M. prostate template
    M. TP-200 applicator
MIC-Key G, J gastrostomy tube
miconazole
Micral urine dipstick test
Micro-6 ureteroscope
microabscess
micro-acini
microadenoma
microaerophilic organism
microalbuminuria
microanastomosis
    laser-assisted m. (LAMA)
microaneurysm
microangiopathic renal injury
microangiopathy
    diabetic m.
    tacrolimus-associated m.
    thrombotic m.
microballoon probe
microbial
    m. approach
    m. ecology
microbiliary inflammation
microbiology
microbiota
microcalcification
microcalculus, pl. microcalculi
microcalix
Microcell chamber
microcephaly
microchimerism
    donor hematopoietic cell m.
    donor-type m.
microchromoendoscopy
microclimate
    acid m.
Micrococcus
Microcoleus
microcolitis
microcolon
microcrystal
microcrystalline material
microcyst
    lymphatic m.
microcystic disease of renal medulla
microdensitometer
    Vickers M85a m.
microdroplet fat deposition

microelectrode
  M. MI-506 small-caliber pH
    electrode
  M. MI-506 small-caliber probe
microemulsion
  cyclosporine for m.
microendoprobe
  Toshiba m.
microenvironment
  gastric m.
microepididymal sperm aspiration (MESA)
microerosion
microexplosive generator
microfibril
microfibrillar
  m. collagen hemostat (MCH)
  m. protein (MP)
microfilament bundle
microfilariasis
microfil-associated glycoprotein (MAGP)
microfilter
  Minnpure m.
microflora
  colonic m.
microfluorometric measurement
microfold (M)
  m. cell
microgastria
microgenitalism
Microglass pH electrode
microgram
micrograph
  low-magnification electron m.
Microgyn II urinary incontinence device
microhamartoma, pl. **microhamartomata, microhamartomas**
  biliary m.
microhematuria
microimplant
  silicone m.
microimplant
microlens cystourethroscope
microlith
microlithiasis
  common bile duct m. (CBDM)
  pulmonary alveolar m.
  testicular m.
microlithiasis-induced pancreatitis
MicroLyzer
  M. Gas analyzer

  M. model 12i
  M. model SC
micromanipulation
  gamete m.
  oocyte m.
micrometastasis
  hematogenous m.
Micronase
microneedle holder
micronidia
micronized
  m. flavonidic fraction
  m. purified flavonoid fracture
    (MPFF)
micronodular cirrhosis
microparticle enzyme immunoassay (MEIA)
micropenis
microperforation
microperfusion study
microphallus
micropipette
micropuncture
  epididymis m.
  m. technique
microrchidia
micros
  Peptostreptococcus m.
microsatellite instability (MSI)
microscope
  ELMISKOP 101 electron m.
  JEM-100B and 100S electron m.
  JEOL 100 CX electron m.
  JEOL JSM 35 CF scanning
    electron m.
  laser m.
  Olympus BH2-epifluorescence m.
  Olympus BH2-RFCA reflecting m.
  Olympus BHT-2 m.
  Olympus CBK fluorescence m.
  Phillips CM 12 electron m.
  real-time confocal scanning
    laser m.
  scanning electron m.
  Zeiss IDO3 phase-contrast m.
  Zeiss S9 electron m.
microscopic
  m. colitis
  m. colitis syndrome
  m. epididymal sperm aspiration
  m. hematuria

M

NOTES

microscopic *(continued)*
  m. polyangiitis (MPA)
  m. urine examination
microscopy
  electron m.
  epifluorescence m.
  immune electron m.
  immunofluorescence m.
  light m.
  paraffin-section light m.
  polarization m.
  rotary shadowing electron m.
  scanning electron m.
  scanning force m. (SFM)
  transmission electron m. (TEM)
  urinalysis sediment m.
  in vivo m.
microseminoprotein
  beta m.
MicroSkin ostomy pouch
microsomal
  m. damage
  m. ethanol oxidizing system
    (MEOS)
microsome
  m. antibody (MCHA)
  liver-kidney m. (LKM)
microsome antibody (MCHA)
microsphere
  biodegradable m.
  Super-Bright m.
  ^{99m}Tc albumin m.
Microspike approximator clamp
Microsporidia
microsporidian
microsporidiosis
microsurgery
  rectal-expander-assisted transanal
    endoscopic m. (RE-TEM)
  transanal endoscopic m. (TEM)
microsurgical
  m. denervation of the spermatic
    cord
  m. epididymal sperm aspiration
    (MESA)
  m. epididymal sperm aspiration
    procedure
  m. epididymovasostomy (MSEV)
  m. extraction of ductal sperm
    (MEDS)
  m. extraction of sperm from
    epididymis (MASE)
  m. inguinal varicocelectomy
microsuture
  Sharpoint m.
microtelangiectasia
microtendon

microtip
  m. sensor catheter
  m. transducer catheter
microtitration plate reader
microtrabecular hepatocellular carcinoma
microtransducer
  imbedded m.
  Konigsberg m.
  m. technique
microtubule (MT)
microtubulotomy technique
microvascular
  m. clamp
  m. flap
  m. needle holder
Microvasive
  M. Altertome
  M. angled hydrophilic guidewire
  M. ASAP 18
  M. balloon catheter
  M. biliary stent system
  M. CRE esophageal dilator
  M. disposable alligator-shaped
    forceps
  M. 5F mini-snare
  M. Geenen Endotorque guidewire
  M. Glidewire guidewire
  M. Gold probe bipolar
    electrocautery device
  M. instrumentation
  M. papillotome
  M. radial jaw 3 biopsy forceps
  M. retrieval balloon
  M. Rigiflex balloon dilator
  M. Rigiflex through-the-scope
    balloon
  M. sclerotherapy needle
  M. Ultraflex esophageal stent
    system
  M. ultratome
microvesicular
  m. fat
  m. steatosis
microvillous membrane
microvillus, pl. **microvilli**
  m. inclusion disease
microvolt (μV)
microwave
  m. antenna design
  m. applicator
  m. coagulation
  endoscopic m.
  m. hyperthermia
  m. nonsurgical treatment
  m. thermotherapy
microwave-assisted streptavidin-biotin peroxidase method
microwell plate

miction
MIC-TJ transgastric jejunal tube
micturating
    m. cystogram
    m. cystourethrogram
    m. cystourethrography (MCU)
micturition
    m. cystourethrogram
    m. phase
    m. problem
    m. reflex
    m. reflex inhibition
    m. reflex manual initiation
midabdominal
    m. abscess
    m. transverse incision
    m. wall
midaxillary line
midazolam
    m. conscious sedation
    m. hydrochloride
midclavicular line (MCL)
midcolon
middle
    m. colic artery (MCA)
    m. extrahepatic bile duct
    m. gland
    m. hemorrhoidal artery
    m. hepatic vein (MHV)
    m. hypospadias
    m. rectal fold
    m. rectal vein
    m. rectal venous plexus
    m. stomach
    m. ureter
midepigastric area
midepigastrium
midesophageal diverticulum
midesophagus
midgastric electrode
midgut
    m. ischemia
    m. volvulus
    m. volvulus with malrotation
midline
    m. abdominal crease
    m. lower abdominal incision
    m. upper abdominal incision
midodrine
midrectal area
midregion PTH
midsigmoid colon

midstomach
midstream
    m. specimen of urine (MSU)
    m. urinalysis
midureteral calculus
MIE
    meconium ileus equivalent
Miescher cheilitis granulomatosa
MIF
    migration inhibition factor
mifepristone
miglitol
migraine
    abdominal m.
migrating
    m. motor complex (MMC)
    m. myoelectric complex
migration
    aboral m.
    calculus m.
    electrode m.
    gallstone m.
    gastrostomy tube m.
    m. inhibition factor (MIF)
    intravesical m.
    lymphocyte m.
    metallic biliary stent m.
    stent m.
    tube m.
Mik
    Mikulicz
Mikulicz (Mik)
    M. bag
    M. clamp
    M. colostomy
    M. drain
    M. drain technique
    M. gastroscope
    M. gastrostomy tube
    M. operation
    M. packing
    M. pad
    M. peritoneal forceps
    M. procedure
    M. pyloroplasty
    M. retractor
mil
    delta per m.
mild
    m. distress
    m. hyperoxaluria

M

NOTES

Miles
    M. abdominoperineal resection
    M. operation
    M. V.I.P. 300 vacuum infiltration
      processor
milia (*pl. of* milium)
miliaria rubra
miliary tuberculosis
milium, pl. **milia**
milk
    acidophilus m.
    m. diet
    m. of magnesia (MOM)
    m. protein antibody
    m. sickness
    m. thistle
milk-alkali syndrome
milking of intestine
Milkinol
milkman's line
milk-of-calcium bile
milk-sensitive colitis
milky
    m. ascites
    m. fluid
    m. urine
Millard mouth gag
Millar urodynamic catheter
**Millen technique retropubic
prostatectomy**
Miller
    M. cystoscope
    M. Fisher syndrome
    M. rectal forceps
    M. rectal scissors
Miller-Abbott intestinal tube
milleri
    Streptococcus m.
Miller-Senn retractor
Millex-GS 0.22-mm pore-size filter
Millex-GV 0.22-mm filter
Millie female urinal
Milligan-Morgan
    M.-M. hemorrhoidectomy
    M.-M. operation
    M.-M. technique for hemorrhoid
      treatment
millijoule (mJ)
milliliter (mL, ml)
millimeter of mercury (mmHg, mm Hg)
millimolar concentration
millimole per liter (mmol/L)
Millin
    M. bladder retractor
    M. forceps
    M. T-clamp
milliosmole/kilogram (mosm/kg)

Millipore filter
milliwatt (mW)
Mill-Rose
    M.-R. flexible endoscopic overtube
    M.-R. RiteBite biopsy forceps
milrinone
Milroy disease
MILTS
    Multicentre International Liver Tumor
      Study
mimic
    endocrine m.
mind-bladder syndrome
mineral
    divalent m.
mineralocorticoid
mineralocorticoid-independent factor
Ming gastric carcinoma classification
miniature
    m. probe
    m. ultrasound suction device
miniaturized ultrasound catheter probe
MiniBard catheter
Miniguard adhesive patch
mini-helical basket
minilaparatomy approach
minilaparoscope
    m. cholecystectomy
    Storz m.
minilaparotomy
    m. incision
    m. pelvic lymph node dissection
    m. restorative proctocolectomy
    m. staging pelvic lymphadenectomy
mini-loop
    m.-l. ligation
    Olympus HX-21L detachable m.-l.
minimal
    m. access surgery
    m. change disease
    m. inhibitory concentration (MIC)
    m. transurethral resection of
      prostate (M-TURP)
minimal-change nephrotic syndrome
minimal-lesion nephrotic syndrome
minimally invasive treatment
minimicrosphere
minimum daily requirement (MDR)
minipapillotome
mini-perc technique
mini-Pfannenstiel incision
Minipress
miniprobe
    high-frequency m.
minipump
    Alzer Model 2001 osmotic m.
Miniscope

miniscope
    Candela M.
    Circon-ACMI m.
    Wolfe m.
mini-snare
    Microvasive 5F m.-s.
mini-VAB
    vinblastine, actinomycin D, bleomycin
mink cell bioassay
Minnesota
    M. antilymphocyte globulin
    M. Multiphasic Personality
    Inventory
    M. tube
Minnpure microfilter
Minocin
minocycline
minor
    curvatura gastrica m.
    curvatura ventriculi m.
    globus m.
    m. papilla
    papilla duodeni m.
    m. papilla sphincterotomy
minoxidil
Mintezol
minus
    omentum m.
minute
    m. bleeding
    count per m. (cpm, CPM)
    m. polypoid lesion
    30-m. transurethral microwave
    thermotherapy
    30-m. TUMT
minutissimum
    Corynebacterium m.
MIP
    megameatus-intact prepuce
mirabilis
    Proteus m.
MiraLax
Mirizzi syndrome
mirror-image artifact
misakiensis
    Streptomyces m.
mismatch
    HLA m.
    V/Q m.
misonidazole
misoprostol protection

misperfusion
    gastroduodenal m.
misplaced gland
missense mutation
Mission
    M. vacuum constriction device
    M. vacuum erection device
    M. VCD
    M. VED
Missouri catheter
**Misstique female external urinary
    collector**
mistletoe
MIT
    mean input time
Mitchell technique for epispadias repair
Mitek bone anchor
Mithracin
Mithramycin
mithramycin
mitis
    nephritis m.
mitochondria
    giant m.
mitochondrial
    m. antibody
    m. complex
    m. ethanol oxidase system
    m. fatty acid beta-oxidation
    m. glutamate dehydrogenase
    pathway
    m. immunological study
    m. neurogastrointestinal
    encephalomyopathy (MNGIE)
    m. phosphate-dependent glutaminase
mitogen
**mitogen-activated protein kinase
    (MAPK)**
mitogenic
    m. effect
    m. stimulation
    m. stimulus
mitomycin
    m. adsorbed onto activated
    charcoal (M-CH)
    m. C
    fluorouracil, Adriamycin, m. C
    (FAMe)
    5-fluorouracil, Adriamycin, m. C
    (FAM)
    m. transarterial embolization
    treatment

M

NOTES

mitosis count
mitosis-karyorrhexis index (MKI)
mitotane
mitotic
    m. activity
    m. index
mitoxantrone
Mitrofanoff
    M. appendicovesicostomy
    M. catheterizable channel
    M. conduit
    M. continent urinary diversion technique
    M. continent urinary stoma
    M. mechanism
    M. neourethra
    M. principle
    M. procedure
    M. solution
    M. tube
    M. valve
Mitrolan
Mitscherlich test
mittelschmerz
mivacurium chloride
MIVOD
    mesenteric inflammatory venoocclusive disease
mixed
    m. cirrhosis
    m. connective tissue disease (MCTD)
    m. connective tissue disorder
    m. essential cryoglobulinemia
    m. germ cell-sex cord stromal tumor
    m. germ cell tumor
    m. gonadal dysgenesis
    m. growth on culture
    m. hemorrhoids
    m. hyperlipidemia
    m. hyperplastic-adenomatous gastric polyp
    m. incontinence
    m. intralobular fibrosis
    m. leukocyte culture (MLC)
    m. rhabdomyosarcoma
    m. structure
mixed-cholesterol gallstone
Mixter
    M. clamp
    M. dilating probe
    M. dissector
    M. gallstone forceps
    M. hemostat
mixture
    amino acid-glucose m.
    citric acid bladder m.

    eutectic m.
    eutectic m. of local anesthetics (EMLA)
    sodium citrate and potassium citrate m.
Miyazaki-Bonney test for stress incontinence
mizoribine
mJ
    millijoule
MK
    menaquinone
MK801
MK886
MKI
    mitosis-karyorrhexis index
MKII automated scanner
MKIII
    Digitrapper M.
mL, ml
    milliliter
MLC
    mixed leukocyte culture
    allogeneic MLC
MLH1 gene
MLN
    mesenteric lymph node
MLP
    multiple lymphomatous polyposis
MM
    measuring-mounting
    MM catheter
MMAP
    Maine Medical Assessment Program
    MMAP index
MMC
    migrating motor complex
    murine mesangial cell
MMD
    intramural microvessel density
MMF
    mycophenolate
    mycophenolate mofetil
mmHg, mm Hg
    millimeter of mercury
MMK
    Marshall-Marchetti-Krantz
mmol/L
    millimole per liter
MMP
    matrix metalloproteinase
MMR
    mutation mismatch repair
MMUA
    macromolecular uronate
MN
    mononuclear

MN cell
MN infiltrate

MNB
monomicrobial nonneutrocytic
bacterascites

MNE
monosymptomatic nocturnal enuresis

MNGIE
mitochondrial neurogastrointestinal
encephalomyopathy

MNTI
melanotic neuroectodermal tumor of
infancy

M-O
Haley's M-O

MoAb
monoclonal antibody

Moban

Mobigesic

mobile gallbladder

mobilis
lien m.
ren m.

mobility
electrophoretic m.

mobilization
anorectal m.

Mobin-Uddin umbrella

Moctanin

modality
dialysis m.
therapeutic m.

Modane
M. Soft
M. Versabran

mode
autosomal recessive m.
linear m.
radial m.

model
Cox regression m.
M. 500F electromagnetic flowmeter
M. IL 750, AA spectrophotometer
Markov m.
M. 3-60 mass spectroscopy
m. 440 M1.5, M4 electrode
M. 5500 vapor pressure osmometer

modeling
penile m.
urea kinetic m. (UKM)

moderate distress

moderately differentiated adenoma

modification
Al-Ghorab m.
M. of Diet in Renal Disease
(MDRD)
M. of Diet in Renal Disease trial
Goligher m.
high-energy m.
Kelly-Kennedy m.
lifestyle m. (LSM)
Muzsnai m.
posttranslational m.
pylorus-preserving Whipple m.
(PPW)
Raz m.
Walsh surgical m.

modified
m. barium swallow (MBS)
m. Barthel degree of disability
index
m. Cantwell technique
m. caulking gun
m. Essed-Schroeder corporoplasty
m. Gibson incision
m. Hassan open technique
m. ileocecal valve
m. Ingelman-Sundberg procedure
m. Lich-Gregoir
ureteroneocystostomy
m. liver diet
m. Lloyd Davies position
m. method of Pugh
m. Minnesota tube
m. Nesbit procedure
m. Norfolk procedure
m. penectomy
m. Pereyra bladder neck suspension
m. polyethylene dilator
m. Sacks-Vine push-pull technique
m. sham feeding
m. Thiersch-Duplay technique
m. transduodenal rendezvous
procedure
m. Vest technique
m. Whitehead hemorrhoidectomy
m. Young-Dees-Ledbetter technique
m. Young urethroplasty
m. Z-stent

modifier
biologic response m. (BMR)

modulation
antigenic m.

M

NOTES

modulation *(continued)*
    obstruction-induced m.
    pressure amplitude m.
Modulith
    M. SL 20 device for ESWL
    M. SL 20 lithotriptor
Moduretic
MODY
    maturity-onset diabetes of the young
Moersch esophagoscope
MOF
    MeCCNU, Oncovin, fluorouracil
    multiple organ failure
mofetil
    mycophenolate m. (MMF)
Mogen clamp
Mohr test
Mohs microsurgery technique
moiety
    steroid m.
moist
    m. laparotomy pack
    m. mucous membrane
    m. necrosis
    m. papule
Moi-Stir
molar pregnancy
mole
    hydatidiform m.
    repeated complete m.
Molectron Nd:YAG laser
molecular
    m. adsorbents recirculating system
      (MARS)
    m. cloning
    m. cloning and sequencing
    m. genetic alteration
    m. marker
    m. study
    m. typing
    m. weight (mol wt)
molecule
    adhesion m.
    CD4 m.
    CD8 m.
    cell-adhesion m.
    class I, II MHC m.
    HLA-DQ2 m.
    immunoglobulin superfamily
      adhesion m.
    lithostathine m.
    lymphocyte costimulatory m.
    messenger RNA m.
    monocyte adhesion m.
    neural cell-adhesive m. (NCAM,
      N-CAM)

molecule-1
    endothelial leukocyte adhesion m.-1
      (ELAM-1)
    intercellular adhesion m.-1 (ICAM-
      1)
    vascular cell adhesion m.-1
      (VCAM-1)
molgramostim
molimen, pl. **molimina**
molindone
molluscum
    m. contagiosum
    m. contagiosum virus (MCV)
molluscum contagiosum virus (MCV)
Molnar disk
mol wt
MOM
    milk of magnesia
Mondor phlebitis
Monfort
    M. abdominoplasty
    M. operation
mongolian spot
Monilia **esophagitis**
monilial
    m. esophagitis
    m. infection
moniliasis
Monistat
monitor
    Contimed II pelvic floor
      muscle m.
    Dinamap Plus m.
    Dobbhoff biofeedback m.
    gastric pH m.
    Gould pressure m.
    24-hour ambulatory gastric pH m.
    Ingold M3, M4 glass electrode
      pH m.
    in-line blood gas m.
    Interceptor M3 triple-channel, solid
      state m.
    m. peptide
    return electrode m. (REM)
    RigiScan penile tumescence and
      rigidity m.
    television m.
    video m.
monitoring
    ambulatory intraesophageal
      bilirubin m.
    ambulatory intraesophageal pH m.
    ambulatory urodynamic m.
    clinical m.
    cystometrographic m.
    endoscopic m.
    esophageal pH m.
    fluoroscopic m.

heart rate m.
24-hour ambulatory esophageal
  pH m.
intracranial pressure m.
intraesophageal pH m. (EpHM)
nocturnal penile tumescence m.
NPT m.
pH m.
self blood glucose m. (SBGM)
tumescence m.
monitor/recorder
Gastroreflex ambulatory pH m./r.
monoamine oxidase inhibitor
monocapsule
bismuth triple m.
monoclonal
m. antibody (MAb, mAb, MoAb)
m. antibody BR96
m. antibody ED1
m. antibody MIB-1
m. antibody scintigraphic scan
m. antibody therapy
m. antigen
m. anti-HBc
4B4 m. antibody
19B7 m. antibody
m. gammopathy
m. IgM
4KB5 m. antibody
m. light chain
m. proliferation
monoclonality by genetic analysis
Monocryl suture
monocyte
m. adhesion molecule
m. chemoattractant protein
m. chemoattractant protein-1 (MCP-
  1)
m. chemotactic protein (MCP)
WBC m.
monocytes/macrophages
monocytogenes
Listeria m.
Monodox
Monodral
monoethanolamine oleate
monoethylglycinexylidide (MEGX)
m. liver function tests
monofilament
m. absorbable suture
m. nylon suture
m. snare wire

monofocal papillary carcinoma
Mono-Gesic
monohydrate
cefadroxil m.
doxycycline m.
sodium phosphate monobasic m.
monohydroxy bile salt
monokine
monolayer
cobblestone-like m.
**MonoLith single-piece mechanical
  lithotriptor**
**monomicrobial nonneutrocytic
  bacterascites (MNB)**
mononephrous
mononuclear (MN)
m. cell recruitment
m. dyspepsia
m. histiocytic portal infiltrate
mononucleotide
flavin m.
monooctanoin infusion
monooxygenase pathway
monophosphate
5′-m.
adenosine m. (AMP)
cyclic adenosine m. (cAMP)
5′-cyclic adenosine m. (cAMP)
cyclic guanosine m. (cGMP)
5′-cyclic guanosine m. (cGMP)
guanosine m.
guanosine 5′-m. (GMP)
monopodial
monopolar
BICAP m.
m. coagulation
m. electrocautery
m. electrocoagulation
m. probe
m. triple-hook active needle
monopole
monosaccharide
monosialoganglioside
monosialosyl Lea
monosodium urate
Monospot
**monosymptomatic nocturnal enuresis
  (MNE)**
monoterpene
monotherapy
androgen ablative m.

M

NOTES

monotherapy *(continued)*
    bicalutamide m.
    nonsteroidal antiandrogen m.
mons
    m. plasty
    m. veneris
Montague
    M. proctoscope
    M. sigmoidoscope
Montezuma revenge
Montgomery
    M. abdominal strap
    M. salivary bypass tube
    M. strap dressing
    M. tape
Monurol
Mood Adjective Check List
moon
    m. facies
    M. rectal retractor
Moore
    M. classification for vascular
      anomalies of the gastrointestinal
      tract
    M. gallstone scoop
MOP-Videoplan morphometric system
Moraxella
    M. bovis
    M. nonliquefaciens
morbidity
    febrile m.
    maternal m.
    operative m.
    postoperative m.
    reflux m.
    m. risk
    treatment m.
    uncorrected maternal m.
    uncorrected reflux m.
morbid obesity
morbus
    cholera m.
morcellated nephrectomy
morcellation
    m. technique
    vaginal m.
morcellator
    Cook tissue m.
    electric tissue m.
    high-speed electrical tissue m.
    tissue m.
morcellement operation
Moreno gastroenterostomy clamp
Morgagni
    M. appendix
    M. caruncle
    column of M.
    M. crypt

    foramen of M.
    M. fovea
    frenulum of M.
    M. hernia
    M. hydatid
    M. lacunae
    M. retinaculum
    M. valve
Morganella morganii
morganii
    Morganella m.
    Proteus m.
Morganstern
    M. aspiration/injection system
    M. continuous-flow operating
      cystoscope
moribund
moricizine
Mori knife
Morison
    hepatorenal space of M.
    M. method
    M. pouch
morning diarrhea
Moro-Heisler diet
Moro reflex
morphea
morphine
    m. cholescintigraphy
    m. narcotic analgesic therapy
morphine-neostigmine test
morphogenesis
morphogenetic process
morphologic stage
morphology
    chromosome m.
    closed m.
    Dogiel type I, II m.
    filamentous m.
    glomerular m.
    Gram-stain m.
    open m.
morphometric criteria
morphometry
    nuclear m.
morrhuate
    m. sclerosant
    sodium m.
mortality
    cardiovascular m.
    intraoperative m.
    overall m.
    risk-adjusted m.
mortar kidney
mortis
    livor m.
    rigor m.
mosaic duodenal mucosal pattern

mosaicism
    XX male m.
Moschcowitz
    M. operation
    M. procedure
    M. vaginal prolapse repair
Moscontin
MOSD
    multiple organ system dysfunction
MOSF
    multiple organ system failure
Mosher
    M. bag
    M. dilator
    M. esophagoscope
mosm/kg
    milliosmole/kilogram
900 mOsmolar amino acid-glucose solution (P-900)
mosquito
    m. forceps
    m. hemostat
    m. hemostatic clamp
Moss
    M. gastrostomy tube
    M. G-tube
    M. G-tube PEG kit
    M. Mark IV tube
    M. T-anchor introducer gun
Mosse syndrome
Mostofi grade prostate cancer
mother
    m. cyst
    m. endoscopic retrograde cholangiopancreatoscopy system
mother-baby endoscope system
mother-baby-scope system
mother-daughter endoscope
mother-infant dyad
mother-to-infant transmission of hepatitis C virus
motif
    coiled coil m.
    Patterson-Parker m.
motilide
motilin
    basal release of m.
    m. plasma level
motility
    m. agent
    altered sperm m.
    colonic m.

    colorectal m.
    m. disorder
    disordered m.
    esophageal m.
    gastrointestinal m.
    ineffective esophageal m. (IEM)
    interdigestive antroduodenal m.
    neurohumoral control of m.
    prefreeze m.
    reduced m.
    sequential m.
    spermatozoon m.
    m. test
Motilium
motion
    brownian m.
    full range of m.
    limited range of m.
    paradoxic m.
    passive range of m.
    m. picture camera
    range of m.
    m. sickness
motogenesis
motogenic
motoneuron
    enteric excitatory m.
    enteric inhibitory m.
motor
    m. activity
    m. endplate
    m. examination
    m. meal barium GI series
    m. neuron
    m. oil peritoneal fluid
    m. quiescence
    m. syringe
    m. test meal
    m. unit action potential
    m. urgency
Moto-Tool
    Dremel M.-T.
Motrin
mottled testis
moulage sign
mound
    infraumbilical m.
Moure esophagoscope
mouse
    peritoneal m.
Mousseau-Barbin prosthetic tube

M

NOTES

mouth
> m. breathing
> Ceylon sore m.
> m. gag
> m. guard

mouthguard
> oxygenating m.
> Oxyguard oxygenating m.

movable testis

movement
> bowel m. (BM)
> dyscoordinate hyoid m.
> pelvic floor m.
> periodic leg m. (PLM)
> segmentation m.
> symmetric face m.
> tongue m.
> vermicular m.

moxalactam

moxisylyte injection

MOX TM-100 portable renal preservation machine

Moynihan
> M. artery forceps
> M. bile duct probe
> M. clamp
> M. gall duct forceps
> M. gallstone probe
> M. gallstone scoop
> M. technique
> M. test

MP
> mesenteric panniculitis
> microfibrillar protein

6-MP
> 6-mercaptopurine

MPA
> microscopic polyangiitis

MPD
> main pancreatic duct
> MPD stent

MPEC
> multipolar electrocoagulation

MPFF
> micronized purified flavonoid fracture

MPGN
> membranoproliferative glomerulonephritis (type I, II)

M-phase

MP-RAGE
> magnetization prepared-rapid gradient echo

MRA
> magnetic resonance angiography

MRC
> magnetic resonance cholangiography
> magnetic resonance colonography

MRCC
> metastatic renal cell carcinoma

MRCP
> magnetic resonance cholangiopancreatography
>   MRCP using HASTE with a phased array coil

MRDM
> malnutrition-related diabetes mellitus

MR hydrography

MRI
> magnetic resonance imaging
>   endorectal surface coil MRI
>   fast spin-echo acquisition MRI
>   rectal coil MRI
>   MRI scan
>   ultrafast MRI

mRNA
> messenger ribonucleic acid
> messenger RNA
>   AR mRNA
>   beta-actin mRNA
>   clusterin mRNA
>   cotransporter mRNA
>   COX mRNA
>   cyclooxygenase messenger ribonucleoprotein acid
>   gastrin mRNA
>   glomerular fibronectin mRNA
>   HSP-70 mRNA
>   IGF-binding protein-1 mRNA
>   IGF-1R mRNA
>   preproEt-1 mRNA
>   taurine cotransporter mRNA
>   TCT mRNA

MRP
> magnetic resonance pancreatography
> maximum (anal) resting pressure

MRS
> magnetic resonance spectroscopy

MRSA
> methicillin-resistant *Staphylococcus aureus*

MRT
> mean resistance time

MRU
> magnetic resonance urography

MS-8
> Pancrecarb M.

MSAO
> meal-stimulated acid output

MS Classique balloon dilatation catheter

MSEV
> microsurgical epididymovasostomy

MSH2 **gene**

MS-1, -2 hepatitis

MSI
> microsatellite instability
>> MSI nylon membrane

MSOF
> multiple system organ failure
> multisystem organ failure

MSP
> maximum squeeze pressure

MSU
> midstream specimen of urine

MSUD
> maple-syrup urine disease

MT
> malignant teratoma
> maximal toleration
> microtubule

MT12
>> Ultrase M.

MT20

MT24

MTAC
> mass transfer area coefficient

MTBE
> methyl tert-butyl ether
> methyl tertiary butyl ether
>> MTBE gallstone dissolution
>> MTBE therapy

MTHFR
> 5,10-methylene-tetrahydrofolate reductase

m-THP-Chlorin

MTI
> malignant teratoma, intermediate

MTPT
> 1-methyl-4-phenyl-1,2,3,6-
> tetrahydropyridine

MTS1 **gene**

MTS2 **gene**

Mt. Sinai classification

MTT
> malignant teratoma, trophoblastic
> mean transit time

M-TURP
> minimal transurethral resection of
> prostate

MTV
> maximal toleration volume
> maximum tolerable volume

MTX
> methotrexate

MU-3 monoclonal antibody

MUC
> mucosal ulcerative colitis

MUC-1 **gene**

mucilaginous

mucin
> intracytoplasmic m.

mucin-hypersecreting
> m.-h. carcinoma
> m.-h. tumor

mucinous
> m. adenocarcinoma
> m. adenoma
> m. carcinoma
> m. cystadenoma
> m. cystic neoplasm
> m. cystic tumor
> m. ductal ectasia (MDE)
> m. pancreatic tumor
> m. tumor nodule

mucin-producing
> m.-p. adenocarcinoma
> m.-p. cancer
> m.-p. tumor

mucin-type glycolipid

Muckle-Wells syndrome

mucocele
> appendiceal m.
> m. of gallbladder

mucociliary clearance

mucocolitis

mucocutaneous
> m. hemorrhoid
> m. pigmentation of Peutz-Jeghers
> syndrome

mucoenteritis

mucoepidermoid carcinoma

mucoid
> m. secretion
> m. stool

mucolipidosis, pl. **mucolipidoses**

mucolytic agent

mucolytic-antifoam solution

mucomembranous enteritis

Mucomyst

mucopolysaccharide

mucoprotein
> Tamm-Horsfall m. (THM)

mucopurulent
> m. cervicitis
> m. exudate

Mucorales

Mucor corymbifera

Mucoreae

M

NOTES

mucormycosis
   m. esophagitis
   gastric m.
   isolated renal m.
   pulmonary m.
mucorrhea
mucosa, pl. mucosae
   antral m.
   antral-type m.
   antrofundal m.
   biopsy of gastric m.
   blanching of m.
   buccal m.
   burned-out m.
   cardiac stomach m.
   cardiac-type m.
   cobblestone m.
   cobblestoning of m.
   colitic m.
   colorectal m.
   columnar m.
   congested m.
   corpus gastric m.
   denuded m.
   duodenal m. (DM)
   dysplastic m.
   ectopic gastric m.
   edematous hyperemic m.
   esophageal m.
   foveolar gastric m.
   friable m.
   frog-spawn-like m.
   fundic m.
   gastric muscularis m.
   gastroduodenal m.
   gastrosuccorrhea m.
   heterotopic gastric m.
   hyperemic m.
   inflamed m.
   inlet patch m.
   intestinal m.
   lamina muscularis mucosae
   multifocal ectopic gastric m.
   muscularis m.
   neoanal m.
   normal-appearing m.
   oxyntic m.
   pyloric m.
   rectal m.
   rose thorn ulcer of m.
   sloughing of m.
   tethering of m.
   thumbprinting of m.
   tunica m.
   urothelial m.
   vaginal m.

mucosa-associated
   m.-a. lymphoid tissue (MALT, MALToma)
   m.-a. lymphoid tissue lymphoma
mucosal
   m. abnormality
   m. abrasion
   m. adenocarcinoma
   m. aneuploidy
   m. angiography
   m. atrophy
   m. background
   m. barrier maturation
   m. biopsy
   m. bleeding
   m. blood flow
   m. blood hemoglobin
   m. border
   m. break
   m. bridge
   m. bridging
   m. cell proliferation
   m. cobblestoning
   m. detachment
   m. disease
   m. diverticulum
   m. dysplasia
   m. electrosensitivity (MES)
   m. elevation
   m. erosion
   m. esophageal ring
   m. fatty acid
   m. fold
   m. gastric ulcer
   m. graft
   m. guideline pattern
   m. hexosamine content
   m. homogenate
   m. ileal diaphragm
   m. ileostomy
   m. injury
   m. integrity
   m. ischemia
   m. island
   m. junction
   m. lesion
   m. line
   m. lymphoid follicle
   m. nodularity
   m. pallor
   m. pit
   m. plexus
   m. PMN grade
   m. polyp
   m. proctectomy
   m. prolapse
   m. prolapse syndrome
   m. prostaglandin synthesis

m. sleeve resection
m. stripping
m. suspensory ligament
m. tear
m. tongue
m. ulcerative colitis (MUC)
m. urease
m. vaccine
m. vascular dilation
m. vascular permeability
m. washout
m. web

mucosanguineous
mucosa-to-mucosa anastomosis
mucosectomy
aspiration m.
endoanal m.
endoscopic m.
endoscopic aspiration m. (EAM)
negative pressure method
ambulatory endoscopic
esophageal m.
rectal m.
suck and cut m.

mucoserous
mucositis
mucous
m. colic
m. colitis
m. crypt
m. crypt of duodenum
m. depletion
m. diarrhea
m. enteritis
m. fistula
m. gel thickness
m. gland
m. lake of the stomach
m. membrane
m. membrane pemphigoid
m. neck cell
m. papule
m. patch
m. stool
m. tunic

mucoviscidosis
MUCP
maximum urethral closure pressure
mucus
excess m.
extruding m.
gastric m.

mucus-secreting
m.-s. cell
m.-s. gland
mud
biliary m.
Mueller-Hinton-supplemented agar plate
muelleri
ductus m.
Muir hemorrhoid forceps
Muir-Torre syndrome
Mui Scientific pressurized capillary infusion system
mulberry
m. calculus
m. gallstone
m. lesion
m. stone
Mulholland sphincterotomy
muliebris
hydrocele m.
orificium urethrae externum m.
testis m.
urethra m.
mulleri
Streptococcus m.
müllerian
m. capsule
m. duct
m. duct cyst
m. duct derivation syndrome
m. duct, unilateral renal agenesis, and anomalies of the cervicothoracic somites (MURCS)
m. inhibiting factor
m. remnant
Müller maneuver
Multi-12
multiacinar regenerative nodule
multiband ligating device
multicenter study
Multicentre International Liver Tumor Study (MILTS)
multicentricity
multicentric lesion
multichannel cystometry
multicystic
m. dysplastic kidney (MCDK)
m. kidney (MCK)
m. kidney disease
m. renal dysplasia
multidrug regimen
multidrug-resistance gene

M

NOTES

multifiber catheter
Multifire
    M. clip applicator
    M. Endo GIA stapling device
Multi-Flex stent
multifocal
    m. atrophic gastritis (MAG)
    m. bladder tumor
    m. ectopic gastric mucosa
    m. involvement
multiforme
    erythema m. (EM)
    glioblastoma m.
Multifunctional Opus surgical table
Multikine
multiligand receptor
multiloaded clip applier
multiload occlusive clip applicator
multilobar kidney
multilobular
    m. cirrhosis
    m. kidney
multilocular
    m. crypt
    m. cyst
    m. cystic nephroma
multilocularis
    Echinococcus m.
multiloculated cyst
multilumen
    m. manometric catheter
    m. probe
multimodal protocol
multinucleated giant cell
multiorgan
    m. hernia
    m. system failure
multiple
    m. acute rejection episode
    m. anal sphincterotomies (MAS)
    m. band ligator
    m. biopsy
    m. calices
    m. concentric ring sign
    m. endocrine adenomatosis type I
      (MEA-I)
    m. endocrine adenomatosis type II
      (MEA-II)
    m. endocrine neoplasia (MEN)
    m. endocrine neoplasia 1
    m. endocrine neoplasia 2A (MEN
      2A)
    m. endocrine neoplasia 2B (MEN
      2B)
    m. endocrine neoplasia syndrome
      (MENS)
    m. familial polyposis
    m. hamartoma syndrome

    m. hepatitis virus infection
    m. intraluminal impedancometry
    m. lymphomatous polyposis (MLP)
    m. myeloma
    m. nodule
    m. organ failure (MOF)
    m. organ failure syndrome
    m. organ system dysfunction
      (MOSD)
    m. organ system failure (MOSF)
    m. polyp
    m. recurrent renal colic
    m. sclerosis
    m. stone
    m. surgical procedure
    m. system atrophy
    m. system organ failure (MSOF)
    m. vasovasotomy
    m. vitamin for infusion
multiplication
    countercurrent m.
multiplier
    countercurrent m.
multipolar
    m. coagulation
    m. electrocautery
    m. electrocoagulation (MPEC)
    m. neuron
Multipulse laser system
multiseptate gallbladder
multishot speedbander
multisynaptic pathway
multisystem organ failure (MSOF)
multitargeted antifolate
multocida
    Pasteurella m.
mumps
    m. epididymitis
    m. pancreatitis
Munchausen syndrome
Munich inclusion criteria
Munk disease
Munro point
mural
    m. kidney
    m. thrombus
MURCS
    müllerian duct, unilateral renal agenesis,
    and anomalies of the cervicothoracic
    somites
      MURCS association
murine
    m. B16 cell
    m. hepatitis
    m. kidney
    m. lymphoid cell
    m. mesangial cell (MMC)
    m. mesangial cell line

m. proximal tubule cell
3T3 m. fibroblast

muris

Cryptosporidium m.
Trichuris m.

murmur

continuous m.
diastolic m.
systolic m.

muromonab-CD3

Murphy

M. button
M. common duct dilator
M. drip
M. gallbladder retractor
M. kidney punch
M. sign
M. treatment

muscarinic

m. activity
m. blockade
m. cholinergic agonist
m. receptor

muscle

adductor brevis m.
adductor longus m.
aryepiglottic m.
m. atrophy
Bell m.
bladder neck detrusor m.
bladder smooth m.
Braune m.
bulbospongiosus m.
circular m.
coccygeus m.
colonic circular m.
cremaster m.
cremasteric m.
cricopharyngeus m.
dartos m.
diaphragmatic m.
digastric anterior m.
digastric posterior m.
electromyography of penile corpus
  cavernosum m.
external anal sphincter m.
external oblique m.
external sphincter ani profundus m.
m. filling
gastrointestinal smooth m.
Gavard m.
geniohyoid m.

gracilis m.
m. guarding
Houston m.
m. hypertrophy
ileococcygeus m.
iliacus m.
iliococcygeus m.
interfoveolar m.
internal oblique m.
ischiocavernosus m.
labium majus m.
labium minus m.
lacuna of m.
latissimus dorsi m.
m. layer disease
levator ani m.
levator veli palatini m.
lower esophageal sphincter
  circular m.
mylohyoid m.
oblique arytenoid m.
obturator internus m.
Ochsner m.
organic m.
palatoglossus m.
palatopharyngeus m.
paraspinous m.
pectoralis m.
pelvis m.
perineal m.
periurethral striated m.
piriformis m.
pleuroesophageal m.
psoas m.
puboanalis m.
pubococcygeus m.
puborectal m.
puborectalis m.
pubovisceral m.
pyramidal m.
rectococcygeus m.
rectourethral m.
rectourethralis m.
rectus abdominis m.
rhabdosphincter m.
sacrospinalis m.
m. sensory receptor
serratus posterior m.
smooth m.
m. spasm
styloglossus m.
stylohyoid m.

M

NOTES

muscle *(continued)*
    stylopharyngeus m.
    submucosal vaginal m.
    superficial trigonal m.
    suspensory m.
    tendinous arch of levator ani m.
    tensor veli palatini m.
    thyroarytenoid m.
    thyrohyoid m.
    transverse abdominis m.
    transversus abdominis m.
    transversus perinei m.
    urogenital sphincter m.
    vascular smooth m.
    visceral m.
    m. wasting
    Wilson m.
muscle-alginate complex
muscle-brain isoenzyme of creative kinase (CK-MB)
muscle-cutting incision
muscle-filling procedure
muscle-splitting
    m.-s. incision
    m.-s. technique
muscular
    m. coat
    m. dystrophy
    m. esophageal ring
    m. tunic
muscularis
    m. externa
    m. mucosa
    m. propria
    tunica m.
    m. tunnel closure
muscularization of vein
musculature
    electrophysiology of the gastric m.
    paraspinal m.
musculocutaneous flap
musculotropic relaxant
MUSE
    Medicated Urethral System for Erection
    MUSE urethral suppository
mushroom
    Amanita m.
    m. catheter
    m. poisoning
mushroom-and-stem appearance
mushroom-shaped mass
mushy stool
musical bowel sounds
Musshoff modification of the Ann Arbor classification
mustard
    m. seed

Mustarde
    M. hypospadias repair
    M. procedure
mutagenic effect
Mutamycin
mutated colorectal carcinoma (MCC)
mutation
    C282Y m.
    deletion m.
    endogenous m.
    germline m.
    H63D m.
    insertion m.
    Ki-*ras* gene m.
    Kirsten-*ras* oncogen m.
    Liddle m.
    m. mismatch repair (MMR)
    missense m.
    nontruncating m.
    p53 m.
    splice-cite m.
    transition m.
    transversion m.
MutL **gene**
MutS **gene**
Muzsnai modification
muzzled sperm
MVAC, M-VAC
    methotrexate, vinblastine, Adriamycin, cisplatin
M-VEC
    methotrexate, vinblastine, epirubicin, cisplatin
MVO
    mean venous outflow
MVP
    maximum vasal pressure
MVT
    mesenteric vein thrombosis
    acute MVT
mW
    milliwatt
Mya disease
myalgia
    tension m.
myasthenia
    m. gastrica
    m. gravis
mycelial
    m. antibody
    m. phase
mycetism, mycetismus
    m. gastrointestinalis
Mycin
    E.P. M.
mycobacteria
    Runyon group III m.

mycobacterial
    m. antibody
    m. disease
    m. spheroplast
mycobacteriology
Mycobacterium
    M. avium
    M. avium complex
    M. avium-intracellulare (MAI)
    M. bovis
    M. bovis BCG
    M. fortuitum
    M. gordonae
    M. infection
    M. intracellulare
    M. kansasii
    M. leprae
    M. paratuberculosis
    M. smegmatis
    M. tuberculosis
    M. xenopi
mycogastritis
Mycolog-II
mycology
mycophenolate (MMF)
    m. mofetil (MMF)
    m. mofetil capsule
    m. mofetil intravenous for injection
    m. mofetil oral suspension
    m. mofetil tablet
Mycoplasma
    M. hominis
mycoplasma
    m. urethritis
mycoplasmal
mycosis, pl. **mycoses**
    endemic deep m.
    m. fungoides
    gastric m.
    m. intestinalis
Mycostatin
mycotic
    m. aneurysm
    m. gastritis
    m. prostatitis
Mycotrim triphasic culture system
MycroMesh
myectomy
    anorectal m.
    detrusor m.
myelin kidney
myelocele

myelocystocele
myelodysplasia
myelography
myeloid
    m. dentritic cell
    m. metaplasia
myelolipoma
    adrenal gland m.
myeloma
    IgA kappa chain m.
    m. kidney
    multiple m.
    plasmablastic m.
    m. protein
myelomeningocele
myelomonocytic cell line
myelopathy
    HTLV-I-associated m.
myeloperoxidase
myeloperoxidase-H2O2-halide system
myelophthisic splenomegaly
myeloproliferative
    m. disease
    m. disorder
myelosuppression
myenteric
    m. ganglion cell
    m. plexus
    m. potential oscillation
    m. reflex
myentericus
    plexus m.
Myers
    M. bunching technique
Myers-Fine test
Mygel
    M. II
myiasis
    intestinal m.
Mylanta
    M.-II
Myles hemorrhoidal clamp
Mylicon
Mylius test
mylohyoid muscle
myoblastic myoma
myoblastoma
    bladder granular cell m.
    granular cell m.
myocardial
    m. infarction

M

NOTES

myocardial *(continued)*
    m. ischemia
    m. revascularization
myocelialgia
myoclonic encephalopathy
myoclonus
myoclonus-opsoclonus syndrome
myocutaneous flap
myoelectric activity
myoelectrical
myofibroblast
myofibroma
myogenic tumor
myoglobinuria
myointimal hyperplasia
Myojector
myolysis
myoma
    ball m.
    myoblastic m.
    red degeneration of uterine m.
myoneurosis
    colic m.
    intestinal m.
myopathy
    childhood visceral m. (CVM)
    familial visceral m. (FVM)
    hereditary internal anal
      sphincter m.
    ipecac-induced m.
    nemaline m.
    nonfamilial visceral m.
    schistosomal pelvic floor m.
    sporadic hollow visceral m.
myoplasty
    latissimus dorsi detrusor m.

myorrhaphy
myosin
    m. crossbridge
    detrusor muscle m.
    m. light-chain kinase
myotomy
    circular m.
    cricoid m.
    cricopharyngeal m.
    esophageal m.
    Heller m.
    laparoscopic Heller m.
    laser-assisted endoscopic m.
    Livaditis circular m.
    longitudinal m.
Myotonachol
myotonic muscular dystrophy
MyoTrac EMG
Myotrophin
Myphentol
Myriadlase Side-Fire laser
myringotomy tube
Mytelase
myxedema ascites
myxocystitis
myxofibroma
myxoglobulosis appendicitis
myxomembranous
    m. colitis
    m. enteritis
myxoneurosis
    intestinal m.
myxorrhea
    m. gastrica
    m. intestinalis

N
  ammonia
    N loop
¹³N
  ammonia-13
NA
  nalidixic acid
Nabi-HB
NABS
  normoactive bowel sounds
nabumetone
NABX
  needle aspiration biopsy
N-acetyl-5-ASA (Ac-5-ASA)
N-acetylated alpha-linked dipeptidase
N-acetyl-beta-D-glucosaminidase
N-acetyl-beta-glucosaminidase (NAG)
N-acetylcysteine
N-acetyl-p-benzoquinoneimine (NAPQI)
Nachlas gastrointestinal tube
Nachlas-Linton esophagogastric balloon
  tamponade device
Naclerio
    N. sign
    V sign of N.
NADH
  nicotinamide adenine dinucleotide
nadolol
NADPH
  nicotinamide adenine dinucleotide
    phosphate
    NADPH diaphorase stain
    NADPH oxidase
NAE
  net acid excretion
naeslundii
    Actinomyces n.
NaF
  sodium fluorescein
nafamostat mesylate
nafcillin
NAFLD
  nonalcoholic fatty liver disease
nafoxidine
NAG
  N-acetyl-beta-glucosaminidase
  nonagglutinable
    NAG lysosomal marker enzyme
nagging pain
NA+-glucose cotransporter
Na+/H+
    amiloride-sensitive, electroneutral N.
      antiporter
    N. antiporter
    NA+/H+ antiporter activity

nail
    n. bed
    thickened n.
nail-patella syndrome
naive B and T lymphocyte
Nakao snare (I, II)
Na/K-ATPase
    N.-A. activity
NaK-ATPase membrane
Nakayama test
naked fat sign
nalbuphine
Naldecon
nalidixic acid (NA)
NA+-linked cotransport system
Nallpen
nalmefene
naloxone hydrochloride
NAMI DDV ligator
nana
    Hymenolepis n.
NANB
    non-A, non-B
    NANB hepatitis
NANC
    nonadrenergic noncholinergic
    NANC inhibitory transmitter
nandrolone decanoate
NaP
    sodium phosphate
naphazoline
naphthylamine
naphthylurea
    polysulfonated n.
napkin-ring annular lesion
nappe
    polyadenomes en n.
nappy
    electronic recording n.
NAPQI
    N-acetyl-p-benzoquinoneimine
Naprosyn
naproxen sodium
Naqua
Narath operation
Narcan
Narco
    N. Bio-Systems MMS 200
      physiograph tracing
    N. Bio-Systems rectilinear recorder
    N. esophageal motility machine
narcotic
    n. analgesic
    n. bowel syndrome
Nardil

Nardi test
naris, pl. **nares**
narrow
    n. albumin gradient ascites
    n. lens
narrow-caliber duct
narrowing
    bird-beak n.
    discrete n.
    hourglass n.
    luminal n.
nasal
    Concentraid N.
    n. deformity
    n. discharge
    n. feeding
    n. intubation
    n. polyp
    n. trumpet
Nasalcrom
Nasalide
nascent macula densa
NASH
    nonalcoholic steatohepatitis
nasobiliary
    n. catheter (NBC)
    n. drain (NBD)
    n. drainage
    n. drainage catheter
    n. drain cholangiography
    n. tube
nasocystic
    n. catheter
    n. catheter lavage
    n. drain
    n. drainage tube
nasoduodenal feeding tube
nasoenteric
    n. feeding
    n. feeding tube
nasogastric (NG)
    n. aspirate
    n. decompression
    n. drainage
    n. feeding tube
    n. intubation
    n. lavage
    n. suction
    n. tube (NGT)
nasoileal tube
nasojejunal (NJ)
    n. feeding
    n. feeding tube
nasopancreatic
    n. catheter
    n. drainage

nasopharyngeal
    n. angiofibroma
    n. reflux
nasotracheal intubation
nasovesicular
    n. catheter
    n. catheter technique
NAT
    nucleic acid testing
nateglinide
national
    N. Association of Anorexia
      Nervosa and Associated Disorders
    N. Cooperative Dialysis Study
    N. general purpose cystoscope
    N. Health and Nutrition
      Examination Survey (NHANES)
    N. Institute of Diabetes, Digestive
      and Kidney Disease (NIDDK)
    N. Institutes of Health (NIH)
    N. Institutes of Health Chronic
      Prostatitis Symptom Index (NIH-
      CPSI)
    N. Kidney Foundation-Data
      Outcomes Quality Initiative (NKF-
      DOQI)
    N. Prostatic Cancer Project
    N. Prostatic Cancer Treatment
      Group (NPCTG)
    N. Wilms Tumor Study Group
      (NWTSG)
native
    n. kidney function
    n. pancreatic secretin receptor
    n. renal biopsy
    n. urethra
    n. valve bacterial endocarditis
NA+ transport system
natriuresis
    pressure n.
natriuretic peptide receptor (NPR)
natural
    n. immunity
    n. killer (NK)
    n. killer cell
    N. stool formula
nature
    Gentle N.
Naturetin
nausea
    chemotherapy-induced n.
    epidemic n.
    postprandial n.
    n. and vomiting (N&V)
    n., vomiting, diarrhea (NVD)
nauseant
nauseate
nauseous

Navane
navel
> blue n.

navicular
> n. abdomen
> fossa of Morgagni n.

navicularis
> fossa n.
> valvula fossae n.

Navigator flexible endoscope
Navy single-layer everting anastomosis
NBC
> nasobiliary catheter
> nephroblastomatosis complex
> nonbacterial cystitis

NBD
> nasobiliary drain
> nucleotide-binding domain

N-benzoyl-L-tyrosyl-P-aminobenzoic
> N-b.-L-t.-P-a. acid
> N-b.-L-t.-P-a. acid excretion test

NBNC CLD
> HBsAg-negative, anti-HCV-negative
> chronic liver disease

NBP
> nonbacterial prostatitis

NBT
> nitroblue tetrazolium

NBT-PABA
> nitroblue tetrazolium-paraaminobenzoic
> acid
> NBT-PABA test

N-butyl cyanoacrylate
NBVV
> nonbleeding visible vessel

NC
> nephrocalcin

N-cadherin
NCAM, N-CAM
> neural cell-adhesive molecule

NCB
> needle core biopsy

NCCT
> noncontrast helical computed tomography

NCGN
> necrotizing crescentic glomerulonephritis

NCPF
> noncirrhotic portal fibrosis

NCT
> number connection test

N-deethylation

NDF
> new differentiation factor

NDI
> Nepean Dyspepsia Index
> nephrogenic diabetes insipidus
> X-linked recessive NDI

Nd:YAG
> neodymium:yttrium-aluminum-garnet
> Nd:YAG laser
> Nd:YAG laser irradiation
> Nd:YAG laser photoablation
> Nd:YAG laser therapy

near-infrared electronic endoscope
nebulizer
> jet n.

nebulous urine
NEC
> necrotizing enterocolitis

Necator americanus
necatoriasis
neck
> bladder n.
> humeral n.
> n. of pancreas
> tonic n.
> transurethral incision of the
> bladder n. (TUIBN)
> vesical n.

necroinflammation
> lobular n.

necroinflammatory activity
necrolysis
> toxic epidermal n. (TEN)

necrolytic
> n. migratory erythema
> n. migratory erythema syndrome

necropsy
necropurulent appendicitis
necrosectomy
necrosis, pl. **necroses**
> acute sclerosing hyaline n. (ASHN)
> acute tubular n. (ATN)
> avascular n.
> Balser fatty n.
> biliary piecemeal n.
> bowel n.
> bridging n.
> calpain in acute tubular n.
> caseating n.
> cecal n.
> cell n.
> central n.

N

NOTES

necrosis *(continued)*
    centrilobular acidophilic n.
    centrizonal n.
    cheesy n.
    coagulation n.
    coagulative n.
    colliquative n.
    colonic n.
    distal renal tubular n.
    drug-induced acute tubular n.
    electrocoagulation n.
    enzymatic fat n.
    ethanol-induced tumor n. (ETN)
    fatty n.
    fibrinoid n.
    fibrosing piecemeal n.
    gangrenous n.
    glomerular n.
    gummatous n.
    heme pigment-induced acute
      tubular n.
    hepatocellular n.
    hepatocyte n.
    icteric n.
    infected n.
    infected pancreatic n. (IPN)
    infectious pancreatic n.
    intestinal n.
    ischemia n.
    laminar cortical n.
    liquefactive n.
    massive hepatic n.
    maximum coagulative n.
    metastatic fat n.
    moist n.
    nephrotoxic tubule n.
    pancreatic glandular n.
    papillary n.
    patchy n.
    penile n.
    pericentral n.
    peripancreatic n.
    peripheral n.
    perivenular confluent n.
    piecemeal n.
    postischemic tubular n.
    pressure n.
    progressive emphysematous n.
    puromycin aminonucleoside n.
    renal coagulation n.
    renal cortical n.
    n. of renal papilla
    renal papillary n. (RPN)
    renal tubular n.
    scrotal fat n.
    septic n.
    spinal cord n.
    spontaneous penile ischemic n.

    sterile pancreatic n.
    strangulation n.
    subacute hepatic n.
    submassive hepatic n.
    tissue n.
    tubular n.
    tumor n.
necrospermia
necrotic
    n. cirrhosis
    n. hemorrhagic colitis
    n. hemorrhoid
    n. tissue
    n. ulceration
necroticans
    enteritis n.
necrotizing
    n. bowel vasculitis
    n. crescentic glomerulonephritis
      (NCGN)
    n. enterocolitis (NEC)
    n. fasciitis
    n. fasciitis of the scrotum
    n. infection
    n. pancreatitis
    n. vasculitis of bowel
necrozoospermia
needle
    Articulator injection n.
    ASAP channel cut automated
      biopsy n.
    ASAP prostate biopsy n.
    aspirating n.
    n. aspiration biopsy (NABX)
    n. aspiration cytology
    Bassini n.
    B-D Safety-Gard n.
    bi-curved n.
    n. biopsy diagnosis
    Biopty cut n.
    BIP high-speed multi biopsy n.
    n. bladder neck suspension
    blunt n.
    butterfly n.
    CE-24 n.
    Chiba n.
    Childs-Phillips intestinal plication n.
    circle n.
    10-cm n. GIP
    Colapinto n.
    concentric n.
    n. core biopsy (NCB)
    Corson n.
    n. count
    curved transjugular n.
    cutting LR n.
    diathermic precut n.
    n. driver

Durrani dorsal vein complex
  ligation n.
n. electrode
n. electrode electromyography
electrosurgical n.
Ferguson n.
fine n.
flexible aspiration n.
French eye n.
GAN-19 n.
gastrointestinal n.
GIP/Med-Globe n.
Gittes n.
Greenwald n.
Grice suture n.
Hemoject n.
n. holder
Howell n.
n. hydrophone
J n.
Jamshidi liver biopsy n.
Keith n.
KeyMed disposable variceal
  injection n.
Klatskin liver biopsy n.
n. knife
Lahey aneurysm n.
Madayag biopsy n.
Mayo trocar-point n.
Menghini liver biopsy n.
Microvasive sclerotherapy n.
monopolar triple-hook active n.
noncutting n.
Nottingham colposuspension n.
Olympus NM-K-series
  sclerotherapy n.
Olympus NM-L-series n.
Olympus reusable oval cup forceps
  with n.
optical n.
n. papillotome
Pentax prototype n.
Pereyra n.
pneumoperitoneum n.
Promex biopsy n.
PS-2 n.
reusable forceps with n.
Safety AV fistula n.
sclerotherapy n.
Seldinger gastrostomy n.
Silverman n.
Silverman-Boeker n.

single-use maximum capacity radial
  jaw with n.
skinny Chiba n.
smaller gauge n.
Spinelli biopsy n.
Stamey n.
Stifcore transbronchial aspiration n.
Sure-Cut biopsy n.
n. suspension procedure
suture-release n.
swaged n.
swaged-on n.
tapered n.
through-the-scope injection n.
n. tip catheter
n. tracheoesophageal puncture
n. tract
Tru-Cut biopsy n.
Tru Taper Ethalloy n.
TT-3 n.
Turner-Warwick n.
Variject n.
Veress n.
Vim-Silverman biopsy n.
Williams n.
winged steel n.
Yang n.

needle-catheter jejunostomy
needle-knife
  n.-k. electrocautery (NKE)
  n.-k. endoscopic pancreatic
    sphincterotomy
  n.-k. fistulotome
  n.-k. fistulotomy (NKF)
  n.-k. papillotome
  n.-k. papillotomy (NKP)
  n.-k. precut papillotomy (NKPP)
  n.-k. sphincterotome
  n.-k. technique
  n.-k. wire
needleless system
needlescope device
needlescopic adrenalectomy
needle-tip laparoscopic electrode
needle-tipped sphincterotome
needle-track seeding
nefazodone hydrochloride
negative
  n. immunofluorescence
  n. laparotomy
  n. nitrogen balance
  n. predictive value (NPV)

NOTES

negative *(continued)*
    n. pressure-controlled tube
    n. pressure method ambulatory endoscopic esophageal mucoscctomy
    n. pressure overtube
    n. pressure tube
NegGram
negligible blood loss
negro
    vomito n.
Negus rigid esophagoscope
Neil-Moore electrode
Neisseria gonorrhoeae
Neisser syringe
Neivert polyp hook
Nélaton
    N. catheter
    N. fold
    N. rubber tube drain
    N. sphincter
nelfinavir
Nellcor Durasensor adult oxygen transducer
Nelson
    N. forceps
    N. scissors
    N. syndrome
nemaline myopathy
nematode infection
nematodiasis
Nembutal
NEMD
    nonspecific esophageal motility disorder
neoadjuvant
    n. androgen derivation therapy
    n. antiandrogenic treatment
    n. chemoradiation
    n. chemotherapy
    n. hormonal ablation therapy
    n. hormonal deprivation
    n. total androgen ablation
neoanal
    n. function
    n. mucosa
    n. sphincter
neobladder
    Camey n.
    decompensated n.
    gastric n.
    Hautmann ileal n.
    hemi-Kock n.
    ileal n.
    ileocolonic n.
    Kock n.
    Le Bag n.
    Melchior ileal n.
    orthotopic ileal n.

    sigmoid n.
    Studer n.
    W-stapled ileal n.
neobladder-urethra anastomosis
neocholangiole
Neocholex
neocystostomy
    ureteral n.
    ureteroileal n.
neodymium:YAG laser therapy
neodymium:yttrium-aluminum-garnet (Nd:YAG)
neodymium:yttrium garnet laser
neoformans
    Candida n.
    Cryptococcus n.
neointimal hyperplasia
Neo-Lax
Neoloid
neomeatus
Neomed electrocautery
neomembrane
neomycin
neonatal
    n. adrenal gland hemorrhage
    n. arginine vasopressin
    n. cholestasia
    n. conjugated hyperbilirubinemia
    n. exstrophic bladder repair
    n. hepatitis
    n. jaundice
    n. oliguria
neonate
    amino acid excretion in n.
    aminoaciduria in n.
neonatorum
    icterus n.
    melena n.
    volvulus n.
neopenis
neophallus
neoplasia
    anal intraepithelial n. (AIN)
    cervical intraepithelial n. (CIN)
    colonic n.
    intratubular germ cell n. (ITGCN)
    metachronous n.
    multiple endocrine n. (MEN)
    multiple endocrine n. 1
    multiple endocrine n. 2A (MEN 2A)
    multiple endocrine n. 2B (MEN 2B)
    penile intraepithelial n.
    preinvasive urothelial n.
    prostatic intraepithelial n. (PIN)
    n. risk

neoplasm
    anal n.
    bladder n.
    colorectal n.
    extragonadal germ cell n.
    genitourinary n.
    germ cell n.
    intraductal mucin-hypersecreting n.
    intraductal oncocytic papillary n.
      (IOPN)
    intraductal papillary mucinous n.
      (IPMN)
    megacystic mucinous n.
    n. metastasis
    mucinous cystic n.
    nonseminomatous germ cell n.
    paratesticular n.
    periampullary n.
    prostatic n.
    retroperitoneal n.
    n. staging
    stomach n.
    urothelial n.
    vascular n.
neoplastic
    n. cell proliferation
    n. cyst
    n. disease
    n. lesion
    n. origin
    n. polyp
    n. potential
    n. renal mass
    n. tissue
    n. transformation
Neopterin
Neoral
neorectal emptying
neorectum
neoscrotum
neosphincter
    Acticon n.
    gracilis n.
    stimulated gracilis n.
Neosporin G.U. Irrigant
neostigmine methylsulfate
neostomy
neoterminal ileum
neotransformation
    papillomatous n.
neourethra
    Mitrofanoff n.

Neo-Vadrin
neovagina
    n. construction
    gracilis myocutaneous n.
    skin graft n.
neovascular bundle
neovascularization
Nepean Dyspepsia Index (NDI)
nephelometry
nephradenoma
nephralgia
    idiopathic n.
nephralgic
NephrAmine
nephrectomize
nephrectomized
    post n.
nephrectomy
    abdominal n.
    adjunctive n.
    adjuvant n.
    n. allograft
    anterior n.
    apical polar n.
    Balkan n.
    bilateral n.
    extracorporeal partial n.
    extraperitoneal laparoscopic n.
    extraperitoneal supracostal live
      donor n.
    flank n.
    laparoscopic living donor n.
    laparoscopic partial n.
    laparoscopic radical n. (LRN)
    laser partial n.
    live donor n.
    lumbar n.
    morcellated n.
    palliative n.
    paraperitoneal n.
    partial polar n.
    perifascial n.
    polar segmental n.
    posterior n.
    radical n.
    retroperitoneoscopic n.
    simple n.
    transperitoneal laparoscopic n.
      (TLN)
    transplant n.
    unilateral n.
nephredema

N

NOTES

nephrelcosis
nephremia
nephremphraxis
nephric
nephridium
nephrism
nephritic
    n. calculus
    n. edema
    n. sediment
    n. syndrome
nephritis, pl. **nephritides**
    acute focal bacterial n. (AFBN)
    acute interstitial n. (AIN)
    acute serum sickness n.
    albuminous n.
    allergic interstitial n.
    anaphylactoid purpura n.
    antiglomerular basement membrane
      antibody n.
    antiglomerular basement membrane-
      negative crescentric glomerular n.
    anti-Thy-1 n.
    autoimmune interstitial n.
    bacterial n.
    Balkan n.
    capsular n.
    n. caseosa
    caseous n.
    catarrhal n.
    cheesy n.
    chloroazotemic n.
    clostridial n.
    crescentic n.
    croupous n.
    degenerative n.
    diffuse suppurative n.
    n. dolorosa
    dropsical n.
    embolic n.
    epidemic n.
    exudative n.
    fibrolipomatous n.
    fibrous n.
    focal bacterial n.
    glomerulocapsular n.
    n. gravidarum
    hemorrhagic n.
    hereditary n.
    Heymann n.
    hydremic n.
    hydropigenous n.
    hypogenetic n.
    ICR strain-derived glomerular n.
      (ICGN)
    idiopathic hypocomplementemic
      interstitial n.
    immune-mediated interstitial n.

    indurative n.
    infection-related interstitial n.
    interstitial scarlatinal n.
    interstitial syphilitic n.
    Lancereaux n.
    latent n.
    leptospiral n.
    lipomatous n.
    Lohlein n.
    lupus n. (LN)
    Masugi n.
    mercuric chloride-induced n.
    n. mitis
    nephrotoxic n. (NTN)
    nephrotoxic antiglomerular basement
      membrane antibody n.
    nephrotoxic serum n.
    parenchymatous n.
    passive Heymann n. (PHN)
    pauciimmune glomerular n.
    phenacetin n.
    pneumococcus n.
    postinfective glomerular n.
    potassium-losing n.
    n. of pregnancy
    productive n.
    salt-losing n.
    saturnine n.
    scarlatinal n.
    serum n.
    shunt n.
    silent lupus n.
    Steblay n.
    subacute n.
    suppurative cortical n.
    syphilitic n.
    tartrate n.
    transfusion n.
    trench n.
    tuberculous n.
    tubulointerstitial n. (TIN)
    vascular n.
    Volhard n.
    war n.
    water-losing n.
nephritogenic
    n. antigen
    n. epitope
nephroabdominal
nephroangiosclerosis
nephroblastoma
nephroblastomatosis complex (NBC)
nephrocalcin (NC)
nephrocalcinosis
    calcium phosphate n.
nephrocapsectomy
nephrocardiac
nephrocele

nephrocelom
nephrocolic
nephrocolopexy
nephrocoloptosis
nephrocystanastomosis
nephroerysipelas
nephrogastric
nephrogenic, nephrogenetic
    n. adenoma
    n. ascites
    n. cord
    n. diabetes insipidus (NDI)
    n. rest
    n. ridge
    n. zone
nephrogenous
    n. albuminuria
    n. dialysis ascites
    n. proteinuria
nephrogram
    delayed n.
    diffuse patchy n.
    rim n.
    soap-bubble n.
nephrographic
    generalized n. (GNG)
nephrography
    isotope n.
nephrohemia
nephrohydrosis
nephrohypertrophy
nephroid
nephrolith
nephrolithiasis
    autosomally inherited forms of n.
    calcium oxalate n.
    N. Clinical Guidelines Panel
    glucocorticoid-induced
      hypercalcemic n.
    hypercalcemic n.
    iatrogenic hypercalcemic n.
    indinavir-induced n.
    percutaneous n.
    X-linked recessive n. (XRN)
nephrolitholapaxy
    percutaneous n.
nephrolithotomy
    anatrophic n.
    percutaneous n. (PCN, PCNL,
      PNL)
    simultaneous bilateral
      percutaneous n. (SBPN)

nephrolithotripsy
    percutaneous n. (PCNL)
nephrologist
nephrology
nephrolysin
nephrolysis
nephrolytic
nephroma
    cystic n.
    embryonal n.
    kidney n.
    mesoblastic n.
    multilocular cystic n.
nephromalacia
nephromegaly
nephron
    aldosterone-sensitive distal n.
    n. loss
    mesonephric n.
    n. plasma flow
    proximal n.
    n. transport
nephroncus
nephronia
    lobar n.
nephronophthisis
    familial juvenile n.
    juvenile n.
nephron-sparing surgery
nephroomentopexy
nephroparalysis
nephropathia epidemica
nephropathic
nephropathy
    acute hypokalemic n.
    acute urate n.
    Adriamycin n.
    amphotericin B n.
    amyloid n.
    analgesic n.
    Balkan n.
    Berger n.
    bismuth n.
    cadmium n.
    carbon tetrachloride n.
    cast n.
    chronic allograft n.
    chronic hypokalemic n.
    chronic urate n.
    cisplatin n. (CPN)
    copper n.
    C1q n.

N

NOTES

nephropathy *(continued)*
    Danubian endemic familial n.
    diabetic n.
    dropsical n.
    epidemic n.
    gold n.
    HIV-associated n. (HIVAN)
    human immunodeficiency virus-
      associated n. (HIVAN)
    hypazoturic n.
    hypercalcemic n.
    hypochloruric n.
    hypokalemic n.
    IgA n.
    IgM n.
    immunoglobulin A n.
    incipient n.
    iodide n.
    iron n.
    kaliopenic n.
    kanamycin n.
    lead n.
    malarial n.
    membranous n.
    mesangial n.
    nonnephrotic immunoglobulin A n.
    obstructive n.
    overt n.
    oxalate n.
    phenacetin n.
    polymyxin n.
    n. of potassium depletion
    proteinuric n.
    puromycin aminonucleoside n.
      (PAN)
    Ramipril Efficacy in N. (REIN)
    reflux n.
    salt-losing n.
    sickle-cell n.
    silver n.
    sodium wasting n.
    streptomycin n.
    sulfonamide n.
    tetracycline n.
    toxic n.
    tropical n.
    tubular n.
    tubulointerstitial n.
    urate n.
    uric acid n.
    vascular n.
nephropexy
nephrophagiasis
nephrophthisis
    familial juvenile n.
nephropoietic
nephropoietin

nephroptosis, nephroptosia
nephropyelitis
nephropyelography
nephropyelolithotomy
nephropyeloplasty
nephropyosis
nephrorrhagia
nephrorrhaphy
nephrosclerosis
    arteriolar n.
    benign n.
    hyaline arteriolar n.
    hyperplastic arteriolar n.
    hypertensive n. (HN)
    intercapillary n.
    malignant n.
    senile n.
nephroscope
    flexible n.
    rigid n.
    n. sheath
    steerable n.
    Storz n.
    Wolf percutaneous universal n.
nephroscopy
    anatrophic n.
    antegrade n.
    flexible n.
    second-look flexible n.
nephrosis
    acute n.
    Adriamycin-induced n.
    amyloid n.
    cholemic n.
    congenital n.
    Epstein n.
    familial n.
    glycogen n.
    Haymann n.
    hydropic n.
    hypokalemic n.
    infectious avian n.
    larval n.
    lipid n.
    lipoid n. (LN)
    lower nephron n.
    mercurial n.
    osmotic n.
    pure n.
    puromycin aminonucleoside n.
      (PAN)
    steroid-dependent idiopathic n.
    steroid-resistant idiopathic n.
    steroid-sensitive idiopathic n.
    vacuolar n.
    n. with hypovolemia
    n. without hypovolemia

nephrosonephritis
    hemorrhagic n.
    Korean hemorrhagic n.
nephrospasia, nephrospasis
nephrosplenopexy
nephrostogram
nephrostolithotomy
    percutaneous n. (PCNL)
nephrostomy
    n. catheter
    percutaneous n.
    retrograde n.
    n. tube
nephrotic
    n. edema
    n. syndrome
nephrotomic cavity
nephrotomogram
nephrotomography
    infusion n.
nephrotomy
    abdominal n.
    anatrophic n.
    lumbar n.
    n. tube
nephrotoxic
    n. acute renal failure
    n. antiglomerular basement
      membrane antibody nephritis
    n. antiserum
    n. nephritis (NTN)
    n. serum nephritis
    n. tubule necrosis
nephrotoxicity
    cadmium-induced n.
    cyclosporine n.
    mercuric chloride n.
nephrotoxin
nephrotrophic
nephrotropic
nephrotuberculosis
nephrotyphoid
nephrotyphus
nephroureteral stent
nephroureterectasis
nephroureterectomy
    Beer n.
    bilateral n.
    hand-assisted laparoscopic n.
      (HALNU)
    laparoscopic n.
    radical n.

    transperitoneal laparoscopic n.
    n. with en bloc removal of cuff
      of bladder
nephroureterocystectomy
nephroureteroscopy
    virtual n.
nephrourography
nephrovesical stent
Nephrox Suspension
Nepro diet supplement
Neptune girdle
NERD
    nonerosive reflux disease
Nernst equation
nerve
    afferent renal n.
    anterior scrotal n.
    n. block
    cavernosal n.
    cavernous n.
    n. conduction study
    n. cooling
    criminal n.
    dorsal n. of penis
    n. entrapment syndrome
    extrapudendal pelvic n.
    femoral n.
    genitofemoral n.
    gluteal n.
    Grassi n.
    n. growth factor (NGF)
    n. growth factor receptor (NGFR)
    n. hook
    hypogastric n.
    iliohypogastric n.
    ilioinguinal n.
    inferior anal n.
    inferior rectal n.
    intrapancreatic n.
    n. of Latarjet
    noncholinergic n.
    obturator n.
    pelvic autonomic n.
    perineal n.
    posterior scrotal n.
    postganglionic cholinergic n.
    postganglionic sympathetic n.
    pudendal pelvic n.
    rectal n.
    renal afferent n.
    renal sympathetic n.
    saphenous n.

N

NOTES

nerve *(continued)*
    sciatic n.
    somatic peripheral n.
    splanchnic n.
    subcostal n.
    transcutaneous n.
    n. transsection
    vagus n.

nerve-sparing
    n.-s. lymph node dissection
    n.-s. radical retropubic
      prostatectomy

nervi erigentes

nervosa
    anorexia n. (AN)
    bulimia n.
    dysphagia n.

nervosus
    singultus gastricus n.

nervous
    n. bladder
    n. dyspepsia
    n. eructation
    n. gut
    n. indigestion
    n. urine
    n. vomiting

Nesbit
    N. corporeal
    N. cystoscope
    N. operation
    N. plication
    N. technique
    N. technique ureterocolonic
      anastomosis
    N. tuck procedure

nesidiectomy

nesidioblastoma

NESP
    Novel erythropoiesis stimulating protein

nest
    Brunn epithelial n.
    von Brunn epithelial n.

NET
    neuroendocrine tumor

net
    n. acid excretion (NAE)
    rotatable Roth retrieval n.
    Roth polyp retrieval n.
    ureteric retrieval n.

netilmicin

Netromycin

network
    capillary n.
    Pentax EndoNet digital
      endoscopy n.
    trans-Golgi n.
    vascular collateral n.

Neubauer and Fischer test

Neukomm test

Neu-Laxova syndrome

NEU oncoprotein

neural
    n. cell-adhesive molecule (NCAM,
      N-CAM)
    n. control
    n. growth factor receptor (NGFR)
    n. invasion
    n. nodule
    n. pathway
    n. plexus

neuraminidase

neuraminidase-treated sheep erythrocyte

neurasthenia
    gastric n.

neurectomy
    gastric n.

neurinoma

neuroaminidase

neuroanatomy

neuroblastoma
    cervical n.
    metastatic n.
    olfactory bulb n.
    paravertebral n.
    presacral n.
    n. staging
    n. subcutaneous nodule

neuroblockage

neurocutaneous syndrome

neurodegenerative disorder

neuroectodermal dysplasia

neuroendocrine
    n. cell
    n. tumor (NET)

neuroendocrinology
    gastrointestinal n.

neurofibroma
    bladder n.
    duodenal n.
    gastrointestinal n.
    plexiform n.
    Recklinghausen gastric n.

neurofibromatosis (NF)
    familial intestinal n.
    von Recklinghausen n.

neurofilament protein triplet

neurogastroenterology

neurogenic
    n. bladder
    n. diabetes insipidus
    n. dysphagia
    n. erectile dysfunction
    n. hyperreflexia
    n. intestinal obstruction
    n. refractory urge incontinence

n. secretory diarrhea
n. sphincteric incompetence
n. tumor
neurogram
pudendal n.
neurohumoral
n. control of motility
n. disease
n. excitation state
n. factor
neurohumoral-immune axis
neurohypophysis
neuroimmune dysfunction
neurokinin
n. A, B
neurologic
n. complication
n. deficit
n. disorder
neurolysis
celiac plexus n. (CPN)
CT-guided celiac plexus n.
endosonography-guided celiac
plexus n.
neurolytic
n. celiac plexus block
n. drug
neuroma
neuromedin U
neuromodulation
chronic sacral n.
sacral root n.
subchronic sacral n.
neuron
adrenergic n.
afferent n.
alpha motor n.
argyrophilic and argyophobic n.
bipolar n.
cholinergic n.
enteric vasodilator n.
final motor n.
gamma aminobutyric acidergic n.
intestinofugal n.
motor n.
multipolar n.
nonadrenergic n.
noncholinergic n.
parasympathetic postganglionic n.
parasympathetic preganglionic n.
peptidergic n.
S n.

sensory n.
serotoninergic n.
unipolar n.
upper motor n.
vagal input n.
vagal preganglionic n.
neuronal cell line
neuronoma
VIP-secreting n.
neuron-specific enolase (NSE)
neuroparacrine mechanism
neuropathic
n. bladder
n. cystinosis
n. voiding dysfunction
neuropathy
autonomic n.
cyclosporine-induced optic n.
diabetic autonomic n.
familial visceral n. (FVN)
IgA n.
immunoglobulin n.
membranous n.
optic n.
pigment n.
polyradicular n.
pudendal n.
reflux n.
topical n.
vasculitic n.
visceral n.
neuropeptide Y (NPY)
neuropharmacology
neurophysiologic recording
neurophysiology
pelvic floor n.
neuroplasticity
neuropraxia
neuropsychotropic drug
neurosis
bladder n.
neurospinal dysraphism
neurosteroid
neurostimulation
sacral n.
transcutaneous sacral n.
neurotensin
neurotransmitter
noncholinergic n.
neurotrophin
neurotropic
neuroureterectomy

N

NOTES

neurourological
neurturin
neutral
    n. endopeptidase
    K-Phos N.
neutralophile
Neutra-Phos
Neutra-Phos-K
Neutrexin
neutrocytic ascites
neutron
neutropenia
neutropenic
    n. colitis
    n. typhlitis
neutrophil
    n. chemotactic peptide
    n. dysfunction
    n. elastase
    polymorphonuclear n. (PMNN)
    WBC n.
neutrophil-activating protein of
   Helicobacter pylori **(HP-NAP)**
neutrophilia
neutrophilic
    n. cryptitis
    n. dermatosis
    n. gastroduodenitis
    n. infiltration
neutropic virus
nevi (*pl. of* nevus)
Neville tracheal reconstruction prosthesis
nevirapine
nevus, pl. nevi
    n. flammeus
    inguinal crease compound n.
    pigmented n.
    spider n.
newborn
    n. hepatitis
    n. jaundice
newcastle
    Shigella n.
new differentiation factor (NDF)
Newman proctoscope
newport
    Salmonella n.
Nexium
nexus
Nezhat-Dorsey irrigator/aspirator
NF
    neurofibromatosis
NF-KB
    nuclear factor kappa B
N-formyl-methyonyl-leucyl-phenylalanine
   (fMLP)

NG
    nasogastric
    NG suction
NGD-95-1 antiobesity compound
NGF
    nerve growth factor
NGFR
    nerve growth factor receptor
    neural growth factor receptor
^{15}**N-glutamine**
NGT
    nasogastric tube
NH2-terminal SH2 domain
NHANES
    National Health and Nutrition
    Examination Survey
NHL
    non-Hodgkin lymphoma
niacin deficiency
nialamide
Niblitt dissector
nicardipine
niche sign
Nichols-Condon bowel preparation
Nichols IRMA kit
niclosamide
Nicolet SM-300 stimulator
Nicorette
nicotinamide
    n. adenine dinucleotide (NADH)
    n. adenine dinucleotide phosphate
    (NADPH)
nicotine
nicotinic
    n. agonist
    n. receptor
    n. receptor blocker
NIDDK
    National Institute of Diabetes, Digestive
    and Kidney Disease
NIDDM
    non-insulin-dependent diabetes mellitus
nidogen
Niemann-Pick disease
Niemeier gallbladder perforation
nifedipine
    n. extended release
    n. ointment
    topical n.
Niferex-150
nifurtimox
nigericin
nightly intermittent peritoneal dialysis
   (NIPD)
nighttime polyuria
nigra
    linea n.

nigricans
>> acanthosis n.
>> malignant acanthosis n.

NIH
> National Institutes of Health
>> NIH Classification Category I
>> acute bacterial prostatitis
>> NIH Classification Category II
>> chronic bacterial prostatitis
>> NIH Classification Category III
>> inflammatory and noninflammatory
>> chronic pelvic pain
>> NIH Classification Category (I–IV)
>> NIH Classification Category IV
>> asymptomatic inflammatory
>> prostatitis
>> NIH Classification System for
>> Prostatitis

NIH-CPSI
> National Institutes of Health Chronic
> Prostatitis Symptom Index
>> NIH-CPSI prostatitis classification
>> NIH-CPSI (type I–IV)

NIHF
> nonimmune hydrops fetalis

Nihon tocodynamometer
Nilandron
nil disease
Nilstat
nilutamide
nimesulide
nimodipine
Ninhydrin
Niopam contrast medium
NIPD
> nightly intermittent peritoneal dialysis

nipple
>> antireflux n.
>> antirefluxing n.
>> continence n.
>> n. discharge
>> ileum n.
>> intussuscepted ileal triple n.
>> Kock n.
>> pigmented n.
>> split-cuff n.
>> ureteral split-cuff n.
>> n. valve

nippled stoma
Nippostrongylus brasiliensis
Nipride
niridazole

Nisbet
>> N. chancre
>> N. disease

nisoldipine
N-isopropyl-p-iodoamphetamine
> biodistribution of N.-i.-p.-i.

Nissen
>> N. antireflux operation
>> N. 360-degree wrap fundoplication
>> N. fundoplication wrap
>> N. gall duct forceps
>> lap N.
>> N. laparoscopic fundoplication
>> N. repair

Nissenkorn stent
nitazoxanide
nitecapone
nitidus
>> lichen n.

nitinol
>> n. basket
>> n. mesh-covered frame
>> n. mesh stent
>> n. wire

Niti-S stent
nitrate
>> gallium n.
>> intravesical silver n.
>> methylatropine n.
>> organic n.
>> silver n.

nitrate-induced venodilation
nitrazepam
nitrendipine
nitric
>> n. oxide (NO)
>> n. oxide blocked sphincter
>> relaxation
>> n. oxide donor
>> n. oxide-releasing NSAID (NO-
>> NSAIDs)
>> n. oxide synthase inhibitor
>> n. oxide synthetase

nitrite
>> amyl n.
>> dietary n.
>> n. test

4-nitrobiphenyl
nitroblue
>> n. tetrazolium (NBT)
>> n. tetrazolium-paraaminobenzoic acid
>> (NBT-PABA)

N

NOTES

nitrofurantoin hepatotoxicity
nitrofurazone
nitrogen
  n. balance
  blood urea n. (BUN)
  glutamine n.
  high n. (HN)
  high calorie and n. (HCN)
  n. overload
  n. partition test
  n. retention test
  serum urea n. (SUN)
  total body n. (TBN)
  urea n. (UN)
  urine urea n. (UUN)
nitrogenous waste
nitroglycerin
  intravenous n.
  vasopressin with n.
nitroimidazole
2-nitropropane hepatotoxicity
nitroprusside
  sodium n. (SNP)
4-nitroquinolin-1-oxide-induced tumor
  (4NOQ)
nitrosamine
  carcinogenic n.
nitroso compound
nitrosourea
Nitrostat
nitrous
  n. oxide
  n. oxide insufflator
nizatidine
Nizoral
NJ
  nasojejunal
  NJ feeding tube
NK
  natural killer
  NK cell
NKE
  needle-knife electrocautery
NKF
  needle-knife fistulotomy
NKF-DOQI
  National Kidney Foundation-Data
  Outcomes Quality Initiative
NK1, NK2 tachykinin receptor
NKP
  needle-knife papillotomy
NKPP
  needle-knife precut papillotomy
NLH
  nodular lymphoid hyperplasia
N-linked glycoprotein
NLV
  Norwalk-like virus

NM
  nuclear medicine
NM23 **gene**
N-methyl-D-glucamide (NMG)
NMG
  N-methyl-D-glucamide
N^G-monomethyl-L-arginine (L-NMMA)
NMP
  nuclear matrix protein
NMP-22
  nuclear matrix protein
    NMP-22 test
NMR
  nuclear magnetic resonance
N-*myc* oncogene
N^G-nitro-L-arginine methyl ester (L-NAME)
N-nitrosamine
NO
  nitric oxide
Noble
  N. bowel plication
  N. surgical plication of bowel
Nocardia otitidis-caviarum
nociceptive
  n. sensory input
  n. stimulation
  n. structure
nociceptor
nocte
  ranitidine n.
nocturia
  age-related n.
nocturnal
  n. acid reflux
  n. diarrhea
  n. emission
  n. enuresis
  n. erection
  n. gastric reflux
  n. heartburn
  n. hemodialysis
  n. incontinence
  n. pain
  n. penile tumescence (NPT)
  n. penile tumescence monitoring
  n. polyuria
  n. regurgitation
  n. tumescence self-monitoring
node
  celiac lymph n.
  n. of Cloquet
  n. dissection
  n. distribution
  Ewald n.

hypogastric n.
inguinal lymph n.
intermediate mesenteric lymph n.
juxtaposed mesenteric lymph n.
juxtaregional n.
lymph n.
matted n.
mesenteric lymph n. (MLN)
obturator lymph n.
Osler n.
pelvic lymph n.
perigastric n.
retrorectal lymph n.
sentinel n.
shotty lymph n.
Sister Mary Joseph lymph n.
subcarinal n.
succulent mesenteric lymph n.
Troisier n.
Virchow sentinel n.
Virchow-Troisier n.
nodosa
periarteritis n.
polyarteritis n.
vasitis n.
nodose ganglia
nodosum
erythema n.
nodular
n. hyperplasia
n. hyperplasia of prostate
n. lesion
n. liver
n. lymphoid hyperplasia (NLH)
n. lymphoma
n. pancreatitis
n. regenerative hyperplasia (NRH)
n. transformation
n. transitional cell carcinoma
nodularity
antral n.
coarse n.
mucosal n.
surface n.
nodulated
nodulation
nodule
cecal mucosal n.
colonic lymphoid n.
daughter n.
discrete n.

Gamna n.
Gandy-Gamna n.
gelatinous n.
hyperplastic n.
liver n.
lymphoid n.
lymphomatous n.
macroregenerative n.
mucinous tumor n.
multiacinar regenerative n.
multiple n.
neural n.
neuroblastoma subcutaneous n.
pentastomum denticulatum n.
peritoneal n.
prostatic n.
regenerative cirrhotic n.
siderotic n.
Sister Mary Joseph n.
spindle cell n.
surface n.
thyroid n.
yellow n.
nodule-in-nodule pattern
Nolvadex
nomenclature
anorectal n.
nomogram
A Bayesian n.
Abrams-Griffith n.
Schäfer n.
Siroky n.
non-A
n.-A., non-B (NANB)
n.-A., non-B hepatitis
n.-A., non-B, non-C hepatitis
n.-A., non-B posttransfusion
hepatitis
nonabsorbable
n. disaccharide
n. suture
nonadherent clot
nonadhesive dressing
nonadrenergic
n. neuron
n. noncholinergic (NANC)
n. noncholinergic inhibitory
transmitter
**nonadrenergic noncholinergic inhibitory
transmitter**
non-A–E hepatitis

N

NOTES

non-A–G
    n.-A–G chronic liver disease
    n.-A–G fulminant hepatitis
nonagglutinable (NAG)
nonalcoholic
    n. fatty liver disease (NAFLD)
    n. steatohepatitis (NASH)
non-alpha, non-beta pancreatic islet cell
nonamyloid glomerulopathy
nonaneuploid tumor
non-anion-gap metabolic acidosis
nonantibiotic colitis
non-antigen-expressing target cell
nonantral endocrine cell hyperplasia
nonapoptotic pathway
NO-naproxen
nonatrophic pangastritis
nonautoimmune fundic atrophic gastritis
nonazotemic cirrhosis
non-B
    n.-B islet cell tumor
    non-A, n.-B (NANB)
    n.-B, non-C chronic liver disease
      (NBNC CLD)
nonbacterial
    n. cystitis (NBC)
    n. gastroenteritis
    n. prostatitis (NBP)
nonbench surgery
nonbilious vomitus
nonbiodegradable
nonbleeding visible vessel (NBVV)
nonbloody stool
non-breath-hold MR cholangiography
nonbuckling erection
noncalcareous renal calculus
noncalcified stone
noncalculous disease
noncardiac chest pain
noncaseating tubercle-like granuloma
noncerebral vasculopathy
non-CH4 excretor
noncholecystokinin substance
noncholinergic
    n. nerve
    n. neuron
    n. neurotransmitter
    nonadrenergic n. (NANC)
nonchylous ascites
noncirrhotic
    n. liver
    n. portal fibrosis (NCPF)
    n. portal hypertension
noncleaved B cell
noncollagen protein
noncommunicating
    n. biliary cyst

    n. diverticulum
    n. hydrocele
    n. polycystic disease
noncompliance
nonconductive guidewire
nonconfluent
noncontrast helical computed
    tomography (NCCT)
noncontributory
noncrushing bowel clamp
noncutting needle
nondiabetic
    n. gastroparesis
    n. neurogenic erectile dysfunction
    n. proteinuric renal disease
nondilating reflux
nondismembered anastomosis
nondisseminated intestinal threadworm
nondistended abdomen
nondistensible
nonenzymatic glycosylation
nonenzymic reaction
nonepithelial cyst
nonerosive
    n. esophagitis
    n. gastric mucosal lesion
    n. gastroesophageal reflux disease
    n. nonspecific gastritis
    n. reflux disease (NERD)
nonestrogen-supplemented
nonfamilial
    n. gastrointestinal polyposis
    n. intestinal pseudoobstruction
    n. visceral myopathy
nonferromagnetic MR endoscope XGIF-
    MR30
nonfixed cancer
nonfluctuant
nonfunction
    primary graft n.
nonfunctional pituitary tumor
nonfunctioning gallbladder
nonfusion
nonganglionated plexus
nongangrenous sigmoid volvulus
non-gas-forming liver abscess
nongene carrier
nongenomic
non-germ-cell carcinoma
nonglomerular hematuria
nonglycated albumin
nongonococcal urethritis
nongranulomatous
    n. jejunitis
    n. ulcerative jejunoileitis
nonhealing ulcer
non-heart-beating donor protocol

nonhemolytic
    n. jaundice
    n. *Streptococcus*
nonhemolyzed blood
non-Hodgkin lymphoma (NHL)
nonhyperfunctioning adrenocortical
  adenoma
nonicteric
    n. sclerae
    n. skin
nonimmune
    n. hydrops
    n. hydrops fetalis (NIHF)
nonimmunocompromised
nonimmunologic immunity
nonimmunosuppressed
noninflamed peripheral tissue
non-insulin-dependent diabetes mellitus
  (NIDDM)
nonintussuscepted valve
noninvasive
    n. assessment of urinary flow
    n. diagnosis
    n. diagnostic test
    n. intra-anal electromyography
    n. method
    n. tumor
nonionizing radiation
nonirrigating
    n. descending colostomy
    n. patient
nonischemic tubule
nonkeratinizing squamous epithelium
nonliquefaciens
    Moraxella n.
nonmalleable pelvis
nonmalodorous fluid
nonmetallic
nonnecrotizing granuloma
nonnegligible number
Nonnenbruch syndrome
nonneoplastic
    n. lesion
    n. polyp
nonnephrotic immunoglobulin A
  nephropathy
nonnephrotoxic drug
nonneurogenic
    n. neurogenic bladder
    n. voiding dysfunction
NONOate
    spermine N.

nonobstructive
    n. hepatic parenchymal disease
    n. jaundice
nonocclusive
    n. intestinal infarction
    n. mesenteric ischemia
    n. mesenteric thrombosis
nonoliguric acute renal failure
nonorgan confined disease
nonorganic dyspepsia
nonoxynol-9
nonpalpable cryptorchidism
nonparametric
    n. Wilcoxon statistics
nonparasitic
    n. cyst of liver
    n. splenic cyst
nonparticulate radiation
nonpathogenic *Escherichia coli*
nonpeptidyl agonist
nonperforated
    n. appendicitis
    n. appendix
nonpitting
nonpliable
nonplicated appendicocystostomy
nonpolar region
nonpolypoid adenoma
nonpolyposis colorectal cancer
nonpruritic
nonradioactive ^{13}C test
nonreactive pupil
nonreflux esophagitis
nonrefluxing colon conduit
nonrehydrated
    n. guaiac examination
    n. guaiac examination of rectum
nonrosetted cell
NO-NSAIDs
    nitric oxide-releasing NSAID
nonsecreting pituitary tumor
nonsecretory sigmoid cystoplasty
nonseminomatous
    n. germ cell neoplasm
    n. germ cell tumor (NSGCT)
    n. testicular carcinoma
nonskin malignancy
nonspecific
    n. colitis
    n. erosive gastritis
    n. esophageal motility disorder
    (NEMD)

N

NOTES

nonspecific *(continued)*
n. esophagitis
n. gas pattern
n. reactive hepatitis
n. ulcerative proctitis
n. urethritis (NSU)
nonsteroidal
n. antiandrogen monotherapy
n. antiinflammatory agent (NSAIA)
n. antiinflammatory drug (NSAID)
n. antiinflammatory drug
gastropathy
n. antiinflammatory drug-induced
intestinal stricture
nonstructural protein 4 (NSP4)
nonstruvite
n. calculus
n. stone
nonsulfated bile acid
nonsuppurative destructive cholangitis
non–swallow-associated relaxation
nontarget tissue
non-T-cell fraction
nontoxic goiter
nontransected pancreatic duct
nontropical sprue
nontruncating mutation
nontuberculous mycobacteria-associated
enterocolitis
nontumorous epithelia
nontyphoidal
n. *Salmonella*
n. salmonellosis
nonulcer
n. dyspepsia (NUD)
n. dysplasia
nonvariceal upper GI hemorrhage
nonvenereal bubo
nonviable tissue
nonvisualization of gallbladder
nonvoiding patient
Noonan syndrome
noose
Dormia n.
4NOQ
4-nitroquinolin-1-oxide-induced tumor
noradrenaline
serum n.
no rejection (NR)
norepinephrine lavage
norethandrolone
Norflex
norfloxacin
Norfolk technique
normal
n. appendix
bowel sounds n. (BSN)
n. carrier hepatitis

n. detrusor contractility
eversion n.
n. flora
n. maturation
palpably n.
n. saline meal
n. saline solution
visibly n.
normal-appearing mucosa
normal-caliber duct
normalized
n. protein catabolic rate (NPCR)
n. protein nitrogen appearance
(nPNA)
normal-pressure hydrocephalus
normeperidine
Nor-Mil
normoacidity
normoactive bowel sounds (NABS)
normocephalic
normochlorhydria
normochromic
normocytic
Normodyne
normoglycemia
normoproliferative
normospermatogenic sterility
normotensive
Normotest test
normothermia
normothermic effect
Noroxin
Norplant
Norpramin
Nortech SLED electrode
Nor-tet Oral
North American Medical Incorporated
deep dorsal vein
Northern blot analysis
Northgate
N. SD-3 dual-purpose lithotriptor
N. SD-100 EHL generator
nortriptyline
Norvasc
Norwalk
N. agent
N. gastroenteritis
N. virus
Norwalk-like virus (NLV)
Norwegian cholestasia
Norwich
Norwood rectal snare
NOS
induced nitric oxide synthase
no-scalpel vasectomy
nosocomial
n. fungal infection
n. urinary tract infection

nostras
    cholera n.
nostril blood
notch
    n. of gallbladder
    gastric n.
    splenic n.
note
    percussion n.
Nottingham
    N. colposuspension needle
    N. Key-Med introducer
    N. Key-Med introducing device
    N. One-Step tapered dilator
    N. semirigid introducer
    N. ureteral dilator
Nourse syringe
Nova II machine
Novamine amino acid
Novantrone
Novel erythropoiesis stimulating protein (NESP)
novo
    de n.
Novocain
NovolinPen device
NPCR
    normalized protein catabolic rate
NPCTG
    National Prostatic Cancer Treatment Group
NPH insulin
nPNA
    normalized protein nitrogen appearance
NPR
    natriuretic peptide receptor
NPT
    nocturnal penile tumescence
    NPT monitoring
NPV
    negative predictive value
NPY
    neuropeptide Y
NR
    no rejection
NRH
    nodular regenerative hyperplasia
NS3/NS4 junction
NS4/NS5 junction
NSAIA
    nonsteroidal antiinflammatory agent

NSAID
    nonsteroidal antiinflammatory drug
    NSAID gastropathy
    nitric oxide-releasing NSAID (NO-NSAIDs)
NSAID-induced
    NSAID-i. gastric injury
    NSAID-i. intestinal injury
NSE
    neuron-specific enolase
NSGCT
    nonseminomatous germ cell tumor
N-shaped sigmoid loop
NS2, NS3, NS4, NS5 protein
NSP4
    nonstructural protein 4
NSU
    nonspecific urethritis
NT
    nucleation time
N-terminal
    N-t. fragment
    N-t. propeptide of type III procollagen
NTN
    nephrotoxic nephritis
N-trimethylsilylimidazole
NTS
    nucleus tractus solitarius
NTZ Long Acting Nasal Solution
nuchal rigidity
Nuck
    canal of N.
    diverticulum of N.
    N. hydrocele
nuclear
    n. bleeding scan
    n. enema
    n. factor kappa B (NF-KB)
    n. factor kappa B transcription factor protein
    n. fragment
    n. hepatobiliary imaging
    n. hyperchromasia and pleomorphism
    n. isotope scan
    n. magnetic resonance (NMR)
    n. matrix
    n. matrix alteration
    n. matrix protein (NMP, NMP-22)
    n. medicine (NM)
    n. medicine scan

N

NOTES

nuclear *(continued)*
n. membrane
n. morphometry
n. protein cyclin proliferating cell nuclear antigen
n. roundness factor
n. sclerosis
n. transcriptional activation
nuclear-tagged
n.-t. cell
n.-t. red blood cell bleeding study
nuclear-to-cytoplasmic size ratio
nucleation
epitaxial n.
homogenous n.
n. time (NT)
nucleic
n. acid
n. acid hybridization
n. acid testing (NAT)
nucleocapsid
n. antigen-specific
n. antigen-stimulated interferon-gamma
nucleoside
nucleosome
nucleotide
adenosine n.
guanine n.
nucleotide-binding domain (NBD)
nucleus
n. ambiguus
cigar-shaped hyperchromatic n.
elongated, pseudostratified n.
hyperchromatic n.
Onuf n.
pyknotic n.
n. raphe obscurus
n. solitarius
n. of the solitary tract
n. tractus solitarius (NTS)
NUD
nonulcer dyspepsia
Nu-Hope
N.-H. Adhesive waterproof skin barrier
N.-H. cleaning solvent
N.-H. Convex insert
N.-H. hole cutter
N.-H. ileostomy pouch
N.-H. karaya powder
N.-H. neonatal and premie pouch
N.-H. Nu-Self drainable pouch
N.-H. pouch cover
N.-H. Protective Skin Barrier
N.-H. tubing
N.-H. urinary pouch

N.-H. urine collection bottle
N.-H. urostomy pouch
null cell tumor
Nullo deodorant tablet
NuLytely enema
number
n. connection test (NCT)
nonnegligible n.
shock n.
numbness
Nupercainal ointment
Nuport PEG tube
Nursoy formula
Nussbaum
N. experiment
N. intestinal clamp
N. intestinal forceps
nutcracker esophagus
Nu-Tetra
Nu-Tip laparoscopic scissors
nutmeg liver
nutraceutical
Nutramigen formula
Nutricia
nutrient enema
nutrition
enteral n. (EN)
home parenteral n. (HPN)
intradialytic parenteral n. (IDPN)
intravenous n. (IVN)
Jevity isotonic liquid n.
luminal n.
Nutri-Vent liquid n.
parenteral n.
Peptamen liquid n.
perioperative n.
Replete liquid n.
support parenteral n. (SPN)
total enteral n. (TEN)
total parenteral n. (TPN)
total peripheral parenteral n. (TPPN)
nutritional
n. assessment
n. cirrhosis
n. deficiency
n. dropsy
n. index
n. pancreatitis
n. status
n. support
n. therapy
nutritive
nutriture
Nutri-Vent liquid nutrition
Nutromat Pad S feeding pump
Nutropin
Nuttall liver retractor

nux vomica
N&V
    nausea and vomiting
NVD
    nausea, vomiting, diarrhea
NWTSG
    National Wilms Tumor Study Group
nycturia
Nyhus-Nelson gastric decompression and
    jejunal feeding tube

nylidrin
nylon tissue biopsy bag
Nymox urinary test
nystagmus
nystatin suspension
Nystex
Nytilax

NOTES

N

O₂

O$_2$
    oxygen
        fMLP-stimulated O$_2$
        PMA-stimulated O$_2$

OA-519 prognostic prostate carcinoma marker

OAC
    omeprazole, amoxicillin, clarithromycin

OAE
    open access endoscopy

OAI
    Ostomy Assessment Inventory

OAM
    omeprazole, amoxicillin, metronidazole

O antigen

OASIS
    One Action Stent Introduction System

oasis
    O. pusher tube system
    O. stent

oasthouse urine disease

oat
    o. cell
    o. cell carcinoma
    Lactobacillus plantarum-fermented o.

oatmeal
    colloidal o.

OB-10 Comfort bite block

OBA
    oral bile acid

O'Beirne sphincter

obesity
    adult-onset o.
    alimentary o.
    endogenous o.
    exogenous o.
    hyperplasmic o.
    hyperplastic o.
    hypertrophic o.
    o. hypoventilation syndrome (OHS)
    o. index
    lifelong o.
    morbid o.

OB gene

object
    foreign o.
    ingested foreign o.
    irretrievable o.
    radiolucent o.

objective
    o. lens
    o. vertigo

OBK
    obstructed kidney

obligate anaerobe

obligatory dialysate protein loss

oblique
    aponeurosis of external o.
    aponeurosis of internal o.
    o. arytenoid muscle
    external o.
    o. fibers of stomach
    o. fluoroscopy
    o. forward-viewing instrument
    o. gastric fiber
    o. incision
    internal o.
    o. obturator

oblique-viewing
    o.-v. echoendoscope
    o.-v. endoscope

obliterans
    appendicitis o.
    arteriosclerosis o.
    balanitis xerotica o. (BXO)
    endophlebitis hepatica o.

obliterated varix

obliteration
    balloon-occluded retrograde transvenous o. (B-RTO)
    endoscopic extirpation cicatricial o.
    percutaneous transhepatic o.
    o. of psoas shadow

obscurus
    nucleus raphe o.

observation
    electron immunoperoxidase o.
    light and electron immunoperoxidase o.

observational followup study

obsolescent glomerulus

obstetric injury

obstipation

obstipum
    abdomen o.

obstructed
    o. kidney (OBK)
    o. pelvis
    o. perineal testis

obstructing
    o. cancer
    o. rectosigmoidal carcinoma

obstruction
    acquired ureteropelvic junction o.
    acute extrarenal o.
    adynamic intestinal o.
    airflow o.
    airway o.
    benign prostatic o. (BPO)

O

obstruction *(continued)*
    bilateral ureteral o. (BUO)
    o. of bile flow
    biliary tract o.
    bladder neck o.
    bladder outflow o.
    bladder outlet o. (BOO)
    bowel o.
    bronchial o.
    Brugia lymphatic o.
    calix o.
    cerumen o.
    closed-loop intestinal o.
    clot-induced urinary tract o.
    colonic o.
    common bile duct o.
    complete bowel o.
    congenital ureteropelvic junction o.
    ductal o.
    duodenal o.
    o. duodenum
    ejaculatory duct o.
    epididymis o.
    esophageal o.
    extrahepatic bile duct o.
    extrahepatic biliary o.
    extrahepatic portal vein o.
     (EHPVO)
    extrinsic ureteral o.
    extrinsic ureteropelvic junction o.
    false colonic o.
    fecal o.
    food bolus o.
    functional cystic duct o.
    gastric outlet o. (GOO)
    hepatic venous outflow o. (HVOO)
    high-grade o.
    high small bowel o.
    idiopathic o.
    o. index
    infravesical prostatic o.
    intermittent o.
    intestinal o. (IO)
    intrahepatic portal o.
    intratubular o.
    intrinsic ureteropelvic junction o.
    large bowel o.
    low small bowel o.
    lymphatic o.
    malignant biliary o.
    mechanical biliary o.
    mechanical duct o.
    mechanical extrahepatic o.
    mechanical intestinal o.
    mechanical small bowel o.
    neurogenic intestinal o.
    oliguric o.
    outflow o.
    outlet o.
    palliation of malignant large
     bowel o.
    paralytic colonic o.
    paralytic intestinal o.
    partial bile outflow o.
    partial bowel o.
    partial ureteral o.
    portal vein o.
    postoperative ureteral o.
    prostatic outlet o. (POO)
    pyloric outlet o.
    pyloroduodenal o.
    renovascular o.
    secondary o.
    seminal vesicle o.
    shrapnel-induced biliary o.
    simple mechanical o.
    small bowel o. (SBO)
    splenic vein o. (SVO)
    strangulated bowel o.
    tubular o.
    unilateral ureteral o. (UUO)
    ureteral o.
    ureteric o.
    ureteropelvic junction o.
    ureterovesical o.
    urethral o.
    urinary o.
    urodynamic o.
    vas deferens o.

obstruction-induced modulation

obstructive
    o. anuria
    o. appendicitis
    o. biliary cirrhosis
    o. cholangitis
    o. defecation
    o. dysfunctional ileitis
    o. gastroduodenal Crohn disease
    o. jaundice
    o. megaureter
    o. nephropathy
    o. pancreatitis
    o. sleep apnea
    o. uropathy

obtunded

obturation

obturator
    Alcock-Timberlake o.
    o. artery
    blunt-tipped o.
    Endopath Optiview laparoscopic o.
    o. hernia
    o. internus muscle
    o. lymphatic chain
    o. lymph node
    o. nerve

oblique o.
Optiview o.
o. shelf cystourethropexy
o. sign
o. test
Timberlake o.
o. vein
obtuse margin
OCBF
    outer cortical blood flow
occipital
occiput
occluded shunt
occludens
    zona o.
    zonulae o.
occlusion
    o. balloon
    balloon ureteral o.
    o. cholangiogram
    enteromesenteric o.
    hepatic vein o.
    mesenteric vascular o.
    portal triad o.
    retinal artery o.
    retinal vein o.
    o. of TIPS
    tourniquet o.
    urethral o.
occlusive
    o. azoospermia
    o. clamp
    o. collodion dressing
    o. ileus
    o. infarction
occult
    o. blood
    o. filariasis
    o. gastrointestinal bleeding
    o. hepatitis
    o. levator ani hernia
    o. spinal dysraphism
occupational
    o. toxin
    o. toxin exposure
OCG
    oral cholecystogram
Ochoa syndrome
Ochsner
    O. clamp
    O. flexible spiral gallstone probe
    O. forceps

O. gallbladder probe
O. gallbladder trocar
O. hemostat
O. muscle
O. retractor
O. ring
O. treatment
Ockerblad-Boari flap
OCL bowel preparation
OCLG
    osteoclast-like giant cell
10 o'clock selector catheter
O'Connor drape
OCP
    ova, cysts, and parasites
OCT
    optical coherence tomography
    OCT medium
octahedral-shaped dihydrate
Octamide
octanoic acid breath test
octapeptide
    cholecystokinin o. (CCK-8, CCK-OP)
OctreoScan
    O. kit
    O. scintigraphy
octreotide
    o. acetate
    o. acetate for injectable suspension
    o. effect
    somatostatin analog o.
octreotide-induced hepatic toxicity
OCTT
    orocecal transit time
Ocuflox
ocular
    o. abnormality
    o. lesion
oculocerebrorenal
    o. dystrophy
    o. syndrome
oculopharyngeal muscular dystrophy
OD
    outer diameter
    overdose
ODC
    ornithine decarboxylase
Oddi
    denervated sphincter of O.
    sphincter of O. (SO)
O'Donoghue cystourethroscope

O

NOTES

odor
>   breath o.
>   foul-smelling o.
>   fruity o.

odorant
O'Duffy criteria
odynophagia
OEC-Diasonics 9400 fluoroscopy C-arm system
OEIS
>   omphalocele, exstrophy of the bladder, imperforate anus, and spinal
>>   OEIS abnormalities
>>   OEIS complex

Oerskovia
OES
>   Olympus endoscopy system
>>   OES 4000 resectoscope

Oettingen abdominal retractor
offset lens ureteroscope
ofloxacin
Ogen
Ogilvie syndrome
O'Hanlon intestinal clamp
Ohara disease
O'Hara forceps
25(OH)D3
>   25-hydroxyvitamin D3

OHS
>   obesity hypoventilation syndrome

oil
>   arachis o.
>   castor o.
>   cottonseed o.
>   fish o.
>   Fleet Enema Mineral O.
>   Fleet Flavored Castor O.
>   Kellogg's Castor O.
>   Lorenzo o.
>   olive o.
>   pennyroyal o.
>   peppermint o.
>   o. red O stain
>   o. retention enema
>   seabuckthorn seed o.

oily stool
ointment
>   Calmoseptine o.
>   Ethezyme debriding o.
>   nifedipine o.
>   Nupercainal o.
>   Panafil o.
>   Pazo Hemorrhoidal O.
>   Tucks o.

OK432 streptococcal suspension
Okamoto method
OK cell

OKT3
>   OKT3 anti-T-cell antibody
>   OKT3 monoclonal antibody
>   Orthoclone OKT3

OKT4 cell
OKT8 cell
Okuda transhepatic obliteration of varix
Olbert balloon dilator
Oldfield syndrome
Olean
oleandomycin
oleate
>   ethanolamine o.
>   intravariceal ethanolamine o.
>   monoethanolamine o.

oleic acid
olestra
>   O. fat substitute

olfactory bulb neuroblastoma
oligoasthenospermia
oligoasthenoteratospermia
oligoasthenoteratozoospermia
oligoazoospermia
oligocholia
oligochylia
oligochymia
oligocilia
oligohydramnios complex
oligohydruria
oligomeganephronia
oligomerize
oligometric complex
oligonecrospermia
oligonephronic hypoplasia
oligonucleotide
>   antisense o.
>   o. probe
>   specific o.

oligopepsia
oligopeptide
oligophosphaturia
oligosaccharidase
oligosaccharide
oligosaccharide-binding membrane protein
oligospermatic
oligospermia, oligospermatism
oligosymptomatic ADPKD
oligosynaptic pathway
oligoteratoasthenozoospermia (OTA)
oligozoospermatism, oligozoospermia
oliguresia, oliguresis
oliguria
>   neonatal o.

oliguric
>   o. obstruction
>   o. renal failure

olive
>Eder-Puestow o.
>expandable o.
>metal o.
>o. oil
>o. over guidewire
>palpable pyloric o.
>Savary-Gilliard metal o.
>o. shaped

olive-tipped
>o.-t. catheter
>o.-t. plastic dilator

OLS
>ouabainlike substance

olsalazine-S
olsalazine sodium
Olsen cholangiogram clamp
OLT
>orthotopic liver transplant

oltipraz
Olympus
>O. adapter
>O. A5256 laparoscope
>O. alligator-jaw endoscopic forceps
>O. Aloka EU-MI ultrasound gastrointestinal fiberscope
>O. Aloka GF-EU-series endoscope
>O. automatic reprocessor
>O. basket-type endoscopic forceps
>O. BH2-epifluorescence microscope
>O. BH2-RFCA reflecting microscope
>O. BHT-2 microscope
>O. BML-3Q, -4Q lithotriptor
>O. CBK fluorescence microscope
>O. CD-20Z heater probe
>O. CD-Z-series heat probe thermocoagulator
>O. CF-20 fibercolonoscope
>O. CF-HM-series magnifying colonoscope
>O. CF-L-series flexible sigmoidoscope
>O. CF-MB/LB colonoscope
>O. CF-MB-M colonoscope
>O. CF-MB-series colonoscope
>O. CF-OSF-series flexible sigmoidoscope
>O. CF-PL-series colonoscope
>O. CF-P20S fiberoptic colonoscope
>O. CF100S sigmoidoscope
>O. CF100TL

>O. CF-TL-series forward-viewing video colonoscope
>O. CF-1T100L video colonoscope
>O. CF-T-series colonoscope
>O. CF-TVL-series colonoscope
>O. CF-UHM-series colonoscope
>O. CF-UM3 colonoscope
>O. CF-UM3 flexible echocolonoscope
>O. CF-UM-series echoendoscope
>O. CF-UM20 ultrasound endoscope
>O. CF-VL-series colonoscope
>O. CF-200Z colonoscope
>O. CF-200Z endoscope
>O. CG-P-series colonofiberscope
>O. CHF-P20 choledochoscope
>O. CHF-Q10 cholangioscope
>O. clip-fixing device
>O. CLV10 fiberscope light source
>O. CLV-series fiberoptic system
>O. CLV-U 20 endoscopic halogen light source
>O. continuous flow resectoscope
>O. CV-series colonoscope
>O. CV-series endoscope
>O. CYF-3 OES cystofiberscope
>O. cytology brush
>O. DES-series endoscope
>O. EF-series esophagoscope
>O. endoscopy system (OES)
>O. Endo-Therapy disposable biopsy forceps
>O. ENF-P-series laryngoscope
>O. EUM-20 endoscope
>O. EU-M-series endosonography image processor
>O. Europe ETD automated endoscope washer
>O. EUS-series endoscope
>O. EVIS 140
>O. EVIS color computer chip system
>O. EVIS Q-series endoscope
>O. EVIS 140 Q video endoscope
>O. EVIS video colonoscope
>O. EW-series fiberoptic duodenoscope
>O. FB 20C endoscopic forceps
>O. FB 25K endoscopic forceps
>O. FBK 13 forceps
>O. FG-12U wide mouth forceps
>O. fiberoptic cystoscope

O

NOTES

Olympus *(continued)*

O. FK-13-1 biopsy forceps
O. FS-K-series endoscopic suture-cutting forceps
O. gastrostomy
O. GF-EU1 gastrointestinal fiberscope
O. GF-series video endoscope
O. GF-UC30P echoendoscope
O. GF-UCT30P linear array echoendoscope
O. GF-UM30P echoendoscope
O. GF-UM30P endoscope
O. GF-UM30P linear scanning probe
O. GF-UM29 radial scanner echoendoscope
O. GF-UM20 radial scanning endoscope
O. GF-UM20 ultrasound endoscope
O. GF-UM3, -UM20 system
O. GIF-D2 endoscope
O. GIF-D-series panendoscope
O. GIF20 echoendoscope
O. GIF-EUM2 echoendoscope
O. GIF-HM-series endoscope
O. GIF-J-series endoscope
O. GIF-K-series gastroscope
O. GIF-P endoscope
O. GIF-Q200 endoscope
O. GIF-Q30 fiberscope
O. GIF-series double-channel therapeutic videoendoscope
O. GIF-series echoendoscope
O. GIF-SQ-series videoendoscope
O. GIF-1T10 echoendoscope
O. GIF-2T200 endoscope
O. GIF-T-series endoscope
O. GIF-T-series videoendoscope
O. GIF-XP-series endoscope
O. GIF-XQ30 flexible gastroscope
O. GIF-XQ-series panendoscope
O. GIF-XV-series endoscope
O. grasping rat-tooth forceps
O. GTF-A gastrocamera
O. heat probe
O. hot biopsy forceps
O. HX-21L detachable mini-loop
O. injector
O. intracavity transducer
O. JF-series video duodenoscope
O. JF-series video endoscope
O. JF1T endoscope
O. JF1T10 fiberoptic duodenoscope
O. JF-T-series endoscope
O. JF-TV-series endoscope
O. JF-UM20 echoendoscope
O. JF-V-series endoscope

O. JF-V-series video duodenoscope
O. JT-series video duodenoscope
O. large-channel endoscope GIF1T130
O. linear array echoendoscope
O. magnetic extractor forceps
O. MAJ363 FNA needle system
O. mini-snare forceps
O. monopolar cannula
O. Nd:YAG laser
O. needle-knife papillotome
O. NM-K-series sclerotherapy needle
O. NM-L-series needle
O. OES fiberscope
O. OM-2 camera with SM-45 enlarging adapter
O. OM-1 reflex camera
O. OM-series endoscopic camera
O. one-step button gastrostomy tube
O. OSF flexible sigmoidoscope
O. OSP fluorescence measuring system
O. OTV-S-series miniature camera
O. P20
O. PCF-series pediatric colonoscope
O. pelican-type endoscopic forceps
O. PJF endoscope
O. PJF-series pediatric duodenoscope
O. PJF-series pediatric endoscope
O. PSD-10 electrosurgical blend current
O. P-series endoscope
O. PW-1L wash catheter
O. Q200 video endoscope
O. rat-tooth endoscopic forceps
O. reusable oval cup forceps
O. reusable oval cup forceps with needle
O. rubber-tip endoscopic forceps
O. SCA-series endoscopic camera
O. SD-5L semicircular snare
O. shark-tooth endoscopic forceps
O. SIF-10 enteroscope
O. SIF-M magnifying colonoscope
O. SIF-M-series video enteroscope
O. SIF-Q240 enteroscope
O. SIF-SW fiberoptic endoscope
O. SIF-SW-series video enteroscope
O. SIF-100 video push endoscope
O. SIF-100 video push enteroscope
O. sphincterotome
O. spray catheter PW-5V
O. SP-series image analyzer
O. S-20-20R probe
O. SSIF-series video enteroscope

O. SSIF-VI KAI fiberoptic
endoscope
O. stone retrieval basket
O. 2T100 endoscope
O. TJF-10, -100, -200
duodenoscope
O. tripod-type endoscopic forceps
O. 2T-2000 twin-channel
therapeutic gastroscope
O. UES-series snare cautery device
O. ultrasonic esophagoprobe
O. ultrathin balloon-fitted ultrasound
probe
O. UM-F30-20R probe
O. UM-20 radial echoendoscope
O. UM-2R, -3R probe
O. UM-R-series miniature ultrasonic
probe
O. UM-series endoscope
O. UM-S30-25R probe
O. UM-W-series endoscopic probe
O. URF-P2 translaparoscopic
choledochofiberscope
O. URF type P2 flexible
ureteroscope
O. video endoscopy system
O. video urology procedure system
O. V-series endoscope
O. VU-M2 echoendoscope
O. W-shaped endoscopic forceps
O. XCF-XK-series endoscope
O. XCHF-37 choledochoscope
O. XGF-UCT30 endoscope
O. XIF-UM3 echoendoscope
O. XK-series oblique-viewing
flexible fiberscope
O. XMP-U2 catheter echoprobe
O. XP-series endoscope
O. XQ-200, XQ-230 video
endoscope
O. XSIF-series video enteroscope
omapatrilat
Ombrédanne
O. forceps
O. operation
OMC
omeprazole, metronidazole,
clarithromycin
OME
omeprazole
OmegaPort access port
omega-shaped incision

omenta (*pl. of* omentum)
omental
o. adhesion
o. band
o. bursitis
o. cyst
o. enterocleisis
o. foramen
o. hammock
o. infarction
o. interposition
o. J-pexy
o. patch
o. pedicle
o. pedicle flap
o. pedicle flap graft
o. plug
o. studding
o. tuberosity
o. vein
o. wrapping
omentale
foramen o.
omentalis
taenia o.
tenia o.
omentectomy
omentitis
omentofixation
omentopexy
omentoplasty
pedicled o.
pelvic o.
omentorrhaphy
omentovolvulus
omentum, pl. **omenta**
bowel adherent to o.
colic o.
gastric o.
gastrocolic o.
gastrohepatic o.
gastrosplenic o.
greater o.
incarcerated o.
interposition flap of o.
lesser o.
o. majus
o. majus flap procedure
o. minus
pancreaticosplenic o.
pedicled o.
splenogastric o.

O

NOTES

omentumectomy
omeprazole (OME)
    o., amoxicillin, clarithromycin (OAC)
    o., amoxicillin, metronidazole (OAM)
    o., metronidazole, clarithromycin (OMC)
    o. test
    o. therapy
omeprazole/amoxicillin
omeprazole-clarithromycin-amoxicillin therapy
Omnicide disinfectant
Omni-LapoTract support system
Omnipaque
Omnipen
Omnipen-N
OmniPhase penile prosthesis
OMNI Prep
OmniPulse MAX holmium laser
Omnitract retractor
omphalectomy
omphalocele
    o., exstrophy of the bladder, imperforate anus, and spinal (OEIS)
    o., exstrophy of the bladder, imperforate anus, and spinal abnormalities
Onchocerca volvulus
onchocerciasis
oncoantigen 519
oncocytoma
    kidney o.
    renal o.
oncocytomatosis
oncofetal protein
oncogene
    c-*jun* o.
    c-*met* o.
    c-*myc* o.
    Her-2/neu o.
    o. inactivation
    Kirsten-*ras* o.
    K-*ras* o.
    N-*myc* o.
    polyoma middle T o.
    ras p21 o.
    sarcoma virus o.
oncogene-induced carcinogenesis
oncological radicality
oncologic principle
On-Command catheter
oncoprotein
    c-ErbB-2/NEU o.
    NEU o.

OncoScint
    O. colorectal/ovarian carcinoma localization scintigraphy (OncoScint CR/OV)
    O. CR103
    O. CR/OV
OncoSeed
OncoSpect
ondansetron
    metoclopramide, dexamethasone, lorazepam, o. (MDLO)
one
    O. Action Stent Introduction System (OASIS)
    O. Touch blood glucose meter
one-handed knot
one-hour office pad test
oneirogmus
one-minute endoscopy room test
one-piece
    Bard regular o.-p.
    o.-p. disposable plug
    o.-p. ostomy pouch
one-session crossover study
one-shot
    o.-s. intravenous urography
    o.-s. IVU
one-stage
    o.-s. hypospadias repair
    o.-s. procedure
    o.-s. reaction
one-step
    Surgitek O.-s. (SOS)
One-Step gastric button
onlay
    o. island flap
    o. island flap urethroplasty
    o. technique
onlay-tube-onlay urethroplasty technique
online hemodiafiltration
onset of pain
ontogeny
Onuf nucleus
Oochoristica
oocyst
    Cryptosporidium o.
oocyte micromanipulation
oolemma
oophorectomy
ooplasm
ooze
oozing blood
O&P
    ova and parasites
    O&P test
opacification
opacify

opaque
    o. meal
    Sur-Fit Natura closed-end pouch, o.
open
    o. access endoscopy (OAE)
    o. adrenalectomy
    o. biopsy
    bowels not o. (BNO)
    o. cystotomy
    o. drainage
    o. electrocautery snare
    o. end flow-through radiopaque tip
    o. hemorrhoidectomy
    o. injury
    o. mesh-plug hernioplasty
    o. morphology
    o. prostatectomy
    o. pyelolithotomy
    o. pyelotomy
    o. renal descent
    o. retroperitoneal high ligation
    o. sphincterotome
    o. transurethral resection
    o. ulcer
    o. wound
open-ended
    o.-e. ostomy pouch
    o.-e. ureteral catheter
    o.-e. vasectomy
opener
    potassium channel o.
opening
    appendiceal o.
    epispadiac o.
open-label Gelusil
operating
    10-degree o. laparoscope
    o. frequency
operation (*See also* procedure, repair)
    Abbe small bowel o.
    Aldridge o.
    Alexander-Adams o.
    Allingham o.
    Amussat o.
    Andrews o.
    antireflux o.
    Aylett o.
    Bacon-Babcock rectovaginal
      fistula o.
    Ball o.
    bariatric o.
    Bassini o.

Bates o.
Battle o.
Belfield o.
Belsey Mark IV antireflux o.
Belsey Mark V o.
Bennett o.
Bergenhem o.
Best o.
Bevan o.
Bevan-Rochet o.
Bigelow o.
Bloch-Paul-Mikulicz o.
Bloodgood o.
Boari o.
Bottini o.
bottle o.
Bozeman o.
Bricker o.
Browne o.
Brunschwig o.
Calot o.
Camey I, II o.
Cecil o.
Child o.
Civiale o.
Clark o.
Cock o.
Collis antireflux o.
Crespo o.
Davat o.
Delorme rectal prolapse o.
Deming o.
Denis Browne o.
Dittel o.
Doppler o.
Doyen o.
Duhamel o.
Duplay o.
Edebohls o.
Everett-TeLinde o.
eversion o.
Finney o.
Foley o.
Franco o.
Frank o.
Fredet-Ramstedt o.
Freyer o.
Fuller o.
Furlow-Fisher modification of Virag
  1 o.
Gauderer-Ponsky PEG o.
Gil-Vernet o.

O

NOTES

operation *(continued)*

Hagner o.
Halsted o.
Hartmann o.
Heineke-Mikulicz o.
Heller o.
Hess o.
Hill antireflux o.
Hochenegg o.
Hofmeister o.
Horton-Devine o.
Huggins o.
interposition o.
Israel o.
Ivalon sponge-wrap o.
Jaboulay-Doyen-Winkleman o.
Jonnesco o.
Kader o.
Kasai o.
Kelly o.
Kelly-Deming o.
Kelly-Stoeckel o.
kidney sparing o.
Kocher o.
Kraske o.
Kropp o.
Ladd o.
Lane o.
Lester Martin modification of
  Duhamel o.
Longmire o.
Lowsley o.
Macewen hernia o.
MAGPI o.
Mainz pouch o.
Makkas o.
Manchester-Fothergill o.
Mann-Williamson o.
Mansson o.
Marian o.
Marshall-Marchetti-Birch o.
Marshall-Marchetti-Krantz o.
Martin o.
Martius o.
Martius-Harris o.
Mason o.
Matson o.
Maunsell-Weir o.
Maydl o.
Mayo o.
Mays o.
McVay o.
Mercier o.
Merindino o.
mica o.
Mikulicz o.
Miles o.
Milligan-Morgan o.

Monfort o.
morcellement o.
Moschcowitz o.
Narath o.
Nesbit o.
Nissen antireflux o.
Ombrédanne o.
orthotopic hemi-Kock o.
Palomo o.
Payne o.
Petersen o.
Pickrell o.
Pólya o.
pubovaginal o.
Puestow-Gillesby o.
Ramstedt o.
Raz sling o.
Rigaud o.
Ripstein rectal prolapse o.
Roux-en-Y o.
Rovsing o.
sacrofixation o.
Scott o.
scrotal pouch o.
second-look o.
sling o.
Smith-Boyce o.
Soave o.
sphincter-preserving o. (SPO)
Spivack o.
Ssabanejew-Frank o.
staging o.
Steinach o.
Stoppa o.
string o.
Swenson o.
Tanner o.
Thal fundic patch o.
Thiersch anal incontinence o.
Torek o.
transection and devascularization o.
Tuffier o.
Turnbull multiple ostomy o.
Turner-Warwick o.
van Hook o.
Vidal o.
Virag o.
Vogel o.
Volkmann o.
Voronoff o.
Wangensteen o.
Waugh-Clagett o.
Wheelhouse o.
Whipple o.
White o.
Whitehead o.
Wood o.
Young o.

Young-Dees o.
Young-Dees-Leadbetter o.
operative
o. cholangiogram
o. cholangiography
o. choledochoscopy
o. decompression
o. laparoscope
o. morbidity
o. mortality rate
o. staging
ophthalmoplegia
internuclear o.
opiate
o. antagonist
o. receptor
opioid
o. antagonist
o. antidiarrheal
antisecretory o.
endogenous o.
o. peptide
o. receptor agonist (ORA)
opioid-mediated pruritus
opisthorchiasis
Opisthorchis
O. felineus
O. sinensis
O. viverrini
Opitz-Frias syndrome
opium
deodorized tincture of o. (DTO)
Opmilas 144 Plus laser system
opportunistic
o. complication
o. infection
opposure
Op-Site dressing
opsonic activity
opsonization
opsonized zymosan
optical
o. coherence tomography (OCT)
o. crystallography
o. esophagoscope
o. fiber
o. laser knife
o. multichannel analyzer system
o. needle
o. switch
o. ureterotome
o. urethrotome knife

optic neuropathy
optics
Wappler cystoscope with microlens o.
Optilume prostate balloon dilator
Optimal Regimen Cures *Helicobacter-* **Induced Dyspepsia (ORCHID)**
Optimental
optimization
optimizing
o. HLA matching
o. human leukocyte antigen matching
optimum cooling range
Optiray
Optiview obturator
Opti-Vue plastic barrel
OPUS-1
Ausonics O.
ORA
opioid receptor agonist
Oracit
orad propagation
Oragrafin contrast medium
oral
o. barium suspension
o. bile acid (OBA)
o. cholecystogogic
o. cholecystogram (OCG)
o. cholecystography
o. disease
o. intubation
o. iron
o. iron preparation
o. lavage
o. leukoplakia
Nor-tet O.
Permitil O.
Protostat O.
o. purge
o. rehydration
o. rehydration solution (ORS)
o. rehydration therapy (ORT)
o. suction catheter
Sumycin O.
o. thermometer
o. thrush
o. tolerance
o. transmission
o. ulcer
Oralgen
Oramide

O

NOTES

Orandi
O. knife
O. technique
orange bezoar
orange-colored tonsil
Orasone
OraSure salivary collection device
OraVax vaccine
orbiculare
Pityrosporon o.
orbital
o. depression
o. exenteration gastroscopic access
technique
Orcein stain
orchalgia
orchalis
adiposis o.
orchectomy
orchialgia
orchiatrophy
orchichorea
ORCHID
Optimal Regimen Cures *Helicobacter*-
Induced Dyspepsia
ORCHID study
orchid
calix o.
orchidalgia
orchidectomy
partial o.
radical o.
orchidic
orchiditis
orchidocelioplasty
orchidoepididymectomy
orchidometer
Prader o.
punched-out o.
Test-Size o.
orchidopexy
Fowler-Stephens o.
prophylactic o.
orchidoptosis
orchidorrhaphy
orchidotherapy
orchidotomy
orchiectomy
prophylactic o.
radical inguinal o.
orchiencephaloma
orchiepididymitis
orchilytic
orchiocatabasis
orchiocele
orchiococcus
orchiodynia
orchiomyeloma

orchioncus
orchioneuralgia
orchiopathy
orchiopexy
Bevan o.
Cabot-Nesbit o.
eversion o.
Fowler-Stephens o.
laparoscopic o.
Prentiss o.
scrotal pouch o.
staged o.
standard o.
Torek o.
transseptal o.
two-step o.
vasal pedicle o.
orchioplasty
orchiorrhaphy
orchiotherapy
orchiotomy
orchis
orchitic
orchitis
filarial o.
metastatic o.
o. parotidea
Salmonella enteritidis o.
spermatogenic granulomatous o.
traumatic o.
o. variolosa
orchitolytic
orchotomy
orciprenaline
O'Regan
O. hemorrhoid ligator
O. procedure
Oresus Potentest test
Oretic
Oreticyl
organ
o. allocation policy
artificial o.
o. donation
o. of Giraldes
O. Procurement Program
radiosensitive o.
o. transplantation
well-matched o.
o. of Zuckerkandl
organelle
organic
o. conditioning film
o. impotence
o. muscle
o. neurologic disease
o. nitrate

organism
    Campylobacter-like o. (CLO)
    enteropathic o.
    gram-positive o.
    Helicobacter pylori-like o. (HPLO)
    microaerophilic o.
    pyogenic o.
    terrestrial o.
    urea-splitting o.
organized germinal center
organoaxial gastric volvulus
organogenesis
organomegaly
organoscopy
orgastic impotence
Oriental
    O. cholangiohepatitis
    O. schistosomiasis
orienting reflex
orifice
    appendiceal o.
    bell-shaped o.
    biliary o.
    duodenal o.
    epispadiac o.
    fistulous o.
    pancreatic o.
    papillary o.
    sharp-edged o.
    ureteral o.
orificial
orificium, pl. **orificia**
    o. urethrae externum internum
    o. urethrae externum muliebris
    o. urethrae externum virilis
origin
    neoplastic o.
    O. trocar
original endowment
O-ring
Orion model AE 940 ion analyzer
orlistat
Ormond
    O. disease
    O. syndrome
ornidazole
ornithine
    o. carbamoyl transferase deficiency
    o. decarboxylase (ODC)
ornithine-aspartate
orocecal transit time (OCTT)
oroesophageal overtube

orogastric Ewald tube
oropharyngeal
    o. carcinoma
    o. damage
    o. dysphagia
    o. tube
ororespiratory tract
orosomucoid
orotracheal intubation
orphanin FQ
orphenadrine
Orr
    O. automatic reprocessor
    O. gall duct forceps
    O. rectal prolapse repair
Orr-Loygue transabdominal proctopexy
ORS
    oral rehydration solution
ORT
    oral rehydration therapy
Ortho
    O. Diagnostic System
    O. HCV 2.0 ELISA test system
    for hepatitis C
    O. HCV ELISA test system
    second generation
orthochromatic dye
Orthoclone OKT3
Orthohepadnavirus
Orthopara-DDD
orthophosphate
orthoplasty
    penile o.
orthostatic
    o. change
    o. proteinuria
orthostatism
orthotopic
    o. appendicocystostomy
    o. bladder
    o. bladder augmentation
    o. bladder substitution
    o. colonic reservoir
    o. continent reservoir
    o. hemi-Kock operation
    o. ileal neobladder
    o. liver transplant (OLT)
    o. liver transplantation
    o. reconstruction
    o. remodeled ileocolonic reservoir
    o. ureterocele

O

NOTES

orthotopic *(continued)*
    o. urinary diversion
    o. voiding
Orthotripter
    OssaTron O.
orthovoltage teletherapy
Orthoxine
Orudis
OS
    overall survival
OSB gastrostomy device
Osbon
    O. ErecAid VCD
    O. pressure-point tension ring
Os-Cal
oscheal
oscheitis
oschelephantiasis
oscheocele
oscheohydrocele
oscheolith
oscheoma
oscheoncus
oscheoplasty
oscillation
    myenteric potential o.
oscillatory potential
oscilloscope
    Tektronix digital o.
Osler
    O. node
    O. syndrome II
Osler-Weber-Rendu
    O.-W.-R. disease
    O.-W.-R. syndrome
    O.-W.-R. telangiectasia
Osmette osmometer
osmium tetroxide
Osmoglyn
osmolality
    body fluid o.
    diurnal urine o.
    medullary interstitial o.
    plasma o.
    urine o.
osmolar clearance
osmolarity
    o. gap
    o. of the ink
    serum o.
    urine o. (Uosm)
Osmolite HN enteral feeding
osmolyte
osmometer
    Model 5500 vapor pressure o.
    Osmette o.
osmoreceptor
OSMO reverse osmosis unit

osmotherapy
osmotic
    o. cathartic
    o. demyelination syndrome
    o. diarrhea
    o. diuresis
    o. diuretic
    o. laxative
    o. load
    o. nephrosis
    o. stimulus
OssaTron Orthotripter
osseous metaplasia
ossification
    metaplastic o.
osteitis pubis
osteoarthropathy
    hypertrophic o.
osteoblast-derived
osteoblast-like proliferation
osteocalcin
osteoclast
    acid phosphate o.
    o. maturation
osteoclast-activating factor
osteoclast-like giant cell (OCLG)
osteodystrophy
    Albright hereditary o. (AHO)
    azotemic o.
    hepatic o.
    renal o.
osteogenic
    o. differentiation
    o. sarcoma
osteomalacia
    dialysis o.
    low turnover o. (LTOM)
osteoonychodysplasia
    hereditary o.
osteopenia
osteophyte
    esophageal o.
osteopontin
osteoporosis
osteosarcoma
    bladder o.
osteotomy
    anterior innominate o.
    Dickson o.
    pelvic o.
ostia (*pl. of* ostium)
ostial
    o. artery atherosclerosis
    o. atherosclerotic plaque
ostiomeatal
ostium, pl. **ostia**
    o. appendicis vermiformis
    o. ileocecale

o. pyloricum
o. urethrae externum feminae
o. urethrae externum masculinae
o. urethrae internum
o. valvae ilealis

ostomate
ostomy
o. appliance
O. Assessment Inventory (OAI)
o. bag
ConvaTec Durahesive Wafer o.
o. loop
o. skin
o. takedown

ostreotoxism
O'Sullivan-O'Connor abdominal retractor
O'Sullivan scoring system
OTA
oligoteratoasthenozoospermia
12-O-tetradecanoylphorbol-13-acetate (TPA, tPA)
phorbol ester 12-O.-t.-a. (phorbol ester TPA)
Otis
O. anoscope
O. sound
O. urethrotome
O. urethrotomy

otitidis-caviarum
Nocardia o.-c.
otolaryngologic manifestation
Otrivin
Ott/Mayo Channel Sampling kit
ouabain
ouabainlike substance (OLS)
out
coring o.
outcome
health o.
long-term o.
poor long-term o.
o. predictor
o. and process assessment
short-term survival o.
outer
o. cortical blood flow (OCBF)
o. crossbar
o. diameter (OD)
o. inflammatory protein
o. medulla

o. medullary collecting duct
o. medullary ischemia
outflow
hepatic venous o.
mean venous o. (MVO)
o. obstruction
pulmonary o.
o. tract
vagal efferent o.
outlet
bladder o.
o. delay
o. dysfunction
gastric o.
o. obstruction
o. obstruction constipation
pyloric o.
outlier syndrome
outline
gastric o.
out-of-scope lithotriptor
outpatient endoscopy
output
basal acid o. (BAO)
bile phospholipid o. (BPO)
bile salt o. (BSO)
biliary cholesterol o. (BCO)
cardiac o.
intake and o. (I&O)
maximal acid o. (MAO)
meal-stimulated acid o. (MSAO)
peak acid o. (PAO)
urinary o.
ova (*pl. of* ovum)
oval
o. esophagoscope
o. fat body
o. snare
ovalbumin
oval-form colonic groove
ovalis
fossa o.
oval-open esophagoscope
ovaria (*pl. of* ovarium)
ovarian
o. artery
o. cancer
o. carcinoma
o. dermoid cyst
o. disease
o. endometrioma
o. enlargement

O

NOTES

537

ovarian *(continued)*
  o. fibroma
  o. hyperstimulation syndrome
  o. overstimulation syndrome
  o. remnant syndrome
  o. teratoma
  o. vein syndrome
ovarii
  stroma o.
  struma o.
  tunica albuginea o.
ovarium, pl. **ovaria**
  o. masculinum
ovary
  streak o.
ovatus
  Bacteroides o.
overactive bladder
overactivity
  detrusor muscle o.
overall
  o. mortality
  o. survival (OS)
over-and-over suture
overdistention, overdistension
  bladder o.
overdose (OD)
  acetaminophen o.
overdosing
overexpression
  p53 o.
overflow
  o. aminoaciduria
  o. fecal incontinence
  o. proteinuria
  o. theory
overgrowth
  bacterial o.
  candidal o.
  gastric bacterial o. (GBO)
  small intestinal bacterial o. (SIBO)
  tube o.
  tumor o.
  yeast o.
overlap
  o. syndrome
  o. system n
overlapping sphincteroplasty
overload
  African iron o.
  hepatic copper o.
  nitrogen o.
  transfusional iron o.
  volume o.
overlying clot
overproduction
  oxalate o.
overreactive puborectalis

oversedation
over-the-endoscope Witzel dilator
over-the-wire
  o.-t.-w. balloon catheter
  o.-t.-w. set
  o.-t.-w. technique
overt nephropathy
overtube
  Christopher-Williams o.
  flexible endoscopic o.
  Mill-Rose flexible endoscopic o.
  negative pressure o.
  oroesophageal o.
  rotational colonoscope o.
  o. sheath
  split o.
  Steigmann-Goff endoscopic ligature o.
  Williams varix injection o.
oviductal fluid
oviduct epithelia
ovoid fungus
ovum, pl. **ova**
  ova, cysts, and parasites (OCP)
  ova and parasites (O&P)
oxacillin
oxacillin-associated anicteric hepatitis
oxalate
  calcium o.
  o. calculus
  o. crystal
  dietary o.
  o. intestinal absorption
  o. metabolism
  o. nephropathy
  o. overproduction
  urinary o.
oxalic acid
oxaliplatin
oxaloacetate
Oxalobacter formigenes
oxalosis
  primary o.
oxaluria
  calcium o.
  enteric o.
oxamniquine
oxandrolone treatment
oxaprozin
oxatomide
oxazepam
oxcarbazepine
oxidant
  o. injury
  iron-dependent o.
oxidant-trapping potential
oxidase
  o. cytosolic factor

diamine o.
NADPH o.
xanthine o.

oxidation
arachidonic acid o.
substrate o.
xanthine o.

oxidative
o. burst
o. cell injury
o. phosphorylation
slow-twitch o.
o. stress

oxidative-glycolytic fiber

oxide
deuterium o.
donor of nitric o.
endothelium-derived nitric o.
(EDNO)
ethylene o.
magnesium o.
mercuric o.
nitric o. (NO)
nitrous o.
propylene o.
ultrasmall superparamagnetic iron o.
(USPIO)

oxidized
o. LDL
o. lipoprotein
o. low density lipoprotein (Ox-
LDL)

oxidoreductase activity

oxime
sugar o.

oximetry
pulse o.

oxine

Ox-LDL
oxidized low density lipoprotein

oxocortisol-18

oxybutynin
o. chloride
intravesical o.

Oxycel cotton

oxychlorosene sodium

oxycodone

oxygen (O_2)
blood gas on o.
o. desaturation
fractional percentage of inspired o.
(FIO_2)
hyperbaric o.
o. radical
o. saturation
o. saturation index (ISO_2)

oxygen-15

oxygenating mouthguard

oxygenation
medullary o.

oxygenator
membrane o.

oxygen-derived free radical

oxygen-free radical

Oxyguard oxygenating mouthguard

oxymorphone

oxyntic
o. cell
o. gland
o. mucosa
o. mucosal gastritis

oxyphenbutazone

oxyphencyclimine hydrochloride

oxyphenonium

oxytoca
Klebsiella o.

oxytocin

Oxyuris

NOTES

O

P

P blood group system
P cell

P-32, ^{32}P

phosphorus-32

P-900

900 mOsmolar amino acid-glucose
solution

p21

p53

p53 allelotyping
p53 antibody
p53 assay
p53 expression
p53 gene
p53 immunohistochemical stain
p53 immunohistochemistry
p53 mutation
p53 nuclear protein
p53 nuclear staining
p53 overexpression
p53 protein
p53 protooncogene
p53 reactivity
p53 tumor suppressor gene analysis

p15 **gene**
P15/INK4B **gene**
p16 **gene**
p18 **gene**
P21/WAF1 **gene**
P23b Statham pressure transducer
P24 antigen
P27Kip1 **gene**
P450 function
PA

plasminogen activator

PAA

periampullary adenoma

10Pa Amicon chamber
PAb

protein antibody
PAb 1801 monoclonal antibody

PABA

paraaminobenzoic acid
PABA test

P-A-C
PACAP

pituitary adenylate cyclase activating
polypeptide

paced rhythm
pacemaker

p. cell
Enterra gastrointestinal p.

pachycholia
pachychymia

pacinian corpuscle
**Pacis BCG bladder cancer
immunotherapy**
pack

gauze p.
laparotomy p.
moist laparotomy p.
petrolatum gauze p.

package

lymphatic p.

Packard Auto-Gamma 5650 analyzer
packed red blood cells
packing

Adaptic p.
p. forceps
p. fraction
gelatin sponge p.
Mikulicz p.

paclitaxel
Pacquin ureterolysis
pad

abdominal fat p.
abdominal laparotomy p.
Active Living incontinence p.
antimesenteric fat p.
bed p.
bulbocavernosus fat p.
p. cover
dinner p.
esophagogastric fat p.
fat p.
ileocecal fat p.
lap p.
laparotomy p.
Martius fat p.
Mikulicz p.
perineal p.
Sani Pads medicated cleansing p.
p. testing
p. test for urinary incontinence
p. urinary incontinence test

padding

absorbent p.
Spenco p.

Padua bladder urinary pouch
Paecilomyces
PAF

platelet-activating factor

Pagano

P. technique ureterocolonic
anastomosis
P. ureteral anastomosis

PAGE

polyacrylamide gel electrophoresis

Page kidney

P

Pagenstecher circle
Paget
      P. disease of perianal area
      P. extramammary disease
      P. perianal disease
pagetoid
Pagitane
PAH
    paraaminohippurate
    paraaminohippuric
      PAH acid
      PAH clearance
PAI
    plasminogen activator inhibitor
PAI-1
    plasminogen activator inhibitor type 1
PAI-2
    plasminogen activator inhibitor type 2
pain
      abdominal p.
      acute flank p.
      biliary p.
      biliary tract p. (BTP)
      bladder p.
      boring p.
      burning p.
      chest p.
      colicky abdominal p.
      constricting p.
      p. control
      crampy abdominal p.
      deep p.
      diffuse p.
      drug-induced p.
      dull p.
      epicritic p.
      epigastric p.
      exacerbation of p.
      exertion-induced p.
      exquisite p.
      p. fiber
      flank p.
      functional p.
      gnawing p.
      hunger p.
      intermittent p.
      knife-like p.
      lancinating p.
      localized p.
      loin p.
      nagging p.
      NIH Classification Category III
        inflammatory and noninflammatory
        chronic pelvic p.
      nocturnal p.
      noncardiac chest p.
      onset of p.
      palliation of p.

      parietal p.
      perianal p.
      perirectal p.
      poorly localized p.
      postligation p.
      postprandial p.
      posture-dependent p.
      protopathic p.
      radiating p.
      rebound p.
      recurrent abdominal p. (RAP)
      referred p.
      remission of p.
      retrosternal chest p.
      scrotal p.
      severe p.
      somatic p.
      steady p.
      sudden onset of p.
      tearing p.
      testicular p.
      triangle of p.
      unrelenting p.
      unrelieved p.
      unremitting p.
      visceral p.
painful
      p. defecation
      p. hematuria
painless
      p. hematuria
      p. jaundice
      p. rectal bleeding
**pain-predominant irritable bowel
  syndrome**
paint
      Castellani p.
painter's colic
Pak
      Trovan/Zithromax Compliance P.
palate
      cleft p.
      smoker's p.
palatine pillar
palatinus
      torus p.
palatoglossus muscle
palatopharyngeal fold
palatopharyngeus muscle
Palco enuretic alarm system
pale
      p. cell
      p. stool
Paleolithic diet
palindrome
palindromic rheumatism
palisade-type vein

palladium-103
>p. seed implant
>transperineal p.

palliation
>p. of malignant large bowel obstruction
>p. of pain

palliative
>p. cystectomy
>p. decompression
>p. exeresis
>p. nephrectomy
>p. surgery
>p. therapy

pallidum
>*Treponema p.*

pallidus
>raphe p.

pallor
>mucosal p.

palmar
>p. erythema
>p. grasp

palmaris
>tylosis p.

palmatus
>penis p.

Palmaz
>P. balloon-expandable stent
>P. Corinthian biliary stent and delivery system

Palmaz-Schatz biliary stent
Palmer acid test for peptic ulcer
palmin test
palmitin test
Palomo
>P. operation
>P. procedure
>P. technique

palonosetron
palpable
>p. adenopathy
>p. cord
>p. gallbladder
>p. kidney
>p. mass
>p. pyloric olive
>p. rib diastasis
>p. stool

palpably normal
palpating probe

palpation
>bladder p.
>p. tenderness

palpatory proteinuria
palpebrae
>paraphimosis p.

palsy
>cerebral p.

PAM
>pancreatic acinar metaplasia

Pamelor
Pamine
Pamisyl
pamoate
>pyrantel p.

pampiniformis
>plexus p.

pampiniform plexus
pampinocele
PAN
>puromycin aminonucleoside nephropathy
>puromycin aminonucleoside nephrosis

panacinar
>p. disease
>p. emphysema

Panafil ointment
pan-bud anomaly
p-ANC
>perinuclear antineutrophil cytoplasmic
>p-ANC genetic marker

p-ANCA
>perinuclear antineutrophil cytoplasmic antibody

pancake kidney
pancolectomy
pancolitis
>steroid responsive p.

pancolonoscopy
pancreas
>aberrant p.
>p. accessorium
>accessory p.
>acinarization of p.
>anlage of p.
>annular p.
>Aselli p.
>capsule of p.
>Christmas tree appearance of p.
>divided p.
>p. divisum (PD)
>ectopic p.

NOTES

P

pancreas *(continued)*
    endoscopic retrograde
      parenchymography of p. (ERPP)
    exocrine p.
    fibrofatty infiltration of the p.
    head of p.
    heterotopic p.
    intraductal papillary and mucinous
      tumors of p. (IPMY)
    p. lesion
    lesser p.
    lobule of p.
    neck of p.
    solid and cystic tumor of the p.
      (SCTP)
    tail of p.
    p. transplantation
    unciform p.
    uncinate process of p.
    Willis p.
    Winslow p.
Pancrease
    P. MT 4, 10, 16, 20
pancreas-kidney
    simultaneous p.-k. (SPK)
    p.-k. transplant
pancreatalgia
pancreatectomy
    distal p.
    en bloc distal p.
    left-to-right subtotal p.
    partial p.
    subtotal p.
    total p.
    Whipple p.
pancreatic
    p. acinar cell
    p. acinar cell carcinoma
    p. acinar metaplasia (PAM)
    p. acinus
    p. alpha-amylase
    p. amylase
    p. ascariasis
    p. ascites
    p. bladder
    p. blood flow
    p. calcification
    p. calculus
    p. cancer (PC)
    p. cancer marker
    p. carcinoma (PCA)
    p. cholera
    p. cholera syndrome
    p. colic
    p. cutaneous fistula
    p. cyst
    p. diabetes
    p. diastase

p. disease
p. diverticulum
p. duct
p. ductal hypertension
p. ductal morphological change
p. duct-choledochus channel
p. duct disruption
p. duct encasement
p. duct manipulation
p. ductogram
p. duct pressure (PDP)
p. duct sphincter (PDS)
p. duct sphincterotomy
p. duct stent
p. duct stone
p. duct stricture
p. endopeptidase
p. endoprosthesis
p. enema
p. enzyme
p. enzyme replacement therapy
p. exocrine dysfunction
p. exocrine insufficiency
p. exopeptidase
p. fibrosis
p. flare
p. fluid collection (PFC)
p. glandular necrosis
p. hamartoma
p. injury
p. intraluminal radiation therapy
p. islet cell
p. islet cell carcinoma
p. islet cell transplantation
p. islet cell tumor
p. juice
p. lesion
p. lipase
p. lipase deficiency
p. lymphangiectasia
p. mucinous cystadenocarcinoma
p. oncofetal antigen (POA)
p. orifice
p. papillary stenosis
p. parenchyma
p. phlegmon
p. polypeptide (PP)
p. polypeptide-secreting tumor
  (PPoma)
p. polypeptide stain
p. pseudocyst
p. pseudocyst abscess
p. pseudocystogastrostomy
p. rendezvous
p. rest
p. sarcoidosis
p. secretory flow rate (PSFR)
p. secretory test

p. secretory trypsin inhibitor (PSTI)
p. sepsis
p. sepsis in acute pancreatitis
p. sphincteroplasty
p. steatorrhea
p. stone protein (PSP)
p. tail resection
p. transpapillary stenting
p. trauma
p. tree
p. tumor diagnosis
p. tumor localization

pancreatica
achylia p.
ansa p.
diarrhea p.
p. magna artery
sialorrhea p.

pancreaticobiliary
p. common channel
p. disease
p. ductal junction
p. ductal system
p. endoscopy
p. malignancy
p. maljunction
p. reflux
p. septum
p. sphincter
p. stricture
p. tract
p. tree

pancreaticocholedochoductal junction
pancreaticocystostomy
pancreaticoduodenal
anterior superior p. (ASPD)
p. arteriography
p. transplantation
p. vein
p. venous drainage

pancreaticoduodenectomy
pyloric-sparing p.
Whipple p.

pancreaticoduodenostomy
Child p.
Dennis-Varco p.
Waugh-Clagett p.
Whipple p.

pancreaticogastric anastomosis
pancreaticogastrostomy
pancreaticohepatic syndrome

pancreaticojejunostomy
caudal p.
Duval distal p.
lateral p.
longitudinal p.
Puestow p.
Roux-en-Y p.
p. stenosis

pancreaticopleural fistula
pancreaticosplenic omentum
pancreatic-portal vein fistula
pancreaticus
ansa p.
ductus p.
hemosuccus p.
liquor p.
succus p.

pancreatin
pancreatis
arteria caudae p.
caput p.
corpus p.
facies anterior p.
facies inferior p.
facies posterior p.

pancreatitis
acquired p.
acute edematous p. (AEP)
acute gallstone p. (AGP)
acute hemorrhagic p.
acute recurrent p. (ARP)
acute relapsing p.
alcoholic p.
alcohol-induced p.
biliary p.
calcareous p.
calcific p.
calcifying p.
capsula p.
centrilobular p.
chronic p. (CP)
chronic alcoholic p. (CAP)
chronic calcifying p. (CCP)
chronic relapsing p.
coagulopathy p.
diffuse p.
drug-induced acute p.
edematous p.
endoscopic sphincterotomy-
  induced p.
familial p.
focal p.

NOTES

P

pancreatitis *(continued)*
    fulminating p.
    gallstone p.
    Glasgow criteria for severity of p.
    groove p.
    hemoductal p.
    hemorrhagic necrotizing p.
    hereditary p. (HP)
    idiopathic fibrosing p.
    idiopathic recurrent p. (IRP)
    inflammatory p.
    interstitial p.
    microlithiasis-induced p.
    mumps p.
    necrotizing p.
    nodular p.
    nutritional p.
    obstructive p.
    pancreatic sepsis in acute p.
    pentamidine-induced p.
    perilobar p.
    phlegmonous p.
    post-ERCP-induced p.
    postprocedure p.
    purulent p.
    Ranson criteria for severity of p.
    recurrent p.
    relapsing acute p.
    segmentary p.
    tropical calcific p.
    ventral chronic calcific p.
pancreatitis-related
    p.-r. bleeding
    p.-r. hemorrhage
pancreatobiliary
    p. canal
    p. region
pancreatocholangiography
    retrograde p.
pancreatocholecystostomy
pancreatoduodenal cancer
pancreatoduodenectomy
    pylorus-preserving p. (PPPD)
pancreatoduodenostomy
pancreatogastrostomy
pancreatogenic, pancreatogenous
    p. diarrhea
pancreatogram
    rat-tail appearance on p.
pancreatography
    endoscopic digital p. (EDP)
    endoscopic retrograde p. (ERP)
    magnetic resonance p. (MRP)
    retrograde p.
    three-dimensional CT p. (3D-CTP)
pancreatojejunostomy
    cystolateral p.
    retrocolic end-to-end p.

pancreatolith
pancreatolithectomy
pancreatolithiasis
pancreatolithotomy
pancreatolysis
pancreatolytic
pancreatomegaly
pancreatomy
pancreatopathy
pancreatoscope
    peroral electronic p. (PEPS)
    ultrathin p.
pancreatoscopic laser lithotripsy (PSLL)
pancreatoscopy
    peroral p. (POPS)
pancreatotomy
Pancrecarb MS-8
pancreectomy
pancrelipase
pancreolith
pancreopathy
pancreoprivic
pancreoscopy
    infragastric p.
pancreozymin
Pancrex
pancuronium
pandysautonomia
panel
    Nephrolithiasis Clinical
      Guidelines P.
panel-reactive antibody (PRA)
panendoscope
    cap-fitted p.
    flexible forward-viewing p.
    Olympus GIF-D-series p.
    Olympus GIF-XQ-series p.
    Storz p.
    Wolf rigid p.
panendoscopy
    fiberoptic p.
    lower p.
    primary p.
    upper gastrointestinal p.
panenteroscopy
    laparoscopically assisted p.
Paneth cell
pangastritis
    atrophic p.
    nonatrophic p.
panlobular emphysema
panmalabsorption
panmucosal inflammatory cell
  infiltration
panmural cystitis
Panmycin
panniculalgia
panniculectomy

panniculitis
    mesenteric p. (MP)
    scrotal p.
panniculus, pl. **panniculi**
    hanging p.
pannus
Panoview rod-lens ureteroscope
panproctocolectomy
pantaloon hernia
Pantoloc tablet
Pantopaque
pantoprazole
    p. sodium
    p. sodium tablet
pantothenic
    p. acid
    p. acid deficiency-induced colitis
pants
    Ashton p.
    Dignity incontinence p.
    Endo p.
    Holyoke p.
    Kleinert p.
    Suretys p.
    Ultrafem p.
pants-over-vest
    p.-o.-v. hernial repair
    p.-o.-v. herniorrhaphy
Panzer gallbladder scissors
PAO
    peak acid output
PAOGRP
    peak acid output after gastrin-releasing
      peptide
PAOPg
    peak acid output after pentagastrin
      stimulation
PAP
    prostatic acid phosphatase
    pulmonary artery pressure
Pap
    Papanicolaou
      Pap smear
      Pap test
papain
Papanicolaou (Pap)
    P. method
    P. stain
papaverine
    p. hydrochloride
    p. injection

paper
    theoretical p.
PAP-HT25 cell
papilla, pl. **papillae**
    balloon dilation of the p.
    ballooning of p.
    bile p.
    bulging p.
    duodenal p.
    p. duodeni major
    p. duodeni minor
    foliate p.
    frenulum of duodenal p.
    fungiform p.
    glans penis p.
    ileal p.
    p. ilealis
    p. ileocaecalis
    ileocecal p.
    intradiverticular p.
    laparoscopic transcystic duct
      stenting of p.
    major p.
    minor p.
    necrosis of renal p.
    patulous p.
    renal p.
    p. of Santorini
    sloughed p.
    Suda classification of p. (type I,
      II, III)
    vallate p.
    p. of Vater
papillary
    p. adenocarcinoma
    p. adenoma
    p. cystitis
    p. gastric carcinoma
    p. hyperplasia
    p. lesion
    p. manometry
    p. necrosis
    p. orifice
    p. renal cancer
    p. renal cell carcinoma
    p. stenosis
    p. tip
    p. transitional cell carcinoma
papillate
papillation
papilledema
papilliferous

NOTES

P

papilliform
papillitis
papilloma
    bladder inverted p.
    esophageal squamous p.
    gingival p.
    hirsutoid p.
    inverted p.
    p. of renal pelvis
    sporadic gingival p.
    squamous cell p. (SCP)
    p. venereum
    villous p.
papilloma-carcinoma sequence
papillomatosis
    biliary p.
    p. coronae
    p. of intrahepatic bile duct
papillomatous neotransformation
papillomavirus
    genital human p.
    human p. (HPV)
    human p. 16 (HPV 16)
papillotome
    30-30 p.
    Accuratome pre-curved p.
    Bard Companion p.
    Bilisystem wire-guided p.
    Classen-Demling p.
    Cremer-Ikeda p.
    double-lumen tapered-tip p.
    dual-lumen p.
    Erlangen p.
    Frimberger-Karpiel 12 o'clock p.
    Howell Rotatable BII p.
    Huibregtse-Katon p.
    Microvasive p.
    needle p.
    needle-knife p.
    Olympus needle-knife p.
    Piggyback needle-knife p.
    precut p.
    shark fin p.
    Swenson p.
    Wilson-Cook p.
    Wiltek p.
papillotome/sphincterotome
    Zimmon p./s.
papillotomy
    access p.
    endoscopic p. (EPT)
    Erlangen pull-type precut p.
    laparoscopic transcystic p.
    needle-knife p. (NKP)
    needle-knife precut p. (NKPP)
    precut p.
Pap-Kaps

papule
    Bowen p.
    moist p.
    mucous p.
    pearly penile p.
papulosis
    bowenoid p.
    malignant atrophic p.
papulosquamous disorder
papulous gastropathy
Paque
    E-Z P.
Paquin
    P. repair
    P. technique
    P. ureteral reimplantation
PAR
    postanesthesia recovery
paraaminobenzoic acid (PABA)
paraaminohippurate (PAH)
    p. clearance
paraaminohippuric (PAH)
    p. acid
    p. acid synthetase
paraaminosalicylate hypersensitivity
para-ANC antibody
paraaortic
    p. lymphadenectomy
    p. region
parabola
paracancerous tissue
paracecal appendix
paracellular
    p. pathway
    p. route
paracentesis
    abdominal p.
    diagnostic p.
    large-volume p. (LVP)
paracervical tenderness
paracetamol
    p. absorption
    p. absorption test
parachute reflex
Paracoccidioides brasiliensis
paracoccidioidomycosis
paracolic
    p. abscess
    p. groove
    p. gutter
paracollicular biopsy
paracolostomy
    p. hernia
    p. herniation
paraconal fascia
paracrine
    p. cell

p. factor
p. peptide
paradigm
Sternberg p.
paradoxical
p. diarrhea
p. incontinence
p. puborectalis contraction
p. renal response
p. sphincter reaction
paradoxic motion
paradoxus
pulsus p.
paraductal adenopathy
paraduodenal
p. fold
p. hernia
p. pseudocyst
paradysenteriae
Shigella p.
paraesophageal
p. collateral vein
p. diaphragmatic hernia
p. hernia (type I, II)
p. hiatal hernia
p. varix
paraesophagogastric devascularization
paraexstrophy skin flap
paraffin-embedded
p.-e. specimen
p.-e. tissue
paraffinoma
paraffin-section light microscopy
paraformaldehyde
parafrenal abscess
paraganglioma
paragastric pseudocyst
paragenitalis
paraglobulinuria
paraglomerular space
parahaemolyticus
Vibrio p.
parahiatal hernia
paraileostomal hernia
paraisopropyliminodiacetic acid (PIPIDA)
parakeratosis
parallel plate dialyzer
paralysis, pl. **paralyses**
esophageal p.
paralytic
p. colonic obstruction
p. ileus

p. incontinence
p. intestinal obstruction
p. secretion
paralytica
dysphagia p.
paralyticus
ileus p.
parameatal-based flap
paramedian incision
parameter
anthropomorphic p.
chronobiological p.
clinical p.
clotting p.
DIC p.
kinetic p.
prostate-specific antigen-based p.
PSA-based p.
paraneoplastic
p. dermatomyositis
p. syndrome
paranephric abscess
paranephritis
lipomatous p.
paranephroma
paranitroaniline release
paraparesis
spastic p.
tropical spastic p.
parapelvic cyst
paraperitoneal nephrectomy
paraphimosis palpebrae
paraplegia
paraproctitis
paraprostatitis
paraproteinemia
parapubic hernia
paraquat
paraquat-induced upper gastrointestinal injury
pararectal
p. abscess
p. fistula
p. line
p. pouch
pararectus incision
parasagittal plane
parasite
p. examination
hemoflagellate p.
intestinal p.
isosporan p.

NOTES

P

549

parasite *(continued)*
    ova and p.
    ova, cysts, and p.'s (OCP)
    protozoan p.
    stool for ova and p.'s
    urinalysis sediment microscopy p.
parasitemia
parasitic
    p. chylocele
    p. cyst
    p. infection
    p. infestation
    p. leiomyoma
    p. liver disease
    p. peritonitis
    p. prostatitis
parasitizing macrophage
parasitology
paraspadia, paraspadias
paraspinal musculature
paraspinous
    p. aspect
    p. muscle
parastomal hernia
parasympathetic
    p. postganglionic neuron
    p. preganglionic neuron
    p. projection
parasympatholytic drug
parasympathomimetic
    p. agent
    p. anticholinesterase
    p. drug
paratesticular
    p. fat
    p. leiomyosarcoma
    p. malignancy
    p. neoplasm
    p. rhabdomyosarcoma
    p. tumor
parathyroid
    p. disease
    p. hormone (PTH)
    p. hormone-related polypeptide
    p. hyperplasia
    p. imaging
paratuberculosis
    Mycobacterium p.
paratyphi
    Salmonella p.
paraumbilical
    p. vein
    p. vein tumor (PUVT)
paraureteric
paraurethra
paraurethral
    p. cyst
    p. gland

paraurethrales
    ductus p.
paraurethritis
paravaginal
    p. fascial repair
    p. pedicle
paravariceal
    p. fibrosis
    p. injection
    p. sclerotherapy
paravertebral neuroblastoma
paravesical
    p. fossa
    p. pouch
paregoric
parenchyma
    allograft p.
    hepatic p.
    inhomogeneity of p.
    liver p.
    pancreatic p.
    renal p.
parenchymal
    p. atrophy
    p. collapse
    p. hematoma
    p. inflammation
    p. jaundice
    p. liver disease
    p. sparing surgery
    p. tissue
    p. tumor
parenchymatous
    p. acute renal failure
    p. nephritis
parenchymography
    endoscopic retrograde p. (ERP)
parenteral
    p. alimentation
    p. diarrhea
    p. feeding
    p. guanethidine
    p. hyperalimentation
    p. immunization
    p. methyldopa
    p. nutrition
paresthesia
    lateral cutaneous p.
paretic impotence
pargyline
paries, pl. **parietes**
parietal
    p. cell
    p. cell index
    p. cell vagotomy (PCV)
    p. epithelium
    p. fistula
    p. hernia

p. pain
p. peritoneum
**Parietex composite mesh for hernia
  surgery**
parietitis
parietocolic fold
parietography
  gastric p.
parietosplanchnic
Paris renal adenocarcinoma
Parker-Kerr
  P.-K. closed method
  P.-K. closed method of end-to-end
    enteroenterostomy
  P.-K. suture
Parker retractor
Parkinson disease
parkinsonian gait
Parks
  P. ileal reservoir
  P. ileoanal anastomosis
  P. ileoanal reservoir
  P. ileostomy pouch
  P. method of anal fistulotomy
  P. partial sphincterotomy
  P. retractor
  P. staged fistulotomy
Parnate
paromomycin
paromphalocele
paronychia
parorchidium
parotidea
  orchitis p.
parotid gland enlargement
parovarian
  p. cyst
  p. mass
paroxetine
paroxysmal
  p. anal hyperkinesis
  p. motor disease
  p. nocturnal hemoglobinemia
  p. nocturnal hemoglobinuria (PNH)
Parsidol
partial
  p. adrenalectomy
  p. bile outflow obstruction
  p. bladder denervation
  p. bowel obstruction
  p. cystectomy
  p. enterocele

p. external biliary diversion
p. fasting
p. fundoplication
p. gastrectomy
p. hepatectomy
p. hood assisted lift-and-cut method
p. ileal bypass
p. nephrogenic diabetes insipidus
  phenotype
p. orchidectomy
p. pancreatectomy
p. penectomy
p. polar nephrectomy
p. thromboplastin time (PTT)
p. ureteral obstruction
p. villous atrophy (PVA)
p. water bath and water cushion
p. zonal dissection (PZD)
partial-occlusion clamp
particle
  Dane p.
  food p.
  virus-like p. (VLP)
particulate
  p. radiation
  p. silicone
  p. stool
Partington-Rochelle procedure
Partin table
partition
  gastric p.
partitioning
  abdominal p.
paruresis
parvum
  Corynebacterium p.
  Cryptosporidium p.
  Diphyllobothrium p.
PAS
  periodic acid-Schiff
  PAS stain
  PAS test
PAS-AB
  periodic acid-Schiff-Alcian blue
passage
  biliary p.
  P. biliary dilatation catheter
  p. of flatus per vagina
  guidewire p.
  incomplete p.
  p. pressure

NOTES

P

passage *(continued)*
>   spontaneous fragment p.
>   p. of stool

passer
>   Carter-Thomason suture p.
>   Protect-a-Pass suture p.

passion flower

passive
>   p. chest drainage
>   p. congestion
>   p. Heymann nephritis (PHN)
>   p. incontinence
>   p. range of motion

Passport Balloon-on-a-Wire dilatation catheter

paste
>   Anatrast barium sulfate p.
>   barium p.
>   Coloplast skin barrier p.
>   Hollister Premium p.
>   iLEX skin protectant p.
>   Karaya 5 p.
>   sandy skin prepping p.
>   Stomahesive p.

Pasteurella multocida

past pointing

PAT
>   prophylactic antibiotic treatment

patch
>   Androderm testosterone
>   transdermal p.
>   aortic p.
>   bladder p.
>   Bowen p.
>   Carrel aortic p.
>   p. clamp technique
>   colic p.
>   colonic p.
>   estradiol transderm p.
>   Gore-Tex soft tissue p.
>   p. graft
>   p. graft urethroplasty
>   herald p.
>   inlet p.
>   Kugel hernia p.
>   Miniguard adhesive p.
>   mucous p.
>   omental p.
>   Peyer p.
>   Rutkow sutureless plug and p.
>   schistosomiasis sandy p.
>   Testoderm p.
>   testosterone p.
>   vein p.
>   white p.

patchiness
>   endoscopic p.
>   histologic p.

patchy
>   p. colitis
>   p. colonic ulceration
>   p. necrosis

patella disease

patency
>   biliary stent p.
>   p. rate
>   stent p.

patent
>   p. airway
>   p. processus vaginalis
>   p. urachus

Paterson-Brown-Kelly syndrome

Paterson-Kelly syndrome

pathergy phenomenon

Pathfinder
>   P. exchange guidewire
>   P. wire

Pathibamate-200

Pathilon

pathogen
>   blood-borne p.
>   enteric p.
>   invasive enteric p.
>   prokaryotic p.
>   protozoan p.

pathogenesis
>   bacterial p.

pathogenetic factor

pathogenic bacterium

pathogenicity

pathognomonic feature

pathologic
>   p. reflux
>   p. substaging

pathological
>   p. diagnosis
>   p. hypersecretory condition

pathology
>   renal p.
>   thoracic aortic p.

pathophysiology

pathway
>   antigen-dependent p.
>   antigen-independent p.
>   beta-oxidation p.
>   cholehepatic shunt p.
>   cyclooxygenase p.
>   gluconeogenic p.
>   glutamine aminotransferase p.
>   guanosine monophosphate p.
>   lipoxygenase p.
>   mitochondrial glutamate
>   dehydrogenase p.
>   monooxygenase p.
>   multisynaptic p.
>   neural p.

nonapoptotic p.
oligosynaptic p.
paracellular p.
polyol p.
receptor-mediated endocytosis p.
renal transduction p.
signal transduction p.
transduction p.

PATI
Penetrating Abdominal Trauma Index

patient
p. analgesia
asymptomatic hemodialysis p.
Child (class A,B,C) p.
cholestasia p.
diabetic p.
endoscopically normal p.
gastrectomized p.
hemodialysis p.
hypoalbuminemic p.
hypochondriacal p.
immunosuppressed p.
irrigating p.
Medicare p.
nonirrigating p.
nonvoiding p.
p. positioning
posttransplant p.
renal transplant p.
shock p.
stone-forming p.
tube-fed p.

pattern
abdominal wall venous p.
anhaustral colonic gas p.
circadian testosterone p.
cobblestone p.
colonic mucosal p.
crow's foot p.
cytometric p.
DNA ploidy p.
echo p.
fasted-to-fed p.
fasting motor p.
fed motor p.
fine gastric mucosal p.
fine reticular p.
fold p.
gallstone p.
gas p.
haustral p.
hindgut p.

histochemical p.
honeycomb p.
irregular amputated mucosal p.
manometric p.
mendelian p.
mesangial p.
mosaic duodenal mucosal p.
mucosal guideline p.
nodule-in-nodule p.
nonspecific gas p.
propulsive motor p.
Quimby p.
reticulonodular p.
rugal p.
snake-skin mucosal p.
sonographic gallstone p.
spongy p.
trabecular sinusoidal p.
vascular p.
venous p.
Wilms tumor tubuloglomerular p.

Patterson-Parker
P.-P. method
P.-P. motif

patulous
p. anus
p. cardia
p. gastroesophageal junction
p. hiatus
p. papilla
p. pylorus

Pauchet procedure
pauciimmune
p. antineutrophil cytoplasmic antibody-associated glomerulonephritis
p. crescentic glomerulonephritis
p. glomerular nephritis

paucity
bile duct p.

Paul-Mikulicz resection
Paul-Mixter tube
pause-squeeze method
Pavabid
Pavacap
Pavacen
Pavatine
PAX
PAX2 gene
PAX8 gene
Payne-DeWind jejunoileal bypass
Payne operation

NOTES

P

Payr
P. disease
P. method
P. pyloric clamp
P. pyloric forceps
P. syndrome
Pazo Hemorrhoidal Ointment
PBC
primary biliary cirrhosis
PBC-associated antibody
PBD
percutaneous biliary drainage
PBG
porphobilinogen
PBG-D
porphobilinogen deaminase
PBI
penile-brachial index
PBL
peripheral blood lymphocyte
PBMC
peripheral blood mononuclear cell
interphase PBMC
PBNS
percutaneous bladder neck stabilization
percutaneous bladder neck suspension
PBPI
penile-brachial pressure index
PBS
phosphate-buffered saline
PBS-Tween buffer
PBTE
percutaneous transhepatic liver biopsy
with tract embolization
PC
pancreatic cancer
principal cell
PC Polygraf HR device
PC10 monoclonal antibody
PCA
pancreatic carcinoma
PCa
prostate cancer
P-Cadherin
PCAR
presumed circle area ratio
PCC
peripheral cholangiocarcinoma
pneumatosis cystoides coli
PCCL
percutaneous cholecystolithotomy
PCD
pneumatic compression device
postparacentesis circulatory dysfunction
PCDAI
Pediatric Crohn Disease Activity Index
PCF20

PCF-140L pediatric colonoscope
PCI
pneumatosis cystoides intestinalis
PCIVOT
Prostate Cancer Intervention Versus
Observation Trial
PCLD
polycystic liver disease
PCM
pericellular matrix
protein-calorie malnutrition
PCN
percutaneous nephrolithotomy
PCNA
proliferating cell nuclear antigen
PCNA-labeling index (PCNA-LI)
PCNA-LI
PCNA-labeling index
PCNL
percutaneous nephrolithotomy
percutaneous nephrolithotripsy
percutaneous nephrostolithotomy
PCP
Pneumocystis carinii pneumonia
PCPS
peroral cholangiopancreatoscopy
PCR
polymerase chain reaction
protein catabolic rate
PCRC
primary colorectal cancer
PCS
peroral cholangioscopy
portacaval shunt
postcholecystectomy syndrome
PCT
porphyria cutanea tarda
portacaval transposition
proximal convoluted tubule
PCTCL
percutaneous transhepatic
cholecystolithotomy
PCV
parietal cell vagotomy
PCWP
pulmonary capillary wedge pressure
PD
pancreas divisum
peritoneal dialysis
potential difference
prostatodynia
PDAI
Perianal Crohn Disease Activity Index
PDB
preperitoneal distention balloon
PDC
peritoneal dialysis catheter

PDE
  peritoneal dialysis effluent
  phosphodiesterase
PDE5 inhibitor
PDG
  phosphate-dependent glutaminase
PDGF
  platelet-derived growth factor
PDH
  pyruvate dehydrogenase
PDL
  polycystic disease of liver
PDP
  pancreatic duct pressure
PDS
  pancreatic duct sphincter
    PDS Vicryl suture
PDT
  photodynamic therapy
PE
  pharyngoesophageal
  platinum, etoposide
  portal embolization
peak
  p. acid output (PAO)
  p. acid output after gastrin-
    releasing peptide (PAOGRP)
  p. acid output after pentagastrin
    stimulation (PAOPg)
  p. flow
  p. flow rate (PFR)
  p. pressure
  pressure p.
  p. response
  p. secretory flow rate (PSFR)
  p. secretory flow rate test
  p. urinary flow study
  p. uroflow
Péan
  P. clamp
  P. forceps
peanut
  p. agglutinin (PNA)
  p. dissector
  p. sponge
pearly
  p. papule of penis
  p. penile papule
Pearson-product correlation
Pearson syndrome
pea soup stool
peau d'orange

PEB
  platinum, etoposide, bleomycin
Pecqueti
  receptaculum P.
pecten
  anal p.
  p. of anal canal
  p. analis
  p. band
pectenitis
pectenotomy
pectin
pectinate line
pectin-base skin barrier
pectiniforme
  septum p.
pectoralis muscle
pectorlloquy
  whispered p.
pectus excavatum
pedal
  p. control venography
  p. edema
  suction foot p.
Pedialyte RS electrolyte solution
Pediapred
pediatric
  p. carcinoma
  p. colonoscope
  p. colonoscopy
  P. Crohn Disease Activity Index
    (PCDAI)
  p. cryptococcal epididymoorchitis
  p. endoscope
  p. endoscopy
  p. esophagogastroduodenoscopy
  p. feeding tube
  p. fiberscope
  p. gastroscope
  p. nasogastric tube
  P. Peritoneal Dialysis Study
    consortium
  p. stirrups
  p. urinary lithiasis
  p. urinary tract infection
  p. urology
  p. voiding dysfunction
Pediazole
pedicle
  p. clamp
  p. flap urethroplasty
  p. graft

NOTES

P

pedicle *(continued)*
  p. island flap
  kidney vascular p.
  p. muscle flap
  omental p.
  paravaginal p.
  renal p.
  vascular p.
pedicled
  p. omental graft
  p. omentoplasty
  p. omentum
  p. penile skin urethroplasty
pediculicide
pediculosis pubis
Pedi PEG tube
pedunculated polyp
pedunculation
peel-away sheath
peeping testis
Pee Wee low profile gastrostomy tube
pefloxacin
PEG
  percutaneous endoscopic gastrostomy
  polyethylene glycol
    Bard PEG
    PEG bumper
    complete replacement PEG
    CT PEG
    20F PEG tube
    PEG insertion
    PEG lavage
    Ponsky-Gauderer type PEG
    PEG pull
    PEG push
    replacement PEG
    Sacks-Vine type PEG
    Sandoz Caluso 22F, 28F super
      PEG
    PEG tube
peg
  rete p.
PEG-400 tube
PEG-assisted decompression
Pegasys
PEG-ELS
  polyethylene glycol electrolyte lavage
  solution
PEG-interferon
  P.-i. alfa-2a
  P.-i. alfa-2b powder for injection
PEG-Intron powder for injection
PEG-J
  percutaneous endoscopic
  gastrojejunostomy

PEG-JET
  percutaneous endoscopic gastrostomy and
  jejunal extension tube
    PEG-JET placement
PEG-LES
  polyethylene glycol electrolyte lavage
  solution
pegylated interferon
PEI
  percutaneous ethanol injection
  polyethylenimine
    PEI therapy
PEJ
  percutaneous endoscopic jejunostomy
    PEJ tube
pelican biopsy forceps
Pelikan brand India ink
peliosis
  bacillary p.
  hepatic p.
  p. hepaticus
  p. hepatis
pellagra
  infantile p.
pellagroid
pellagrous
pellet
  p. artifact
  radiopaque p.
  ^{99m}Tc-labeled Amberlite p.
pelleted stool
pellicular enteritis
pellucida
  zona p. (ZP)
pelves (*pl. of* pelvis)
pelvic
  p. abscess
  p. adhesion
  p. appendicitis
  p. autonomic nerve
  p. brim
  p. colon
  p. colonic surgery
  p. colon of Waldeyer
  p. diaphragm
  p. discontinuity
  p. dissection
  p. evisceration
  p. exenteration
  p. fascia
  p. floor
  p. floor descent
  p. floor disorder
  p. floor dysfunction
  p. floor dyssynergia
  p. floor electrical stimulation (PFS)
  p. floor electromyography
  p. floor exercise (PFE)

p. floor movement
p. floor neurophysiology
p. floor relaxation
p. floor syndrome
p. girdle relaxation (PGR)
p. ileal reservoir construction
p. ileal reservoir volume
p. inflammatory disease (PID)
p. kidney
p. lipomatosis
p. lymphadenectomy
p. lymph node
p. lymphocelectomy
p. malleability
p. muscle training
p. nerve plexus
p. omentoplasty
p. osteotomy
p. peritoneum
p. phased-array coil (PPA)
p. pole
p. pouch
p. pouchoscopy
p. pouch procedure
p. prolapse
p. sepsis
p. sidewall
p. stimulation
p. stone
p. ureter

pelvicaliceal
p. stasis
p. system

pelvicus
plexus p.

pelviectasis
pelvilithotomy, pelviolithotomy
pelvioileoneocystostomy
pelviolithotomy
pelvioneocystostomy
pelvioneostomy
pelvioperitonitis
pelvioplasty
pelvioradiography
pelviostomy
pelviotomy, pelvitomy
pelviperitonitis
pelviradiography
pelvirectal
p. abscess
p. achalasia
p. fistula

pelviroentgenography
pelvis, pl. **pelves**
arcus tendineus fascia p.
bifid renal p.
bony p.
cavum p.
coccygeal p.
extrarenal renal p.
fascia p.
female p.
p. fracture
p. innervation
male p.
p. muscle
nonmalleable p.
obstructed p.
papilloma of renal p.
pseudospider p.
renal p.
spider p.
split p.
subepithelial hematoma of the
renal p.
p. of ureter

pelviscope
pelviscopic clip ligation technique
pelvitomy (*var. of* pelviotomy)
pelviureteroradiography
pelvocaliectasis
Pemberton sigmoid clamp
pemoline
pemphigoid
benign mucous membrane p.
(BMMP)
bullous p.
mucous membrane p.

pemphigus
benign familial p.
p. foliaceus
p. vulgaris

PE-MV balloon dilatation catheter
pen
Intron A multidose p.

penbutolol
pencil
cautery p.
electrocautery p.

pencil-like stool
pencil-tipped electrode
pendetide
satumomab p.

NOTES

P

pendulous
    p. abdomen
    p. urethra
penectomy
    modified p.
    partial p.
penes (*pl. of* penis)
Penetrak
penetrans
    ulcus p.
penetrating
    p. abdominal trauma
    P. Abdominal Trauma Index
      (PATI)
    p. pancreatic trauma
    p. ulcer
    p. wound
penetration
    capsular p.
    splenic p.
Penetrex
Pen-F half-frame camera
penial
penicillamine
D-penicillamine
penicilli (*pl. of* penicillus)
penicilliary
penicillin
    benzathine p.
    beta-lactamase-resistant p.
    procaine p.
penicillin-streptomycin
Penicillium
    P. citrinum
    P. marneffei
penicillus, pl. **penicilli**
    penicilli arteriae lienalis
    penicilli arteriae splenicae
penile
    p. amputation
    p. arteriography
    p. artery
    p. biothesiometry
    p. blood pressure
    p. body
    p. carcinoma
    p. clamp
    p. crus
    p. curvature
    p. cyst
    p. deformity
    p. Doppler
    p. duplex ultrasonography
    p. edema
    p. epispadias
    p. erection
    p. extensibility
    p. fibromatosis

    p. fibrosis
    p. hypospadias
    p. implant
    p. incarceration
    p. injection testing
    p. injection therapy
    p. intraepithelial neoplasia
    p. island flap
    p. kraurosis
    p. lesion
    p. melanosis
    p. modeling
    p. necrosis
    p. orthoplasty
    p. plethysmography
    p. prosthesis
    p. prosthesis mechanical problem
    p. prothesis reliability
    p. pulse volume recording
    p. raphe
    p. reflex
    p. revascularization
    p. root
    p. rupture
    p. schwannoma
    p. sensitivity
    p. shaft degloving
    p. synechia
    p. torsion
    p. tuberculosis
    p. turgescence
    p. urethra
    p. vascular function assessment
    p. vein ligation
    p. vein occlusion therapy
    p. venous ligation surgery
    p. vibratory stimulation
penile-brachial
    p.-b. index (PBI)
    p.-b. pressure index (PBPI)
penis, pl. **penes**
    adolescent p.
    albuginea p.
    angiofibroma of p.
    bifid p.
    bulbus p.
    buried p.
    p. captivus
    carcinoma in situ of the glans p.
    chordeic p.
    clubbed p.
    collum glandis p.
    concealed p.
    corona glandis p.
    corpus spongiosum p.
    crus p.
    cutaneous horn of p.
    dorsum of p.

double p.
dystrophic p.
emissary vein of p.
flaccid p.
p. fracture
frenulum preputii p.
glans p.
hirsute papilloma of p.
inconspicuous p.
leukoplakia of p.
p. lunatus
p. lymphoma
micaceous growth of p.
p. palmatus
pearly papule of p.
p. plastica
preputium p.
prosthetic p.
pseudoepitheliomatous micaceous
  growths of p.
psoriasis of the p.
radix p.
raphe p.
p. reconstruction
p. reflex
retractile concealed p.
p. sarcoma
scapus p.
p. sclerosing lymphangitis
septum p.
septum glandis p.
septum of glans p.
p. syringoma
trabeculae of corpora cavernosa
  of p.
trabeculae corporis spongiosi p.
trabeculae corporum
  cavernosorum p.
trabeculae of corpus spongiosum
  of p.
trapped p.
venae cavernosae p.
ventrum of p.
webbed p.
penischisis
penitis
Penn
  P. pouch
  P. umbilical scissors
Pennington
  P. clamp

P. forceps
P. rectal speculum
pennyroyal oil
penoplasty
penopubic
  p. epispadias
  p. junction
penoscrotal
  p. hypospadias
  p. junction
  p. transposition
  p. transposition complex
  p. trapping
  p. webbing
penotomy
Penrose
  P. seton
  P. sump drain
pentagastrin (PG)
  p. gastric secretory test
  p. infusion
  p. infusion test
  p. provocative test
  p. stimulated analysis
  p. stimulated analysis test
pentamidine-induced pancreatitis
pentamidine isethionate
pentane excretion level
pentapiperium
Pentasa
pentastomiasis
pentastomum
  p. denticulatum
  p. denticulatum nodule
Pentax
  P. EC-series video endoscope
  P. EG-2901,-2940,-3800 endoscope
  P. EG-2900 videogastroscope
  P. EndoNet
  P. EndoNet digital endoscopy
    network
  P. endoscopic camera
  P. ESI-2000 fiberoptic endoscope
  P. EUP-EC124 ultrasound
    gastroscope
  P. FC-series colonoscope
  P. FD-series video endoscope
  P. FG-32UA
  P. FG-36-UX linear array
    echoendoscope
  P. FG-38X endoscope
  P. fiberscope

NOTES

P

Pentax *(continued)*
    P. FS-series flexible fiberoptic
      video sigmoidoscope
    P. linear array echoendoscope
    P. prototype needle
    P. VSB-2000 fiberoptic endoscope
    P. VSB-P2900 pediatric
      colonoscope
    P. VSB-P-series enteroscope
Pentax/Hitachi FG-32UA
pentazocine
pentetreotide
    indium-111 p.
penthienate
pentolinium
pentopril
pentosan
    p. polysulfate sodium
    p. sodium polysulfate
    p. sulfate
pentose phosphate shunt
pentosuria
pentoxifylline
Pento-X syndrome
pentretreotide
    In-111 p.
Pen-Vee K
peotomy
Pepcid
    P. AC
    P. Complete
    P. I.V.
    P. RPD
PEPCK
    phosphoenolpyruvate carboxykinase
peplomycin
pepo
    Cucurbita p.
peppermint oil
PEPS
    peroral electronic pancreatoscope
pepsic
pepsin
    inactivated p. (IP)
    p. secretion
pepsinogen
    p. A-C ratio
    p. I
    p. level (A, B, C)
pepstatin
Peptamen liquid nutrition
Peptavlon stimulation test
peptic
    p. cell
    p. cell receptor
    p. esophageal stricture
    p. esophagitis
    p. reflux

    p. reflux disease
    p. ulcer
    p. ulcer bleeding
    p. ulcer disease (PUD)
peptidase
peptide
    adrenomedullin 52-amino acid p.
    28-amino acid p.
    antral p.
    atrial natriuretic p. (ANP)
    brain-gut p.
    brain natriuretic p. (BNP)
    calcitonin gene-related p. (CGRP)
    cellular p.
    chemotactic p.
    C-type atrial natriuretic p. (C-ANP)
    C-type natriuretic p. (CNP)
    gastrin-releasing p. (GRP)
    gastrointestinal regularity p.
    glucose-dependent insulinotropic p.
    p. HI
    p. histidine isoleucine (PHI)
    p. hormone
    intestinal p.
    10-kd p.
    p. mass fingerprinting
    met-enkephalin p.
    monitor p.
    neutrophil chemotactic p.
    opioid p.
    paracrine p.
    peak acid output after gastrin-
      releasing p. (PAOGRP)
    plasma atrial natriuretic p.
    posttranslational processing of
      the p.
    regulatory p.
    somatostatin p.
    trefoil p.
    p. tyrosine
    vasoactive intestinal p. (VIP)
    vasoconstrictor p.
    p. YY (PYY)
peptide/bombesin
    gastrin-releasing p./b.
peptidergic
    p. mechanism
    p. neuron
Pepto-Bismol
peptone
Peptostreptococcus micros
per
    p. anum
    p. anum bleeding
    p. anum intersphincteric rectal
      dissection
    p. rectal portal scintigraphy
    p. rectum

percent
>p. reduction in urea (PRU)
>p. transferrin saturation

percentage of hypochromic red cell (%HYPO)

Percival gastric balloon

Percodan

Percoll
>P. bead
>P. filter

Percufix catheter cuff kit

Percuflex
>P. Amsterdam stent
>P. biliary stent
>P. catheter
>P. endopyelotomy stent
>P. Plus ureteral stent

percussion
>dullness to p.
>p. note
>p. tenderness

percutaneous
>p. abscess drainage
>p. antegrade biliary drainage
>p. antegrade pyelography
>p. antegrade urography
>p. bacille Calmette-Guérin administration
>p. balloon aspiration
>p. balloon dilation
>p. biliary bypass
>p. biliary drainage (PBD)
>p. bladder neck stabilization (PBNS)
>p. bladder neck suspension (PBNS)
>p. catheter cecostomy
>p. cholecystolithotomy (PCCL)
>p. choledochoscopy
>p. CT-guided aspiration
>p. debulking
>p. drainage of epididymal abscess
>p. embolization therapy
>p. endopyeloureterotomy
>p. endoscopic cecostomy
>p. endoscopic gastrojejunostomy (PEG-J)
>p. endoscopic gastrostomy (PEG)
>p. endoscopic gastrostomy and jejunal extension tube (PEG-JET)
>p. endoscopic gastrostomy and jejunal extension tube placement
>p. endoscopic jejunostomy (PEJ)

>p. endoscopic placement of jejunal tube
>p. endoscopic removal
>p. epididymal sperm aspiration
>p. ethanol injection (PEI)
>p. ethanol injection therapy
>p. femoral vein catheter
>p. fetal cystoscopy
>p. fine-needle pancreatic biopsy
>p. gastroenterostomy (PGE)
>p. gastrostomy (PG)
>p. hepatobiliary cholangiography
>p. image-guided thermal ablation of hepatic metastasis
>p. liver biopsy (PLB)
>p. native renal biopsy
>p. needle aspiration
>p. nephrolithiasis
>p. nephrolitholapaxy
>p. nephrolithotomy (PCN, PCNL, PNL)
>p. nephrolithotripsy (PCNL)
>p. nephrostolithotomy (PCNL)
>p. nephrostomy
>p. nephrostomy Malecot catheter
>p. nephrostomy tube placement
>p. pancreas biopsy
>p. pressure ureteral perfusion test
>p. radical cryosurgical ablation of prostate
>p. removal of bezoar
>p. resection
>p. sampling method
>p. stent
>P. Stoller Afferent Nerve Stimulation System (PerQ SANS)
>p. stone removal
>p. testosterone gel
>p. transcatheter perfusion
>p. transhepatic approach
>p. transhepatic biliary drainage (PTBD)
>p. transhepatic biliary drainage catheter
>p. transhepatic cholangio-drainage (PTCD)
>p. transhepatic cholangiogram (PTC, PTHC)
>p. transhepatic cholangiography (PTC, PTHC)
>p. transhepatic cholangioscopy (PTCS)

NOTES

percutaneous *(continued)*
    p. transhepatic cholecystolithotomy (PCTCL)
    p. transhepatic cholecystoscopy (PTCC)
    p. transhepatic cholecystostomy
    p. transhepatic choledochoscopic electrohydraulic
    p. transhepatic decompression
    p. transhepatic drainage (PTD)
    p. transhepatic liver biopsy with tract embolization (PBTE)
    p. transhepatic obliteration
    p. transhepatic obliteration of esophageal varix
    p. transhepatic pigtail catheter
    p. transhepatic portography (PTP)
    p. transluminal angioplasty (PTA)
    p. transluminal balloon angioplasty
    p. transluminal renal angioplasty (PTRA)
    p. transperineal seed implantation
    p. ultrasonic lithotriptor
    p. vasectomy
    p. vasography
Percy intestinal forceps
Percy-Wolfson gallbladder retractor
Perdiem Plain
perendoscopic manometry
Pereyra
    P. bladder neck suspension
    P. ligature carrier
    P. needle
    P. procedure
Pereyra-Raz cystourethropexy
PerFix Marlex mesh plug
perflubron
perforate
perforated
    p. acid peptic ulcer
    p. appendicitis
    p. appendix
    p. carcinoma
    p. cholecystitis
    p. diverticulum
    p. nasal septum
    p. ulcer disease
    p. viscus
perforating
    p. aneurysm
    p. diverticulitis
    p. forceps
    p. ulcer
perforation
    appendiceal p.
    barogenic p.
    bladder p.
    bowel p.

    cecal p.
    p. of colon
    colonic p.
    ductal system p.
    duodenal p.
    duodenal ulcer p. (DUP)
    endoscopic sphincterotomy-induced duodenal p.
    eosinophilic ileal p.
    esophageal p.
    p. of gallbladder
    gastric p.
    iatrogenic tumor p.
    intestinal p.
    intraperitoneal p.
    Niemeier gallbladder p.
    peritoneal p.
    polyethylene p.
    prepyloric p.
    pyloroduodenal p.
    retroduodenal p.
    retroperitoneal p.
    stercoral p.
perforin
Performa ultrasound system
perfringens
    Clostridium p.
perfusate
    p. bag
    esophageal p.
    hyperosmolar p.
    p. solution
perfusion
    allogenic liver p.
    p. cannula
    CCD p.
    con A/anti-con A p.
    continuous hypothermic pulsatile p.
    p. cooling
    extracorporeal liver p. (ECLP)
    extracorporeal whole organ p.
    ex vivo p.
    heterologous liver p.
    p. hypothermia technique
    hypothermic pulsatile p.
    intestinal p.
    intraperitoneal hyperthermic p. (IPHP)
    isolated hepatocyte p.
    p. machine
    percutaneous transcatheter p.
    plasma p.
    skin p.
    p. study
    transcatheter p.
    transvenous p.
    trickle p.
pergolide dopaminergic medication

perhexiline maleate
Periactin
periadvential tissue
periampullary
    p. adenoma (PAA)
    p. carcinoma
    p. duodenal diverticulum
    p. duodenal tumor
    p. malignancy
    p. mass
    p. neoplasm
    p. pseudotumor
perianal
    p. anorectal space
    p. area
    p. condyloma
    p. Crohn disease
    P. Crohn Disease Activity Index
      (PDAI)
    p. edema
    p. fistula
    p. fistula abscess
    p. hematoma
    p. hygiene
    p. infection
    p. lesion
    p. pain
    p. region
    p. sepsis
    p. skin tag
    p. soak
    p. wart
periappendicitis decidualis
periarteritis
    p. gummosa
    p. nodosa
pericapillary diffusion
pericardial
    p. air-fluid level
    p. decompression
    p. knock
pericarditis
    constrictive p.
pericecal abscess
pericellular matrix (PCM)
pericentral
    p. cholestasia
    p. fibrosis
    p. hypoxia
    p. necrosis
    p. pyridine nucleotide fluorescence
pericholangiolar

pericholangitis
pericholecystic
    p. abscess
    p. edema
    p. stranding
pericholecystitis
    gaseous p.
perichromatin granule
Peri-Colace
pericolic
    p. abscess
    p. membrane syndrome
    p. phlegmon
pericolitis
pericolonic fat
pericolostomy area
pericostal suture
pericrypt eosinophilic enterocolitis
pericystitis
perididymis
perididymitis
peridiverticular
peridiverticulitis
    phlegmonous p.
periductal
    p. fibrosis
    p. gland
periesophageal collateral vein
periesophagitis
    chronic p.
periesophagogastric lymph node
    metastasis
perifascial nephrectomy
perigastric node
periglandular nonspecific inflammatory
    reaction
periglomerular
perihepatic
    p. adhesion
    p. lymphadenopathy
perihepatitis syndrome
perihilar cholangiocarcinoma
periileal
perikaryon
perilobar pancreatitis
perilobular
    p. duct
    p. fibrosis
perimedial fibroplasia
perimesangial GBM
perimolysis
perimylolysis

NOTES

P

perinatal
 p. hemochromatosis
 p. torsion
 p. urology
perindopril
perinea (*pl. of* perineum)
perineal
 p. abscess
 p. body
 p. Crohn disease
 p. descent
 p. drain
 p. fascia
 p. flexure
 p. hypospadias
 p. impact trauma
 p. incision
 p. infection
 p. lithotomy
 p. muscle
 p. nerve
 p. nerve terminal motor latency test
 p. pad
 p. polyp
 p. pouch
 p. prostatectomy
 p. raphe
 p. rectosigmoidectomy
 p. region
 p. section
 p. sensation
 p. sinus
 p. sinus tract
 p. skin tag
 p. tendon
 p. ulcer
 p. urethrostomy
 p. urethrotomy
 p. urinary fistula
perinealis
 raphe p.
perinei
 raphe p.
perineobulbar
 p. detrusor facilitative reflex
 p. detrusor inhibitory reflex
perineodetrusor inhibitory reflex
perineometer
 Peritron Precision P.
perineometry
perineorrhaphy
perineostomy
perineotomy
perinephric
 p. abscess
 p. fat
 p. fluid collection

 p. hematoma
 p. stranding
 p. tissue
perinephrium
perineum, pl. **perinea**
 anterior p.
 bulging of the p.
 female p.
 male p.
 posterior p.
 raphe of p.
 watering-can p.
 water pot p.
perinuclear
 p. antineutrophil cytoplasmic (p-ANC)
 p. antineutrophil cytoplasmic antibody (p-ANCA)
period
 dwell p.
 intradialytic p.
periodic
 p. abdominalgia
 p. acid-Schiff (PAS)
 p. acid-Schiff-Alcian blue (PAS-AB)
 p. acid-Schiff-Alcian blue combination stain
 p. acid-Schiff stain
 p. acid-Schiff test
 p. leg movement (PLM)
 p. peritonitis
 p. polyserositis
 p. vomiting
periodicity
 circadian p.
perioperative
 p. antibiotic
 p. data
 p. nutrition
 p. risk
 p. vomiting
periotic vomiting
peripancreatic
 p. area
 p. fibrosis
 p. fluid
 p. fluid collection
 p. necrosis
peripapillary diverticulum
peripartum
 p. endoscopy
 p. symphysis separation
peripelvic
 p. cyst
 p. extravasation
 p. fat
peripenial

peripheral
- p. acinar vein
- p. adrenergic agent
- p. arterial vasodilation theory
- p. arthritis
- p. bile duct
- p. bladder denervation
- p. blood lymphocyte (PBL)
- p. blood mononuclear cell (PBMC)
- p. capillary filtration slit length
- p. cholangiocarcinoma (PCC)
- p. extremity edema
- p. hyperalimentation
- p. intrahepatic cholangiocarcinoma
- p. intravenous alimentation
- p. leukocyte count
- p. loading
- p. necrosis
- p. nerve evaluation (PNE)
- p. nerve evaluation test
- p. T cell
- p. vascular
- p. vascular resistance
- p. vasodilatation
- p. venous thrombosis
- p. zone

periphery
- hypoechoic p.

Periplast sealant
periportal
- p. area
- p. cirrhosis
- p. fibrosis
- p. hepatocyte
- p. inflammation
- p. invasion
- p. pyridine nucleotide fluorescence
- p. sinusoidal dilation

periportal-perisinusoidal fibrosis
periprandial
periprostatic
- p. block
- p. tissue

perirectal
- p. abscess
- p. fat
- p. fat infiltration
- p. fistula
- p. mass
- p. pain

perirenal
- p. abscess

- p. fascia
- p. fat
- p. hematoma

perisigmoid colon
perisinusoidal
- p. cell
- p. fibrin deposition
- p. fibrosis
- p. space

perispermatitis serosa
perisplenitis
- fibropurulent p.

peristalsis
- absent p.
- antral p.
- decreased p.
- esophageal p.
- high-amplitude p. (HAP)
- mass p.
- retrograde p.
- reversed p.
- secondary p.
- visible p.

peristaltic
- p. anastomosis
- p. contraction
- p. pump
- p. reflex
- p. rush
- p. unrest
- p. wave

peristomal
- p. area
- p. infection
- p. skin
- p. varix

peritomy
peritoneal
- p. access
- p. adenocarcinoma
- p. adhesion
- p. anatomy
- p. aspiration
- p. attachment
- p. autoplasty
- p. band
- p. biopsy
- p. blastomycosis
- p. button
- p. carcinoma
- p. carcinomatosis
- p. cavity

NOTES

P

peritoneal *(continued)*
    p. cavity abscess
    continuous ambulatory p.
    p. deposit
    p. dialysate
    p. dialysis (PD)
    p. dialysis catheter (PDC)
    p. dialysis creatinine clearance
      target
    p. dialysis effluent (PDE)
    p. dialysis urea removal
    p. dropsy
    p. encapsulation
    p. equilibration test (PET)
    p. fluid
    p. friction rub
    p. fungal infection
    p. lavage
    p. leukocyte
    p. lymphangiectasia
    p. macrophage
    p. malignancy
    p. membrane permeability
    p. membrane solute transport
      capacity
    p. membrane transport
    p. mesothelioma
    p. mouse
    p. nodule
    p. perforation
    p. reflection
    p. sac
    p. seeding
    p. sign
    p. soilage
    p. solute transport
    p. space
    p. studding
    p. tap
    p. toilet
    p. transfusion
    p. tuberculosis
    p. vein
    p. window
peritoneal-anal distance
peritoneal-atrial shunt
peritonealgia
peritonealis
    cavitas p.
peritonealize
peritonectomize
peritonei
    carcinomatosis p.
    pseudomyxoma p.
peritoneocaval shunt
peritoneocentesis
peritoneoclysis
peritoneogram

peritoneography
peritoneojugular shunt
peritoneopathy
peritoneopexy
peritoneoplasty
peritoneoscope
peritoneoscopy
peritoneotomy
    inverted-V p.
peritoneovenous
    p. shunt (PVS)
    p. shunt patency scan
peritoneum
    abdominal p.
    p. lateral umbilical fold
    p. medial fold
    p. median fold
    parietal p.
    pelvic p.
    visceral p.
peritonism
peritonitis
    bacterial p.
    barium p.
    benign paroxysmal p.
    bile p.
    Candida p.
    chemical p.
    chylous p.
    coccidioidal p.
    Coccidioides immitis p.
    p. deformans
    exudative p.
    fecal p.
    fungal p.
    generalized p.
    granulomatous p.
    meconium p.
    parasitic p.
    periodic p.
    postsclerotherapy bacterial p.
    primary p.
    sclerosing encapsulating p.
    secondary bacterial p.
    Sgambati test for p.
    spontaneous bacterial p. (SBP)
    starch granulomatous p.
    sterile p.
    subacute nonspecific p.
    tuberculous p.
peritonize
Peritron Precision Perineometer
peritubular
    p. capillary
    p. fluid
    p. HCO_3^-
    p. myoid cell
    p. sodium

perityphlitis actinomycotica
periumbilical
    p. port
    p. region
periureteral
    p. abscess
    p. fibrosis
    p. stone
    p. stranding
periureteric
periureteritis plastica
periurethral
    p. abscess
    p. bulking agent
    p. collagen injection
    p. gland
    p. injection therapy
    p. ligament
    p. spongiofibrosis
    p. striated muscle
    p. transurethral microwave
      thermotherapy (P-TUMT)
    p. vein
periurethritis
perivascular
    p. fibroblast
    p. plexus
    p. sheath
perivascularis
    capsula fibrosa p.
peri-Vaterian therapeutic endoscopic
  procedure
perivenular
    p. confluent necrosis
    p. fibrosis
perivesical fat
perivesicular
perivesiculitis
Perkin-Elmer model 5000 atomic
  absorption spectrophotometer
Perls
    P. reaction
    P. stain
Perma-hand silk suture
Permalume covering
permanent
    p. end colostomy
    p. loop ileostomy
    p. section
    p. stoma
permanganate
    potassium p.

PermCath
    P. dual lumen catheter
    Quinton P.
permeability
    capillary p.
    colonic p.
    intestinal p.
    membrane p.
    mucosal vascular p.
    peritoneal membrane p.
    tight junction p.
    transurothelial p.
    urea p.
    water p.
permeable
permeation
    lymphovascular p.
permethrin
Permitil Oral
permselectivity
Permutit method
pernasal cholangiogram
pernicious
    p. anemia
    p. malaria
    p. vomiting
    p. vomiting of pregnancy
peroral
    p. approach
    p. bougienage
    p. cholangiopancreatoscopy (PCPS)
    p. cholangioscopy (PCS)
    p. electronic pancreatoscope (PEPS)
    p. endoprosthesis
    p. endoscopy
    p. esophageal dilation
    p. gastroscope
    p. jejunal biopsy
    p. maneuver
    p. pancreatoscopy (POPS)
    p. pneumocolon examination
    p. retrograde pancreaticobiliary
      ductography
    p. shock wave lithotripsy (PSWL)
peroxidase
    endogenous p.
    glutathione p.
    p. stain
peroxidase-conjugated streptavidin
peroxidation
    lipid p.
    membrane p.

NOTES

P

peroxide
hydrogen p.
peroxisome proliferator-activated receptor (PPAR)
peroxynitrite-induced colitis
perphenazine
PerQ SANS
Perry bag
Persantine
persimmon bezoar
persistent
p. chronic hepatitis
p. cloaca
p. müllerian duct syndrome
p. postmolar gestational trophoblastic tumor
p. proteinuria
p. pylorospasm
p. viral hepatitis (PVH)
p. viral hepatitis, non-A, non-B (PVH-NANB)
p. viral hepatitis, type B (PVH-B)
p. vomiting
Personal EMG trainer
personality
histrionic p.
ulcer-prone p.
personalized program
pertechnetate
^{99m}Tc sodium p.
technetium-99m p.
Pertik diverticulum
Pertofrane
pertussin
p. toxin
p. toxin-sensitive G protein
pertussis
PERV
porcine endogenous retrovirus
perversion
taste p.
perversus
situs p.
perverted appetite
pessary
bladder neck support p.
Gellhorn p.
Smith-Hodge p.
pestis
Yersinia p.
PET
peritoneal equilibration test
positron emission tomography
PET dialysate volume
PET scan
petal-fugal flow
petechia, pl. **petechiae**
gastric p.

petechial
p. angioma
p. rash
Petersen
P. bag
P. operation
pethidine premedication
Petit triangle
petrificans
urethritis p.
petrolatum gauze pack
Pettenkofer test
Petz clamp
Peutz-Jeghers
P.-J. gastrointestinal polyposis
P.-J. hamartoma
P.-J. polyp
P.-J. syndrome (PJS)
Peyer patch
Peyronie
P. disease
P. plaque
Pezzer
P. catheter
P. drain
Pfannenstiel incision
PFC
pancreatic fluid collection
PFE
pelvic floor exercise
PFGE
pulsed field gel electrophoresis
PFIC
progressive familial intrahepatic cholestasia
PFR
peak flow rate
PFS
pelvic floor electrical stimulation
pressure-flow study
Adriamycin PFS
Pfuhl sign
PFV
portal-vein blood flow velocity
PG
pentagastrin
percutaneous gastrostomy
prostaglandin
pyoderma gangrenosum
Amogel PG
serum PG
PGE
percutaneous gastroenterostomy
PGE2
prostaglandin E2
exogenous PGE2
ratio of PGF2-alpha PGE2

PGE₁
    intraurethral PGE₁
PGE1 injection
PGF2-alpha
    prostaglandin F2-alpha
PGG
    prostaglandin G
PGG2 endoperoxide
PGH
    prostaglandin H
PGH2 endoperoxide
PGI2
    prostaglandin I2
PGR
    pelvic girdle relaxation
        symptom-giving PGR
PGV
    proximal gastric vagotomy
PGWBI
    Psychological General Well Being Index
pH
    blood pH
    pH electrode placement
    gastric luminal pH
    pH holding time
    intracellular pH
    intraesophageal pH
    intragastric pH
    pH monitoring
    pH probe
    pH recording
    pH standardized meal
    pH test
    pH threshold
    urinalysis pH
    urinary pH
pH4
    area under pH4 (AU4)
PH30 protein
Phadebas angiotensin-I test
phage type
phagocyte
    bactericidal function of p.
    p. respiratory burst
phagocytic stellate cell
phagocytosis
phagosome
phallalgia
phallanastrophe
phallaneurysm
phallectomy
phalli (*pl. of* phallus)

phallic construction
phallitis
phalloarteriography
phallocampsis
phallocrypsis
phallodynia
phalloncus
phalloplasty
    reconstructive p.
phalloplethysmography (PPG)
phallorrhagia
phallorrhea
phallotomy
phallus, pl. **phalli**
phantom
    P. 5 Plus ST balloon dilatation
    catheter
    p. ulcer
pharmacoangiography
pharmacoarteriography
pharmacocavernosogram
pharmacocavernosography
pharmacocavernosometry
pharmaco-duplex ultrasonography
pharmacodynamic
pharmacokinetics
    famotidine p.
pharmacological
    p. agent
    p. treatment
pharmacologically induced erection
pharmacomechanical coupling
PharmaSeed
    P. iodine-125 seed
    P. palladium-103 seed
pharyngeal
    p. anesthesia
    p. diverticulum
    p. exudate
    p. pouch
    p. pouch syndrome
    p. tear
    p. tunic
    p. wall
pharyngeal-UES incoordination
pharyngitis
    herpes p.
pharyngobasilar tunic
pharyngoesophageal (PE)
    p. diverticulectomy
    p. diverticulum
    p. function

NOTES

P

pharyngoesophageal *(continued)*
    p. junction
    p. sphincter
    p. tear
pharyngoesophagogastroduodenoscopy
pharyngolaryngoesophagectomy
pharynx
phase
    complement-independent
      autologous p.
    hepatic arterial-dominant p. (HAP)
    p. II contraction
    p. II, III marrow transplant
      recipient
    lag p.
    micturition p.
    mycelial p.
    predialysis p.
    pre-S p.
    prolonged expiratory p.
    reservoir p.
    skin graft imbibition p.
    skin graft inosculation p.
phasic
    p. contractile activity
    p. contraction
    p. fluctuation on squeeze
    p. wave duration
    p. wave sequence
phasic-free tone variation
Phazyme
Phazyme-95
Phazyme-125
Phazyme-PB
PHBD
    predominant hyperparathyroid bone
    disease
PHC-821505
pHCV31 antigen
pHCV34 antigen
phenacetin
    p. nephritis
    p. nephropathy
phenazopyridine
    p. hydrochloric acid
    p. hydrochloride
    sulfamethoxazole and p.
    sulfisoxazole and p.
phencyclidine abuse
phendimetrazine
phenelzine
Phenergan
phen-fen diet
phenindamine
phenindione hypersensitivity
phenmetrazine
phenobarbital

phenol
    aqueous p.
    p. II
    p. red chromoendoscopy
Phenolax
phenolphthalein
phenolsulfonphthalein
phenoltetrachlorophthalein test
phenomenon, pl. **phenomena**
    bicalutamide withdrawal p.
    capillary-leak p.
    cloud p.
    common cavity p.
    disappearing p.
    dystonic p.
    first-set p.
    Goldblatt p.
    Hayflick p.
    jet stream p.
    J-wave p.
    Kanagawa p.
    mask p.
    pathergy p.
    Schramm p.
    second-set p.
    walking stick p.
    yo-yo weight fluctuation p.
phenothiazine
phenotype
    antigenic p.
    B-cellular p.
    CD4 p.
    CD8 p.
    HLA class II p.
    partial nephrogenic diabetes
      insipidus p.
    Potter p.
    replication error p.
    slow bilirubin glucuronidation p.
    ZZ p.
phenotypic
    p. sex
    p. study
Phenoxine
phenoxybenzamine hydrochloride
phenoxymethylpenicillin
phenprocoumon
phentermine
phentolamine
    p. methylate
    p. test
phentosanpolysulfate
phenylacetate
phenylalanine
ʟ-phenylalanine mustard (L-PAM)
phenylbutazone hepatotoxicity
phenylephrine

phenylethyl alcohol agar
phenylethylamine N-methyl transferase
 (PNMT)
phenylhydrazine
phenyl-methane-sulfonyl fluoride
phenylpropanolamine
phenylpropylmethylamine
phenytoin
pheochromocytoma
  bilateral p.
  bladder p.
  ectopic p.
  familial p.
  malignant p.
PHG
  portal hypertensive gastropathy
PHI
  peptide histidine isoleucine
PH-I
  primary hyperoxaluria type I
Philadelphia chromosome
philippinensis
  Capillaria p.
Phillips
  P. catheter
  P. CM 12 electron microscope
  P. LaxCaps
  P. Milk of Magnesia
  P. rectal clamp
  P. ultrasound machine
phimosiectomy
phimosis, pl. phimoses
  adult p.
phimotic
pHisoHex scrub
PHIV
  portal hypertensive intestinal
  vasculopathy
PHLA
  postheparin lipolytic activity
phlebectasia
phlebitis
  Mondor p.
phlebography
  intraoperative p.
phlebolith
phleborheography
phleborrheograph
  Cranley p.
phlebosclerosis
  chronic ischemic colonic lesion
  caused by p. (CICLP)

phlegmon
  diverticular p.
  pancreatic p.
  pericolic p.
phlegmonous
  p. abscess
  p. adenitis
  p. alcoholic fatty liver
  p. change
  p. enteritis
  p. gastritis
  p. mass
  p. pancreatitis
  p. peridiverticulitis
phlorizin
pH-manometry probe
pH-meter
  intragastric continuous pH-m.
pH-metric testing
pH-metry
  esophagogastric pH-m.
  24-hour ambulatory pH-m.
  24-hour home pH-m.
PHN
  passive Heymann nephritis
pholedrine
phonoenterography
  computerized p.
phonorenogram
phorbol
  p. ester 12-O-tetradecanoylphorbol-
   13-acetate (phorbol ester TPA)
  p. ester TPA
  p. myristate acetate (PMA)
PhosLo
Phosphaljel
phosphatase
  alkaline p. (ALP, AP)
  alkaline phosphatase antialkaline p.
   (APAAP)
  Bessey-Lowry unit for alkaline p.
  bone alkaline p. (BAP)
  bone-specific alkaline p. (BALP)
  leukocyte alkaline p. (LAP)
  phosphorylase p.
  placental alkaline p. (PIAP)
  prostate-specific acid p.
  prostatic acid p. (PAP)
  protein p.
  protein tyrosine p.
  total serum prostatic acid p.
   (TSPAP)

NOTES

P

phosphate
aluminum p.
p. binder therapy
p. buffered saline solution
calcium hydrogen p.
cellulose p.
chloroquine p.
p. crystal
dexamethasone sodium p.
dietary p.
disopyramide p.
elemental p.
p. enema
estramustine p.
fludarabine p.
p. ion (PI)
p. ion-urea (PI-urea)
magnesium ammonium p.
nicotinamide adenine dinucleotide p.
(NADPH)
phosphatidylinositol p. (PI4P)
potassium p.
potassium-titanyl p. (KTP)
pyridoxal p.
renal p.
sodium p. (NaP)
sodium cellulose p.
phosphate-buffered saline (PBS)
phosphate-dependent glutaminase (PDG)
phosphate-independent glutaminase (PIG)
phosphatidylethanolamine
phosphatidylinositol (PI)
p. phosphate (PI4P)
**phosphatidylinositol-4,5-bisphosphate
(PI4,5P2)**
phosphatidylserine
phosphaturia
phosphodiester
phosphodiesterase (PDE)
p. inhibitor
p. type 5 inhibitor (PDE5 inhibitor)
**phosphoenolpyruvate carboxykinase
(PEPCK)**
phosphofructokinase
phosphoglucomutase
phosphoinositide
phosphokinase
creatine p. (CPK)
phospholipase
p. A2 (PLA2)
p. A2 catalytic activity
p. C (PLC)
p. D
phospholipid
p. bilayer
p. ratio
serum p.
phospholipidase A

phospholipid-bound choline concentration
phospholipidosis
phosphonoformate
phosphoramidite chemistry
phosphoribosyltransferase
adenine p. (APRT)
**phosphorous-31 magnetic resonance
spectroscopy**
phosphorus
dietary p.
p. metabolism
p. poisoning
serum p.
tubular reabsorption of p.
phosphorus-32 (P-32, ^{32}P)
phosphorylase
brain-type glycogen p. (BGP)
glycogen p.
p. phosphatase
uridine p.
phosphorylated growth factor receptor
phosphorylation
oxidative p.
protein p.
p. protein
src p.
tyrosine p.
phosphorylcholine
Phospho-Soda
P.-S. enema
Fleet P.-S.
**phosphotungstic acid-magnesium chloride
precipitation method**
phosphotyrosine antibody
phosphotyrosine-SH2 binding
phosphotyrosyl protein profile
photoablation
laser p.
Nd:YAG laser p.
photoaffinity
photochemical ablation
photochemotherapy
photocoagulation
infrared p. (IRC)
laser p.
transendoscopic laser p.
p. treatment
photodestruction
laser p.
photodiode
photodocumentation
photodynamic
p. diagnosis (PPD)
p. therapy (PDT)
photodynamic therapy (PDT)
Photofrin derivative
photogastroscope

photography
  endoscopic p.
  instant p.
  laparoscopic p.
  television p.
photoirradiation
photometer
  TUR-Cue photometer
photometry
  flame p.
photomicrograph
  high-power p.
  low-power p.
  medium-power p.
photomicrography
photomultiplier
  EMI 9813B p.
  p. tube
photon-deficient lesion
photophobia
photoradiation therapy
photoscan
photosensitivity
photosensitizer
  porphyrin p.
**photosensitizing hemoporphyrin
  derivative**
photothermal laser ablation
PHP
  pseudohypoparathyroidism
phrenalgia
phrenectomy
phrenemphraxis
phrenic artery
phrenicectomize
phrenicectomy
phreniclasia
phreniclasis
phrenicocolic, phrenocolic
  p. ligament
phrenicoesophageal ligament
phrenicoexeresis
phreniconeurectomy
phrenicotomy
phrenicotripsy
phrenocolic (*var. of* phrenicocolic)
phrenocolopexy
phrenodynia
phrenoesophageal membrane
phrenogastric
phrenoglottic
phrenohepatic

phrenoplegia
phrenoptosis
phrenospasm
phrenosplenic
phrygian
  p. cap
  p. cap deformity
pH-sensitive radiotelemetry capsule
PHSL
  primary hepatosplenic lymphoma
    B-cell PHSL
PHT
  portal hypertension
phthiriasis
Phthirus pubis
phycomycetes
phycomycosis
phyllodes
  cystosarcoma p.
phylloquinone
phylogenetic tree
physalopteriasis
physic
physical inactivity
Physicians'
  P. Health Study I
  P. Health Study II (PSH II)
Physick pouch
**physicochemical basis of gallstone
  formation**
physiograph
physiologic
  p. gastrectomy
  p. jaundice
  p. measurement
  p. pH solution
  p. reflux test (PRT)
  p. role in acid secretion
  p. salt solution (PSS)
  p. scaling
  p. testosterone-replacement therapy
physiological
  p. condition
  p. trophic effect
physiology
  anorectal p.
  p. testing
physiotherapy
  chest p.
physostigmine
phytobezoar
phytochemical

NOTES

P

phytoestrogen
phytoestrogen-induced menstrual cycle
  disturbance
phytohemagglutinin
phytonadione
phytopharmaceutical
phytosterolemia
phytotherapy
phytyl group
PI
    phosphate ion
    phosphatidylinositol
      PI 3-kinase
      PI surgical stapler
pi
      glutathione S-transferase p.
PI-30 stapler
PI90 double-headed stapler
PIAP
    placental alkaline phosphatase
pica
Picchini syndrome
pick
      P. cell
    tubular adenoma of P.
      P. tubular adenoma
Picker Vista MagnaScanner
picket fence appearance
Pickrell operation
pickwickian syndrome
picobirnavirus
picosulfate
    sodium p.
picture-frame vertebra
PID
    pelvic inflammatory disease
piecemeal
      p. necrosis
      p. polypectomy
      p. resection
Piersol point
piezoelectric
      p. crystal
      p. generator
      p. lithotripsy
      p. shock wave lithotriptor
      p. transducer
piezoelectrically generated ultrasound
Piezolith
      P. EPL
      P. EPL lithotriptor
      P. 2300, 2500 model lithotriptor
PIG
    phosphate-independent glutaminase
piggyback
      p. liver transplantation
      P. needle-knife papillotome
piggybacking of IV

pigment
      p. gallstone
    gastric p.
      p. neuropathy
      p. stone
pigmentary cirrhosis
pigmentation
pigmented
      p. gallstone
      p. histiocyte
      p. nevus
      p. nipple
pigment-laden Kupffer cell
pigmentosa
    urticaria p.
pigmenturia
pIgR
    polyimmunoglobulin receptor
pigtail
      p. biliary stent
      p. catheter
      p. endoprosthesis
      p. nephrostomy tube
      3/4-p. plastic endoprosthesis
PIL
    primary intestinal lymphangiectasia
pile, pl. **piles**
    bleeding p.
    prostatic p.
    sentinel p.
    thrombosed p.
pileuse
    tumeur p.
pilimiction
pili torti et canaliculus
pillar
    palatine p.
pill esophagitis
pill-induced
    p.-i. esophageal injury
    p.-i. esophagitis
pillow
    Bedge p.
    Sand-Eze EGD p.
    p. sign
pilonidal
      p. cyst
      p. cystectomy
      p. perirectal abscess
      p. sinus
      p. sinus disease
pilosicoli
    Serpulina p.
pimagedine
pimelorrhea
PIN
    prostatic intraepithelial neoplasia
pinacidil

pinch
>p. biopsy
>diaphragmatic p.
>p. forceps
>p. injury

pinchcock
>diaphragmatic p.
>p. effect
>p. mechanism

pindolol
pineapple test
pine cone appearance of bladder
pineoblastoma
pinguecula
pinocytosis
>fluid-phase p.
>p. vacuole

pinpoint pupil
pinwheel appearance
pinworm
PIP
>pressure inversion point
>>PIP on esophageal manometry

PI4P
>phosphatidylinositol phosphate

PI4,5P2
>phosphatidylinositol-4,5-bisphosphate

pipe
>endoscopic washing p.
>Mauch double-sheathed plastic wash p.

pipecuronium
pipenzolate
piperacillin sodium
piperazine citrate
piperidolate
piperoxan
pipestem
>p. cirrhosis
>p. stool

PIPIDA
>paraisopropyliminodiacetic acid
>>PIPIDA hepatobiliary scan
>>^{99m}Tc PIPIDA

^{99m}Tc PIPIDA

Pippi-Salle technique
Pipracil
PIR
>pressure increment rate

pirenzepine
piretanide
piriform
>p. fossa

>p. pooling
>p. sinus

piriformis
>p. artery
>p. muscle

piritramide
piritrexim
piroxicam
piston-type syringe
pit
>anal p.
>p. cell
>clathrin-coated p.
>colonic p.
>Frey gastric p.
>gastric p.
>mucosal p.
>postanal p.

pitfall
>potential p.

Pitres sign
Pitressin
pitting
>anal p.
>colonic p.
>p. edema
>gastric p.

pituitary
>p. adenoma
>p. adenylate cyclase activating polypeptide (PACAP)
>p. tumor

pituitary-gonadal axis
pityriasis
>p. lingua
>p. rotunda

Pityrosporon orbiculare
PI-urea
>phosphate ion-urea

pivalate derivative
PIVKA
>protein in vitamin K absence

PIVKA-II
>prothrombin induced by vitamin K absence or antagonist-II
>>PIVKA-II antagonist
>>PIVKA-II EIA kit for hepatocellular carcinoma

PIVOT
>Prostate Cancer Intervention Versus Observation Trial

PiZZ alpha-1-antitrypsin deficiency

NOTES

P

PJS
    Peutz-Jeghers syndrome
PKC
    protein kinase C
PKD1, PKD2 **gene**
PLA2
    phospholipase A2
placebo
    p. effect
    p. therapy
placement
    band p.
    dilator p.
    electrode p.
    endoscopic biliary stent p.
    endotracheal tube p.
    feeding tube p.
    five-port fan p.
    four-port diamond p.
    graft p.
    intestinal sling p.
    laparoscopy trocar p.
    metallic stent p.
    PEG-JET p.
    percutaneous endoscopic gastrostomy
      and jejunal extension tube p.
    percutaneous nephrostomy tube p.
    pH electrode p.
    posttreatment p.
    radiologic biliary stent p.
    tube p.
    ultrasound-assisted PEG p.
    ureteral stent p.
    wire-guided p.
placental alkaline phosphatase (PIAP)
Placer guidewire
plain
    p. catgut suture
    p. film
    p. film of abdomen
    p. gut
    p. gut suture
    Perdiem P.
    p. radiograph
planar
    p. imaging
    p. xanthoma
plane
    Addison p.
    Camper p.
    cleavage p.
    p. of dissection
    intersphincteric p.
    ischiorectal fossa p.
    parasagittal p.
    p. of Treves
planimeter
planimetric measurement

planimetry
    impedance p.
    rectal impedance p.
planning
    preintervention p.
Plantago ovata **seed**
plantar grasp
plantaris
    hyperkeratosis palmaris et p.
    tylosis palmaris et p.
plantarum
    Lactobacillus p.
planuria
planus
    lichen p.
plaque
    atherosclerotic p.
    augmentation p.
    Hollenhorst p.
    p. incision
    ostial atherosclerotic p.
    Peyronie p.
    Randall p.
    stone p.
plaquelike
    p. lesion
    p. linear defect
    p. thickening
plasma
    p. albumin
    p. ammonia
    p. androgen
    p. apo B48
    p. atrial natriuretic peptide
    p. bile acid measurement
    p. bubble
    p. caffeine concentration
    p. catecholamine
    p. cell
    p. cell balanitis
    p. cell granuloma
    p. cell hepatitis
    p. cell portal infiltration
    p. clearance
    p. cloud
    p. cortisol
    p. creatinine
    cryoprecipitated p.
    dialysis to p.
    p. enzyme
    p. exchange
    p. fibronectin
    p. flow
    fresh frozen p. (FFP)
    gastric p.
    p. gastrin concentration
    p. homocysteine
    p. inulin

p. ionized calcium
p. kallikrein
p. membrane marker
p. met-enkephalin
p. norepinephrine concentration
p. oncotic pressure
p. osmolality
p. parathyroid hormone (PTH)
p. perfusion
p. protein
p. protein fraction
p. renin
p. renin activity (PRA)
p. renin activity captopril test
p. renin concentration
p. ultrafiltrate
p. urea
p. urea concentration
p. viscosity
p. volume
p. volume depletion
p. volume expansion

plasma-activated
p.-a. complement 3 (C3a)
p.-a. complement 4 (C4a)
p.-a. complement 5 (C5a)

plasmablastic myeloma
plasmacellularis
balanitis circumscripta p.

plasmacytoma
bladder p.
extramedullary p.
gastric p.
radioresistant gastric p.

plasmacytosis
plasma-free choline concentration
PlasmaKinetic
P. radiofrequency energy delivery
P. surgery

plasmalogen
Plasma-Lyte
Plasmanate
plasmapheresis
therapeutic p.

plasmid
p. mediated
p. profile
p. profile role

plasminogen
p. activator (PA)
p. activator inhibitor (PAI)

p. activator inhibitor type 1 (PAI-1)
p. activator inhibitor type 2 (PAI-2)
functional p.

Plasmodium
P. falciparum
P. malariae

plasmodium
encapsulated p.

Plastibell circumcision
plastic
p. endoprosthesis

plastica
linitis p.
penis p.
periureteritis p.
rectal linitis p. (RLP)

plasty
bladder neck Y-V p.
Foley Y-V p.
mons p.
posterior bladder flap p.
V-Y p.
Y-V p.

plate
anal p.
bladder p.
blood agar p.
bowel p.
cloacal p.
exstrophic bladder p.
hilar p.
levator p.
limiting p.
liver cell p.
Maxisorb test p.
microwell p.
Mueller-Hinton-supplemented agar p.
Skirrow agar p.
Sur-Fit Natura irrigation adapter face p.
trigonal p.
urethral p.

plateau
dieting p.
p. response

platelet
p. abnormality
p. activation
p. count
p. dysfunction

NOTES

P

platelet (*continued*)
    p. factor 4
    p. glycoprotein 2b3a receptor
      antagonist
    p. transfusion
platelet-activating factor (PAF)
platelet-derived growth factor (PDGF)
Platinol
    etoposide, Adriamycin, P. (EAP)
    5-fluorouracil, Adriamycin, P.
      (FAP)
    fluorouracil, leucovorin rescue,
      Adriamycin, P. (FLAP)
    Ifex, Taxol, P. (ITP)
    VePesid, ifosfamide (with mesna
      rescue), P. (VIP)
platinum
    cyclophosphamide, Velban,
      actinomycin-D, bleomycin, p.
      (VAB-VI)
    p., etoposide (PE)
    p., etoposide, bleomycin (PEB)
    Velban, actinomycin-D,
      bleomycin, p. (VAB-II)
    p., Velban, bleomycin (PVB)
platinum-based consolidation
  chemotherapy
platysma
PLB
    percutaneous liver biopsy
PLC
    phospholipase C
PLC-50 linear stapler
PLC-PRF 5 cell
PLD
    polycystic liver disease
pleating of small bowel
Pleatman sac
Plegine
pleiotropic
pleomorphic
    p. destructive cholangitis
    p. rhabdomyosarcoma
pleomorphism
    nuclear hyperchromasia and p.
Plesiomonas shigelloides
plethora
plethoric
plethysmography
    impedance p. (IPG)
    penile p.
pleural
    p. mass
    p. rub
    p. tube
pleuritis
    bile p.
pleurobiliary fistula

pleurocholecystitis
pleuroesophageal muscle
pleuroperitoneal
    p. canal
    p. foramen
    p. sinus
pleurovisceral
plexiform neurofibroma
plexus
    Auerbach and Meissner p.
    Auerbach mesenteric p.
    biliary p.
    celiac p.
    colonic myenteric p.
    cystic p.
    deep muscular p.
    distal venous p.
    esophageal p.
    extrapancreatic nerve p.
    fundic p.
    ganglionated p.
    gastric p.
    gastroesophageal variceal p.
    gastrointestinal myenteric p.
    hemorrhoidal p.
    hypogastric p.
    ileocolic p.
    inferior anal p.
    inferior hypogastric p.
    longitudinal subepithelial venous p.
    lumbar p.
    lumbosacral p.
    Meissner p.
    middle rectal venous p.
    mucosal p.
    myenteric p.
    p. myentericus
    neural p.
    nonganglionated p.
    pampiniform p.
    p. pampiniformis
    pelvic nerve p.
    p. pelvicus
    perivascular p.
    preprostatic p.
    prostaticovesical p.
    p. prostaticus
    proximal venous p.
    rectal p.
    p. renalis
    sacral p.
    Santorini venous p.
    spermatic p.
    p. spermaticus
    submucosal venous p.
    submucous p.
    submuscular p.
    suburothelial nerve p.

superior hypogastric nerve p.
superior rectal venous p.
suprarenal p.
testicular p.
p. testicularis
thyreoideus impar p.
ureteric p.
p. uretericus
vascular p.
p. venosus
vesical p.
p. vesicale
p. vesicalis
vesicoprostatic p.

pliable lesion
plica, pl. **plicae**
plicae circulares
p. duodenalis
p. epigastrica
p. ileocecalis
p. longitudinalis
p. pubovesicalis
Rathke p.
p. umbilicalis
p. vesicalis transversa

plicamycin
plicated appendicocystostomy
plication
Child-Phillips bowel p.
dorsal curve p.
fundal p.
Graham p.
Kaliscinski p.
Kelly p.
Nesbit p.
Noble bowel p.
Rehne-Delorme p.
Starr p.
p. suture
suture p.
transgastric p.
transmesenteric p.
tunica albuginea p.

PLM
periodic leg movement
ploidy
p. analysis
chromosome p.
plot
Eadie-Hofstee p.
plug
bile p.

canalicular bile p.
Coloplast conseal p.
p. gastrostomy
meconium p.
omental p.
one-piece disposable p.
PerFix Marlex mesh p.
protein p.
urethral p.
plugged liver biopsy
plumbism
plume
laser p.
Plummer
P. bag
P. dilator
P. treatment
Plummer-Vinson syndrome
plus
Candela Miniscope P.
Charcoal P.
Ensure P.
Lithostar P.
Losotron P.
Maalox P.
Pyridium P.
Riopan P.
Therevac P.
Titralac P.
PMA
phorbol myristate acetate
PMA-stimulated O_2
PMC
pontine micturition center
pseudomembranous colitis
PMMA
polymethylmethacrylate
PMMA bead
PMME
primary malignant melanoma of the
esophagus
PMN
polymorphonuclear
PMN cell
PMN chemotaxis assay
PMN infiltrate
PMN leukocyte
PMN oxidative burst capacity
uremic PMN
PMN-elastase
fecal PMN-e.

NOTES

P

PMNL
    polymorphonuclear leukocyte
PMN-mediated endothelial cell injury
PMNN
    polymorphonuclear neutrophil
P-Mod-S factor
PN
    pyelonephritis
PNA
    peanut agglutinin
PNCA
    proliferating nuclear cell antigen
PNE
    peripheral nerve evaluation
        PNE test
PNET
    primitive neuroectodermal tumor
pneumatic
        p. bag
        p. bag dilation of esophagus
        p. bag esophageal dilation
        p. balloon catheter dilation
        p. balloon dilator
        p. compression device (PCD)
        p. endoscopic lithotriptor
        p. leg pump
        p. lithotripsy
pneumatinuria
pneumatocele
        scrotal p.
pneumatosis
        p. coli
        p. cystoides coli (PCC)
        p. cystoides intestinalis (PCI)
        p. cystoides intestinorum
        intestinal p.
        p. intestinalis
pneumaturia
pneumobilia
pneumocholecystitis
pneumococcal infection
pneumococcus nephritis
pneumocolon
        spiral computed tomography p.
Pneumocystis
        P. carinii
        P. carinii pneumonia (PCP)
pneumocystosis
        gastric p.
pneumodissection
pneumoenteritis
pneumogastrography
pneumography
        retroperitoneal p.
pneumohydraulic capillary infusion system
pneumohydroperitoneum

pneumokidney
pneumomediastinum
pneumonectomy
pneumonia
        aspiration p.
        lymphoid interstitial p.
        Pneumocystis carinii p. (PCP)
        Proteus p.
        Pseudomonas aeruginosa p.
        Pseudomonas pseudomallei p.
pneumoniae
        Klebsiella p.
pneumonitis
        radiation p.
pneumopenis
pneumopericardium
pneumoperitoneum
        benign p.
        p. needle
        stent-induced p.
        tension p.
pneumoperitonitis
pneumophila
        Legionella p.
pneumopyelography
pneumoradiography
        retroperitoneal p.
pneumoretroperitoneum
pneumoscrotum
Pneumo Sleeve
pneumostatic dilation
pneumothorax
        iatrogenic p.
        tension p.
PNH
        paroxysmal nocturnal hemoglobinuria
PNI
        prognostic nutritional index
PNL
        percutaneous nephrolithotomy
PNMT
        phenylethylamine N-methyl transferase
POA
        pancreatic oncofetal antigen
        POA test
Pockel cell
pocketed calculus
podagra
podocalyxin
podocin
podocyte
        glomerular p.
        p. glycocalyx
podocyte-specific protein
podofilox solution
podophyllin
podophyllotoxin

POEMS
    polyneuropathy, organomegaly,
     endocrinopathy, monoclonal (M-)
     protein, and skin changes
      POEMS syndrome
poikilocyte
    teardrop p.
point
    Addison p.
    APACHE-II p.
    bleeding p.
    Boas p.
    Brewer p.
    Cannon p.
    Chauffard p.
    Desjardins p.
    dorsal p.
    F2 focal p.
    Griffith p.
    Halle p.
    Hartmann p.
    Lanz p.
    Mackenzie p.
    McBurney p.
    Munro p.
    Piersol p.
    pressure inversion p. (PIP)
    Ramond p.
    respiratory inversion p. (RIP)
    p. of respiratory reversal on
     esophageal manometry
    Robson p.
    Sudeck critical p.
    p. tenderness
    Voillemier p.
point-counting image
pointed condyloma
pointer
    LaserMed laser p.
POINTER computer program
pointing
    past p.
Poiseuille-Hagen law
Poiseuille law
poison
poisoning
    ackee fruit p.
    acute lead p.
    acute mercury p.
    Amanita phalloides mushroom p.
    bacterial food p.
    chronic lead p.

    chronic mercury p.
    excitotoxic food p.
    ferrous salt p.
    food p.
    iron p.
    lead p.
    mercury p.
    mushroom p.
    phosphorus p.
    Salmonella food p.
    Staphylococcus food p.
    thallium p.
Poisson regression
Polachrome 35-mm slide system
Poland syndrome
polar
    p. artery
    p. body
    P. enteral feeding bag
    p. region
    p. segmental nephrectomy
    p. sheathed flagella
Polaris grasper
polarization microscopy
polarized
    p. glucose transporter
    p. standing reflex
polarographic study
Polaroid
    P. camera
    P. endocamera EC-3
    P. SX-70 with ACMI adapter
pole
    caudal p.
    cranial p.
    inferior p.
    p. of kidney
    pelvic p.
Polhemus-Schafer-Ivemark syndrome
policy
    organ allocation p.
polidocanol
    p. injection
    p. injection therapy
    p. sclerosant
poliomyelitis
POLIP
    polyneuropathy, ophthalmoplegia,
     leukoencephalopathy, and intestinal
     pseudoobstruction
      POLIP syndrome

NOTES

P

Politano-Leadbetter
- P.-L. anastomosis
- P.-L. technique
- P.-L. tunnel creation
- P.-L. ureterolysis
- P.-L. ureteroneocystostomy

polka fever
Pollack ureteral catheter
pollakiuria
pollen extract
Pólya
- P. anastomosis
- P. gastrectomy
- P. gastroenterostomy
- P. operation
- P. technique

polyacrylamide
- p. gel
- p. gel electrophoresis (PAGE)

polyadenomes en nappe
polyamine
- p. level
- p. spermine

polyangiitis
- microscopic p. (MPA)

polyanion
- GBM p.

polyantibiotic chemotherapy
polyarteritis nodosa
polyarthritis
- seronegative p.

polycationic
- p. histochemical probe
- p. marker

polychemotherapy
polychloruria
Polycillin-N
Polycitra
Polycitra-K
Polycitra-LC
polyclonal
- p. epidermal growth factor antibody
- p. IgG

Polycose glucose supplement
polycystic
- p. chronic esophagitis
- p. disease of liver (PDL)
- p. kidney disease
- p. liver
- p. liver disease (PCLD, PLD)

polycystin-1, -2
polycythemia vera
Polydek suture
polydimethylsiloxane
polydioxan
polydioxanone suture

polydipsia
- psychogenic p.

polyester-reinforced Dacron tape
polyestradiol phosphate therapy
polyethylene
- p. balloon dilator
- p. cannula
- p. catheter
- p. endoprosthesis
- p. glycol (PEG)
- p. glycol 600
- p. glycol-based lavage
- p. glycol electrolyte lavage solution (PEG-ELS, PEG-LES)
- p. glycol electrolyte solution
- p. glycol lavage solution
- p. perforation
- p. stent
- p. tube

polyethylenimine (PEI)
polyglactin
- p. monofilament loop
- p. suture

polyglecaprone 25 suture
polyglutamate folate
polyglycolic
- p. acid
- p. acid collar
- p. acid suture

polyglyconate
- p. monofilament loop
- p. staple
- p. suture

polygonal hepatocyte
polyhydramnios
polyimmunoglobulin receptor (pIgR)
poly-L-lysine-coated glass slide
polylobar liver
polymer
- silicone p.

polymerase
- p. chain reaction (PCR)
- p. chain reaction technology
- DNA p.
- HBV-associated DNA p.
- Taq p.

polymerization
- IgA p.

polymethylmethacrylate (PMMA)
- p. m. membrane

polymicrobial
- p. bacterascites
- p. infection

polymorphic
- p. gene
- p. reticulosis

polymorphism
- ACE gene p.

aldosterone synthase p.
angiotensin-converting enzyme
   gene p.
angiotensin I-converting enzyme
   insertion/deletion p.
deletion p.
DNA p.
restriction fragment length p.
   (RFLP, RLP)
polymorphonuclear (PMN)
   p. cell
   p. inflammatory infiltrate
   p. leukocyte (PMNL)
   p. neutrophil (PMNN)
Polymox
polymyositis
polymyositis-dermatomyositis
polymyxin
   p. B
   p. nephropathy
polyneuropathy
   familial amyloid p. (FAP)
   p., ophthalmoplegia,
      leukoencephalopathy, and intestinal
      pseudoobstruction (POLIP)
   p., organomegaly, endocrinopathy,
      monoclonal (M-) protein, and
      skin changes (POEMS)
polyol pathway
polyoma middle T oncogene
polyomavirus
Polyomavirus **infection**
polyorchism, polyorchidism
polyp
   adenomatous p. (AP)
   adenomatous colorectal p.
   adenomatous gastric p.
   antral p.
   benign adenomatous p.
   bleeding p.
   broad-based p.
   cervical p.
   cholesterol p.
   cloacogenic p.
   colonic p.
   colorectal p.
   diminutive p. (DP)
   diminutive adenomatous p.
   diminutive colonic p.
   diminutive hyperplastic p.
   duodenal p.
   elusive p.

eroded p.
esophageal p.
fibroid p.
fibrovascular p.
filiform p.
fundic gland p.
gastric p.
gastric antral sessile p.
gastric hyperplastic p.
gastric inflammatory fibroid p.
gastrointestinal hamartomatous p.
p. grasper
hamartomatous gastric p.
hyperplasiogenic p.
hyperplastic p. (HP)
hyperplastic adenomatous p.
hyperplastic epithelial gastric p.
hyperplastic gastric p.
inflammatory fibroid p. (IFP)
invasive colorectal p.
juvenile retention p.
lymphoid p.
malignant p.
metaplastic p.
mixed hyperplastic-adenomatous
   gastric p.
mucosal p.
multiple p.
nasal p.
neoplastic p.
nonneoplastic p.
pedunculated p.
perineal p.
Peutz-Jeghers p.
polypoid p.
postinflammatory p.
prepyloric p.
prostatic urethral p.
rectal p.
p. relocation
retention p.
sentinel hyperplastic p.
sessile p.
p. stalk
synchronous p.
tuberculosis p.
tubular p.
tubulovillous p.
villoglandular p.
villous p.
polypectomized

NOTES

P

polypectomy
  colonoscopic p.
  duodenal endoscopic p.
  electrosurgical snare p.
  endoscopic sessile p.
  gastric p.
  incomplete p.
  piecemeal p.
  saline-assisted p. (SAP)
  snare p.
  p. snare
  p. stump
polypeptide
  gastric inhibitory p. (GIP)
  p. growth factor
  islet amyloid p.
  pancreatic p. (PP)
  parathyroid hormone-related p.
  pituitary adenylate cyclase
    activating p. (PACAP)
  vasoactive intestinal p. (VIP)
polypeux
polyphagia
polyphosphate
  ^{99m}Tc p.
polyphosphoinositide
polypiform
polypoid
  p. cancer
  p. carcinoma
  p. colorectal cavernous hemangioma
  p. dysplasia
  p. excrescence
  p. exophytic nonulcerating
    carcinosarcoma
  p. filling defect
  p. gastric rugal hyperplasia
  p. lesion
  p. lymphoid hyperplasia
  p. lymphoma
  p. lymphomatous hyperplasia
  p. mass
  p. polyp
  p. tumor
  p. urethritis
  p. vascular malformation
polyposa
  colitis p.
  enteritis p.
  gastritis cystica p.
polyposis
  adenomatous p.
  cap p.
  p. coli
  colonic p.
  dense p.
  diffuse hyperplastic p.
  diffuse mucosal p.

  duodenal p.
  familial adenomatous p. (FAP)
  familial colorectal p.
  familial gastrointestinal p.
  familial hamartomatous p.
  familial intestinal p.
  familial juvenile p. (FJP)
  filiform p.
  florid p.
  gastric p.
  gastrointestinal p. (GIP)
  hamartomatous p.
  hyperplastic p.
  intermediate p.
  intestinal p.
  juvenile p. (JP)
  lymphomatous p. (LP)
  multiple familial p.
  multiple lymphomatous p. (MLP)
  nonfamilial gastrointestinal p.
  Peutz-Jeghers gastrointestinal p.
  sparse p.
  p. syndrome
  p. ventriculi
polypous gastritis
polyprenoic acid
Polyprep centrifugation
polypropylene
  p. mesh
  p. suture
polypus
  p. cysticus
  p. hydatidosus
polyradicular neuropathy
polyribosome
polysaccharide
  p. antigen
  p. capsule
  p. Kreha (PSK)
polysaccharide-iron complex
polyserositis
  familial paroxysmal p. (FPP)
  familial recurrent p.
  periodic p.
polysome
  endoplasmic reticulum-bound p.
polysomnography
polyspermy, polyspermia
polysplenia syndrome
polystyrene sodium sulfonate
polysulfate
  pentosan sodium p.
  sodium pentosan p. (PPS)
polysulfonated naphthylurea
polysulfone
  760 p. dialyzer
  F60S p.

high-flux p.
p. membrane
polysynaptic reflex
Polytef injection
polytetrafluoroethylene (PTFE)
p. mesh
p. paste injection
p. periurethral injection
p. sock
Polytrac Gomez retractor
polytropous enteronitis
polyunsaturated lecithin
polyurethane
p. nasoenteric catheter
p. stent
polyurethane-covered metallic stent
polyuria
nighttime p.
nocturnal p.
polyvinyl
p. alcohol
p. alcohol sponge
p. alcohol sponge hysterosacropexy
p. bougie
p. chloride (PVC)
p. chloride catheter
p. dilator
p. tubing
POMC
proopiomelanocortin
Pompe disease
Pondimin
Ponka
P. herniorrhaphy
P. technique herniorrhaphy
anesthesia
P. technique for local anesthesia
pons hepatis
Ponsky
P. pull
P. technique
Ponsky-Gauderer type PEG
ponticulus, pl. ponticulie
p. hepatis
pontine micturition center (PMC)
pontine-sacral reflex
POO
prostatic outlet obstruction
pool
abdominal p.
bile acid p.
gastric p.

pooled saliva
Poole suction tube
pooling
piriform p.
vallecular p.
venous p.
poor
p. long-term efficacy
p. long-term outcome
p. risk
p. surgical risk case
poorly
p. compliant bladder
p. differentiated adenoma
p. localized pain
popliteal
p. swelling
p. tenderness
pop-off suture
Poppel sign
POPS
peroral pancreatoscopy
population
gluten-dependent p.
hemodialysis p.
porcelain gallbladder
porcine
p. carboxypeptidase B
p. dermis for pubovaginal sling
p. endogenous retrovirus (PERV)
p. hepatocyte
pore
shuntlike p.
porfimer sodium
Porges catheter
pori (*pl. of* porus)
porin channel protein
pork tapeworm
porotomy
porous filter membrane
porphobilinogen (PBG)
p. deaminase (PBG-D)
porphyria
acute p.
acute intermittent p. (AIP)
p. cutanea tarda (PCT)
hepatic p.
variegate p. (VP)
porphyrin photosensitizer
porphyrinuria
porphyruria

NOTES

P

port
 BardPort implanted p.
 inlet p.
 MCL p.
 OmegaPort access p.
 periumbilical p.
 p. site metastasis
 subcostal p.
 suprapubic p.
 umbilical p.
porta
 p. hepatis
 p. renis
portable
 p. digital data recorder
 p. perfused manometric system
 p. renal preservation machine
Port-A-Cath catheter
portacaval
 p. anastomosis
 p. H graft
 p. H-graft shunt
 p. shunt (PCS)
 p. transposition (PCT)
Portagen
 P. diet
 P. feeding
 P. formula
Port-A-Germ anaerobic transport vial
portal
 p. azygous collateral
 p. block
 p. blood velocity
 p. canal
 p. cannula
 p. catheter
 p. circulation
 p. cirrhosis
 p. decompression
 p. embolization (PE)
 p. eosinophilic inflammation
 p. fissure
 p. hypertension (PHT)
 p. hypertensive gastropathy (PHG)
 p. hypertensive intestinal
  vasculopathy (PHIV)
 p. lobulation
 p. lobule
 p. perfusion defect
 p. plasma cell infiltration
 p. portography
 p. pyemia
 p. shunt index (PSI)
 p. tract
 p. tract fibrosis
 p. tract inflammation
 p. triad
 p. triaditis
 p. triad occlusion
 p. trunk
 p. vascular bed
 p. vein (PV)
 p. vein congestive index (PVCI)
 p. vein obstruction
 p. vein thrombosis (PVT)
 p. venous pressure (PVP)
 p. venous system
 p. venous velocity (PVV)
 p. venule
 p. zone
 p. zone granuloma
portal-collateral circulation
portal-systemic (*var. of* portosystemic)
portal-to-portal
 p.-t.-p. bridging
 p.-t.-p. fibrosis
portal-vein blood flow velocity (PFV)
Porter duodenal forceps
portoenterostomy
 Kasai p.
portography
 arterial p.
 computed tomography arterial p.
  (CTAP)
 computed tomography during
  arterial p. (CT-AP)
 CT during arterial p. (CTAP)
 percutaneous transhepatic p. (PTP)
 portal p.
 splenic p.
 transhepatic p.
 umbilical p.
portopulmonary shunt
portosystemic, portal-systemic
 p. encephalopathy (PSE)
 p. shunt
 p. shunting (PSS)
 p. shunt surgery
PortSaver PercLoop device
Portsmouth predictor equation
porus, pl. **pori**
 p. galeni
position
 anterooblique p.
 body p.
 Buie p.
 cervical p.
 curved flank p.
 decubitus p.
 dorsal lithotomy p.
 dorsosacral p.
 Edebohls p.
 Elliot p.
 final p.
 flank p.
 Fowler p.

frog leg p.
Gil-Vernet p.
greater curve p.
jackknife p.
knee-chest p.
knee-elbow p.
Kraske p.
lateral decubitus p.
left decubitus p.
left lateral decubitus p.
lithotomy p.
Lloyd Davies Trendelenburg p.
Lloyd Davis p.
Mayo-Robson p.
modified Lloyd Davies p.
prone p.
prone split leg p.
reverse Trendelenburg p.
right antero-oblique p.
Robson p.
Scultetus p.
semioblique p.
Sims p.
ski p.
subclavian p.
supine p.
Trendelenburg p.

positional obstructive uropathy
positioner
gallbladder bag p.
positioning
automated endoscopic system for
optimal p. (AESOP)
flank roll p.
patient p.
positive
antigen p.
p. bowel sounds
extradomain A p. (EDA+)
p. family history
p. nitrogen balance
p. predictive value (PPV)
p. secretin stimulation study
positive-pressure urethrography
Positrap
P. mini-retrieval basket
P. retriever
P. three prong non-retracting
grasping forceps
positron
p. camera
p. emission tomography (PET)

p. emission tomography scan
P. Plus cushion
Posner attention test
post
p. jejunoileal bypass hepatic
disease
p. nephrectomized
p. rubber band sepsis
status p. (S/P)
postage stamp penile tumescence test
postanal
p. dimpling
p. pit
p. repair
postanesthesia recovery (PAR)
postatrophic hyperplasia
postauricular Wolfe graft
postautoclave contamination
postbiopsy
p. fistula
p. vascular complication
postbulbar duodenal ulcer
postcaval ureter
postcecal abscess
postcholecystectomy
p. flatulent dyspepsia
p. syndrome (PCS)
postcholecystitis adhesion
postcibal symptom
postcoagulation syndrome
postcoital test
postcolonoscopy distention syndrome
postcricoid
p. area
p. web
postdialysis urea rebound
postdilation meglumine diatrizoate
postdystrophic scarring
postendoscopic cholangitis
postendoscopy
postenteritis syndrome
post-ERCP-induced pancreatitis
posterior
p. abdominal wall
anterior and p. (A&P)
arteria caecalis p.
arteria gastrica p.
arteria pancreaticoduodenalis
superior p.
p. bladder flap plasty
p. duodenal ulcer
p. extremity

NOTES

P

posterior *(continued)*
    p. fissure
    p. flap vaginoplasty
    p. hypospadias
    p. lumbar approach
    p. nephrectomy
    p. pararenal compartment
    p. pelvic exenteration
    p. perineum
    p. rectopexy
    p. rectus sheath
    p. renal fascia
    p. sagittal anorectoplasty
    p. scrotal nerve
    p. superior pancreaticoduodenal
        artery
    p. transthoracic incision
    p. urethra
    p. urethral valve (type I–IV)
        (PUV)
posterolateral
postevacuation
    p. film
    p. view
post-fatty meal cholecystography
postfundoplication syndrome
postganglionic
    p. cholinergic nerve
    p. sympathetic nerve
postgastrectomy
    p. bleed
    p. cancer
    p. dysfunction
    p. gastritis
    p. hemorrhage
    p. stasis
    p. syndrome
postglomerular arteriole
postheparin lipolytic activity (PHLA)
posthepatic, posthepatitic
    p. cirrhosis
posthepatitis aplastic anemia
posthetomy
posthioplasty
posthitis
posthoc test
postholith
postictal
postinfectious glomerulonephritis
postinfective glomerular nephritis
postinflammatory
    p. contracture
    p. polyp
    p. traction
postischemic
    p. acute renal failure
    p. tubular necrosis

postligation
    p. discomfort
    p. pain
    p. ulcer
postmenopausal
postmicturition
    p. continuous leakage
    p. dribble
postmortem intussusception
postmyotomy reflux
postnasal drip
postnecrotic
    p. cirrhosis
    p. scarring
postobstructive diuresis
postoperative
    p. abscess
    p. adhesion
    p. anticoagulation therapy
    p. autologous transfusion
    p. biliary leakage
    p. cholangiography
    p. choledochoscopy
    p. cholesterol embolism
    p. complication
    p. gastritis
    p. hydrocele
    p. ileus
    p. irrigation-suction
    p. irrigation-suction drainage
    p. morbidity
    p. pleurobiliary fistula
    p. reflux
    p. regimen for oral early feeding
        (PROEF)
    p. retroperitoneal fibrosis
    p. stricture
    p. ureteral obstruction
    p. urinary retention
    p. vomiting
postparacentesis circulatory dysfunction (PCD)
postpartum constipation
postperfusion
postpolypectomy
    p. bleed
    p. coagulation syndrome
    p. hemorrhage
postprandial
    p. distention
    p. fullness
    p. hypoglycemia
    p. nausea
    p. pain
    p. portal hyperemia
    p. vomiting
postprocedure pancreatitis
postprostatectomy incontinence

postpyloric feeding tube
postreceptor signaling of parietal cell
postrema
    area p.
postrenal
    p. albuminuria
    p. anuria
    p. proteinuria
postsclerotherapy bacterial peritonitis
postsecretory processing
postshunt encephalopathy
postsphincterotomy
    p. ductography
    p. ERCP cannulation
postsplenectomy infection
poststreptococcal
    p. acute glomerulonephritis
    p. glomerulonephritis (PSGN)
postsurgical
    p. change
    p. endoscopy
    p. gastric stasis
    p. recurrent ulcer
postthaw sperm motility index
postthrombotic syndrome
post-TNM stage (I, II, III, IV)
posttransfusion hepatitis
posttranslational
    p. modification
    p. processing of the peptide
posttransplant
    p. antiglomerular basement
      membrane
    p. diabetes mellitus (PTDM)
    p. immunosuppression
    p. immunosuppression therapy
    p. lymphoproliferative disorder
      (PTLD)
    p. patient
    p. renal dysfunction
posttransplantation cholangitis
posttransurethral microwave
  thermotherapy prostatitis-like
  syndrome
posttraumatic
    p. autotransplantation
    p. incontinence
    p. pancreatic-cutaneous fistula
    p. urethral stricture
posttreatment
    p. discomfort
    p. placement

post-TUMT prostatitis-like syndrome
posttussive vomiting
postulate
    Koch p.
postural
    p. quantitative analysis of acid
      exposure
    p. regurgitation
    p. stimulation test (PST)
posture-dependent pain
postureteral ligation
postureteroscopic manipulation
posture test
posturing
    decerebrate p.
    decorticate p.
posturography
    computerized dynamic p. (CDP)
post-UUO time
Pos-T-Vac
    P.-T-V. vacuum erection device
    P.-T-V. VCD
postvagotomy
    p. diarrhea
    p. dysphagia
    p. gastroparesis
    p. syndrome
postvoid
    p. dribble
    p. dribbling of urine
    p. incontinence
    p. radiography
    p. residual (PVR)
    p. residual urine
postvoiding cystogram (PVC)
Potaba
potassium
    aminobenzoate p.
    p. balance
    p. bicarbonate
    p. binding resin
    p. channel
    p. channel opener
    p. chloride (KCl)
    p. citrate
    p. conductance
    p. cyanide
    p. deficiency
    p. depletion
    dietary p.
    p. electrolyte
    extracellular p.

NOTES

P

potassium (*continued*)
    fractional excretion of p. (FEFEK)
    p. hydroxide smear
    intracellular p.
    p. permanganate
    p. phosphate
potassium-canrenoate antagonist
potassium-losing nephritis
potassium-sparing diuretic
potassium-titanyl phosphate (KTP)
potato liver
potency
    erectile p.
potential
    p. difference (PD)
    evoked p.
    excitatory junction p. (EJP)
    excitatory postsynaptic p. (EPSP)
    inhibitory postsynaptic p. (IPSP)
    malignant p.
    motor unit action p.
    neoplastic p.
    oscillatory p.
    oxidant-trapping p.
    p. pitfall
    pudendal evoked p.
    redox p.
    resting membrane p.
    short-lasting afterhyperpolarizing p.'s
    spike p.
    stromal tumor of unknown
      malignant p. (STUMP)
    threshold p.
    visual evoked p.
potentiation
    alcohol p.
    p. of drug hepatotoxicity
Potter
    P. disease
    P. facies
    P. phenotype
    P. syndrome
Potts
    P. forceps
    P. scissors
Potts-Smith
    P.-S. forceps
    P.-S. scissors
pouch
    abdominovesical p.
    anal p.
    Assura closed mini p.
    Assura convex drainable p.
    Assura convex urostomy p.
    Assura pediatric p.
    Assura standard drainable p.
    banded gastroplasty with a
      divided p.

Bard closed-end adhesive p.
Bard drainage adhesive p.
Bard Extra Ileo B p.
Bard Integrale p.
Bard security p.
Barnett p.
Benchekroun p.
p. biopsy
bladder replacement urinary p.
blind upper esophageal p.
Bricker p.
bulky colonic p.
Camey urinary p.
catheterization p.
closed-end ostomy p.
colonic p.
Coloplast closed p.
Coloplast drainable p.
Coloplast flange p.
Coloplast mini p.
coloplasty p.
p. configuration
continent ileal reservoir
  catheterization p.
ConvaTec colostomy p.
ConvaTec Little One Sur-Fit p.
ConvaTec Sur-Fit two-piece p.
Cymed Micro Skin one-piece
  drainage p.
Dansac Karaya Seal one-piece
  drainage p.
Dansac Standard Ileo p.
Denis Browne p.
double loop p.
Douglas p.
drainable ostomy p.
Duke p.
endorectal ileal p.
p. excision
p. failure
First-Choice drainable p.
p. fistula
Florida urinary p.
Fobi p.
p. former
fundal p.
gastric p.
Graham closure with omental p.
Greer EZ Access drainage p.
Hartmann p.
haustral p.
Heidenhain p.
hemi-Kock p.
hernia p.
Hollister First Choice p.
Hollister Holligard p.
Hollister Karaya 5 ostomy p.
Hollister Karaya Seal p.

Hollister Premium p.
Hunt-Lawrence p.
ileal J-p.
ileal low-pressure bladder
  substitute p.
ileal neobladder urinary p.
ileal S-p.
ileal W-p.
p. ileitis
ileoanal p.
ileocecal p.
ileocolonic p.
Indiana urinary p.
inlet p. (IP)
intraluminal p.
inverted-U p.
jejunal p.
J pelvic ileal p.
J-shaped ileal p.
Kock urinary p.
lateral-lateral p.
Le Bag ileocolonic p.
Le Bag urinary p.
low-pressure p.
Mainz p. II
Mainz urinary p.
Mansson urinary p.
Marlen Gas Relief drainage p.
Marlen Odor-Ban ileostomy p.
Marlen Solo ileostomy p.
Marlen Zip Klosed p.
Miami p.
MicroSkin ostomy p.
Morison p.
Nu-Hope ileostomy p.
Nu-Hope neonatal and premie p.
Nu-Hope Nu-Self drainable p.
Nu-Hope urinary p.
Nu-Hope urostomy p.
one-piece ostomy p.
open-ended ostomy p.
Padua bladder urinary p.
pararectal p.
paravesical p.
Parks ileostomy p.
pelvic p.
Penn p.
perineal p.
pharyngeal p.
Physick p.
rectal p.
rectouterine p.

rectovaginal p.
rectovesical p.
renal p.
right colon p.
Rowland p.
sigma rectum p.
sigmoid p.
sigmoid-rectum p.
S pelvic ileal p.
S-shaped p.
Studer p.
superficial inguinal p.
Sur-Fit Mini p.
Sur-Fit Natura flexible wafer and
  drainable p.
Sur-Fit Natura urostomy p.
Tena p.
terminal ileal p.
three-loop ileal p.
triple loop p.
two-loop J-shaped ileal p.
two-piece ostomy p.
U p.
UCLA catheterization p.
p. ulceration
United Bongort Life-style p.
United Max-E drainable p.
United Surgical Bongort Life-
  style p.
United Surgical Featherlite
  ileostomy p.
United Surgical Shear Plus
  drainable p.
United Surgical Soft & Secure p.
vesica ileale p.
vesicouterine p.
VPI nonadhesive open-end p.
W p.
Willis p.
W pelvic ileal p.
W-shaped p.
Zenker p.
pouch-anal anastomosis
pouched ileostomy
pouchitis
  chronic active p.
  refractory p.
  wastebasket p.
pouchocele
pouchogram
pouchography
  evacuation p.

NOTES

P

pouchoscopy
pelvic p.
Poupart
P. ligament
P. ligament shelving edge
P. line
povidone-iodine
p.-i. enema
p.-i. wash
powder
BC Cold P.
Karaya p.
Nu-Hope karaya p.
p. pyelogram
Secretin-Ferring P.
Seidlitz p.
Sween Micro Guard p.
power
p. Doppler ultrasound
p. grip
PP
pancreatic polypeptide
PP65
PP65 antigenemia
PP65 antigenemia assay
PPA
pelvic phased-array coil
PPAF
progressive perivenular alcoholic fibrosis
PPAR
peroxisome proliferator-activated receptor
PPC
prostatic pressure coefficient
p47, p67 cytosolic protein
PPD
photodynamic diagnosis
purified protein derivative test
PPD immunological study
p_2 penile brachial index
PPG
phalloplethysmography
PPI
proton pump inhibitor
PPI triple therapy
PP-immunoreactive cell
PPJ
pure pancreatic juice
PPoma
pancreatic polypeptide-secreting tumor
pure PPoma
PPPD
pylorus-preserving
pancreatoduodenectomy
PPS
sodium pentosan polysulfate
PPTT
prepubertal testicular tumor

PPV
positive predictive value
PPW
pylorus-preserving Whipple modification
PRA
panel-reactive antibody
plasma renin activity
Prader orchidometer
Prader-Willi syndrome
praeacutus
Bacteroides p.
praecox
ejaculatio p.
icterus p.
praeputii
smegma p.
pralidoxime
pramlintide
pramoxine hydrochloride
Prandase
Prandin
Pratt
P. anoscope
P. bivalve retractor
P. crypt hook
P. rectal hook
P. rectal probe
P. rectal scissors
P. rectal speculum
pravastatin
praziquantel
prazosin hydrochloride
PRCA
pure red cell aplasia
preampullary portion of bile duct
preauricular
prebiotic
precaliceal canalicular ectasia
precancerous lesion
prechylomicron transport vesicle
precipitancy
precipitant
p. leakage
p. urination
precipitation
glucagon p.
precirrhosis
precirrhotic hemochromatosis
precision
p. grip
intraassay p.
P. Isotein HN powdered feeding
P. Isotonic powdered feeding
P. LR powdered feeding
P. QID glucose monitoring system
P. Tack Transvaginal anchor
system
Precision-HN

Precision-LR
Precisor
    P. Direct Bite biopsy forceps
    P. disposable biopsy forceps
Preclude peritoneal membrane
precordium
    hyperdynamic p.
precore mutant strain
Precose
precursor
    androgen p.
    benign neoplastic p.
    T-helper p.
precut
    p. incision
    p. papillotome
    p. papillotomy
    p. sphincterotome
    p. sphincterotomy
Pred
    Liquid Pred
predialysis
    p. phase
    p. plasma phosphate concentration
Predicta TGF-β1 kit
predictive value
predictor
    independent p.
    metabolic p.
    outcome p.
predigested protein formula
predigestion
    diastase p.
predisposition
    familial p.
    genetic p.
prednisolone
    p. enema
    p. metasulfobenzoate
prednisone
prednisone-colchicine combination
predominant
    p. hyperparathyroid bone disease
      (PHBD)
    p. median lobe
preeclamptic liver disease
preendoscopy
preesophageal dysphagia
preexisting
    p. discomfort
    p. disease
preferential heating

prefreeze
    p. motility
    p. semen analysis
Pregestimil formula
preglomerular
    p. arteriole
    p. vasculature
pregnancy
    abdominal ectopic p.
    acute fatty liver of p. (AFLP)
    ectopic sigmoid p.
    fatty liver of p.
    heartburn of p.
    intrahepatic cholestasia of p. (ICP)
    molar p.
    nephritis of p.
    pernicious vomiting of p.
    pyelonephritis of p.
    recurrent molar p.
    subacute fatty liver of p.
    toxemia of p.
    tubal ectopic p.
    ureteral calculi in p.
    voluntary interruption of p. (VIP)
    p. wastage
pregnant uterus
pregnenolone
Prehn sign
preintervention planning
preinvasive urothelial neoplasia
prekallikrein
Prelone
Preludin
Premarin
premature
    p. ejaculation
    p. stop codon
prematurity
    retinopathy of p.
premedication
    metoclopramide p.
    pethidine p.
    viscous lidocaine p.
premenarchal
premicturition pressure
premier
    P. Platinum HpSA
    P. Platinum HpSA test
Premium
    P. Barrier
    P. CEEA circular stapler
    P. Plus CEEA disposable stapler

NOTES

P

Premix-Slip
Prempree modification staging system
prenatal
    p. diagnosis
    p. fetal hydronephrosis
Prentice-Wilcoxon test
Prentiss
    P. maneuver
    P. orchiopexy
preoperative
    p. antibiotic
    p. lesion
    p. tumor treatment
prep
    preparation
      OMNI Prep
      Sween Prep
      United Skin Prep
prepancreatic anlagen
prepapillary bile duct
preparation (prep)
    bowel p.
    Brown dietary method for colon p.
    colonic purge p.
    Colonlite bowel p.
    CoLyte bowel p.
    cytocentrifuge p.
    Dulcolax bowel p.
    electrolyte p.
    Emulsoil bowel p.
    Evac-Q-Kit bowel p.
    Evac-Q-Kwik bowel p.
    Fleet bowel p.
    galenic p.
    GoLYTELY bowel p.
    P. H
    inadequate bowel p.
    lactobacilli p.
    lavage bowel p.
    Nichols-Condon bowel p.
    OCL bowel p.
    oral iron p.
    renal proximal tubule p.
    Touch p.
    Tridrate bowel p.
    X-Prep bowel p.
prepatent period filariasis
prepenile dislocation of scrotum
preperfusion
preperitoneal
    p. abscess
    p. anesthesia
    p. approach
    p. distention balloon (PDB)
    p. fat
    p. space
    transabdominal p. (TAPP)
preproenkephalin

preproEt-1 mRNA
preprostatic
    p. plexus
    p. sphincter
    p. urethra
prepubertal testicular tumor (PPTT)
prepuce
    frenulum of p.
    hooded p.
    megameatus-intact p. (MIP)
    ventral apron p.
preputial
    p. adhesion
    p. calculus
    p. collar
    p. continent vesicostomy
    p. gland
    p. stenosis
    p. transverse island flap and glans
      channel
preputiotomy
preputium
    p. clitoridis
    p. penis
prepyloric
    p. antral diaphragm
    p. antrum
    p. atresia
    p. gastric ulcer
    p. perforation
    p. polyp
    p. sphincter
prerectal lithotomy
prerenal
    p. anuria
    p. azotemia
presacral
    p. cyst
    p. ectopic kidney
    p. neuroblastoma
    p. rectopexy
    p. space
    p. teratoma
    p. tumor
presbyacousia
presbyesophagus
prescribed clearance
presentation
    rectocele p.
    trismus p.
preservation
    bladder p.
    cadaver renal p.
    extracorporeal renal p.
    renal p.
    simple cold storage p.
    p. time
    p. times effect

presinusoidal intrahepatic portal hypertension
pre-S phase
pressure
    abdominal p.
    abdominal leak-point p. (ALPP)
    ambulatory blood p.
    p. amplitude modulation
    anal sphincter squeeze p.
    basal anal canal p.
    basal anal sphincter p.
    bile duct p.
    biliary tract p.
    bladder p. (BP)
    bladder intravesical p.
    blood p. (BP)
    cavernosal systolic p.
    cavernous artery occlusion p.
    central venous p. (CVP)
    cerebral perfusion p. (CPP)
    choledochal basal p.
    closing p.
    colloid osmotic p.
    cybernetic regulation of blood p.
    detrusor muscle leak-point p.
    p. diverticulum
    p. dressing
    dynamic closure p.
    end-expiratory intragastric p.
    end-filling p.
    esophageal peristaltic p.
    p. flow analysis
    free hepatic venous p. (FHVP)
    glomerular capillary p.
    hepatic vein wedge p.
    hepatic venous p.
    hepatic wedge p.
    high intraluminal p.
    high resting anal p.
    hydrostatic p.
    p. increment rate (PIR)
    intraabdominal p.
    intraanal p.
    intraballoon p.
    intracavernosal p.
    intracholedochal p.
    intraductal p.
    intraesophageal peristaltic p.
    intraesophageal variceal p.
    intragastric p.
    intraglomerular p.
    intraluminal esophageal p.

    intraluminal urethral p.
    intraurethral p.
    intravariceal p.
    intravesical p.
    p. inversion point (PIP)
    leak p.
    leak-point p. (LPP)
    LES p.
    lower esophageal sphincter p. (LESP)
    low urethral p. (LUP)
    maximum (anal) resting p. (MRP)
    maximum squeeze p. (MSP)
    maximum urethral closure p. (MUCP)
    maximum vasal p. (MVP)
    mean arterial p. (MAP)
    mean arterial blood p. (MABP)
    p. measurement
    melanoma intratumor p.
    p. natriuresis
    p. necrosis
    pancreatic duct p. (PDP)
    passage p.
    p. peak
    peak p.
    penile blood p.
    plasma oncotic p.
    portal venous p. (PVP)
    premicturition p.
    proximal p.
    pulmonary artery p. (PAP)
    pulmonary capillary wedge p. (PCWP)
    p. regulated electrohydraulic lithotripsy
    renal profusion p.
    resting anal sphincter p.
    sinusoidal capillary p.
    p. sore
    sphincter of Oddi p. (SOP)
    splanchnic capillary p.
    squeeze p.
    static closure p.
    p. study
    systemic arterial p.
    p. transducer
    transglomerular hydrostatic filtration p.
    transmembrane hydraulic p.
    p. transmission ratio (PTR)
    ureteral p.

NOTES

P

pressure *(continued)*
  urethral closure p.
  Valsalva leak point p. (VLPP)
  variceal p.
  wedge p.
  wedged hepatic venous p. (WHVP)
  Whitaker perfusion p.
pressure-flow
  p.-f. electromyography study
  p.-f. micturition study
  p.-f. study (PFS)
pressure-point tension ring
pressure-specific bladder capacity
prestomal ileitis
presumed circle area ratio (PCAR)
presurgical medical evaluation
presynaptic inhibition
preternatural anus
pretransplant evaluation
preureteral iliac artery
preurethritis
Prevacare total solution skin care spray
Prevacid
Prevail protective underwear
prevalence
  cholelithiasis p.
prevention
  Centers for Disease Control and P.
    (CDC)
  somatostatin p.
preventive intravesical therapy
prevertebral fascia
Prevpac triple therapy
PRF
  pulse repetition frequency
PrHPT
  primary hyperparathyroidism
priapism
  arterial p.
  drug-induced p.
  high-flow p.
  low-flow p.
  secondary p.
  stuttering p.
  Winter shunt for p.
priapitis
priapus
prilocaine
Prilosec
primaquine
primary
  p. adrenal insufficiency
  p. anastomosis
  p. antiphospholipid syndrome
  p. arteriovenous fistula
  p. B-cell lymphoma
  p. biliary cirrhosis (PBC)
  p. ciliary dyskinesia

  p. closure
  p. colorectal cancer (PCRC)
  p. contraction
  p. diagnostic endoscopy
  p. fistulotomy
  p. gastric lymphoma staging
  p. glomerular disease
  p. glomerular lesion
  p. graft nonfunction
  p. hepatosplenic lymphoma (PHSL)
  p. hyperaldosteronism
  p. hyperoxaluria type I (PH-I)
  p. hyperoxaluria type II
  p. hyperparathyroidism (PrHPT)
  p. indication
  p. intestinal lymphangiectasia (PIL)
  p. malignant melanoma of the
    esophagus (PMME)
  p. obstructive megaureter
  p. oxalosis
  p. panendoscopy
  p. perineal hypospadias surgery
  p. peristaltic wave
  p. peritonitis
  p. procedure
  p. prophylaxis
  p. pseudoobstruction syndrome
  p. refluxing megaureter
  p. renal calculus
  p. sclerosing cholangitis (PSC)
  p. spermatocyte
  p. sterility
  p. suture
  p. syphilis
  p. transitional cell carcinoma
  p. tuberculosis
  p. urinary diversion
  p. vesicoureteral reflex
primed cell
primidone
priming
  androgen p.
**primitive neuroectodermal tumor
  (PNET)**
primordial kidney
Primus
  P. Prostate Machine
  P. transrectal thermography
principal cell (PC)
Principen
principle
  Boari-Ockerblad p.
  countercurrent multiplier p.
  Goodwin cup-patch p.
  Heineke-Mikulicz p.
  Mitrofanoff p.
  oncologic p.

Sarfeh p.
Seldinger p.
Pringle maneuver
printer
Mavigraph color video p.
Priscoline
privilege
bathroom p.
proband
Pro-Banthine
probe
Aloka MP-PN ultrasound p.
ambulatory p.
antisense RNA p.
Bakes p.
Barr fistula p.
Beckman 39042 pH p.
beta-actin cDNA p.
BICAP bipolar hemostasis p.
BICAP electrocoagulation p.
BICAP electrode p.
BICAP endoscopic p.
biliary balloon p.
Bilitec 2000 intraluminal
  fiberoptic p.
biotinylated DNA p.
biplane sector p.
Bipolar Circumactive P. (BICAP)
Bipolar EndoStasis p. (BESP)
bipolar hemostasis p.
blunt p.
Buie fistula p.
bullet p.
caliber p.
Cameron-Miller monopolar p.
catheter p.
catheter-based ultrasound p.
cDNA p.
8-channel cross-sectional anal
  sphincter p.
coagulation p.
CO_2 laser p.
contact p.
continuously perfused p.
Corson needle electrosurgical p.
C-Trak p.
cystic fibrosis gene p.
Desjardins gallbladder p.
Desjardins gall duct p.
Desjardins gallstone p.
p. dilator
Dobbhoff bipolar coagulation p.

Doppler p.
dot-plotted p.
Earle rectal p.
EHL p.
electrode p.
electrohydraulic lithotripsy p.
electrosurgical monopolar spatula p.
end-fire transrectal p.
endoanal p.
endorectal p.
endoscopic BICAP p.
endoscopic Doppler p.
endoscopic heat p.
EndoSound ultrasound p.
Fenger gallbladder p.
FIDUS p.
fistula p.
Fluhrer rectal p.
Fogarty biliary p.
front-loading ultrasound p. (FLUP)
gallstone p.
galvanic p.
genomic DNA p.
Gold p.
p. gorget
G3PDH CDNA p.
p. and groove director
heat p.
heater p. (HP)
24-hour esophageal pH p.
human apo A-I DNA p.
human fibronectin cDNA p.
human gastrin p.
injection gold p. (IGP)
intraductal ultrasound p.
intraluminal p.
KTP laser p.
lacrimal duct p.
large-bore heat p.
Larry rectal p.
laser-Doppler Periflux PF-3 p.
light monitoring p.
linear p.
Mayo common duct p.
Meadox Surgimed Doppler p.
mechanical rotating p.
Medi-Tech bipolar p.
Medrad Mrinnervu endorectal
  colon p.
20-MHz endoscopic ultrasound p.
microballoon p.

NOTES

P

probe *(continued)*

Microelectrode MI-506 small-caliber p.
miniature p.
miniaturized ultrasound catheter p.
Mixter dilating p.
monopolar p.
Moynihan bile duct p.
Moynihan gallstone p.
multilumen p.
Ochsner flexible spiral gallstone p.
Ochsner gallbladder p.
oligonucleotide p.
Olympus CD-20Z heater p.
Olympus GF-UM30P linear scanning p.
Olympus heat p.
Olympus S-20-20R p.
Olympus ultrathin balloon-fitted ultrasound p.
Olympus UM-F30-20R p.
Olympus UM-2R, -3R p.
Olympus UM-R-series miniature ultrasonic p.
Olympus UM-S30-25R p.
Olympus UM-W-series endoscopic p.
palpating p.
pH p.
pH-manometry p.
polycationic histochemical p.
Pratt rectal p.
Radiometer GK2803C pH p.
rectal p.
reflectance spectrophotometric p.
RNA p.
Sandhill P32 pH antimony p.
silver p.
Sonoblate P.
Sonocath ultrasound p.
stimulation p.
tactile p.
through-the-scope catheter p.
Transonics Systems 0.5-mm flow p.
transrectal p.
triple balloon p.
tumor p.
ultrasonic lithotriptor p.
ultrasound catheter p. (UCP)
V33W high-density endocavity p.
water p.

probenecid
probenecid-containing solution
probenecid-inhibited organic anion transport system
Probiotica
probiotic therapy

problem

bone marrow transplantation-related p.
clinical p.
micturition p.
penile prosthesis mechanical p.

probucol
procainamide
procainamide-induced systemic lupus erythematosus
procaine

p. hydrochloride
p. penicillin

Pro-Cal-Sof
Procaltrol
procarbazine
Procardia XL
procedural amnesia
procedure *(See also* operation, repair)

abdominal p.
Acucise retrograde p.
Acucise RP outpatient p.
Al-Ghorab p.
antegrade continence enema p.
antiincontinence p.
antireflux p.
Asopa p.
Ball p.
Barcat p.
basket p.
Belsey Mark IV p.
bladder chimney p.
Bloodgood p.
Boari bladder flap p.
bowel refashioning p.
Boyce-Vest p.
Burch p.
bypass p.
Camey p.
Campbell p.
CaverMap p.
cecal imbrication p.
Cecil p.
Chester-Winter p.
Cleveland Clinic weighted scale of endoscopic p.'s
Cohen antireflux p.
colon p.
coring-out p.
corporal plication p.
corporeal rotation p.
dartos pouch p.
Datta p.
DAWG p.
Delorme p.
Devine-Devine p.
Duckett p.
Duval p.

Ebbehoj p.
endoscopy p.
esophageal sling p.
Essed surgical p.
flap valve antireflux p.
flip-flap p.
Fowler-Stephens p.
Frykman-Goldberg p.
Fungi-Fluor p.
gastric neobladder p.
Gilchrist p.
Gil-Vernet p.
Gittes-Loughlin p.
Gittes urethral suspension p.
glans approximation p. (GAP)
Goulding p.
Gregoir-Lich p.
Halban p.
Hanley rectal bladder p.
Harewood suspension p.
Hartmann p.
Heitz-Boyer p.
Heller-Dor p.
hemi-Kock p.
Hinman p.
Hodgson technique of modified
   Lich p.
Hodgson XX p.
Hofmeister p.
hydrocelectomy bottle p.
hydrocelectomy dartos pouch p.
ileoanal pull-through p.
infrarenal template p.
intraparavariceal p.
invasive p.
island flap p.
Jaboulay p.
Johnston buttonhole p.
Kasai p.
Kelling-Madlener p.
Kelly plication p.
Kocher ureterosigmoidostomy p.
Kock pouch modified p.
Kropp p.
Ladd p.
laparoscopic bladder neck suture
   suspension p.
laparoscopic urinary diversion p.
Leadbetter p.
LeFort p.
Lewis-Tanner esophagectomy p.
Lich p.

Malone antegrade colonic enema
   stoma p.
Marshall-Marchetti-Krantz p.
Mathieu p.
Maydl p.
McIndoe p.
Michal p. (I, II)
microsurgical epididymal sperm
   aspiration p.
Mikulicz p.
Mitrofanoff p.
modified Ingelman-Sundberg p.
modified Nesbit p.
modified Norfolk p.
modified transduodenal
   rendezvous p.
Moschcowitz p.
multiple surgical p.
muscle-filling p.
Mustarde p.
needle suspension p.
Nesbit tuck p.
omentum majus flap p.
one-stage p.
O'Regan p.
Palomo p.
Partington-Rochelle p.
Pauchet p.
pelvic pouch p.
Pereyra p.
peri-Vaterian therapeutic
   endoscopic p.
primary p.
ProstRcision p.
Puestow p.
Puestow-Gillesby p.
pull-through p.
Ransley p.
Raz p.
repeat p.
retropubic needle suspension p.
Richardson p.
Righini p.
Ripstein p.
Rives-Stoppa p.
Rossetti-Nissen p.
Roux-en-Y p.
Salle p.
Schoemaker p.
sling p.
Snow p.
Soave abdominal pull-through p.

NOTES

P

procedure *(continued)*
    Spence p.
    sphincter-saving p.
    Stamey p.
    Stamey-Martius p.
    Sting p.
    Stretta p.
    Studer pouch p.
    suburethral rectus fascial sling p.
    Sugiura p.
    surgical p.
    takedown of pelvic sling p.
    tension-free vaginal tape p.
    Thiersch p.
    Thiersch-Duplay proximal tube p.
    Thompson p.
    TIPS p.
    Toupet p.
    transhepatic antegrade biliary
      drainage p.
    transjugular intrahepatic portacaval
      shunt p.
    transvaginal Burch p.
    TVT p.
    untethering p.
    upper gastrointestinal p.
    ureteral patch p.
    vaginal flap reconstruction and
      pubovaginal sling p.
    vaginal needle suspension p.
    vaginal wall sling p.
    Van de Kramer fecal fat p.
    Vesica sling p.
    Walsh p.
    Whipple p.
    Winter p.
    Womack p.
    York-Mason p.
    Young-Dees p.
process
    fingerlike epithelial p.
    foot p. (FP)
    glycosylation p.
    juxtacapillary p.
    knobby p.
    morphogenetic p.
    signal transduction p.
    sodium-linked p.
    spinous p.
    transverse p.
    uncinate p.
processing
    image p.
    postsecretory p.
    swim-up p.
processor
    Miles V.I.P. 300 vacuum
      infiltration p.

    Olympus EU-M-series
      endosonography image p.
    real-time video p.
    ThinPrep P.
    video p.
processus vaginalis
prochlorperazine 25-mg suppository
ProCide disinfectant
procidentia
    anal p.
    internal p.
    rectal p.
    p. recti
procoagulant
procollagen
    C-terminal propeptide of type I p.
    N-terminal propeptide of type
      III p.
Procrit
proctalgia fugax
proctectasia
proctectomy
    mucosal p.
proctitis
    acute p.
    allergic p.
    bleeding p.
    chronic radiation p.
    chronic ulcerative p.
    Dean stage I, II radiation p.
    diversion p.
    epidemic gangrenous p.
    factitial p.
    glutaraldehyde-induced p.
    gonococcal p.
    gonorrheal p.
    idiopathic p.
    nonspecific ulcerative p.
    radiation p.
    traumatic p.
    ulcerative p.
proctoclysis
proctocolectomy
    minilaparotomy restorative p.
    restorative p. (RP, RPC)
    single-stage total p.
    totally stapled restorative p.
      (TSRPC)
proctocolitis
    aphthoid p.
    idiopathic p.
    radiation p.
    venereal p.
proctocolonoscopy
ProctoCream-HC
proctocystocele
proctocystoplasty
proctocystotomy

proctoelytroplasty
Proctofoam
Proctofoam-HC
proctogram
 balloon p.
 defecating p.
proctography
 dynamic p.
 evacuation p.
 quantitative scintigraphic
  evacuation p.
proctoperineoplasty
proctopexy
 Orr-Loygue transabdominal p.
proctoplasty
proctoptosis
Proctor-Livingston
 P.-L. endoprosthesis
 P.-L. tube
proctorrhaphy
proctoscope
 Boehm p.
 Gabriel p.
 Kelly p.
 Lieberman p.
 Montague p.
 Newman p.
 Salvati p.
 Vernon-David p.
proctoscopy
 rigid p.
proctosigmoidectomy
proctosigmoiditis
 refractory p.
proctosigmoidoscope
 ACMI fiberoptic p.
proctosigmoidoscopy
 rigid p.
proctostenosis
proctotomy
 external p.
 internal p.
 linear p.
proctovalvotomy
procyclidine
Prodium
prodromal symptom
prodrome
prodrug
 GSH p.
product
 Amadori p.

fibrin/fibrinogen degradation p.
 (FDP)
fibrinogen degradation p.
fibrin split p. (FSP)
mechanical p.
secretory p.
thermodynamic solubility p.
production
 ammonia p.
 autoantibody p.
 chylomicron p.
 creatinine p.
 hydrogen ion p.
 lymphokine p.
 spermatozoon p.
 superoxide p.
 unilateral renin p.
productive nephritis
prodynorphin gene
PROEF
 postoperative regimen for oral early
 feeding
proenkephalin gene
profile
 ASTRA p.
 gut-hormone p.
 liver function p.
 P. pediatric polypectomy snare
 phosphotyrosyl protein p.
 plasmid p.
 resting urethral pressure p.
 sickness impact p.
 spicule in p.
 StoneRisk diagnostic p.
 stress urethral pressure p.
 urethral closure pressure p.
 urethral pressure p. (UPP)
profiled dialysis
profilometry
 urethral pressure p.
profound acid reduction
profunda
 colitis cystica p. (CCP)
 fascia penis p.
 gastritis cystic p.
profuse vomiting
progenitalis
 herpes p.
progesteronal agent
progesterone
progesterone-associated colitis

NOTES

P

prognostic
    p. factor
    p. indicator
    p. nutritional index (PNI)
    p. significance
prograde technique
Prograf
program
    CLIM computer p.
    low-energy p.
    Maine Medical Assessment P.
      (MMAP)
    Organ Procurement P.
    personalized p.
    POINTER computer p.
    Stat-View computer p.
    Synectics computer p.
programming
    in utero p.
progression
    p. factor
    renal p.
progressive
    p. diet
    p. dysphagia
    p. emphysematous necrosis
    p. familial cirrhosis
    p. familial intrahepatic cholestasia
      (PFIC)
    p. intrahepatic cholestasia
    p. perivenular alcoholic fibrosis
      (PPAF)
    p. renal dysfunction
    p. renal insufficiency
    p. suppurative cholangitis
    p. systemic sclerosis (PSS)
    p. toxicity
Prohibit anti-fog face mask
proinflammatory cytokine
project
    Captopril Prevention P. (CAPPP)
    National Prostatic Cancer P.
projectile vomiting
projection
    afferent p.
    Chassard-Lapiné p.
    parasympathetic p.
    single-shot voxel p.
    sympathetic p.
prokaryotic pathogen
prokinetic
    p. agent
    p. drug
    p. effect
    p. therapy
prolactin
Prolamine

prolapse
    anal p.
    bladder p.
    buttonpexy fixation of stomal p.
    external anorectal mucosal p.
    gastric mucosal p.
    p. gastropathy
    genitourinary p.
    hemorrhoidal p.
    incarcerated p.
    incomplete rectal p.
    intestinal p.
    mucosal p.
    pelvic p.
    rectal p.
    stomal p.
    sudden valve p.
    ureterocele p.
    urethral p.
    urogenital p.
    valve p.
prolapsed
    p. bowel
    p. internal hemorrhoid
    p. rectum
    p. stoma
prolapsing fourth-degree hemorrhoid
Prolase
    Cytocare P. II
    P. II lateral firing Nd:YAG laser
Pro-Lax
Prolene suture
Proleukin aldesleukin
proliferans
    angiocholitis p.
    cholecystitis glandularis p.
proliferating
    p. cell nuclear antigen (PCNA)
    p. tubular cell
proliferation
    bile duct p.
    cell p.
    cellular p.
    colonic epithelial p.
    cystic epithelial p.
    diffuse mesangial p.
    DNA p.
    extraglandular endocrine cell p.
    p. of the gastric epithelium
    glomerular cell p.
    index of cell p.
    intracystic epithelial p.
    intraluminal p.
    mesangial p.
    monoclonal p.
    mucosal cell p.
    neoplastic cell p.

osteoblast-like p.
rectal cell p.
proliferative
p. glomerulonephritis
p. hypertrophic gastritis
p. inflammatory atrophy
ProLine endoscopic instrument
prolinuria
glycyl p.
Prolixin
prolonged expiratory phase
Proloprim
promazine
promethazine
Promex biopsy needle
promontory
sacral p.
promulgated
Pronase
pronation
pronator drift
prone
p. position
p. split leg position
pronephros
Pronestyl
pronucleus, pl. **pronuclei**
proopiomelanocortin (POMC)
p. gene
propafenone
propagated antroduodenal contraction
propagation
p. of contraction
orad p.
propantheline bromide
propendens
venter p.
proper
p. hepatic artery
p. lamina
p. tunic
properitoneal
p. fat
p. flank stripe
p. hernia
prophecy
self-fulfilling p.
propHiler urinary pH testing kit
prophylactic
p. antibiotic
p. antibiotic treatment (PAT)
p. cephalosporin

p. cholecystectomy
p. device
p. gamma globulin
p. lymphadenectomy
p. orchidopexy
p. orchiectomy
p. sclerotherapy
p. urethritis
prophylaxis
antibiotic p.
antimicrobial p.
continuous p.
primary p.
secondary p.
stress ulcer p.
stricture p.
propidium iodide
propionate
testosterone p.
Propionibacterium acnes
propiverine
propofol
proporphyria
erythropoietic p. (EPP)
propoxyphene hydrochloride
propranolol
propria
arteria hepatica p.
intestinal lamina p.
lamina p.
muscularis p.
ratio of mucosa to submucosa to
muscularis p.
tunica p.
proprioception
intact p.
Propulsid
propulsion
colonic p.
ineffective colonic p.
propulsive
p. motor pattern
p. wave
propylene oxide
propylhexedrine
propylthiouracil (PTU)
prorenin
serine protease-activated p.
Proscan
P. ultrasound imaging system
P. ultrasound unit
Proscar

NOTES

Pros-Check
 P.-C. kit
 P.-C. PSA assay
Prosed/DS
Proshield Plus skin protectant
ProSobee liquid formula
prospective
 p. clinical trial
 p. comparison
 p. multicenter study
prospermia
Prostacoil stent
prostacyclin
prostaglandin (PG)
 p. 1
 p. analog
 colonic p.
 cytoprotective p.
 p. E
 p. E1
 p. E2 (PGE2)
 p. F
 p. F2-alpha (PGF2-alpha)
 p. G (PGG)
 p. H (PGH)
 p. I2 (PGI2)
 renal p.
 renal vasodilator p.
 p. supplementation
 p. synthesis
Prostakath urethral stent
prostanoid synthesis
ProstaScint scan
ProstaSeed
 P. I-125
 P. I-125 seed
prostata (*pl. of* prostate)
prostatae
 isthmus p.
prostatalgia
prostate, pl. **prostata**
 atypical small acinar proliferation
  of p. (ASAP)
 p. balloon dilator
 boggy p.
 p. cancer (PCa)
 P. Cancer Intervention Versus
  Observation Trial (PCIVOT,
  PIVOT)
 carcinoma of p. (CAP)
 coagulation and hemostatic
  resection of the p. (CHRP)
 contact laser vaporization of the p.
  (CLVP)
 Costello laser ablation of p.
 cryosurgical ablation of the p.
  (CSAP)
 enlarged p.

funnel-neck p.
p. gland benign hyperplasia
p. gland biopsy
p. gland C3 complement
p. gland color flow Doppler
 examination
p. gland cross section
p. gland cytoskeleton
p. gland electrovaporization
p. gland hypoplasia
p. gland innervation
p. gland involution
p. gland leiomyosarcoma
p. gland lymphoma
p. gland needle ablation
p. gland peripheral zone
p. gland periurethral zone
p. gland prostate-specific membrane
 antigen
p. gland sarcoma
p. gland secretion
p. gland small cell carcinoma
p. gland stroma
p. gland stromal cell
p. gland tissue matrix
p. gland transition zone
p. gland transurethral balloon
 dilation
p. gland transurethral resection
holmium laser resection of the p.
 (HoLRP)
median furrow of the p.
minimal transurethral resection
 of p. (M-TURP)
nodular hyperplasia of p.
percutaneous radical cryosurgical
 ablation of p.
prostatisme sans p.
p. rhabdomyosarcoma
salvage cryoablation of the p.
thick loop transurethral resection of
 the p.
total transurethral resection of p.
 (T-TURP)
transurethral electrovaporization
 of p. (TUVP, TVP)
transurethral evaporation of p.
 (TUEP)
transurethral grooving of p.
transurethral incision of p. (TUIP)
transurethral laser incision of
 the p.
transurethral needle ablation of
 the p.
transurethral resection of p.
 (TURP)
transurethral vaporization of p.
 (TUVP)

transurethral vaporization-resection
of p. (TUVRP)
visual laser ablation of p. (VLAP)
p. volume
prostatectomy
anatomical radical retropubic p.
cavernosal nerve-sparing radical p.
KTP laser p.
laparoscopic radical p.
laser p.
Madigan p.
Millen technique retropubic p.
nerve-sparing radical retropubic p.
open p.
perineal p.
radical p. (RP)
radical perineal p.
radical retropubic p. (RRP)
radical transcoccygeal p.
retropubic ascending radical p.
salvage p.
Stanford radical retropubic p.
suprapubic p.
total perineal p.
transurethral ablative p.
transurethral balloon
Laserthermia p.
transurethral ultrasound-guided laser-
induced p. (TULIP)
visual laser-assisted p. (VLAP)
Walsh radical retropubic p.
prostate-specific
p.-s. acid phosphatase
p.-s. antigen (PSA)
p.-s. antigen-based parameter
p.-s. antigen bound to alpha-1
antichymotrypsin (PSA-ACT)
p.-s. antigen density (PSAD)
p.-s. antigen density of the
transition zone (PSA-TZ)
p.-s. antigen velocity (PSAV)
p.-s. membrane (PSM)
p.-s. membrane antigen (PSMA)
Prostathermer
Biodan P.
P. 99D
P. device
P. prostatic hyperthermia system
prostatic
p. abscess
p. acid phosphatase (PAP)
p. adenocarcinoma

p. adenoma
p. antibacterial factor
p. artery
p. calculus
p. capsule
p. catheter
p. chip
p. cryptococcosis
p. fascia
p. fossa
p. hyperplasia
p. hypertrophy
p. intraepithelial neoplasia (PIN)
p. massage
p. mesonephric remnant
p. neoplasm
p. nodule
p. outlet obstruction (POO)
p. pile
p. pressure coefficient (PPC)
p. sinus
p. stent
p. thermal treatment
p. tuberculosis
p. urethra
p. urethral polyp
p. urethral transitional cell
carcinoma
p. utricle
p. volume
prostatica
ductuli p.
vesica p.
prostatici
ductus p.
prostaticovesical plexus
prostaticovesiculectomy
prostaticus
plexus p.
utriculus p.
prostatism
silent p.
vesical p.
prostatisme sans prostate
prostatitic
prostatitis
bacterial p.
chemical p.
chronic abacterial p.
chronic bacterial p. (CBP)
chronic nonbacterial p. (CNP)
granulomatous p.

NOTES

P

prostatitis *(continued)*
    mycotic p.
    NIH Classification Category I
      acute bacterial p.
    NIH Classification Category II
      chronic bacterial p.
    NIH Classification Category IV
      asymptomatic inflammatory p.
    NIH Classification System for P.
    nonbacterial p. (NBP)
    parasitic p.
    tuberculous p.
prostatocystitis
prostatocystotomy
prostatodynia (PD)
prostatography
prostatolith
prostatolithotomy
prostatomegaly
prostatometer
prostatomy
    lateral p.
prostatomyomectomy
prostatorrhea
prostatoseminal vesiculectomy
prostatoseminalvesiculectomy
prostatotomy
prostatotoxin
prostatourethral fistula
prostatourethral-rectal fistula
prostatovesical junction
prostatovesiculectomy
prostatovesiculitis
Prostatron transurethral thermotherapy device
prostatropin
prosthesis
    Alpha I inflatable penile p.
    Ambicor penile p.
    AMS Hydroflex penile p.
    AMS 700 inflatable penile p.
    AMS 600 malleable penile p.
    Amsterdam-type p.
    AMS three-piece inflatable
      penile p.
    AMS Ultrex penile p.
    Angelchik antireflux p.
    Angelchik ring p.
    antireflux p.
    Atkinson p.
    balloon tamponade p.
    biliary p.
    bilioduodenal p.
    bladder neck support p.
    Celestin p.
    covered self-expanding p.
    CXM p.
    CX Plus p.

    Dacron p.
    Dilamezinsert penile p.
    double-pigtail p.
    Dura-II positionable penile p.
    Duraphase inflatable penile p.
    Dynaflex penile p.
    ERCP conventional p.
    EsophaCoil p.
    esophageal p.
    Finney Flexirod penile p.
    Flexi-Flate I, II penile p.
    Flexirod penile p.
    GFS Mark II inflatable penile p.
    Gianturco expandable (self-
      expanding) metallic biliary p.
    glass penile p.
    hydraulic hinge penile p.
    Hydroflex penile p.
    inflatable penile p. (IPP)
    Introl bladder neck support p.
    iridium p.
    Jonas penile p.
    malleable p.
    Mentor Alpha 1 inflatable
      penile p.
    Mentor GFS penile p.
    Mentor IPP penile p.
    Mentor malleable penile p.
    Mentor Mark II penile p.
    mesh stent p.
    Neville tracheal reconstruction p.
    OmniPhase penile p.
    penile p.
    Scott AMS inflatable penile p.
    silicone donut p.
    silicone self-expanding p.
    Small-Carrion penile p.
    Subrini penile p.
    testicular p.
    Ultraflex esophageal p.
    Ultrex Plus penile p.
    Uni-Flate 1000 penile p.
    Unitary inflatable penile p.
    urethral stent p.
    UroLume Endourethral Wallstent p.
    UroLume urethral p.
    valved voice p.
    Wallstent esophageal p.
    Wilson-Cook plastic p.
prosthetic
    p. arterial graft
    p. bladder
    p. penis
    p. testis
    p. utricle cyst
    p. valve click
prosthetist
Prosthex sponge

Prostigmin
ProstRcision
    P. procedure
    P. treatment
ProTack
    P. stapler
    P. tacking device
Protalba-R
protamine
    p. sulfate
    p. zinc insulin
protease
    p. inhibitor
    serine p.
    V8 p.
proteasome
protectant
    Proshield Plus skin p.
Protect-a-Pass suture passer
protection
    gastroduodenal mucosal p.
    misoprostol p.
protective probiotic flora
protector plus wire
protein
    A-4 p.
    acute phase p.
    adenovirus-12 viral p.
    aldosterone-induced p. (AIP)
    androgen-binding p.
    p. antibody (PAb)
    antibody to c100 p.
    anti-Tamm-Horsfall p.
    ascitic fluid total p. (AFTP)
    band 3 p.
    basement membrane p.
    Bence Jones p.
    bone morphogenic p.
    p. C
    cagA p.
    calcium binding p.
    calcium-regulated p.
    calcium-specific binding p.
    p. catabolic rate (PCR)
    CD3 p.
    CD4 p.
    CD8 p.
    CD2-associated p.
    CDC42 p.
    p. C deficiency
    cholesterol ester transfer p. (CETP)
    c-MET p.

    complement regulatory p.
    copper-binding p. (CBP)
    C-reactive p. (CRP)
    CSF p.
    p. C, S level
    cytoplasmic adaptor p.
    cytotoxin-associated gene A p.
    p. depletion
    dietary p.
    dipstick p.
    downstream signaling p.
    E1b p.
    E1, E2, E6 p.
    E2F p.
    enzymic p.
    eosinophil cationic p. (ECP)
    eosinophilic major basic p.
    eosinophil p. X (EPX)
    EP2-EP3 p.
    estramustine binding p. (EMBP)
    fatty acid binding p. (FABP)
    fibronectin-binding p.
    fyn p.
    G p.
    Gal 4 p.
    GTPase activating p.
    GTP-dependent signaling p.
    GTP-regulatory p.
    guanine nucleotide-regulatory p.
    HCV p.
    heat shock p. (HSP)
    helix-loop-helix p.
    helix-turn-helix p.
    hepatocellular p.
    heptahelical receptor p.
    heterodimeric p.
    heterotrimeric G p.
    H-related p.
    IkBa p.
    intestinal fatty acid-binding p. (I-FABP)
    87kDa p.
    p. kinase A
    p. kinase C (PKC)
    lck p.
    liver-specific p.
    low molecular weight p.
    MAGP microfibrillar p.
    membrane cofactor p. (MCP)
    membrane transport p.
    mesenchymal p.
    p. metabolism

NOTES

P

protein *(continued)*
  microfibrillar p. (MP)
  monocyte chemoattractant p.
  monocyte chemotactic p. (MCP)
  myeloma p.
  noncollagen p.
  Novel erythropoiesis stimulating p.
    (NESP)
  NS2, NS3, NS4, NS5 p.
  nuclear factor kappa B
    transcription factor p.
  nuclear matrix p. (NMP, NMP-22)
  oligosaccharide-binding membrane p.
  oncofetal p.
  outer inflammatory p.
  p53 p.
  pancreatic stone p. (PSP)
  pertussin toxin-sensitive G p.
  PH30 p.
  p. phosphatase
  p. phosphorylation
  phosphorylation p.
  plasma p.
  p. plug
  p53 nuclear p.
  podocyte-specific p.
  porin channel p.
  p47, p67 cytosolic p.
  PTH-related p. (PTH-rP)
  rac p.
  ras-related p.
  Rb p.
  receptor-associated p. (RAP)
  p. restriction
  retinoid-binding p.
  retinol-binding p. (RBP)
  rho p.
  p. S
  S-100 p.
  scrapie p.
  p. S deficiency
  p. serine kinase
  p. serine/threonine kinase activity
  serum p.
  serum core p.
  p. solder
  STAR p.
  steroidogenic acute regulatory p.
  stress p.
  p. supplement
  surface p.
  p. synthesis
  Tamm-Horsfall p. (THP)
  TATA-binding p.
  T cell-specific p.
  testicular androgen-binding p.
  p. threonine kinase
  tight-junction p.

  total p.
  transmembrane p.
  triglyceride-rich p. (TRL)
  p. tubular reabsorption
  p. tyrosine kinase
  p. tyrosine phosphatase
  urinary marker p.
  uronic acid-rich p.
  vitamin-D-binding p. (DBP)
  p. in vitamin K absence (PIVKA)
protein-1
  insulinlike growth factor-binding p.
    (IGFBP-1)
  monocyte chemoattractant p. (MCP-
    1)
proteinaceous
  p. cast
  p. cast material
proteinase
  p. enzyme
  p. inhibitor
protein-bound homocysteine
protein-calorie malnutrition (PCM)
protein-energy malnutrition
protein-glutathione-S-transferase
  receptor-associated p.-g.-S.-t.
protein-losing
  p.-l. enteropathy
  p.-l. gastroenteropathy
  p.-l. gastropathy
protein-mediated tubular toxicity
protein-overload proteinuria
protein-protein assay
proteinuria
  asymptomatic p.
  Bence Jones p.
  BSA-induced overload p.
  cardiac p.
  colliquative p.
  cyclic p.
  emulsion p.
  enterogenic p.
  febrile p.
  globular p.
  glomerular p.
  gouty p.
  hematogenous p.
  incipient p.
  intermittent p.
  intrinsic p.
  nephrogenous p.
  orthostatic p.
  overflow p.
  palpatory p.
  persistent p.
  postrenal p.
  protein-overload p.
  residual p.

p. test
transient p.
tubular p.
proteinuric
  p. glomerulopathy
  p. nephropathy
  p. state
proteoglycan
  p. biglycan
  p. decorin
  heparan sulfate p. (HSPG)
proteolysis
proteolytic
  p. degradation
  p. digestion
  p. enzyme
Proteus
  P. mirabilis
  P. morganii
  P. pneumonia
  P. rettgeri
  P. vulgaris
proteus
  Vibrio cholerae biotype p.
prothrombin
  des-gamma-carboxy p. (DCP)
  p. induced by vitamin K absence
    or antagonist-II (PIVKA-II)
  p. time (pro time, PT)
  p. time/partial thromboplastin time
    (PT/PTT)
Protilase
pro time
protocol
  p. biopsy
  CISCA p.
  clinical p.
  Costello p.
  ELF chemotherapy p.
  Eulexin plus LHRH-A
    chemotherapy/radiation therapy p.
  high-energy p.
  low-energy p.
  multimodal p.
  non-heart-beating donor p.
  salvage p.
  software characteristics of the
    treating p.
  Stanford p.
  surveillance p.
  treatment p.
  VAB-6 chemotherapy p.

Protocult test
proton
  p. flux
  p. magnetic resonance spectroscopy
  p. pump
  p. pump blocker
  p. pump inhibition therapy
  p. pump inhibitor (PPI)
protonated
proton-induced release of secretin
Protonix
protooncogene
  c-fos p.
  c-jun p.
  c-myc p.
  p53 p.
  RET p.
protopathic pain
protoporphyria
  erythropoietic p.
protoporphyrin-9
Protostat Oral
prototype cholangioscope
protozoa
  intestinal p.
protozoal
  p. abscess
  p. disease
  p. dysentery
protozoan
  p. enteritis
  p. parasite
  p. pathogen
protriptyline
protruding fat
protrusion
  anal p.
protuberant
  p. abdomen
  p. carcinoma
Provera
Providencia
  P. alcalifaciens
  P. rettgeri
  P. stuartii
Provir
provocation
  edrophonium p.
provocative
  P. sensitivity balloon

NOTES

P

609

provocative *(continued)*
    p. test
    p. testing
provoked cystometry
proxetil
    cefpodoxime p.
proximal
    p. bile duct
    p. convoluted tubule (PCT)
    p. gastrectomy
    p. gastric vagotomy (PGV)
    p. human colonic flora
    p. muscle weakness
    p. nephron
    p. pouch leak
    p. pressure
    p. splenorenal shunt
    p. straight tubule (PST)
    p. superior mesenteric artery
    p. tubule (PT)
    p. tubule function
    p. venous plexus
proximate
    P. flexible linear stapler
    P. ILS SDH circular stapler
    P. intraluminal stapler
    P. linear cutter
Prozac
PRT
    physiologic reflux test
PRU
    percent reduction in urea
prucalopride
Prudoxin cream
Pruitt anoscope
Prulet
prune-belly syndrome (category I, II, III)
prune juice peritoneal fluid
prunetin
pruning
    p. abnormality
    p. sign
pruritic
pruritus
    p. ani
    opioid-mediated p.
    p. scroti
    uremic p.
PS-2 needle
PSA
    prostate-specific antigen
    PSA doubling time
    free to total PSA
    PSA free/total index
    F:T PSA
        free to total prostate-specific antigen
    PSA RT-PCR
    total PSA
PSA4 prostate cancer test
PSA-ACT
    prostate-specific antigen bound to alpha-1 antichymotrypsin
PSA-based parameter
PSAD
    prostate-specific antigen density
PSA-TZ
    prostate-specific antigen density of the transition zone
PSAV
    prostate-specific antigen velocity
PSC
    primary sclerosing cholangitis
PSE
    portosystemic encephalopathy
Pseudallescheria boydii
pseudoachalasia
    malignant p.
pseudoalcoholic liver disease
pseudoallergy
pseudoaneurysm
    p. formation
    ruptured p.
pseudoaneurysmal roof
pseudobile canaliculus
pseudo-Billroth I appearance
pseudocapsule
pseudocholangiocarcinoma sign
pseudochylous ascites
pseudocirrhosis
    cholangiodysplastic p.
pseudocolitis
pseudocryptorchism
pseudo-Cushing syndrome
pseudocyst
    p. communication
    drainage-resistant p.
    endosonography-guided drainage of pancreatic p.
    extramural p.
    extrapancreatic p.
    heterogenous p.
    infected p.
    intrasplenic p.
    pancreatic p.
    paraduodenal p.
    paragastric p.
    p. puncture
    retrogastric p.
    uriniferous p.
pseudocystobiliary fistula
pseudocystogastrostomy
    pancreatic p.
pseudodefecation
pseudodeficiency rickets

pseudodiverticulosis
    esophageal intramural p.
pseudodiverticulum
    urethral p.
pseudoductular transformation of hepatocyte
pseudodysentery
pseudodyssynergia
pseudoephedrine hydrochloride
pseudoepitheliomatous micaceous growths of penis
pseudoesophageal colic
pseudoexstrophy
pseudogout
pseudohermaphroditism
pseudohydronephrosis
pseudohypha, pl. **pseudohyphae**
pseudohypoaldosteronism
    type I, II p.
pseudohyponatremia
pseudohypoparathyroidism (PHP)
pseudoileus
pseudoleukemia gastrointestinalis
pseudolipomatosis
pseudolithiasis
    ceftriaxone p.
pseudolymphoma
    gastric p.
pseudomelanosis
pseudomembrane
pseudomembranous
    p. colic
    p. colitis (PMC)
    p. enteritis
    p. enterocolitis
    p. gastritis
pseudomicrolithiasis
pseudomigration
Pseudomonas
    P. aeruginosa
    P. aeruginosa pneumonia
    P. exotoxin A
    P. pseudomallei pneumonia
pseudomononucleosis
pseudomyxoma peritonei
pseudoneurogenic bladder
pseudoobstruction
    acute colonic p.
    bowel p.
    chronic idiopathic intestinal p. (CIIP)
    chronic intestinal p. (CIP, CIPO)

    colonic p.
    dolichocolon with p.
    familial intestinal p.
    idiopathic intestinal p.
    intestinal p.
    nonfamilial intestinal p.
    polyneuropathy, ophthalmoplegia, leukoencephalopathy, and intestinal p. (POLIP)
    p. syndrome
pseudopancreatic cholera syndrome
pseudoparallel channel sign
pseudopelade
pseudoperoxidase
pseudophimosis
pseudophytobezoar
pseudopodia
    tumorous p.
pseudopolyp
    chili-bean p.
pseudopolyposis medicamentosus
pseudo-prune-belly syndrome
pseudo-pseudohypoparathyroidism
pseudoresistance
pseudosac
pseudosacculation
pseudosarcoid
pseudosarcoma
    bladder p.
pseudospider pelvis
pseudostone
pseudostricture
pseudotubercle
pseudotuberculosis
    Yersinia p.
pseudotumor
    p. appearance
    helminthic p.
    inflammatory p.
    kidney p.
    periampullary p.
    urethral p.
pseudovaginal perineoscrotal hypospadias
pseudowatermelon esophagus
pseudo-Whipple disease
pseudoxanthoma elasticum
PSFR
    pancreatic secretory flow rate
    peak secretory flow rate
    PSFR test
PSGN
    poststreptococcal glomerulonephritis

NOTES

P

PSH II
   Physicians' Health Study II
PSI
   portal shunt index
psittaci
      Chlamydia p.
PSK
   polysaccharide Kreha
PSLL
   pancreatoscopic laser lithotripsy
PSM
   prostate-specific membrane
PSMA
   prostate-specific membrane antigen
psoas
     p. abscess
     p. fascia
     p. hitch
     p. loss
     p. muscle
     p. shadow
     p. sign
psorenteritis
psoriasis of the penis
psoriatic arthropathy
Psorospermium haeckelii
PSP
   pancreatic stone protein
PSS
   physiologic salt solution
   portosystemic shunting
   progressive systemic sclerosis
PST
   postural stimulation test
   proximal straight tubule
PSTI
   pancreatic secretory trypsin inhibitor
PSWL
   peroral shock wave lithotripsy
psychic
     p. dysuria
     p. impotence
psychogenic
     p. constipation
     p. erectile dysfunction
     p. erection
     p. impotence
     p. polydipsia
     p. vomiting
     p. water drinking
psychologic
     p. dysfunction
     p. enuresis
     p. nonneuropathic bladder
psychological
     p. disorder
     p. factor

P. General Well Being Index
   (PGWBI)
     p. support
psychometric test
psychometry
psychopharmacologic medication
psychophysiologic testing
psychosexual
     p. history
     p. support
     p. therapy
psychosis
psychosomatic disorder
psychotropic
     p. drug
     p. medication
psychrophore
psyllium husk fiber
PT
   prothrombin time
   proximal tubule
PTA
   percutaneous transluminal angioplasty
PTBD
   percutaneous transhepatic biliary drainage
     PTBD catheter
PTC
   percutaneous transhepatic cholangiogram
   percutaneous transhepatic
     cholangiography
PTCC
   percutaneous transhepatic
     cholecystoscopy
PTCD
   percutaneous transhepatic cholangio-
     drainage
PTC-guided biopsy
PTCS
   percutaneous transhepatic cholangioscopy
PTD
   percutaneous transhepatic drainage
PTDM
   posttransplant diabetes mellitus
pteroylglutamic acid
pterygium
pterygoid depression
PTFE
   polytetrafluoroethylene
PTH
   parathyroid hormone
   plasma parathyroid hormone
     carboxyterminal PTH
     intact PTH
     midregion PTH
PTHC
   percutaneous transhepatic cholangiogram

percutaneous transhepatic
  cholangiography
    PTHC catheter
PTH-related protein (PTH-rP)
PTH-rP
  PTH-related protein
    PTH-rP by immunoradiometric
      assay
PTLD
  posttransplant lymphoproliferative
    disorder
ptosis
    renal p.
PTP
  percutaneous transhepatic portography
PT/PTT
  prothrombin time/partial thromboplastin
    time
PTR
  pressure transmission ratio
PTRA
  percutaneous transluminal renal
    angioplasty
PTT
  partial thromboplastin time
PTU
  propylthiouracil
P-TUMT
  periurethral transurethral microwave
    thermotherapy
ptyocrinous cell
P-type amylase
puberty
pubes, pl. pubes
pubic
    p. arch
    p. diastasis
    p. fixation
    p. hair line
    p. ramus
    p. symphysis
    p. tubercle
pubis
    body of p.
    osteitis p.
    pediculosis p.
    Phthirus p.
    symphysis ossium p.
puboanalis muscle
pubocervical
    p. fascia
    p. ligament

pubococcygeal
    p. line
    p. muscle training
pubococcygeus muscle
puboprostatic
    p. ligament
    p. sling
puborectalis
    p. dysfunction
    dyskinetic p.
    p. loop
    p. muscle
    p. muscle function
    overreactive p.
    p. sling
    p. syndrome
puborectal muscle
pubosacral line
pubourethral
    p. ligament
    p. sling
pubovaginal
    p. operation
    p. sling
pubovesicalis
    plica p.
pubovesical ligament
pubovesicocervical fascia
pubovisceral muscle
Pucci-Seed
    P.-S. hook
    P.-S. spatula
PUD
    peptic ulcer disease
pudding
    Ensure p.
    Sustacal p.
puddle sign
puddling on barium enema
pudenda (*pl. of* pudendum)
pudendal
    p. artery
    p. canal
    p. evoked potential
    p. nerve function
    p. nerve terminal motor latency
    p. nerve terminal motor latency
      test
    p. neurogram
    p. neuropathy
    p. pelvic nerve

NOTES

P

pudendal *(continued)*
    p. vein
    p. vessel
pudendal-anal reflex
pudendum, pl. **pudenda**
    rima pudenda
puerperal septic pelvic vein
  thrombophlebitis
puerperium
Puestow
    P. pancreaticojejunostomy
    P. procedure
Puestow-Gillesby
    P.-G. operation
    P.-G. procedure
Pugh
    P. classification
    P. modification of Child criteria
    modified method of P.
Pugh-Child scoring system
pull
    complete PEG p.
    p. method
    PEG p.
    Ponsky p.
pull-apart introducer
pull-enteroscopy
pull-through
    Duhamel p.-t.
    endorectal ileal p.-t.
    ileal p.-t.
    ileoanal endorectal p.-t.
    p.-t. manometry
    p.-t. procedure
    rapid p.-t. (RPT)
    sacroabdominoperineal p.-t.
    Soave endorectal p.-t.
    station p.-t. (SPT)
    Swenson abdominal p.-t.
    p.-t. technique
pull-type sphincterotomy
pulmonary
    p. alveolar microlithiasis
    p. arteriovenous malformation
    p. artery pressure (PAP)
    p. aspiration
    p. capillaritis
    p. capillary wedge pressure
    (PCWP)
    p. cavitation
    p. complication
    p. disorder
    p. edema
    p. embolism
    p. embolus
    p. gas embolism during
    laparoscopy
    p. granuloma

    p. methane excretion
    p. mucormycosis
    p. outflow
pulp
    splenic p.
pulpa
    p. lienis
    p. splenica
pulpar cell
pulpy testis
pulsatile
    p. hematoma
    p. mass
pulsatility index
pulse
    abdominal p.
    abrupt p.
    Altmann p.
    atrial liver p.
    Corrigan p.
    p. dye laser
    intermittent p.
    p. oximetry
    Quincke p.
    p. repetition frequency (PRF)
    p. spray catheter
    thready p.
    p. volume recording
pulsed
    p. Doppler
    p. Doppler ultrasound
    p. dye laser therapy
    p. dye neodymium:YAG laser
    p. field gel electrophoresis (PFGE)
    p. irrigation
    p. Solu-Medrol
Pulse-Pak infusion kit
pulse-width analysis
pulsion
    enterocele p.
Pulsolith laser
pulsus
    p. abdominalis
    p. paradoxus
pulverizer
    Thermovac tissue p.
Pulvules
    Cinobac P.
pump
    Abbott LifeCare p.
    AS-800 p.
    ASID Bonz PP infusion p.
    bile salt export p. (BSEP)
    Biosearch 7000 enteral feeding p.
    Bluemle p.
    calcium ATPase p.
    centrifugal p.
    Companion feeding p.

Compat 199205 enteral feeding p.
Cub R-200 enteral feeding p.
Endolav lavage p.
Enteroport feeding p.
Flexiflo Companion enteral
   feeding p.
Flexiflo II enteral feeding p.
Flocare 500 feeding p.
Flo-Gard p.
Frenta Mat feeding p.
Frenta System II feeding p.
Harvard p.
hepatic artery infusion p.
H-K-ATPase proton p.
Holter Pediatric P. 903, 907
IMED 430 enteral feeding p.
Infusaid chemotherapy
   implantable p.
Infusaid hepatic p.
infusion p. (IP)
Kangaroo 200, 330 enteral
   feeding p.
Kangaroo 324 feeding p.
Keofeed 500 enteral feeding p.
Keofeed II enteral feeding p.
KMI 60 enteral feeding p.
MasterFlex p.
McGaw volumetric p.
Nutromat Pad S feeding p.
peristaltic p.
pneumatic leg p.
proton p.
retroperistaltic p.
reverse osmosis p.
roller p.
Sarns Siok II blood p.
sodium p.
Space Saver volumetric p.
stomach p.
subcutaneous morphine p. (SQMP)
suction p.
Tonkaflo p.
VTR-300 enteral feeding p.
xenobiotic p.
pumped-dye laser
punch
aortic p.
biopsy p.
p. biopsy
kidney p.
Murphy kidney p.
Turkel p.

punched-out
p.-o. orchidometer
p.-o. ulcer
p.-o. ulceration
punctata
Aeromonas p.
punctate
p. area
p. ulcer
puncture
caliceal p.
calix p.
cystic p.
diathermic p.
direct cautery p.
endoscopic fine-needle p.
epididymis percutaneous p.
epigastric p.
Marfan epigastric p.
needle tracheoesophageal p.
pseudocyst p.
suprapubic p.
tracheoesophageal p. (TEP)
pupil
asymmetric p.'s
blown p.
dilated p.
irregular p.
nonreactive p.
pinpoint p.
pure
p. cholestasia
p. cutting current
p. nephrosis
p. pancreatic juice (PPJ)
p. PPoma
p. red cell aplasia (PRCA)
purgation
purge
oral p.
purging
bingeing and p.
self-induced p.
purified
p. HBeAg
p. protein derivative test (PPD)
p. T cell
Purilon
Comfeel P.
purine
dietary p.
p. synthesis inhibitor

NOTES

P

puromycin
    p. aminonucleoside
    p. aminonucleoside necrosis
    p. aminonucleoside nephropathy
      (PAN)
    p. aminonucleoside nephrosis (PAN)
purpura
    p. abdominalis
    anaphylactoid p.
    Echinacea p.
    Henoch-Schönlein p.
    idiopathic thrombocytopenic p.
    lung p.
    Schönlein-Henoch p.
    thrombocytopenic p.
    thrombotic thrombocytopenic p.
      (TTP)
purpureum
    tinea p.
purse-string, pursestring
    p. ligature
    p. suture
pursestringed
pursuer
    P. CBD helical stone basket
    P. mini-helical stone basket
purulent
    p. appendicitis
    p. debris
    p. discharge
    p. gastritis
    p. material
    p. pancreatitis
puruloid
pus
    p. collection
    frank p.
push
    complete PEG p.
    p. enteroscope
    p. enteroscopy
    PEG p.
    p. technique
pusher
    p. catheter
    Clarke-Reich knot p.
    Endo-Assist reusable knot p.
    Gazayerli knot p.
    metal-tipped stent p.
    p. tube
push-pull T technique
push-type enteroscopy
pustule
putative
    p. hepatotrophic factors
      insulin/glucagon
    p. host restriction
    p. transmitter

putredinis
    Bacteroides p.
putrefactive diarrhea
putrescine
putty kidney
PUV
    posterior urethral valve (type I–IV)
PUVT
    paraumbilical vein tumor
PV
    portal vein
P&V
    pyloroplasty and vagotomy
PVA
    partial villous atrophy
PVB
    platinum, Velban, bleomycin
PVC
    polyvinyl chloride
    postvoiding cystogram
    PVC catheter
PVCI
    portal vein congestive index
PVH
    persistent viral hepatitis
PVH-B
    persistent viral hepatitis, type B
PVH-NANB
    persistent viral hepatitis, non-A, non-B
PVP
    portal venous pressure
PVR
    postvoid residual
PVS
    peritoneovenous shunt
PVT
    portal vein thrombosis
PVV
    portal venous velocity
PW-5V
    Olympus spray catheter P.
pyelectasis, pyelectasia
pyelic
pyelitic
pyelitis
    calculous p.
    p. cystica
    defloration p.
    encrusted p.
    p. glandularis
    hematogenous p.
    urogenous p.
pyelocalicotomy
pyelocaliectasis
pyelocystanastomosis
pyelocystitis
pyelocystostomosis
pyelofluoroscopy

pyelogenic renal cyst
pyelogram
    antegrade p.
    dragon p.
    hydrated p.
    intravenous p. (IVP)
    powder p.
    retrograde p. (RPG)
pyelography
    air p.
    antegrade p.
    ascending p.
    p. by elimination
    excretion p.
    infusion p.
    intravenous p.
    lateral p.
    percutaneous antegrade p.
    respiration p.
    respiratory p.
    retrograde p.
    washout p.
pyeloileocutaneous anastomosis
pyelointerstitial
pyelolithotomy
    coagulum p.
    extended p.
    Gil-Vernet extended p.
    laparoscopic p.
    open p.
    standard p.
pyelolymphatic backflow
pyelolysis
pyelometer
pyelometry
pyelonephritis (PN)
    acute nonobstructive p.
    ascending p.
    asymptomatic p.
    chronic p. (CP, CPN)
    chronic bacterial p.
    cryptococcal p.
    emphysematous p.
    fungal p.
    hematogenous p.
    p. of pregnancy
    xanthogranulomatous p. (XGP)
pyelonephrosis
pyelopathy
pyeloplasty
    Anderson-Hynes dismembered p.
    capsular flap p.

    Culp-DeWeerd spiral flap p.
    Culp spiral flap p.
    disjoined p.
    dismembered p.
    Foley Y-plasty p.
    Foley Y-V p.
    laparoscopic dismembered p.
    Scardino-Prince vertical flap p.
    Scardino vertical flap p.
    Thompson capsule flap p.
pyeloplication
pyelorenal
    p. backflow
    p. reflux
pyeloscopy
pyelosinus
    p. backflow
    p. extravasation
pyelostomy
    cutaneous p.
pyelotomy
    p. closure
    extended p.
    p. incision
    open p.
    slash p.
pyelotubular
    p. backflow
    p. reflux
pyeloureteral catheter
pyeloureterectasis
pyeloureteritis cystica
pyeloureterogram
pyeloureterography
    antegrade p.
pyeloureterolysis
pyeloureteroplasty
pyeloureterostomy
pyelovenous backflow
pyelovesical stent
pyelovesicostomy
pyemesis
pyemia
    portal p.
Pygeum
    P. africanum
pygeum extract
pyknotic nucleus
pylephlebitis
pyloralgia
pylorectomy
    Kocher p.

NOTES

P

pylori
  cagA-negative *Helicobacter p.*
  cagA-positive *Helicobacter p.*
  Campylobacter p.
  coccoid form of *Helicobacter p.*
  Helicobacter p. (HP)
  intrafamilial clustering of
    Helicobacter p.
  neutrophil-activating protein of
    Helicobacter p. (HP-NAP)
  P. Stat assay test
  taeniae p.
pyloric
  p. atresia
  p. autotransplantation
  p. canal
  p. cap
  p. channel
  p. channel ulcer
  p. dilation
  p. fullness
  p. gland
  p. insufficiency
  p. intubation
  p. mucosa
  p. outlet
  p. outlet obstruction
  p. pressure wave
  p. ring
  p. sphincter
  p. spreader
  p. stenosis
  p. stricture
  p. string sign
  p. tone
pyloric-sparing pancreaticoduodenectomy
pyloricum
  antrum p.
  ostium p.
Pylorid
PyloriScreen test
Pyloriset EIA-G test
pyloristenosis
PyloriTek
  P. *Helicobacter pylori* test kit
  P. rapid urease test
  P. reagent strip
pylorodiosis
pyloroduodenal
  p. junction
  p. obstruction
  p. perforation
  p. segment
pylorogastrectomy
pyloromyotomy
  Fredet-Ramstedt p.
  Ramstedt p.
  Ramstedt-Fredet p.

pyloroplasty
  double p.
  Finney p.
  Heineke-Mikulicz p.
  Horsley p.
  Jaboulay p.
  Judd p.
  Mikulicz p.
  Ramstedt p.
  reconstructive p.
  truncal vagotomy and p.
  p. and vagotomy (P&V)
  vagotomy and p. (V&P)
  Weinberg modification of p.
pyloroptosis, pyloroptosia
pyloroscopy
pylorospasm
  congenital p.
  persistent p.
  reflex p.
pylorostenosis
pylorostomy
pylorotomy
pylorus
  closed p.
  double p.
  hypertrophic p.
  patulous p.
pylorus-preserving
  p.-p. pancreatoduodenectomy (PPPD)
  p.-p. Whipple modification (PPW)
PyNPase activity
pyocalix
pyocele
pyochezia
pyocystis
pyoderma gangrenosum (PG)
pyogenes
  Streptococcus p.
pyogenic
  p. bacterium
  p. cholangitis
  p. granuloma
  p. liver
  p. liver abscess
  p. meningitis
  p. organism
pyohydronephrosis
pyonephritis
pyonephrolithiasis
pyonephrosis
pyonephrotic
pyopneumocholecystitis
pyopneumohepatitis
pyopneumoperitoneum
pyopneumoperitonitis
pyopyelectasis
pyosemia

pyospermia
pyostomatitis vegetans
pyoureter
pyovesiculosis
PYP
　　pyrophosphate
　　^{99m}Tc PYP
pyramid
　　base of renal p.
　　p. of kidney
　　Malpighi p.
　　medullary p.
　　renal p.
pyramidal
　　p. muscle
　　p. trocar
Pyraminyl
pyramis
pyrantel pamoate
pyrazinamide
pyrazinoisoquinoline
pyrexia
pyrexial
Pyribenzamine
pyridinoline
　　serum p.
Pyridium
　　P. Plus
　　P. test of vaginal drainage
Pyridorin XR

pyridostigmine
pyridoxal
　　p. phosphate
　　p. 5′-phosphate deficiency
pyridoxamine
pyridoxine
pyrilamine
Pyrilinks-D urinary assay
pyrimethamine
pyrimidine synthesis
pyrogen
　　endogenous p.
pyrophosphate (PYP)
　　stannous p. (SPP)
pyrosis
pyrrolidinedithiocarbamate
pyruvate
　　p. dehydrogenase (PDH)
　　p. kinase
PYtest urea breath test
pyuria
　　abacterial p.
pyxigraphic
　　p. device
　　p. sampling capsule
PYY
　　peptide YY
PYY-like immunoreactivity
PZD
　　partial zonal dissection

NOTES

Q
- Q cell
- Q fever

QAD-1
- Doppler QAD-1
- QAD-1 sonography unit

QDR 1000 densitometer absorptiometer
QHS
- quantitative hepatobiliary scintigraphy

QID
- Quantum inflation device

Q-Maxx side-firing laser device
QOL
- quality of life

Q-switched
- Q-s. alexandrite laser
- Q-s. Nd:YAG laser

Q-tip test
Q-TWIST
- quality-adjusted time without symptoms or toxicity

Quad-Lumen drain
QuadraCoil stent
quadrant
- all four q.'s
- both lower q.'s (BLQ)
- both upper q.'s (BUQ)
- left lower q. (LLQ)
- left upper q. (LUQ)
- right lower q. (RLQ)
- right upper q. (RUQ)
- q. sampling technique

quadrate
- q. lobe
- q. lobe of liver

quadriplegia
quadruple therapy
qualitative
- q. fecal fat test
- q. microculture assay

quality-adjusted time without symptoms or toxicity (Q-TWIST)
quality of life (QOL)
quantified protein excretion
Quantikine quantitative immunoenzymatometric sandwich technique
quantitative
- q. angiography
- q. fecal fat test
- q. hepatobiliary scintigraphy (QHS)
- q. liquid hybridization
- q. scintigraphic evacuation proctography

- q. stool collection
- q. ultrasound (QUS)

quantum
- Q. inflation device (QID)
- Q. TTC balloon dilator
- Q. TTC biliary balloon

quartan malaria
Quartey technique
quartz waveguide
Quarzan
quasispecies
quatro therapy
quazepam
queasiness
queasy
quercetin
Quervain abdominal retractor
query
questionnaire
- Bowel Disease Q.
- Inflammatory Bowel Disease Q. (IBDQ)
- McGill pain q.
- Sexual Function Inventory Q. (SFIQ)
- Short Inflammatory Bowel Disease Q. (SIBDQ)
- The Bowel Disease Q.

Questran
Quetelet BMI index
Queyrat
Quick test
QuickVue one-step *Helicobacter pylori* test
Quidel-QuickVue *Helicobacter pylori* test
quiescence
- motor q.

quiescent
- q. hepatitis
- q. human fibroblast

Quiess
quiet bowel sounds
quill sheath
quilted suture
Quimby
- Q. method
- Q. pattern

quinacrine
Quinaglute
quinapril
Quincke
- Q. pulse
- Q. triad

quinidine
- q. gluconate

quinidine *(continued)*
    q. intoxication
    q. sulfate
quinine urea hydrochloride
Quinlan test
quinolone
Quinton
    Q. catheter
    Q. PermCath
    Q. single port scissor-valve

    Q. suction biopsy instrument
    Q. tube
Quinton-Mahurkar dual-lumen peritoneal catheter
Quinton-Scribner shunt
Quintron
    Q. AlveoSampler
    Q. Microlyzer 12 chromatograph
QUS
    quantitative ultrasound

R
    resistance
R5
    Salmonella typhimurium R5
RA
    renal artery
RAAA
    ruptured abdominal aortic aneurysm
RAAS
    renin-angiotensin-aldosterone system
rabbit stool
rabeprazole sodium
Rabuteau test
RAC
    ranitidine bismuth citrate, amoxicillin,
        clarithromycin
racephedrine
RackBeta scintillation counter
Racobalamin-57 radioactive agent
rac protein
RAD
    reactive airway disease
radial
    r. groove
    r. immunodiffusion
    r. incision
    r. jaw bladder biopsy forceps
    r. jaw hot biopsy forceps
    r. jaw 3 Max Capacity with
        needle biopsy forceps
    r. jaw 3 single-use biopsy forceps
    r. mode
    r. Ro-resection
    r. sector scanning echoendoscope
    r. suture track
radiata
    coronal r.
radiating pain
radiation
    r. cystitis
    r. dosage
    effective dose equivalent r.
    endocavitary r.
    r. enteritis
    r. enterocolitis
    r. enteropathy
    r. esophagitis
    r. exposure
    5-fluorouracil, mitomycin C r.
        (FUMIR)
    r. gastritis
    r. hepatopathy
    r. injury
    ionizing r.
    nonionizing r.

    nonparticulate r.
    particulate r.
    r. pneumonitis
    r. proctitis
    r. proctocolitis
    radiotracer half-life r.
    rectosigmoid r.
    r. sensitizer
    r. stenosis
    r. telangiectasia
    r. therapy
radiation-induced
    r.-i. angiosarcoma
    r.-i. angiosclerosis
    r.-i. colitis
    r.-i. disease
    r.-i. obliterative arteritis
    r.-i. sterility
    r.-i. ulceration
    r.-i. ureteral stricture
radical
    r. cystectomy
    r. en bloc removal
    free r.
    r. hemorrhoidectomy
    hydroxyl r.
    hydroxyl-free r.
    r. inguinal orchiectomy
    r. nephrectomy
    r. nephroureterectomy
    r. orchidectomy
    oxygen r.
    oxygen-derived free r.
    oxygen-free r.
    r. perineal prostatectomy
    r. prostatectomy (RP)
    r. resection group
    r. retropubic prostatectomy (RRP)
    superoxide r.
    r. surgery
    r. transcoccygeal prostatectomy
radicality
    oncological r.
radices (*pl. of* radix)
radiciform
radicle
    biliary r.
    intrahepatic r.
    right hepatic r.
    tertiary r.
radiculitis
radii (*pl. of* radius)
radioactive
    r. carbon-14 test
    r. cholesterol

radioactive *(continued)*
    r. detection
    r. iodine-131
    r. seed
    r. seed implantation
radioallergosorbent test (RAST)
radioautography
    thaw-mount r.
radiobiology
radiocephalic fistula
radiochemotherapy
**radiochromium-labeled erythrocyte
  method**
radiocolloid
radiocontrast-induced
    r.-i. acute renal failure
    r.-i. renal vasoconstriction
radiocystitis
radiodensity
radioenzymatic assay
radiograph
    plain r.
radiographic triad
radiography
    barium contrast r.
    calculus r.
    double-contrast r.
    kidneys, ureters, bladder r.
    KUB r.
    postvoid r.
    single-contrast r.
    skeletal r.
radioimmunoassay (RIA)
    Cyclotrac-SP r.
    homogenous r.
    solid-phase r.
    Yang PSA r.
radioimmunodetection
radioimmunoguided surgery (RIGS)
radioimmunoinhibition assay
radioimmunoprecipitation assay
radioimmunoscintimetry
radioiodination
radioisotope
    r. capsule
    r. renal excretion test
    r. renogram test
    r. renography
    r. scan
    r. scanning
    r. scintigraphy
radiolabeled
    r. imaging
    r. leucine
    r. macromolecule
radiologic
    r. biliary stent placement

    r. castration
    r. portacaval shunt
radiological
    r. investigation
    r. study
radiolucent
    r. gallstone
    r. object
radiometer
    R. GK2803C pH probe
    R. 85 instrument
radionecrosis
radionuclide
    r. cholescintigraphy
    r. cystography
    r. esophageal emptying time
    $[^{123}$I]iodoamphetamine r.
    r. renal imaging
    r. scan
    r. scintigraphy
    r. ^{99}Tc scintiscanning
    r. therapy
    r. transit study
    r. voiding cystourethrography
radiopaque
    r. density
    r. dye
    r. ERCP catheter
    r. marker
    r. pellet
radioresistant gastric plasmacytoma
radioscintigraphy
radioscopically
radiosensitive organ
radiotelemetering capsule
radiotherapy
    infradiaphragmatic r.
    intraluminal r.
    intraoperative r. (IORT)
    intraoperative electron beam r.
radiotracer half-life radiation
radius, pl. **radii**
    R. enteral feeding tube
    thrombocytopenia-absent r. (TAR)
    r. of varix
radix, pl. **radices**
    r. penis
RAEB
    refractory anemia with excess of blasts
ragged-red fiber
railroading
railroad track scars
RAIR
    rectoanal inhibitory reflex
rake
    r. retractor
    r. ulcer
Ralks adapter

R

rami (*pl. of* ramus)
ramification
ramipril
R. Efficacy in Nephropathy (REIN)
R. Efficacy in Nephropathy study
Ramirez
R. shunt
R. Silastic cannula
Ramond point
ramosum
Absidia r.
Clostridium r.
ramotomy
superior pubic r.
Rampley sponge-holding forceps
Ramstedt
R. operation
R. pyloric stenosis dilator
R. pyloromyotomy
R. pyloroplasty
Ramstedt-Fredet pyloromyotomy
ramus, pl. **rami**
pubic r.
ranarum
Basidiobolus r.
Randall
R. plaque
R. stone forceps
Randolph abdominoplasty
random
r. bladder biopsy
r. flap
R. Primed DNA Labeling kit
r. stool sample
randomized clinical trial data
Ranfac cholangiographic catheter
range
chromatofocusing pH r.
dilation r.
hapatotoxic r.
metabolic r.
r. of motion
optimum cooling r.
ranitidine
r. bismuth citrate (RBC)
r. bismuth citrate, amoxicillin,
clarithromycin (RAC)
r. bismuth citrate, metronidazole,
tetracycline (RMT)
r. hydrochloride
r. nocte
r. therapy

rank
Spearman r.
Rankin clamp
Ransley-Cantwell repair
Ransley procedure
Ranson
R. acute pancreatitis classification
R. criteria
R. criteria for severity of
pancreatitis
R. grading system
RANTES
regulated upon activation, normal T cell
expressed and secreted
RAP
receptor-associated protein
recurrent abdominal pain
Rapamune
R. oral solution
R. tablet
rapamycin inhibitor
raphe
anococcygeal r.
r. pallidus
penile r.
r. penis
perineal r.
r. perinealis
r. perinei
r. of perineum
scrotal r.
r. scroti
r. of scrotum
rapid
r. acquisition fast spin echo
sequence
r. colonic lavage
r. decrease
r. emptying of dye
r. enzyme immunoassay
r. exchange technique for
therapeutic endoscopy
r. gastric emptying
r. pull-through (RPT)
r. pull-through esophageal
manometry technique
r. serum amylase test
r. urease test (RUT)
r. urease testing kit
RapidFire multiple band ligator

NOTES

Rapid-hyb buffer
rapidly progressive glomerulonephritis (RPGN)
Rapoport test
Rappaport classification
Rapunzel syndrome
RARS
    refractory anemia with ringed sideroblast
RAS
    renin-angiotensin system
        RAS blocker
rash
        butterfly r.
        discoid r.
        genital r.
        petechial r.
        scarlatiniform r.
raspatory
    Doyen r.
***ras* p21 oncogene**
ras-related protein
RAST
    radioallergosorbent test
rate
        albumin excretion r. (AER)
        allograft survival r.
        amphotericin B-induced reduction glomerular filtration r. (AmB-induced reduction GFR)
        average flow r.
        basal carbohydrate oxidation r.
        basal metabolic r. (BMR)
        basal secretory flow r. (BSFR)
        blood flow r. (BFR)
        erythrocyte sedimentation r. (ESR)
        exponential r.
        flow r.
        gallbladder ejection r. (GBER)
        glomerular filtration r. (GFR)
        kidney electrolyte clearance r.
        kidney electrolyte excretion r.
        lipid oxidation r.
        logarithmic r.
        maximum free flow r.
        maximum urinary flow r.
        mean TIMP-1/GAPDH r.
        metabolic r.
        normalized protein catabolic r. (NPCR)
        operative mortality r.
        pancreatic secretory flow r. (PSFR)
        patency r.
        peak flow r. (PFR)
        peak secretory flow r. (PSFR)
        pressure increment r. (PIR)
        protein catabolic r. (PCR)
        r. ratio (RR)
        rebleeding r.
        recurrence r.
        reoperation r.
        respiratory r.
        seroconversion r.
        seroprevalence r.
        single-nephron glomerular filtration r. (SNGFR)
        stone-free r.
        survival r.
        transcapillary escape r.
        urine flow r.
        voiding flow r.
Rathke
    R. duct
    R. plica
ratio
        adenoma-hyperplastic polyp r.
        adenoma-nonadenoma r.
        aldosterone-to-renin r.
        amylase/creatinine clearance r.
        androstenedione-to-testosterone r.
        apolipoprotein CII-CIII r.
        AST/ALT r.
        BCAA/AAA plasma r.
        bile salt-phospholipid r.
        BUN-to-creatinine r.
        calcium-creatinine r.
        CD4+–CD8+ T-cell r.
        chloride-to-phosphate r.
        CO_2-CO_2 abundance r.
        dialysate-to-plasma r.
        dialysis-to-plasma urea r.
        D-P urea r.
        foveola-gland r.
        free-to-total PSA r.
        G:D-cell r.
        ketone body r. (KBR)
        lactulose-mannitol r.
        LCA-DCA r.
        likelihood r.
        lipid-to-protein r.
        lithocholic acid-deoxycholic acid r.
        lithocolic acid-deoxycholic acid r. (LCA-DCA)
        mean TIMP-3/GAPDH r.
        r. of mucosa to submucosa to muscularis propria
        nuclear-to-cytoplasmic size r.
        pepsinogen A-C r.
        r. of PGF2-alpha PGE2
        phospholipid r.
        pressure transmission r. (PTR)
        presumed circle area r. (PCAR)
        rate r. (RR)
        renal vein renin r.
        serum pepsinogen I/II r.
        signal-to-cutoff r.

somatostatin mRNA-D-cell
density r.
standardized incidence r. (SIR)
surface-to-volume r.
UA/C r.
urea reduction r. (URR)
urinary protein-urinary creatinine r.
urine-plasma r. (U/P)
Valsalva r.
Xc/R r.
rationing
Ratliff-Blake gallstone forceps
Ratliff-Mayo forceps
rat-tail
r.-t. appearance on pancreatogram
r.-t. configuration
r.-t. sign
rat-tooth
r.-t. Olympus FG 8L grasping
forceps
Rauber
hepatic funiculus of R.
Raudixin
Rautlna
Rauval
Rauwolfia
Rauzide
raw
r. milk-associated diarrhea
r. surface of liver bed
Rayer disease
Raz
R. anterior vaginal wall sling
R. bladder neck suspension
R. double-prong ligature carrier
R. four-corner vaginal wall sling
R. four-quadrant suspension
R. modification
R. needle bladder suspension
R. procedure
R. sling operation
R. urethral suspension
R. vaginal wall sling
razor
r. blade
r. blade ingestion
Rb
Rb gene
Rb influx
Rb protein
RBC
ranitidine bismuth citrate

red blood cell
technetium-99m pyrophosphate-
tagged RBC
RBF
renal blood flow
RBL
rubber band ligation
rubber band ligator
RBP
retinol-binding protein
RC
retrograde cystogram
RCC
renal cell carcinoma
RCF
Ross carbohydrate free
RCF formula
RCRC
recurrent colorectal cancer
RCS
red color sign
RCS sign
RCT
rectal carcinoid tumor
RCU
recurrent calcium urolithiasis
RDA
recommended daily allowance
RDG
retrograde duodenogastroscopy
RDW
red cell distribution width
RE
reflux esophagitis
regional enteritis
Reabilan HN tube feeding formula
reabsorption
fractional proximal r.
HCO^{3-} r.
protein tubular r.
sodium r.
spontaneous cyst r.
tubular sodium r.
reactance (Xc)
r. and resistance (Xc/R)
reaction
acrosome r.
allergic r.
amplification refractory mutation
system-polymerase chain r.
(ARMS-PCR)
anaphylactic r.

NOTES

reaction *(continued)*
>> Bittorf r.
>> cholestatic r.
>> desmoplastic r.
>> diazo r.
>> drug r.
>> Feulgen r.
>> fixed drug r.
>> foreign body r.
>> hypersensitivity r.
>> immune-mediated r.
>> insulin r.
>> Jaffe picrate r.
>> lichenoid r.
>> nonenzymic r.
>> one-stage r.
>> paradoxical sphincter r.
>> periglandular nonspecific
>> inflammatory r.
>> Perls r.
>> polymerase chain r. (PCR)
>> reversed passive hemagglutination r.
>> (RPHA)
>> reverse transcriptase r.
>> reverse transcriptase-polymerase
>> chain r.
>> reverse transcription-polymerase
>> chain r. (RT-PCR)
>> scar tissue r.
>> Schmorl r.
>> sphincter r.
>> T-lymphocyte-mediated cytotoxic r.
>> urticarial r.
>> van der Bergh r.
>> Weiss r.

reactive
>> r. airway disease (RAD)
>> r. arthritis
>> r. hyperemia
>> r. inflammatory vascular dermatosis
>> r. oxygen metabolite
>> r. oxygen species (ROS)

reactivity
>> Goodpasture r.
>> lectin r.
>> p53 r.

reader
>> microtitration plate r.

reagent
>> ABC r.
>> Chemstrip bG r.
>> CHOD-PAP cholesterol r.
>> Ehrlich r.
>> Folin phenol r.
>> lipofection r.
>> SAB r.
>>> streptavidin-biotin peroxidase
>>> complex

real focus shock wave
real-time
>> r.-t. confocal scanning laser
>> microscope
>> r.-t. 3-D biplanar transperineal
>> prostate implantation
>> r.-t. endoscopic ultrasound-guided
>> fine-needle aspiration
>> r.-t. fine-needle aspiration (RTFNA)
>> r.-t. gallbladder ultrasound
>> r.-t. sonographic unit
>> r.-t. spectral analysis
>> r.-t. ultrasonography (RUS)
>> r.-t. video processor

reanastomosis
>> end-to-end branch r.
>> laparoscopic ureteral r.
>> Roux-en-Y r.

reapproximate
reassignment
>> gender r.

Rebetol with Intron
Rebetron Combination therapy
rebleeding rate
rebound
>> gastric acid r.
>> r. pain
>> postdialysis urea r.
>> r. sign
>> r. tenderness

recanalization
>> r. of clogged biliary stent
>> endoscopic laser r.
>> spontaneous r.
>> umbilical vein r.

receiver-operating characteristic (ROC)
receptaculum, pl. **receptacula**
>> r. chyli
>> r. Pecqueti

receptive
>> r. anal intercourse
>> r. relaxation

receptor
>> adhesive protein r.
>> adrenergic r.
>> alpha-adrenergic r.
>> alpha-1-adrenergic r.
>> alpha-2-adrenergic r.
>> androgen r.
>> angiotensin II r.
>> ANP r.
>> antidiuretic arginine vasopressin
>> V2 r. (AVPR2)
>> asialoglycoprotein r.
>> beta-adrenergic r.
>> bladder muscarinic r.
>> bombesin r.

C3 r.
C5 r.
cardiac beta r.
C3b, C4b r.
cell surface r.
chemokine r.
cholinergic r.
ciliary-derived neurotrophic factor r.
  (CDNF)
c-*met* r.
complement r. type 1 (CR1)
corpus cavernosum muscarinic r.
r. cross talk
endothelin r.
endothelin A r.
epidermal growth factor r. (EGFR)
estrogen r. (ER)
EtA, EtB r.
fMLP chemoattractant r.
formyl peptide r.
gastric mucosal laminin r.
gastric oxyntic cell r.
gastrin r.
gp330 r.
H2 r.
high-affinity r.
histaminergic type 2 r.
hormone r.
5-HT3 r.
5HTM3 r. antagonist
human motilin r.
human PDGF r.
IL-2 r.
IL-3 r.
IL-4 r.
IL-6 r.
IL-8 r.
insulin receptor-related r.
32/67-kD laminin r.
killer-activating r. (KAR)
laminin r.
liver Ah r.
mesenteric sensory r.
multiligand r.
muscarinic r.
muscle sensory r.
native pancreatic secretin r.
natriuretic peptide r. (NPR)
nerve growth factor r. (NGFR)
neural growth factor r. (NGFR)
nicotinic r.
NK1, NK2 tachykinin r.

opiate r.
peptic cell r.
peroxisome proliferator-activated r.
  (PPAR)
phosphorylated growth factor r.
polyimmunoglobulin r. (pIgR)
recombinant pancreatic secretin r.
retinoid X r. (RXR)
sensory r.
serotonergic type 3 r.
r. and signal transduction
smooth muscle motilin r.
soluble recombinant complement r.
  1
soluble transferrin r. (sTf-R)
somatostatin r. (SSR)
steroid r.
stretch r.
T-cell r. (TCR)
tyrosine kinase growth factor r.
uroepithelial glycoid r.
vasopressin type 2 r.
vitamin D r. (VDR)
receptor-associated
  r.-a. protein (RAP)
  r.-a. protein-glutathione-S-transferase
receptor-blocker
  H2 r.-b.
receptor-mediated endocytosis pathway
recess
  splenorenal r.
recession
  clitoral r.
recessive polycystic kidney disease
recessus, pl. **recessus**
recipient
  r. hepatectomy
  kidney transplant r.
  marrow transplant r.
  phase II, III marrow transplant r.
  renal allograft r.
  renal transplant r.
recipient-derived anti-HLA antibody
reciprocal ligand
Recklinghausen
  R. disease
  R. gastric neurofibroma
  R. tumor
Reclomide
recognition
  ligand r.

NOTES

recombinant
  r. capsid protein of Norwalk virus
    (rNV)
  r. erythropoietin
  r. HBcAg (rHBcAg)
  r. hepatitis C antigen
  r. HGF
  r. human alpha interferon
  r. human erythropoietin (rh-EPO)
  r. human gelsolin
  r. human relaxin
  r. IL-10
  r. immunoblot assay (RIBA)
  r. immunoblot assay-2
  r. immunoblot assay-2 test
  r. interferon-alfa (rIFN-alpha)
  r. interferon alfa-2a
  r. interleukin-2
  r. pancreatic secretin receptor
  recombinant interferon alfa-2b,
  r. tissue transglutaminase
    radioligand assay
  r. tTG radioligand assay
recombination fraction
Recombivax HB
recommended daily allowance (RDA)
reconstruction
  anal sphincter r.
  biliary r.
  Billroth I, II r.
  bladder r.
  bladder neck r.
  bladder outlet r.
  corporeal r.
  3-D computer r.
  dural patch r.
  genital r.
  Kropp bladder neck r.
  orthotopic r.
  penis r.
  Roux-en-Y r.
  sphincter r.
  synchronous bladder r.
  Tanagho bladder neck r.
  r. technique
  total anorectal r.
  tubularized bladder neck r.
  urethral surgical r.
  Young-Dees bladder neck r.
  Young-Dees-Leadbetter bladder
    neck r.
reconstructive
  r. endourology
  r. phalloplasty
  r. pyloroplasty
record
  intragastric pH monitor r.

recorder
  Narco Bio-Systems rectilinear r.
  portable digital data r.
  Rectigraph-8K r.
  rectilinear r.
  Sandhill-800 TDS chart r.
  Sekomic SS-100F r.
  Toshiba ERVF 1A video floppy r.
  video r.
recording
  bipolar esophageal r.
  intraluminal pressure r.
  neurophysiologic r.
  penile pulse volume r.
  pH r.
  pulse volume r.
recovery
  postanesthesia r. (PAR)
recreational drug
recrudescence
recruitment
  mononuclear cell r.
recta
  vasa r.
rectal
  r. abscess
  r. akinesia
  r. alimentation
  r. ampulla
  r. amyloidosis
  r. artery
  r. augmentation
  r. balloon
  r. barostat
  r. biopsy
  r. bladder urinary diversion
  r. bleeding
  r. cancer
  r. capacity
  r. carcinoid tumor (RCT)
  r. carcinoma
  r. cell proliferation
  r. cisapride
  r. coil MRI
  r. column
  r. compliance
  r. compliance measurement
  r. cream
  r. descensus
  r. dilation
  r. dilator
  r. disease
  r. dissection
  r. distention
  r. emptying
  r. endoscopic ultrasonography
    (REU, REUS)
  r. endosonography

r. epithelial cell
r. evacuation
r. evacuatory disorder (RED)
r. examination
r. expander
r. fascia
r. feedback trigger
r. filling
r. fistula
r. fold
r. foreign body
r. fossa
r. gluten challenge
r. gonorrhea
r. hypotonia
r. impaction
r. impedance
r. impedance planimetry
r. incontinence
r. inhibitory reflex
r. injury
r. innervation
r. intussusception
r. laceration
r. leiomyosarcoma
r. linitis plastica (RLP)
r. linitis plastica colorectal
   carcinoma
r. lumen
r. mass
r. motor complex
r. mucosa
r. mucosectomy
r. muscle cuff
r. myogenic tumor
r. nerve
r. plexus
r. polyp
r. pouch
r. probe
r. probe electroejaculation
r. procidentia
r. prolapse
r. pulsed irrigation
r. reservoir
r. sensation
r. shelf
r. sinus
r. snare
r. sparing
r. spasm
r. speculum

r. sphincter
r. stenosis
r. stricture
r. stump
r. suppository
r. tenderness
r. tenesmus
r. thermometer
r. trauma
r. tube
r. ulcer
r. valve
r. valvotomy
r. varix
r. vault
r. vein
r. villous adenoma
r. visceral sensitivity

rectales
columnae r.

rectal-expander-assisted transanal endoscopic microsurgery (RE-TEM)

recti
flexura perinealis r.
flexura sacralis r.
folliculi lymphatici r.
procidentia r.

Rectigraph-8K recorder
rectilinear recorder
rectoabdominal
rectoanal
r. dyssynergia
r. function
r. inhibitor
r. inhibitory reflex (RAIR)
r. reflex

rectocele presentation
rectoclysis
rectococcygeus muscle
rectocystotomy
rectogenital septum
rectoischiadic excavation
rectolabial fistula
rectoneovaginal fistula
rectopexy
abdominal r.
anterior r.
Ivalon sponge r.
laparoscopic suture r.
Marlex mesh abdominal r.
posterior r.
presacral r.

R

NOTES

rectopexy *(continued)*
    Ripstein anterior sling r.
    suture r.
    Teflon sling r.
    Wells posterior r.
rectoplasty
    vertical reduction r.
rectorrhagia
rectosacral
    r. fascia
    r. ligament
rectosigmoid
    r. anastomosis
    r. cancer
    r. colon
    r. function
    r. junction
    r. manometry
    r. radiation
    r. region
    r. varix
rectosigmoidectomy
    Altemeier perineal r.
    perineal r.
rectosigmoidoscopy
rectosphincteric
    r. abnormality
    r. dyssynergia
    r. reflex (RSR)
rectosphincter manometric study
rectotomy
rectourethral
    r. fistula
    r. muscle
rectourethralis muscle
rectourinary fistula
rectouterina
    excavatio r.
rectouterine
    r. pouch
    r. pouch of Douglas
rectovaginal
    r. fistula
    r. pouch
    r. septum
    r. surgery
    r. surgical treatment
rectovesical
    r. center
    r. fascia
    r. fistula
    r. lithotomy
    r. pouch
    r. septum
rectovesicalis
    excavatio r.
rectovestibular fistula
rectovulvar fistula

rectum
    augmented valved r.
    bleeding per r.
    blood per r. (BPR)
    bright red blood per r. (BRBPR)
    r. digital stimulation
    gastric mucosal ectopia in r.
     (GMER)
    Hartmann closure of r.
    horizontal folds of r.
    r. irrigation
    nonrehydrated guaiac examination
     of r.
    per r.
    prolapsed r.
    transverse folds of r.
    valved r.
    watermelon r.
rectus
    r. abdominis
    r. abdominis hematoma
    r. abdominis muscle
    r. abdominis musculocutaneous flap
    r. diastasis
    r. fascia
    r. fascial wrap
    r. fascia sling
    r. femoris flap
    r. sheath
    r. sheath hematoma (RSH)
recurrence
    anastomotic r.
    local r.
    r. rate
    varicocelectomy r.
    Wilms tumor r.
recurrent
    r. abdominal pain (RAP)
    r. appendicitis
    r. bouts of vomiting
    r. calcium stone formation
    r. calcium urolithiasis (RCU)
    r. cholestasia
    r. colonic histoplasmosis
    r. colorectal cancer (RCRC)
    r. cystitis
    r. focal sclerosing
     glomerulonephritis
    r. molar pregnancy
    r. pancreatitis
    r. pyogenic cholangiohepatitis
     (RPC)
    r. stress incontinence
    r. stricture
    r. ulcer
    r. urinary tract infection
RED
    rectal evacuatory disorder

red
- r. blood cell (RBC)
- r. blood cell cast
- r. blood cell count
- r. blood cell extravasation
- r. blood cell folate
- r. blood cell folate level
- r. cell distribution width (RDW)
- r. color sign (RCS)
- r. degeneration of uterine myoma
- r. flag sign
- r. ring sign
- r. rubber Robinson catheter
- ruthenium r.
- r. wale marking

Reddick cystic duct cholangiogram catheter

Reddick-Saye
- R.-S. method
- R.-S. screw

Redfield infrared coagulator

Redivac suction drain

Rediwash skin cleanser

Redman approach

redness
- diffuse r. (DR)

Redo intestinal clamp

Redon drain

red-out

redox potential

reduced
- r. liver transplant (RLT)
- r. motility

reduced-size
- r.-s. graft
- r.-s. liver transplant (RSLT)

reducible hernia

reducing
- r. diet
- r. substance
- r. substances test

reductase
- aldose r. (AR)
- hepatic 3-methylglutaryl coenzyme A r. (HMG-CoA)
- 5,10-methylene-tetrahydrofolate r. (MTHFR)

reduction
- air pressure enema r.
- barium enema r.
- dissimilatory sulfate r.
- gastric acidity r.

- hemorrhoid r.
- hepatic venous pressure gradient r.
- profound acid r.
- sigmoid loop r.
- volvulus r.

redundant sac tissue

Redux

Redy hemodialysis system

REE
- resting energy expenditure

reefing
- stomach r.

reentry

re-examined
- retrospectively r.-e.

reexploration

refeeding
- casein r.
- r. syndrome

reference value

referred pain

refill
- capillary r.
- delayed capillary r.

refined carbohydrate complex

reflectance
- r. analysis
- endoscopic r.
- r. spectrophotometer
- r. spectrophotometric probe
- r. spectrophotometry
- r. spectroscopy
- r. TS-200 spectrum analyzer

reflecting edge of ligament

reflection
- colon medial r.
- hepatoduodenal r.
- hepatoduodenal-peritoneal r.
- peritoneal r.
- total internal r.

reflex
- absent gag r.
- anal r.
- anocutaneous r.
- axon r.
- Babinski r.
- Barrington third r.
- bladder cooling r.
- blinking r.
- r. bradycardia
- bulbocavernosus r. (BCR)
- cardioesophageal r.

NOTES

reflex *(continued)*
celiac plexus r.
consensual r.
corneal r.
cremasteric r.
cutaneous r.
deep tendon r.
deglutition r.
descending inhibitory r.
detrusodetrusor facilitative r.
r. detrusor contraction
detrusosphincteric inhibitory r.
detrusourethral inhibitory r.
diminished gag r.
r. dyspepsia
emetic r.
enteric neuronal r.
enterogastric r.
r. erection
esophagosalivary r.
fencing r.
gag r.
Galant r.
gastrocolic r.
gastroileal r.
gastroiliac r.
gastropancreatic r.
glabella r.
guarding r.
gustatory-salivary r.
r. HPV test
ileogastric r.
r. incontinence
infant r.
inhibitory intestinointestinal r.
intestinogastric r.
intramural secretory r.
intrinsic r.
Landau r.
light r.
masticatory-salivary r.
micturition r.
Moro r.
myenteric r.
r. neurogenic bladder
r. neuropathic bladder
orienting r.
parachute r.
penile r.
penis r.
perineobulbar detrusor facilitative r.
perineobulbar detrusor inhibitory r.
perineodetrusor inhibitory r.
peristaltic r.
polarized standing r.
polysynaptic r.
pontine-sacral r.
primary vesicoureteral r.

pudendal-anal r.
r. pylorospasm
rectal inhibitory r.
rectoanal r.
rectoanal inhibitory r. (RAIR)
rectosphincteric r. (RSR)
renal r.
renointestinal r.
renorenal r.
Roger r.
rooting r.
scrotal r.
secondary vesicoureteral r.
secretory r.
sexual r.
single lens r. (SLR)
skin-CNS-bladder r.
somatointestinal r.
spinobulbospinal micturition r.
r. splanchnic vasoconstriction
stepping r.
swallowing r.
r. sympathetic dystrophy
sympathetic enteroenteric
   inhibitory r.
sympathetic sphincter constrictor r.
thermal sphincteric r.
urethral sphincter recruitment r.
urethrodetrusor facilitative r.
urethrosphincteric guarding r.
urethrosphincteric inhibitory r.
urinary continence r.
vasovagal r.
vesicoanal r.
vesicointestinal r.
virile r.
visceral traction r.
viscerosensory r.
r. voiding
r. voiding dysfunction
von Mering r.
wake r.
wink r.
reflexogenic erection
reflux
acid r.
antiperistaltic r.
bile r.
r. bile gastritis
cecoileal r.
cholangiovenous r.
contralateral r.
delayed vesicoureteral r.
r. disease
duodenal r.
duodenobiliary r.
duodenogastric r. (DGR)
duodenogastroesophageal r. (DGER)

R

duodenopancreatic r.
r. dyspepsia
ejaculatory duct r.
esophageal r.
r. esophagitis (RE)
r. esophagitis classification (I–IV)
free r.
gastroesophageal r. (GER)
gastrointestinal r.
hepatojugular r.
Hinman r.
ileal r.
intrarenal r.
r. laryngitis
r. morbidity
nasopharyngeal r.
r. nephropathy
r. neuropathy
nocturnal acid r.
nocturnal gastric r.
nondilating r.
pancreaticobiliary r.
pathologic r.
peptic r.
postmyotomy r.
postoperative r.
pyelorenal r.
pyelotubular r.
Roux gastric r.
scintigraphic r.
r. small bowel examination
ureterorenal r.
urethrovesiculodifferential r.
vesicoileal r.
vesicoureteral r. (VUR)
vesicoureteric r.
vesicourethral r.

refluxant
refluxate
refluxlike dyspepsia
reflux-related stricture
refraction
refractory
r. anemia with excess of blasts
(RAEB)
r. anemia with ringed sideroblast
(RARS)
r. ascites
r. duodenal ulcer
r. esophagitis
r. hypertension
r. pouchitis

r. proctosigmoiditis
r. sideroblastic anemia
r. sprue
r. variceal hemorrhage
refrigerant diuretic
Regan isoenzyme
regeneration
bladder r.
carbon tetrachloride-induced liver r.
tubular r.
regenerative cirrhotic nodule
regimen
antireflux r.
bismuth triple r.
bowel emptying r.
dietetic r.
immunosuppressive r.
multidrug r.
sequential quadruple drug r.
Shorr r.
three-drug r.
region
antropyloroduodenal r.
capsid-encoding r.
choledochal r.
floor of inguinal r.
gastric pacemaker r.
genitourinary r.
hepatic hilar r.
hydrophobic binding r.
hypervariable r. 1 (HVR1)
hypochondriac r.
hypogastric r.
ileocecal r.
inframammary r.
r. of interest
interpolar r.
intertriginous r.
ischiorectal r.
lateral abdominal r.
nonpolar r.
pancreatobiliary r.
paraaortic r.
perianal r.
perineal r.
periumbilical r.
polar r.
rectosigmoid r.
retroperitoneal r.
suprainguinal r.
suprapubic r.

NOTES

region (*continued*)
    umbilical r.
    urogenital r.
regional
    r. colitis
    r. enteritis (RE)
    r. enterocolitis
    r. heparinization
    r. ileitis (RI)
    R. Organ Procurement Agency
      (ROPA)
registration
    transcutaneous r.
registry
    Michigan Kidney R.
Regitine
Reglan
Regressin
regression
    r. analysis
    linear r.
    lymphocele spontaneous r.
    Poisson r.
    spontaneous r.
Regroton
regucalcin
regular diet
regularly
    bowels open r. (BOR)
regulated upon activation, normal T cell expressed and secreted (RANTES)
regulation
    autocrine r.
    follicle-stimulating hormone
      inhibin r.
    growth r.
regulator
    cystic fibrosis transductance r.
    cystic fibrosis transmembrane
      conductance r. (CFTR)
regulatory
    r. peptide
    steroidogenic acute r. (STAR)
Regulax SS
regurgitant
regurgitation
    acid r.
    chronic r.
    r. jaundice
    nocturnal r.
    postural r.
    vesicoureteral r.
Regutol
rehabilitation
    renal r.
    sexual r.

Rehfuss
    R. duodenal tube
    R. method
    R. stomach tube
    R. test
Rehne abdominal retractor
Rehne-Delorme plication
Rehydralyte
rehydrating solution (RS)
rehydration
    oral r.
    r. therapy
Reichel-Pólya stomach resection
Reichert
    R. FLPS-series flexible fiberoptic
      sigmoidoscope
    R. MH-series flexible fiberoptic
      sigmoidoscope
    R. MS-series flexible fiberoptic
      sigmoidoscope
    R. SC-series flexible fiberoptic
      sigmoidoscope
Reichmann
    R. disease
    R. rod
    R. syndrome
Reich-Nechtow forceps
Reifenstein syndrome
reimplantation
    aortorenal r.
    Cohen cross-trigonal r.
    end-to-side r.
    extravesical r.
    Leadbetter-Politano r.
    Paquin ureteral r.
    ureteral r.
    ureteric r.
REIN
    Ramipril Efficacy in Nephropathy
      REIN study
reinforcement
    Gore-Tex sling r.
    responsibility r.
reinforcing suture
Reinke crystal
reinsertion
reintubation
Reitan trail making test
Reiter
    R. disease
    R. syndrome
Reitman-Frankel test
rejection
    accelerated transplant r.
    acute cellular r.
    acute vascular r.
    allograft r.
    r. cholangitis

chronic transplant r.
clinical r.
delayed hyperacute transplant r.
ductopenic r.
hyperacute r.
interstitial r.
no r. (NR)
renal allograft r.
renal transplantation r.
subclinical r.
transplant r.
tubulointerstitial r.
vascular r.
xenograft r.

relapsing
r. acute pancreatitis
r. appendicitis
related living donor (RLD)
relationship
dyadic r.
endoscope-body position r.
intraluminal pH-pressure r.
relative
first-degree r.
r. sterility
r. supersaturation (RSs)
relaxant
cGMP-mediated r.
musculotropic r.
smooth muscle r.
relaxation
adaptive r.
bladder stress r.
cardioesophageal r.
endothelial-dependent r.
esophageal sphincter r.
incomplete r.
LES r.
lower esophageal sphincter r.
(LESR)
nitric oxide blocked sphincter r.
non–swallow-associated r.
pelvic floor r.
pelvic girdle r. (PGR)
receptive r.
stress r.
r. suture
r. technique
transient LES r.
transient lower esophageal r.
(TLESR)

upper esophageal sphincter r.
(UESR)
vagovagally mediated receptive r.
relaxatory response
relaxin
recombinant human r.
relaxing incision
Relay suture delivery system
release
G-cell gastrin r.
nifedipine extended r.
paranitroaniline r.
renin r.
stimulated r.
tethered-cord r.
twin pulse shock wave r.
reliability
penile prothesis r.
Reliance urinary control insert
ReliaSeal skin barrier
Relia-Vac drain
Reliquet lithotrite
relocation
polyp r.
REM
return electrode monitor
Remegel Soft Chewable Antacid
remethylation
Remicade
R. infliximab
R. IV infusion
remission of pain
remnant
cloacal r.
gastric r.
mesonephric r.
müllerian r.
prostatic mesonephric r.
removal
colonoscopic r.
endoscopic stone r.
forceps r.
foreign body r.
gastric coin r.
percutaneous endoscopic r.
percutaneous stone r.
peritoneal dialysis urea r.
radical en bloc r.
small polyp r.
through-the-scope balloon r.
tube r.
ureteral stoma r.

R

NOTES

remover
>Detachol adhesive r.
>Macaluso stent r.

ren
>r. mobilis
>r. unguliformis

Renacidin irrigation
Renaflo hollow-fiber dialyzer
Renagel tablet
renal
>r. absorption of calcium
>r. acid excretion
>r. adenocarcinoma
>r. afferent arteriolar resistance
>r. afferent nerve
>r. agenesis
>r. allograft
>r. allograft infection
>r. allograft recipient
>r. allograft rejection
>r. allograft rupture
>r. aminoaciduria
>r. ammonium excretion
>r. amyloidosis
>r. angiography
>r. angiomyolipoma
>r. anuria
>r. arterial occlusive disease
>r. arteriography
>r. arteriole
>r. arteriovenous fistula
>r. artery (RA)
>r. artery aneurysm
>r. artery cholesterol embolization
>r. artery diameter
>r. artery embolism
>r. artery embolism embolectomy
>r. artery graft
>r. artery stenosis
>r. artery stent
>r. artery thrombosis
>r. autoregulation
>r. autoregulatory ability
>r. autoregulatory mechanism
>r. autotransplantation
>r. baroreceptor
>r. biopsy
>r. blastema
>r. blood flow (RBF)
>r. bone disease
>r. calcium leak
>r. capsular flap
>r. capsule
>r. capsulotomy
>r. carbuncle
>r. carcinosarcoma
>r. cell carcinoma (RCC)
>r. cholesterol embolus

>r. clearance
>r. coagulation necrosis
>r. colic
>r. collecting duct cell
>r. complication
>r. concentrating defect
>r. congestion
>r. corpuscle
>r. cortex
>r. cortical abscess
>r. cortical adenoma
>r. cortical malondialdehyde content
>r. cortical necrosis
>r. cortical scintigraphy
>r. cortical tubule cell
>r. corticoadrenal
>r. cryoablation
>r. cryptococcosis
>r. cyst decortication
>r. cyst hemorrhage
>r. cystic disease
>r. cyst infection
>r. cyst marsupialization
>r. descensus
>r. dialysis
>r. duplication
>r. ectopia
>r. endarterectomy
>r. endothelin
>r. epistaxis
>r. epithelial cell
>r. excretion of acid
>r. excretion of calcium
>r. exploration
>r. failure
>r. failure index
>r. Fanconi-like syndrome
>r. fascia
>r. fibroma
>r. fibromuscular disease
>r. function
>r. function study (RFS)
>r. gallium-67 scintigraphy
>r. glomerulus
>r. glucosuria
>r. hamartoma
>r. helical CT (RHCT)
>r. helical CT imaging
>r. hemangioma
>r. hematoma
>r. hematuria
>r. hemodynamics
>r. hemophilia
>r. hilar dissection
>r. hilum
>r. hilus
>r. histologic section
>r. histopathology

r. homotransplantation
r. hydatid disease
r. hydatidosis
r. hypercalciuria
r. hyperfiltration
r. hypertension
r. hypertrophy
r. hypoperfusion
r. hyposthenuria
r. hypothermia
r. impression
r. impression on liver
r. injury repair
r. insufficiency
r. interstitium
r. ischemia
r. kallikrein-kinin system
r. labyrinth
r. lithiasis
r. lobe
r. lymphoblastoma
r. mass
r. medulla
r. medullary carcinoma
r. messenger ribonucleic acid
r. morphometric analysis
r. oncocytoma
r. osteodystrophy
r. papilla
r. papillary necrosis (RPN)
r. parenchyma
r. pathology
r. pedicle
r. pelvic transitional cell carcinoma
r. pelvis
r. pelvis calculus
r. percutaneous transluminal angioplasty
r. perfusion pressure-flow study
r. perfusion scintigraphy
r. phosphate
r. phosphate excretion
r. plasma flow (RPF)
r. pouch
r. preservation
r. preservation perfusion system
r. profusion pressure
r. progression
r. prostaglandin
r. proximal tubular cell
r. proximal tubule preparation
r. ptosis

r. pyramid
r. reflex
r. rehabilitation
r. replacement therapy
r. resistive index
r. revascularization
r. rhabdosarcoma
r. rickets
r. sarcoidosis
r. scan
r. scarring
r. segmental renal dysplasia
r. sinus
r. sinus cyst
r. sodium
r. sodium excretion
r. sodium retention
r. sodium wasting
r. sonography
r. stab wound
r. stone
r. structural damage
r. sympathetic activity
r. sympathetic nerve
r. sympathetic nerve activity recording electrode
R. System HF250 filter
r. thromboendarterectomy
r. tissue kallikrein expression
r. toxicity
r. transduction pathway
r. transplant
r. transplantation
r. transplantation rejection
r. transplant patient
r. transplant recipient
r. trauma
r. tuberculosis
r. tubular acidosis (RTA)
r. tubular acidosis I (RTA-I)
r. tubular acidosis (type I–IV)
r. tubular cell
r. tubular fluid
r. tubular metabolic acidosis
r. tubular necrosis
r. tubular sodium handling
r. tubule
r. tubule epithelial cell
r. ultrasonogram
r. vascular injury
r. vascular resistance (RVR)
r. vascular resistance index (RVRI)

NOTES

renal *(continued)*
    r. vascular tone
    r. vasculitis
    r. vasoconstriction
    r. vasodilation
    r. vasodilator
    r. vasodilator prostaglandin
    r. vein
    r. vein renin
    r. vein renin activity (RVRA)
    r. vein renin assay (RVRA)
    r. vein renin concentration (RVRC)
    r. vein renin ratio
    r. vein thrombosis
    r. venogram
    r. venography
    r. venous outflow compression
    vertebral, anal, tracheoesophageal
      fistula, r. (VATER)
    r. volume
    r. xanthine oxidase-xanthine
      dehydrogenase activity
renale
    hilum r.
renales
    columnae r.
renal-hepatic steal syndrome
Renalin dialyzer
renalis
    fascia r.
    hilum r.
    plexus r.
renal-ocular syndrome
renal-retinal syndrome
renal-sparing surgery
Renalyzer
Renatron dialyzer
rendezvous
    pancreatic r.
Rendu-Osler-Weber
    R.-O.-W. disease
    R.-O.-W. syndrome
Renese
renewal
    epithelial restitution and r.
    tissue r.
renicapsule
renicardiac
reniculus, pl. **reniculi**
renin
    active r.
    r. inhibition
    plasma r.
    r. release
    renal vein r.
    r. secreting juxtaglomerular cell
      tumor
    r. secretion

    r. stimulation test
    r. synthesis
renin-aldosterone system
renin-angiotensin
    r.-a. system (RAS)
    r.-a. system blocker
renin-angiotensin-aldosterone
    r.-a.-a. axis
    r.-a.-a. system (RAAS)
renin-angiotensin system (RAS)
renin-mediated renovascular
    hypertension
reninoma
renipelvic
reniportal anastomosis
renipuncture
renis
    capsula adiposa r.
    capsula fibrosa r.
    porta r.
    venulae rectae r.
Rennes variant galactosemia
renocortical
renogastric fistula
Renografin
renogram
    captopril r.
    furosemide washout r.
    isotope r.
    MDT r.
renography
    captopril r.
    captopril-enhanced r.
    diethylenetriamine pentaacetic
      acid r.
    diuretic nuclear r.
    DTPA r.
    isotope r.
    radioisotope r.
renointestinal reflex
Reno-M contrast medium
renomedullary interstitial cell (RMIC)
renomegaly
renopathy
renoprival
renopulmonary
Renoquid
renorenal reflex
renorrhaphy
renotrophic
renotropic
renotropin
renovascular
    r. disease
    r. hypertension
    r. hypertrophy
    r. obstruction
Renovist Injection

Renovue 65
Renu enteral feeding
renzapride
reoperation rate
reoperative ureteroneocystostomy
reovirus
reoxygenation
repaglinide
repair (*See also* operation, procedure)
    Alliston GE reflux r.
    Altemeier r.
    anal sphincter r.
    Asopa hypospadias r.
    Barcat-Redman hypospadias r.
    Bassini inguinal hernia r.
    Belsey Mark IV r.
    Belt-Fuqua hypospadias r.
    Bengt-Johanson r.
    Boari ureteral flap r.
    Boerema hernia r.
    Cantwell-Ransley epispadias r.
    Cecil r.
    cloacal exstrophy one-stage r.
    cloacal exstrophy two-stage r.
    Collis r.
    cross-trigonal r.
    Devine-Horton flip flap for
      hypospadias r.
    Devine hypospadias r.
    double-faced island flap for
      hypospadias r.
    DualMesh hernia r.
    epispadias r.
    extracorporeal r.
    first-stage r.
    Halsted-Bassini hernia r.
    hernia r.
    hernial r.
    Hill esophageal antireflux r.
    Hill hiatus hernia r.
    Hill median arcuate r.
    Horton-Devine flip-flap
      hypospadias r.
    hydrocele r.
    intraperitoneal mesh r.
    intraperitoneal onlay mesh hernia r.
      (IPOM)
    Judd ventral hernia r.
    Koyanagi technique for
      hypospadias r.
    laparoscopic varicocele r.
    LaRoque r.

    Lich-Gregoire r.
    Lichtenstein hernial r.
    Madden r.
    Marlex hernial r.
    McVay inguinal hernial r.
    Mitchell technique for epispadias r.
    Moschcowitz vaginal prolapse r.
    Mustarde hypospadias r.
    mutation mismatch r. (MMR)
    neonatal exstrophic bladder r.
    Nissen r.
    one-stage hypospadias r.
    Orr rectal prolapse r.
    pants-over-vest hernial r.
    Paquin r.
    paravaginal fascial r.
    postanal r.
    Ransley-Cantwell r.
    renal injury r.
    reverse sigma penoscrotal
      transposition r.
    Rodney Smith biliary stricture r.
    slipped Nissen r.
    sphincter r.
    Stoppa r.
    TAPP hernia r.
    TEP hernia r.
    Thal esophageal stricture r.
    Theirsch-Duplay r.
    tight Nissen r.
    totally extraperitoneal hernia r.
    transabdominal preperitoneal
      hernia r.
    two-stage r.
    vascular laceration r.
    vest-over-pants hernial r.
    VVF r.
    Young epispadias r.
repeat
    long terminal r. (LTR)
    r. procedure
    terminal r. (TR)
repeated complete mole
repens
    Serenoa r.
reperfusion injury
reperitonealization
replaced hepatic vessel
replacement
    bladder r.
    buccal mucosal urethral r.
    gastric bladder r.

R

NOTES

replacement *(continued)*
    intestinal ureteral r.
    r. PEG
    tube r.
    tunica r.
    volume r.
Replete liquid nutrition
replication
    r. error phenotype
    gastric epithelial cell r.
    viral r.
replicator
    Steers r.
Repliform dermal allograft
Replogle tube
repopulation
    clonogenic r.
Rep-Pred
repreparation
reprocessor
    American Endoscopy automatic r.
    automatic endoscopic r. (AER)
    Bard automatic r.
    Custom Ultrasonic automatic r.
    ECI automatic r.
    KeyMed automatic r.
    Lutz automatic r.
    Medivator automatic r.
    Olympus automatic r.
    Orr automatic r.
    Steris automatic r.
reproduction
    assisted r.
reproductive
    r. axis
    r. system
reptilase acid
requirement
    analgesic r.
    minimum daily r. (MDR)
re-reflux
rescinnamine
rescue
    fluorouracil, Adriamycin,
      methotrexate with leucovorin r.
      (FAMTX)
    leucovorin r.
    r. therapy
    uridine r.
research
    r. application
    biomedical r.
resectable
resection
    abdominoperineal r. (APR)
    abdominosacral r.
    anterior r.
    antral r.

bladder neck transurethral r.
bowel r.
cap-assisted r.
cold cup r.
colon cancer r.
colorectal r.
colosigmoid r.
continence-preserving r.
curative r.
cutting endoscopic mucosal r. (C-EMR)
cylindrical mucosal r.
diathermic r.
duodenum-preserving pancreatic head r.
ejaculatory duct transurethral r.
elective r.
electrocautery r.
en bloc vein r.
endoscopic mucosal r. (EMR)
endoscopic snare r.
esophageal r.
free r.
gastric r. (GR)
hepatic r.
ileal r. (IR)
ileocecal r.
ileocolic r.
intersphincteric r.
laparoscopic abdominoperineal r.
laparoscopically assisted colorectal r.
laparoscopic ultralow anterior r.
lift-and-cut endoscopic mucosal r. (LC-EMR)
liver r.
Lortat-Jacob hepatic r.
low anterior r. (LAR)
Mason abdominotranssphincteric r.
Miles abdominoperineal r.
mucosal sleeve r.
open transurethral r.
pancreatic tail r.
Paul-Mikulicz r.
percutaneous r.
piecemeal r.
prostate gland transurethral r.
Reichel-Pólya stomach r.
segmental colonic r.
snare r.
spermatocele r.
strip r.
suture rectopexy with sigmoid r.
terminal ileal r.
thick loop transurethral r. of the prostate
total transurethral r. of prostate (T-TURP)

transanal endoscopic
  microsurgical r.
transhiatal r.
transurethral r. (TUR)
transurethral r. of prostate (TURP)
transverse r.
wedge r.
Whipple r.
resective colostomy
resectoscope
continuous-flow r.
Foroblique r.
Iglesias fiberoptic r.
r. loop
OES 4000 r.
Olympus continuous flow r.
Richard Wolf video r.
r. sheath
Storz r.
transurethral r.
Wolf r.
resectoscopy
resedation
reserpine
hydrochlorothiazide and r.
reserpine-induced ulcer
reservoir
Camey r.
colonic J-pouch r.
continent cutaneous r.
continent ileal r.
detubularized right colon r.
double-barrel r.
double J-shaped r.
double-stapled ileal r.
fecal r.
Florida pouch urinary r.
Hoffmann-Steinberg gastric r.
Hunt-Limo-Basto gastric r.
ileal r.
ileoanal r.
ileocecal continent urinary r.
Indiana continent r.
intraabdominal ileal r.
inverted U-pouch ileal r.
isoperistaltic ileal r.
J r.
J-shaped ileal r.
J-Vac suction r.
Kock r.
lateral internal pelvic r.
Lawrence gastric r.

Le Bag pouch r.
Mainz pouch urinary r.
r. mucosal absorption
orthotopic colonic r.
orthotopic continent r.
orthotopic remodeled ileocolonic r.
Parks ileal r.
Parks ileoanal r.
r. phase
rectal r.
sigmoid colon r.
spherical r.
S-shaped r.
Studer cross-folded ileal r.
W-stapled urinary r.
reset osmostat syndrome
Resident Assessment Protocol for incontinence
residua (*pl. of* residuum)
residual
r. albuminuria
r. barium
r. chordee
r. fragment
postvoid r. (PVR)
r. proteinuria
r. rectoperineal fistula
r. stone
r. stool
r. urine
r. urine volume (RUV)
residue
dibasic amino acid r.
fecal r.
food r.
sialic acid r.
sialyl r.
residuum, pl. **residua**
gastric r.
resin
anion exchange r.
bile-salt binding r.
Epon 812 r.
potassium binding r.
resinifera
Euphorbia r.
resiniferatoxin therapy
resipump
resistance (R)
activated protein C r. (APCR)
amphotericin B r.
antimicrobial r

NOTES

resistance *(continued)*
    basal renal vascular r.
    cancer drug r.
    drug r.
    hepatic arterial vascular r.
    insulin r.
    peripheral vascular r.
    reactance and r. (Xc/R)
    renal afferent arteriolar r.
    renal vascular r. (RVR)
    R-factor in bacterial
      antimicrobial r.
    systemic vascular r. (SVR)
    tissue r.
    transhepatic vascular r.
    urethral r.
    vesical neck r.
    vitamin D r.
resistant ascites
resistin
resistive index (RI)
Resol electrolyte solution
resolution
    spatial r.
    spontaneous r.
resonance
    endoscopic magnetic r. (EMR)
    hydatid r.
    magnetic r.
    nuclear magnetic r. (NMR)
    tympanitic r.
    vesiculotympanitic r.
    wooden r.
resonant abdomen
resorbable thread clip applicator
resorption
    tubular r.
resorptive hypercalciuria
Resource enteral feeding
respiration pyelography
respiratory
    r. acidosis
    r. alkalosis
    r. burst
    r. burst activity
    r. depression
    r. distress
    r. distress syndrome
    r. embarrassment
    r. excursion
    r. failure
    r. inversion point (RIP)
    r. pyelography
    r. rate
    r. symptom (RS)
respiratory-esophageal fistula
response
    alloantigen r.

ameliorated vasodilating r.
antibody directed cytotoxic r.
apoptotic r.
bellow r.
cell-mediated immunohistological r.
cellular immune r.
cytotoxic T-cell r.
desmoplastic r.
desmopressin r.
effector r.
fed r.
gag r.
hypercontractile external sphincter r.
immune r.
inflammatory r.
macrophage-rich inflammatory r.
maladaptive r.
paradoxical renal r.
peak r.
plateau r.
relaxatory r.
sacral evoked r.
skin sympathetic r.
sympathetic skin r.
responsibility reinforcement
responsiveness
    vasculature r.
rest
    adrenal r.
    bowel r. (BR)
    ectopic adrenal r.
    gut r.
    Krause arm r.
    nephrogenic r.
    pancreatic r.
    testicular adrenal r.
    total bowel r.
restaging of cancer
restenosis
resting
    r. anal sphincter pressure
    r. energy expenditure (REE)
    r. membrane potential
    r. tremor
    r. urethral pressure profile
restless leg syndrome
restoration
    foreskin r.
    voice r.
restorative proctocolectomy (RP, RPC)
Restoril
restricted
    HLA class II r.
restriction
    dietary protein r.
    r. endonuclease
    r. enzyme
    fluid r.

r. fragment length polymorphism
(RFLP, RLP)
intrauterine growth r. (IUGR)
protein r.
putative host r.
sodium r.

result
medium-term r.
Surveillance, Epidemiology, and
End R.'s (SEER)
transurethral microwave
thermotherapy functional r.
transurethral resection of the
prostate functional r.
TUMT functional r.
TURP functional r.

resuscitation
fluid r.

retained
r. antrum
r. antrum syndrome
r. barium
r. bladder syndrome
r. feces
r. foreign body (RFB)
r. gallstone
r. testicle
r. testis

retainer
Mectra tissue sample r.

retardata
ejaculatio r.

retardation
triad of adenoma sebaceum,
epilepsy, and mental r.

retch
retching
rete, pl. **retia**
r. peg
r. ridge
r. testis
r. testis adenocarcinoma

RE-TEM
rectal-expander-assisted transanal
endoscopic microsurgery

retention
acute urinary r. (AUR)
r. band
barium r.
BSP r.
chronic urinary r. (CUR)
crystal r.

r. cyst
r. enema
r. esophagitis
gastric r.
r. jaundice
r. meal
r. polyp
postoperative urinary r.
renal sodium r.
sodium r.
stool r.
r. suture
r. uremia
urinary r.
r. vomiting

re-tethering
retia (*pl. of* rete)
retial
reticularis
formatio r.
zona r.
reticulin antigen
reticulocyte hemoglobin content
reticuloendothelial system
reticulonodular pattern
reticulosis
polymorphic r.
reticulum
endoplasmic r.
sarcoplasmic r.
retinaculum
Morgagni r.
retinal
r. artery occlusion
r. vein occlusion
retinitis
albuminuric r.
retinoblastoma
retinoic acid
retinoid
acylic r.
r. chaperone
r. transport
r. X receptor (RXR)
retinoid-binding protein
retinol-binding protein (RBP)
retinol concentration
retinopathy of prematurity
retinyl ester clearance
RET protooncogene
retracted stoma

R

NOTES

retractile
    r. concealed penis
    r. mesenteritis
    r. testis
retraction
    bladder r.
    foreskin manual r.
retractor
    Army-Navy r.
    Aronson esophageal r.
    baby Balfour r.
    Balfour abdominal r.
    Balfour self-retaining r.
    Barr rectal r.
    Beardsley esophageal r.
    B.E. Glass abdominal r.
    Berens esophageal r.
    Berkeley-Bonney r.
    Bookwalter-Goulet r.
    Bookwalter-Hill-Ferguson rectal r.
    Bookwalter ring r.
    Bookwalter-St. Mark deep pelvic r.
    Breisky-Navratil straight r.
    Buie-Smith r.
    Christie gallbladder r.
    Cole duodenal r.
    Collin abdominal r.
    Collin intestinal r.
    Crile angle r.
    Crile malleable r.
    Cushing vein r.
    Deaver r.
    DeBakey-Cooley r.
    Denis Browne abdominal r.
    Deucher abdominal r.
    Doyen abdominal r.
    fan elevator r.
    fan-type laparoscopic r.
    Farabeuf r.
    Ferguson anal r.
    Ferguson-Moon rectal r.
    Finochietto r.
    fixed ring r.
    Foerster abdominal ring r.
    Forder r.
    Foss bifid gallbladder r.
    Foss biliary duct r.
    Franz abdominal r.
    Friedman perineal r.
    Fritsch r.
    gallows-type r.
    Gazayerli endoscopic r.
    Gelpi self-retaining r.
    Gibson-Balfour abdominal r.
    Gil-Vernet r.
    Goelet r.
    Goligher r.
    Gosset appendectomy r.

    Grant gallbladder r.
    Greene r.
    Greishaber self-retaining r.
    hand-held r.
    Haney r.
    Harrington Deaver r.
    Harrington splanchnic r.
    Heaney r.
    hilar r.
    Hill-Ferguson rectal r.
    Hill rectal r.
    illuminated St. Mark's r.
    Israel r.
    Jansen r.
    Johns Hopkins gallbladder r.
    Kelly abdominal r.
    Kirschner abdominal r.
    Kocher gallbladder r.
    Lone Star r.
    Lowsley r.
    malleable r.
    Mayo abdominal r.
    Mayo-Adams appendectomy r.
    McBurney r.
    Mediflex-Gazayerli r.
    metal bar r.
    Mikulicz r.
    Miller-Senn r.
    Millin bladder r.
    Moon rectal r.
    Murphy gallbladder r.
    Nuttall liver r.
    Ochsner r.
    Oettingen abdominal r.
    Omnitract r.
    O'Sullivan-O'Connor abdominal r.
    Parker r.
    Parks r.
    Percy-Wolfson gallbladder r.
    Polytrac Gomez r.
    Pratt bivalve r.
    Quervain abdominal r.
    rake r.
    Rehne abdominal r.
    ribbon r.
    Richards abdominal r.
    Richardson appendectomy r.
    Rigby appendectomy r.
    ring abdominal r.
    Robin-Masse abdominal r.
    Roux r.
    Sawyer rectal r.
    Scott r.
    self-retaining ring r.
    Senn r.
    Senn-Kanavel r.
    Smith-Buie rectal r.
    Smith rectal r.

Space-OR flexible internal r.
spoon r.
spring-wire r.
Stamey dorsal vein apical r.
T-bar r.
Theis self-retaining r.
Tuffier abdominal r.
Upper Hands r.
U.S. Army double-ended r.
vein r.
Volkmann rake r.
Walker gallbladder r.
Webb-Balfour abdominal r.
Weinberg vagotomy r.
Weitlaner r.
Wesson perineal r.
Wexler r.
Wickham r.
Wilkinson abdominal r.
Wishbone Omni-Track r.
Wolfson gallbladder r.
Wylie splanchnic r.
Young prostatic r.
Yu-Holtgrewe prostatic r.

retransplantation
retreatment
lithotripsy r.
retrieval
r. balloon
r. basket
spermatozoon r.
retriever
Entract stone r.
Positrap r.
snail-headed catheter r.
Soehendra stent r.
stone r.
three-pronged polyp r.
retrocaval ureter
retrocecal
r. abscess
r. appendicitis
r. appendix
retrocecalis tumor thrombus
retrocolic
r. anastomosis
r. end-to-end pancreatojejunostomy
r. end-to-side choledochojejunostomy
r. fossa
retroduodenal
r. artery

r. artery severance
r. perforation
retroesophageal abscess
retroflexed
r. cystoscopy sheath
r. scope
r. uterus
r. view
retroflexion
endoscopic r.
intrarectal r.
retrogastric pseudocyst
retrograde
r. amnesia
r. approach
r. balloon rupture
r. cannulation
r. cholangiography
r. contrast study
r. cystogram (RC)
r. cystography
r. cystourethrogram
r. duodenogastroscopy (RDG)
r. ejaculation
r. endopyelotomy
r. fashion
r. flow on barium enema
r. genitography
r. hernia
r. intrarenal surgery
r. intussusception
r. loopography
r. nephrostomy
r. occlusion balloon catheter
r. pancreatocholangiography
r. pancreatography
r. peristalsis
r. pyelogram (RPG)
r. pyelography
r. small bowel examination
r. sphincterotomy
r. technique
r. ureteropyelogram
r. ureteropyelography
r. urethrogram (RUG)
r. urethrography (RUG)
r. urogram (RU)
r. urography
r. vascularization of superior mesenteric artery
retrohepatic vena cava

NOTES

R

retroileal
    r. appendicitis
    r. appendix
retroiliac ureter
Retromax endopyelotomy stent
retropancreatic tunnel
retroperistaltic pump
retroperitoneal
    r. abscess
    r. approach
    r. area
    r. calcification
    r. carbon dioxide insufflation study
    r. cavity
    r. cutaneous ureterostomy
    r. fat
    r. fibrosis
    r. fistula
    r. hematoma
    r. hemorrhage
    r. hernia
    r. infection
    r. lymphadenectomy
    r. lymph node dissection (RPLD)
    r. lymphoma
    r. neoplasm
    r. perforation
    r. pneumography
    r. pneumoradiography
    r. region
    r. seminoma
    r. space
    r. surgery
    r. tumor
    r. varicocelectomy
retroperitoneal-iliopsoas abscess
retroperitoneoscopic
    r. adrenalectomy
    r. nephrectomy
    r. vein ligature
retroperitoneoscopy
retroperitoneum sarcoma
retroperitonitis
    idiopathic fibrous r.
retropexy
    abdominal r.
retropneumoperitoneum
retropubic
    r. ascending radical prostatectomy
    r. implant
    r. Lapides-Ball bladder neck suspension
    r. needle suspension procedure
    r. space
    r. urethrolysis
    r. urethroscopy
retrorectal
    r. cyst

    r. lymph node
    r. space
retrospectively re-examined
retrospective nature of the study
retrosternal
    r. chest pain
    r. hernia
retrourethral catheterization
retroversion
retroverted uterus
retrovesical vesiculectomy
retroviral genome
retrovirus
    r. infection
    porcine endogenous r. (PERV)
retrusive meatus
rettgeri
    Proteus r.
    Providencia r.
return
    r. electrode monitor (REM)
    total predicted r.
retzii
    cavum r.
Retzius
    space of R.
    R. space
    R. vein
REU
    rectal endoscopic ultrasonography
REUS
    rectal endoscopic ultrasonography
reusable
    r. forceps with needle
    r. laparoscopic electrode
reuse syndrome
reuteri
    Lactobacillus r.
Reuter suprapubic trocar and cannula system
revascularization
    myocardial r.
    penile r.
    renal r.
revenge
    Montezuma r.
reverberation artifact
Reverdin abdominal spatula
reversal
    r. jejunoileal bypass surgery
    jejunoileal fold pattern r.
    vasectomy r.
reverse
    r. alpha sigmoid loop
    r. cystotome
    r. dot hybridization
    r. osmosis pump

r. sigma penoscrotal transposition repair

r. sphincterotome

r. transcriptase (RT)

r. transcriptase-polymerase chain reaction

r. transcriptase reaction

r. transcription

r. transcription-polymerase chain reaction (RT-PCR)

r. Trendelenburg position

reversed

r. anorexia syndrome

r. Mercedes Benz sign

r. passive hemagglutination reaction (RPHA)

r. peristalsis

r. reimplanted appendicocystostomy

reversible

r. blockade

r. vasectomy

review

metaanalytic r.

Rex-Cantli-Serege line

Reye syndrome

Rezipas

Rezulin

R-factor in bacterial antimicrobial resistance

RFB

retained foreign body

RFLP

restriction fragment length polymorphism

RFS

renal function study

RFS2000

rhabdoid Wilms tumor

rhabdomyoblastic differentiation

rhabdomyolysis

exertional r.

hypoxia-induced r.

rhabdomyoma

rhabdomyomatous

rhabdomyosarcoma (RMS)

alveolar r.

bladder r.

interlabial r.

kidney r.

mixed r.

paratesticular r.

pleomorphic r.

prostate r.

rhabdosarcoma

renal r.

rhabdosphincter

r. electromyography

r. muscle

rhagades

rhamnosus

Lactobacillus r.

rHBcAg

recombinant HBcAg

RHCT

renal helical CT

RHCT imaging

Rheaban

Rhein anthrone

rhenium 186

Rheomacrodex

rh-EPO

recombinant human erythropoietin

rhesus rotavirus-tetravalent vaccine (RRV-TV)

rheumatica

scarlatina r.

rheumatic disease

rheumatism

palindromic r.

rheumatoid

r. arthritis

r. vasculitis

rhinosporidiosis

Rhinosporidium seeberi

rhizopidoformis

Rhizopus r.

Rhizopus

R. rhizopidoformis

R. species

rhizotomy

dorsal r.

sacral posterior root r.

selective sacral r.

rhodamine

alexandrite and r.

r. 6G dye

r. 6G dye laser

r. stain

Rhodesian trypanosomiasis

rhodesiense

Trypanosoma r.

Rhodes Inventory of Nausea and Vomiting

rhonchus, pl. **rhonchi**

rho protein

NOTES

rhubarb test
RHV
    right hepatic vein
rhythm
    biphasic diurnal r.
    circadian r.
    gallop r.
    irregular r.
    paced r.
    r. strip
    ultradian r.
rhythmicity
    circadian r.
rhythmometry
    cosinor-r.
RI
    regional ileitis
    resistive index
RIA
    radioimmunoassay
    RIA kit
RIBA
    recombinant immunoblot assay
    RIBA test
RIBA-2 test
ribavirin
ribbon
    iridium r.
    r. retractor
    r. stool
rib cutter
riboflavin deficiency
ribonuclease
    low molecular weight protein r.
ribonucleic acid (RNA)
ribonucleoprotein (RNP)
riboprobe
    complementary, single-stranded, anti-sense r.
    ^{35}S antisense fibronectin r.
ribose-1-phosphate
ribose-5-phosphate
ribosome
    free r.
rice-flour breath test
rice-fruit diet
Rice-Lyte
rice-water stool
Richard
    R. Wolf Piezolith lithotriptor
    R. Wolf video resectoscope
Richards abdominal retractor
Richardson
    R. appendectomy retractor
    R. procedure
Richet fascia umbilicus
Richner-Hanhart syndrome
Richter hernia

Richter-Monroe line
ricin
rickets
    celiac r.
    hypophosphatemic r.
    pseudodeficiency r.
    renal r.
Rickettsia conorii
Rider-Moeller
    R.-M. dilator
    R.-M. glossitis
ridge
    interureteric r.
    nephrogenic r.
    rete r.
    ureteric r.
ridged-convoluted villus
Riedel lobe
Riegel test meal
Rieger syndrome
Riepe-Bard gastric balloon
Rieux hernia
rifabutin
rifampicin
rifampin
rifamycin
rifaximin
rIFN-alpha
    recombinant interferon-alfa
Rigaud operation
Rigby appendectomy retractor
Righini procedure
right
    r. anterior pararenal space
    r. antero-oblique position
    r. colon
    r. colonic flexure
    r. colon pouch
    r. gastroomental artery
    r. gutter
    r. hepatic duct
    r. hepatic radicle
    r. hepatic vein (RHV)
    r. inguinal hernia (RIH)
    r. kidney (RK)
    r. lobe
    r. lower quadrant (RLQ)
    r. ovarian vein syndrome
    r. upper quadrant (RUQ)
    r. ureter
right-angle
    r.-a. clamp
    r.-a. electrode
    r.-a. lens
right-angled end-to-side anastomosis
right-sided
    r.-s. clonus
    r.-s. lesion

R

rigid
>r. abdomen
>r. endoscope
>r. esophagoscopy
>r. nephroscope
>r. proctoscopy
>r. proctosigmoidoscopy
>r. scoop
>r. sigmoidoscope
>r. ureteroscope
>r. ureteroscopy

rigidity
>abdominal r.
>boardlike r.
>involuntary reflex r.
>nuchal r.

Rigiflator hand-held inflation/deflation device

Rigiflex
>R. ABD balloon dilatation catheter
>R. achalasia balloon
>R. achalasia dilator
>R. biliary balloon dilatation catheter
>R. esophageal TTS balloon catheter
>R. OTW balloon dilatation catheter
>R. TTS balloon
>R. TTS balloon dilatation catheter
>R. TTS balloon dilator

RigiScan
>R. device
>R. measurement
>R. penile tumescence and rigidity monitor
>R. testing

Rigler sign
rigor mortis
RIGS
>radioimmunoguided surgery

RIGScan
>R. CR49 test for colorectal cancer detection

RIH
>right inguinal hernia

Riley-Day
>R.-D. syndrome
>R.-D. syndrome of familial dysautonomia

rim
>r. of fascia

>r. nephrogram
>r. sign

rima, pl. **rimae**
>r. pudenda
>r. vulva

rind
ring
>A r.
>abdominal inguinal r.
>r. abdominal retractor
>anorectal r.
>apex of external r.
>B r.
>R. biliary drainage catheter
>biofragmentable anastomotic r. (BAR)
>Cannon r.
>Coloplast skin barrier r.
>confidence r.
>constriction r.
>continence r.
>distal esophageal r.
>elastic O r.
>esophageal A, B r.
>esophageal contractile r.
>esophageal mucosal r.
>esophageal muscular r.
>estradiol releasing silicone vaginal r.
>Estring estradiol vaginal r.
>external inguinal r.
>finger r.
>r. forceps
>ilioinguinal r.
>iliopsoas r.
>inguinal r.
>inositol r.
>internal abdominal r.
>internal inguinal r.
>intrahaustral contraction r.
>Kayser-Fleischer r.
>lower esophageal B r.
>lower esophageal contraction r.
>lower esophageal mucosal r.
>Lyon r.
>Maclet magnetic r.
>mucosal esophageal r.
>muscular esophageal r.
>Ochsner r.
>Osbon pressure-point tension r.
>pressure-point tension r.
>pyloric r.

NOTES

ring *(continued)*
    rust r.
    Schatzki r.
    Silastic r.
    silicone elastomer r.
    Smith r.
    sphincter contraction r.
    sutureless biofragmentable r.
Ringer lactate
ringlike
    r. contraction
    r. lesion
    r. stricture
ring-type rigidity measuring device
rinse
    SaliCept oral r.
Riopan Plus
RIP
    respiratory inversion point
Ripstein
    R. anterior sling rectopexy
    R. procedure
    R. rectal prolapse operation
risedronate
risk
    r. adjustment
    r. evaluation
    Goldman classification of
      operative r.
    morbidity r.
    neoplasia r.
    perioperative r.
risk-adjusted mortality
Ritalin
RiteBite biopsy forceps
ritonavir
river blindness
Rives-Stoppa
    R.-S. procedure
    R.-S. technique
RJL Model 10 bioelectrical impedance analyzer
RK
    right kidney
RLD
    related living donor
RLP
    rectal linitis plastica
    restriction fragment length polymorphism
      RLP colorectal carcinoma
RLQ
    right lower quadrant
RLT
    reduced liver transplant
RMIC
    renomedullary interstitial cell
RMS
    rhabdomyosarcoma

Ruvalcaba-Myhre-Smith
    RMS syndrome
    RMS voltage
RMT
    ranitidine bismuth citrate, metronidazole, tetracycline
RNA
    ribonucleic acid
    albumin messenger RNA
    HCV RNA
    hepatitis C virus RNA
    IGF-1R RNA
    messenger RNA (mRNA)
    RNA probe
RNA-based finding
RNAse digestion
RNP
    ribonucleoprotein
rNV
    recombinant capsid protein of Norwalk virus
Roadmapper
    FluoroPlus R.
Roadrunner wire
Robaxisal
Robbers forceps
Robengatope radioactive agent
Roberts
    R. folding esophagoscope
    R. oval esophagoscope
    R. syndrome
Roberts-Jesberg esophagoscope
Robertson
    R. sign
    R. TM urethroscope
Robin-Masse abdominal retractor
Robinow syndrome
robin's egg-blue gallbladder
Robinson catheter
Robinson-Kepler-Power water test
Robinul
Robinul Forte
Roboprep G instrument
robotic-automated assist device
Robson
    R. intestinal forceps
    R. point
    R. position
ROC
    receiver-operating characteristic
    ROC XS suture fastener
Rocaltrol
Rocephin IM
Roche sign
Rochester-Carmalt forceps
Rochester gallstone forceps
Rochester-Mixter forceps
Rochester-Ochsner forceps

Rochester-Péan
    R.-P. forceps
    R.-P. hemostat
Rockey-Davis incision
rod
    colostomy r.
    gram-negative r.
    ileostomy r.
    Meckel r.
    Reichmann r.
    Sur-Fit Natura loop ostomy r.
rod-lens system
rodless end-loop stoma
Rodney Smith biliary stricture repair
Roeder
    R. loop
    R. loop knot
Roenigk
    R. grade
    R. score
roentgen finding
roentgenography
    double-contrast r.
rofecoxib
Roferon-A
Roger
    R. reflex
    R. syndrome
Rokitansky
    R. disease
    R. diverticulum
    R. hernia
    R. kidney
Rokitansky-Aschoff
    R.-A. sinus
    R.-A. sinus hyperplasia
Rokitansky-Cushing ulcer
Rokitansky-Kuster-Hauser syndrome
Rolaids
role
    additional unproven r.
    plasmid profile r.
roll
    iliac r.
    Kraske r.
rollerball electrode
roller pump
rolling hiatal hernia
Romazicon
Rome criteria (I, II)
Rommelaere sign

roof
    pseudoaneurysmal r.
    r. strip
rooperi
    Hypoxis r.
Roosevelt clamp
root
    ginger r.
    r. mean square voltage
    penile r.
    sacral nerve r.
rooting reflex
rootlet
    ventral sacral r.
ROPA
    Regional Organ Procurement Agency
Ro-resection
    radial R.-r.
ROS
    reactive oxygen species
Rosch-Uchida transjugular liver access set
rose
    r. bengal sodium ^{131}I biliary scan
    r. bengal sodium ^{131}I radioactive agent
    r. bengal test
    r. thorn ulcer
    r. thorn ulcer of mucosa
Rose-Bradford kidney
rosebud stoma
Rosenbach-Gmelin test
Rosenbach sign
Rosen cyst
Rosenthal test
rosette
    r. appearance of anus
    Homer Wright r.
rosetted
Rosetti-Nissen procedure
Rosewater syndrome
Rossbach disease
Ross carbohydrate free (RCF)
Rosser crypt hook
Rossetti
    R. modification of Nissen fundoplication
    R.-Nissen procedure
rotary shadowing electron microscopy
RotaShield
rotatable Roth retrieval net
rotating
    r. endoprobe

NOTES

rotating *(continued)*
    r. endo-scissors
    r. sphincterotome
rotation
    external r.
    internal r.
rotational colonoscope overtube
rotator
    Jarit r.
Rotator polypectomy snare
rotavirus
    r. diarrhea
    r. gastroenteritis
    group C r.
    r. infection
    r. tetravalent vaccine
rotavirus-associated diarrhea
Rotazyme test
Roth
    R. Grip-Tip suture guide
    R. polyp retrieval net
    R. spot
Rothmund-Thomson syndrome
roticulator stapling device
Rotolith lithotrite
Rotor syndrome
rotunda
    pityriasis r.
rotund abdomen
roughage
round
    r. ligament
    r. ulcer
roundworm
route
    fecal-oral r.
    paracellular r.
routine neonatal circumcision
Roux
    R. gastric reflux
    R. limb
    R. limb emptying
    R. retractor
    R. stasis syndrome
Roux-en-Y
    R.-e.-Y anastomosis
    R.-e.-Y biliary bypass with antrectomy
    R.-e.-Y chimney surgical technique
    R.-e.-Y choledochojejunostomy
    R.-e.-Y cystojejunostomy
    R.-e.-Y distal jejunoileostomy
    R.-e.-Y esophagojejunostomy
    R.-e.-Y gastric bypass
    R.-e.-Y gastroenterostomy
    R.-e.-Y hepaticojejunostomy
    R.-e.-Y jejunal limb
    R.-e.-Y jejunostomy

    R.-e.-Y limb enteroscopy
    R.-e.-Y loop
    R.-e.-Y loop of jejunum
    R.-e.-Y operation
    R.-e.-Y pancreaticojejunostomy
    R.-e.-Y procedure
    R.-e.-Y procedure with vagotomy
    R.-e.-Y reanastomosis
    R.-e.-Y reconstruction
Roux-limb stasis
Roux-type gastroduodenal anastomosis
Rovighi sign
Rovsing
    R. operation
    R. sign
    R. syndrome
Rowasa enema
Rowland pouch
roxatidine acetate
Roxicodone
roxithromycin
RP
    radical prostatectomy
    restorative proctocolectomy
RP3 stain
RPC
    recurrent pyogenic cholangiohepatitis
    restorative proctocolectomy
RPD
    Pepcid RPD
RPF
    renal plasma flow
RPG
    retrograde pyelogram
RPGN
    rapidly progressive glomerulonephritis
RPHA
    reversed passive hemagglutination reaction
RPLD
    retroperitoneal lymph node dissection
RPMI-1640 medium
RPN
    renal papillary necrosis
RPT
    rapid pull-through
    RPT technique
RR
    rate ratio
RRP
    radical retropubic prostatectomy
RRV-TV
    rhesus rotavirus-tetravalent vaccine
RS
    rehydrating solution
    respiratory symptom
    RS associated with GERD

RSH
rectus sheath hematoma
RSLT
reduced-size liver transplant
RSR
rectosphincteric reflex
RSs
relative supersaturation
RT
reverse transcriptase
RTA
renal tubular acidosis
RTA-I
renal tubular acidosis I
RTFNA
real-time fine-needle aspiration
RT-PCR
reverse transcription-polymerase chain
reaction
PSA RT-PCR
RU
retrograde urogram
rub
friction r.
peritoneal friction r.
pleural r.
rubber
r. band ligation (RBL)
r. band ligation of hemorrhoid
r. band ligator (RBL)
r. dam
rubber-sheathed clamp
rubber-shod clamp
rubella
rubeola
Rubin-Quinton small-bowel biopsy tube
Rubinstein-Taybi syndrome
Rubin tube
rubitecan
rubor
dependent r.
rubra
miliaria r.
Rubratope-57 radioactive agent
rubrum
tinea r.
Trichophyton r.
ructus
Rudd
R. Clinic hemorrhoidal forceps
R. Clinic hemorrhoidal ligator

rudiment
hepatic r.
rudimentary testis syndrome
Rud syndrome
RUG
retrograde urethrogram
retrograde urethrography
ruga, pl. **rugae**
rugae gastricae
rugae of stomach
r. of urinary bladder
rugae zone
rugal
r. fold
r. hypertrophy
r. pattern
rugate
rugitus
rugose, rugous
rule
Goodsall r.
Weigert-Meyer r.
ruler catheter
Rulox No. 1, 2
rumble
rumbling bowel sounds
Rumel tourniquet
rumen
rumination
runner's diarrhea
running suture
runny stool
runting syndrome
Runyon group III mycobacteria
rupture
acute hepatic r.
bladder r.
catheterization pouch r.
duodenopancreaticocholedochal r.
ERCP-induced splenic r.
esophageal r.
gastric r.
hepatic r.
hydatid cyst intrahepatic r.
Mallory-Weiss mucosal r.
mesenteric r.
penile r.
renal allograft r.
retrograde balloon r.
splenic r.
spontaneous r.
traumatic r.

R

NOTES

rupture *(continued)*
    umbilical hernia r.
    uterine r.
ruptured
    r. abdominal aortic aneurysm (RAAA)
    r. appendiceal cystadenoma
    r. appendix
    r. hepatic tumor
    r. peliotic lesion
    r. pseudoaneurysm
    r. sigmoid diverticulum
RUQ
    right upper quadrant
RUS
    real-time ultrasonography
Rusch stent
Rusconi anus
rush
    peristaltic r.
rushing
Russell
    R. gastrostomy kit
    R. peel-away sheath dilator
    R. percutaneous endoscopic gastrostomy
    R. sign
    R. technique
    R. viper venom test
    R. viper venom time
Russell-Silver syndrome
Russian tissue forceps
rust ring

RUT
    rapid urease test
    RUT kit
ruthenium red
Rutkow sutureless plug and patch
RUV
    residual urine volume
Ruvalcaba-Myhre-Smith (RMS)
    R.-M.-S. syndrome
Ruysch
    R. disease
    R. glomerulus
    R. vein
RVR
    renal vascular resistance
RVRA
    renal vein renin activity
    renal vein renin assay
RVRC
    renal vein renin concentration
RVRI
    renal vascular resistance index
R-wave
    R-w. coordination
    R-w. triggering
RWG
    rye whole-grain
RX Herculink 14 biliary stent system
RXR
    retinoid X receptor
ryanodine binding
rye whole-grain (RWG)
Ryle tube

S

S cell
S neuron
S pelvic ileal pouch

S-100

S-100 immunohistochemical stain
S-100 protein

S 10036
S100 super family
S3 segment
SAA

serum amyloid A
splenic artery aneurysm

SAAG

serum-ascites albumin gradient

Saathoff test
saber stroke
Sabouraud glucose agar
sabre

coup de s.
en coup de s.

SAB reagent
saburra
saburral colic
sac

enterocele s.
fluid-filled s.
greater peritoneal s.
hernia s.
high ligation of hernia s.
indirect hernial s.
lesser peritoneal s.
peritoneal s.
Pleatman s.
wide-mouth s.
yolk s.

saccharate
saccharin
saccharomyces

yeast s.

Saccharomyces boulardii
sacciform kidney
Saccomanno

S. fixative
S. solution

saccular

s. aneurysm
s. colon

sacculated

s. bladder

sacculation

cecal s.
colic s.
s. of colon
tubular narrowing and s.

saccule
sacculiform
sacculus, pl. **sacculi**

sacculi of Beale

Sachse

S. urethrotome
S. urethrotomy

Sachs solution
sack

entrapment s.

Sacks

S. QuickStick catheter
S. Single-Step catheter

Sacks-Vine

S.-V. feeding gastrostomy tube
S.-V. gastrostomy kit
S.-V. PEG system
S.-V. PEG tube
S.-V. technique
S.-V. type PEG

sacral

s. afferent fiber
s. agenesis
s. artery
s. edema
s. evoked response
s. nerve root
s. nerve stimulation (SNS)
s. nerve stimulation therapy
s. neurostimulation
s. plexus
s. posterior root rhizotomy
s. promontory
s. reflex arc
s. root neuromodulation
s. vein

sacroabdominoperineal pull-through
sacrococcygeal

s. pilonidal cyst
s. pilonidal sinus tract
s. region germ cell tumor
s. teratoma

sacrocolpopexy
sacrofixation operation
sacroiliac joint
sacroiliitis
sacrospinalis

s. ligament vaginal fixation
s. muscle

sacrospinous

s. ligament
s. ligament vaginal fixation

sacrotuberous ligament
sacrouterine ligament
sacrum

SAD
 sinoaortic denervation
S-adenosylmethionine (SAMe)
 S-a. deficiency
Saeed
 S. multiband ligator
 S. multiple ligator
 S. 10-shooter
 S. six-shooter
 S. six-shooter ligator
 S. technique
safe
 S. and Dry panty and pad system
 s. gastrocutaneous fistulous tract
Safe-T-Flex enteral feeding container
safe-tract technique
safety
 S. AV fistula needle
 s. pin ingestion
 s. wire
saffron stain
SAGB
 Swedish Adjustable Gastric Band
SAGES
 Society of American Gastrointestinal
 Endoscoping Surgeons
saginata
 Taenia s.
sagittal
 s. fissure of liver
 s. image
sago-grain stool
sagrada
 cascara s.
Sahli glutoid test
Sahli-Nencki test
Saint triad
Salem
 S. duodenal sump tube
SALF
 subacute liver failure
Salflex
SaliCept
 S. freeze-dried dressing
 S. oral rinse
salicylate
 s. abuse
 methyl s.
salicylazosulfapyridine
saline
 buffered s.
 s. cleansing enema
 s. continence test
 s. cystometry
 s. flush
 half-normal s.
 heparinized s.
 hypertonic s.

iced s.
indigo carmine-stained normal s.
s. infusion
s. injection therapy
isotonic s.
s. laxative
s. load test
phosphate-buffered s. (PBS)
s. slush
s. suppression test
saline-assisted polypectomy (SAP)
saline-epinephrine
 hypertonic s.-e. (HSE)
saline-filled cholangiocatheter
saline-moistened sponge
saliva
 s. bicarbonate
 pooled s.
 s. substitute
salivarius
 Streptococcus s.
Salivart
salivary
 s. amylase
 s. calculus
 s. epidermal growth factor (sEGF)
 s. epidermal growth factor-1
 s. gland enlargement
 s. gland scan
 s. hypersecretion
 s. mass
 s. tenderness
 s. testing
salivation
Salkowski-Schipper test
Salle procedure
salmon
 S. backcut incision
 S. law
Salmonella
 S. agona
 S. choleraesuis
 S. colitis
 S. enteritidis
 S. enteritidis orchitis
 S. hartford
 S. heidelberg
 S. hirschfeldii
 S. infantis
 S. newport
 nontyphoidal *S.*
 S. paratyphi
 S. paratyphi A
 S. paratyphi B
 S. paratyphi C
 Salmonella food poisoning
 S. typhi
 S. typhimurium

S. typhimurium enterocolitis
S. typhimurium R5
salmonellosis
    nontyphoidal s.
salmonicida
    Aeromonas s.
Salomon test
salpingitis
salpinx
salt
    bile s. (BS)
    bismuth s.
    s. consumption
    dihydroxy s.
    fura-2, pentapotassium s.
    gold s.
    low s. (LNaCl)
    magnesium s.
    monohydroxy bile s.
    s. and pepper duodenal erosion
    trihydroxy s.
salt-losing
    s.-l. nephritis
    s.-l. nephropathy
salt-sensitive hypertension
saluresis
Saluron
Salutensin
salvage
    s. brachytherapy
    s. cryoablation
    s. cryoablation of the prostate
    s. cystectomy
    s. cystoprostatectomy
    s. cytology
    s. cytology technique
    s. prostatectomy
    s. protocol
    s. surgery
    s. therapy
Salvati proctoscope
Salzer test meal
samarium
SAMe
    S-adenosylmethionine
sample
    arterial blood s.
    aspirated s.
    Bethesda System for
      cervicovaginal s.
    blood s.
    random stool s.

stool s.
urine s.
venous blood s.
sampling
    adrenal vein aldosterone s.
    arterial stimulation venous s.
    (ASVS)
    s. gate
    mediastinal lymph node s.
    tissue s.
    transhepatic portal venous s.
Sam Roberts esophagoscope
sand
    hydatid s.
    urinary s.
sandbag
Sanders incision
Sand-Eze EGD pillow
Sandhill-800 TDS chart recorder
Sandhill P32 pH antimony probe
Sandifer syndrome
Sandimmune
Sandostatin LAR Depot
Sandoz
    S. Caluso 22F, 28F super PEG
    S. Caluso PEG gastrostomy tube
    S. 22F balloon replacement tube
    S. feeding/suction tube
sandwich
    s. staghorn calculus therapy
    s. technique
sandy skin prepping paste
sanguineous
    s. drainage
    s. fluid
sanguis
    Streptococcus s.
Sani Pads medicated cleansing pad
Sani-Supp
Sanorex
SANS
    Stoller afferent nerve stimulation
      PerQ SANS
        Percutaneous Stoller Afferent
        Nerve Stimulation System
Sansert
Santiani-Stone classification
^{35}S antisense fibronectin riboprobe
santonin test
Santorini
    S. canal
    duct of S.

S

NOTES

Santorini *(continued)*
  S. labyrinth
  papilla of S.
  S. sphincter
  S. venous plexus
santorinicele
SAP
  saline-assisted polypectomy
  serum amyloid P
saphenofemoral junction
saphenous
  s. nerve
  s. vein
saponifiable fecal bile acid
saponification
Sappey
  accessory portal system of S.
Sapporo virus
saprophyticus
  Staphylococcus s.
saprophytism
SAPS
  single-action pumping system
saquinavir
saralasin
sarcocele
sarcoidosis
  epididymal s.
  hepatic s.
  pancreatic s.
  renal s.
  urethral s.
sarcoma
  appendiceal Kaposi s.
  bladder s.
  Boeck s.
  botryoid s.
  clear cell s.
  Ewing s.
  gastric Kaposi s.
  gastrointestinal Kaposi s.
  granulocytic s.
  hemangioendothelial s.
  intracolonic Kaposi s.
  Ito cell s.
  Kaposi s. (KS)
  kidney clear cell s.
  kidney osteogenic s.
  Kupffer cell s.
  lipoblastic s.
  osteogenic s.
  penis s.
  prostate gland s.
  retroperitoneum s.
  seminal vesicle s.
  testis s.
  vasoablative endothelial s. (VABES)
  s. virus oncogene

sarcomatoid squamous cell carcinoma
sarcomatous
sarcomphalocele
sarcoplasmic reticulum
Sarcoptes scabiei
Sarfeh principle
Sarisol No. 2
Sarns Siok II blood pump
Sarot needle holder
SART
  standard acid reflux test
satellite lesion
satiety
  early s.
  s. test
Satinsky clamp
satumomab pendetide
saturated fatty acid (SFA)
saturation
  arterial s.
  s. index (SI)
  oxygen s.
  percent transferrin s.
  transferrin s.
saturnine
  s. colic
  s. nephritis
saturnism
saucerization
saucerized biopsy
Saundby test
Saunders disease
sausage digit
sausagelike appearance
Savage perineal body
Savary
  S. bougie
  S. bronchoscope
  complete S.
  S. tapered thermoplastic dilator
Savary-Gilliard
  S.-G. esophagitis (grade I, II)
  S.-G. metal olive
  S.-G. over-the-wire dilator
  S.-G. Silastic flexible bougie
  S.-G. wire-guided bougie
Savary-Miller
  S.-M. criteria
  S.-M. II grade
saver
  Cell S.
sawtooth
  s. appearance sign
  s. irregularity of bowel contour
sawtoothed appearance
Sawyer
  S. rectal retractor
  S. rectal speculum

S-B
Sengstaken-Blakemore
S-B tube
SBE
small bowel enteroscopy
SBFT
small bowel followthrough
SBGM
self blood glucose monitoring
SBO
small bowel obstruction
SBP
spontaneous bacterial peritonitis
SBPN
simultaneous bilateral percutaneous
nephrolithotomy
SBT
skin bleeding time
SC
secretory component
sieving coefficient
subcutaneous
sulfur colloid
^{99m}Tc SC
scabiei
Sarcoptes s.
scabies
genital s.
scale
Charrière s.
children's coma s.
ECOG performance status s.
Flint Colon Injury S. (FCIS)
French s.
Gastrointestinal Symptom Rating S.
(GSRS)
Glasgow coma s.
Goldberg Anorectic Attitude s.
gray s.
Hetzel-Dent s.
Karnofsky performance status s.
Kodsi s.
Lanza s.
Likert s.
Madsen-Iversen s.
scaling
physiologic s.
scalloped
s. antimesenteric border
s. bowel lumen
scalpel
s. blade

harmonic s.
ultrasonic s.
scan
acetyltriglycine renal s.
bone s.
colloid shift on liver-spleen s.
CT s.
diethylenetriamine pentaacetic acid
renal s.
dimercaptosuccinic acid renal s.
dimethyl iminodiacetic acid s.
DISIDA s.
DMSA s.
DTPA renal s.
dual-energy CT s.
endoanal ultrasound s.
esophageal transit s.
fluorescence-activated cell sorter s.
(FACScan)
gallbladder s.
gallium s.
gastric emptying s.
gastroesophageal reflux s.
GI bleeding s.
hepatic blood pool s.
hepatobiliary s.
HIDA s.
Hybritech PSA s.
indium-labeled leukocyte s.
indium 64-labeled white blood
cell s.
indium leukocyte s.
intercostal s.
iodine s.
iodocholesterol s.
isotope renal s.
isotropic s.
labeled red blood cell s.
liver s.
liver-spleen s.
MAG-3 renal s.
Meckel s.
monoclonal antibody scintigraphic s.
MRI s.
nuclear bleeding s.
nuclear isotope s.
nuclear medicine s.
peritoneovenous shunt patency s.
PET s.
PIPIDA hepatobiliary s.
positron emission tomography s.
ProstaScint s.

S

NOTES

scan *(continued)*
    radioisotope s.
    radionuclide s.
    renal s.
    rose bengal sodium ^{131}I biliary s.
    salivary gland s.
    SPECT s.
    splenic perfusion measurement by dynamic CT s.
    sulfur colloid liver s.
    tagged red blood cell bleeding s.
    ^{99m}Tc-DTPA renal s.
    Tc-HIDA s.
    ^{99m}Tc HMPAO-labeled leukocyte s.
    ^{99m}Tc IDA s.
    ^{99m}Tc MDP nuclear isotope bone s.
    ^{99m}Tc pertechnetate s.
    ^{99m}Tc RBC bleeding s.
    ^{99m}Tc sulfur colloid s.
    technetium-labeled autologous red blood cell s.
    technetium-labeled red blood cell s.
    technetium-99m diethylenetriamine pentaacetic acid s.
    technetium-99m IDA s.
    technetium radionuclide s.
    s. test
    transabdominal s.
    transrectal s.
    transvesical s.
    UJ13A nuclear isotope bone s.
    ultrasound s.
scan-directed biopsy
scanner
    Bruel-Kjaer s.
    conventional static s.
    high-resolution real-time s.
    Kretz Combison 330 ultrasound s.
    Kretz 311 ultrasound s.
    linear convex array s.
    Lunar DPX total-body s.
    7.5 MHz sector s.
    MKII automated s.
    Tesla GE Signa whole body s.
scanning
    captopril-DTPA s.
    s. electron microscope
    s. electron microscopy
    endoscopic magnetic resonance s.
    fluorescent gene s.
    s. force microscopy (SFM)
    iodine hippurate s.
    radioisotope s.
    transrectal ultrasound s. (TRUS)
scaphoid abdomen
scapus penis

scar
    Billroth II anastomotic s.
    chest tube s.
    episiotomy s.
    iridectomy s.
    railroad track s.'s
    sternotomy s.
    thoracotomy s.
    s. tissue formation
    s. tissue reaction
scarce bowel sounds
Scardino
    S. flap
    S. ureteropelvioplasty
    S. vertical flap pyeloplasty
Scardino-Prince
    S.-P. ureteropelvioplasty
    S.-P. vertical flap pyeloplasty
scarified duodenum
scarlatinal nephritis
scarlatina rheumatica
scarlatiniform rash
Scarpa
    S. fascia
    S. triangle
scarring
    duodenum deformed by s.
    gastrostomy s.
    kidney s.
    local s.
    postdystrophic s.
    postnecrotic s.
    renal s.
scatoma
scattered fluorescein
scatter factor
scattering
scavenger
    free radical s.
    hydroxyl radical s.
SCC
    squamous cell carcinoma
S-CCK-Pz
    secretin-cholecystokinin-pancreatozymin
    S-CCK-Pz stimulation
    S-CCK-Pz test
SCE
    specialized columnar epithelium
SCFA
    short-chain fatty acid
Schachowa spiral tube
Schäfer nomogram
Schatzki ring
Schaumann body
Scheffe-F test
schenckii
    Sporothrix s.

Schiff
- S. biliary cycle
- S. stain
- S. test

Schilder disease
Schiller-Duval body
Schilling test
Schindler
- S. disease
- S. esophagoscope
- S. peritoneal forceps
- S. semiflexible gastroscope

Schistosoma
- S. haematobium
- S. intercalatum
- S. japonica
- S. japonicum
- S. mansoni
- S. mekongi

schistosomal
- s. cervicitis
- s. dysentery
- s. liver disease
- s. pelvic floor myopathy

schistosomiasis
- active s.
- acute s.
- Asiatic s.
- bladder s.
- colon s.
- colonic s.
- ectopic s.
- hepatic s.
- inactive s.
- intestinal s.
- Japanese s.
- Manson s.
- Oriental s.
- s. sandy patch
- ureteral s.
- urinary s.
- vesical s.

Schmidt
- S. diet
- S. syndrome

Schmitz bacillus
schmitzii
- *Shigella s.*

Schmorl reaction
Schneider stent

Schnidt
- S. gall duct forceps
- S. thoracic forceps

Schoemaker
- S. anastomosis
- S. gastroenterostomy
- S. procedure

Schoemaker-Billroth II technique
Schoenberg intestinal forceps
Schönlein-Henoch
- S.-H. disease
- S.-H. purpura

Schramm phenomenon
Schuchardt relaxing incision
Schultz
- S. angina
- S. disease
- S. syndrome

Schwachman syndrome
Schwann
- S. cell
- S. cell lipidosis

schwannian spindle cell
schwannoma
- penile s.

Schwartz
- S. clamp
- S. method
- S. test

Schwartz-Jampel syndrome
Schweizer-Foley Y-plasty
SCI
- spinal cord injury

ScI-70 autoantibody
sciatic
- s. hernia
- s. nerve

sciatica
SCID
- severe combined immunodeficiency

science
- biomedical s.

scintigram
- ^{99m}technetium-dimercaptosuccinic acid s.

scintigraph
scintigraphic
- s. balloon
- s. balloon topography
- s. diagnosis
- s. emptying study
- s. reflux

NOTES

S

scintigraphy
adrenal s.
antral s.
dimercaptosuccinic acid s.
direct vesicoureteral s. (DVS)
diuretic renal s.
DMSA s.
gastric emptying s.
gastroesophageal s.
hepatobiliary s.
OctreoScan s.
OncoScint colorectal/ovarian
  carcinoma localization s.
  (OncoScint CR/OV)
per rectal portal s.
quantitative hepatobiliary s. (QHS)
radioisotope s.
radionuclide s.
renal cortical s.
renal gallium-67 s.
renal perfusion s.
somatostatin receptor s. (SRS)
somatostatin receptor s. (SRS)
tagged erythrocyte s.
^{99m}Tc-GSA s.
^{99m}Tc-HMPAO-labeled leukocyte s.
^{99m}Tc pertechnetate s.
technetium-99m red cell s.
whole-gut transit s. (WGTS)
scintillation vial
scintiphotosplenoportography
scintirenography
scintiscan
biliary s.
false-positive s.
gastroesophageal s.
scintiscanning
radionuclide ^{99}Tc s.
scintography
leukocyte s.
scirrhous
s. adenocarcinoma
s. carcinoma
s. lesion
scissors
Buie rectal s.
Busch umbilical s.
Church deep surgery s.
cold s.
Crafoord thoracic s.
curved Mayo s.
Deaver operating s.
diathermy s.
dissection s.
s. dissection
Doyen abdominal s.
Duffield deep surgery s.
electrosurgical curved s.

endoscopic s.
Ferguson abdominal s.
Graham deep surgery s.
Harrington-Mayo s.
hook s.
Hooper deep surgery s.
insulated curved s.
insulated straight s.
Kelly fistula s.
Lincoln deep surgery s.
Mayo s.
Mayo-Noble dissecting s.
meatotomy s.
Metzenbaum s.
Miller rectal s.
Nelson s.
Nu-Tip laparoscopic s.
Panzer gallbladder s.
Penn umbilical s.
Potts s.
Potts-Smith s.
Pratt rectal s.
Snowden-Pencer s.
strabismus s.
Strulle s.
Super-Cut s.
surgical s.
suture s.
Sweet esophageal s.
Thorek-Feldman gallbladder s.
Thorek gallbladder s.
umbilical s.
Vezien abdominal s.
Westcott tenotomy s.
Willauer thoracic s.
scissor-valve
Quinton single port s.-v.
Scivoletto test
SCIWOA
spinal cord injury without radiographic
  abnormality
sclera, pl. **sclerae**
anicteric sclerae
icteric sclerae
nonicteric sclerae
scleral icterus
sclerodactyly
scleroderma
s. bowel disease
esophageal s.
s. of esophagus
s. renal crisis
scleroderma sine s.
Scleromate sclerosant
sclerosant
absolute alcohol s.
bucrylate s.

s. dosage
esophageal variceal s.
ethanolamine oleate s.
s. injection
Krazy Glue s.
latex s.
morrhuate s.
polidocanol s.
Scleromate s.
sodium tetradecyl sulfate s.
s. solution
Sotradecol s.
variceal s.

sclerosant-contrast solution
sclerose
sclerosing
s. adenosis
s. agent
s. cholangitis
s. encapsulating peritonitis
s. hepatic carcinoma (SHC)
s. lymphangitis
s. mesenteritis
s. solution
s. therapy

sclerosis
alcohol s.
biliary s.
central hyaline s.
diffuse mesangial s. (DMS)
endoscopic injection s.
esophageal variceal s.
focal s.
gastric s.
global s.
glomerular s.
hepatic s.
hepatoportal s.
injection s.
laser s.
multiple s.
nuclear s.
progressive systemic s. (PSS)
systemic s. (SSc)
systemic duodenal s.
tetracycline s.
tuberous s.
variceal s.

sclerosus
lichen s.

sclerotherapist

sclerotherapy
antegrade scrotal s.
bismuth s.
colonoscopic s.
s. complication
endoscopic s. (ES)
endoscopic injection s. (EIS)
endoscopic retrograde s.
endoscopic variceal s.
esophageal variceal s. (EVS)
ethanol s.
fiberoptic injection s. (FIS)
hemorrhoidal s.
injection s.
intravariceal injection s.
low-volume s.
s. needle
paravariceal s.
prophylactic s.
ultra-low-volume s.
variceal s.

sclerotic
s. atrophy
s. kidney
s. stomach
s. tuft

SCO
Sertoli-cell-only
SCO syndrome

scolex, pl. **scoleces**
scoliosis
scoop
Beck abdominal s.
Desjardins gallbladder s.
Desjardins gallstone s.
Ferguson gallstone s.
Ferris common duct s.
gallbladder s.
Klebanoff gallstone s.
malleable s.
Mayo common duct s.
Mayo gallstone s.
Mayo-Robson gallstone s.
Moore gallstone s.
Moynihan gallstone s.
rigid s.

scope
baby s.
J-turn of the s.
retroflexed s.
torquing of s.

Scopinaro pancreaticobiliary bypass

S

NOTES

scopolamine
scorbutic dysentery
S-cord
score
    activity s.
    APACHE-II s.
    Baylor bleeding s.
    Beppu s.
    Boyarsky BPH symptom s.
    CCKNOW s.
    Child-Pugh s.
    Cleveland Clinic Incontinence S.
    Danish Prostate Symptom S.
      (DAN-PSS)
    DeMeester acid s.
    fibrin s.
    fibrosis s.
    Glasgow Dyspepsia Severity S.
      (GDSS)
    Gleason s.
    Hetzel s.
    hostility s.
    incontinence s.
    International Autoimmune Hepatitis
      Group s.
    International Prognostic Index s.
    International Prostate Symptom S.
      (IPSS)
    Karnofsky s.
    Knodell s.
    linear analog pain s.
    Madsen symptom s.
    Roenigk s.
    sexual function s. (SFI)
    symptom s.
    total corrected incremental s.
      (TCIS)
Scott
    S. AMS inflatable penile prosthesis
    S. jejunoileal bypass
    S. operation
    S. retractor
SCP
    squamous cell papilloma
SCr
    serum creatinine
scrapie protein
scraping brush
screen
    Biosafe PSA4 s.
    ChemTrak AccuMeter s.
    ENA s.
screening
    cancer s.
    catatonic trypsinogen DNA s.
    colon cancer s.
    colonoscopy s.
    colorectal cancer s.

    s. cystometry
    endocrine s.
    s. endoscopy
screw
    Reddick-Saye s.
Scribner shunt
scrota (pl. of scrotum)
scrotal
    s. agenesis
    s. angiokeratoma
    s. arteriovenous malformation
    s. calcification
    s. encroachment
    s. fat necrosis
    s. hemangioma
    s. hernia
    s. hypospadias
    s. lymphangioma
    s. mass
    s. pain
    s. panniculitis
    s. pneumatocele
    s. pouch operation
    s. pouch orchiopexy
    s. raphe
    s. reflex
    s. septum
    s. swelling
    s. tenderness
    s. varicocelectomy
    s. violation
scrotal-perineal artery
scrotectomy
    total s.
scrotitis
scrotocele
scrotoplasty
scrotoscopy
scrotum, pl. scrota, scrotums
    acute s.
    angiokeratoma of s.
    bifid s.
    s. calcification
    s. cyst
    ectopic s.
    elephantiasis scroti
    lymph s.
    necrotizing fasciitis of the s.
    prepenile dislocation of s.
    pruritus scroti
    raphe scroti
    raphe of s.
    sebaceous cyst of s.
    septum of s.
    watering-can s.
scrub
    Betadine s.
    pHisoHex s.

SCTAT
> sex cord tumors with annular tubules

SCTP
> solid and cystic tumor of the pancreas

Scudder
>> S. intestinal clamp
>> S. intestinal forceps

SCUF
> slow continuous ultrafiltration

Scultetus position

scybalous stool

scybalum, pl. **scybala**

SDB
> sleep-disordered breathing

SDH
> sorbitol dehydrogenase
> succinate dehydrogenase activity
>> SDH enzyme

SDS
> sodium dodecyl sulfate

SEA
> soluble egg antigen

sea anemone ulcer

sea-blue histiocyte syndrome

seabuckthorn seed oil

seal
>> fibrin s.
>> Karaya 5 s.
>> long s. (LS)

sealant
>> Beriplast fibrin s.
>> fibrin s.
>> Hemaseel APR kit fibrin s.
>> Periplast s.
>> Tisseel fibrin s.

Seal-tight adhesive gasket

searcher
>> stone s.

Sears Wee Alert

sebaceous
>> s. cyst
>> s. cyst of scrotum

sebaceum
>> adenoma s.

seborrheic
>> s. dermatitis
>> s. keratitis

SEC
> sinusoidal endothelial cell
> superficial esophageal carcinoma

secalin

Seckel syndrome

secobarbital

secoisolariciresinol

secondary
>> s. achalasia
>> s. amyloidosis
>> s. bacterial peritonitis
>> s. bile acid
>> s. biliary cirrhosis
>> s. biliary fibrosis
>> s. closure
>> s. contraction
>> s. cyst
>> s. enterocele
>> s. hyperaldosteronism
>> s. hyperparathyroidism
>> s. hypertension
>> s. impotence
>> s. incontinence
>> s. jejunal ulcer
>> s. metastatic carcinoma
>> s. obstruction
>> s. peristalsis
>> s. peristaltic wave
>> s. priapism
>> s. prophylaxis
>> s. pseudoobstruction syndrome
>> s. refluxing megaureter
>> s. renal calculus
>> s. sclerosing cholangitis
>> s. spermatocyte
>> s. sterility
>> s. surgery
>> s. suture
>> s. syphilis
>> s. tumor
>> s. vesicoureteral reflex
>> s. volvulus

second-cuff implantation

second-generation
>> s.-g. cephalosporin
>> s.-g. enzyme immunoassay (EIA-2)
>> s.-g. lithotriptor
>> s.-g. recombinant immunoblot assay

second-line drug

second-look
>> s.-l. flexible nephroscopy
>> s.-l. laparotomy
>> s.-l. operation

second-set phenomenon

secosteroid hormone

NOTES

S

secretagogue
luminal s.
somatostatin s.
secreted
regulated upon activation, normal T
cell expressed and s. (RANTES)
secretin
proton-induced release of s.
s. provocation test
s. stimulation
s. stimulation test
s. ultrasonography
secretin-CCK stimulation test
secretin-cholecystokinin-pancreatozymin
(S-CCK-Pz)
Secretin-Ferring Powder
secretin-glucagon-vasoactive intestinal
peptide family
secretin-pancreozymin stimulation test
secretion
acid s.
basal acid s.
biliary cholesterol s.
chloride s.
chylomicron s.
epididymis s.
estrogen testicular s.
expressed prostatic s.'s (EPS)
follicle-stimulating hormone s.
gastric acid s.
gonadotropin-releasing hormone
pulsatile s.
hydrochloric acid s.
idiopathic gastric acid s.
intrinsic factor s.
Leydig cell s.
macromolecular s.
meal-stimulated pancreatic s.
medication-associated suppression of
gastric s.
mucoid s.
paralytic s.
pepsin s.
physiologic role in acid s.
prostate gland s.
renin s.
syndrome of inappropriate
antidiuretic hormone s. (SIADH)
toxin-mediated intestinal s.
urinalysis sediment microscopy
prostatic s.
vas deferens s.
secretory
s. canaliculus
s. cell
s. coil
s. component (SC)
s. diarrhea

s. IgA (sIgA)
s. immunoglobulin A
s. product
s. reflex
section
abdominal s.
adrenal gland microscopic s.
distal shave s.
frozen s.
Giemsa-stained s.
perineal s.
permanent s.
prostate gland cross s.
renal histologic s.
ultrathin araldite s.
sectioning
celiac plexus s.
thin shave s.
7.5-MHz sector scanner
Sectral
sedation
benzodiazepine conscious s.
conscious s.
IV s.
meperidine conscious s.
midazolam conscious s.
terminal s. (TS)
sedation-induced hypoventilation
sedative
anxiolytic s.
gastric s.
intestinal s.
sediment
nephritic s.
spun urine s.
urinary s.
sedimentation
Ficoll-Hypaque gradient s.
sedoanalgesia
seeberi
Rhinosporidium s.
seed
BrachySeed brachytherapy s.
I-Plant brachytherapy s.
iridium s.
mustard s.
PharmaSeed iodine-125 s.
PharmaSeed palladium-103 s.
L-phenylalanine mustard (L-PAM)
Plantago ovata s.
ProstaSeed I-125 s.
radioactive s.
Symmetra I-125 brachytherapy s.
seeding
instrument-track s.
malignant s.
needle-track s.

peritoneal s.
tumor s.

SeedNet system
seepage
    fecal s.
SEER
    Surveillance, Epidemiology, and End
    Results
sEGF
    salivary epidermal growth factor
segment
    afferent tubular isoperistaltic s.
    Ask-Upmark renal s.
    Barrett s.
    demucosalized augmentation with
      gastric s. (DAWG)
    ileal s. (IS)
    ileocecal s.
    pyloroduodenal s.
    S3 s.
    tumor-bearing s.
segmenta (*pl. of* segmentum)
segmental
    s. appendicitis
    s. bile duct fibrosis
    s. change
    s. colectomy
    s. colonic adenomatous polyposis
      syndrome
    s. colonic resection
    s. colonic tuberculosis
    s. enteritis
    s. glomerulosclerosis
    s. ileal infarction
    s. intestine
    s. ischemic colitis
    s. liver graft
    s. testicular infarction
    s. ureterectomy
segmentary pancreatitis
segmentation movement
segmentectomy
    hepatic s.
    s. of liver
segmented neutrophil
segmentum, pl. **segmenta**
segregator
    Cathelin s.
    Harris s.
    Luy s.
Segura basket
Segura-Dretler laser basket

SeHCAT
    selenium-labeled homocholic acid
    conjugated with taurine
    SeHCAT test
Seidlitz powder
Seitzinger tripolar cutting forceps
seizure disorder
Sekomic SS-100F recorder
^{75}Se-labeled bile acid test
SelCID
Seldinger
    S. cystic duct catheterization
    S. gastrostomy needle
    S. principle
    S. technique
selectin
selective
    s. bladder activation
    s. catheterization
    s. ductal cannulation
    s. endothelin A
    s. intestinal decontamination (SID)
    s. jejunal hyperalgesia
    s. left gastric arteriography
    s. mesenteric angiography
    s. proximal vagotomy (SPV)
    s. sacral rhizotomy
    s. targeting
    s. vagotomy
selectivity
    charge s.
selenite
    insulin-transferrin-sodium s.
Selenite-F enrichment medium
selenium-75
selenium-labeled homocholic acid
    conjugated with taurine (SeHCAT)
selenomethionine radioactive agent
self-antigen
self blood glucose monitoring (SBGM)
self-bougienage treatment
self-catheterization
    intermittent s.-c. (ISC)
self-drainage catheter
self-expandable
    s.-e. metal stent
    s.-e. stainless steel braided
      endoprosthesis
self-expanding
    s.-e. biliary metal stent
    s.-e. coil stent
    s.-e. metallic stent (SEMS)

S

NOTES

self-fulfilling prophecy
self-induced
    s.-i. purging
    s.-i. vomiting
self-injection therapy
self-MHC
self-monitoring
    nocturnal tumescence s.-m.
self-obturation
    intermittent s.-o.
self-poisoning
self-retaining
    s.-r. catheter
    s.-r. coil stent
    s.-r. ring retractor
self-retractor
    Lone Star s.-r.
self-tightening slip knot
Seltzer
    Bromo S.
SELU
    seromuscular enterocystoplasty lined with
    urothelium
semantic conditioning
Semb ligature carrier
semen
    s. analysis
    s. analysis test
    s. for assisted reproductive
    technique
    s. coagulation
    s. collection
    s. liquefaction
    s. round cell
    s. sperm concentration
    s. viscosity
    s. volume
semenuria
semicircular line of Douglas
semielemental
    s. diet
    s. enteral feeding
semiflexible endoscope
semiformed stool
Semilente insulin
semilunar-shaped fold
seminal
    s. colliculus
    s. fluid
    s. plasma C3
    s. plasma cholesterol
    s. plasma choline
    s. plasma citrate
    s. plasma citric acid
    s. plasma fructose
    s. plasma Zn-α2-glycoprotein
    s. tract washout
    s. vesicle

    s. vesicle abscess
    s. vesicle adenocarcinoma
    s. vesicle agenesis
    s. vesicle amyloid deposit
    s. vesicle aplasia
    s. vesicle aspiration
    s. vesicle atrophy
    s. vesicle calculus
    s. vesicle carcinoid
    s. vesicle hydatid cyst
    s. vesicle infection
    s. vesicle innervation
    s. vesicle lymphoma
    s. vesicle obstruction
    s. vesicle sarcoma
    s. vesicle weight
    s. vesiculography (SVG)
    s. vesiculotomy
seminalis
    colliculus s.
    ductus excretorius vesiculae s.
    vesicula s.
semination
seminiferous
    s. tubule
    s. tubule blood-testis barrier
    s. tubule epithelium
    s. tubule gonocyte
    s. tubule peritubular structure
    s. tubule Sertoli cell
seminis
    liquor s.
seminogelin
seminologist
seminology
seminoma
    anaplastic s.
    retroperitoneal s.
    testicular s.
seminomatous
seminome
seminoprotein
    gamma s.
seminuria
semioblique position
semiopen hemorrhoidectomy
semipedunculated lesion
semiquantitative
    s. agglutination SERA-TEK Ames
    s. culture
semirigid
    s. endoscope
    s. fiberoptic ureteroscope
    s. Nottingham introducer
    s. sigmoidoscope
semisolid stool
Semken tissue forceps

SEMS
    self-expanding metallic stent
      membrane-coated SEMS
SEM stent
Senecio
senescence
    accelerated s.
senescent cell
Sengstaken-Blakemore (S-B)
    S.-B. esophageal balloon
    S.-B. method
    S.-B. tamponade
    S.-B. tube
    S.-B. tube insertion
senile nephrosclerosis
Senior-Loken syndrome
senktide
senna
    extractum s.
Senn-Kanavel retractor
Senn retractor
Senokot-S
Senokot X-Prep
SENSA
    Hemoccult SENSA
sensation
    bladder s.
    burning s.
    esophageal globus s.
    foreign body s.
    perineal s.
    rectal s.
    threshold of rectal s.
Sensation Short Throw snare
SensiCare synthetic powder-free surgical glove
sensitive and specific ELISA
sensitivity
    anaphylactoid food s.
    culture and s. (C&S)
    gluten s.
    interpersonal s.
    penile s.
    rectal visceral s.
    soy protein s.
sensitizer
    radiation s.
sensor
    anal EMG PerryMeter s.
    anterior esophageal s. (AES)
    bladder pressure s.

    fiberoptic s.
    manometric s.
    S. Medics pressure transducer
    sleeve s.
    ultrasonic tactile s.
sensorium change
sensory
    s. biofeedback
    s. finding
    s. loss
    s. nervous terminal
    s. neuron
    s. receptor
    s. urgency
    s. voiding dysfunction
sentinel
    s. clot
    s. fold
    s. hyperplastic polyp
    s. loop
    s. node
    s. pile
    s. tag
sentry system
separation
    peripartum symphysis s.
separator
    Benson pylorus s.
Sephacryl S-300 HR gel
Sepharose 4B-coupled-protein-A column
Seprafilm bioresorbable membrane
Sepramesh
sepsis
    anal s.
    anorectal s.
    biliary s.
    enterococcal s.
    gram-negative s.
    gram-positive s.
    s. intestinalis
    intraabdominal s. (IAS)
    pancreatic s.
    pelvic s.
    perianal s.
    post rubber band s.
    staphylococcal s.
    s. syndrome
septa (*pl. of* septum)
septal hematoma
Septata intestinalis
septate vagina

S

NOTES

septation
    cloaca s.
    internal s.
septectomy
septic
    s. cholangitis
    s. necrosis
    s. shock
    s. wound
septicemia
Septisol
Septopal bead
Septra DS
septulum, pl. **septula**
    septula testis
septum, pl. **septa**
    s. bulbi urethra
    cloacal s.
    deviated s.
    s. glandis penis
    s. of glans penis
    interhaustral s.
    pancreaticobiliary s.
    s. pectiniforme
    s. penis
    perforated nasal s.
    rectogenital s.
    rectovaginal s.
    rectovesical s.
    scrotal s.
    s. of scrotum
    s. of testis
    tracheoesophageal s.
    transverse vaginal s.
    urethrovaginal s.
    urorectal s.
sequela, pl. **sequelae**
    clinical s.
sequence
    adenoma-carcinoma s.
    adenomatous polyp-cancer s.
    contrast-enhanced fast s. (CE-FAST)
    dysplasia-to-carcinoma s.
    esophageal manometric s. (EMS)
    flanking s.
    FLASH pulse s.
    genomic s.
    HASTE s.
    leucine zipper s.
    metaplasia-dysplasia-carcinoma s.
    papilloma-carcinoma s.
    phasic wave s.
    rapid acquisition fast spin echo s.
    turbo spin-echo s.
sequence-sequence oligonucleotide hybridization

sequencing
    s. analysis
    molecular cloning and s.
sequential
    s. motility
    s. multiple analyzer (SMA)
    s. quadruple drug regimen
    s. ultrafiltration hemodialysis
    s. video converter
sequestrant
    bile acid s.
sequestration
    fluid s.
sera (*pl. of* serum)
Seraflo blood line
Serenoa
    S. repens
    S. repens extract
Serentil
Sergent white adrenal line
serial
    s. cholangiograms
    s. dilution
series
    acute abdominal s. (AAS)
    gallbladder s. (GBS)
    Gastrografin GI s.
    liver function s. (LFS)
    motor meal barium GI s.
    upper GI s.
serine
    s. protease
    s. protease-activated prorenin
    s. threonine kinase gene 11 (*STK11*)
seroconversion rate
Serodia commercial kit
seroepidemiological study
seroepidemiology
serologic
    s. diagnosis
    s. marker
    s. test
    s. test for syphilis (STS)
serology
    IgG s.
    specific anti-Hp s.
seromuscular
    s. colocystoplasty
    s. enterocystoplasty lined with urothelium (SELU)
    s. intestinal patch graft
    s. layer
    s. Lembert suture
seromyectomy
    duodenal s.
seromyotomy
    laparoscopic s.

seronegative polyarthritis
seropositive
seroprevalence
    s. rate
seroprotection
serosa
    cecal s.
    gastric s.
    perispermatitis s.
    tunica s.
serosal
    s. afferent innervation
    s. blood vessel
    s. creeping fat
    s. infiltration
    s. surface
    s. tear
serosanguineous
    s. drainage
    s. fluid
serositis
    uremic s.
serotonergic
    s. drug
    s. type 3 receptor
serotonin (5-HT)
    s. antagonist treatment
    s. cell
    s. receptor antagonist
    s. reuptake transporter (SERT)
    serum s.
    s. stain
serotoninergic neuron
serous
    s. diarrhea
    s. membrane
Serpasil-Esidrix
serpiginous
    s. microcystic duct
    s. ulcer
    s. ulceration
Serpulina
    S. hyodysenteria
    S. innocens
    S. pilosicoli
serrated adenoma
Serratia
    S. liquefaciens
    S. marcescens
serratum
    Lycopodium s.
serratus posterior muscle

serrefine clamp
SERT
    serotonin reuptake transporter
Sertina
Sertoli
    S. cell
    S. cell secretory function
    S. cell tumor
Sertoli-cell-only (SCO)
    S.-c.-o. syndrome
Sertoli-Leydig cell
sertraline serotonin reuptake inhibitor
serum, pl. **sera**
    s. albumin
    s. alpha$_1$-protease inhibitor
    s. ammonia
    s. amylase
    s. amylase test
    s. amyloid A (SAA)
    s. amyloid P (SAP)
    s. amyloid P component
    s. bicarbonate
    s. bile acid measurement
    s. bilirubin
    s. bilirubin test
    s. blocking factor
    s. calcitonin
    s. calcium
    s. calcium concentration
    calibrator s.
    s. carotene
    s. ceruloplasmin
    s. chloride
    s. cholesterol
    s. cholinesterase activity
    s. chromogranin A
    s. core protein
    s. creatinine (SCr)
    s. creatinine test
    s. cytokine analysis
    s. elastase 1
    s. electrophoresis
    familial nephritis s.
    s. ferritin
    fetal calf s.
    s. folate
    s. gamma glutamyltransferase
    s. gastrin
    s. gastrin level
    s. glutamic-oxaloacetic transaminase
    (SGOT)

S

NOTES

serum *(continued)*
s. glutamic-pyruvic transaminase (SGPT)
s. haptoglobin
heat-inactivated fetal calf s.
s. hepatitis
s. hyaluronic acid
immune s. (IS)
s. interleukin-2
s. interleukin-6
s. iron (SI)
s. iron test
s. leptin level
s. lipase
s. marker
s. metabolic evaluation
s. nephritis
s. noradrenaline
s. osmolarity
s. pepsinogen I/II ratio
s. pepsinogen isoenzyme (I, II)
s. PG
s. phospholipid
s. phosphorus
s. protein
s. protein electrophoresis (SPEP)
s. protein test
s. pyridinoline
s. RIBA-2 test
s. serotonin
s. sickness
s. testosterone
s. thrombotic accelerator
s. transferrin
s. triglyceride
s. urate level
s. urea nitrogen (SUN)
s. uric acid
s. virus antibody
serum-ascites albumin gradient (SAAG)
Serutan
servo-mechanism sphincter
sesquioxide
chromium s.
sessile
s. adenoma
endoscopic s.
s. lesion
s. nodular carcinoma
s. polyp
set
Assura deluxe irrigation s.
Assura economy irrigation s.
Boehm rectal diagnostic and treatment s.
Brunner ligature s.
Coloplast ostomy irrigation s.
Conseal ostomy irrigation s.

Criticare HN-Isocal tube feeding s.
cytocentrifuge s.
Dansac ostomy irrigation s.
dilating s.
Eliminator nasal biliary catheter s.
Freiburg biopsy s.
French introducer s.
Heyer-Schulte Small-Carrion sizing s.
Hulbert endo-electrode s.
introducer s.
Jeffrey introducer s.
KeyMed advanced esophageal dilator s.
Lipshultz urology microsurgical s.
mandril s.
over-the-wire s.
s. point theory
Rosch-Uchida transjugular liver access s.
Sur-Fit Natura night drainage container s.
Sur-Fit Natura Visi-Flow irrigation starter s.
United Ostomy irrigation s.
urology s.
Setguard antireflux valve
Sethotope radioactive agent
seton
s. management
Penrose s.
silk s.
s. treatment of high anal fistula
setophobia
sevelamer
s. hydrochloride
s. hydrochloride tablet
severance
retroduodenal artery s.
severe
s. combined immunodeficiency (SCID)
s. erosive esophagitis
s. gastritis
s. macrovesicular steatosis
s. pain
s. reflux esophagitis
s. secretory diarrhea
severity
Crohn Disease Endoscopic Index of S. (CDEIS)
sex
s. accessory tissue
s. assignment by fetal ultrasonography
s. cord-mesenchyme tumor
s. cord tumors with annular tubules (SCTAT)

s. hormone binding globulin (SHBG)
phenotypic s.
s. reversal syndrome
s. therapy
sextant technique
sexual
s. abuse
s. differentiation
s. evaluation
s. function
S. Function Inventory Questionnaire (SFIQ)
s. function score (SFI)
s. infantilism
s. reflex
s. rehabilitation
s. stimulation testing
sexually
s. related intestinal disease
s. transmitted colitis
s. transmitted disease (STD)
s. transmitted disease contact tracing
Scyd-Neblett perineal template
Sézary syndrome
SF
sucrose-free
Isomil SF
SF-9 baculovirus-insect cell system
SFA
saturated fatty acid
SFI
sexual function score
SFIQ
Sexual Function Inventory Questionnaire
SFM
scanning force microscopy
Sgambati
S. reaction test
S. test for peritonitis
SGOT
serum glutamic-oxaloacetic transaminase
SGOT test
SGP-2
sulfated glycoprotein-2
SGPT
serum glutamic-pyruvic transaminase
SGPT test
SH2
src-homology 2
SH2-binding domain

shadow
dumbbell-shaped s.
obliteration of psoas s.
psoas s.
shadowing
hyperechoic s.
shaft
Eder-Puestow dilator s.
shaggy tumor
sham
s. feeding
s. feeding test
s. injection
s. surgery
s. treatment
Shambaugh fistula hook
shape
s. memory alloy (SMA)
s. memory alloy stent
shaped
olive s.
sharing
United Network for Organ S. (UNOS)
shark
s. fin papillotome
The S. disposable biopsy forceps
s. tooth forceps
sharp
s. dissection
s. spoon
sharp-edged
s.-e. orifice
s.-e. tip
Sharpoint
S. cutting instrument
S. microsuture
shave biopsy
SHBG
sex hormone binding globulin
SHC
sclerosing hepatic carcinoma
SHE
subclinical hepatic encephalopathy
shears
Bethune s.
harmonic scalpel coagulating s.
LaparoSonic coagulating s.
Lebsche s.
UltraCision harmonic laparoscopic cutting s.

S

NOTES

sheath
> Amplatz s.
> anterior rectus s.
> fibrous s.
> Futura resectoscope s.
> nephroscope s.
> overtube s.
> peel-away s.
> perivascular s.
> posterior rectus s.
> quill s.
> rectus s.
> resectoscope s.
> retroflexed cystoscopy s.
> sport s. (SS)
> Teflon s.
> Universal s.
> ureterorenoscope procedure s.
> ureteroscope s.
> Waldeyer s.
> water-filled balloon s.
> working s.

sheathed
> s. cytology brush
> s. flexible sigmoidoscope

shedding
> virus s.

sheet
> Dacron-impregnated Silastic s.

sheet-like adenoma

shelf
> Blumer rectal s.
> mesocolic s.
> rectal s.

shell vial culture

shelving edge of Poupart ligament

shepherd's hook catheter

shield
> Active Living incontinence s.
> CapSure continence s.
> Fuller rectal s.
> syringe s.

shift
> fluid s.
> mediastinal s.

shifting dullness

Shiga
> S. bacillus
> S. dysentery
> S. toxin (Stx)
> S. toxin-producing *Escherichia coli* (STEC)

shigae
> *Shigella* s.

Shiga-like toxin (SLT)

Shigella
> S. ambigua
> S. arabinotarda type A, B

> S. boydii
> S. colitis
> S. dysenteriae
> S. dysentery
> S. flexneri
> S. newcastle
> S. paradysenteriae
> S. schmitzii
> S. shigae
> S. sonnei

shigelloides
> *Plesiomonas* s.

shigellosis

shim
> step-up s.

Shimadzu RF-5301 PC spectrometer

Shiner tube

Shirodkar cervical cerclage

shock
> hypovolemic s.
> s. liver
> s. number
> s. patient
> septic s.
> spinal s.
> s. wave
> s. wave lithotripsy (SWL)
> s. wave lithotripsy cavitation component
> s. wave lithotripsy failure
> s. wave lithotriptor
> s. wave treatment

Shoemaker intestinal clamp

Shohl-Pedley method

Shohl solution

shooter

6-shooter
> Wilson-Cook 6-s.

10-shooter
> Saeed 10-s.
> Wilson-Cook 10-s.

Shorr regimen

short
> s. band stenosis
> s. daily at home
> s. daily dialysis
> s. daily in-center
> s. incubation hepatitis
> S. Inflammatory Bowel Disease Questionnaire (SIBDQ)
> s. urethra

short-bowel syndrome

short-chain fatty acid (SCFA)

short-dwell hypertonic exchange

short-gut syndrome

short-lasting afterhyperpolarizing potentials

short-segment
> s.-s. Barrett epithelium
> s.-s. Barrett esophagus (SSBE)
> s.-s. CLE
> s.-s. lesion

short-term survival outcome

shot
> flat low-angle s. (FLASH)

shotty lymph node

shoulder
> s. girdle
> s. shrug

Shouldice inguinal herniorrhaphy

shower
> uric acid s.

shrapnel-induced
> s.-i. biliary obstruction
> s.-i. obstructive jaundice

shrug
> shoulder s.

shrunken liver

shunt
> Al-Ghorab modification s.
> Allen Brown s.
> angiographic portacaval s.
> arterioportal venous s.
> arteriovenous s.
> AV shunt
> biliopancreatic s.
> Brescia-Cimino s.
> Buselmeier s.
> caval-atrial s.
> cavernospongiosum s.
> cerebral fluid s.
> chloride s.
> congenital portacaval s.
> Cordis-Hakim s.
> cystoperitoneal s.
> Denver peritoneovenous s.
> Denver pleuroperitoneal s.
> dialysis s.
> distal splenorenal s. (DSRS)
> Drapanas s.
> end-to-side portacaval s.
> esophageal s.
> extrahepatic s.
> gastric venacaval s.
> gastrorenal s.
> Gott s.
> Hashmat s.
> Hashmat Waterhouse s
> hepatofugal arterioportal s.

> hepatofugal portosystemic venous s.
> Hyde s.
> s. index via the inferior mesenteric vein (SI-I)
> s. index via the superior mesenteric vein (SI-S)
> intrahepatic s.
> intrahepatic artery-systemic s.
> jejunoileal s.
> Kasai peritoneal venous s.
> LeVeen ascites s.
> LeVeen peritoneal s.
> LeVeen peritoneovenous s.
> Linton s.
> mesocaval H-graft s.
> mesocaval interposition s.
> s. nephritis
> occluded s.
> pentose phosphate s.
> peritoneal-atrial s.
> peritoneocaval s.
> peritoneojugular s.
> peritoneovenous s. (PVS)
> portacaval s. (PCS)
> portacaval H-graft s.
> portopulmonary s.
> portosystemic s.
> proximal splenorenal s.
> Quinton-Scribner s.
> radiologic portacaval s.
> Ramirez s.
> Scribner s.
> side-to-side s.
> small bowel s.
> splenorenal bypass s.
> spontaneous portal-systemic s. (SPSS)
> stenotic s.
> Thomas s.
> transhepatic portacaval s.
> transjugular intrahepatic portosystemic s. (TIPS)
> transjugular intrahepatic portosystemic stent s. (TIPSS)
> s. tubing
> ventriculoperitoneal s.
> vesicoamniotic s.
> VP s.
> Warren splenorenal s.
> Winter s.

shunting
> arterioportal vein s. (APS)

S

NOTES

shunting *(continued)*
    intrapulmonary s.
    portosystemic s. (PSS)
    surgical portosystemic s.
shuntlike pore
Shwachman-Diamond syndrome
Shwachman syndrome
Shy-Drager syndrome
SI
    saturation index
    serum iron
    sucrase-isomaltase
        SI of bile
SIADH
    syndrome of inappropriate antidiuretic
      hormone secretion
sialic
    s. acid
    s. acid residue
sialidase
sialoadenectomy
sialoglycoprotein
sialomucin
    acidic s.
sialorrhea pancreatica
sialosyl-Tn antigen
sialyl
    s. Lewis A
    s. Lewis A antigen
    s. residue
sialylated
    s. derivative
    s. lacto-N-fucopentaose
sialylation
sialyllactose
sialyl-Tn antigen
SIBDQ
    Short Inflammatory Bowel Disease
      Questionnaire
sibling
    HLA-identical s.
SIBO
    small intestinal bacterial overgrowth
sibutramine HCl
sicca
    cholera s.
    s. syndrome
sicchasia
sick
    s. cell syndrome
    s. euthyroid state
sickle
    s. cell anemia
    s. cell disease
    s. hemoglobinopathy
sickle-cell nephropathy
sickling
    erythrocyte s.

sickness
    black s.
    Gambian sleeping s.
    s. impact profile
    Indian s.
    Jamaican vomiting s.
    milk s.
    motion s.
    serum s.
SID
    selective intestinal decontamination
side
    s. branch
    high-lying s.
Side-Fire
    S.-F. laser
    S.-F. reflecting dish
sideroblast
    refractory anemia with ringed s.
      (RARS)
sideropenic dysphagia
siderotic
    s. nodule
    s. splenomegaly
side-to-side
    s.-t.-s. anastomosis
    s.-t.-s. isoperistaltic strictureplasty
      (SSIS)
    s.-t.-s. shunt
side-viewing
    s.-v. endoscope
    s.-v. fiberoptic duodenoscope
    s.-v. fiberscope
    s.-v. video duodenoscope
sidewall
    pelvic s.
Siegel-Cohen dilating catheter
Siegel stent
Sielaff gastroscope
Siemens
    S. Endo-P endodrectal transducer
    S. Lithostar
    S. Lithostar Plus System C
      lithotriptor
    S. MRI unit
    S. Somatom DRH CT analyzer
    S. Somatom DRH CT analyzer
      unit
    S. Sonoline ultrasonography
sieving
    s. coefficient (SC)
    dextran s.
    s. effect
    s. function
    Keller hydrodynamic hypothesis
      of s.
    s. of solid food

sIgA
    secretory IgA
sigma
    S. 34 monoplace hyperbaric
      chamber
    s. rectum pouch
    s. type I
sigmoid
    s. colon
    s. colon carcinoma
    s. colon reservoir
    s. colon volvulus
    s. conduit
    s. curve
    s. cystoplasty
    s. disease
    s. diverticulitis
    s. diverticulum
    s. enterocystoplasty
    s. flexure
    s. fold
    s. kidney
    s. loop
    s. loop reduction
    s. neobladder
    s. pouch
    s. ulcer
    s. valve
sigmoideae
    arteriae s.
sigmoidectomy
sigmoid-end colostomy
sigmoideum
    colon s.
sigmoid-loop rod colostomy
sigmoidoanal intussusception
sigmoidocele
sigmoidocystoplasty
sigmoidopexy
    endoscopic s.
sigmoidoproctostomy
sigmoidorectostomy
sigmoidoscope
    ACMI T-915, TX-915 fiberoptic s.
    adult s.
    American ACMI (S3565, TX-915)
      flexible fiberoptic s.
    Boehm s.
    Buie s.
    disposable sheathed flexible s.
    ESI fiberoptic s
    fiberoptic s.

    flexible s.
    Fujinon ES-200ER s.
    Fujinon FS-100ER s.
    Fujinon PRO-PC flexible
      fiberoptic s.
    Fujinon SIG-E2 fiberoptic s.
    Fujinon SIG-EK-series flexible
      fiberoptic s.
    Fujinon SIG-E-series flexible
      fiberoptic s.
    Fujinon SIG-ET-series flexible
      fiberoptic s.
    Kelly s.
    Lieberman s.
    Lloyd-Davis s.
    Montague s.
    Olympus CF-L-series flexible s.
    Olympus CF-OSF-series flexible s.
    Olympus CF100S s.
    Olympus OSF flexible s.
    Pentax FS-series flexible fiberoptic
      video s.
    Reichert FLPS-series flexible
      fiberoptic s.
    Reichert MH-series flexible
      fiberoptic s.
    Reichert MS-series flexible
      fiberoptic s.
    Reichert SC-series flexible
      fiberoptic s.
    rigid s.
    semirigid s.
    sheathed flexible s.
    Vernon-David s.
    Vision System s.
    VSI 2000 s.
    Welch Allyn flexible s.
sigmoidoscopy
    fiberoptic s.
    flexible s.
    s. table
sigmoidostomy
sigmoidotomy
sigmoidovesical fistula
sigmoid-rectum pouch
sign
    Aaron s.
    accordion s.
    arrowhead s.
    auscultatory s.
    Babinski s.
    Ballance s.

NOTES

S

sign *(continued)*

barber pole s.
Battle s.
beading s.
Bergman s.
Blatin s.
blue dot s.
Blumberg s.
Boas s.
bowler hat s.
Boyce s.
Brodie s.
Brudzinski s.
Carman s.
Carman-Kirklin meniscus s.
Carnett s.
catheter coiling s.
chain-of-lakes s.
Chilaiditi s.
Christmas tree s.
Clark s.
Claybrook s.
closed eyes s.
cobblestoning s.
cobra-head s.
coiled spring s.
Cole s.
colon cutoff s.
colon single-stripe s.
comblike redness s.
comet s.
Cope s.
Courvoisier s.
Cruveilhier s.
Cullen s.
cushion s.
Dance s.
Dew s.
double-bubble duodenal s.
double duct s.
drooping lily s.
Duroziez s.
E s.
echo s.
Federici s.
flapping tremor s.
flush-tank s.
Fothergill s.
four lines s.
Fournier s.
Fraley s.
Frostberg reversed 3 s.
Gilbert s.
Gottron s.
Gowers s.
Grey Turner s.
Grocco s.
guarding s.

Guyon s.
Hampton s.
Haudek s.
heliotrope s.
Henning s.
histologic s.
Horn s.
Howship-Romberg s.
iliopsoas s.
inverted-V s.
Kantor string s.
Kehr s.
Kelly s.
Kernig s.
Klemm s.
Lennhoff s.
Leser-Trélat s.
lifting s.
ligature s.
liver flap s.
Lloyd s.
lollipop tree s.
malignant meniscus s.
McBurney s.
McCormack gastric mucosal s.
McCort s.
Meltzer s.
meniscus s.
Mercedes Benz s.
Mexican hat s.
moulage s.
multiple concentric ring s.
Murphy s.
Naclerio s.
naked fat s.
niche s.
obturator s.
peritoneal s.
Pfuhl s.
pillow s.
Pitres s.
Poppel s.
Prehn s.
pruning s.
pseudocholangiocarcinoma s.
pseudoparallel channel s.
psoas s.
puddle s.
pyloric string s.
rat-tail s.
RCS s.
rebound s.
red color s. (RCS)
red flag s.
red ring s.
reversed Mercedes Benz s.
Rigler s.
rim s.

s. of the rising tide
Robertson s.
Roche s.
Rommelaere s.
Rosenbach s.
Rovighi s.
Rovsing s.
Russell s.
sawtooth appearance s.
Sister Mary Joseph s.
snow-white duodenum s.
Stierlin s.
Stransky s.
Strauss s.
string s.
string-of-beads s.
string-of-pearls s.
Sumner s.
tail s.
tenting s.
Terry fingernail s.
tethered-bowel s.
Thornton s.
thread-and-streaks s.
thumbprinting s.
tissue rim s.
Toma s.
Trimadeau s.
Troisier s.
Turner s.
Uhthoff s.
ureterocele drooping lily s.
vital s.
white ball s.
white nipple s.
Zugsmith s.

Signa Dress Hydrocolloid dressing
signal
adenosine s.
adrenergic s.
beta-actin mRNA s.
sodium s.
s. transduction pathway
s. transduction process
transmembrane s.
signaling cascade
signal-to-cutoff ratio
signet-ring
s.-r. cell
s.-r. cell carcinoma
s.-r. pattern of gastric carcinoma

significance
atypical glandular cells of
unknown s. (AGUS)
atypical squamous cells of
undetermined s. (ASCUS)
prognostic s.
visible vessel s.
significant reported complication
SIHC
surgically implanted hemodialysis
catheter
SI-I
shunt index via the inferior mesenteric
vein
Silain-Gel
Silastic
S. catheter
S. collar-reinforced stoma
S. indwelling ureteral stent
S. ring
S. ring vertical gastroplasty
S. silo reduction of gastroschisis
S. sling
Silber
S. technique
S. vasoepididymostomy
sildenafil citrate
silent
s. abdomen
s. aspiration
s. autonephrectomy
s. belch
s. gallstone
s. lupus nephritis
s. prostatism
s. stone
s. thrombosis
s. ulcer
silicate
s. calculus
s. urinary lithiasis
silicone
s. balloon
s. donut prosthesis
s. elastomer band
s. elastomer ring
s. elastomer ring vertical
gastroplasty (SRVG)
s. microimplant
particulate s.
s. polymer
s. pressure sensor device

NOTES

silicone *(continued)*
    s. rubber Dacron-cuffed catheter
    s. self-expanding prosthesis
    s. sizer
silicone-coated metallic self-expanding stent
Silipos
    S. arthritic/diabetic gel sock
    S. soft walk gel sock
Silitek Uropass stent
silk
    S. Bullet feeding tube
    s. ligature
    s. Mersilene suture
    S. Pill feeding tube
    s. pop-off suture
    s. seton
    S. Tip feeding tube
    s. traction suture
Silon tent
silver
    s. catheter
    s. cell
    s. clip
    s. nephropathy
    s. nitrate
    s. probe
    s. stain
    s. stool
silver-coated stent
Silverman-Boeker needle
Silverman needle
Silybum marianum
Silymarin
SIM
    small intestine mesentery
    specialized intestinal metaplasia
    SIM 2 catheter
Simaal
    S. Gel
    S. Gel 2
simethicone
    aluminum hydroxide, magnesium hydroxide, and s.
    calcium carbonate and s.
Similac PM 60/40 low-iron formula
Simmons catheter
Simplastic catheter
simple
    s. cold storage preservation
    s. cystectomy
    s. enterocele
    s. hydrocele
    s. mechanical obstruction
    s. nephrectomy
    s. renal cyst

simplex
    exulceratio s.
    herpes s.
simplified nocturnal home hemodialysis (SNHHD)
Simpson endoscope
Sims
    S. anoscope
    S. position
    S. rectal speculum
simulation
    computer graphic s. (CGS)
simulator
    flexible bronchocopy s.
Simulect
simultaneous
    s. bilateral extracorporeal shock waves
    s. bilateral percutaneous nephrolithotomy (SBPN)
    s. hemodialysis and hemofiltration
    s. pancreas-kidney (SPK)
    s. urethral cystometry
simvastatin
sincalide
Sinemet
sinensis
    Clonorchis s.
    Opisthorchis s.
Sinequan
Singer-Blom endoscopic tracheoesophageal puncture technique
single
    s. beta-actin mRNA species
    s. cell keratinization
    s. gamma wrap
    s. lens reflex (SLR)
    s. loop tourniquet
    s. lumen
    s. potential analysis of cavernous electrical (SPACE)
    s. potential analysis cavernous electrical activity
    s. stapling
    s. strand conformation polymorphism analysis
single-action pumping system (SAPS)
single-channel
    s.-c. colonoscope
    s.-c. in vivo light dosimeter
    s.-c. wire-guided sphincterotome
single-color direct immunofluorescence study
single-contrast
    s.-c. barium enema
    s.-c. radiography
single-dose I.V. Timentin
single-drug therapy

single-fiber
 s.-f. EMG electrode
 s.-f. needle electromyography
single-layer continuous intestinal anastomosis
single-lens reflex camera
single-lumen Broviac silicone catheter
single-nephron
 s.-n. GFR
 s.-n. glomerular filtration rate (SNGFR)
 s.-n. glomerular transport
single-parameter
 s.-p. DNA
 s.-p. DNA analysis
single-pass hemodialysis
single-photon
 s.-p. emission computed tomography (SPECT)
 s.-p. emission computerized tomography (SPECT)
single-pigtail stent
single-puncture laparoscopy
single-shot voxel projection
single-stage total proctocolectomy
single-stripe colitis (SSC)
single-system ureterocele
single-use maximum capacity radial jaw with needle
Singley
 S. intestinal forceps
 S. intestinal ring clamp
Singular Oval polypectomy snare
singultation
singultus gastricus nervosus
sinister
 ductus hepaticus s.
 ductus lobi caudati s.
sinistra
 arteria gastrica s.
 arteria gastroomentalis s.
 flexura coli s.
sink-trap malformation
sinoaortic
 s. baroreceptor
 s. denervation (SAD)
sinogram
sinus
 anal s.
 s. anales
 s. bradycardia
 coronary s.

 draining s.
 s. excision
 Forssell s.
 perineal s.
 pilonidal s.
 piriform s.
 pleuroperitoneal s.
 prostatic s.
 rectal s.
 renal s.
 Rokitansky-Aschoff s.
 splenic s.
 subpubic s.
 s. tachycardia
 s. tenderness
 s. tract
 urachal s.
 urogenital s.
sinusoid
 corporeal s.
 erectile s.
 hepatic s.
 liver s.
sinusoidal
 s. capillary pressure
 s. endothelial cell (SEC)
 s. endothelium
 s. endothelium cornucopia
 s. fibrosis
 s. lymphocyte
 s. wall
sinusoid-lining cell
siphonage
Sipple syndrome
Sippy
 S. diet
 S. esophageal dilator
SIR
 standardized incidence ratio
Siroky
 S. nomogram
 S. nomogram for uroflowmetry
sirolimus
 s. oral solution
 s. tablet
SIRS
 systemic inflammatory response syndrome
SI-S
 shunt index via the superior mesenteric vein

NOTES

S

Sister
- S. Mary Joseph lymph node
- S. Mary Joseph nodule
- S. Mary Joseph sign

site
- bleeding s.
- crypt-villus s.
- endoscopic biopsy s.
- entry s.
- estrogen binding s. (EBS)
- exit s.
- genomic s.
- injection s.
- internal ribosome entry s. (IRES)
- s. specificity
- stoma s.
- vascular access s.

sitophobia
sitosterolemia
- beta s.

situ
- adenocarcinoma in s.
- bladder carcinoma in s.
- carcinoma in s. (CIS)
- in s.
- squamous cell carcinoma in s.

situs
- s. inversus
- s. inversus viscerum
- s. perversus

sitz bath
Sitzmarks radiopaque marker in gelatin capsule
Siurala classification
six-shooter
- Saeed s.-s.

six-wire spiral tip Segura basket
size
- inoculum s.
- kidney s.
- large needle s.
- spot s.
- uterine s.

sizer
- silicone s.

Sjögren syndrome (SS)
Sjöqvist method
SJS
- Stevens-Johnson syndrome

skatole
Skelaxin
skeletal
- s. muscle disease
- s. radiography

skeletonize
Skene
- S. duct
- S. gland

skin
- anicteric s.
- s. atrophy
- s. bleeding time (SBT)
- s. crease
- s. dimpling
- s. disease
- dry s.
- s. fold thickness test
- s. graft
- s. graft imbibition phase
- s. graft inosculation phase
- s. graft neovagina
- icteric s.
- jaundiced s.
- s. knife
- s. line
- nonicteric s.
- ostomy s.
- s. perfusion
- peristomal s.
- s. staple
- s. stapling
- s. sympathetic response
- s. tag
- s. tube
- s. turgor
- s. xanthoma

skin-CNS-bladder reflex
skinny Chiba needle
skinny-needle biopsy
skip
- s. appendicitis
- s. area
- s. lesion

ski position
skipping
- exon s.

Skirrow
- S. agar plate
- S. medium

skullcap
SL
- standard laparoscopy

SL20
- Storz Modulith SL20

SLA
- soluble liver antigen

slash pyelotomy
SLC
- sodium-lithium countertransporter

SLE
- systemic lupus erythematosus

SLED
- slow low-efficiency dialysis
- sustained low-efficiency dialysis

sleep
    s. apnea syndrome
    s. enuresis
sleep-disordered breathing (SDB)
sleeve
    s. advancement
    Assura irrigation s.
    Bard irrigation s.
    Coloplast transparent irrigation s.
    Dent s.
    ileal s.
    laparoscopic trocar s.
    Pneumo S.
    s. sensor
    Sur-Fit Natura irrigation s.
    s. technique
    Watzki s.
    Williams overtube s.
sleeve-multiple sidehole manometric assemble
sleeve-type circumcision
slide
    gelatin-subbed s.
    guaiac-impregnated s.
    Hemoccult SENSA s.
    poly-L-lysine-coated glass s.
    s. system
slide-by view
sliding
    s. esophageal hiatal hernia
    s. filament model of contraction
    s. tube
SlimSIGHT gastrointestinal videoscope
sling
    autologous rectus fascia s.
    Brigham s.
    Burch-Cooper ligament s.
    Cooper ligament s.
    fascia lata suburethral s.
    intestinal s.
    lyophilized dura mater for pubovaginal s.
    Martius fascial s.
    Mersilene for pubovaginal s.
    s. muscle fiber
    s. operation
    porcine dermis for pubovaginal s.
    s. procedure
    puboprostatic s.
    puborectalis s.
    pubourethral s.
    pubovaginal s.

    Raz anterior vaginal wall s.
    Raz four-corner vaginal wall s.
    Raz vaginal wall s.
    rectus fascia s.
    Silastic s.
    Stratasis urethral s.
    suburethral s.
    Suspend s.
    triangular vaginal patch s.
    Vesica s.
sling-and-blanket technique
sling/mesh
    SurgiSis s./m.
sling-ring complex
Slip-Coat tip
slipped
    s. fundoplication wrap
    s. Nissen fundoplication
    s. Nissen repair
slipper-tipped guidewire
slit
    Cheatle s.
    s. diaphragm
    dorsal s.
    s. lamp
    s. pore length density
SLM-8000 fluorescence spectrophotometer
Slo-bid
slotted
    s. anoscope
    s. instrument
    s. nerve clamp
    s. speculum
sloughed
    s. papilla
    s. urethra syndrome
sloughing of mucosa
slow
    s. bilirubin glucuronidation phenotype
    s. colonic transit
    s. continuous ultrafiltration (SCUF)
    S. Fe
    s. low-efficiency dialysis (SLED)
    s. phasic contraction
    s. transit constipation (STC)
    s. twitch striated muscle fiber
    s. wave
Slow-K
slow-twitch oxidative

S

NOTES

SLR
single lens reflex
SLT
Shiga-like toxin
SLT contact MTRL laser
SLT 7 laser fiber
sludge
biliary s.
gallbladder s.
slurry of stool
slush
ice s.
saline s.
SMA
sequential multiple analyzer
shape memory alloy
smooth muscle antibody
superior mesenteric artery
Doppler sonography of the SMA
SMA formula
SMA spiral stent
small
s. bowel
s. bowel anastomosis
s. bowel biopsy
s. bowel continuity
s. bowel enema
s. bowel enteroclysis
s. bowel enteroscopy (SBE)
s. bowel followthrough (SBFT)
s. bowel infarct
s. bowel meal
s. bowel obstruction (SBO)
s. bowel shunt
s. bowel thickening
s. bowel transit time
s. bowel transplantation
s. bowel tube
s. dissecting sponge
s. granule cell
s. intestinal bacterial overgrowth (SIBO)
s. intestinal Crohn disease
s. intestinal enterocyte
s. intestinal infarction
s. intestinal malignant lymphoma
s. intestinal membrane
s. intestinal stenosis
s. intestinal submucosa
s. intestinal ulcer
s. intestinal villus
s. intestine
s. intestine leiomyosarcoma
s. intestine mesentery (SIM)
s. intestine trauma
s. non-cleaved-cell lymphoma
s. polyp removal
s. stomach syndrome

small-caliber esophagogastroduodenoscopy
Small-Carrion penile prosthesis
small-cell tumor
small-diameter endosonographic instrument
small-droplet fatty liver
small-duct primary sclerosing cholangitis
smaller gauge needle
SmallHand polpypectomy snare
SMA-portogram
SMART
sperm microaspiration retrieval technique
SMAS
superior mesenteric artery syndrome
Smead-Jones closure
smear
buccal s.
KOH s.
low-grade positive s.
Pap s.
potassium hydroxide s.
smegma praeputii
smegmatis
Mycobacterium s.
smiley face knotting technique
smiling incision
Smith
S. electrode
S. method of silver staining
S. rectal retractor
S. ring
S. test
Smith-Boyce operation
Smith-Buie rectal retractor
Smith-Hodge pessary
smithii
Methanobrevibacter s.
Smith-Lemli-Opitz syndrome
smoker's
s. palate
s. tongue
smooth
s. diet
s. muscle
s. muscle antibody (SMA)
s. muscle isoform actin
s. muscle motilin receptor
s. muscle relaxant
s. tissue forceps
s. urethral sphincter
smooth-muscle immunological study
SMV
superior mesenteric vein
SMV thrombosis
SMX/TMP
sulfamethoxazole and trimethoprim
SMZ/TMP
sulfamethoxazole and trimethoprim

snail-headed catheter retriever
snake-skin mucosal pattern
snake venom converting enzyme
    inhibiting action
snap
        s. gauge
        s. gauge band
        s. gauge test
snap-frozen biopsy
Snap-Gauge
Snap-It lubricating jelly
snare
        barbed s.
        Captiflex polypectomy s.
        Captivator polypectomy s.
        s. cautery
        coaxial s.
        colorectal s.
        crescent s.
        diathermal s.
        Douglas rectal s.
        s. electrocoagulation
        electrosurgical s.
        endoscopic s.
        s. excision biopsy
        Frankfeldt rectal s.
        hexagon s.
        incarcerated s.
        lasso s.
        long-nosed retriever s.
        s. loop biopsy
        Nakao s. (I, II)
        Norwood rectal s.
        Olympus SD-5L semicircular s.
        open electrocautery s.
        oval s.
        s. polypectomy
        polypectomy s.
        Profile pediatric polypectomy s.
        rectal s.
        s. resection
        Rotator polypectomy s.
        Sensation Short Throw s.
        Singular Oval polypectomy s.
        SmallHand polpypectomy s.
        standard endoscopy polypectomy s.
        UroSnare cystoscopic tumor s.
        Weston rectal s.
        wire s.
SNGFR
        single-nephron glomerular filtration rate

SNHHD
        simplified nocturnal home hemodialysis
Sn-mesoporphyrin (SnMP)
SnMP
        Sn-mesoporphyrin
Snodgrass technique
Snowden-Pencer scissors
Snow procedure
snowstorm effect
snow-white duodenum sign
SNP
        sodium nitroprusside
Sn-protoporphyrin
SNS
        sacral nerve stimulation
        sympathetic nervous system
            SNS therapy
SO
        sphincter of Oddi
soak
        perianal s.
soap-bubble nephrogram
soapsuds enema (SSE)
soap-sudsy appearance
soapy kidney
soar-crash effect
Soave
        S. abdominal pull-through procedure
        S. endorectal pull-through
        S. operation
sobria
        Aeromonas s.
society
        S. of American Gastrointestinal
            Endoscoping Surgeons (SAGES)
        International Continence S. (ICS)
sock
        polytetrafluoroethylene s.
        Silipos arthritic/diabetic gel s.
        Silipos soft walk gel s.
SOD
        sphincter of Oddi dysfunction
        superoxide dismutase
sodium
        s. acid urate
        acyclovir s.
        s. anion diarrhea
        s. azide
        s. balance
        s. bicarbonate
        brequinar s.
        s. butyrate concentration

NOTES

687

sodium (*continued*)
    cefazolin s.
    ceftriaxone s.
    s. cellulose phosphate
    s. chloride
    s. citrate
    s. citrate and potassium citrate
      mixture
    s. cromoglycate
    cromolyn s.
    dalteparin s.
    dantrolene s.
    s. deficiency
    s. deoxycholate
    diclofenac s.
    dietary s.
    docusate s.
    s. dodecyl sulfate (SDS)
    s. electrolyte
    enoxaparin s.
    epoprostenol s.
    estramustine phosphate s.
    s. exchange
    s. fluorescein (NaF)
    s. flux
    fractional excretion of s. (FENa)
    s. homeostasis
    s. hyaluronate
    s. hyaluronate injection
    s. iodipamide
    s. iodipamide contrast medium
    s. iothalamate
    latamoxef s.
    low s. (LNa)
    luminal s.
    s. meclofenamate
    s. meclofenamate-induced
      esophageal ulcer
    mesalamine s.
    s. methylglucamine diatrizoate
    s. morrhuate
    s. morrhuate injection
    naproxen s.
    s. nitroprusside (SNP)
    olsalazine s.
    oxychlorosene s.
    pantoprazole s.
    s. pentosan polysulfate (PPS)
    pentosan polysulfate s.
    peritubular s.
    s. phosphate (NaP)
    s. phosphate-based laxative
    s. phosphate dibasic anhydrous
    s. phosphate monobasic
      monohydrate
    s. picosulfate
    piperacillin s.
    s. polystyrene sulfonate

    porfimer s.
    s. pump
    rabeprazole s.
    s. reabsorption
    renal s.
    s. restriction
    s. retention
    s. signal
    sterile ceftriaxone s.
    sulbactam s.
    s. taurocholate
    s. tauroglycocholate
    s. tetradecyl injection
    s. tetradecyl sulfate
    s. tetradecyl sulfate sclerosant
    s. thiosulfate solution spray
    s. transport
    tyropanoate s.
    s. valproate
    s. wasting nephropathy
sodium-linked process
sodium-lithium countertransporter (SLC)
sodium-loading test
Soehendra
    S. catheter dilator
    S. catheter system
    S. dilating catheter
    S. stent extractor
    S. stent retrieval device
    S. stent retriever
soft
    s. abdomen
    s. bland diet
    s. food dysphagia
    S. Guard XL Skin Barrier
    Modane S.
    s. rubber string
    s. stool
    s. tissue
    s. tissue mass
    s. tissue stranding
    s. x-ray film
softener
    stool s.
SofTouch vacuum erection device
Softpatch
    Impress S.
soft-tipped wire guide
software
    s. characteristics of the treating
      protocol
    CODAS s.
    Cytologic s.
    Medtrax urology s.
    SPOT mobile 3D ultrasound
      system and s.
    t-EASE s.

soilage
    peritoneal s.
soiling
    colostomy s.
    fecal s.
solani
    Fusarium s.
solar fever
Solcia classification
solder
    laser tissue welding s.
    protein s.
solid
    s. bolus challenge
    s. and cystic tumor of the
      pancreas (SCTP)
    s. egg white meal
    s. emptying
    s. evidence
    s. food
    s. food digestion
    s. food dysphagia
    s. sphere test
    s. teratoma
    s. tumor
solid-column esophagogram
solid-phase
    s.-p. extraction chromatography
    s.-p. radioimmunoassay
solid-state
    s.-s. esophageal manometry catheter
    s.-s. pressure transducer
solitarius, pl. **solitarii**
    folliculi lymphatici s.
    nucleus s.
    nucleus tractus s. (NTS)
solitary
    s. diverticulum
    s. hepatic cyst
    s. kidney
    s. rectal ulcer syndrome (SRUS)
    s. testis
    s. ulcer
    s. ulcer syndrome
solium
    Taenia s.
SoloPass Percuflex biliary stent
SOLO-Surg Colo-Rectal self-retaining
  retractor system
solubility
solubilization
    micellar s.

solubilize
solubilized
    s. HLA
    s. human leukocyte antigen
      (solubilized HLA)
Solu-Biloptin contrast medium
soluble
    s. egg antigen (SEA)
    s. liver antigen (SLA)
    s. recombinant complement receptor
    1
    s. transferrin receptor (sTf-R)
Solu-Medrol
    pulsed S.-M.
solute
    s. equilibrium
    s. removal index
    s. transport
solution
    Adcon-P adhesion barrier s.
    AIO parenteral s.
    Albright s.
    amino acid-based dialysate s.
    Aminofusin L Forte amino acid s.
    BA-EDTA s.
    balanced electrolyte s.
    balanced salt s. (BSS)
    Balance lavage s.
    barium sulfate s.
    Belzer UW liver preservation s.
    bile acid-EDTA solution
    Block-Ace s.
    Bouin fixative s.
    Bretschneider histidine tryptophan s.
    buffer s.
    Burrow s.
    Cidex activated dialdehyde s.
    Cidex Plus s.
    Collins indigo carmine s.
    Collins intracellular electrolyte s.
    colloid s.
    colonic lavage s.
    commercial dialysis s. (CDS)
    crystalloid s.
    Delflex peritoneal dialysis s.
    Denhardt s.
    diphosphate buffer s.
    Domeboro s.
    Earle s.
    electrolyte flush s.
    electrolyte-polyethylene glycol
      lavage s.

S

NOTES

solution *(continued)*
    Euro-Collins s.
    ferumoxides injectable s.
    formaldehyde s.
    FreAmine amino acid s.
    Gastrolyte oral s.
    gelatin Hank buffered salt s.
      (GHBSS)
    gluten s.
    GoLYTELY s.
    Hank balanced salt s. (HBSS)
    Hank buffer s.
    Hartmann s.
    HepatAmine amino acid s.
    HEPES s.
    Hibidil s.
    Hollande s.
    HSE s.
    s. hybridization RNAse protection
      assay
    hypertonic saline-epinephrine s.
    iced lactated Ringer s.
    inulin s.
    Krebs s.
    Krebs-Ringer s.
    lactated Ringer s.
    lactulose s.
    lavage s.
    Liposyn II fat emulsion s.
    Lugol iodine s.
    Lytren electrolyte s.
    Mayer hematoxylin s.
    Mefoxin-saline s.
    Mitrofanoff s.
    900 mOsmolar amino acid-
      glucose s. (P-900)
    mucolytic-antifoam s.
    normal saline s.
    NTZ Long Acting Nasal S.
    oral rehydration s. (ORS)
    Pedialyte RS electrolyte s.
    perfusate s.
    phosphate buffered saline s.
    physiologic pH s.
    physiologic salt s. (PSS)
    podofilox s.
    polyethylene glycol electrolyte s.
    polyethylene glycol electrolyte
      lavage s. (PEG-ELS, PEG-LES)
    polyethylene glycol lavage s.
    probenecid-containing s.
    Rapamune oral s.
    rehydrating s. (RS)
    Resol electrolyte s.
    Saccomanno s.
    Sachs s.
    sclerosant s.
    sclerosant-contrast s.

    sclerosing s.
    Shohl s.
    sirolimus oral s.
    Soyalac fat emulsion s.
    Sporox disinfectant s.
    Suby G s.
    Synthamin amino acid s.
    taurocholate s.
    Tolerex feeding s.
    Travamulsion fat emulsion s.
    University of Wisconsin s.
    UW s.
    Vamin amino acid s.
    warm saline s.
    whole-gut lavage s.
    Wisconsin s.
    Y-type Dianeal peritoneal
      dialysis s.
solution-diluted India ink
Solutrast 300 contrast
Soluvite
solvent
    s. drag
    s. infusion
    Nu-Hope cleaning s.
    stone s.
SOM
    somatostatin
    sphincter of Oddi manometry
Soma
somatic
    s. allelic deletion
    s. growth
    s. pain
    s. peripheral nerve
    s. teniasis
somatization
somatointestinal reflex
somatomedin C
Somatome DRG CT technique
somatostatin (SOM, SS)
    s. analog
    s. analog octreotide
    s. analog therapy
    antral s.
    s. cell
    s. infusion therapy
    ^{125}I-Tyr1-s.
    s. mRNA-D-cell density ratio
    s. MRNA level
    s. peptide
    s. prevention
    s. receptor (SSR)
    s. receptor scintigraphy (SRS)
    s. secretagogue
    s. stain
somatostatin-14
somatostatin-28

somatostatinoma syndrome
somatotropin release-inhibiting factor
 (SRIF)
somatropin injection
somite
> müllerian duct, unilateral renal
> agenesis, and anomalies of the
> cervicothoracic s.'s (MURCS)

Somogyi unit
Sonablate 200 system
Sonazoid
Sonde
> S. enteroscope
> S. enteroscopy

Song stent
sonicated albumin
Sonicath endoluminal ultrasound
 catheter
Sonne-Duval bacillus
Sonne dysentery
sonnei
> *Shigella s.*

Sonnenberg classification
Sonoblate
> S. ablation device
> S. Probe

Sonocath ultrasound probe
sonoelasticity imaging
sonogram
> fatty meal s. (FMS)
> transverse s.

sonographic
> s. gallstone pattern
> s. planning of oncology treatment
> (SPOT)

sonography
> amplitude coded-color Doppler s.
> catheter s.
> colonic transabdominal s. (CTAS)
> color-coded Doppler s.
> color-coded duplex s.
> 3-D s.
> duplex s.
> endoureteral ultrasound s.
> gray scale s.
> high-frequency s.
> high-frequency ultrasound probe s.
> (HFUPS)
> high-resolution endoluminal s.
> (HRES)
> intraaortic endovascular s.
> renal s.

> transabdominal hydrocolonic s.
> transrectal s.

sonography-guided aspiration
sonoguided biopsy
Sonoline SI-200/250 ultrasound imaging
 system
Sonoprobe Endoscopic Ultrasonography
 System
Sonotrode
> S. channel
> S. lithotriptor

sonourethrography
Sony Promavica still capture device
SOP
> sphincter of Oddi pressure

sorbent
> s. dialysate regeneration system
> s. hemodialysis

sorbitol
> s. dehydrogenase (SDH)
> s. diarrhea
> s. enema

sorbitol-MacConkey
> s.-M. agar
> s.-M. medium

sordes, pl. **sordes**
> s. gastricae

sore
> canker s.
> pressure s.
> venereal s.

Soreson pressure transducer
sorter
> fluorescence-activated cell s.
> (FACS)

SOS
> Surgitek One-Step

sotalol
soterenol
Sotradecol sclerosant
souffle
> splenic s.

sound
> absent bowel s.'s
> active bowel s.'s
> apical s.
> auscultation of bowel s.'s
> auscultatory s.
> Béniqué s.
> bowel s.'s
> breath s.
> bronchial s.

NOTES

S

691

sound (*continued*)
    Campbell s.
    common duct s.
    crescendoing bowel s.
    Davis interlocking s.
    diminished bowel s.'s
    distant heart s.
    Dittel s.
    esophageal s.
    extra heart s.
    Greenwald s.
    gurgling bowel s.'s
    Guyon s.
    high-pitched bowel s.'s
    hyperactive bowel s.'s
    hypoactive bowel s.'s
    Jewett s.
    Klebanoff common duct s.
    Le Fort s.
    low-pitched bowel s.'s
    McCrea s.
    metal s.
    musical bowel s.'s
    normoactive bowel s.'s (NABS)
    Otis s.
    positive bowel s.'s
    quiet bowel s.'s
    rumbling bowel s.'s
    scarce bowel s.'s
    succussion s.
    tinkling bowel s.'s
    van Buren s.
    Walther s.
sour
    s. brash
    s. stomach
source
    discrete bleeding s.
    endoscopic light s.
    Olympus CLV10 fiberscope light s.
    Olympus CLV-U 20 endoscopic
      halogen light s.
    xenon light s.
South American trypanosomiasis
Southern
    S. blot
    S. blot analysis
    S. blot hybridization
Souttar tube
soya-induced enteropathy
Soyalac
    S. fat emulsion solution
    S. formula
soy-based formula
soy protein sensitivity
SP
    substance P

S/P
    status post
SP-303
**SP-501 gastric lesion staging by
   endoscopic ultrasonography**
SPA
    sperm penetration assay
SPACE
    single potential analysis of cavernous
      electrical
space
    anorectal s.
    Bogros s.
    Bowman s.
    Courtney s.
    dead s.
    deep perineal s.
    deep postanal anorectal s.
    s. of Disse
    Disse s.
    epidural s.
    extravascular s.
    intercellular s.
    intercostal s.
    intermediate s.
    intersphincteric anorectal s.
    ischiorectal anorectal s.
    Kiernan s.
    lateral fossa of preputial s.
    Lesgaft s.
    s. of Mall
    paraglomerular s.
    perianal anorectal s.
    perisinusoidal s.
    peritoneal s.
    preperitoneal s.
    presacral s.
    retroperitoneal s.
    retropubic s.
    retrorectal s.
    Retzius s.
    s. of Retzius
    right anterior pararenal s.
    S. Saver volumetric pump
    subarachnoid s.
    subhepatic s.
    subperitoneal s.
    subphrenic s.
    subumbilical s.
    superficial perineal s.
    suprahepatic s.
    supralevator anorectal s.
    supraomental s.
    Traube semilunar s.
    vesicovaginal s.
Spacemaker balloon dissector

space-occupying
    s.-o. disease
    s.-o. lesion
Space-OR flexible internal retractor
span
    hepatic s.
    levator s.
    liver s.
spansule
sparfloxacin
sparing
    rectal s.
spark-gap shock wave generator
sparse
    s. inflammatory infiltrate
    s. polyposis
sparteine
spasm
    acid-provoked s.
    bladder s.
    cervical s.
    cricopharyngeal s.
    diffuse esophageal s. (DES)
    esophageal s.
    experienced rectal s.
    fecal paradoxical puborectalis s.
    glottic s.
    muscle s.
    rectal s.
spasmodic stricture
Spasmolin
spasmolytic
spastic
    s. bowel syndrome
    s. colon
    s. constipation
    s. esophagus
    s. gait
    s. ileus
    s. motor disorder
    s. paraparesis
    s. pelvic floor syndrome
spastica
    cholepathia s.
    dysphagia s.
    urina s.
spasticity
spatial
    s. change
    s. resolution
spatula
    Davis s.

electrosurgical s.
    Haberer abdominal s.
    Pucci-Seed s.
    Reverdin abdominal s.
    Tuffier abdominal s.
spatulated overlap anastomosis
spatulation
    graft s.
    ureteral s.
spatula-tip laparoscopic electrode
Spearman
    S. rank
    S. rank correlation
    S. test
specialized
    s. columnar epithelium (SCE)
    s. intestinal metaplasia (SIM)
species
    Cryptosporidium s.
    gastrin mRNA s.
    G3PDH mRNA s.
    reactive oxygen s. (ROS)
    Rhizopus s.
    single beta-actin mRNA s.
    Vibrionaceae s.
specific
    s. activity
    s. algorithm
    antigen s.
    s. anti-Hp serology
    s. gastritis
    s. gravity test
    s. immunotherapy
    s. oligonucleotide
    s. organic acidopathy
    s. red cell adherence test
    s. urethritis
specificity
    LKM s.
    site s.
specimen
    clean-catch urine s.
    clean-voided s. (CVS)
    cytologic s.
    intraurethral swab s.
    paraffin-embedded s.
    s. trap
    yarn-collected s.
speck
    hemorrhagic s.

S

NOTES

SPECT
single-photon emission computed
tomography
single-photon emission computerized
tomography
SPECT scan
spectinomycin
spectometry
time-of-flight mass s. (TOFMS)
spectral
s. analysis
s. broadening
Spectramed transducer
spectrometer
liquid scintillation s.
Shimadzu RF-5301 PC s.
spectrometry
gas isotope ratio mass s.
laser desorption/ionization mass s.
spectrophotometer
atomic absorbance s.
Genetics Systems microplate
reader s.
Hitachi F-2000 fluorescence s.
Model IL 750, AA s.
Perkin-Elmer model 5000 atomic
absorption s.
reflectance s.
SLM-8000 fluorescence s.
spectrophotometric analysis
spectrophotometry
endoscopic reflectance s.
reflectance s.
spectroscopy
elastic scattering s.
Fourier transform infrared s.
(FTIR)
gas chromatography/mass s.
(GC/MS)
^{1}H magnetic resonance s.
infrared s.
laser-induced fluorescence s. (LIFS)
magnetic resonance s. (MRS)
Model 3-60 mass s.
phosphorous-31 magnetic
resonance s.
proton magnetic resonance s.
reflectance s.
steady-state autofluorescence s.
x-ray photoelectron s.
Spectrum silicone Foley catheter
speculum
Barr rectal s.
Barr-Shuford rectal s.
beveled s.
Bodenhammer rectal s.
Brinkerhoff rectal s.
Chelsea-Eaton anal s.

Cook rectal s.
Czerny rectal s.
David rectal s.
Hinkle-James rectal s.
Hirschmann s.
Kelly rectal s.
Killian rectal s.
Martin-Davis rectal s.
Mathews rectal s.
Pennington rectal s.
Pratt rectal s.
rectal s.
Sawyer rectal s.
Sims rectal s.
slotted s.
Vernon-David rectal s.
speech
garbled s.
speedbander
multishot s.
Speedband Superview ligator
Speed Lok soft stent
Spence procedure
Spencer disease
Spenco padding
SPEP
serum protein electrophoresis
sperm
s. aspiration
s. cryopreservation
extracted ductal s.
s. granuloma
s. immunobead coincubation
s. microaspiration retrieval
technique (SMART)
microsurgical extraction of
ductal s. (MEDS)
s. motility-inhibiting factor
muzzled s.
s. penetration assay (SPA)
s. survival factor
s. yield
spermacrasia
spermagglutination
Sperma-Tex preshaped mesh
spermatic
s. abscess
s. artery
s. calculus
s. cord
s. cord leiomyosarcoma
s. cord liposarcoma
s. cord torsion
s. fascia
s. fistula
s. plexus
s. vein

s. vein ligation
s. vesicle
spermatica
chorda s.
spermaticide
spermaticus
funiculus s.
plexus s.
spermatid
spermatin
spermatoblast
spermatocele
alloplastic s.
autogenous s.
s. resection
spermatocelectomy
spermatocidal
spermatocyst
spermatocystectomy
spermatocystitis
spermatocystotomy
spermatocytal
spermatocyte
primary s.
secondary s.
spermatocytic
spermatocytogenesis
spermatogenesis depression
spermatogenic
s. arrest
s. epididymitis
s. granulomatous orchitis
spermatogenous
spermatogeny
spermatogone
spermatogonia
s. dark type A
s. pale type A
s. type B
spermatogonium
spermatogram
spermatoid
spermatology
spermatolysin
spermatolysis
spermatolytic
spermatopoietic
spermatorrhea
spermatoschesis
spermatozoa
acrosome-reacted s.
disordered acrosome reaction of s.

spermatozoal
spermatozoon, pl. **spermatozoa**
s. concentration
s. cryopreservation
double-head s.
double-tail s.
s. motility
s. production
s. retrieval
s. volume
spermaturia
SpermCheck test
spermectomy
spermia
spermiation
spermicidal jelly
spermicide
spermidine
spermiduct
sperm-immunobead binding
spermine
s. NONOate
polyamine s.
spermiogenesis
spermoblast
spermoculture
spermolith
spermolytic
spermophlebectasia
spermosphere
spermotoxic
spermotoxin
SP-101 gastric lesion staging by endoscopic ultrasonography
spherical reservoir
spheroplast
mycobacterial s.
sphincter
AMS artificial s.
AMS 700-series double-cuff Silastic artificial urinary s.
AMS 800-series double-cuff Silastic artificial urinary s.
anal s. (AS)
anal ileostomy with preservation of s.
anorectal s.
artificial genitourinary s.
artificial urethral s. (AUS)
artificial urinary s.
AS-800 artificial s.
s. atony

S

NOTES

sphincter *(continued)*
    biliary s.
    Boyden s.
    cardiac s.
    cardioesophageal s.
    choledochal s.
    s. contraction ring
    cricopharyngeal s.
    double-cuff urinary s.
    s. dysfunction
    s. EMG
    esophageal s.
    external anal s. (EAS)
    external rectal s.
    external striated urinary s.
    external urethral s.
    s. function
    gastroesophageal s.
    Giordano s.
    Glisson s.
    Henle s.
    Hydroflex s.
    hypertensive lower esophageal s.
    Hyrtl s.
    ileocecal s.
    incompetent s.
    inguinal s.
    internal anal s. (IAS)
    internal rectal s.
    intrinsic striated s.
    intrinsic urethral s.
    lesser esophageal s. (LES)
    long anal s.
    lower esophageal s. (LES)
    Lütkens s.
    Nélaton s.
    neoanal s.
    O'Beirne s.
    s. of Oddi (SO)
    s. of Oddi ablation
    s. of Oddi dysfunction (SOD)
    s. of Oddi homogenate
    s. of Oddi manometry (SOM)
    s. of Oddi pressure (SOP)
    pancreatic duct s. (PDS)
    pancreaticobiliary s.
    pharyngoesophageal s.
    preprostatic s.
    prepyloric s.
    pyloric s.
    s. reaction
    s. reconstruction
    rectal s.
    s. repair
    Santorini s.
    servo-mechanism s.
    smooth urethral s.
    stomach s.

    striated detrusor s.
    striated urethral s.
    threshold of internal s.
    s. tone
    upper esophageal s. (UES)
    urethral s.
    urethrovaginal s.
    Wirsung s.
sphincteral achalasia
sphincterectomy
    endoscopic s.
sphincteric
    s. construction
    s. disobedience syndrome
    s. incontinence
    s. mechanism
    s. squeeze
sphincterismus
sphincteritis
sphincteroplasty
    overlapping s.
    pancreatic s.
    transduodenal s.
sphincteroscope
    Kelly s.
sphincteroscopy
sphincterotome
    bipolar s.
    Bitome bipolar s.
    Cotton s.
    Demling-Classen s.
    Doubilet s.
    double-channel s.
    ERCP s.
    Fluorotome double-lumen s.
    long-nosed s.
    needle-knife s.
    needle-tipped s.
    Olympus s.
    open s.
    precut s.
    reverse s.
    rotating s.
    single-channel wire-guided s.
    Ultratome double-lumen s.
    Ultratome XL triple-lumen s.
    Wilson-Cook double-channel s.
    Wilson-Cook (modified) wire-
      guided s.
    wire-guided s.
sphincterotomy
    s. basket
    biliary s.
    biliary endoscopic s.
    choledochal s.
    Doubilet s.
    endoscopic s. (ES, EST)
    endoscopic biliary s.

endoscopic pancreatic s. (EPS)
endoscopic pancreatic duct s.
Erlangen pull-type s.
external s.
guidewire s.
internal s.
lateral s.
minor papilla s.
Mulholland s.
multiple anal s.'s (MAS)
needle-knife endoscopic
  pancreatic s.
pancreatic duct s.
Parks partial s.
precut s.
pull-type s.
retrograde s.
stenosed s.
s. stenosis
stent-guided s.
transduodenal s.
transendoscopic s.
transpancreatic sphincter precut
  approach to biliary s.
transurethral s.
urethral s.

sphincter-preserving operation (SPO)
sphincter-saving procedure
sphingolipid derivative
sphingomyelin
SPI
symptom problem index
spiculated appearance
spiculation on colon
spicule
bony s.
s. in profile
spider
s. angioma
arterial s.
colonic arterial s.
s. nevus
s. pelvis
s. telangiectasia
spigelian hernia
spike
s. burst on electromyogram of
  colon
s. potential
spike-burst electrical activity
spiking fever

spillage
fecal s.
tumor s.
s. of tumor cells
spina bifida
spinach stool
spinal
s. anesthesia
s. cord compression
s. cord electric stimulation
s. cord injury (SCI)
s. cord injury without radiographic
  abnormality (SCIWOA)
s. cord necrosis
s. dysraphism
s. fluid finding
s. hemangioblastoma
omphalocele, exstrophy of the
  bladder, imperforate anus, and s.
  (OEIS)
s. shock
s. stenosis
spindle
s. cell
s. cell nodule
s. colonic groove
spine
s. dysraphism
iliac s.
s. stenosis
spin-echo
fat-suppressed s.-e. (FSSE)
half-Fourier acquisition single-shot
  turbo s.-e. (HASTE)
Spinelli biopsy needle
spinning
s. top deformity of the bladder
s. top urethra
spinobulbospinal
s. micturition reflex
s. micturition reflex inhibition
spinous
s. aspect
s. process
s. tenderness
spiral
s. bacterium
s. basket
s. computed tomography
s. computed tomography
  pneumocolon
s. CT

S

NOTES

spiral *(continued)*
 s. CT technique
 s. fold
 s. fold of cystic duct
 s. gallstone forceps
 intraprostatic s.
 s. stent
 s. tip catheter
 s. valve
 s. valve of Heister
spiralis
 Trichinella s.
 valvula s.
spiramycin
SpiraStent ureteral stent
spirillar dysentery
spirochetal dysentery
spirochete
 intestinal s.
spirochetosis
SpiroFlo prostate stent
spirometry
 incentive s.
spironazide
spironolactone
 hydrochlorothiazide and s.
Spirozide
Spirulina Pacifica nutritional supplement
Spitzer-Weinstein syndrome
Spivack
 S. operation
 S. valve
SPK
 simultaneous pancreas-kidney
 SPK transplantation
splanchna
splanchnectopia
splanchnemphraxis
splanchnic
 s. afferent fiber
 s. AV fistula
 s. blood flow
 s. capillary pressure
 s. hyperemia
 s. nerve
 s. primary afferent
 s. vasoconstriction
 s. vein
splanchnicectomy
 chemical s.
splanchnicus
 Bacteroides s.
splanchnocele
splanchnodiastasis
splanchnolith
splanchnopathy
splanchnoptosis, splanchnoptosia
splanchnotomy

splanchnotribe
splash
 succussion s.
S-plasty
spleen
 accessory s.
 s. index
 kidneys, liver, s. (KLS)
 s. tip
 trabeculae of s.
splenalgia
splenectomy
 incidental s.
splenic
 s. abscess
 s. agenesis syndrome
 s. angiogram
 s. anlage
 s. arterial embolization
 s. artery
 s. artery aneurysm (SAA)
 s. atrophy
 s. AV fistula
 s. avulsion
 s. capillary hemangiomatosis
 s. capsule
 s. dullness
 s. flexure
 s. flexure carcinoma
 s. flexure colonoscopy
 s. flexure syndrome
 s. function
 s. hilum
 s. injury
 s. laceration
 s. notch
 s. penetration
 s. perfusion measurement by dynamic CT scan
 s. portography
 s. pulp
 s. rupture
 s. sinus
 s. souffle
 s. tissue
 s. trauma
 s. vein
 s. vein obstruction (SVO)
 s. vein thrombosis
 s. venography
 s. venous blood flow
splenica
 arteria s.
 pulpa s.
splenicae
 penicilli arteriae s.
 trabeculae s.

splenici
  folliculi lymphatici s.
  lymphonoduli s.
splenobronchial fistula
splenocele
splenocleisis
splenocolic ligament
splenodynia
splenogastric omentum
splenography
splenolaparotomy
splenomegaly, splenomegalia
  congenital s.
  congestive s.
  Egyptian s.
  fibrocongestive s.
  Gaucher s.
  hemolytic s.
  infectious s.
  infective s.
  myelophthisic s.
  siderotic s.
  spodogenous s.
  tropical s.
splenonephroptosis
splenopancreatic ligament
splenopathy
splenopexy
splenoportal
  s. hypertension
  s. venography
splenoportography
splenorenal
  s. angle
  s. bypass
  s. bypass graft
  s. bypass shunt
  s. ligament
  s. recess
  s. venous anastomosis
splenorrhagia
splenorrhaphy
splenosis
splice-cite mutation
splicing
  aberrant mRNA s.
  alternate mRNA s.
splinting of abdomen
splint/stent
  kidney internal s./s. (KISS)
split
  s. ileostomy

  s. overtube
  s. pelvis
  s. renal function
  s. renal function study (SRFS)
  s. renal function test
  s. sheath introducer
split-and-roll technique
split-beam coupler for TURP
split-cuff
  s.-c. nipple
  s.-c. nipple technique
split-liver transplant
split-nipple
  s.-n. technique
  s.-n. technique urinary diversion
splitter
  Syn-Optics video image s.
split-thickness skin graft
SPN
  support parenteral nutrition
SPO
  sphincter-preserving operation
spodogenous splenomegaly
spondylitis
  ankylosing s.
sponge
  absorbable gelatin s.
  cherry s.
  s. count
  s. dissector
  Endozime s.
  fibrin s.
  s. forceps
  gauze s.
  gelatin s.
  Ivalon s.
  lap s.
  laparotomy s.
  Lapwall laparotomy s.
  peanut s.
  polyvinyl alcohol s.
  Prosthex s.
  saline-moistened s.
  small dissecting s.
  s. stick
  Weck-cel s.
sponge-holding forceps
sponge-tent
spongiofibrosis
  periurethral s.
spongioplasty
spongiosa

S

NOTES

spongiosal
spongiosi
>tunica albuginea corporis s.

spongiositis
spongiosum
>corpus s.

spongy pattern
spontaneous
>s. ascites filtration
>s. bacterial peritonitis (SBP)
>s. cystometry
>s. cyst reabsorption
>s. dialytic ultrafiltration
>s. dissection
>s. fragment passage
>s. partial elimination
>s. penile ischemic necrosis
>s. portal-systemic shunt (SPSS)
>s. reactivation of hepatitis
>s. recanalization
>s. regression
>s. resolution
>s. rupture

spoon
>Falk appendectomy s.
>s. forceps
>gall duct s.
>Mayo common duct s.
>s. retractor
>sharp s.
>Volkmann pancreatic calculus s.

spoon-tip laparoscopic electrode
Sporacidin disinfectant
sporadic
>s. dysentery
>s. gingival papilloma
>s. hollow visceral myopathy
>s. (nonfamilial) clear cell carcinoma

spore
>fungal s.

sporocyst
Sporothrix schenckii
Sporox disinfectant solution
sporozoites
sport sheath (SS)
sporulation
>coccidian s.

SPOT
>sonographic planning of oncology treatment
>>SPOT mobile 3D ultrasound system and software

spot
>central s.
>cherry red s. (CRS)
>cold s.
>cotton-wool s. (CWS)

dark s.
S. endoscopic marker
epigastric s.
Fordyce s.
gastric red s.
hematocystic s. (HCS)
hot s.
hyperechoic s.
Koplik s.
mongolian s.
Roth s.
s. size

S-pouch
>three-limb S-p.

spout
>ileal s.

SPP
>stannous pyrophosphate
>^{99m}Tc SPP

Spratt curette
spray
>alginate s.
>DDAVP nasal s.
>Maalox s.
>Prevacare total solution skin care s.
>sodium thiosulfate solution s.
>thrombin s.

spray-fixed
spraying
>dye s.
>fibrin s.

spreader
>meatal s.
>pyloric s.

spreading fistulation
spring-loaded
>s.-l. biopsy gun
>s.-l. type biopsy instrument

spring-wire
>s.-w. coil
>s.-w. retractor

Sprinz-Dubin syndrome
Sprinz-Nelson syndrome
sprue
>celiac s.
>collagenous s.
>nontropical s.
>refractory s.
>subclinical s.
>tropical s.

SPSS
>spontaneous portal-systemic shunt

SPT
>station pull-through
>>SPT technique

spun urine sediment

spuria
> hemospermia s.
> melena s.

spurious calculus

spurting blood

sputum, pl. **sputa**
> s. aerogenosum
> green s.

SPV
> selective proximal vagotomy

SQMP
> subcutaneous morphine pump

squamocolumnar mucosal junction

squamous
> s. cell
> s. cell cancer
> s. cell carcinoma (SCC)
> s. cell carcinoma antigen
> s. cell carcinoma in situ
> s. cell papilloma (SCP)
> s. epithelium

square knot

squeeze
> hot s.
> phasic fluctuation on s.
> s. pressure
> s. pressure profile of anal sphincter test
> sphincteric s.

src-**homology 2 (SH2)**
> s.-h. domain

src **phosphorylation**

S-reservoir

SRFS
> split renal function study

SRH
> stigmata of recent hemorrhage

SRIF
> somatotropin release-inhibiting factor

SRS
> somatostatin receptor scintigraphy

SRUS
> solitary rectal ulcer syndrome

SRVG
> silicone elastomer ring vertical gastroplasty

SRY **gene**

SS
> Sjögren syndrome
> somatostatin
> sport sheath
> > Regulax SS

Ssabanejew-Frank
> S.-F. gastrostomy
> S.-F. operation

SSBE
> short-segment Barrett esophagus

SSC
> single-stripe colitis

SSc
> systemic sclerosis

SSE
> soapsuds enema

SSE2-L electrosurgical unit

S-shaped
> S-s. body
> S-s. ileal pouch-anal anastomosis
> S-s. pouch
> S-s. reservoir

SSI
> symptom severity index

SSIAM
> Structured and Scaled Interview to Assess Maladjustment
> SSIAM interview

SSIS
> side-to-side isoperistaltic strictureplasty

SSR
> somatostatin receptor

ST
> heat-stable enterotoxin

St.
> St. John's wort
> St. Mark pudendal electrode

stab
> s. incision
> s. wound

stability
> detrusor s.
> detrusor muscle s.
> structural s.

stabilization
> percutaneous bladder neck s. (PBNS)
> Vesica percutaneous bladder neck s.

stabilizer

stable face

stab-wound drain

staccato voiding

Stacke meatoplasty

stack-of-coins appearance

Stadol

S

NOTES

stage
  s. B, C carcinoma
  Dean s.
  Dukes s.
  Hoehn and Yahr s.
  s. III papillary serous
    cystadenocarcinoma
  morphologic s.
  post-TNM s. (I, II, III, IV)
  Tanner s.
  tumor s.
staged orchiopexy
stage-specific embryonic antigen
staghorn
  s. calculus
  s. stone
  s. urinary lithiasis
staging
  Ann Arbor cancer s.
  Boden-Gibb tumor s.
  s. of cancer
  clinicopathologic s.
  endosonographic s.
  Marshall and Tanner pubertal s.
  neoplasm s.
  neuroblastoma s.
  s. operation
  operative s.
  primary gastric lymphoma s.
  Stanford s.
  TNM system for tumor s.
  transrectal ultrasound s.
  tumor s.
stagnant
  s. bile
  s. loop syndrome
stain
  19A2 s.
  acid-Schiff s.
  Alcian blue s.
  anti-Schiff s.
  argentaffin s.
  azan s.
  Bryan-Leishman s.
  carbolfuchsin s.
  chromogranin s.
  Congo red s.
  Diff-Quik s.
  elastin s.
  eosin s.
  esterase s.
  Fite s.
  Fontana-Masson s.
  Fungi-Fluor chitin s.
  gastrin s.
  Genta s.
  Giemsa s.
  Glaxo s.

  glucagon s.
  Gram s.
  Grimelius silver s.
  Grocott methenamine silver s.
  Hale colloidal iron s.
  Hansel s.
  H&E s.
  hematological s.
  hematoxylin and eosin s.
  immunocytochemical s.
  immunohistochemical s.
  immunoperoxidase s.
  indigo carmine s.
  insulin s.
  Jones silver s.
  Ki-67 s.
  Kossa s.
  lead citrate s.
  Lendrum s.
  Lugol solution s.
  Mallory-Azan s.
  Martius scarlet blue s.
  Masson-Fontana s.
  Masson trichrome s.
  Mayer acid alum hematoxylin s.
  May-Grünwald-Giemsa s.
  methylene blue s.
  NADPH diaphorase s.
  oil red O s.
  Orcein s.
  pancreatic polypeptide s.
  Papanicolaou s.
  PAS s.
  periodic acid-Schiff s.
  periodic acid-Schiff-Alcian blue
    combination s.
  Perls s.
  peroxidase s.
  p53 immunohistochemical s.
  rhodamine s.
  RP3 s.
  saffron s.
  Schiff s.
  serotonin s.
  silver s.
  S-100 immunohistochemical s.
  somatostatin s.
  Steiner s.
  Sternheimer-Malbin s.
  Sudan black B fat s.
  Sudan-III s.
  sulfated mucin s.
  toluidine blue s.
  trichrome s.
  uranyl acetate s.
  vasoactive intestinal polypeptide s.
  VIP s.
  von Kossa s.

Warthin-Starry silver s.
Wright s.
Wright-Giemsa s.
Ziehl-Neelsen s.
staining
Berlin blue s.
BrDu s.
cytokeratin s.
cytoplasmic s.
endoscopy with iodine s.
ethidium bromide s.
Feulgen s.
Grimelius s.
immunohistochemical s.
immunoperoxidase s.
iodine s.
lectin s.
MIB-1 s.
p53 nuclear s.
Smith method of silver s.
Steiner modification of Warthin-
Starry s.
vimentin s.
vital s.
stainless
s. steel mesh stent
s. steel suture
stairstep air-fluid level
stalk
polyp s.
Stamey
S. classification
S. colosuspension
S. dorsal vein apical retractor
S. needle
S. needle bladder neck suspension
S. open tip ureteral catheter
S. procedure
S. test
S. tube
S. urethropexy
Stamey-Malecot catheter
Stamey-Martius procedure
Stamm
S. gastroplasty
S. gastrostomy
S. gastrostomy tube
stammering bladder
stand
Mayo s.
standard
s. acid reflux test (SART)

Aub-Dubois s.
s. colonoscope
s. duodenoscope
s. endoscopy polypectomy snare
s. ERCP catheter
s. fatty meal
s. hemodialysis
s. laparoscopy (SL)
s. orchiopexy
s. pyelolithotomy
s. radioenzymatic method
standardized
s. incidence ratio (SIR)
s. instrument
Stanford
S. protocol
S. radical retropubic prostatectomy
S. staging
Stanley bacillus
stanniocalcin
stannous pyrophosphate (SPP)
stanolone
stanozolol
staphylococcal sepsis
Staphylococcus
S. albus
S. aureus
coagulase-negative *S.*
S. epidermidis
S. saprophyticus
Staphylococcus food poisoning
S. viridans
staple
absorbable s.
s. line dehiscence
metallic s.
polyglyconate s.
skin s.
stapled
s. closure
s. end-to-end ileoanal anastomosis
s. hemorrhoidectomy
s. intestinal anastomosis
s. pouch-anal anastomosis
s. strictureplasty
stapler
anvil portion of EEA s.
Auto Suture Multifire Endo GIA
30 s.
Auto Suture Premium CEEA s.
CEEA s.
circular s.

S

NOTES

stapler *(continued)*
    Cobe s.
    double-headed P190 s.
    s. doughnut
    EEA AutoSuture s.
    end-end s.
    Endo-Babcock s.
    Endo GIA 30, 60 s.
    Endo GIA suture s.
    Endo Hernia s.
    Endopath 30, 60 s.
    Endopath EMS hernia s.
    Ethicon CDH29 s.
    Ethicon TLH30 s.
    EZ vascular 35 linear s.
    GIA s.
    hernia s.
    ILA surgical s.
    intraluminal s. (ILS)
    laparoscopic s.
    LDS s.
    ligating and dividing s. (LDS)
    linear s.
    PI-30 s.
    PI90 double-headed s.
    PI surgical s.
    PLC-50 linear s.
    Premium CEEA circular s.
    Premium Plus CEEA disposable s.
    ProTack s.
    Proximate flexible linear s.
    Proximate ILS SDH circular s.
    Proximate intraluminal s.
    TA90-BN s.
    TA30, TA55 s.
    TL90 Ethicon s.
    vascular s.

stapling
    gastric s.
    single s.
    skin s.
    surgical s.

STAR
    steroidogenic acute regulatory
    STAR protein

starch
    amylase-resistant s. (ARS)
    s. blocker
    s. granulomatous peritonitis
    wheat s.

Starck dilator
star construction test
Starlix
Starr
    S. plication
    S. technique

stasis
    antral s.

    bile s.
    biliary s.
    s. cirrhosis
    s. esophagitis
    fecal s.
    gallbladder s.
    s. gallbladder
    gastric s.
    ileal s.
    intestinal s.
    s. liver
    pelvicaliceal s.
    postgastrectomy s.
    postsurgical gastric s.
    Roux-limb s.
    s. syndrome
    s. ulceration
    venous s.

stasis-induced ulceration
STAT!
    ImmunoCard S.

Stat
    S. Simple whole-blood antibody
    test

state
    S. end-to-end anastomosis
    gradient-recalled acquisition in a
    steady s. (GRASS)
    hypercoagulable s.
    hypermetabolic s.
    hypogonadal s.
    neurohumoral excitation s.
    proteinuric s.
    sick euthyroid s.

Statham
    S. external transducer
    S. P23 strain gauge

statherin
static
    s. closure pressure
    s. cystogram
    s. cytophotometry
    s. image DNA cytometry

station
    s. pull-through (SPT)
    s. pull-through esophageal
    manometry technique

statistics
    nonparametric Wilcoxon s.

status
    apical biopsy s.
    s. evaluation
    fertility s.
    s. gastricus
    Karnofsky performance s.
    nutritional s.
    s. post (S/P)
    ureteroenteric s.

Stat-View computer program
Stauffer syndrome
stavudine
StayErec system
stay suture
STC
   slow transit constipation
STD
   sexually transmitted disease
STDS
   stone-tissue detection system
steady pain
steady-state autofluorescence
   spectroscopy
steakhouse syndrome
steal
   arterial s.
steam autoclave
stearrhea
steatohepatitis
   nonalcoholic s. (NASH)
steatorrhea
   biliary s.
   idiopathic s.
   intestinal s.
   pancreatic s.
steatosis
   drug-induced s.
   hepatic s.
   macrovesicular s.
   microvesicular s.
   severe macrovesicular s.
   toxic s.
Steblay nephritis
STEC
   Shiga toxin-producing *Escherichia coli*
   Stx 2-producing *Escherichia coli* strain
steely-hair disease
steerable
   s. cystoscopy
   s. nephroscope
Steers replicator
stegnosis
stegnotic
Steigmann-Goff
   S.-G. endoscopic ligator kit
   S.-G. endoscopic ligature overtube
Steinach operation
Steiner
   S. modification of Warthin-Starry
   staining
   S. stain

Steinert
   S. disease
   S. myotonic dystrophy
Stein-Leventhal syndrome
Steinmann intestinal forceps
steinstrasse
Stelazine
stellate
   s. cell
   s. venule
stem cell
Stemetic
stemline
   DNA s.
stenosed sphincterotomy
stenosis, pl. **stenoses**
   afferent limb nipple s.
   ampullary s.
   anal s.
   anorectal s.
   antral s.
   aortic valvular s.
   atherosclerotic renal artery s.
   benign papillary s.
   bile duct s.
   canal s.
   choledochoduodenal junctional s.
   congenital esophageal s.
   congenital hypertrophic pyloric s.
   cystic duct s.
   delayed ureteral anastomotic s.
   diaphragm-like s.
   distal esophageal s.
   duodenal s.
   esophageal s.
   hypertrophic pyloric s. (HPS)
   idiopathic hypertrophic pyloric s.
   ileoureteric s.
   infantile hypertrophic pyloric s.
    (IHPS)
   infundibular s.
   infundibulopelvic s.
   intestinal s.
   Klatskin s.
   luminal s.
   malignant s.
   meatal s.
   pancreaticojejunostomy s.
   pancreatic papillary s.
   papillary s.
   preputial s.
   pyloric s.

NOTES

stenosis *(continued)*
    radiation s.
    rectal s.
    renal artery s.
    short band s.
    small intestinal s.
    sphincterotomy s.
    spinal s.
    spine s.
    stomal s.
    s. of TIPS
    transplant renal artery s. (TRAS)
    tubular s.
    unilateral renal artery s.
    ureteral reimplantation s.
    ureteroileal s.
    urethral s.
    vesical neck s.
    vesicoureteric s.
stenotic
    s. cancer
    s. lesion
    s. shunt
    s. stoma
stenotogram
Stenotrophomonas maltophilia
Stensen duct
stent
    Amsterdam biliary s.
    Angiomed blue s.
    Angiomed Puroflex s.
    antibiotic-coated s.
    antireflux double-J s.
    ASI prostatic s.
    ASI Titan s.
    Bard Memotherm colorectal s.
    Beamer ejection s.
    Beamer injection s.
    biliary s.
    Biliary Spiral Z s.
    Biofix s.
    bioresorbable s.
    BioSorb resorbable urology s.
    Black Beauty ureteral s.
    Braun s.
    Carson internal/external
      endopyelotomy s.
    C-Flex Amsterdam s.
    C-Flex ureteral s.
    coil s.
    colonic s.
    common bile duct s.
    conventional s.
    Cook s.
    Cotton-Huibregtse double pigtail s.
    Cotton-Leung biliary s.
    covered biliary metal s.
    Cragg Endopro System I s.

    crutched stick-type biliary duct s.
    Cysto Flex s.
    s. deployment
    Diamond s.
    digestive-respiratory fistula s.
    double-J indwelling catheter s.
    double-J silicone s.
    double-J Surgitek catheter s.
    double-J ureteral s.
    double-pigtail s.
    DoubleStent biliary
      endoprosthesis s.
    Elastalloy esophageal s.
    Eliminator biliary s.
    Eliminator pancreatic s.
    encrustation of s.
    endobronchial s.
    EndoCoil biliary s.
    EndoCoil esophageal s.
    endopyelotomy s.
    endoscopic biliary s.
    Entract s.
    EsophaCoil self-expanding
      esophageal s.
    esophageal I s.
    esophageal Strecker s.
    s. exchange
    expandable esophageal s. (EES)
    expandable intrahepatic portacaval
      shunt s.
    expandable metallic s.
    Fader Tip ureteral s.
    Firlit-Kluge s.
    Flexima biliary s.
    floating s.
    forgotten s.
    French double-J ureteral s.
    s. funnel
    Gianturco expandable (self-
      expanding) metallic biliary s.
    Gianturco metal urethral s.
    Gianturco-Rosch self-expandable Z-
      stent s.
    Gianturco-Roubin flexible coil s.
    Gianturco-Z s.
    Gibbon indwelling ureteral s.
    Greenen pancreatic s.
    helical-ridged ureteral s.
    Herculink Plus biliary s.
    Heyer-Schulte s.
    Horizon prostatic s.
    Huibregtse biliary s.
    Hydromer coated polyurethane s.
    Hydro Plus s.
    ileal artery s.
    s. incrustation
    InStent EsophaCoil s.
    intracholedochal s.

IntraCoil nitinol s.
intraesophageal s.
intraluminal Silastic esophageal s.
intraprostatic s.
iridium-192-loaded s.
J-Maxx s.
large-bore double-pigtail s.
Lubri-flex ureteral s.
magnetic internal ureteral s.
main pancreatic duct s.
Mardis soft s.
Megalink biliary s.
membrane-covered s.
Memotherm colorectal s.
Memotherm Flexx biliary s.
Memotherm nitinol s.
mesh s.
metal s.
metallic biliary s.
Metal Z s.
s. migration
MPD s.
Multi-Flex s.
nephroureteral s.
nephrovesical s.
Nissenkorn s.
nitinol mesh s.
Niti-S s.
Oasis s.
Palmaz balloon-expandable s.
Palmaz-Schatz biliary s.
pancreatic duct s.
s. patency
Percuflex Amsterdam s.
Percuflex biliary s.
Percuflex endopyelotomy s.
Percuflex Plus ureteral s.
percutaneous s.
pigtail biliary s.
polyethylene s.
polyurethane s.
polyurethane-covered metallic s.
Prostacoil s.
Prostakath urethral s.
prostatic s.
pyelovesical s.
QuadraCoil s.
recanalization of clogged biliary s.
renal artery s.
Retromax endopyelotomy s.
Rusch s.
Schneider s.

self-expandable metal s.
self-expanding biliary metal s.
self-expanding coil s.
self-expanding metallic s. (SEMS)
self-retaining coil s.
SEM s.
shape memory alloy s.
Siegel s.
Silastic indwelling ureteral s.
silicone-coated metallic self-
  expanding s.
Silitek Uropass s.
silver-coated s.
single-pigtail s.
SMA spiral s.
SoloPass Percuflex biliary s.
Song s.
Speed Lok soft s.
spiral s.
SpiraStent ureteral s.
SpiroFlo prostate s.
stainless steel mesh s.
straight s.
Strecker s.
Surgitek Tractfinder ureteral s.
Surgitek Uropass s.
Tannenbaum s.
Teflon s.
thermoexpandable s.
thermosensitive s.
s. through wire mesh technique
Titan s.
titanium urethral s.
tracheobronchial Z s.
transhepatic biliary s.
transpapillary cystopancreatic s.
transpapillary insertion of self-
  expanding biliary metal s.
T-tube s.
Ultraflex Diamond s.
Ultraflex Microvasive s.
Ultraflex nitinol expandable
  esophageal s.
Ultraflex tracheobronchial s.
uncoated mesh s.
Universal s.
ureteral s.
urethral s.
UroCoil self-expanding s.
Uro-Guide s.
UroLume prostate s.
UroLume urethral s.

S

NOTES

stent *(continued)*
    UroLume Wallstent s.
    Urosoft s.
    Urospiral urethral s.
    U-tube s.
    s. and vent system
    Vistaflex biliary s.
    Wallstent s.
    Wallstent-covered SEM s.
    whistle s.
    Wilson-Cook French s.
    Z s.
    Za-Stent endoscopic biliary s.
    Zimmon biliary s.
stent-guided sphincterotomy
stent-induced pneumoperitoneum
stenting
    biliary s.
    s. catheter
    endoscopic pancreatic s. (EPS)
    endoscopic papillotomy and s.
    endoscopic retrograde biliary s.
    endovascular s.
    hilar bile duct s.
    pancreatic transpapillary s.
    tumor s.
    ureteral s.
stepladder incision technique
steppage gait
stepping reflex
step-up shim
step-wise regression analysis
steradian
Sterapred
stercolith
stercoraceous
    s. abscess
    s. vomiting
    s. vomitus
stercoral
    s. abscess
    s. appendicitis
    s. colic
    s. diarrhea
    s. fistula
    s. perforation
    s. ulcer
    s. ulceration
stercoralis
    Strongyloides s.
stercoroma
stercorous
stercus
stereocilium, pl. **stereocilia**
stereognost-3-alpha enzymatic test
StereoGuide
    Lorad S.

sterile
    s. abscess
    s. ceftriaxone sodium
    s. cyst
    s. dressing
    s. pancreatic necrosis
    s. peritonitis
sterility
    absolute s.
    aspermatogenic s.
    chemotherapy-induced s.
    dysspermatogenic s.
    male s.
    normospermatogenic s.
    primary s.
    radiation-induced s.
    relative s.
    secondary s.
sterilization
    ETO s.
    gas s.
sterilize
sterilized
    autoclave s.
Steris automatic reprocessor
Steri-Strip
steri-stripped incision
Sternberg paradigm
Sternheimer-Malbin stain
sternocleidomastoid
sternotomy scar
sternum
    bowed s.
steroid
    adrenal s.
    anabolic s.
    s. foam enema
    high-dose pulse s.
    s. moiety
    s. receptor
    s. responsive pancolitis
    s. therapy
    s. withdrawal
steroid-dependent
    s.-d. Crohn disease
    s.-d. diet
    s.-d. idiopathic nephrosis
steroid-induced azoospermia
steroidogenic
    s. acute regulatory (STAR)
    s. acute regulatory protein
steroid-refractory
    s.-r. Crohn disease
    s.-r. diet
steroid-resistant
    s.-r. idiopathic nephrosis
    s.-r. nephrotic syndrome
steroid-sensitive idiopathic nephrosis

sterol
stethoscope
 esophageal s.
Stetten intestinal clamp
Stevens-Johnson syndrome (SJS)
Stewart crypt hook
Stewart-Treves syndrome
sTf-R
 soluble transferrin receptor
stick
 sponge s.
 s. tie
Stiegmann-Goff
 S.-G. Clearvue endoscopic ligator
 S.-G. technique
 S.-G. variceal ligator
Stierlin sign
Stifcore transbronchial aspiration needle
stiffening
 s. tube
 s. wire
stiff-man syndrome
stigma, pl. **stigmata, stigmas**
 endoscopic s.
 stigmata of recent hemorrhage
 (SRH)
 syphilitic s.
 Turner s.
stigmatic
stigmatism
stigmatization
still camera
Stille
 S. clamp
 S. elevator
 S. gallstone forceps
Stille-Barraya intestinal forceps
Stilphostrol
stimulant laxative
stimulated
 s. gastric secretion test
 s. gracilis neosphincter
 s. gracilis neosphincter technique
 s. graciloplasty
 s. release
stimulation
 adenyl cyclase s.
 anal electrical s.
 anocutaneous s.
 antigen s.
 central vagal nerve s.
 chronic low-frequency electrical s.

 chronic sacral spinal nerve s.
 cutaneous electrical field s.
 electrogalvanic s. (EGS)
 extradural electrical s.
 s. fork
 gastric electrical s.
 hilum s.
 interferential electrical s.
 interferon-gamma s.
 intraoperative cavernous nerve s.
 intravaginal electrical s.
 magnetic s.
 mitogenic s.
 nociceptive s.
 peak acid output after
  pentagastrin s. (PAOPg)
 pelvic s.
 pelvic floor electrical s. (PFS)
 penile vibratory s.
 s. probe
 rectum digital s.
 sacral nerve s. (SNS)
 S-CCK-Pz s.
 secretin s.
 spinal cord electric s.
 Stoller afferent nerve s. (SANS)
 s. test
 testosterone s.
 transcranial magnetic s. (TCMS)
 transcutaneous electrical nerve s.
  (TENS)
 transurethral electrical bladder s.
  (TEBS)
 vagal s.
 vaginal electrical s.
stimulator
 EGS Model 100 electrogalvanic s.
 electrogalvanic s.
 Grass Model S9 s.
 Nicolet SM-300 s.
 URYS 800 nerve s.
stimulus, pl. **stimuli**
 external s.
 mitogenic s.
 osmotic s.
 symbolic s.
STING
 subureteric Teflon injection
Sting procedure
stirrups
 Allen s.
 Allyn s.

S

NOTES

stirrups *(continued)*
    Lloyd Davies s.
    pediatric s.
stitch
    baseball s.
    cobbler's s.
    Connell s.
    Gambee s.
    intersymphyseal s.
    lock s.
    marker s.
    tagging s.
    tilt s.
STK11
    serine threonine kinase gene 11
    STK11 gene
stochastic knotting
Stockholm trial (I, II)
stoichiometry
    coupling s.
Stokvis
    S. disease
    S. test
Stokvis-Talma syndrome
Stoller
    S. afferent nerve stimulation
      (SANS)
    S. scoring system
Stoll test
stoma, pl. **stomas, stomata**
    abdominal s.
    anastomotic s.
    appendicoumbilical s.
    bowel s.
    s. caps
    concealed umbilical s.
    continent abdominal wall s.
    diverting s.
    dusky s.
    end s.
    end-loop s.
    flush s.
    gastrointestinal s.
    Gomez horizontal gastroplasty with
      reinforced s.
    ileostomy s.
    Laws gastroplasty with Silastic
      collar-reinforced s.
    loop s.
    maturing the s.
    Mitrofanoff continent urinary s.
    nippled s.
    permanent s.
    prolapsed s.
    retracted s.
    rodless end-loop s.
    rosebud s.
    Silastic collar-reinforced s.

    s. site
    stenotic s.
    Turnbull loop s.
    ureteral s.
    ureteric s.
stomach
    aberrant umbilical s.
    acid-suppressed s.
    adenomyoepithelioma of s.
    anacidic s.
    angular notch of s.
    angulus of s.
    antrum of s.
    s. bed
    bilocular s.
    butterflies in the s.
    s. calculus
    caliber-persistent artery of the s.
    cardia of s.
    cardiac s.
    cascade s.
    cirrhosis of s.
    cup-and-spill s.
    curvature of s.
    dilation of the s.
    distal blind s.
    dumping s.
    functional disorder s.
    fundus of s.
    granulocytic sarcoma of s.
    greater curvature of s.
    hourglass s.
    insufflation of s.
    intrathoracic s.
    s. lavage
    leather-bottle s.
    lesser curvature of s.
    middle s.
    mucous lake of the s.
    s. neoplasm
    oblique fibers of s.
    s. pump
    s. reefing
    rugae of s.
    sclerotic s.
    sour s.
    s. sphincter
    thoracic s.
    trifid s.
    s. tube
    tympany of the s.
    upset s.
    upside down s.
    vascular coat of s.
    villous folds of s.
    watermelon s. (WS)
    water-trap s.
stomachalgia

stomachodynia
Stomahesive
    S. paste
    S. skin barrier wafer
stomal
    s. aperture
    s. bag
    s. duskiness
    s. invagination
    s. prolapse
    s. stenosis
    s. ulcer
stomalike channel
stomas (*pl. of* stoma)
stomata (*pl. of* stoma)
Stomate
    S. decompression tube
    S. extension tube
stomatitis
    aphthous s.
    herpetic s.
stomatoscopy
    diagnostic fiberoptic s.
stone
    ampullary s.
    s. and basket impaction
    bile duct s.
    biliary tract s.
    bilirubinate s.
    black faceted s.
    black pigment s.
    bladder s.
    brown pigment s.
    s. burden
    calcium bilirubinate s.
    calcium oxalate dihydrate s.
    calcium oxalate monohydrate s.
    carbonate apatite s.
    cholesterol s.
    S. clamp applier
    s. clearance
    s. comminution
    common bile duct s.
    common duct s.
    complex s.
    s. cup
    cystic duct s.
    cystine s.
    s. disease
    s. dislodger
    endoscopic extraction pancreatic
      duct s.

    s. extraction
    extraction bile duct s.
    extraction pancreatic s.
    s. former
    s. fragmentation
    gallbladder s.
    s. granuloma
    s. granuloma formation
    hepatic duct s.
    hyperoxaluric s.
    impacted ampullary s.
    s. impactor
    infection s.
    S. intestinal clamp
    intrahepatic s.
    intraluminal s.
    kidney s.
    large common duct s.
    s. management
    s. maturation
    metabolic s.
    mulberry s.
    multiple s.
    noncalcified s.
    nonstruvite s.
    pancreatic duct s.
    pelvic s.
    periureteral s.
    pigment s.
    s. plaque
    s. recognition system
    renal s.
    residual s.
    s. retrieval balloon
    s. retrieval basket
    s. retriever
    s. searcher
    silent s.
    s. solvent
    staghorn s.
    struvite s.
    s. surgery
    ureteral s.
    ureteric s.
    uric acid s.
    urinary s.
stone-forming patient
stone-free rate
stone-grasping forceps
Stone-Holcombe intestinal clamp
stone-holding basket forceps
stonelike debris

NOTES

S

StoneRisk
  S. citrate test
  S. cystine test
  S. diagnostic monitoring kit
  S. diagnostic profile
  S. diagnostic test
  S. profile test
stone-tissue
  s.-t. detection system (STDS)
  s.-t. recognition system (STR)
stool
  acholic s.
  s. antigen assay
  bilious s.
  black tarry s.
  blood in s.
  blood admixed with s.
  blood on surface of s.
  blood passed with s.
  blood-streaked s.
  bloody s.
  brown s.
  bulky s.
  butter s.
  caddy s.
  s. chromatography
  clay-colored s.
  Clinitest-negative s.
  Clinitest-positive s.
  s. colonization
  s. color
  continent of s.
  s. culture
  currant jelly s.
  s. cytotoxin test
  dark s.
  diarrhea s.
  s. electrolyte
  s. electrolyte test
  s. elimination
  s. evacuation
  fatty s.
  floating s.
  foamy s.
  formed s.
  foul-smelling s.
  frank blood in s.
  frequency of s.
  Gram stain of s.
  green s.
  guaiac-negative s.
  guaiac-positive s.
  hard s.
  heme-negative s.
  heme-positive s.
  impacted s.
  s. incontinence
  lienteric s.

liquid s.
loose s.
mahogany-colored s.
malodorous s.
maroon-colored s.
melenic s.
mucoid s.
mucous s.
mushy s.
nonbloody s.
s. for occult blood
oily s.
s. osmolality test
s. osmotic gap
s. osmotic gap test
s. for ova and parasites
pale s.
palpable s.
particulate s.
passage of s.
pea soup s.
pelleted s.
pencil-like s.
pipestem s.
rabbit s.
residual s.
s. retention
ribbon s.
rice-water s.
runny s.
sago-grain s.
s. sample
scybalous s.
semiformed s.
semisolid s.
silver s.
slurry of s.
soft s.
s. softener
spinach s.
straining at s.
tarry black s.
s. toxin assay
Trélat s.
undigested food in s.
unformed s.
watery s.
Wright stain of s.
stooling
stool-softening laxative
stop-cock
  three-way s.-c.
Stoppa
  S. operation
  S. repair
storage
  cold s.
  hypothermic s.

store

    hepatic glycogen s.
    iron s.
    liver iron s.
    liver protein s.

Storz

    S. cholangiograsper
    S. cystoscope
    S. esophagoscope
    S. minilaparoscope
    S. Modulith SL20
    S. Monolith lithotriptor
    S. multifunction valve
        trocar/cannula system
    S. nephroscope
    S. panendoscope
    S. resectoscope
    S. 27022 SK ureteroscope
    S. syringe
    S. urethrotome

STR

    stone-tissue recognition system

strabismus scissors
Strachan

    S. disease
    S. syndrome

Strachan-Scott syndrome
straddle injury
straight

    s. endoprosthesis
    s. intestine
    s. Maryland forceps
    s. mosquito clamp
    s. stent
    s. venule

straightener

    colonoscopy technique with an
        external s.
    external s.

straightening maneuver
Straight-In

    S.-I. male sling system
    S.-I. surgical system

strain

    Bio-Tract proprietary s.
    Cowan 1 s.
    eubacterial s.
    s. gauge transducer
    metronidazole-resistant s.
    precore mutant s.
    Statham P23 s. gauge

    Stx 2-producing *Escherichia coli* s.
        (STEC)

straining

    s. at stool
    defecatory s.
    excessive s.
    s. for urination

strand

    Billroth s.
    fibrin s.
    internodal s.

stranding

    fascial s.
    hyperechoic s.
    mesenteric s.
    pericholecystic s.
    perinephric s.
    periureteral s.
    soft tissue s.

strands
strangulated

    s. bowel
    s. bowel obstruction
    s. hemorrhoid
    s. hernia
    s. viscus

strangulation

    s. of bladder
    s. necrosis

stranguria
strangury
S-transferase

    glutathione S-t. (GST)

Stransky sign
strap

    Allen s.
    Montgomery abdominal s.

Strassburg test
strata (*pl. of* stratum)
Stratagene SCS-96 thermocycler
Stratasis urethral sling
strategy

    antisense s.

stratiform
Stratte needle holder
stratum, pl. **strata**

    s. malpighii
    submucous s.

Strauss sign
strawberry

    s. gallbladder
    s. hemangioma

S

NOTES

straw-colored
    s.-c. ascites
    s.-c. fluid
streak
    erythematous s.
    s. gonad
    lymphangitic s.
    s. ovary
stream
    curve of s.
Strecker stent
Strelinger colon clamp
strength
    artery weld s.
    detrusor contraction s.
    hemostatic bond s.
    masseter s.
    tensile s.
streptavidin
    peroxidase-conjugated s.
streptavidin-biotin peroxidase complex (SAB reagent)
streptococcal esophagitis
Streptococcus
    S. agalactiae
    alpha-hemolytic *S.*
    anhemolytic *S.*
    beta-hemolytic *S.*
    S. bovis
    S. bovis bacteremia
    S. bovis endocarditis
    S. faecalis
    S. milleri
    S. mulleri
    nonhemolytic *S.*
    S. pyogenes
    S. salivarius
    S. sanguis
    S. thermophilus
    S. viridans
streptococcus
    group B s. (GBS)
    hemolytic s.
Streptococcus **enteritis**
streptokinase
Streptomyces misakiensis
streptomycin nephropathy
streptozocin, streptozotocin
streptozotocin-induced diabetes mellitus
stress
    s. cystogram
    s. erosion
    s. erythrocytosis
    s. gastritis
    s. hematuria
    s. incontinence (type 0, I, II, III)
    s. lesion
    oxidative s.

    s. protein
    s. relaxation
    surgical s.
    s. testing
    s. ulcer
    s. ulceration
    s. ulcer hemorrhage
    s. ulcer prophylaxis
    s. urethral pressure profile
    s. urinary incontinence (SUI)
stress-induced gastric ulceration
stress-related
    s.-r. erosive syndrome
    s.-r. mucosal injury
Stresstein liquid feeding
stretch receptor
stretch-sensitive ion channel
Stretta
    S. procedure
    S. system
stria, pl. **striae**
    epidermal s.
    Looser-Milkman s.
striated
    s. detrusor sphincter
    s. muscle innervation
    s. urethral sphincter
Strickler
    S. technique ureterocolonic anastomosis
    S. ureteral anastomosis
strict implementation
stricture
    anal s.
    anastomotic s.
    annular esophageal s.
    antral s.
    benign bile duct s. (BBDS)
    benign biliary s.
    bile duct s.
    biliary tract s.
    bulbomembranous s.
    bulbourethral s.
    s. cannulation
    caustic s.
    cicatricial s.
    colorectal s.
    complete ureteral s.
    congenital ureteral s.
    congenital urethral s.
    contractile s.
    corrosive esophageal s.
    diaphragm-like s.
    distal esophageal s.
    ductal s.
    esophageal s.
    extrahepatic biliary s.
    filiform s.

focal s.
hourglass s.
Hunner s.
intestinal s.
intrahepatic biliary s.
intrinsic ureteral s.
irritable s.
left hepatic duct s.
longitudinal esophageal s.
malignant rectal s.
nonsteroidal antiinflammatory drug-
  induced intestinal s.
pancreatic duct s.
pancreaticobiliary s.
peptic esophageal s.
postoperative s.
posttraumatic urethral s.
s. prophylaxis
pyloric s.
radiation-induced ureteral s.
rectal s.
recurrent s.
reflux-related s.
ringlike s.
spasmodic s.
upper tract s.
ureteral s.
ureterocolic s.
ureteroenteric s.
ureteroileal s.
urethral s.
vas deferens s.
vesicourethral anastomotic s.
strictured esophagus
strictureplasty (SXPL)
Finney s.
Heineke-Mikulicz s.
side-to-side isoperistaltic s. (SSIS)
stapled s.
stricturoplasty
endoscopic s.
Thal s.
stricturotomy
endoscopic s.
stridor
string
s. guideline
s. method for treatment of penile
  incarceration
s. operation
s. sign
soft rubber s.

swallowed s.
s. test
string-of-beads
s.-o.-b. appearance
s.-o.-b. appearance of renal medial
  fibroplasia
s.-o.-b. sign
string-of-pearls
s.-o.-p. appearance of gastric body
s.-o.-p. sign
strip
Ames Hemastix reagent s.
Bio-Gen urine test s.
s. biopsy
s. biopsy resection technique
DisIntek reagent s.
ganglion-free muscle s.
Gore-Tex s.
PyloriTek reagent s.
s. resection
rhythm s.
roof s.
stripe
s. interstitial fibrosis
properitoneal flank s.
stripping
mucosal s.
urethral s.
stroke
saber s.
stroma, pl. **stromata**
fibroelastic connective tissue s.
fibrous s.
hyalinized s.
s. ovarii
prostate gland s.
stromal
s. invasion
s. tumor of unknown malignant
  potential (STUMP)
Strongyloides
S. stercoralis
S. venezuelensis
strongyloidiasis
strongyloid infection
strongyloma
strontium-89 chloride
structural
s. fatigue
s. stability
structure
biliary s.

S

NOTES

structure *(continued)*
 cord s.
 ductular s.
 glandular s.
 insular s.
 malignant nuclear s.
 mixed s.
 nociceptive s.
 seminiferous tubule peritubular s.
 trabecular s.
 undifferentiated s.
Structured and Scaled Interview to Assess Maladjustment (SSIAM)
Strulle scissors
struma, pl. **strumae**
 Hashimoto s.
 s. ovarii
strumous bubo
strut
 Mersilene s.
struvite
 s. calculus
 s. crystal formation
 s. stone
 s. urinary lithiasis
Stryker frame
STS
 serologic test for syphilis
 STS lithotripsy system
stuartii
 Providencia s.
Stucker bile duct dilator
studding
 omental s.
 peritoneal s.
Studer
 S. bladder substitute
 S. cross-folded ileal reservoir
 S. neobladder
 S. pouch
 S. pouch procedure
 S. reservoir urinary diversion
study
 AEC S.
 A28 immunological s.
 American Endosonography Club S.
 antegrade contrast s.
 anti-DNA immunological s.
 anti-ENA immunological s.
 antihepatitis A-IgM immunological s.
 antinuclear antibody immunological s.
 anti-SSA immunological s.
 anti-SSB immunological s.
 barium s.
 bead chain s.
 B12 immunological s.

 bladder outlet kinesiologic s.
 bulb-tip retrograde s.
 Candida immunological s.
 Celecoxib Long-Term Arthritis Safety S. (CLASS)
 C3 immunological s.
 cinefluorographic s.
 circulating immunocomplexes immunological s.
 Collaborative Transplant S. (CTS)
 colonic transit s.
 colon transit marker s.
 colorectal physiologic s.
 dark adaptation s.
 detrusor muscle pressure-flow micturition s.
 diisopropyliminodiacetic acid enterogastroesophageal reflux s.
 DISIDA enterogastroesophageal reflux s.
 diuretic renal quantitative camera s.
 DNCB immunological s.
 double-blind randomized s.
 dynamic urethral profile s.
 ESR immunological study immunological s.
 flow cytometric s.
 gene-blotting s.
 genitocerebral evoked potential s.
 HALT-C s.
 HBeAg immunological s.
 HBsAg immunological s.
 hematologic s.
 HLA typing immunological s.
 HOPE s.
 24-hour ambulatory manometry s.
 24-hour intraesophageal pH s.
 IgA immunological s.
 IgG immunological s.
 IgM immunological s.
 immunological s.
 Intergroup Rhabdomyosarcoma S. (IRS)
 intestinal transit s.
 isotope s.
 kinetic gallbladder s.
 light micrographic s.
 luminal contrast s.
 MACH1 s.
 manometric s.
 marker transit s.
 microperfusion s.
 mitochondrial immunological s.
 molecular s.
 multicenter s.
 Multicentre International Liver Tumor S. (MILTS)
 National Cooperative Dialysis S.

nerve conduction s.
nuclear-tagged red blood cell
  bleeding s.
observational followup s.
one-session crossover s.
ORCHID s.
peak urinary flow s.
perfusion s.
phenotypic s.
Physicians' Health S. I
Physicians' Health S. II (PSH II)
polarographic s.
positive secretin stimulation s.
PPD immunological s.
pressure s.
pressure-flow s. (PFS)
pressure-flow electromyography s.
pressure-flow micturition s.
prospective multicenter s.
radiological s.
radionuclide transit s.
Ramipril Efficacy in
  Nephropathy s.
rectosphincter manometric s.
REIN s.
renal function s. (RFS)
renal perfusion pressure-flow s.
retrograde contrast s.
retroperitoneal carbon dioxide
  insufflation s.
retrospective nature of the s.
scintigraphic emptying s.
seroepidemiological s.
single-color direct
  immunofluorescence s.
smooth-muscle immunological s.
split renal function s. (SRFS)
^{99m}Tc-phytate liquid state
  esophageal transit s.
Treponema immunofluorescence s.
T-tube s.
upper gastrointestinal barium
  roentgenographic s.
urodynamic flow s.
videoendoscopic swallowing s.
  (VESS)
videofluoroscopic swallow s.
videofluorourodynamic s.
voiding s.
Stühmer disease

STUMP
  stromal tumor of unknown malignant
    potential
stump
  appendiceal s.
  blind s.
  dehiscence of cystic s.
  duodenal s.
  funicular s.
  gastric s.
  s. invagination
  s. ligation
  polypectomy s.
  rectal s.
Sturge-Weber syndrome
stuttering
  s. priapism
  urinary s.
  s. urination
Stx
  Shiga toxin
  Stx 2-producing *Escherichia coli*
    strain (STEC)
Stylet internal esophageal MRI coil
styloglossus muscle
stylohyoid muscle
stylopharyngeus muscle
S-type amylase
Stypven time test
subacute
  s. abscess
  s. atrophy of liver
  s. cystitis
  s. fatty liver of pregnancy
  s. hepatic necrosis
  s. hepatitis
  s. liver disease
  s. liver failure (SALF)
  s. nephritis
  s. nonspecific peritonitis
subadventitial fibroplasia
subaponeurotic abscess
subarachnoid space
subareolar
subcapsular
  s. hematoma
  s. hemorrhage
  s. hepatic abscess
subcarinal node
subcecal appendix
subcholangiopancreatoscope

NOTES

S

subchronic
    s. atrophy of liver
    s. sacral neuromodulation
subcitrate
    colloidal bismuth s. (CBS)
subclavian
    s. catheter
    s. catheter insertion
    s. position
    s. vein
    s. vein catheterization
subclinical
    s. hepatic encephalopathy (SHE)
    s. hepatitis
    s. rejection
    s. sprue
subconjunctival hemorrhage
subcoronal hypospadias
subcostal
    s. flank incision
    s. margin
    s. nerve
    s. port
    s. transperitoneal incision
subcu, subq
    subcutaneous
subcutaneous (SC, subcu, subq)
    s. EGF
    s. emphysema
    s. fat
    s. layer
    s. morphine pump (SQMP)
    s. tissue
    s. urinary diversion
subcuticular suture
subdeterminant
    hepatitis B surface antigen s.
subdiaphragmatic abscess
subendoscope
subendothelial deposit
subepithelial
    s. deposit
    s. hematoma of the renal pelvis
    s. hemorrhage
subfertile
subfraction
    uremic serum s.
subfulminant liver failure
subglottic lesion
subhepatic
    s. abscess
    s. area
    s. space
subinguinalis
    fossa s.
subinguinal microsurgical
   varicocelectomy
subjective vertigo

sublingual hyoscyamine
submassive hepatic necrosis
submucosa
    small intestinal s.
submucosal
    s. arterial malformation
    s. artery
    s. calculus
    s. dissection
    s. endothelial angiodysplasia
    s. fat
    s. fibromuscular angiodysplasia
    s. gastric hemorrhage
    s. ileal lipoma
    s. mass
    s. saline injection
    s. saline injection technique
    s. tattoo
    s. Teflon injection
    s. thickening
    s. track
    s. upper gastrointestinal tract lesion
    s. vaginal muscle
    s. vaginal smooth musculofascial
    layer
    s. vascular dilation
    s. vascular malformation
    s. venous plexus
    s. wound
submucous
    s. cystitis
    s. layer
    s. plexus
    s. stratum
    s. ulcer
submuscular plexus
subparta
    ileus s.
subperitoneal
    s. abscess
    s. appendicitis
    s. fascia
    s. space
subphrenic
    s. abscess
    s. space
subpubic sinus
subq (var. of subcu)
Subrini penile prosthesis
subsalicylate
    bismuth s.
subscapular
subsegmentectomy
    hepatic s.
subserosal
    s. calbindin
    s. disease
    s. layer

subserous
    s. fascia
    s. ganglia
    s. tunnel
subsigmoid fossa
substaging
    pathologic s.
substance
    s. abuse
    s. A, K, S
    caustic s.
    hepatic stimulatory s. (HSS)
    noncholecystokinin s.
    ouabainlike s. (OLS)
    s. P (SP)
    reducing s.
substitute
    ileal orthotopic bladder s.
    low pressure bladder s.
    Olestra fat s.
    saliva s.
    Studer bladder s.
substituted benzimidazole
substitution
    bladder s.
    ileal ureteral s.
    orthotopic bladder s.
    s. urethroplasty
substrate
    copolymerized s.
    s. oxidation
substratum
    cell s.
subsymphyseal epispadias
subtotal
    s. colectomy
    s. gastrectomy
    s. gastric exclusion
    s. pancreatectomy
    s. villous atrophy (SVA)
subtraction angiography
subtrigonal cystectomy
subtunical venule
subtype
    HBsAg s.
subtyping
    HLA-DR2 s.
subumbilical space
subureteric Teflon injection (STING)
suburethral
    s. rectus fascial sling procedure
    s. sling

suburothelial
    s. infiltrative cancer
    s. nerve plexus
    s. vascular bed
subvesical duct
subxiphoid
Suby G solution
subzonal insemination (SUZI)
succagogue
succimer
succinate
    s. dehydrogenase activity (SDH)
    sumatriptan s.
succinylcholine
succorrhea
succulent mesenteric lymph node
succus
    s. entericus
    s. gastricus
    s. pancreaticus
succuss
succussion
    hippocratic s.
    s. sound
    s. splash
suck-and-cut
    s.-a.-c. method
    s.-a.-c. mucosectomy
    s.-a.-c. technique
sucker
    tonsil s.
sucralfate
    s. retention enema
    s. therapy
sucrase-isomaltase (SI)
sucrose-free (SF)
sucrose-isomaltase deficiency
sucrose tolerance test
suction
    s. banding
    s. biopsy
    bulb s.
    S. Buster catheter
    s. channel
    continuous NG s.
    s. cylinder
    s. drain
    s. drainage
    flexible dental s.
    s. foot pedal
    Gomco s.
    Harris tube s.

S

NOTES

suction *(continued)*
>lavage and s.
>low intermittent s.
>nasogastric s.
>NG s.
>S. oral brush
>s. pump
>s. tip
>s. tube
>Wangensteen s.

suction-coagulator
>Cameron-Miller s.-c.

suctioning
>intermittent s.

Suda classification of papilla (type I, II, III)

Sudan
>S. black B fat stain

Sudan-III stain

sudden
>s. onset of pain
>s. valve prolapse

Sudeck
>S. atrophy
>S. critical point

sufentanil

sugar
>s. oxime
>s. test

Sugarbaker technique

sugar-free
>Citrucel s.-f.

Sugiura
>S. esophageal variceal transection
>S. paraesophagogastric
>devascularization
>S. procedure

SUI
>stress urinary incontinence

suite
>endoscopy s.

sulbactam
>s. sodium

sulciform

sulcus, pl. **sulci**
>coronal s.
>costovertebral s.
>intersphincteric s.
>s. of umbilical vein

sulfa

sulfacytine

sulfadiazine

sulfamethizole

sulfamethoprim

sulfamethoxazole
>s. and phenazopyridine

>s. and trimethoprim (SMX/TMP, SMZ/TMP)
>trimethoprim-s. (TMP-SMX)

Sulfamylon

sulfanilamide

sulfasalazine enema

sulfasalazine-induced oxidative hemolysis

sulfasoxazole

sulfate
>atropine s.
>barium s.
>bleomycin s.
>dehydroepiandrosterone s. (DHAS)
>dermatan s.
>dextran sodium s. (DSS)
>ephedrine s.
>ferrous s.
>gentamicin s.
>hydrazine s.
>hyoscyamine s.
>pentosan s.
>protamine s.
>quinidine s.
>sodium dodecyl s. (SDS)
>sodium tetradecyl s.
>tetradecyl s.

sulfated
>s. glycoprotein-2 (SGP-2)
>s. mucin stain

sulfation
>tyrosine s.

Sulfatrim DS

sulfhydryl

sulfinpyrazone

sulfisoxazole and phenazopyridine

sulfolithocholylglycine

sulfolithocholyltaurine

sulfomucin
>acidic s.

sulfonamide nephropathy

sulfonate
>mercaptoethane s.
>polystyrene sodium s.
>sodium polystyrene s.

sulfone syndrome

sulfoxide
>dimethyl s. (DMSO)

sulfur
>s. amino acid metabolism
>s. colloid (SC)
>s. colloid liver scan

sulfuric acid

sulglycotide

sulindac

Sulkowitch test

sulmarin

sulotroban

sulphydryl donor

sulpiride
sumatriptan succinate
Sumikoshi classification
summer
    s. cholera
    s. diarrhea
summit of bladder
Sumner
    S. method
    S. sign
sump
    s. drain
    s. nasogastric tube
    s. syndrome
    s. ulcer
Sumycin Oral
SUN
    serum urea nitrogen
superantigen
Super-Bright microsphere
SuperChar
Super-Cut scissors
superfibronectin
superficial
    s. bladder cancer
    s. depressed cancer
    s. esophageal carcinoma (SEC)
    s. fascia
    s. fluorescein
    s. gastric carcinoma
    s. gastritis
    s. inguinal pouch
    s. linear ulcer
    s. perineal aponeurosis
    s. perineal space
    s. trigonal muscle
    s. tumor
superficialis
    arteria epigastrica s.
    colitis cystica s.
    esophagitis dissecans s.
    fascia penis s.
superficially spreading carcinoma
superimposed alcoholic hepatitis
superinfection
    delta hepatitis s.
    hepatitis D s.
superior
    arteria epigastrica s.
    arteria mesenterica s.
    arteria rectalis s.
    ductulus aberrans s.

    s. duodenal fold
    s. extremity
    fascia diaphragmatis pelvis s.
    flexura duodeni s.
    s. hemorrhoidal artery
    s. hypogastric nerve plexus
    s. margin
    s. mesenteric angiography
    s. mesenteric arteriogram
    s. mesenteric artery (SMA)
    s. mesenteric artery syndrome
      (SMAS)
    s. mesenteric-to renal artery
      saphenous vein bypass graft
    s. mesenteric vein (SMV)
    s. mesenterorenal bypass
    s. mesenterorenal bypass technique
    s. pubic ramotomy
    s. rectal vein
    s. rectal venous plexus
    s. vesical artery
supernatant
supernumerary kidney
superoxide
    s. dismutase (SOD)
    extracellular s.
    s. production
    s. radical
Super PEG tube
supersaturated bile
supersaturation
    cystine s.
    relative s. (RSs)
    urine s.
superselective
    s. arteriography
    s. transcatheter embolization
    s. vagotomy
supination
supine position
supper
    fat-free s. (FFS)
supplement
    caloric s.
    Cal Power calorie s.
    Casec calcium s.
    Case Power protein s.
    Dent s.
    Enrich protein and calorie s.
    food s.
    Hy-Cal calorie s.
    Impact nutritional s.

S

NOTES

supplement *(continued)*
    keto acid-amino acid s.
    Nepro diet s.
    Polycose glucose s.
    protein s.
    Spirulina Pacifica nutritional s.
    Travasorb MCT s.
supplementation
    calcium s.
    citrate s.
    dietary s.
    fish oil s.
    prostaglandin s.
    vitamin D s.
support
    artificial hepatic s.
    bladder s.
    nutritional s.
    s. parenteral nutrition (SPN)
    psychological s.
    psychosexual s.
supportive treatment
suppository
    alprostadil urethral s.
    B&O s.
    Canasa s.
    Compro s.
    glycerin s.
    intraurethral prostaglandin s. (IPS)
    mesalamine rectal s.
    MUSE urethral s.
    prochlorperazine 25-mg s.
    rectal s.
    vaginal s.
suppression
    acid s.
    androgen s.
    cell-mediated s.
    hypothalamic s.
    immune s.
    metastasis s.
    s. treatment
    urinary tract infection s.
suppressive
    s. anuria
    s. maneuver
suppressor
    s. gene
    s. T cell
suppuration
suppurativa
    hidradenitis s.
suppurative
    s. appendicitis
    s. appendix
    s. cholangitis
    s. cortical nephritis
    s. gastritis

supraceliac aorta
supraclavicular
supracolic compartment
supracostal incision
supradiaphragmatic diverticulum
supraduodenal approach
Supra-Foley catheter
supragastric bursoscopy
supraglottic squamous cell carcinoma
suprahepatic
    s. abscess
    s. caval cuff
    s. space
    s. vena cava
suprahilar
    s. disease
    s. lymph node dissection
suprainguinal region
supralevator
    s. anorectal space
    s. pelvic exenteration
    s. perirectal abscess
Supramid suture
supraomental space
suprapapillary
    s. fistula
    s. Roux-en-Y duodenojejunostomy
supraphysiological fundoplication
supraprostatectomy
suprapubic
    s. aspiration
    s. aspiration of the bladder
    s. cystography
    s. cystostomy
    s. cystotomy
    s. cystotomy tract urethral atresia
    s. lithotomy
    s. port
    s. prostatectomy
    s. puncture
    s. region
    s. tube
suprarenal
    s. area of liver
    s. gland
    s. Greenfield filter
    s. impression
    s. medulla
    s. plexus
suprarenale
    melasma s.
suprarenalectomy
suprarenalis
    cortex glandulae s.
    medulla glandulae s.
suprarenalism
suprarenalopathy
suprarenogenic syndrome

suprasphincteric fistula
supratrigonal cystectomy
supravesical urinary diversion
suprazonal part of anal canal
sural nerve graft
suramin
SureBite biopsy forceps
Sure-Cut biopsy needle
Sureseal pressure bandage
Suretys
    S. incontinence brief
    S. pants
    S. panty system
surface
    antimesenteric s.
    biomaterial s.
    bosselated s.
    cholesterolosis of mucosal s.
    colonic mucosal s.
    s. cooling
    s. cooling technique
    depression s.
    s. electrode
    s. epithelium
    s. nodularity
    s. nodule
    s. pelvic floor electromyography
    s. protein
    serosal s.
    s. thermometer
    urethral-cooling s.
    ventral s.
surface-to-volume ratio
surfactant laxative
Surfak
Sur-Fit
    S.-F. auto lock closed-end pouch with filter
    S.-F. Mini pouch
    S.-F. Natura closed-end pouch, opaque
    S.-F. Natura disposable convex insert
    S.-F. Natura flange cap
    S.-F. Natura flexible wafer and drainable pouch
    S.-F. Natura irrigation adapter face plate
    S.-F. Natura irrigation sleeve
    S.-F. Natura irrigation sleeve tail closure
    S.-F. Natura loop ostomy rod

    S.-F. Natura night drainage container set
    S.-F. Natura night drainage container tubing
    S.-F. Natura opaque closed-end pouch with filter
    S.-F. Natura urostomy pouch
    S.-F. Natura Visi-Flow irrigation
    S.-F. Natura Visi-Flow irrigation starter set
    S.-F. Pouch cover
    S.-F. stoma cap
Surgaloy suture
Surgenomic endoscope
surgeon
    genitourinary s.
    Society of American Gastrointestinal Endoscoping S.'s (SAGES)
surgeon's knot
surgery
    adrenal-sparing s.
    anal s.
    anorectal s.
    antireflux s.
    bariatric s.
    bench s.
    biliopancreatic obesity s.
    colorectal s. (CRS)
    concomitant antireflux s.
    cytoreductive s.
    diagnostic s.
    dialysis access s.
    extracorporeal s.
    feminizing s.
    flank s.
    gastric bypass s.
    hand-assisted laparoscopic s. (HALS)
    intestinal s.
    jejunoileal bypass s.
    laparoscopic adrenal gland s.
    laparoscopic antireflux s. (LARS)
    laparoscopic colorectal cancer s.
    laser s.
    major GI s.
    minimal access s.
    nephron-sparing s.
    nonbench s.
    palliative s.
    parenchymal sparing s.

S

NOTES

surgery *(continued)*
   Parietex composite mesh for
      hernia s.
   pelvic colonic s.
   penile venous ligation s.
   PlasmaKinetic s.
   portosystemic shunt s.
   primary perineal hypospadias s.
   radical s.
   radioimmunoguided s. (RIGS)
   rectovaginal s.
   renal-sparing s.
   retrograde intrarenal s.
   retroperitoneal s.
   reversal jejunoileal bypass s.
   salvage s.
   secondary s.
   sham s.
   stone s.
   TAAA s.
   telerobotic-assisted laparoscopic s.
   thoracoabdominal aortic aneurysm s.
   transsexual s.
   urologic s.
   vascular s.
   video-assisted thoracic s. (VATS)
   weight reduction s.
surgical
   s. abdomen
   s. care
   s. cystgastrostomy
   s. decompression
   s. drain
   s. drape
   s. extirpation
   s. flap
   s. incision
   s. loupe
   s. portosystemic shunting
   s. procedure
   s. scissors
   s. stapling
   s. stress
   s. therapy
   s. vagotomy
**surgically implanted hemodialysis
   catheter (SIHC)**
Surgicel gauze
Surgilube lubricant
**Surgi-PEG replacement gastrostomy
   feeding system**
Surgipro
   S. mesh
   S. suture
SurgiSis sling/mesh
Surgitek
   S. button
   S. catheter

   S. Flexi-Flate II penile implant
   S. graduated cystocope GC-16
   S. graduated cystoscope
   S. One-Step (SOS)
   S. One-Step percutaneous
      endoscopic gastrostomy
   S. Tractfinder ureteral stent
   S. Uropass stent
Surgitite ligating loop
Surgiwip suture ligature
surreptitious vomiting
surrogate marker
surveillance
   s. colonoscopy
   s. cystogram
   endoscopic s.
   s. endoscopy
   S., Epidemiology, and End Results
      (SEER)
   s. protocol
survey
   metabolic bone s.
   National Health and Nutrition
      Examination S. (NHANES)
survival
   allograft s.
   s. analysis
   graft s.
   improved graft s.
   mean allograft s. (MAS)
   overall s. (OS)
   s. rate
Susano Elixir
susceptibility
   genetic s.
   higher host s.
   LDL s.
   low-density lipoprotein s.
Suspend sling
suspension
   barium sulfate for s.
   bladder neck s. (BNS)
   Burch iliopectineal ligament
      urethrovesical s.
   charcoal s.
   colloidal bismuth s.
   extraperitoneal laparoscopic bladder
      neck s. (ELBNS)
   Gadolite oral s.
   Gittes bladder neck s.
   Gittes-Loughlin bladder neck s.
   laparoscopic bladder neck s.
   modified Pereyra bladder neck s.
   mycophenolate mofetil oral s.
   needle bladder neck s.
   Nephrox S.
   nystatin s.
   octreotide acetate for injectable s.

OK432 streptococcal s.
oral barium s.
percutaneous bladder neck s.
 (PBNS)
Pereyra bladder neck s.
Raz bladder neck s.
Raz four-quadrant s.
Raz needle bladder s.
Raz urethral s.
retropubic Lapides-Ball bladder
 neck s.
Stamey needle bladder neck s.
urethral s.
vesicoureteral s.
vesicourethral s.

suspensory
s. bandage
s. ligament
s. muscle

Sustacal
S. HC liquid feeding
S. pudding

Sustagen liquid feeding
sustained low-efficiency dialysis (SLED)
suture
absorbable s.
Albert s.
Albert-Lembert s.
anastomotic s.
anchoring s.
Appolito s.
approximation s.
atraumatic s.
Bell s.
black silk s. (BSS)
bolster s.
s. bridge
buried s.
button s.
cardinal s.
chain s.
chromic catgut s.
chromic gut s.
circular s.
Connell s.
continuous s.
corner s.
cotton s.
Cushing s.
s. cutter
Czerny s.
Czerny-Lembert s.

Dacron s.
dermal s.
Dermalene s.
Dermalon s.
Dexon s.
Dupuytren s.
Endoloop s.
Ethibond s.
Ethiflex s.
Ethilon s.
everting s.
s. fatigue
figure-of-eight s.
furrier s.
Gambee s.
Gould inverted mattress s.
s. granuloma
green Mersilene s.
s. guide
Gussenbauer s.
Halsted interrupted mattress s.
Halsted interrupted quilt s.
heavy silk s.
hemostatic s.
horizontal mattress s.
Horsley s.
interrupted manual mucomucosal
 absorbable s.
interrupted seromuscular s.
intracuticular s.
intradermal s.
inverting s.
Ivalon s.
Jobert de Lamballe s.
Kessler-Kleinert s.
Lembert inverting seromuscular s.
s. ligated
s. ligature
s. line
s. line dehiscence
s. line ulceration
locking s.
lock-stitch s.
loop s.
Marshall U-stitch s.
s. material
mattress s.
Maxon s.
Mersilene s.
Monocryl s.
monofilament absorbable s.
monofilament nylon s.

NOTES

suture *(continued)*
    nonabsorbable s.
    over-and-over s.
    Parker-Kerr s.
    PDS Vicryl s.
    pericostal s.
    Perma-hand silk s.
    plain catgut s.
    plain gut s.
    s. plication
    plication s.
    Polydek s.
    polydioxanone s.
    polyglactin s.
    polyglecaprone 25 s.
    polyglycolic acid s.
    polyglyconate s.
    polypropylene s.
    pop-off s.
    primary s.
    Prolene s.
    purse-string, pursestring s.
    quilted s.
    s. rectopexy
    s. rectopexy with sigmoid resection
    reinforcing s.
    relaxation s.
    retention s.
    running s.
    s. scissors
    secondary s.
    seromuscular Lembert s.
    silk Mersilene s.
    silk pop-off s.
    silk traction s.
    stainless steel s.
    stay s.
    subcuticular s.
    Supramid s.
    Surgaloy s.
    Surgipro s.
    swaged-on s.
    Teflon-coated Dacron s.
    Tevdek s.
    Ti-Cron s.
    Tom Jones s.
    traction s.
    transition s.
    s. ulcer
    vascular s.
    vertical mattress s.
    vertical plication s.
    Vicryl s.
    Z s.
sutured hemorrhoidectomy
sutureless
    s. biofragmentable ring

    s. bowel anastomosis
    s. colostomy closure
suture-release needle
suturing
    transoral endoscopic s.
    transvaginal s. (TVS)
SUZI
    subzonal insemination
SVA
    subtotal villous atrophy
SVG
    seminal vesiculography
SVO
    splenic vein obstruction
SVR
    systemic vascular resistance
SVRI
    systemic vascular resistance index
swab
    urethral s.
swaged needle
swaged-on
    s.-o. needle
    s.-o. suture
swallow
    s. apraxia
    barium s.
    dry s.
    Gastrografin s.
    Hypaque s.
    ice-water s.
    modified barium s. (MBS)
    water-soluble contrast esophageal s.
    wet s.
swallowed string
swallowing
    air s.
    s. center
    four phases of s.
    s. mechanism
    s. reflex
    s. threshold
Swan-Ganz pulmonary artery catheter
swan-neck
    s.-n. deformity
    s.-n. Missouri catheter
    s.-n. pediatric Coil-Cath catheter
SW 480 cell
sweating
    gustatory s.
sweat test
Swedish
    S. Adjustable Gastric Band
      (SAGB)
    S. Rectal Cancer Trial
Sween
    S. Cream

S. Micro Guard powder
S. Prep
Sween-A-Peel skin barrier
sweep
    duodenal s.
Sweet
    S. esophageal scissors
    S. syndrome
swelling
    cell s.
    external s.
    genital s.
    lysosomal s.
    popliteal s.
    scrotal s.
    testicular s.
    uvular s.
Swenson
    S. abdominal pull-through
    S. operation
    S. papillotome
swimmer's itch
swim-up processing
Swiss
    S. Lithoclast
    S. lithoclast lithotriptor
    S. roll embedding technique
switch
    duodenal s.
    optical s.
swivel adapter
SWL
    shock wave lithotripsy
swollen
    s. tongue
    s. turbinate
Swyer syndrome
SXPL
    strictureplasty
Sydney
    S. classification of gastritis
    S. system
    S. system gastritis classification
Syllact
sylvian fistula
symbolic stimulus
Syme external urethrotomy
Symington body
Symlin
Symmetra I-125 brachytherapy seed
symmetric face movement
Symmetry endo-bipolar generator

sympathetic
    s. chain
    s. cystitis
    s. enteroenteric inhibitory reflex
    s. nervous system (SNS)
    s. nervous system activity
    s. projection
    s. response to vasodilation
    s. skin response
    s. sphincter constrictor reflex
symphyseal bar
symphysis
    s. ossium pubis
    pubic s.
    s. pubica syndrome
Symphytum
symptom
    alarm s.
    alcohol-induced gastrointestinal s.
    Candida s.
    chronic functional gastrointestinal s.
    s. control
    extraesophageal s.
    s. free
    head s.
    incarceration s.
    intradialytic s.
    irritative s.
    lower urinary tract s. (LUTS)
    postcibal s.
    s. problem index (SPI)
    prodromal s.
    respiratory s. (RS)
    s. score
    s. sensitivity index
    s. severity index (SSI)
    target s.
    tuberculosis s.
    urinary urge s.
    urologic s.
symptomatic
    s. benign prostatic hyperplasia
    s. benign prostatic hypertrophy
    s. fluid gain
    s. gallstone
    s. impotence
    s. varicocele
symptomatology
    chronic functional s.
symptom-giving PGR
Syms tractor
Synalar Topical

S

NOTES

Synalgos-DC Capsules
synapse
  axoaxonic s.
synaptic transmission
synaptogenesis
synchondroseotomy
SynchroMed infusion system intraspinal catheter
SYNCHRON CX-5, CX-7 automated analyzer
synchronous
  s. adenoma
  s. bladder reconstruction
  s. inferior cavography
  s. lesion
  s. neonatal torsion
  s. polyp
  s. superior cavography
  s. urinary tract infection
syncongestive appendicitis
syncope
  defecation s.
syncytia
Synder drain
syndrome
  Aagenaes s.
  Aarskog s.
  Aarskog-Scott s.
  abdominal compartment s. (ACS)
  abdominal cutaneous nerve entrapment s.
  abdominal muscle deficiency s.
  acquired immunodeficiency s. (AIDS)
  acute flank pain s.
  acute urethral s.
  Adamantiades-Behçet s.
  Addison s.
  addisonian s.
  adrenogenital s.
  adult respiratory distress s.
  afferent loop s.
  Alagille s.
  Alagille-Watson s.
  Albright s.
  Alcock s.
  Allemann s.
  Allen-Masters s.
  Alport s.
  Alstrom-Edwards s.
  Andersen s.
  androgen insensitivity s.
  androgenital s.
  anorexia-cachexia s.
  anterior abdominal wall s.
  anterior cord s.
  anterior rib impingement s.
  anterior spinal artery s.

antiandrogen withdrawal s.
anticardiolipin antibody s.
antimüllerian derivative s.
antiphospholipid s.
Apert s.
apparent mineral corticoid excess s.
apple-peel bowel s.
Arias s.
Asherson s.
asplenia s.
autoimmune deficiency s.
autosomal-recessive Alport s.
bacterial overgrowth s.
Bannayan-Zonana s.
Banti s.
Bardet-Biedl s.
Barrett s.
Barsony-Polgar s.
Bartter s.
basal cell nevus s.
Bassen-Kornzweig s.
Baumgarten s.
Bazex s.
Bearn-Kunkel-Slater s.
Beckwith-Wiedemann s.
Behçet s.
bent nail s.
Bernard-Sergent s.
Bernard-Soulier s.
Bessauds-Hilmand-Augier s.
bilharzial bladder cancer s.
Blatin s.
bleomycin-associated adult respiratory distress s.
blind loop s. (BLS)
blue diaper s.
blue rubber bleb nevus s.
blue toe s.
Boerhaave s.
Bouveret s.
bowel bypass s.
branchio-oto-renal s. (BOR)
Brennemann s.
brown bowel s. (BBS)
Budd-Chiari s.
Bürger-Grütz s.
buried bumper s.
Burnett s.
burning feet s.
burning mouth s. (BMS)
Byler s.
Bywaters s.
Cacchi-Ricci s.
cafe coronary s.
Canada-Cronkhite s.
cancer family s.
carcinoid s.
Carignan s.

Carney s.
Caroli s.
Carpenter s.
Carter-Horsley-Hughes s.
cast s.
cat-eye s.
cauda equina s.
caudal regression s.
Cecil urethral stricture s.
cerebrohepatorenal s. (CHRS)
cerebrooculofacial s.
Charcot s.
CHARGE s.
Cheek-Perry s.
Chilaiditi s.
Chinese restaurant s. (CRS)
s. of chloride depletion
cholestatic s.
cholesterol emboli s.
cholinergic s.
chronic intestinal ischemic s.
chronic intestinal
  pseudoobstruction s.
chronic pelvic pain s. (CPPS)
chronic prostate pain s. (CPPS)
chronic prostatitis/pelvic pain s.
  (CPPS)
chronic urethral s.
Churg-Strauss s.
Clarke-Hadfield s.
Cohen s.
colonic polyposis s.
colonic pseudo-obstruction s.
colonic solitary ulcer s.
colorectal cancer s.
compression s.
congenital nephrotic s. (CNS)
Conn s.
constipation predominant irritable
  bowel s.
constipation-predominant irritable
  bowel s.
Cooke-Apert-Gallais s.
Cornelia de Lange s.
Courvoisier-Terrier s.
couvade s.
Cowden s.
Cowen s.
CREST s.
cri du chat s.
Crigler-Najjar s. (type I, II)
Cronkhite-Canada s.

CRST s.
crush s.
Cruveilhier-Baumgarten s.
Curran s.
Cushing medicamentosus s.
cyclic vomiting s. (CVS)
Danbolt-Closs s.
Debré-de Toni-Fanconi s.
Degos s.
Dejerine-Sottas s.
del Castillo s.
Denys-Drash s. (DDS)
descending perineum s.
de Toni-Debré-Fanconi s.
de Toni-Fanconi-Debré s.
dialysis disequilibrium s.
dialysis encephalopathy s.
dialysis equilibrium s.
diarrhea-predominant irritable
  bowel s.
diencephalic s.
diffuse alveolar hemorrhage s.
DiGeorge s.
Diogenes s.
Down s.
Drash s.
Dubin-Johnson s.
Dubin-Sprinz s.
Dubowitz s.
dumping s.
dyskinetic cilia s.
dysmetabolic s.
dysuria-pyuria s.
Eagle-Barrett s.
Edwards s.
efferent loop s.
Ehlers-Danlos s.
Ellis-van Creveld s.
empty sella s.
encephalotrigeminal s.
eosinophilic gastroenteritis s.
Epstein s.
Faber s.
faciodigital s.
familial atypical multiple mole
  melanoma s.
familial polyposis s.
FAMM s.
Fanconi s.
Fanconi-de Toni-Debre s.
fatty liver and kidney s. (FLKS)
Fechtner s.

S

NOTES

729

syndrome *(continued)*

Felty s.
female urethral s.
fertile eunuch s.
Fiessinger-Leroy-Reiter s.
Fitz s.
Fitz-Hugh and Curtis s.
Flood s.
flulike s.
flushing s.
Fraley s.
Fraser s.
frequency-urgency-pain s.
Friderichsen-Waterhouse s.
Fröhlich s.
functional bowel s.
G s.
Galloway-Mowat s. (GMS)
Gardner s. (GS)
Gardner-Diamond s.
gas-bloat s.
Gasser s.
gasserian s.
gastrocardiac s.
gastrointestinal immunodeficiency s.
gastrojejunal loop obstruction s.
GAVE s.
gay bowel s.
Gee-Herter-Heubner s.
Gianotti-Crosti s.
Gilbert s.
Gilbert-Behçet s.
Gilbert-Dreyfus s.
Gitelman s.
Glenard s.
glioma-polyposis s.
glucagonoma s.
Goldenhar s.
Goldston s.
Goodpasture s.
Gopalan s.
Gordon s.
Gorlin basal cell nevus s.
Gorlin-Chaudhry-Moss s.
Gowers s.
Guillain-Barré s.
gynecomastia-aspermatogenesis s.
Hadefield-Clarke s.
Hadju-Cheney acroosteolysis s.
Hanot s.
Hanot-Chauffard s.
Hanot-Rössle s.
Hartnup s.
Hawes-Pallister-Landor s.
Heller-Nelson s.
HELLP s.
hematuria-dysuria s.
hemolytic-uremic s. (HUS)

hepatonephoric s.
hepatopulmonary s. (HPS)
hepatorenal s. (HRS)
hereditary flat adenoma s. (HFAS)
hereditary nonpolyposis colorectal
    cancer s.
Hermansky-Pudlak s.
Heyde s.
Hinman s.
Hinman-Allen s.
Hippel-Lindau s.
Holt-Oram s.
hormone-secreting tumor s.
Horner s.
Howel-Evans s.
HPRC s.
hungry bone s.
hyperammonemic s.
hyperdynamic s.
hypereosinophilia s.
hypertensive lower esophageal
    sphincter s.
hypoperistalsis s.
iatrogenic immunodeficiency s.
idiopathic hypereosinophilic s.
    (IHES)
idiopathic nephrotic s.
ileocecal s.
Imerslund s.
immotile cilia s.
impaired regeneration s. (IRS)
s. of inappropriate antidiuretic
    hormone secretion (SIADH)
infantile nephrotic s.
inflammatory bowel s. (IBS)
infrequent voider-lazy bladder s.
inhibitory s.
inspissated bile s.
inspissated sump s.
insulin resistance s.
intestinal polyposis-cutaneous
    pigmentation s.
irrigation fluid absorption s.
irritable bowel s. (IBS)
irritable colon s.
irritable gut s.
isolated retained antrum s.
Ivemark s.
Jadassohn s.
Jamaican vomiting s.
jejunal s.
Jeune s.
Job s.
Johanson-Blizzard s.
Joseph s.
Joubert s.
juvenile polyposis s. (JPS)
Kallmann s.

Karroo s.
Kartagener s.
Katayama s.
Kaufman s.
Kawasaki s.
Kearns-Sayre s. (KSS)
Kimmelstiel-Wilson s.
Klinefelter s.
Klippel-Trenaunay-Weber s.
Koenig s.
Koro s.
Korsakoff s.
Kunkel s.
Labbe s.
Ladd s.
Lambert-Eaton myasthenic s.
late dumping s.
Laubry-Soulle s.
Launois-Cléret s.
Laurence-Moon-Bardet-Biedl s.
Laurence-Moon-Biedl s.
lazy bladder s.
LEOPARD s.
Leriche s.
Lesch-Nyhan s.
levator ani s.
Liddle s.
Li-Fraumeni s.
Lightwood s.
Lignac s.
Lignac-Fanconi s.
locker room s.
Loeffler s.
loin pain hematuria s. (LPHS)
Lowe s.
Lubb s.
Lucey-Driscoll s.
Luder-Sheldon s.
Lyell s.
lymphadenopathy s. (LAS)
lymphoproliferative s.
Lynch s. (I, II)
Mad Hatter s.
Maffucci s.
malabsorption s.
maldigestion-absorption s.
male Turner s.
malignant B-cell s.
malignant carcinoid s.
Mallory-Weiss s.
Maranon s.
Marchiafava-Micheli s.

Marfan s.
Marinesco-Sjögren s.
massive bowel resection s.
Mayer-Rokitansky s.
Mayer-Rokitansky-Kuster-Hauser s.
McArdle s.
McCune-Albright s.
Meckel s.
Meckel-Gruber s.
meconium plug s.
megacystic s.
megacystis-megaureter s.
megacystis-microcolon-intestinal
    hypoperistalsis s.
megasigmoid s.
Meigs s.
Melkersson-Rosenthal s.
MEN I s.
Menkes s.
mesenteric steal s.
metastatic carcinoid s.
microscopic colitis s.
milk-alkali s.
Miller Fisher s.
mind-bladder s.
minimal-change nephrotic s.
minimal-lesion nephrotic s.
Mirizzi s.
Mosse s.
Muckle-Wells s.
mucocutaneous pigmentation of
    Peutz-Jeghers s.
mucosal prolapse s.
Muir-Torre s.
müllerian duct derivation s.
multiple endocrine neoplasia s.
    (MENS)
multiple hamartoma s.
multiple organ failure s.
Munchausen s.
myoclonus-opsoclonus s.
nail-patella s.
narcotic bowel s.
necrolytic migratory erythema s.
Nelson s.
nephritic s.
nephrotic s.
nerve entrapment s.
Neu-Laxova s.
neurocutaneous s.
Nonnenbruch s.
Noonan s.

NOTES

S

syndrome *(continued)*

obesity hypoventilation s. (OHS)
Ochoa s.
oculocerebrorenal s.
Ogilvie s.
Oldfield s.
Opitz-Frias s.
Ormond s.
Osler s. II
Osler-Weber-Rendu s.
osmotic demyelination s.
outlier s.
ovarian hyperstimulation s.
ovarian overstimulation s.
ovarian remnant s.
ovarian vein s.
overlap s.
pain-predominant irritable bowel s.
pancreatic cholera s.
pancreaticohepatic s.
paraneoplastic s.
Paterson-Brown-Kelly s.
Paterson-Kelly s.
Payr s.
Pearson s.
pelvic floor s.
Pento-X s.
pericolic membrane s.
perihepatitis s.
persistent müllerian duct s.
Peutz-Jeghers s. (PJS)
pharyngeal pouch s.
Picchini s.
pickwickian s.
Plummer-Vinson s.
POEMS s.
Poland s.
Polhemus-Schafer-Ivemark s.
POLIP s.
polyposis s.
polysplenia s.
postcholecystectomy s. (PCS)
postcoagulation s.
postcolonoscopy distention s.
postenteritis s.
postfundoplication s.
postgastrectomy s.
postpolypectomy coagulation s.
postthrombotic s.
posttransurethral microwave
  thermotherapy prostatitis-like s.
post-TUMT prostatitis-like s.
postvagotomy s.
Potter s.
Prader-Willi s.
primary antiphospholipid s.
s. of primary biliary cirrhosis
primary pseudoobstruction s.

prune-belly s. (category I, II, III)
pseudo-Cushing s.
pseudoobstruction s.
pseudopancreatic cholera s.
pseudo-prune-belly s.
puborectalis s.
Rapunzel s.
refeeding s.
Reichmann s.
Reifenstein s.
Reiter s.
renal Fanconi-like s.
renal-hepatic steal s.
renal-ocular s.
renal-retinal s.
Rendu-Osler-Weber s.
reset osmostat s.
respiratory distress s.
restless leg s.
retained antrum s.
retained bladder s.
reuse s.
reversed anorexia s.
Reye s.
Richner-Hanhart s.
Rieger s.
right ovarian vein s.
Riley-Day s.
RMS s.
Roberts s.
Robinow s.
Roger s.
Rokitansky-Kuster-Hauser s.
Rosewater s.
Rothmund-Thomson s.
Rotor s.
Roux stasis s.
Rovsing s.
Rubinstein-Taybi s.
Rud s.
rudimentary testis s.
runting s.
Russell-Silver s.
Ruvalcaba-Myhre-Smith s.
Sandifer s.
Schmidt s.
Schultz s.
Schwachman s.
Schwartz-Jampel s.
SCO s.
sea-blue histiocyte s.
Seckel s.
secondary pseudoobstruction s.
segmental colonic adenomatous
  polyposis s.
Senior-Loken s.
sepsis s.
Sertoli-cell-only s.

sex reversal s.
Sézary s.
short-bowel s.
short-gut s.
Shwachman s.
Shwachman-Diamond s.
Shy-Drager s.
sicca s.
sick cell s.
Sipple s.
Sjögren s. (SS)
sleep apnea s.
sloughed urethra s.
small stomach s.
Smith-Lemli-Opitz s.
solitary rectal ulcer s. (SRUS)
solitary ulcer s.
somatostatinoma s.
spastic bowel s.
spastic pelvic floor s.
sphincteric disobedience s.
Spitzer-Weinstein s.
splenic agenesis s.
splenic flexure s.
Sprinz-Dubin s.
Sprinz-Nelson s.
stagnant loop s.
stasis s.
Stauffer s.
steakhouse s.
Stein-Leventhal s.
steroid-resistant nephrotic s.
Stevens-Johnson s. (SJS)
Stewart-Treves s.
stiff-man s.
Stokvis-Talma s.
Strachan s.
Strachan-Scott s.
stress-related erosive s.
Sturge-Weber s.
sulfone s.
sump s.
superior mesenteric artery s.
  (SMAS)
suprarenogenic s.
Sweet s.
Swyer s.
symphysis pubica s.
systemic inflammatory response s.
  (SIRS)
Takayasu s.
TAR s.

terminal reservoir s.
testicular feminization s.
tethered-cord s. (TCS)
Thorn salt-depletion s.
three-week sulfasalazine s.
thrombocytopenia-absent radius s.
tissue matrix s.
Torres s.
Townes-Brocks s.
toxic shock s.
transurethral resection s.
tremor-nystagmus-ulcer s.
triad s.
tropical diarrhea-malabsorption s.
  (TDMS)
Trousseau s.
tubulointerstitial nephritis and
  uveitis s. (TINU)
tumor lysis s.
TUR s.
Turcot s.
Turner s.
Ullrich-Turner s.
uremic s.
urethral s.
urethritis s.
urge s.
urofacial s.
VACTERL s.
vanished testis s.
vanishing bile duct s.
vascular steal s.
VATER s.
venous leak s.
Verner-Morrison s.
vertebral, anal, cardiac,
  tracheoesophageal fistula, renal,
  limb s.
vertebral, anal, tracheoesophageal
  fistula, renal s.
Vinson s.
VIPoma s.
von Hippel-Lindau s.
vulvar vestibulitis s.
WAGR s.
wasting s.
Waterhouse-Friderichsen s.
watery diarrhea s.
Watson-Alagille s.
Weil s.
Weinstein s.
Welt s.

S

NOTES

syndrome *(continued)*
    Wermer s.
    Wernicke s.
    Wernicke-Korsakoff s.
    Whipple s.
    Wiedemann-Beckwith s.
    Williams s.
    Wiskott-Aldrich s.
    Wolfram s.
    X-linked Alport s. (XLAS)
    XX male s.
    XYY male s.
    Young s.
    Youssef s.
    Zanca s.
    ZE s.
    Zellweger s.
    Zieve s.
    Zollinger-Ellison s. (ZES)
synechia, pl. **synechiae**
    penile s.
synectenterotomy
Synectics
    S. computer program
    S. 6000 digital pH-meter meter
Synectics-Dantec
    S.-D. Flo-Lab II uroflowmeter
    S.-D. UD10000 uroflowmeter
synergism
    in vitro s.
Synergist vacuum erection device
synergy
Syn-Optics video image splitter
synorchidism
synorchism
synoscheos
synovial fluid
Synsorb
Synsorb Cd, Pk
Synthamin amino acid solution
synthase
    aldosterone s.
    citrate s.
    induced nitric oxide s. (iNOS, NOS)
synthesis
    albumin s.
    apolipoprotein s.
    collagen s.
    dihydrotestosterone s.
    DNA s.
    eicosanoid s.
    focal collagen s.
    hepatocyte protein s.
    hormone-stimulated cAMP s.
    impaired lecithin s.
    mucosal prostaglandin s.
    prostaglandin s.

    prostanoid s.
    protein s.
    pyrimidine s.
    renin s.
    urea s.
synthesizer
    deoxyribonucleic acid s.
synthetase
    nitric oxide s.
    paraaminohippuric acid s.
synthetic
    s. 5-channel, water-perfused motility catheter
    s. ^{13}C-urea
    s. mesh
    s. vascular graft
Synthetics dual-channel, solid state Digitrapper
Synthroid
syphilis
    anorectal s.
    gastric s.
    primary s.
    secondary s.
    serologic test for s. (STS)
    tertiary s.
syphilitic
    s. gastritis
    s. hepatitis
    s. inguinal adenitis
    s. nephritis
    s. stigma
syphiloma
    Fournier s.
syringe
    Arrow Raulerson s.
    Asepto irrigation s.
    aspiration s.
    Fortuna s.
    LeVeen inflation s.
    Lewy s.
    Luer s.
    Luer-Lok s.
    motor s.
    Neisser s.
    Nourse s.
    piston-type s.
    s. shield
    Storz s.
    Toomey s.
    tuberculin s.
    Wolff s.
syringocele
    Cowper s.
syringoma
    penis s.
syrosingopine

syrup

Calcidrine s.
s. of glycyrrhiza
ipecac s.

system

Abbott Lifeshield needleless s.
Ablatherm HIFU s.
Advantx digital s.
AJCC/UICC staging s.
alimentary s.
Alliance integrated inflation s.
Amplatz TractMaster s.
Ancure abdominal aortic
aneurysm s.
AneuRx stent graft s.
anomalous arrangement of
pancreaticobiliary ductal s.
(AAPBDS)
antigen-antibody s.
APACHE-II, -III scoring s.
AquaSens FMS 1000 fluid
monitoring s.
Arndorfer capillary perfusion s.
Arndorfer pneumohydraulic capillary
infusion s.
Arrow UserGard injection cap s.
ASAP Stacker automated multi-
sample biopsy s.
autofluorescent endsocopic s.
automatic titration s.
autonomic nervous s. (ANS)
Balthazar grading s.
Bard endoscopic suturing s.
Bard Urolase fiber laser s.
Baxter Interline IV s.
Beamer injection stent s.
Bergkvist grading s.
BICAP hemostatic s.
bicarbonate buffer s.
BiliBlanket Phototherapy S.
bioartificial extracorporeal liver
support s. (BELS)
BioLogic-DT s.
BioLogic-DTPF s.
Bitome bipolar s.
B-lymphocyte s.
Bookwalter retractor s.
Boorman gastric cancer typing s.
(type 1–4)
Boyarsky symptom scoring s.
Bridge X3 renal stent s.

Browning and Parks continence
grading s. (category A, B, C, D)
Bruel-Kjaer 1846 ultrasound s.
buffer s.
Can-Opt dual lumen ERCP s.
cell analysis s.
Cell Recovery S. (CRS)
Cell Soft s.
central nervous s. (CNS)
classification s.
Clave needleless s.
closed suction drainage s.
coculture s.
collecting s.
Colormate TLc BiliTest S.
Colour-Quad-System imaging s.
Comhaire grading s.
computer-aided diagnostic s.
computer-controlled sedation
infusion s.
computerized image analysis s.
Conseal one-piece continent
colostomy s.
contact-tip laser s.
Contrajet ERCP contrast delivery s.
core-cut s.
COSTART s.
COX enzyme s.
CS-5 cryosurgical s.
CSM Stretta s.
C-Trak surgical guidance s.
cytochrome P450 enzyme s.
Dantec 12-channel Urocolor
Video s.
Dantec Etude s.
Dantec Menuet s.
daughter endoscopic retrograde
cholangiopancreatoscopy s.
digestive s.
Digitrapper Mark II pH
monitoring s.
DIONEX 2000 s.
Director Guidewire s.
DNA Sequencing S.
Doppler Quantum color flow s.
Dornier MPL 9000 electrohydraulic
lithotriptor ultrasound focusing s.
double-antibody sandwich s.
Drake-Willock delivery s.
Drake-Willock peritoneal dialysis s.
drug carrier s.
Dual-Port s.

S

NOTES

system *(continued)*

ductal s.
Dukes staging s.
Dumon-Gilliard endoprosthesis s.
EdGr s.
Edmondson grading s.
e10 electrosurgery s.
endocrine s.
endoscopic s.
enteric nervous s. (ENS)
ErecAid vacuum s.
EVIS EXERA Video S.
FastPack s.
fiberTome s.
Fisher Capillary S.
Flexiflo Top-Fill Enteral
  Nutrition S.
free-beam laser s.
French Pharmacovigilance s.
Fresenius volumetric dialysate
  balancing s.
Fujinon SP-501 sonoprobe s.
Fujinon video endoscopy s.
Garden prognostic s.
GastrographH ambulatory pH
  monitoring s.
gastrointestinal s. (GIS)
gastrointestinal therapeutic s.
  (GITS)
Gatta prognostic s.
Gleason grading s.
Grabstald (Memorial) staging s.
Gyrus endourology s.
HandPort s.
hemi-Kock s.
HepatAssist Liver Support S.
Hewlett-Packard IVUS imaging s.
high-affinity low-capacity s.
high-affinity sodium-dependent
  phosphate transport s.
Hind-SITE 20/20 s.
H+/K+-ATPase enzyme s.
Hp Chek screening s.
human cytochrome P-450
  enzyme s.
hydraulic capillary infusion s.
Hydra Vision Es urological
  imaging s.
Hydra Vision IV urology s.
Hydra Vision Plus urological s.
illumination s.
immune s.
Impact lithotriptor s.
implantable neuromodulation s.
IMx PSA s.
InCare PRES 9300 s.
Indigo LaserOptic treatment s.
InjecAid s.

Innova home incontinence
  therapy s.
InSIGHT manometry s.
integrated automatic stone-tissue
  detection s.
intensified radiographic imaging s.
  (IRIS)
International Biomedical Mode 745-
  100 microcapillary infusion s.
intracellular signaling s.
intrarenal collecting s.
IsoMed constant flow infusion s.
iterative bifid branching s.
IVAC needleless IV S.
Jackson staging s.
Janus S. III
Jewett staging s.
Jewett-Strong s.
Jewett-Whitmore Cancer Staging S.
Johns Hopkins prostate cancer
  grading s.
Joyce-Loebl Magiscan image
  analysis s.
Kangaroo Delivery S.
Kleinert Safe and Dry panty and
  pad s.
Kretz ultrasound s.
LAGB s.
Lambda Plus PDL 1, 2 laser s.
Laparolift s.
laparoscopic retraction s.
Laparoshield laparoscopic smoke
  filtration s.
Lap-Band adjustable gastric
  banding s. (LAGB)
Laser CHRP rigid fiber scope s.
LifeSite hemodialysis access s.
light induced fluorescence
  endoscopy s. (LIFE-GI)
Lithostar Plus electromagnetic
  lithotriptor bidimensional x-ray
  focusing s.
liver dialysis s.
Lorad StereoGuide prone breast
  biopsy s.
low-affinity, high-capacity s.
low-compliance perfusion s.
low-pressure venous s.
Madsen-Iversen scoring s.
Mayo grading s.
mechanical assist s.
MediClenze hygiene and water
  therapy s.
Mediflex MD-7 endoscopic
  video s.
Medstone IRIS s.
Medstone STS lithotripsy s.
MetaFluor s.

microsomal ethanol oxidizing s.
(MEOS)
Microvasive biliary stent s.
Microvasive Ultraflex esophageal
stent s.
mitochondrial ethanol oxidase s.
molecular adsorbents recirculating s.
(MARS)
MOP-Videoplan morphometric s.
Morganstern aspiration/injection s.
mother-baby endoscope s.
mother-baby-scope s.
mother endoscopic retrograde
cholangiopancreatoscopy s.
Mui Scientific pressurized capillary
infusion s.
Multipulse laser s.
Mycotrim triphasic culture s.
myeloperoxidase-H2O2-halide s.
NA+-linked cotransport s.
NA+ transport s.
needleless s.
Oasis pusher tube s.
OEC-Diasonics 9400 fluoroscopy
C arm s.
Olympus CLV-series fiberoptic s.
Olympus endoscopy s. (OES)
Olympus EVIS color computer
chip s.
Olympus GF-UM3, -UM20 s.
Olympus MAJ363 FNA needle s.
Olympus OSP fluorescence
measuring s.
Olympus video endoscopy s.
Olympus video urology
procedure s.
Omni-LapoTract support s.
One Action Stent Introduction S.
(OASIS)
Opmilas 144 Plus laser s.
optical multichannel analyzer s.
Ortho Diagnostic S.
O'Sullivan scoring s.
Palco enuretic alarm s.
Palmaz Corinthian biliary stent and
delivery s.
pancreaticobiliary ductal s.
P blood group s.
pelvicaliceal s.
Percutaneous Stoller Afferent Nerve
Stimulation S. (PerQ SANS)
Performa ultrasound s.

pneumohydraulic capillary
infusion s.
Polachrome 35-mm slide s.
portable perfused manometric s.
portal venous s.
Precision QID glucose
monitoring s.
Precision Tack Transvaginal
anchor s.
Prempree modification staging s.
probenecid-inhibited organic anion
transport s.
Proscan ultrasound imaging s.
Prostathermer prostatic
hyperthermia s.
Pugh-Child scoring s.
Ranson grading s.
Redy hemodialysis s.
Relay suture delivery s.
renal kallikrein-kinin s.
renal preservation perfusion s.
renin-aldosterone s.
renin-angiotensin s. (RAS)
renin angiotensin-aldosterone s.
(RAAS)
reproductive s.
reticuloendothelial s.
Reuter suprapubic trocar and
cannula s.
rod-lens s.
RX Herculink 14 biliary stent s.
Sacks-Vine PEG s.
Safe and Dry panty and pad s.
SeedNet s.
sentry s.
SF-9 baculovirus-insect cell s.
single-action pumping s. (SAPS)
slide s.
Soehendra catheter s.
SOLO-Surg Colo-Rectal self-
retaining retractor s.
Sonablate 200 s.
Sonoprobe Endoscopic
Ultrasonography S.
sorbent dialysate regeneration s.
StayErec s.
stent and vent s.
Stoller scoring s.
stone recognition s.
stone-tissue detection s. (STDS)
stone-tissue recognition s. (STR)

S

NOTES

system *(continued)*
    Storz multifunction valve
        trocar/cannula s.
    Straight-In male sling s.
    Straight-In surgical s.
    Stretta s.
    STS lithotripsy s.
    Suretys panty s.
    Surgi-PEG replacement gastrostomy
        feeding s.
    Sydney s.
    sympathetic nervous s. (SNS)
    Talent LPS endoluminal stent-
        graft s.
    Targis microwave catheter-based s.
    Technos ultrasound s.
    terminal bifid branching s.
    testosterone transdermal s. (TTS)
    Therasonics Lithotripsy S.
    ThermoChem-HT s.
    ThermoFlex s.
    tissue-stone recognition s. (TSRS)
    Top Notch automated biopsy s.
    transdermal therapeutic s. (TTS)
    transvaginal suturing s.
    Tricomponent Coaxial S. (TCS)
    triple-lumen perfused catheter s.
    Truelove-Witts grading s.
    TVS s.
    Ultrabag dialysis s.
    UltraPak enteral closed feeding s.
    Ultraseed s.
    Ultra Twin bag s.
    Ultra Y-set s.
    United States Renal Data S.
        (USRDS)
    Universal sheath s.
    Urocyte diagnostic cytometry s.
    Uro-jet delivery s.
    Urolab Janus S. III
    Uro-Pak s.
    Urotract x-ray s.
    Urovision ultrasound imaging s.
    UroVive self-contained balloon s.
    Vaccine Adverse Event
        Reporting S.
    vanishing bile duct s.
    varix grading s. F1, F2, F3

    VET-CO vacuum s.
    Virtual Biopsy s.
    Visick gastric cancer grading s.
    Vision Sciences VSI 2000 flexible
        sigmoidoscope s.
    Vivonex Acutrol Enteral
        Feeding S.
    Vocare bladder s.
    Welch Allyn video endoscopy s.
    Whitmore-Jewitt prostate cancer
        classification s.
    Wolf aspiration/injection s.
    Wolf delivery s.
    wolffian ductal s.
    Xillix LIFE-Lung s.
    Y-set s.
    Zenith AAA endovascular graft s.
    Zenith abdominal aortic aneurysm
        endovascular graft s.
    Zieve s.
    Z-stent esophageal endoprosthesis s.
systematic sextant biopsy
systemic
    s. amyloidosis
    s. arterial pressure
    s. *Candida*
    s. duodenal sclerosis
    s. effect
    s. endotoxemia
    s. hypertension
    s. hypotension
    s. inflammatory response syndrome
        (SIRS)
    s. lupus erythematosus (SLE)
    s. lupus erythematosus vasculitis
    s. MAP
    s. mast cell disease
    s. mastocytosis
    s. mercury intoxication
    s. radiation therapy
    s. sclerosis (SSc)
    s. vascular resistance (SVR)
    s. vascular resistance index (SVRI)
    s. venodilation
systolic
    s. click
    s. murmur
Szabo test

T

- T antigen
- T cell
- T-cell antigen receptor/CD3 complex
- T cell-specific protein
- T connector
- T effector cell
- T lymphocyte
- T tube
- T tubogram
- T wave

T138 antigen
T1-weighted image
T2-weighted image
T84 cell
TA90-BN stapler
TAA
- tumor-associated antigen

TAAA
- thoracoabdominal aortic aneurysm
- TAAA surgery

tabes
- t. dorsalis
- t. mesaraica
- t. mesenterica

tabetic
table
- Aub-Dubois t.
- Dornier Urotract cystoscopy t.
- floating t.
- Gerhardt t.
- lithotripsy t.
- Maquet endoscopy t.
- Multifunctional Opus surgical t.
- Partin t.
- sigmoidoscopy t.
- Urodiagnost x-ray t.

tablet
- Asacol delayed-release t.
- Chenix T.
- Dairy-Ease chewable t.
- delayed-release t.
- mycophenolate mofetil t.
- Nullo deodorant t.
- Pantoloc t.
- pantoprazole sodium t.
- Rapamune t.
- Renagel t.
- sevelamer hydrochloride t.
- sirolimus t.
- Urex T.'s
- Visicol t.
- wax-matrix t.

TAC
- total abdominal colectomy

TACE
- transarterial catheter embolization
- transarterial chemoembolization
- transcatheter arterial chemoembolization

tachycardia
- sinus t.
- ventricular t.

tachygastria
tachykinin-bombesin family
tachykinin component
tachyphylaxis
tachypnea
tacked down
tacrolimus
tacrolimus-associated microangiopathy
tactile probe
tactor
Tactyl 1 glove
TACurea
- timed average urea concentration

tadpole-like appearance
TAE
- total abdominal evisceration
- transcatheter arterial embolization

Taenia
- *T. saginata*
- *T. solium*

taenia, pl. taeniae
- t. mesocolica
- t. omentalis
- taeniae pylori
- t. strip of soft tissue
- taeniae of Valsalva

taeniacide
taeniasis
taeniform
taenioides
- *Diphyllobothrium t.*

tag
- edematous t.
- external skin t.
- hemorrhoidal t.
- H-shaped tilt t.
- perianal skin t.
- perineal skin t.
- sentinel t.
- skin t.

TAG-72 glycoprotein
Tagamet HB
tagged
- t. erythrocyte scintigraphy
- t. red blood cell bleeding scan

T

tagging
        fecal t.
        t. stitch
tail
        t. of pancreas
        t. sign
tailgut cyst (TGC)
tailing defect
Tait law
Takayasu
        T. arteritis
        T. disease
        T. syndrome
takedown
        bilateral ureterostomy t.
        t. of colostomy
        ostomy t.
        t. of pelvic sling procedure
taking down of adhesion
TAL
        thick ascending limb
talc embolus
Talent LPS endoluminal stent-graft
  system
talin
talk
        receptor cross t.
TALT
        testicular adrenal-like tissue
Tamm-Horsfall
        T.-H. mucoprotein (THM)
        T.-H. protein (THP)
tamoxifen
tampon
        Corner t.
        t. tube
tamponade, tamponage
        balloon tube t.
        esophageal balloon t.
        esophagogastric t.
        esophagogastric balloon t. (EGBT)
        ferromagnetic t.
        Sengstaken-Blakemore t.
        tract t.
tamponing, tamponment
tamsulosin HCl
Tanagho
        T. bladder flap urethroplasty
        T. bladder neck reconstruction
tandem
        t. colonoscopy (TC)
        t. PSA assay
        t. PSA test
        t. thin-shaft transureteroscopic
          balloon dilatation catheter
        T. XL triple-lumen ERCP cannula
Tandem-E-PSA immunoenzymetric assay

Tandem-ERA PSA immuenzymetric
  assay
Tandem-R
        T.-R assay kit
        T.-R PSA assay
tangential
        t. biopsy
        t. colonic submucosal injection
Tangier disease
tangle of hemorrhoidal veins
Tannenbaum stent
Tanner
        T. operation
        T. stage
tannex
        bisacodyl t.
tannic acid
tantalum-182
TAP
        TAP gene
tap
        abdominal t.
        peritoneal t.
        t. water enema
TAP2 peptide transporter gene
tape
        adhesive t.
        appendectomy t.
        Cath-Secure t.
        circular t.
        Coban t.
        lap t.
        laparotomy t.
        t. marker
        Mersilene t.
        Montgomery t.
        polyester-reinforced Dacron t.
        tension-free vaginal t. (TVT)
        Transpore t.
        umbilical t.
tapered
        t. common bile duct
        t. needle
        t. rubber bougie
tapered-tip
        t.-t. dilator
        t.-t. hydrophilic-coated push catheter
taper-tip catheter
tapeworm
        beef t.
        Cestoda t.
        fish t.
        pork t.
TAPP
        transabdominal preperitoneal
          TAPP hernia repair
Taq polymerase

TAR
    thrombocytopenia-absent radius
    TAR syndrome
tarda
    Edwardsiella t.
    porphyria cutanea t. (PCT)
tardive
    forme t.
target
    t. appearance
    t. area
    t. cell
    t. lesion
    t. localization
    peritoneal dialysis creatinine
      clearance t.
    t. symptom
    t. volume (TV)
targeted
    t. biopsy
    t. cryoablation device
    t. microwave thermotherapy
targeting
    selective t.
Targis microwave catheter-based system
Tarlov cyst
tarry black stool
tartrate
    metoprolol t.
    t. nephritis
    tolterodine t.
    trimeprazine t.
TASI
    transperitoneal anterior subcostal incision
TA stapling device
taste perversion
TATA-binding protein
TA30, TA55 stapler
tattoo
    colonic t.
    colonoscopic t.
    endoscopic four-quadrant t.
    India ink t.
    submucosal t.
tattooing
    four-quadrant t.
taurine
    t. cotransporter (TCT)
    t. cotransporter mRNA
    selenium-labeled homocholic acid
      conjugated with t. (SeHCAT)

taurocholate
    sodium t.
    t. solution
taurocholic acid
tauroglycocholate
    sodium t.
taurolithocholate
Taut cystic duct catheter
Taxol
Taylor
    T. gastric balloon
    T. gastroscope
tazobactam
TBA
    total bile acid
T-bandage
T-bar retractor
TBI
    total body irradiation
T-binder
TBM
    thin basement membrane
    tubular basement membrane
TBMD
    thin basement membrane disease
TBN
    total body nitrogen
TBW
    total body water
TC
    tandem colonoscopy
    therapeutic concentrate
    transhepatic cholangiography
Tc
    technetium
^{99m}Tc, Tc-99m
    technetium-99m
    ^{99m}Tc albumin colloid
    ^{99m}Tc albumin microsphere
    ^{99m}Tc DMSA
    ^{99m}Tc-DPTA
    ^{99m}Tc DTPA aerosol
    ^{99m}Tc GHP
    ^{99m}Tc HIDA
    ^{99m}Tc HMPAO-labeled leukocyte
      scan
    ^{99m}Tc IDA scan
    ^{99m}Tc lidofenin
    ^{99m}Tc MAA
    ^{99m}Tc-MAA
    ^{99m}Tc MDP

NOTES

T

^{99m}Tc *(continued)*
^{99m}Tc MDP nuclear isotope bone scan
^{99m}Tc medronate
^{99m}Tc pertechnetate scan
^{99m}Tc pertechnetate scintigraphy
^{99m}Tc PIPIDA
^{99m}Tc polyphosphate
^{99m}Tc PYP
^{99m}Tc RBC bleeding scan
^{99m}Tc SC
^{99m}Tc sodium pertechnetate
^{99m}Tc SPP
^{99m}Tc sulfur colloid scan
^{99m}Tc tin colloid

TCA
tricarboxylic acid
trichloroacetic acid
trihydrocoprostanic acid

TCBS
thiosulfate-citrate-bile salts-sucrose agar

TCCA

TCCB
transitional cell carcinoma of the bladder

TCD/CBDE
transcystic duct/common bile duct exploration

^{99m}Tc-DISIDA
^{99m}Tc-DISIDA contrast injection

^{99m}Tc-DTPA renal scan

T-cell
T-c. activation
T-c. adhesion
T-c. crossmatch
T-c. cytotoxic therapy
T-c. depletion by elutriation
T-c. epitope
T-c. line
T-c. lymphoma
T-c. receptor (TCR)
T-c. second messenger
T-c. vaccination

T-cell-dependent mechanism

^{99m}Tc-GSA
technetium-99m galactosyl-human serum albumin
^{99m}Tc-GSA scintigraphy

Tc-HIDA scan

^{99m}Tc-HMPAO-labeled leukocyte scintigraphy

TCIS
total corrected incremental score

^{99m}Tc-labeled
^{99m}Tc-l. Amberlite pellet
^{99m}Tc-l. anti-alpha-fetoprotein
^{99m}Tc-l. stannous methylene diphosphonate

T-clamp
Millin T-c.

Tc-99m *(var. of ^{99m}Tc)*

^{99m}Tc-MAG-3 isotope

TCMS
transcranial magnetic stimulation

T-C needle holder

^{99m}Tc-phytate liquid state esophageal transit study

TCR
T-cell receptor

TCS
tethered-cord syndrome
Tricomponent Coaxial System

^{99m}Tc-SC
technetium-99m sulfur colloid

Tc-sulfur colloid

TCT
taurine cotransporter
TCT mRNA

TDMS
tropical diarrhea-malabsorption syndrome

T-drain

TDU
time domain ultrasound

TDX fluorescent polarization immunoassay

TE
tracheoesophageal

TEA
tetraethylammonium

tea
bush t.

Teale gorget

tear
capsular t.
diastatic serosal t.
t. duct
esophageal t.
gastric t.
Mallory-Weiss t.
mesenteric t.
mucosal t.
pharyngeal t.
pharyngoesophageal t.
serosal t.

teardrop
t. bladder
t. incision
t. poikilocyte

tearing
t. pain
t. through

t-EASE software

TEBS
transurethral electrical bladder
stimulation
TEC
transpapillary endoscopic cholecystotomy
teceleukin and interferon alfa-2a
TechneScan
T. MAG-3
technetium (Tc)
t. GSA
t. imaging
t. radionuclide scan
t. Tc 99m Exametazime injection
**99mtechnetium-dimercaptosuccinic acid
scintigram**
technetium-labeled
t.-l. autologous red blood cell scan
t.-l. red blood cell scan
technetium-99m (99mTc, Tc-99m)
t.-99m diethylenetriamine pentaacetic
acid (99mTc-DPTA)
t.-99m diethylenetriamine pentaacetic
acid scan
t.-99m galactosyl-human serum
albumin (99mTc-GSA)
t.-99m IDA scan
t.-99m macroaggregated albumin
(99mTc-MAA)
t.-99m mercaptoacetythiglycine
isotope
t.-99m pentetic acid
t.-99m pertechnetate
t.-99m pyrophosphate-tagged RBC
t.-99m red cell scintigraphy
t.-99m sulfur colloid (99mTc-SC)
t.-99m (Tc-99m) iminodiacetic acid
t.-99m tin colloid
technique
abdominal pressure t.
abdominal-wall lift t.
anthrone colorimetric t.
antiperistaltic t.
antireflux ureteral implantation t.
aseptic t.
assisted reproductive t.
autosuture t.
avascular cuff t.
balloon catheter and basket-
retrieval t.
band and snare t.
band-snare t.
Barcat t.

Belt t.
bench surgical t.
bladder neck preserving t.
blind t.
Brackin ureterointestinal
anastomosis t.
Bricker t.
Buerhenne stone basket t.
bulking t.
buttonhole puncture t.
Campbell t.
Cantwell-Ransley t.
Cape Town t.
capsule flap t.
cavernosal alpha blockade t.
cell separation t.
cephalotrigonal t.
clamshell t.
closed tubule fixation t.
Coffey t.
Cohen cross-trigonal t.
colonic obstruction t.
continuous pull-through t.
Coomassie brilliant blue t.
cup-patch t.
Davis t.
Deisting t.
Denis Browne urethroplasty t.
de novo needle knife t.
diathermy t.
direct fragmentation t.
double-balloon t.
double-folded cup-patch t.
double-staple t.
double stapling t. (DST)
Dufourmentel t.
Eisenberger t.
en bloc t.
end-to-side vasoepididymostomy t.
enuresis alarm t.
esophageal banding t.
extraanatomical renal
revascularization t.
extraction balloon t.
extravesical ureteral
reimplantation t.
Fairley bladder washout
localization t.
fan-shaped biopsy t.
Ferguson t.
finger fracture t.
first-line screening t.

NOTES

T

technique *(continued)*

flap t.
flip-flap t.
flow microsphere fluorescent
  immunoassay t.
full-bladder t.
Gaur balloon distension t.
Gil-Vernet t.
Gittes t.
Glenn t.
Glenn-Anderson t.
Goldschmiedt t.
gold seed implantation t.
Goodwin t.
Goodwin-Hohenfellner t.
Goodwin-Scott t.
Graves t.
gravimetric t.
Grimelius t.
guidewire and mini-snare t.
Hale colloidal iron t.
Hammock t.
Hartmann reconstruction t.
Hauri t.
Hendren t.
Higgins t.
Hippuran clearance t.
histocytochemical t.
Hofmeister t.
hot biopsy t.
hydrocelectomy plication t.
hydrogen gas clearance t.
immunoperoxidase staining t.
immunostaining t.
indirect immunolocalization t.
^{111}In-leukocyte t.
interventional t.
intradermal tattooing t.
invagination t.
Jaboulay-Doyen-Winkleman t.
Jones-Politano t.
Kaliscinski ureteral folding t.
Keystone t.
King t.
Kock t.
Kropp t.
laparoscopic colposuspension t.
LaRoque t.
laryngeal jack t.
laser-assisted tissue welding t.
laser welding t.
lasso t.
lateral bending t.
lateral window t.
Latzko t.
lawn mower t.
Lazarus-Nelson t.
Leach t.

Leadbetter and Clarke t.
Leadbetter modification t.
Leadbetter tunneling t.
LeDuc t.
Lich extravesical t.
Lich-Gregoire t.
lift-and-cut t.
Lotheissen-McVay t.
Madden t.
Marlex plug t.
Masson trichrome staining t.
Mathieu t.
Meares-Stamey t.
membrane catheter t.
Menghini t.
Michal II t.
micropuncture t.
microtransducer t.
microtubulotomy t.
Mikulicz drain t.
mini-perc t.
Mitrofanoff continent urinary
  diversion t.
modified Cantwell t.
modified Hassan open t.
modified Sacks-Vine push-pull t.
modified Thiersch-Duplay t.
modified Vest t.
modified Young-Dees-Ledbetter t.
Mohs microsurgery t.
morcellation t.
Moynihan t.
muscle-splitting t.
Myers bunching t.
nasovesicular catheter t.
needle-knife t.
Nesbit t.
Norfolk t.
onlay t.
onlay-tube-onlay urethroplasty t.
Orandi t.
orbital exenteration gastroscopic
  access t.
over-the-wire t.
Palomo t.
Paquin t.
patch clamp t.
pelviscopic clip ligation t.
perfusion hypothermia t.
Pippi-Salle t.
Politano-Leadbetter t.
Pólya t.
Ponsky t.
prograde t.
pull-through t.
push t.
push-pull T t.
quadrant sampling t.

Quantikine quantitative immunoenzymatometric sandwich t.
Quartey t.
rapid pull-through esophageal manometry t.
reconstruction t.
relaxation t.
retrograde t.
Rives-Stoppa t.
Roux-en-Y chimney surgical t.
RPT t.
Russell t.
Sacks-Vine t.
Saeed t.
safe-tract t.
salvage cytology t.
sandwich t.
Schoemaker-Billroth II t.
Seldinger t.
semen for assisted reproductive t.
sextant t.
Silber t.
Singer-Blom endoscopic tracheoesophageal puncture t.
sleeve t.
sling-and-blanket t.
smiley face knotting t.
Snodgrass t.
Somatome DRG CT t.
sperm microaspiration retrieval t. (SMART)
spiral CT t.
split-and-roll t.
split-cuff nipple t.
split-nipple t.
SPT t.
Starr t.
station pull-through esophageal manometry t.
stent through wire mesh t.
Stiegmann-Goff t.
stimulated gracilis neosphincter t.
strip biopsy resection t.
submucosal saline injection t.
suck-and-cut t.
Sugarbaker t.
superior mesenterorenal bypass t.
surface cooling t.
Swiss roll embedding t.
Thomas t.
Thompson t.

three-loop t.
Traverso-Longmire t.
tube-within-tube t.
tunneled t.
turn-and-suction biopsy t.
Turnbull t.
two-layer latex and Marlex closure t.
two-layer open t.
ultrasound dilution t.
Ussing chamber t.
U-stitch reimplantation t.
ventral bending t.
videofluoroscopic t.
video transurethral resection t.
Vim-Silverman t.
Wallace t.
Warwick and Ashken t.
Wickham t.
xenon-washout t.
Young t.
Young-Dees t.
technology
DNA microarray t.
endoscopic t.
fiberoptic instrument t.
interactive video t. (IVT)
polymerase chain reaction t.
vacuum erection t.
video graphic tool t. (VGTT)
Technomed Sonolith 3000 lithotriptor
Technos ultrasound system
teeth
carious t.
full-surface micro mesh t.
interdigitating t.
TEF
thermic effect of feeding
tracheoesophageal fistula
Teflon
T. ERCP cannula
T. guiding catheter
T. injector
T. nasobiliary drain
T. nasobiliary tube
T. paste injection for incontinence
T. sheath
T. sling rectopexy
T. stent
Teflon-coated
T.-c. Dacron suture
T.-c. guidewire

T

NOTES

Tegaderm dressing
tegaserod
Tegretol
teicoplanin
Teilum tumor
Tektronix digital oscilloscope
tela
    t. subserosa intestini tenuis
    t. subserosa vesicae urinaria
telangiectasia
    calcinosis cutis, Raynaud
      phenomenon, esophageal motility
      disorder, sclerodactyly, and t.
      (CREST)
    calcinosis cutis, Raynaud
      phenomenon, sclerodactyly, and t.
      (CRST)
    duodenal t.
    gastrointestinal t.
    hemorrhagic t.
    hepatic t.
    hereditary hemorrhagic t. (HHT)
    Osler-Weber-Rendu t.
    radiation t.
    spider t.
    t. syndrome
telangiectatic
    t. angioma
    t. vessel
telar vesical tenesmus
Telepaque contrast medium
telerobotic-assisted laparoscopic surgery
telescope
    forward-viewing t.
    t. heater
    Hopkins t.
    Wolff t.
teletherapy
    orthovoltage t.
television
    t. camera
    t. monitor
    t. photography
Telfa dressing
Teline
telomerase
telomere
    t. length
telopeptide
TEM
    transanal endoscopic microsurgery
    transmission electron microscopy
      TEM transanal endoscopy
TEMAC
    tetramethyl ammonium chloride
temafloxacin
Temaril
temazepam

temperature
    actual intraprostatic t.
    core t.
    hand t.
    intraprostatic t.
    laser t.
    urethral t.
template
    Mick prostate t.
    Seyd-Neblett perineal t.
Tempo
temporary
    t. end colostomy
    t. endoprosthetic device
    t. enteroscope
    t. loop ileostomy
temporizing measure
temporomandibular arthritis
TEN
    total enteral nutrition
    toxic epidermal necrolysis
    Vivonex TEN
Tena pouch
Tenckhoff
    T. peritoneal dialysis catheter
    T. two-cuff catheter
tender
    t. liver
    t. thyroid
tenderness
    adnexal t.
    ballottement t.
    bony t.
    cervical motion t.
    costochondral t.
    costovertebral angle t. (CVAT)
    diffuse t.
    exquisite t.
    facial t.
    focal t.
    frontal t.
    localizing t.
    palpation t.
    paracervical t.
    percussion t.
    point t.
    popliteal t.
    rebound t.
    rectal t.
    salivary t.
    scrotal t.
    sinus t.
    spinous t.
    thyroid t.
    uterine t.
tendinous
    t. arc
    t. arch of levator ani muscle

tendon
    conjoined t.
    perineal t.
    t. xanthoma
tenesmic
tenesmus
    rectal t.
    telar vesical t.
Tenex
tenia, pl. **teniae**
    t. coli
    t. libera
    t. omentalis
tenial
teniamyotomy
teniasis
    somatic t.
teniposide (VM-26)
Ten-K
Tenoretic
Tenormin
tenoxicam
TENS
    transcutaneous electrical nerve
    stimulation
      TENS unit
tense ascites
tensile strength
Tensilon test
tensiometer
tension
    t. myalgia
    t. pneumoperitoneum
    t. pneumothorax
    wall t.
tension-free
    t.-f. anastomosis
    t.-f. closure of abdominal cavity
    t.-f. vaginal tape (TVT)
    t.-f. vaginal tape procedure
tensor
    t. fasciae latae flap
    t. veli palatini muscle
tensostat
tent
    Silon t.
tenting
    baseline t.
    t. sign
Tenuate

tenuis
    Corynebacterium t.
    tela subserosa intestini t.
TEP
    totally extraperitoneal
    tracheoesophageal puncture
    TEP hernia repair
TEPA
    thermic effect of physical activity
Tepanil
tepoxalin
teratocarcinoma
teratogenesis
    medication t.
teratogenic medicine
teratoma
    anaplastic malignant t.
    benign cystic t.
    differentiated t.
    gastric t.
    immature t.
    malignant t. (MT)
    mature t.
    ovarian t.
    presacral t.
    sacrococcygeal t.
    solid t.
    testicular t.
    t. testicular cancer
    tropoblastic malignant t.
    undifferentiated malignant t.
teratomatous
teratospermia
teratozoospermia
terazosin
terbutaline hepatitis
teres
    fissure for ligamentum t.
    ligamentum t.
teretis
    fissura ligamenti t.
terfenadine
terlipressin
terminal
    afferent t.
    t. anuria vesical dialysis
    t. bifid branching system
    t. bile duct
    t. colostomy
    t. hematuria
    t. ileal disease
    t. ileal pouch

NOTES

terminal *(continued)*
    t. ileal resection
    t. ileitis
    t. ileostomy
    t. ileum
    t. ileum intubation (TII)
    t. ileus
    t. inner medullary collecting duct
    t. repeat (TR)
    t. reservoir syndrome
    t. sedation (TS)
    sensory nervous t.
    t. uridine deoxynucleotide nick end
      labeling (TUNEL)
terminus
    amino t.
    duodenal t.
    intrapapillary t.
terms
    Coding Symbols for a Thesaurus
    of Adverse Reaction T.
    (COSTART)
terodiline
teroxirone
terrestrial organism
Terry fingernail sign
tert-butyl-ether
    methyl t.-b.-e.
tertiary
    t. contraction
    t. hyperparathyroidism
    t. radicle
    t. syphilis
tertium
    Clostridium t.
Terumo
    T. dialyzer
    T. Glidewire
    T. hydrophilic guidewire
Terumo/Meditech guidewire
Terumo-Radiofocus hydrophilic polymer-
    coated guidewire
Tesberg esophagoscope
TESE
    testicular sperm extraction
Tesla
    T. GE Signa whole body scanner
    T. Signa MR imager
Teslascan
test
    Accu-Dx t.
    acid clearance t. (ACT)
    acid hemolysis t.
    acidification of stool t.
    acid perfusion t.
    acid reflux t.
    adrenocorticotropic hormone
     infusion t.

Advanced Care cholesterol t.
agglutination t.
air tightness t.
Albarran t.
Albustix t.
alkaline phosphatase t.
alkalinization t.
Allen t.
ALT t.
Althausen t.
Ames t.
aminopyrine breath t.
angiotensin II infusion t.
anorectal function t.
antiendomysial antibody t.
antigen stool detection t.
anti-Hu t.
antineuronal enteric antibody t.
anti-SLA t.
APT-Downey alkali denaturation t.
argentaffin reaction t.
artificial erection t.
AST t.
ASTRA profile t.
Aura-Tek FDP t.
Baermann stool t.
balloon expulsion t.
Bard BTA t.
basal secretory flow rate t.
belt t.
bentiromide t.
bentonite flocculation t.
Bernstein acid perfusion t.
beta-2 t.
betazole stimulation t.
bethanechol t.
bile acid breath t.
bile acid tolerance t.
bile solubility t.
BiliCheck t.
bilirubin t.
binder t.
Bio-Enzabead t.
Bio-Gen urine t. strip
biopsy urease t.
Biotel home screening t.
BioWhittaker assay t.
bladder tumor antigen t.
bolus challenge t.
Bonney t.
Bors ice water t.
Bourne t.
Boyden t.
Boyle and Goldstein saline t.
Bozicevich t.
t. breakfast
breath hydrogen excretion t.
breath pentane t.

Breslow-Day t.
brushing urea breath t.
BSFR t.
BSP t.
BTA stat t.
BTA TRAK t.
BT-PABA t.
buckling t.
CA19-9 t.
calcium infusion t.
Campylobacter t.
Campylobacter-like organism t.
 (CLOtest)
cancelling A's t.
captopril plasma renin activity t.
carbon-13 urea breath t. (^{13}C-UBT)
carbon-14 urea breath t.
carbon-14 urinary excretion t.
Carnot t.
Casoni skin t.
catheterization t.
^{13}C-bicarbonate breath t.
CBP t.
C-cholyl-glycine breath excretion t.
CEA t.
cephalin-cholesterol flocculation t.
^{14}C-glycocholate breath t.
C-glycocholic acid breath t.
7C Gold urine t.
chew-and-spit t.
Chiron RIBA HCV t.
Choice2 t.
cholecystokinin t.
C of Hosmer-Lemeshow ratio t.
citrate t.
^{13}C-labeled cholesteryl octanoate
 breath t.
C-lactose t.
Clinitest stool t.
clomiphene t.
clonidine suppression t.
CO_2 breath t.
Cochran-Mantel-Haenszel t.
^{13}C-octanoic acid gastric emptying
 breath t.
Cohen t.
Colaris molecular diagnostic t.
cold stress t.
ColoCARE fecal occult blood t.
colonic transit t.
Coloscreen Self-t.

combined intracavernous injection
 and stimulation t.
complement fixation t.
complete blood count t.
Coombs t.
copper-binding protein t.
cornflake esophageal motility t.
Cortrosyn stimulation t.
cosyntropin stimulation t.
cotton swab t.
cough stress t.
Cox-Mantel t.
CP t.
cracker t.
creatinine t.
C&S t.
CSF glutamine t.
^{14}C-triolein breath t.
culture and sensitivity t.
^{14}C urea breath t. (^{14}C UBT)
C-urea breath t.
deferoxamine mesylate infusion t.
Desican t.
dexamethasone suppression t.
diabetes home screening t.
Diagnex Blue t.
differential renal function t.
differential ureteral catheterization t.
dilute Russell viper venom t.
 (DRVVT)
t. dinner
direct immunobead t.
direct immunofluorescence t. (DIF-
test)
Doppler flow t. (DFT)
duodenal secretin t. (DST)
D-xylose absorption t.
dye-exclusion t.
edrophonium t.
egg yolk-cobalamin absorption t.
 (EYCAT)
Einhorn string t.
Eitest MONO P-II t.
Ektachem slide t.
ELISA-I, -II, -III t.
endomysial antibody t.
Enzygnost antiHIV 1+2 t.
Enzymun t.
ergonovine t.
erythrocyte sedimentation rate t.
esophageal acid infusion t.
esophageal function t.

T

NOTES

test *(continued)*

Fairley bladder washout t.
FDL t.
fecal alpha-1-antitrypsin t.
fecal fat t.
fecal leukocyte count t.
fecal occult blood t. (FEOT, FOBT)
fingerprick latex agglutination t.
Fisher exact probability t.
Fisher two-tailed exact t.
Fishman-Doubilet t.
FlexSure HP t.
FlexSure whole-blood t.
fluorescein dilaurate t.
fluorescein string t.
fluorescent treponemal antibody absorption t.
Fouchet t.
four-glass t.
Fowler-Stephens t.
Francis t.
FTA-ABS t.
gallbladder function t.
GAP t.
gastric accommodation t.
gastric emptying t.
gastric function t.
gastric secretory t.
gastrin stimulation t.
Gastroccult t.
gastrointestinal blood loss t.
Gerhardt t.
GGT t.
GGTP liver function t.
Ghedini-Weinberg serologic t.
Glahn t.
Glazyme APF-EIA-TEST t.
glucose t.
Glucose analyzer II t.
glutamine t.
Gluzinski t.
glycopyrrolate t.
glycyltryptophan t.
Gmelin t.
gonadotropin-releasing hormone t.
graded esophageal balloon distention t.
Graham t.
Gram stain of stool t.
Grassi t.
Griess t.
Gross t.
guaiac t.
Guenzberg t.
Ham t.
Hamel t.
Hanger t.

Harrison spot t.
hatching t.
Hay t.
H2 breath t.
HCV DupliType t.
HCV ELISA t.
Helicobacter pylori breath excretion t.
Helicoblot 2.1 t.
Helisal rapid blood t.
Hematest t.
HemaWipe t.
heme t.
Hemoccult II t.
Hemoccult SENSA t.
HemoQuant fecal blood t.
HemoSelect t.
Hepaplastin t.
hepatitis C virus DupliType t.
Heprofile ELISA t.
Herzberg t.
Histalog stimulation t.
histamine t.
HM-CAP serological t.
Hoesch t.
Hollander t.
home screening t.
HomeSelect t.
24-hour ambulatory pH t.
72-hour fecal fat t.
24-hour gastric acidity t.
12-hour home pad t.
Howard t.
Hpfast rapid urease t.
HpSA t.
5-HT t.
human lymphocyte chromosomal aberration t.
Hunt t.
Huppert t.
Huppert-Cole t.
Hybritech Tandem PSA ratio t.
hydrochloric acid t.
hydrogen breath t.
ICA t.
    islet cell antibody
ice water t.
ICG t.
iliopsoas t.
immunoblot t.
ImmunoCard STAT! Rotavirus t.
ImmunoCyt t.
immunodiffusion t.
immunofluorescent antibody t.
immunological fecal occult blood t. (IFOBT)
immunological rapid urease t.

[111]indium-labeled autologous
  leukocyte t.
intracavernous injection and
  stimulation t.
intraductal secretin t. (IDST)
intraesophageal acid t.
intraesophageal pH t.
intravenous secretin t.
Inutest t.
invasive diagnostic t.
Jacoby t.
Jaffe t.
Jaksch t.
Jatrox *Helicobacter pylori* t.
Jaworski t.
Jolles t.
Kapsinow t.
Kashiwado t.
Kato t.
Kelling t.
ketone body t.
Kinberg t.
Kolmogorov-Smirnov t.
Krokiewicz t.
Kruskal-Wallis t.
Kveim t.
lactose tolerance t.
lactulose hydrogen breath t.
  (LHBT)
lactulose-mannitol permeability t.
Lange t.
LAP t.
Lapides t.
last-generation serologic ELISA t.
latex fixation t.
LDH t.
LDL Direct t.
Leo t.
leucine aminopeptidase t.
leukocyte adherence inhibition t.
leukocyte alkaline phosphatase t.
leukocyte esterase t.
levulose t.
Ligat t.
lipase t.
litmus milk t.
locally made rapid urease t.
  (LRUT)
log-rank t.
Lundh t.
Macdonald t.
Machado-Guerreiro t.

MacLean t.
magnetic susceptibility t.
Maly t.
Mann-Whitney rank sum t.
Mantel-Haenszel t.
Mardi t.
Marechal-Rosen t.
Marshall t.
Marshall-Bonney t.
Marshall-Marchetti t.
Masset t.
McNemar ascites t.
t. meal
measurement t.
Meltzer-Lyon t.
metapyrone stimulation t.
methyl red t.
metyrapone stimulation t.
Micral urine dipstick t.
Mitscherlich t.
Mohr t.
monoethylglycinexylidide liver
  function t.'s
morphine-neostigmine t.
motility t.
Moynihan t.
Myers-Fine t.
Mylius t.
Nakayama t.
Nardi t.
N-benzoyl-L-tyrosyl-P-aminobenzoic
  acid excretion t.
NBT-PABA t.
Neubauer and Fischer t.
Neukomm t.
nitrite t.
nitrogen partition t.
nitrogen retention t.
NMP-22 t.
noninvasive diagnostic t.
nonradioactive [13]C t.
Normotest t.
number connection t. (NCT)
Nymox urinary t.
obturator t.
octanoic acid breath t.
omeprazole t.
one-hour office pad t.
one-minute endoscopy room t.
O&P t.
Oresus Potentest t.
PABA t.

NOTES

T

test *(continued)*
pad urinary incontinence t.
Palmer acid t. for peptic ulcer
palmin t., palmitin t.
pancreatic secretory t.
Pap t.
paracetamol absorption t.
PAS t.
peak secretory flow rate t.
pentagastrin gastric secretory t.
pentagastrin infusion t.
pentagastrin provocative t.
pentagastrin stimulated analysis t.
Peptavlon stimulation t.
percutaneous pressure ureteral
  perfusion t.
perineal nerve terminal motor
  latency t.
periodic acid-Schiff t.
peripheral nerve evaluation t.
peritoneal equilibration t. (PET)
Pettenkofer t.
pH t.
Phadebas angiotensin-I t.
phenoltetrachlorophthalein t.
phentolamine t.
physiologic reflux t. (PRT)
pineapple t.
plasma renin activity captopril t.
PNE t.
POA t.
Posner attention t.
postage stamp penile tumescence t.
postcoital t.
posthoc t.
postural stimulation t. (PST)
posture t.
Premier Platinum HpSA t.
Prentice-Wilcoxon t.
proteinuria t.
Protocult t.
provocative t.
PSA4 prostate cancer t.
PSFR t.
psychometric t.
pudendal nerve terminal motor
  latency t.
purified protein derivative t. (PPD)
PyloriScreen t.
Pyloriset EIA-G t.
Pylori Stat assay t.
PyloriTek rapid urease t.
PYtest urea breath t.
Q-tip t.
qualitative fecal fat t.
quantitative fecal fat t.
Quick t.
QuickVue one-step *Helicobacter
  pylori* t.
Quidel-QuickVue *Helicobacter
  pylori* t.
Quinlan t.
Rabuteau t.
radioactive carbon-14 t.
radioallergosorbent t. (RAST)
radioisotope renal excretion t.
radioisotope renogram t.
rapid serum amylase t.
rapid urease t. (RUT)
Rapoport t.
recombinant immunoblot assay-2 t.
reducing substances t.
reflex HPV t.
Rehfuss t.
Reitan trail making t.
Reitman-Frankel t.
renin stimulation t.
rhubarb t.
RIBA t.
RIBA-2 t.
rice-flour breath t.
Robinson-Kepler-Power water t.
rose bengal t.
Rosenbach-Gmelin t.
Rosenthal t.
Rotazyme t.
Russell viper venom t.
Saathoff t.
Sahli glutoid t.
Sahli-Nencki t.
saline continence t.
saline load t.
saline suppression t.
Salkowski-Schipper t.
Salomon t.
santonin t.
satiety t.
Saundby t.
scan t.
S-CCK-Pz t.
Scheffe-F t.
Schiff t.
Schilling t.
Schwartz t.
Scivoletto t.
secretin-CCK stimulation t.
secretin-pancreozymin stimulation t.
secretin provocation t.
secretin stimulation t.
SeHCAT t.
[75]Se-labeled bile acid t.
semen analysis t.
serologic t.
serum amylase t.
serum bilirubin t.
serum creatinine t.
serum iron t.
serum protein t.

serum RIBA-2 t.
Sgambati reaction t.
SGOT t.
SGPT t.
sham feeding t.
skin fold thickness t.
Smith t.
snap gauge t.
sodium-loading t.
solid sphere t.
Spearman t.
specific gravity t.
specific red cell adherence t.
SpermCheck t.
split renal function t.
squeeze pressure profile of anal
  sphincter t.
Stamey t.
standard acid reflux t. (SART)
star construction t.
Stat Simple whole-blood
  antibody t.
stereognost-3-alpha enzymatic t.
stimulated gastric secretion t.
stimulation t.
Stokvis t.
Stoll t.
StoneRisk citrate t.
StoneRisk cystine t.
StoneRisk diagnostic t.
StoneRisk profile t.
stool cytotoxin t.
stool electrolyte t.
stool osmolality t.
stool osmotic gap t.
Strassburg t.
string t.
Stypven time t.
sucrose tolerance t.
sugar t.
Sulkowitch t.
sweat t.
Szabo t.
tandem PSA t.
Tes-Tape urine glucose t.
TIBC t.
tilt t.
Töpfer t.
Torquay t.
total fecal weight t.
total iron binding capacity t.
Trail t.

Trail Making T.
transferrin t.
transmucosal electrical potential t.
triceps skin fold thickness t.
triolein C-14 breath t.
Trousseau t.
tuberculin t.
tubular reabsorption of phosphate t.
Tukey t.
Tuttle t.
two-stage triolein t.
two-tailed Fisher t.
two-tailed McNemar t.
t. type
Tyson t.
UBT breath t.
Udranszky t.
Uffelmann t.
ultrasound t.
Ultzmann t.
Uni-Gold *Helicobacter pylori* t.
uPM3 urine t.
urea breath t. (UBT)
urea nitrogen t.
urease t.
urecholine supersensitivity t.
uric acid t.
urinary nitrite t.
urine chloride t.
urine concentration t.
Uriscreen t.
van den Bergh t.
ViraPap HPV dot blot
  hybridization t.
vitamin A, B_{12} absorption t.
Voges-Proskauer t.
von Jaksch t.
Wagner t.
washout t.
water-gurgle t.
water-nutrient t.
water-recovery t.
water-restriction t.
water-sipping t.
water-soluble contrast esophageal
  swallow t.
Watson-Schwartz t.
whiff t.
Whipple triad t.
Whitaker pressure-perfusion t.
Winckler t.
Witz t.

T

NOTES

test *(continued)*
    Woldman t.
    Wolff-Junghans t.
    Woolf t.
    xylose absorption t.
    xylose tolerance t.
    Yang Pros-Check PSA t.
    Zappacosta t.
    zona hamster egg t.
testalgia
Tes-Tape urine glucose test
testectomy
testes (*pl. of* testis)
testicle
    maldescended t.
    retained t.
testicular
    t. abscess
    t. adenocarcinoma
    t. adenofibromyoma
    t. adenomatoid tumor vacuole
    t. adrenal-like tissue (TALT)
    t. adrenal rest
    t. androgen-binding protein
    t. angioma
    t. artery
    t. biopsy
    t. carcinoma
    t. cyst
    t. descent
    t. feminization syndrome
    t. fibroma
    t. Hodgkin disease
    t. hypothermia device
    t. implant
    t. interstitial fluid (TIF)
    t. leiomyoma
    t. leukemia
    t. lymphoma
    t. mass
    t. microlithiasis
    t. pain
    t. plexus
    t. prosthesis
    t. seminoma
    t. sperm extraction (TESE)
    t. swelling
    t. teratoma
    t. torsion
    t. tuberculosis
    t. tubular adenoma
    t. tubule
testicularis
    plexus t.
testiculoma
testiculus, pl. **testiculi**
testing
    anorectal physiology t.

    breath alkane t.
    fecal occult blood t.
    goodness-of-fit t.
    histocompatibility t.
    lactose hydrogen breath t. (LHBT)
    nucleic acid t. (NAT)
    pad t.
    penile injection t.
    pH-metric t.
    physiology t.
    provocative t.
    psychophysiologic t.
    RigiScan t.
    salivary t.
    sexual stimulation t.
    stress t.
    urea breath t.
    urodynamic t.
    viability t.
    vibrotactile stimulation t.
    videourodynamic t.
    visual sexual stimulation t.
testis, pl. **testes**
    abdominal t.
    aberratio t.
    adenocarcinoma of infantile t.
    albuginea t.
    appendix t.
    t. cancer
    t. carcinoid
    Cooper irritable t.
    descensus aberrans t.
    descensus paradoxus t.
    dorsum of t.
    dystopia transversa externa t.
    dystopia transversa interna t.
    t. ectopia
    ectopia t.
    ectopic t.
    femoral t.
    fibroma of t.
    fungus t.
    high t.
    interstitial cell tumor of t.
    inverted t.
    irritable t.
    lobuli t.
    mediastinum t.
    mottled t.
    movable t.
    t. muliebris
    obstructed perineal t.
    peeping t.
    prosthetic t.
    pulpy t.
    retained t.
    rete t.
    retractile t.

t. sarcoma
septula t.
septum of t.
solitary t.
torsion t.
torsion of t.
tunica albuginea t.
tunicae t.
undescended t.
vanishing t.
testis-determining factor
testitis
testitoxicosis
Testoderm
T. patch
T. TTS
testoid
testolactone
testopathy
testosterone
basal t.
t. cypionate
t. deficiency
t. enanthate
free t.
t. patch
t. plasma concentration
t. propionate
t. repressed prostate message-2
(TRPM-2)
serum t.
t. stimulation
t. transdermal system (TTS)
t. transdermal therapy
undecenoate of t.
testosterone-binding globulin
testosterone-estrogen-binding globulin
testotoxicosis
Testred C-III
Test-Size orchidometer
test-yolk buffer cryopreservation agent
tetani
Clostridium t.
tetanus globulin
tetany
gastric t.
tether circulating leukocyte
tethered-bowel sign
tethered-cord
t.-c. release
t.-c. syndrome (TCS)
tethered spinal cord

tethering of mucosa
tetracaine lozenge
Tetracap
tetrachloride
carbon t.
tetracycline
bismuth, metronidazole, t. (BMT)
t. hydrochloride
t. nephropathy
ranitidine bismuth citrate,
metronidazole, t. (RMT)
t. sclerosis
tetradecapeptide
tetradecyl sulfate
tetraethylammonium (TEA)
Tetragastrin-NS
tetrahydrocannabinol (THC)
tetrahydrochloride
3′,3-diaminobenzidine t.
tetrahydrozoline
tetralogy
Fallot t.
Tetram
tetramethyl ammonium chloride
(TEMAC)
tetrapalmitate
maltose t.
tetraplegia
tetraploid cell
tetrapyrrol compound
tetrathiomolybdate
tetrazolium
nitroblue t. (NBT)
tetrodotoxin (TTX)
tetroxide
osmium t.
Teucrium chamaedrys
Tevdek suture
Texas
T. style two-piece catheter
T. trauma
texture
heterogeneous t.
homogeneous t.
T-fastener
Brown-Mueller T.-f.
TFE-coated wire guide
TF/UF
tubular fluid:ultrafiltrate
TGC
tailgut cyst

T

NOTES

TGE
transgastrostomic enteroscopy
TG ELISA
TGF
transforming growth factor
tubuloglomerular feedback
human recombinant TGF
TGF-alpha
transforming growth factor alpha
TGF-beta
transforming growth factor beta
TGF-beta-1
transforming growth factor beta-1
TGF-beta-1 gene
TGF-beta-2
transforming growth factor beta-2
TGF-beta-3
transforming growth factor beta-3
TGHA
thyroglobulin antibody
Thal
T. esophageal stricture repair
T. esophagogastroscopy
T. esophagogastrostomy
T. fundic patch operation
T. fundoplasty
T. stricturoplasty
thalidomide
Thalitone
thallium
t. imaging
t. poisoning
thallium-201
thamuria
thaw-mount radioautography
Thaysen disease
THC
tetrahydrocannabinol
transhepatic cholangiography
tHcy
total homocysteine
THE
transhepatic embolization
Theirsch-Duplay repair
Theis self-retaining retractor
thelium, pl. **thelia**
T-helper precursor
thenar eminence
theophylline
t. clearance
t. ethylenediamine
t. level
t. olamine enema
t. toxicity
theoretical paper
theory
Dieulafoy t.
hyperfiltration t.

overflow t.
peripheral arterial vasodilation t.
set point t.
TheraCys
Theradex
Theradigm-HBV
Theragyn
Theralax
therapeutic
t. angiography
t. colonoscopy
t. concentrate (TC)
t. endoscope
t. endourology
t. laparoscopy
t. modality
t. pancreaticobiliary endoscopy
t. plasmapheresis
t. side-viewing duodenoscope
t. upper endoscopy
t. value
therapy
ablative laser t.
acid-suppression t.
adjuvant drug t.
adrenalin injection t.
alarm t.
alimentary t.
alkaline citrate t.
alpha-blocker t.
alpha-interferon t.
alpha-receptor blockade t.
amoxicillin-tinidazole-ranitidine t.
amphotericin B t.
ampullary ablative t.
androgen ablation t. (AAT)
androgen deprivation t.
androgen withdrawal endocrine t.
antibiotic t.
anticholinergic medicine t.
anticoagulation t.
antilymphocyte t.
antimicrobial t.
antioncogene t.
antireflux t.
antisecretory t.
argon laser t.
autolymphocyte t.
Aza-Pred t.
azole t.
balloon photodynamic t.
T. Bayer Caplets
bile acid t.
biofeedback t.
biologic response modifier t.
bismuth-free triple t.
bridging t.
bubble t.

buprenorphine narcotic analgesic t.
chemoradiation t. (CRT)
cholestyramine t.
CIFN t.
clarithromycin triple t.
coagulative laser t.
combined chemoradiation t.
conditioning t.
conformal radiation t.
continuous renal replacement t.
  (CRRT)
corticosteroid t.
cytokine t.
cytolytic t.
debulking t.
dendritic cell t.
diclofenac analgesic t.
diet t.
dilation t.
diltiazem t.
doxycycline-metronidazole-bismuth
  subcitrate triple t.
drug t.
Emitasol nasal t.
endocrine t.
endoscopic hemoclip t.
endoscopic hemostatic t.
endoscopic injection t.
endoscopic laser t. (ELT)
endoscopic pancreatic t.
enterostomal t. (ET)
Enterra t.
enzyme replacement t.
eradication t.
erythropoietin t.
esophageal photodynamic t.
estrogen replacement t. (ERT)
ethanol injection t.
external-beam radiation t. (EBRT)
external vacuum t.
ex vivo liver-directed gene t.
fluid replacement t.
fluoroquinolone t.
flutamide t.
foscarnet t.
gamma globulin t.
gene t.
gene-transfer t.
H2-antagonist t.
heat t.
heater probe t.
Helidac t.

hematoporphyrin derivative t.
hemofiltration t. (HFT)
hemostatic t.
highly active antiretroviral t.
  (HAART)
homeostatic t.
hormonal t.
H2-receptor antagonist t.
hydrocelectomy scleral t.
hydrostatic pressure t.
hyperbaric oxygen t. (HBOT)
hyperfractionated radiation t.
IFN-alpha t.
IFN-alpha-2b t.
immunomodulatory t.
immunomodulatory gene t.
immunosuppressive t.
injection t.
instillation t.
intensity-modulated proton t.
  (IMPT)
intensity-modulated radiation t.
  (IMRT)
interferon alpha t.
interferon alpha-2b t.
intermittent calcitriol t.
International Association for
  Enterostomal T.
interstitial photodynamic t.
intracavernosal injection t. (ICIT)
intracavernous injection t.
intracavitary radiation boost t.
intracavitary topical t.
intracorporeal injection t.
intraoperative radiation t. (IORT)
IV fluid t.
ketoprofen analgesic t.
laser t.
lifestyle t.
medical t.
metabolic t.
methyl-tert-butyl ether t.
metronidazole, amoxicillin,
  clarithromycin, *H. pylori*, one-
  week t. (MACH1)
monoclonal antibody t.
morphine narcotic analgesic t.
MTBE t.
Nd:YAG laser t.
neoadjuvant androgen derivation t.
neoadjuvant hormonal ablation t.
neodymium:YAG laser t.

NOTES

therapy *(continued)*
    nutritional t.
    omeprazole t.
    omeprazole-clarithromycin-
      amoxicillin t.
    oral rehydration t. (ORT)
    palliative t.
    pancreatic enzyme replacement t.
    pancreatic intraluminal radiation t.
    PEI t.
    penile injection t.
    penile vein occlusion t.
    percutaneous embolization t.
    percutaneous ethanol injection t.
    periurethral injection t.
    phosphate binder t.
    photodynamic t. (PDT)
    photoradiation t.
    physiologic testosterone-
      replacement t.
    placebo t.
    polidocanol injection t.
    polyestradiol phosphate t.
    postoperative anticoagulation t.
    posttransplant immunosuppression t.
    PPI triple t.
    preventive intravesical t.
    Prevpac triple t.
    probiotic t.
    prokinetic t.
    proton pump inhibition t.
    psychosexual t.
    pulsed dye laser t.
    quadruple t.
    quatro t.
    radiation t.
    radionuclide t.
    ranitidine t.
    Rebetron Combination t.
    rehydration t.
    renal replacement t.
    rescue t.
    resiniferatoxin t.
    sacral nerve stimulation t.
    saline injection t.
    salvage t.
    sandwich staghorn calculus t.
    sclerosing t.
    self-injection t.
    sex t.
    single-drug t.
    SNS t.
    somatostatin analog t.
    somatostatin infusion t.
    steroid t.
    sucralfate t.
    surgical t.
    systemic radiation t.
    T-cell cytotoxic t.
    testosterone transdermal t.
    TheraSphere t.
    thermal t.
    three-dimensional conformal t. (3-
      DCRT)
    three-dimensional conformal
      radiation t.
    thrombolytic t.
    Trager t.
    transcatheter arterial embolization t.
    transpapillary t.
    transurethral collagen injection t.
    triple t. (TT)
    triple eradication t.
    tumor suppressor gene t.
    ultrasound-guided shock wave t.
    valproic acid t.
    YAG laser t.
TheraSeed
Therasonics
    T. Lithotripsy System
    T. lithotriptor
TheraSphere therapy
Therevac Plus
Therevac-SB
Therma Jaw disposable hot biopsy
    forceps
thermal
    t. ablation
    t. blocking
    t. burn
    t. imaging
    t. sphincteric reflex
    t. therapy
thermally active method
TherMatrx TMx-2000 device
Thermex-II transurethral prostate
    heating device
thermic
    t. effect of feeding (TEF)
    t. effect of physical activity
      (TEPA)
thermoablation
    transurethral t.
ThermoChem-HT system
thermocoagulation
    heater probe t.
    heat probe t.
    HP t.
    KeyMed heater probe t.
    laser t.
thermocoagulator
    Olympus CD-Z-series heat probe t.
thermocycler
    Stratagene SCS-96 t.
thermo-disinfector
    endoscopic t.-d.

thermodynamic solubility product
thermoexpandable stent
ThermoFlex
    T. system
    T. thermotherapy unit
thermogenesis
    adaptive t. (AT)
thermography
    Primus transrectal t.
thermomechanical
thermometer
    air t.
    alcohol t.
    Celsius t.
    centigrade t.
    Fahrenheit t.
    gas t.
    oral t.
    rectal t.
    surface t.
thermophilus
    Streptococcus t.
thermoreceptor
thermosensitive stent
thermosensor
thermotherapy
    cooled catheter transurethral
      microwave t.
    high-energy transurethral
      microwave t. (HE-TUMT)
    low-energy transurethral
      microwave t. (LE-TUMT)
    microwave t.
    30-minute transurethral
      microwave t.
    periurethral transurethral
      microwave t. (P-TUMT)
    targeted microwave t.
    transurethral microwave t. (TUMT)
    Urowave t.
    water-induced t. (WIT)
Thermovac tissue pulverizer
Thermus
    T. aquaticus
    T. aquaticus DNA ligase
thetaiotaomicron
    Bacteroides t.
thiabendazole
thiacetazone
thiamine deficiency
thiazide diuretic
thiazide-induced hyponatremia

thick
    t. adhesion
    t. ascending limb (TAL)
    t. bile
    t. loop transurethral resection of
      the prostate
thickened
    t. gallbladder wall
    t. nail
thickening
    apical t.
    hypoechoic t.
    mediastinal t.
    plaquelike t.
    small bowel t.
    submucosal t.
    wall t.
thickness
    esophageal wall t. (EWT)
    mucous gel t.
    t. of skin fold (TSF)
    triceps skin fold t.
thick-walled gallbladder
Thiersch
    T. anal incontinence operation
    T. graft
    T. procedure
    T. tube
Thiersch-Duplay
    T.-D. proximal tube procedure
    T.-D. tube graft
    T.-D. tubularization
    T.-D. urethroplasty
thiethylperazine
thigh graft arteriovenous fistula
thimble
    bladder t.
    t. bladder
thin
    t. adhesion
    t. basement membrane (TBM)
    t. basement membrane disease
      (TBMD)
    Cutinova hydro t.
    t. glomerular basement membrane
      disease
    t. shave sectioning
thin-layer chromatography (TLC)
thin-needle percutaneous cholangiogram
ThinPrep Processor
thin-walled gallbladder

NOTES

T

thiocyanate
    guanidine t.
thiol
    exogenous t.
    t. intermediate
Thiola
thiopental
Thioplex
thiopropazate
thioridazine hydrochloride
thiosulfate-citrate-bile salts-sucrose agar
   (TCBS)
Thiosulfil
thiotepa
thiothixene
thiourea-resorcinol method
thiphenamil
thiram
third-generation
    t.-g. cephalosporin
    t.-g. lithotriptor
thirst fever
Thiry fistula
Thiry-Vella fistula (TVF)
thistle
    milk t.
THM
    Tamm-Horsfall mucoprotein
Thomas
    T. shunt
    T. technique
Thompson
    T. capsule flap pyeloplasty
    T. lithotrite
    T. procedure
    T. technique
Thomsen-Friedenreich antigen
thoracic
    t. aortic pathology
    t. aortorenal bypass
    t. duct
    t. esophagus
    t. fistula
    t. inlet
    t. kidney
    t. stomach
thoracoabdominal
    t. aortic aneurysm (TAAA)
    t. aortic aneurysm surgery
    t. collateral vein
    t. esophagogastrectomy
    t. extrapleural approach
    t. incision
    t. intrapleural approach
    t. retroperitoneal lymphadenectomy
thoracolaparotomy

thoracotomy
    esophagectomy with t.
    t. scar
Thorazine
Thorek
    T. gallbladder aspirator
    T. gallbladder forceps
    T. gallbladder scissors
Thorek-Feldman gallbladder scissors
Thorek-Mixter gallbladder forceps
thorium
    colloidal t.
    t. dioxide
Thorn salt-depletion syndrome
Thornton sign
Thorotrast contrast medium
THP
    Tamm-Horsfall protein
thread-and-streaks sign
thread-locking device
threadworm
    nondisseminated intestinal t.
thready pulse
three-armed basket forceps
three-dimensional
    t.-d. conformal radiation therapy
    t.-d. conformal therapy (3-DCRT)
    t.-d. CT pancreatography (3D-CTP)
three-drug regimen
three-field
    t.-f. dissection
    t.-f. lymphadenectomy
three-finger grip
three-limb S-pouch
three-loop
    t.-l. ileal pouch
    t.-l. technique
three-pronged
    t.-p. grasper
    t.-p. grasping forceps
    t.-p. polyp retriever
three-quarter circle electrode
three-space dissection
three-way
    t.-w. irrigating catheter
    t.-w. stop-cock
three-week sulfasalazine syndrome
threonine
threshold
    gastric mechanosensory t.
    t. of internal sphincter
    pH t.
    t. potential
    t. of rectal sensation
    swallowing t.
    urethral sensory t.
thrifty colon

thrive
    failure to t.
thrombectomy
thrombi (*pl. of* thrombus)
thrombin
    bovine t.
    t. spray
    topical bovine t.
thrombin-antithrombin
    t.-a. III
    t.-a. III complex
    thrombin-Keflin-sotredechol
Thrombinar
thrombocytopenia
    heparin-induced t. (HIT)
thrombocytopenia-absent
    t.-a. radius (TAR)
    t.-a. radius syndrome
thrombocytopenic purpura
thrombocytosis
thromboelastography
thromboembolic
    t. disease
    t. event
thromboembolism
    venous t. (VTE)
thromboendarterectomy
    renal t.
Thrombogen
thromboglobulin
    beta-t.
thrombolytic
    t. agent
    t. therapy
thrombomodulin
thrombophlebitis
    puerperal septic pelvic vein t.
thrombopoietin (TPO)
thrombosed
    t. internal and external hemorrhoid
    t. pile
thrombosis
    arterial t.
    bilateral renal vein t.
    bland t.
    deep venous t.
    glomerular microvascular t.
    hepatic artery t. (HAT)
    hepatic vein t.
    inferior vena cava t.
    intracapillary t.
    intrarenal vascular t.

    intravascular t.
    mesenteric arterial t.
    mesenteric vein t. (MVT)
    nonocclusive mesenteric t.
    peripheral venous t.
    portal vein t. (PVT)
    renal artery t.
    renal vein t.
    silent t.
    SMV t.
    splenic vein t.
    venous t.
thrombospondin
thrombotic
    t. microangiopathy
    t. thrombocytopenic purpura (TTP)
thromboxane
    t. A_2
thrombus, pl. **thrombi**
    bile t.
    mural t.
    retrocecalis tumor t.
    t. tumor
    white t.
through
    tearing t.
through-and-through appearance
through-the-scope (TTS)
    t.-t.-s. balloon
    t.-t.-s. balloon dilation
    t.-t.-s. balloon removal
    t.-t.-s. bougie
    t.-t.-s. catheter probe
    t.-t.-s. dilator
    t.-t.-s. injection needle
thrush
    t. esophagitis
    oral t.
thumbprinting
    t. of mucosa
    t. sign
thymalfasin
thymic
    t. EC
    t. hypoplasia
thymidine
    [^{3}H]t. uptake
thymidine-labeling index
thymocyte NA+/H+ exchanger
Thymoglobulin
thymol crystal
thymosin

NOTES

thymoxamine
thymus
thymus-derived
    t.-d. cell
    t.-d. lymphocyte
thyreoideus impar plexus
thyroarytenoid muscle
thyroglobulin antibody (TGHA)
thyrohyoid muscle
thyroid
    t. autoimmunity
    t. disease
    t. hormone
    t. hormone response element (TRE)
    t. hormone serum concentration
    medullary carcinoma of t. (MCT)
    t. microsomal antibody
    t. nodule
    tender t.
    t. tenderness
thyroiditis
    autoimmune t.
    Hashimoto t.
thyroidization
thyroid-stimulating hormone level
thyromegaly
thyroplasty
thyrotoxicosis
    gestational t.
thyrotropin-releasing hormone
thyroxine
    free t. (FT4)
thyroxine-binding globulin
TI
    tubulointerstitial
TIBC
    total iron binding capacity
    TIBC test
ticarcillin
tic douloureux of the bladder
Tice
ticklish
ticlopidine
Ti-Cron, Tycron
    T.-C. suture
    T.-C. tie
ticrynafen-induced jaundice
tidal drainage
tide
    sign of the rising t.
tie
    free t.
    stick t.
    Ti-Cron t.
Tielle Plus hydropolymer dressing
tie-over dressing
TIF
    testicular interstitial fluid

Tigan
tight
    t. abdomen
    t. junction permeability
    t. Nissen repair
    t. perirectal adhesion
tight-junction protein
tigroid appearance
TII
    terminal ileum intubation
TIL
    tumor-infiltrating lymphocyte
tilt
    t. stitch
    t. test
Timberlake obturator
time
    abdominopelvic orocecal transit t.
    activated partial thromboplastin t.
     (aPTT)
    activated thromboplastin t.
    ascites euglobulin lysis t. (AELT)
    bleeding t.
    caliceal filling t.
    cancer doubling t.
    clotting t.
    coagulation t.
    cold ischemia t. (CIT)
    colonic transit t.
    dextrinizing t.
    t. domain ultrasound (TDU)
    doubling t.
    duration t.
    esophageal transit t.
    explosive doubling t.
    gastric bleeding t. (GBT)
    gastric emptying t. (GET)
    gastric transit t.
    mean input t. (MIT)
    mean resistance t. (MRT)
    mean transit t. (MTT)
    median operative t.
    nucleation t. (NT)
    orocecal transit t. (OCTT)
    partial thromboplastin t. (PTT)
    pH holding t.
    post-UUO t.
    preservation t.
    pro t.
     prothrombin time
    prothrombin t. (pro time, PT)
    prothrombin time/partial
     thromboplastin t. (PT/PTT)
    PSA doubling t.
    radionuclide esophageal emptying t.
    Russell viper venom t.
    skin bleeding t. (SBT)
    small bowel transit t.

transit t. (TT)
warm ischemia t.
time-activity curve
Timecaps
Levsinex T.
time-concentration curve
timed
t. average urea concentration
(TACurea)
t. voiding
time-dependent variable
Timentin
double-dose I.V. T.
single-dose I.V. T.
time-of-flight mass spectometry
(TOFMS)
timer
video t.
Tim knot
timolol
timori
Brugia t.
TIMP
tissue metalloproteinase
TIMP-2
tissue inhibitor of metalloproteinase-2
TIN
tubulointerstitial nephritis
tincture
t. of belladonna
t. of benzoin
Tindal
tinea
t. cruris
t. purpureum
t. rubrum
tinidazole
tinkling bowel sounds
TINU
tubulointerstitial nephritis and uveitis
syndrome
tiopronin
tip
Andrews suction t.
Buie rectal suction t.
filiform t.
Frazier suction t.
open end flow-through
radiopaque t.
papillary t.
sharp-edged t.
Slip-Coat t.

spleen t.
suction t.
tulip t.
vessel t.
villus t.
weighted t.
TIPPB
transperineal interstitial permanent
prostate brachytherapy
TIPS
transjugular intrahepatic portosystemic
shunt
occlusion of TIPS
TIPS procedure
stenosis of TIPS
TIPSS
transjugular intrahepatic portosystemic
stent shunt
Tis disease
Tisseel
T. fibrin sealant
T. fibrin sealant injection
tissue
acinar t.
adipose t.
ampullary granulation t.
t. approximation
chromaffin t.
cicatricial t.
t. coagulation
connective t.
cryostat t.
t. culture
t. culture assay
t. cushion
t. expansion vaginoplasty
extraperitoneal t.
exuberant granulation t.
fatty t.
fibroadipose t.
fibroelastic t.
fibrous t.
t. fixation
t. forceps
formalin-fixed t.
t. fusion
gastrointestinal-associated
lymphoid t. (GALT)
t. glue
gut-associated lymphoid t. (GALT)
hilar structure scar t.
t. inhibitor of metalloproteinase

T

NOTES

tissue *(continued)*
    t. inhibitor of metalloproteinase-2 (TIMP-2)
    t. kallikrein
    lipoma-like t.
    lipomatous t.
    t. matrix syndrome
    mesorectal t.
    t. metalloproteinase (TIMP)
    t. morcellator
    mucosa-associated lymphoid t. (MALT, MALToma)
    t. necrosis
    necrotic t.
    neoplastic t.
    noninflamed peripheral t.
    nontarget t.
    nonviable t.
    paracancerous t.
    paraffin-embedded t.
    parenchymal t.
    periadvential t.
    perinephric t.
    periprostatic t.
    t. plasminogen activator (TPA, tPA)
    t. polypeptide antigen
    redundant sac t.
    t. renewal
    t. resistance
    t. rim sign
    t. sampling
    sex accessory t.
    soft t.
    t. spectrum analyzer TS-200
    splenic t.
    subcutaneous t.
    taenia strip of soft t.
    T. Tek-II cryostat
    testicular adrenal-like t. (TALT)
    t. transglutaminase (tTG)
    t. transglutaminase ELISA (TG ELISA)
    treated t.
tissue-specific gene expression
tissue-stone recognition system (TSRS)
tissue-type plasminogen activator
Titan
    T. endoprosthesis
    T. stent
titanium
    t. clip
    t. urethral stent
titanous chloride
titer
    anti-HSV IgM Ab t.
    antineutrophil cytoplasmic antibody t.

    antistreptolysin-O t.
    ELISA t.
    end-point dilution t.
    IgM-HEV antibody t.
    viral serologic t.
title peritoneal dialysis (TPD)
Titralac Plus
titratable acidity
TJF-100,-130 large channel duodenoscope
TJF-10,-20 video duodenoscope
TLA
    transperitoneal laparoscopic adrenalectomy
TLC
    thin-layer chromatography
TLESR
    transient lower esophageal relaxation
TL90 Ethicon stapler
TLI
    total lymphoid irradiation
TLN
    transperitoneal laparoscopic nephrectomy
T-lymphocyte activation
T-lymphocyte-mediated cytotoxic reaction
Tm
    tubular maximal
TMD
    transmural drainage
TME
    total mesorectal excision
TMPD
    transmucosal potential difference
TMP-SMX
    trimethoprim-sulfamethoxazole lomefloxacin TMP/SMX
T204N
TNF
    tumor necrosis factor
TNF-alpha
    tumor necrosis factor alpha
        TNF-alpha assay
        TNF-alpha gene
TNM
    tumor, node, metastasis
        TNM carcinoma classification
        TNM classification of carcinoma
        TNM system for tumor staging
TNP-470
TNTC
    too numerous to count
tobramycin
tocainide hydrochloride
tocodynamometer
    guard-ring t.
    Nihon t.
Todd cirrhosis
toddler's diarrhea

toe
> clubbing of the fingers and t.'s

TOFMS
> time-of-flight mass spectometry

Tofranil

Tofranil-PM

toilet
> peritoneal t.

tolazamide

tolazoline hydrochloride

tolbutamide-induced cholestasia

tolcapone

Toldt
> line of T.
> T. membrane
> white line of T.

tolerance
> glucose t.
> oral t.
> transplantation t.

tolerated
> diet as t. (DAT)

toleration
> maximal t. (MT)

Tolerex feeding solution

tolerogenic dendritic cell

tolmetin

tolnaftate

tolterodine
> t. tartrate
> t. tartrate capsule

toluidine
> t. blue
> t. blue stain

Tom
> T. Jones closure
> T. Jones suture

Toma sign

Tomenius gastroscope

Tomocat

tomodensitometric examination

tomography
> computed t. (CT)
> computerized t. (CT)
> contrast-enhanced computed t.
> electron-beam computerized t. (EBCT)
> helical computed t.
> noncontrast helical computed t. (NCCT)
> optical coherence t. (OCT)
> positron emission t. (PET)

> single-photon emission computed t. (SPECT)
> single-photon emission computerized t. (SPECT)
> spiral computed t.
> ultrafast computerized t.
> ultrasonic t.
> unenhanced helical computed t.

tone
> anal sphincter t.
> bowel t.
> cardiac sympathovagal t.
> gastric t.
> lower esophageal sphincter t.
> pyloric t.
> renal vascular t.
> sphincter t.

tongs

tongue
> bifid t.
> black hairy t.
> t. deviation
> fissured t.
> geographic t.
> hairy t.
> t. movement
> mucosal t.
> smoker's t.
> swollen t.
> t. of tumor

tongue-shaped villus

tonic
> t. contraction
> t. neck

Tonkaflo pump

tonometry

tonsil
> t. clamp
> t. forceps
> orange-colored t.
> t. sucker

tonsillar enlargement

tonsillectomy

Toomey
> T. evacuator
> T. syringe

too numerous to count (TNTC)

toothed tissue forceps

TOPA
> topical oropharyngeal anesthesia

Töpfer test

Top-Fill enteral feeding bag

NOTES

T

765

topical
- t. anesthesia
- t. anesthetic
- t. antibiotic
- t. betamethasone
- t. bovine thrombin
- t. neuropathy
- t. nifedipine
- t. oropharyngeal anesthesia (TOPA)
- Synalar T.
- t. treatment
- t. Xylocaine

topic effect

Topicort Cream

Topiglan

topiramate

Top Notch automated biopsy system

topogram
- balloon t.

topography
- scintigraphic balloon t.

topoisomerase I inhibitor

toposcopic catheter

topotecan

Toprol

Toradol

Torbot
- T. cement
- T. faceplate

Torecan

Torek
- T. operation
- T. orchiopexy

toremifene

tori (*pl. of* torus)

Toronto-Western catheter

torovirus

Torquay test

torque
- t. catheter
- translation of t.
- t. vise
- t. wire

torquing of scope

torrential hemorrhage

Torres syndrome

torsemide

torsion
- adnexal t.
- t. of appendage
- appendix testis t.
- biliary tract t.
- cryptorchidism t.
- extravaginal t.
- t. of gallbladder
- gallbladder t.
- intravaginal t.
- penile t.

- perinatal t.
- spermatic cord t.
- synchronous neonatal t.
- testicular t.
- t. testis
- t. of testis
- ureteral t.

torso crease

torticollis

tortuous
- t. esophagus
- t. ureter
- t. venous ectasia

Torulopsis
- *T. glabrata*

torulopsis infection

torus, pl. **tori**
- t. palatinus
- t. ureter

Toshiba
- T. ERVF 1A video floppy recorder
- T. microendoprobe
- T. Sal 38B real-time ultrasonography
- T. Sonolayer SSA250A transrectal ultrasonography
- T. TCE-M-series colonoscope
- T. video endoscope

Tosoh assay

Tostrex

Totacillin

total
- t. abdominal colectomy (TAC)
- t. abdominal evisceration (TAE)
- t. anorectal reconstruction
- t. bilateral vagotomy
- t. bile acid (TBA)
- t. bilirubin
- t. body irradiation (TBI)
- t. body nitrogen (TBN)
- t. body water (TBW)
- t. bowel rest
- t. colonoscopy
- t. corrected incremental score (TCIS)
- t. cystectomy
- t. cystourethrectomy
- t. descent
- t. dose infusion
- t. enteral nutrition (TEN)
- t. fasting
- t. fecal weight test
- t. gastrectomy
- t. gastric wrap
- t. glutathione content
- t. hematuria
- t. hemolytic complement

t. homocysteine (tHcy)
t. homocysteine plasma
 concentration
t. infarction
t. internal reflection
t. iron binding capacity (TIBC)
t. iron binding capacity test
t. lymphocyte (TTL)
t. lymphoid irradiation (TLI)
t. mesorectal excision (TME)
t. pancreatectomy
t. parenteral alimentation
t. parenteral nutrition (TPN)
t. parenteral nutrition line
t. pelvic exenteration
t. perineal prostatectomy
t. peripheral parenteral nutrition
 (TPPN)
t. peroral intraoperative enteroscopy
t. predicted return
t. prostatoseminal vesiculectomy
t. protein
t. protein concentration
t. PSA
t. scrotectomy
t. serum prostatic acid phosphatase
 (TSPAP)
t. slit pore length
t. transurethral resection of prostate
 (T-TURP)

totalis

varicosis coli t.

totally

t. extraperitoneal (TEP)
t. extraperitoneal hernia repair
t. stapled restorative
 proctocolectomy (TSRPC)

touch

t. cytology
T. preparation

Toupet

T. hemifundoplication
T. partial posterior fundoplication
T. procedure

tour de maitre

Tourneux fold

tourniquet

double loop t.
Dupuytren t.
Gill renal t.
t. occlusion

Rumel t.
single loop t.

towel clip

Townes-Brocks syndrome

toxemia

hepatic t.
t. of pregnancy

toxic

t. appearance
t. cirrhosis
t. colitis
t. diarrhea
t. dilatation of bowel
t. dilation of colon
t. epidermal necrolysis (TEN)
t. gastritis
t. glomerulopathy
t. hepatitis
t. megacolon
t. metabolite
t. nephropathy
t. shock syndrome
t. steatosis

toxicity

acetaminophen t.
acute hepatic t.
aluminum t.
ammonia t.
bleomycin t.
calcineurin inhibitor t.
chloroform t.
chlorzoxazone t.
cyclosporine t.
direct tubular t.
hyperbaric oxygen t.
octreotide-induced hepatic t.
progressive t.
protein-mediated tubular t.
quality-adjusted time without
 symptoms or t. (Q-TWIST)
renal t.
theophylline t.
vitamin A t.

Toxicodendron **dermatitis**

toxicosis

toxicum

erythema t.

toxigenic

t. bacterium
t. diarrhea

toxin

t. A, B

NOTES

T

toxin *(continued)*
t. assay
botulinum t. (BTX)
cholera t.
Coley t.
t. exposure
heat-labile t. (LT)
industrial t.
occupational t.
pertussin t.
Shiga t. (Stx)
Shiga-like t. (SLT)
VacA t.
toxin-mediated intestinal secretion
Toxocara canis
toxocariasis
Toxoplasma gondii
toxoplasmosis
TP40 **gene**
TP53 **gene**
TPA, tPA
12-O-tetradecanoylphorbol-13-acetate
tissue plasminogen activator
phorbol ester TPA
phorbol ester 12-O-
tetradecanoylphorbol-13-acetate
TPD
title peritoneal dialysis
TPH
transrectal prostatic hyperthermia
TPN
total parenteral nutrition
TPN line
TPO
thrombopoietin
TPPN
total peripheral parenteral nutrition
TPSV
tumor peak systolic velocity
TR
terminal repeat
trabecula, pl. **trabeculae**
trabeculae of corpora cavernosa of
penis
trabeculae corporis spongiosi penis
trabeculae corporum cavernosorum
penis
trabeculae of corpus spongiosum of
penis
trabeculae lienis
trabeculae of spleen
trabeculae splenicae
trabecular
t. bone fracture
t. sinusoidal pattern
t. structure
trabecularism
trabeculate

trabeculated bladder
trabeculation
t. of bladder dome
detrusor muscle t.
Trabucco double balloon catheter
trace-gas analysis
tracer
focal accumulation of t.
t. Hybrid wire guide
T. ST wire
tracheal
t. bifurcation
t. deviation
t. ulceration
trachelocystitis
tracheobronchial
t. aspiration
t. malacia
t. Z stent
tracheoesophageal (TE)
t. fistula (TEF)
t. junction
t. puncture (TEP)
t. septum
tracheostomy
Trach-Eze closed suction catheter
trachomatis
Chlamydia t.
tracing
Narco Bio-Systems MMS 200
physiograph t.
sexually transmitted disease
contact t.
track
horseshoe t.
radial suture t.
submucosal t.
Tracker catheter
tract
alimentary t.
allantoic t.
benign mesothelioma of genital t.
biliary t.
digestive t.
t. dilation
double-contrast barium examination
of the upper gastrointestinal t.
(DCGI)
drilling t.
fistulous t.
gastrocutaneous fistulous t.
gastrointestinal t. (GIT)
genital t.
genitourinary t.
GI t.
hepatic outflow t.
ileal inflow t.
ileal outflow t.

infected t.
intestinal t.
intramural fistulous t.
Lewis classification for vascular anomalies of the gastrointestinal t.
Moore classification for vascular anomalies of the gastrointestinal t.
needle t.
nucleus of the solitary t.
ororespiratory t.
outflow t.
pancreaticobiliary t.
perineal sinus t.
portal t.
sacrococcygeal pilonidal sinus t.
safe gastrocutaneous fistulous t.
sinus t.
t. tamponade
transsphincteric fistulous t.
T-tube t.
upper gastrointestinal t.
urinary t.
Z t.

traction
caudal t.
cephalad t.
t. diverticulum
enterocele t.
postinflammatory t.
t. suture

tractor
Lowsley t.
Syms t.
Young prostatic t.

trafficking
leukocyte t.
membrane t.

Trager therapy

trail
T. Making Test
T. test

trainer
Personal EMG t.

training
bladder t.
pelvic muscle t.
pubococcygeal muscle t.

trait
X-linked recessive t

tramadol

tramazoline
tram-line calcification
Trandate
tranexamic
t. acid
t. acid enema
tranquilizer
transabdominal
t. Burch urethropexy
t. cholangiography
t. hydrocolonic sonography
t. preperitoneal (TAPP)
t. preperitoneal hernia repair
t. scan
transaminase
glutamate pyruvate t. (GLPT)
glutamic-oxaloacetic t. (GOT)
glutamic-pyruvic t. (GPT)
serum glutamic-oxaloacetic t. (SGOT)
serum glutamic-pyruvic t. (SGPT)
transampullary
transanal
t. anastomosis
t. catheter
t. endoscopic microsurgery (TEM)
t. endoscopic microsurgical resection
t. excision
t. ultrasonography
transaortic endarterectomy
transarterial
t. catheter embolization (TACE)
t. chemoembolization (TACE)
t. perfusion cooling
transballoon cystometry
trans-blotting cell
transcapillary
t. diffusion
t. escape rate
t. hydrostatic pressure gradient
transcarbamylase
heterozygous ornithine t. (HOTC)
transcatheter
t. arterial chemoembolization (TACE)
t. arterial embolization (TAE)
t. arterial embolization therapy
t. arterial infusion
t. embolotherapy
t. hepatic arterial embolization
t. perfusion

T

NOTES

transcatheter *(continued)*
    t. splenic arterial embolization
      (TSAE)
    t. treatment
    t. variceal embolization
transcellular absorption
transcoccygeal vesiculectomy
transcolonic endoscopy
transcranial magnetic stimulation
    (TCMS)
transcriptase
    avian myeloblastosis virus
      reverse t.
    t. polymerase chain reaction assay
    reverse t. (RT)
transcription
    t. factor
    t. factor AP1
    reverse t.
transcutaneous
    t. biopsy
    t. electrical nerve stimulation
      (TENS)
    t. nerve
    t. registration
    t. sacral neurostimulation
    t. sonogram endoscope
    t. ultrasonography
    t. ultrasound
    t. ultrasound imaging
transcystic duct/common bile duct
    exploration (TCD/CBDE)
transdermal therapeutic system (TTS)
Transderm-Nitro
transducer
    antral pressure t.
    bifocal multiplane rectal t.
    Bruel-Kjaer axial t.
    t. catheter
    electromagnetic flow t.
    Elema-Siemens AB pressure t.
    Gould pressure t.
    intracavitary t.
    linear array t.
    linear 35-Mhz t.
    LSC 7000 curved array t.
    3.5–10 MHz curved array t.
    Nellcor Durasensor adult oxygen t.
    Olympus intracavity t.
    P23b Statham pressure t.
    piezoelectric t.
    pressure t.
    Sensor Medics pressure t.
    Siemens Endo-P endorectal t.
    solid-state pressure t.
    Soreson pressure t.
    Spectramed t.
    Statham external t.

    strain gauge t.
    transrectal multiplane three-
      dimensional t.
    ultrasound t.
    volume displacement t.
transductal cystodigestive diversion
transduction
    downstream signal t.
    t. pathway
    receptor and signal t.
transduodenal
    t. approach
    t. drainage
    t. endoscopic decompression
    t. injection
    t. sphincteroplasty
    t. sphincterotomy
transection
    bladder t.
    t. and devascularization operation
    esophageal t.
    high t.
    Sugiura esophageal variceal t.
transendoscopic
    t. electrocoagulation
    t. laser photocoagulation
    t. sphincterotomy
    t. ultrasound
transepithelial tubular transport
transesophageal
    t. endoscopy
    t. ligation
    t. ligation of varix
transfemoral liver biopsy
transfer
    t. dysfunction
    t. dysphagia
    t. factor
    gamete intrafallopian t. (GIFT)
    unidirectional t.
transferase
    aspartate t.
    choline acetyl t. (ChAT)
    gamma-glutamyl t. (GGT)
    glucuronyl t.
    glutathione t.
    phenylethylamine N-methyl t.
      (PNMT)
transferrin
    t. saturation
    t. saturation level
    serum t.
    t. test
transformary mass
transformation
    blastoid t.
    Eadie-Hofstee t.
    giant cell t. (GCT)

neoplastic t.
nodular t.
t. zone
transforming
t. growth factor (TGF)
t. growth factor alpha (TGF-alpha)
t. growth factor beta (TGF-beta)
t. growth factor beta-1 (TGF-beta-1)
t. growth factor beta-2 (TGF-beta-2)
t. growth factor beta-3 (TGF-beta-3)
transfuse
transfusion
autologous t.
blood t.
donor-specific t. (DST)
intraoperative autologous t.
t. nephritis
peritoneal t.
platelet t.
postoperative autologous t.
type-specific blood t.
transfusional iron overload
transfusion-associated hepatitis
transfusion-related chronic liver disease
transfusion-transmitted virus (TTV)
transgastric
t. cholangiogram
t. drainage
t. esophageal bougienage
t. fine-needle aspiration biopsy
t. ligation
t. plication
transgastrostomic enteroscopy (TGE)
transgastrostomy
transgenesis
mammalian t.
transglomerular hydrostatic filtration pressure
transglutaminase
tissue t. (tTG)
trans-Golgi network
transhepatic
t. antegrade biliary drainage procedure
t. biliary drainage
t. biliary stent
t. catheterization
t. cholangiogram

t. cholangiography (TC, THC)
t. embolization (THE)
t. portacaval shunt
t. portal venous sampling
t. portography
t. vascular resistance
transhiatal
t. blunt esophagectomy
t. radical esophagectomy
t. resection
t. simple esophagectomy
transient
t. cholangitis
t. discontinuation
t. gastroparesis
t. LES relaxation
t. lower esophageal relaxation (TLESR)
t. proteinuria
t. relaxations of the LES
transileostomy manometry
transilluminate
transillumination
kidney t.
transilluminator
UV t.
transistor
ion-sensitive field effect t.
transit
delayed colonic t.
gastrointestinal t.
ileocolonic t.
mean colonic t. (MCT)
slow colonic t.
t. time (TT)
whole gut t.
transition
t. mutation
t. suture
t. zone index
t. zone volume
transitional
t. cell
t. cell carcinoma
t. cell carcinoma of the bladder (TCCB)
t. epithelium
t. feeding
t. zone
t. zone biopsy
transitory block

T

NOTES

transjugular
    t. intrahepatic portacaval shunt procedure
    t. intrahepatic portosystemic shunt (TIPS)
    t. intrahepatic portosystemic stent shunt (TIPSS)
    t. liver biopsy
    t. portal venography
translation of torque
translumbar inferior vena cava catheter
transluminal
    t. pseudocyst drainage
    t. ultrasonography
transmembrane
    t. beta-subunit
    t. electrical potential difference
    t. hydraulic pressure
    t. protein
    t. signal
transmesenteric plication
transmission
    blood-borne t.
    t. electron microscopy (TEM)
    fecal t.
    fecal-oral t.
    horizontal t.
    oral t.
    synaptic t.
    vertical t.
transmitter
    NANC inhibitory t.
    nonadrenergic noncholinergic inhibitory t.
    putative t.
transmucosal
    t. electrical potential test
    t. potential difference (TMPD)
transmural
    t. approach
    t. burn
    t. colitis
    t. drainage (TMD)
    t. endoscopy
    t. fibrosis
    t. hydrostatic pressure gradient
    t. ileocolitis
    t. inflammation
transnasal
    t. bile duct catheterization
    t. endoluminal ultrasonography
    t. endoscopy
    t. pancreatico-biliary drain
Transonics
    T. laser-Doppler flowmeter
    T. Systems 0.5-mm flow probe
transoral endoscopic suturing

transpancreatic sphincter precut approach to biliary sphincterotomy
transpapillary
    t. approach
    t. biopsy
    t. cannulation
    t. catheterization
    t. cystopancreatic stent
    t. drain
    t. drainage
    t. endoscopic cholecystotomy (TEC)
    t. endoscopic endoprosthesis
    t. insertion of self-expanding biliary metal stent
    t. therapy
transparent elastic band ligating device
transpeptidase
    gamma-glutamyl t. (GGTP)
    glutamyl t. (GTP)
transperineal
    t. brachytherapy
    t. interstitial permanent prostate brachytherapy (TIPPB)
    t. palladium-103
    t. seed implant
    t. vesiculectomy
transperitoneal
    t. anterior subcostal incision (TASI)
    t. laparoscopic adrenalectomy (TLA)
    t. laparoscopic nephrectomy (TLN)
    t. laparoscopic nephroureterectomy
transplant
    acute rejection of liver t.
    allogenic kidney t.
    auxiliary t.
    cadaveric intestinal t.
    cadaveric renal t.
    combined kidney and pancreas t. (CKPT)
    Domino t.
    failed t.
    Gallie t.
    heart t.
    heart-kidney t.
    hypercholesterolemic cadaveric renal t.
    kidney t.
    liver t.
    living donor t.
    t. nephrectomy
    orthotopic liver t. (OLT)
    pancreas-kidney t.
    reduced liver t. (RLT)
    reduced-size liver t. (RSLT)
    t. rejection
    renal t.

t. renal artery stenosis (TRAS)
split-liver t.

transplantation
anhepatic stage of liver t.
t. antigen
auxiliary heterotopic liver t.
(AHLT)
auxiliary liver t.
auxiliary partial orthotopic liver t.
(APOLT)
auxiliary partial orthotopic living
donor t.
bone marrow t. (BMT)
cadaveric renal t.
en bloc kidney t.
heart t.
hematopoietic cell t.
hepatocyte t.
kidney t.
liver t.
living donor liver t. (LDLT)
organ t.
pancreas t.
pancreatic islet cell t.
pancreaticoduodenal t.
piggyback liver t.
renal t.
small bowel t.
SPK t.
t. tolerance
xenograft t.

transplantectomy
transplanted cancer
Transpore tape
transport
active t.
t. aminoaciduria
bolus t.
cation t.
chyme t.
convective t.
diffusive t.
fluid t.
glucose t.
lymphatic t.
nephron t.
peritoneal membrane t.
peritoneal solute t.
retinoid t.
single-nephron glomerular t.
sodium t.
solute t.

transepithelial tubular t.
urine t.

transporter
glucose t.
low-affinity t.
polarized glucose t.
serotonin reuptake t. (SERT)

transposition
buttonhole preputial t.
gastric t.
gluteus maximus t.
ileocecal segment t.
penoscrotal t.
portacaval t. (PCT)

transpubic incision
transpyloric
t. feeding
t. tube

transrectal
t. multiplane three-dimensional
transducer
t. probe
t. prostatic hyperthermia (TPH)
t. scan
t. sonography
t. ultrasonography (TRUS)
t. ultrasonography-guided biopsy
t. ultrasound (TRUS)
t. ultrasound-guided-sextant biopsy
t. ultrasound scanning (TRUS)
t. ultrasound staging
t. vasography

transscrotal
transsection
nerve t.

transseptal orchiopexy
transsexual surgery
transsphincteric
t. anal fistula
t. fistulous tract

transthoracic
t. esophagectomy
t. resection of esophageal
carcinoma

transthyretin
transudative ascites
transureteropyelostomy
transureteroureteral anastomosis
transureteroureterostomy (TUU)
transurethral
t. ablative prostatectomy
t. balloon dilation

T

NOTES

transurethral *(continued)*
   t. balloon Laserthermia
     prostatectomy
   t. collagen injection therapy
   t. electrical bladder stimulation
     (TEBS)
   t. electrovaporization
   t. electrovaporization of prostate
     (TUVP, TVP)
   t. evaporation of prostate (TUEP)
   t. grooving of prostate
   t. incision (TUI)
   t. incision of the bladder neck
     (TUIBN)
   t. incision of prostate (TUIP)
   t. laser incision of the prostate
   t. microwave thermotherapy
     (TUMT)
   t. microwave thermotherapy
     functional result
   t. needle ablation (TUNA)
   t. needle ablation of the prostate
   t. rectal ultrasound
   t. resection (TUR)
   t. resection of bladder tumor
     (TURBT)
   t. resection of prostate (TURP)
   t. resection of the prostate
     functional result
   t. resection syndrome
   t. resectoscope
   t. sphincterotomy
   t. thermoablation
   t. ultrasound-guided laser-induced
     prostatectomy (TULIP)
   t. unroofing
   t. ureterorenoscopy (URS)
   t. vaporization of prostate (TUVP)
   t. vaporization-resection of prostate
     (TUVRP)
transurothelial permeability
transvaginal
   t. Burch procedure
   t. suturing (TVS)
   t. suturing system
   t. ultrasound (TV-UST)
   t. urethrolysis
transvenous
   t. liver biopsy
   t. perfusion
transversa
   plica vesicalis t.
transversalis fascia
transverse
   t. abdominis muscle
   t. colectomy
   t. colon
   t. colostomy

   t. colostomy effluent
   t. duodenotomy
   t. fissure
   t. folds of rectum
   t. image
   t. loop
   t. process
   t. resection
   t. semilunar skin incision
   t. sonogram
   t. testicular ectopia
   t. ulceration
   t. umbilical line
   t. vaginal septum
   t. view
transverse-loop rod colostomy
transversion mutation
transversostomy
transversourethralis
transversum
   colon t.
transversus
   t. abdominis muscle
   t. perinei muscle
transvesical
   t. scan
   t. vesiculectomy
transwell
   cell culture t.
Tranxene
tranylcypromine
trap
   Endodynamics suction polyp t.
   specimen t.
trapezoid method
trapped
   t. basket
   t. penis
   t. penis after circumcision
   t. prostate gland
trapping
   penoscrotal t.
TRAS
   transplant renal artery stenosis
Tratner catheter
Traube semilunar space
trauma
   autoerotic rectal t.
   bile duct t.
   bladder t.
   blunt abdominal t.
   blunt liver t.
   blunt pancreatic t.
   colonic t.
   colorectal t.
   diaphragmatic hernial t.
   duodenal t.
   esophageal t.

external t.
foreign body t.
gallbladder t.
t. of gallbladder
gastric t.
hepatic t.
homosexual rectal t.
iatrogenic pancreatic t.
liver t.
pancreatic t.
penetrating abdominal t.
penetrating pancreatic t.
perineal impact t.
rectal t.
renal t.
small intestine t.
splenic t.
Texas t.
TraumaCal enteral feeding
Traum-Aid HBC enteral feeding
traumatic
t. appendicitis
t. corporeal veno-occlusive
dysfunction
t. diaphragmatic hernia
t. grasping forceps
t. inflammation
t. lesion
t. locking grasper
t. masturbation
t. orchitis
t. proctitis
t. renal mass
t. rupture
Travamulsion fat emulsion solution
Travasol amino acid
Travasorb
T. Hepatic Diet
T. HN powdered feeding
T. MCT liquid feeding
T. MCT supplement
T. Renal Diet
T. STD liquid feeding
traveler's
t. chemoprophylaxis
t. diarrhea
traverse retubularized ileovesicostomy
Traverso-Longmire technique
tray
Urine Meter Foley t.
trazodone

TRE
thyroid hormone response element
treated tissue
treatment
acorn t.
add-back t.
adjuvant t.
alpha-blocker t.
alpha interferon t.
alternate-day t.
amoxicillin-omeprazole t.
anabolic steroid t.
anoplasty t.
anti-*Helicobacter pylori* t.
t. balloon
behavioral t.
BrachySeed prostate cancer t.
Candida t.
t. channel
cholecystectomy t.
chronic anoplasty t.
corticosteroid t.
CyPat t.
dialytic t.
endoscopic t.
endovascular t.
esophageal dilation t.
t. failure
famotidine maintenance t.
foscarnet t.
Gelfoam particles transarterial
embolization t.
glucocorticoid t.
hemangioma laser t.
Hypertension Optimal T. (HOT)
interferon t.
intracavernosal injection t.
intralesional t.
intraprostatic temperature-guided t.
KTP/Nd:YAG laser t.
lipiodol transarterial embolization t.
maintenance t.
mercury bougienage t.
microwave nonsurgical t.
Milligan-Morgan technique for
hemorrhoid t.
minimally invasive t.
mitomycin transarterial
embolization t.
t. morbidity
Murphy t.
neoadjuvant antiandrogenic t.

T

NOTES

treatment *(continued)*
  Ochsner t.
  oxandrolone t.
  pharmacological t.
  photocoagulation t.
  Plummer t.
  preoperative tumor t.
  prophylactic antibiotic t. (PAT)
  prostatic thermal t.
  ProstRcision t.
  t. protocol
  rectovaginal surgical t.
  self-bougienage t.
  serotonin antagonist t.
  sham t.
  shock wave t.
  sonographic planning of
    oncology t. (SPOT)
  supportive t.
  suppression t.
  topical t.
  transcatheter t.

tree
  biliary t.
  cannulation of the biliary t.
  Croton lechleri t.
  hepatobiliary t.
  pancreatic t.
  pancreaticobiliary t.
  phylogenetic t.

trefoil
  t. deformity
  t. peptide

trehalose

Treitz
  T. arch
  T. fossa
  T. hernia
  ligament of T.

Trélat stool

Trelex mesh

Trelstar depot

tremor
  resting t.

tremor-nystagmus-ulcer syndrome

trench nephritis

Trendelenburg
  T. gait
  T. position

Trental

trephine biopsy

Treponema
  T. immunofluorescence study
  T. pallidum

tretinoin

Treves
  T. fold
  plane of T.

TRI
  intracytoplasmic tuboreticular inclusion
  tubuloreticular inclusion

triad
  t. of adenoma sebaceum, epilepsy,
    and mental retardation
  Andersen t.
  Borchardt t.
  Charcot t.
  Currarino t.
  Dieulafoy t.
  hepatic t.
  portal t.
  Quincke t.
  radiographic t.
  Saint t.
  t. syndrome
  Whipple t.

triaditis
  portal t.

trial
  aggressive therapeutic t.
  AIPRI t.
  Angiotensin-Converting Enzyme
    Inhibition in Progressive Renal
    Insufficiency t.
  Antihypertensive and Lipid-
    Lowering Treatment to Prevent
    Heart Attack T. (ALLHAT)
  Antioxidant Polyp Prevention T.
  clinical t.
  direct current electrotherapy t.
  HOT t.
  Hypertension Optimal Treatment t.
  IRS-IV t.
  Modification of Diet in Renal
    Disease t.
  prospective clinical t.
  Prostate Cancer Intervention Versus
    Observation T. (PCIVOT, PIVOT)
  Stockholm t. (I, II)
  Swedish Rectal Cancer T.
  T. Using Medicinal Microbiotic
    Yogurt (TUMMY)
  VIGOR t.
    Vioxx Gastrointestinal Outcomes
      Research trial
  Vioxx Gastrointestinal Outcomes
    Research t. (VIGOR trial)
  t. without catheter (TWOC)

triamcinolone cream

triamterene
  t. calculus
  hydrochlorothiazide and t.
  t. urinary lithiasis

triangle
  anal t.
  Calot t.

cardiohepatic t.
Charcot t.
cystohepatic t.
digastric t.
t. of doom
femoral t.
T. gelatin-sealed sling material
Grynfeltt t.
Henke t.
Hesselbach t.
iliofemoral t.
inguinal t.
Killian t.
Labbe t.
Lesgaft t.
Livingston t.
lumbocostoabdominal t.
mesenteric t.
t. of pain
Petit t.
Scarpa t.
urogenital t.
triangular
t. ligament
t. vaginal patch sling
triangulation stapling method
triazolam
tricarboxylic
t. acid (TCA)
t. acid cycle
triceps
t. skin fold thickness
t. skin fold thickness test
trichilemmoma
Trichinella spiralis
trichinelliasis
trichinellosis
trichiniasis
trichinosis
trichiura
Trichuris t.
trichlormethiazide
trichloroacetic acid (TCA)
trichloroethylene
trichobezoar
trichocyst
trichomonal balanitis
Trichomonas
T. hominis
T. vaginalis
trichomonas

trichomoniasis
vaginal t.
trichomycosis
trichophagia
trichophytobezoar
Trichophyton
T. mentagrophytes
T. rubrum
Trichosporon
T. beigelli
T. capitatum
trichrome
Masson t.
t. stain
trichuriasis
Trichuris
T. muris
T. trichiura
tricitrate
trick
Hafter diet t.
trickle perfusion
Tricomponent Coaxial System (TCS)
tricyclamol
tricyclic antidepressant
tridecapeptide
tridihexethyl chloride
Tridrate bowel preparation
triene
macrocyclic t.
triethylenethiophosphoramide
trifid stomach
trifluoperazine
triflupromazine
trifurcation variant
trigeminy
Trigesic
trigger
t. point injection
rectal feedback t.
urethral feedback t.
t. voiding
triggering
R-wave t.
triglyceride
t. enzyme deficiency
long-chain t. (LCT)
medium-chain t. (MCT)
serum t.
VLDL t.
triglyceride-rich protein (TRL)
trigona (*pl. of* trigonum)

T

NOTES

trigonal plate
trigone
    bladder t.
    deep t.
    fascia of urogenital t.
trigonitis
trigonotome
trigonum, pl. trigona
    t. urogenitale
    t. vesica
    t. vesicae lieutaudi
trihexyphenidyl
trihydrate
    amoxicillin t.
trihydrocoprostanic acid (TCA)
trihydroxy salt
triiodobenzene
Trilafon
trilobar
    t. hyperplasia
    t. hypertrophy
Trilogy low-profile balloon dilatation catheter
Trimadeau sign
Trimazide
Trimedyne
    T. holmium laser
    T. Optilase 1000 device
trimeprazine tartrate
trimer
trimetaphan
trimethidinium
trimethobenzamide
trimethoprim
    sulfamethoxazole and t. (SMX/TMP, SMZ/TMP)
trimethoprim-sulfamethoxazole (TMP-SMX)
    t.-s. DS
trimethylsilyl ether
trimetrexate glucuronate
Trimox
Trimpex
Trinalin Repetabs
trinitrate
    glyceryl t. (GTN)
Trinovin
Trinsicon
triolein C-14 breath test
triopathy
tripelennamine
tripeptide
    disaccharide t.
triphasic cystometric curve
triphosphatase
    adenosine t. (ATPase)
    hydrogen adenosine t.

triphosphate
    adenosine t. (ATP)
    guanosine t. (GTP)
    inositol t.
1,4,5-triphosphate
    inositol 1,4,5-t. (IP3)
triple
    t. balloon probe
    t. eradication therapy
    t. intussusception
    t. lobe hepatectomy
    t. loop pouch
    t. rubber band ligation
    t. therapy (TT)
triple-lumen
    t.-l. manometry catheter
    t.-l. perfused catheter system
    t.-l. Sengstaken-Blakemore tube
triple-phosphate crystal
triplet
    neurofilament protein t.
triple-voiding cystography
triplication
triploid cell
tripod
    t. grasper
    t. grasping forceps
triprolidine
triptorelin
trip wire
triradiate cecal fold
trisegmentectomy
Tris HCl
tris(hydroxymethyl)aminomethane
trisilicate
    aluminum hydroxide and magnesium t.
    magnesium t.
trismus presentation
trisodium
    mangafodipir t.
trisomy
    t. 13, 18, 21
Tritec
Triton tumor
TRL
    triglyceride-rich protein
trocar
    accessory t.
    Beardsley cecostomy t.
    Campbell t.
    conical t.
    Cook urological t.
    t. cystostomy
    disposable t.
    ensheathing t.
    Ethicon t.
    gallbladder t.

Hasson t.
Landau t.
Ochsner gallbladder t.
Origin t.
pyramidal t.
trochanter
troglitazone
Troisier
T. ganglion
T. node
T. sign
troleandomycin
Trombovar
tromethamine
carboprost t.
fosfomycin t.
ketorolac t.
Tronolane
Trophermyma whipplei
trophic
t. change
t. lesion
trophoblastic
malignant teratoma, t. (MTT)
trophozoite form
tropical
t. calcific pancreatitis
t. diarrhea
t. diarrhea-malabsorption syndrome
(TDMS)
t. hyphemia
t. mesangiocapillary
glomerulonephritis
t. nephropathy
t. spastic paraparesis
t. splenomegaly
t. sprue
tropicalis
Candida t.
tropoblastic malignant teratoma
tropomyosin
troponin
baseline t. T
Trousseau
T. esophageal bougie
T. syndrome
T. test
Troutman rectus forceps
trovafloxacin
Trovan/Zithromax Compliance Pak
TRPM-2
testosterone repressed prostate message-2

Tru-Cut
T.-C. biopsy needle
T.-C. needle biopsy
Truelove-Witts
T.-W. grading system
T.-W. index
trumpet
nasal t.
truncal
t. vagotomy
t. vagotomy and gastroenterostomy
t. vagotomy and pyloroplasty
truncus, pl. **trunci**
t. celiacus
trunci intestinales
trunk
bicarotid t.
celiac t.
lumbosacral t.
portal t.
TRUS
transrectal ultrasonography
transrectal ultrasound
transrectal ultrasound scanning
truss
Tru Taper Ethalloy needle
Trypan blue-stained cell
Trypanosoma
T. congolense
T. cruzi
T. rhodesiense
trypanosomiasis
American t.
Rhodesian t.
South American t.
trypsin
bovine t.
t. inhibitor
trypsinization
trypsinogen
tryptic soy broth
tryptophan metabolism
TS
terminal sedation
TS1
tuberous sclerosis gene TS1
TS2
tuberous sclerosis gene TS2
TS-200
tissue spectrum analyzer T.
TSAE
transcatheter splenic arterial embolization

T

NOTES

TSC
  tuberous sclerosis complex
TSF
  thickness of skin fold
TSPAP
  total serum prostatic acid phosphatase
TSRPC
  totally stapled restorative
    proctocolectomy
TSRS
  tissue-stone recognition system
TT
  transit time
  triple therapy
    TT virus (TTV)
TT-3 needle
TTC
  T-tube cholangiogram
tTG
  tissue transglutaminase
    IgA tTG
      immunoglobulin A
        transglutaminase antibody
t1/2 time of gastric emptying
TTL
  total lymphocyte
TTP
  thrombotic thrombocytopenic purpura
TTS
  testosterone transdermal system
  through-the-scope
  transdermal therapeutic system
    TTS balloon dilation
    TTS dilator
    Testoderm TTS
T-tube
  Cattell T-t.
  T-t. cholangiogram (TTC)
  T-t. cholangiography
  T-t. drain
  T-t. drainage
  French T-t.
  Kehr T-t.
  T-t. stent
  T-t. study
  T-t. tract
  T-t. tract choledochofiberoscopy
  T-t. tract choledochoscopy
T-TURP
  total transurethral resection of prostate
TTV
  transfusion-transmitted virus
  TT virus
TTX
  tetrodotoxin
tuaminoheptane
tubal
  t. ectopic pregnancy

  t. infertility
  t. ligation
tube
  Abbott t.
  Abbott-Miller t.
  Abbott-Rawson double-lumen
    gastrointestinal t.
  Adson suction t.
  All-Silicone Side-Eye EPT
    feeding t.
  Anderson gastric t.
  Argyle chest t.
  Argyle-Salem sump t.
  ascites drainage t.
  aspiration and dissection t.
  Aspisafe nasogastric t.
  Atkinson silicone rubber t.
  Axiom double sump t.
  Baker intestinal decompression t.
  Baker jejunostomy t.
  Bard gastrostomy feeding t.
  Bard PEG t.
  Bilbao-Dotter t.
  Blakemore t.
  Blakemore-Sengstaken t.
  Bower PEG t.
  Boyce modification of Sengstaken-
    Blakemore t.
  Broncho-Cath double-lumen
    endotracheal t.
  Buie rectal suction t.
  Caluso PEG gastrostomy t.
  Cantor t.
  cast-like t.
  t. cecostomy
  Celestin esophageal t.
  Celestin latex rubber t.
  chest t.
  collecting t.
  Compat feeding t.
  conical centrifuge t.
  Cope loop nephrostomy t.
  Corpak feeding t.
  Corpak weighted-tip, self-
    lubricating t.
  Council tip t.
  cuffed endotracheal t.
  cystostomy t.
  Davol colon t.
  Davol feeding t.
  t. decompression
  decompression t.
  Dennis intestinal t.
  Diamond t.
  digestive t.
  direct percutaneous jejunostomy t.
  Dobbhoff gastrectomy feeding t.
  Dobbhoff gastric decompression t.

Dobbhoff PEG t.
double-lumen t.
DPJ t.
drainage t.
Dreiling t.
dual percutaneous gastrostomy t.
Dumon-Gilliard prosthesis
  pushing t.
duodenal t.
Duo-Tube feeding t.
Edlich gastric lavage t.
endoscopic gastrostomy t.
endothelial t.
endotracheal t. (ET)
ENDO-Tube nasal jejunal
  feeding t.
t. enlargement
enteroclysis t.
t. enteroscope
t. enterostomy
EntriStar feeding t.
EntriStar polyurethane PEG t.
ENtube-Pedi feeding t.
Eppendorf t.
ESKA-Buess esophageal t.
esophageal t.
t. esophagogram
Ethox feeding t.
Ewald t.
fallopian t.
t. feeding
feeding gastrostomy t.
Ferrein t.
Flexiflo Inverta-PEG t.
Flexiflo stoma creator t.
Flexiflo Stomate low-profile
  gastrostomy t.
Flexiflo tungsten-weighted
  feeding t.
Flexiflo Versa-PEG t.
Flow-Thru feeding t.
four-lumen t.
20F PEG t.
Frazier suction t.
Frederick-Miller t.
gastric aspiration t.
gastric augment and single
  pedicle t. (GASP)
gastric lavage t.
gastrostomy t.
Gilman-Abrams gastric t.
Glasser gastrostomy t.

Gomco suction t.
Gott t.
t. graft
guttered T t.
Haldane-Priestly t.
Har-el pharyngeal t.
Harris t.
Hodge intestinal decompression t.
insertion t.
jejunal feeding t.
jejunostomy t.
Kangaroo gastrostomy t.
Kaslow intestinal t.
Keofeed II feeding t.
Killian suction t.
large-bore gastric lavage t.
t. leakage
Lepley-Ernst t.
Levin t.
Linton-Nachlas t.
long intestinal t.
Malecot gastrostomy t.
Malecot nephrostomy t.
marked t.
Medena t.
mediastinal t.
Medina t.
Medoc-Celestin pulsion t.
mercury-weighted t.
metal-weighted Silastic feeding t.
MIC gastroenteric t.
MIC gastrostomy t.
MIC-Key G, J gastrostomy t.
MIC-TJ transgastric jejunal t.
t. migration
Mikulicz gastrostomy t.
Miller-Abbott intestinal t.
Minnesota t.
Mitrofanoff t.
modified Minnesota t.
Montgomery salivary bypass t.
Moss gastrostomy t.
Moss Mark IV t.
Mousseau-Barbin prosthetic t.
myringotomy t.
Nachlas gastrointestinal t.
nasobiliary t.
nasocystic drainage t.
nasoduodenal feeding t.
nasoenteric feeding t.
nasogastric t. (NGT)
nasogastric feeding t.

T

NOTES

tube *(continued)*
   nasoileal t.
   nasojejunal feeding t.
   negative pressure t.
   negative pressure-controlled t.
   nephrostomy t.
   nephrotomy t.
   NJ feeding t.
   Nuport PEG t.
   Nyhus-Nelson gastric decompression
     and jejunal feeding t.
   Olympus one-step button
     gastrostomy t.
   orogastric Ewald t.
   oropharyngeal t.
   t. overgrowth
   Paul-Mixter t.
   pediatric feeding t.
   pediatric nasogastric t.
   Pedi PEG t.
   Pee Wee low profile
     gastrostomy t.
   PEG t.
   PEG-400 t.
   PEJ t.
   percutaneous endoscopic gastrostomy
     and jejunal extension t. (PEG-
     JET)
   percutaneous endoscopic placement
     of jejunal t.
   photomultiplier t.
   pigtail nephrostomy t.
   t. placement
   pleural t.
   polyethylene t.
   Poole suction t.
   postpyloric feeding t.
   Proctor-Livingston t.
   pusher t.
   Quinton t.
   Radius enteral feeding t.
   rectal t.
   Rehfuss duodenal t.
   Rehfuss stomach t.
   t. removal
   t. replacement
   Replogle t.
   Rubin t.
   Rubin-Quinton small-bowel
     biopsy t.
   Ryle t.
   Sacks-Vine feeding gastrostomy t.
   Sacks-Vine PEG t.
   Salem duodenal sump t.
   Sandoz Caluso PEG gastrostomy t.
   Sandoz 22F balloon replacement t.
   Sandoz feeding/suction t.
   Schachowa spiral t.

   Sengstaken-Blakemore t.
   Shiner t.
   Silk Bullet feeding t.
   Silk Pill feeding t.
   Silk Tip feeding t.
   skin t.
   sliding t.
   small bowel t.
   Souttar t.
   Stamey t.
   Stamm gastrostomy t.
   stiffening t.
   stomach t.
   Stomate decompression t.
   Stomate extension t.
   suction t.
   sump nasogastric t.
   Super PEG t.
   suprapubic t.
   T t.
   tampon t.
   Teflon nasobiliary t.
   Thiersch t.
   transpyloric t.
   triple-lumen Sengstaken-
     Blakemore t.
   venting percutaneous gastrostomy t.
   Vivonex Moss t.
   Wangensteen suction t.
   Willscher t.
   Wilson-Cook nasobiliary t.
   Wilson-Cook NJFT-series feeding t.
   Wookey skin t.
   woven Dacron t.
   Wurbs-type nasobiliary t.
   Yankauer suction t.
   Young-Dees t.
tubed
   t. free skin graft
   t. groin flap
   t. urethroplasty
tube-fed patient
tubeless lithotriptor
tubercle
   pubic t.
tubercular
   t. diarrhea
   t. involvement
tuberculin
   t. syringe
   t. test
tuberculocele
tuberculoid
tuberculoma
   cavitating t.
tuberculosis
   adrenal t.
   bladder t.

colonic t.
duodenal t.
esophageal t.
gastric t.
genital t.
genitourinary t.
ileocecal t.
intestinal t.
t. of kidney and bladder
miliary t.
Mycobacterium t.
penile t.
peritoneal t.
t. polyp
primary t.
prostatic t.
renal t.
segmental colonic t.
t. symptom
testicular t.
ureteral t.
urethral t.

tuberculous
t. colitis
t. enteritis
t. esophagitis
t. gastritis
t. ileocolitis
t. infectious esophagitis
t. nephritis
t. peritonitis
t. prostatitis

tuberosity
ischial t.
omental t.

tuberous
t. sclerosis
t. sclerosis angiomyolipoma
t. sclerosis complex (TSC)
t. sclerosis gene TS1
t. sclerosis gene TS2

tube-within-tube technique
tubi (*pl. of* tubus)
tubing
t. clamp
large-bore Tygon t.
Nu-Hope t.
polyvinyl t.
shunt t.
Sur-Fit Natura night drainage
  container t.

Tygon venovenous bypass t.
Y-connecting t.

tubogram
T t.

tubular
t. adenoma of Pick
t. atrophy
t. basement membrane (TBM)
t. carcinoma
t. cell desquamation
t. cell dysfunction
t. colonic duplication
t. damage
t. diuresis
t. epithelial cell
t. epithelial cell injury
t. excretory mass
t. fluid:ultrafiltrate (TF/UF)
t. iron accumulation
t. ischemia
t. maximal (Tm)
t. morphologic injury
t. narrowing and sacculation
t. necrosis
t. nephropathy
t. obstruction
t. polyp
t. proteinuria
t. reabsorption of phosphate test
t. reabsorption of phosphorus
t. regeneration
t. resorption
t. sodium handling
t. sodium reabsorption
t. stenosis
t. vertical gastroplasty

tubularization
bladder neck t.
Thiersch-Duplay t.

tubularized
t. bladder neck reconstruction
t. cecal flap

tubule
Albarran t.
Bellini t.
collecting t.
connecting t.
cortical collecting t.
distal t. (DT)
distal convoluted t. (DCT)
epididymal t.
epithelium-lined t.

NOTES

T

tubule *(continued)*
Ferrein t.
Henle t.
human proximal t. (HPT)
isolated cortical t. (ICT)
lumen of seminiferous t.
mesonephric t.
metanephric t.
nonischemic t.
proximal t. (PT)
proximal convoluted t. (PCT)
proximal straight t. (PST)
renal t.
seminiferous t.
sex cord tumors with annular t.'s (SCTAT)
testicular t.
urine-collecting t.
uriniferous t.
uriniparous t.
tubuli (*pl. of* tubulus)
tubulin
tubulitis
tubulocystic
tubulogenesis
vitronectin inhibiting HGF-induced t.
tubulogenic
tubuloglomerular
t. feedback (TGF)
t. feedback mechanism
tubulointerstitial (TI)
t. disease
t. fibrosis
t. inflammation
t. injury
t. nephritis (TIN)
t. nephritis and uveitis syndrome (TINU)
t. nephropathy
t. rejection
tubulointerstitium
tubulopathy
cyclosporine t.
tubuloreticular inclusion (TRI)
tubulorrhexis
tubulosaccular
tubulotoxic effect
tubulous
tubulovesicle
tubulovillar lesion
tubulovillous
t. adenoma
t. polyp
tubulus, pl. **tubuli**
tubus, pl. **tubi**
t. digestorius

tuck
dorsal tunical t.
Tucker
T. esophagoscope
T. spindle-shaped dilator
Tucks ointment
TUEP
transurethral evaporation of prostate
Tuffier
T. abdominal retractor
T. abdominal spatula
T. operation
tuft
t. adhesion
glomerular t.
sclerotic t.
vascular t.
tufting disease
TUI
transurethral incision
TUIBN
transurethral incision of the bladder neck
TUIP
transurethral incision of prostate
Tukey test
TULIP
transurethral ultrasound-guided laser-induced prostatectomy
tulip tip
tumefaction
mesenteric t.
tumescence
t. monitoring
nocturnal penile t. (NPT)
tumeur pileuse
TUMMY
Trial Using Medicinal Microbiotic Yogurt
tumor
abdominal desmoid t.
t. ablation
Abrikosov t.
adenomatoid t.
adnexal t.
adrenal cortex estrogen-secreting t.
adrenal cortex testosterone-secreting t.
adrenal gland metastatic t.
adrenal rest t.
alcohol injection of t.
ampullary t.
anaplastic Wilms t.
t. angiogenesis
angiomatoid t.
benign t.
bifurcation t.
bilateral renal t.
bilateral Wilms t.

biliary tract t.
bismuth t.
bladder t. (BT)
bladder nonepithelial t.
bladder yolk sac t.
bleeding t.
Bolande t.
brain t.
branch duct-type t.
Brenner t.
burned-out t.
Buschke-Löwenstein t.
t. cachexia
carcinoid t.
Castleman t.
celiac t.
t. cell
t. cell lysis
chromophobe cell t.
colorectal t.
core of t.
cystic Wilms t.
debulking of t.
t. debulking
depressed t.
desmoid t.
diploid t.
ductectatic t.
duodenal t.
embryonal t.
encapsulated carcinoid t.
t. encapsulation
epithelial t.
esophageal t.
extracapsular t.
fecal t.
focal t.
t. focus
focus of t.
gastric carcinoid t.
gastrin-secreting non-beta islet
  cell t.
gastroenteropancreatic t.
gastrointestinal autonomic nerve t.
gastrointestinal stromal t.
germ cell t.
gestational trophoblastic t. (GTT)
glomus t.
glycoprotein-producing t.
t. grade
t. grading
granular cell t. (GCT)

granulosa cell t.
granulosa-theca cell t.
Grawitz t.
gritty t.
hepatic t.
high-grade t.
hypersecreting t.
t. infiltration
ingrowth of t.
internist t.
interstitial cell t. of testis
intraabdominal desmoid t.
intractable t.
intraductal mucin-producing t.
intraductal papillary t. (IPT)
intraductal papillary mucinous t.
  (IPMT)
intramesenteric desmoid t.
intraparenchymal t.
islet cell t.
juxtaglomerular apparatus t.
kidney ossifying t.
Klatskin t.
Krukenberg t.
Leydig cell t.
t. location
luteinized granulosa-theca cell t.
lymphoid t.
t. lysis syndrome
malignant mesenchymal t.
t. marker
MCF-7 t.
mediastinal t.
mediastinum germ cell t.
metachronous t.
mixed germ cell t.
mixed germ cell-sex cord
  stromal t.
mucin-hypersecreting t.
mucinous cystic t.
mucinous pancreatic t.
mucin-producing t.
multifocal bladder t.
myogenic t.
t. necrosis
t. necrosis factor (TNF)
t. necrosis factor alpha (TNF-alpha)
t. necrosis factor alpha assay
neuroendocrine t. (NET)
neurogenic t.
4-nitroquinolin-1-oxide-induced t.
  (4NQQ)

NOTES

T

tumor *(continued)*
    t., node, metastasis (TNM)
    nonaneuploid t.
    non-B islet cell t.
    nonfunctional pituitary t.
    noninvasive t.
    nonsecreting pituitary t.
    nonseminomatous germ cell t.
      (NSGCT)
    null cell t.
    t. overgrowth
    pancreatic islet cell t.
    pancreatic polypeptide-secreting t.
      (PPoma)
    paratesticular t.
    paraumbilical vein t. (PUVT)
    parenchymal t.
    t. peak systolic velocity (TPSV)
    periampullary duodenal t.
    persistent postmolar gestational
      trophoblastic t.
    pituitary t.
    polypoid t.
    prepubertal testicular t. (PPTT)
    presacral t.
    primitive neuroectodermal t.
      (PNET)
    t. probe
    t. proliferative index
    Recklinghausen t.
    rectal carcinoid t. (RCT)
    rectal myogenic t.
    renin secreting juxtaglomerular
      cell t.
    retroperitoneal t.
    rhabdoid Wilms t.
    ruptured hepatic t.
    sacrococcygeal region germ cell t.
    secondary t.
    t. seeding
    Sertoli cell t.
    sex cord-mesenchyme t.
    shaggy t.
    small-cell t.
    solid t.
    t. spillage
    t. stage
    t. staging
    t. stenting
    superficial t.
    t. suppressor gene
    t. suppressor gene therapy
    Teilum t.
    thrombus t.
    tongue of t.
    transurethral resection of bladder t.
      (TURBT)
    Triton t.

    upper tract urothelial t.
    ureteral t.
    urethral t.
    urothelial t.
    t. vaccine
    vasoactive intestinal polypeptide t.
      (VIPoma, vipoma)
    villous t.
    virilizing t.
    Wilms t.
    yolk sac t.
    Zollinger-Ellison t.
tumoral calcinosis
tumor-associated antigen (TAA)
tumor-bearing segment
tumor-derived angiogenic inhibitor
tumorigenesis
    t. activity
    colorectal t.
tumorigenic
tumor-infiltrating lymphocyte (TIL)
tumorlet
    Wilms t.
tumorous
    t. epithelia
    t. pseudopodia
tumor-rejection antigen
Tums
TUMT
    transurethral microwave thermotherapy
      cooled catheter TUMT
      TUMT functional result
      high-energy TUMT
      low-energy TUMT
      30-minute TUMT
TUNA
    transurethral needle ablation
tunable
    t. dye laser lithotripsy
    t. pulsed dye laser
TUNEL
    terminal uridine deoxynucleotide nick
      end labeling
tunic
    t. cyst
    epididymal t.
    fibrous t.
    mucous t.
    muscular t.
    pharyngeal t.
    pharyngobasilar t.
    proper t.
    t. of spermatic cord
tunica
    t. adventitia
    t. albuginea
    t. albuginea corporis spongiosi
    t. albuginea corporum cavernosorum

t. albuginea cyst
t. albuginea ovarii
t. albuginea plication
t. albuginea testis
t. fibrosa
t. mucosa
t. muscularis
t. propria
t. replacement
t. serosa
t. spongiosa urethrae feminae
t. vaginalis
t. vaginalis blanket wrap
t. vasculosa

tunicae testis
tunnel
t. creation
t. disease
extravesical seromuscular t.
t. infection
retropancreatic t.
subserous t.
ureteral t.
t. vision
Witzel feeding jejunostomy t.

tunneled
t. technique
t. technique urinary diversion

tunneler
Davol t.

Tuohy-Borst
T.-B. adapter
T.-B. connector

TUR
transurethral resection
TUR syndrome
video monitored TUR

Turapy device
turbid
t. bile
t. peritoneal fluid

turbidity
urinalysis t.
urine t.

turbinate
swollen t.

turbo spin-echo sequence
TURBT
transurethral resection of bladder tumor
turbulent flow
Türck zone
Turcot syndrome

TUR-Cue photometer
turgescence
penile t.

turgor
skin t.

turista
Turkel punch
turn-and-suction
t.-a.-s. biopsy technique
t.-a.-s. method

Turnbull
T. colostomy
T. end-loop ileostomy
T. loop stoma
T. multiple ostomy operation
T. technique

Turner
T. sign
T. stigma
T. syndrome

Turner-Warwick
T.-W. incision
T.-W. inlay
T.-W. needle
T.-W. operation
T.-W. stone forceps
T.-W. urethroplasty

TURP
transurethral resection of prostate
bipolar TURP
direct-beam coupler for TURP
TURP functional result
split-beam coupler for TURP

turpentine enema
Turrell-Wittner rectal forceps
Tuttle test
TUU
transureteroureterostomy
TUVP
transurethral electrovaporization of prostate
transurethral vaporization of prostate
TUVRP
transurethral vaporization-resection of prostate
TV
target volume
TVF
Thiry-Vella fistula
TVP
transurethral electrovaporization of prostate

NOTES

T

TVS
　transvaginal suturing
　TVS system
TVT
　tension-free vaginal tape
　TVT procedure
TV-UST
　transvaginal ultrasound
Tween 20
twin pulse shock wave release
twisted beta-pleated sheet fibril
TWOC
　trial without catheter
two-channel endoscope
two-devices-in-one-channel method
two-dimensional flow cytometric analysis
two-field lymphadenectomy
two-finger grip
two-layer
　t.-l. enteroenterostomy
　t.-l. interrupted intestinal
　　anastomosis
　t.-l. latex and Marlex closure
　　technique
　t.-l. open technique
two-loop J-shaped ileal pouch
two-piece ostomy pouch
two-stage
　t.-s. repair
　t.-s. triolein test
two-step
　Aztec t.-s.
　t.-s. orchiopexy
two-tailed
　t.-t. Fisher test
　t.-t. McNemar test
two-wing Malecot drain
TxA2 receptor antagonist
Tycron (*var. of* Ti-Cron)
Tygon venovenous bypass tubing
Tylenol
tylosis
　t. palmaris
　t. palmaris et plantaris
Tylox
tymazoline
tympanites
　false t.
　uterine t.
tympanitic
　t. abdomen
　t. abscess
　t. dullness
　t. resonance
tympany
　abdominal t. (AT)
　t. of the stomach

type
　t. A, B gastritis
　t. 1, 2 autoimmune hepatitis
　t. B antral gastritis
　biomaterial t.
　blood t.
　t. C cirrhosis
　t. C, D ulcer
　cell t.
　chronic-continuous t.
　t. 2 diabetes mellitus
　diffuse vasculitis of polyarteritis
　　nodosa t.
　DR2 1501 HLA-DRB tissue t.
　DR2 1502 HLA-DRB tissue t.
　DR2 1601 HLA-DRB tissue t.
　DR2 1602 HLA-DRB tissue t.
　DR1 HLA-DRB tissue t.
　DR2 HLA-DRB tissue t.
　DR3 HLA-DRB tissue t.
　DR4 HLA-DRB tissue t.
　DR7 HLA-DRB tissue t.
　DR9 HLA-DRB tissue t.
　DRw8 HLA-DRB tissue t.
　DRw10 HLA-DRB tissue t.
　DRw11 HLA-DRB tissue t.
　DRw12 HLA-DRB tissue t.
　DRw13 HLA-DRB tissue t.
　DRw14 HLA-DRB tissue t.
　t. II cryoglobulinemia
　t. III cholangiocarcinoma
　t. III glycogenosis
　t. I, II pseudohypoaldosteronism
　t. I mesangiocapillary
　　glomerulonephritis
　t. IV amyloidosis
　phage t.
　t. 0–3 stress urinary incontinence
　test t.
typed blood
type-specific blood transfusion
typhi
　Salmonella t.
typhimurium
　Salmonella t.
typhlectasis
typhlectomy
typhlenteritis
typhlitis
　neutropenic t.
typhlodicliditis
typhloempyema
typhlolithiasis
typhlomegaly
typhlopexy, typhlopexia
typhlorrhaphy
typhlostenosis
typhlostomy

typhlotomy
typhloureterostomy
typhoid
    abdominal t.
    t. fever
typing
    HLA t.
    HLA-DQ t.
    HLA-DR t.
    HLA-DR DNA t.
    molecular t.
tyramine
tyremesis
tyropanoate
    t. contrast medium
    t. sodium

tyrosine
    t. kinase activity
    t. kinase growth factor receptor
    peptide t.
    t. phosphorylation
    t. protein kinase
    t. sulfation
tyrosinemia
    hereditary t.
tyrosinuria
tyrosis
Tyshak catheter
Tyson test

NOTES

T

789

U

U pouch

UA

urinalysis

UA/C

urinary albumin to creatinine

UA/C ratio

ubiquitination

UBM

urothelial basement membrane

UBT

urea breath test

UBT breath test

^{14}C UBT

^{14}C urea breath test

UC

ulcerative colitis

urethral catheterization

UCB

unconjugated bilirubin

UCHL-1 monoclonal antibody

UCLA catheterization pouch

UCP

ultrasound catheter probe

UD

urethral discharge

UDC

ursodeoxycholate

UDCA

ursodeoxycholic acid

UDI

Urogenital Distress Inventory

UDP

uridine 5'-diphosphate

UDPGT

uridine diphosphate
glucuronosyltransferase

UDPGT deficiency

Udranszky test

UES

upper esophageal sphincter

UESR

upper esophageal sphincter relaxation

UF

ultrafiltration

Uffelmann test

UG

urogenital

UGI

upper gastrointestinal

UGI endoscope

UGI endoscopy

UGIB

upper gastrointestinal bleeding

UGIE

upper gastrointestinal endoscopy

Uhthoff sign

UICC

Union Internationale Contre le Cancer

UICC tumor classification

UJ13A nuclear isotope bone scan

UKM

urea kinetic modeling

UKTSSA

United Kingdom Transplant Support
Service Authority

ulcer

acid peptic u.

active duodenal u.

agranulocytic u.

Allingham u.

amebic u.

anastomotic u.

anastomotic-stomal u.

anterior duodenal u.

anterior wall antral u.

antral u.

antroduodenal u.

aphthoid u.

aphthous u.

apical duodenal u.

Barrett u.

u. base

bear claw u.

u. bed

benign u.

benign gastric u.

bladder u.

bleeding u.

Bouveret u.

Bouveret-Duguet u.

bulbar peptic u.

Cameron u.

cecal u.

cervical u.

chronic u.

CMV-related u.

coalescent u.

u. collar

collar-button-like u.

colonic u.

colorectal u.

corneal u.

u. crater

Crohn duodenal u.

Cruveilhier u.

Curling u.

Cushing u.

Cushing-Rokitansky u.

ulcer *(continued)*
    cysteamine-induced duodenal u.
    decubitus u.
    Dieulafoy u.
    distention u.
    drug-induced u.
    duodenal u. (DU)
    duodenal ulceroinflammatory u.
    u. duodenum
    u. dyspepsia
    elusive u.
    esophageal u.
    Fenwick-Hunner u.
    flat u.
    focal colonic mucosal u.
    gastric u.
    gastroduodenal double u.
    general peptic u.
    genital u.
    giant gastric u. (GGU)
    giant peptic u.
    greater curvature u.
    healed u.
    herpetic u.
    Hunner u.
    idiopathic esophageal u. (IEU)
    indolent radiation-induced rectal u.
    intractable u.
    jejunal u.
    juxtapyloric u.
    kissing u.'s
    Kocher dilatation u.
    lesser curvature u.
    linear u.
    longitudinal u.
    malignant u.
    Mann-Williamson u.
    marginal u.
    Martorell hypertensive u.
    mucosal gastric u.
    nonhealing u.
    open u.
    oral u.
    penetrating u.
    peptic u.
    perforated acid peptic u.
    perforating u.
    perineal u.
    phantom u.
    postbulbar duodenal u.
    posterior duodenal u.
    postligation u.
    postsurgical recurrent u.
    prepyloric gastric u.
    punched-out u.
    punctate u.
    pyloric channel u.
    rake u.

    rectal u.
    recurrent u.
    refractory duodenal u.
    reserpine-induced u.
    Rokitansky-Cushing u.
    rose thorn u.
    round u.
    sea anemone u.
    secondary jejunal u.
    serpiginous u.
    sigmoid u.
    silent u.
    small intestinal u.
    sodium meclofenamate-induced
      esophageal u.
    solitary u.
    stercoral u.
    stomal u.
    stress u.
    submucous u.
    sump u.
    superficial linear u.
    suture u.
    type C, D u.
    vaginal u.
    u. vessel
    virgin u.
    V-shaped u.
    u. with heaped-up edge

ulcera *(pl. of* ulcus)

ulcerating
    u. adenocarcinoma
    u. carcinoma

ulceration
    anal u.
    anastomotic u.
    ASA-induced gastric u.
    CMV-associated u.
    CMV-induced esophageal u.
    collar-button u.
    duodenal u.
    esophageal u.
    fissure-like u.
    flat polycyclic u.
    gastric u.
    labial u.
    linear u.
    necrotic u.
    patchy colonic u.
    pouch u.
    punched-out u.
    radiation-induced u.
    serpiginous u.
    stasis u.
    stasis-induced u.
    stercoral u.
    stress u.
    stress-induced gastric u.

suture line u.
tracheal u.
transverse u.
ulcerative
    u. colitis (UC)
    u. enteritis
    u. gastritis
    u. jejunitis
    u. jejunitis jejunocecostomy
    u. lymphoma
    u. proctitis
    u. reflux esophagitis
ulcerlike dyspepsia
ulcerogenic fistula
ulcer-prone personality
ulcus, pl. **ulcera**
    u. penetrans
    u. simplex vesica
    u. ventriculi
Uldall subclavian hemodialysis catheter
Ulex europeus I antigen
Ullrich-Turner syndrome
ulnar deviation
ultra
    U. Twin bag system
    U. Y-set system
Ultrabag dialysis system
UltraCision harmonic laparoscopic cutting shears
ultradian rhythm
ultrafast
    u. computerized tomography
    u. MRI
Ultrafem pants
ultrafiltrate
    glomerular u.
    plasma u.
    tubular fluid:u. (TF/UF)
ultrafiltration (UF)
    u. coefficient
    continuous arteriovenous u. (CAVU)
    dialytic u. (DU)
    extracorporeal u. (ECU)
    glomerular u.
    u. hemodialyzer
    slow continuous u. (SCUF)
    spontaneous dialytic u.
Ultraflex
    U. Diamond stent
    U. esophageal prosthesis
    U. Microvasive stent

    U. nitinol expandable esophageal stent
    U. tracheobronchial stent
ultra-high-magnification endoscopy
UltraKlenz skin cleanser
Ultralente insulin
Ultraline
    U. laser
    Lasersonic ACMI U.
UltraLine fiber
ultralow anastomosis
ultra-low-volume sclerotherapy
UltraPak enteral closed feeding system
Ultraseed system
Ultrase MT12
ultrasmall superparamagnetic iron oxide (USPIO)
ultrasonic
    u. aspirator and dissector
    u. cytoreduction
    u. diagnosis
    u. dissection
    u. fragmentation
    u. lithotresis
    u. lithotripsy
    u. lithotriptor
    u. lithotriptor probe
    u. oscillating bur
    u. scalpel
    u. tactile sensor
    u. tomography
ultrasonics
ultrasonogram
    renal u.
ultrasonographic finding
ultrasonography
    abdominal u.
    bladder u.
    B-mode u.
    catheter probe-assisted endoluminal u. (CP-EUS)
    color Doppler u.
    contrast-enhanced endoscopic u. (CE-EUS)
    Doppler u.
    ejaculatory duct u.
    endoluminal rectal u. (ELUS)
    endoscopic u. (EUS)
    endoscopic color Doppler u.
    u. estimate
    EUS-AD gastric lesion staging by endoscopic u.

U

NOTES

793

ultrasonography *(continued)*
    EUS-M gastric lesion staging by endoscopic u.
    EUS-SM gastric lesion staging by endoscopic u.
    gray scale u.
    high-intensity focused u.
    high-resolution 25-megahertz u.
    intraductal u. (IDUS)
    intraoperative u. (IOUS)
    intraportal endovascular u. (IPEUS)
    intrarectal u.
    laparoscopic contact u. (LCU)
    penile duplex u.
    pharmaco-duplex u.
    real-time u. (RUS)
    rectal endoscopic u. (REU, REUS)
    secretin u.
    sex assignment by fetal u.
    Siemens Sonoline u.
    SP-101 gastric lesion staging by endoscopic u.
    SP-501 gastric lesion staging by endoscopic u.
    Toshiba Sal 38B real-time u.
    Toshiba Sonolayer SSA250A transrectal u.
    transanal u.
    transcutaneous u.
    transluminal u.
    transnasal endoluminal u.
    transrectal u. (TRUS)

ultrasound
    BladderScan u.
    U. Bone Analyzer
    u. catheter probe (UCP)
    catheter probe u.
    colonoscopic endoluminal u.
    colorectal endoluminal u.
    compression u. (CUS)
    condom catheter endoscopic u.
    u. dilution technique
    endoanal u. (EAUS)
    endoluminal ureteral u.
    endorectal u. (ERUS)
    u. endoscope
    endoscopic u. (EUS)
    u. gastrointestinal fiberscope
    gray scale u.
    high-frequency intraluminal u.
    high-intensity focused u. (HFU, HIFU)
    hydrogen peroxide u. (HPUS)
    intraductal u. (IDUS)
    intraluminal u. (ILUS)
    intravascular u. (IVUS)
    laparoscopic u. (LUS)
    laparoscopic intracorporal u. (LICU)

    piezoelectrically generated u.
    power Doppler u.
    pulsed Doppler u.
    quantitative u. (QUS)
    real-time gallbladder u.
    u. scan
    u. test
    time domain u. (TDU)
    transcutaneous u.
    u. transducer
    transendoscopic u.
    transrectal u. (TRUS)
    transurethral rectal u.
    transvaginal u. (TV-UST)
    u. wand

ultrasound-assisted
    u.-a. PEG placement
    u.-a. percutaneous endoscopic gastrostomy

ultrasound-guided
    u.-g. anterior subcostal liver biopsy
    u.-g. laser
    u.-g. shock wave therapy
    u.-g. systematic sextant biopsy

ultrastiff wire

ultrastructural basket-weave change

UltraTag RBC kit

ultrathin
    u. araldite section
    u. endoscope
    u. endoscopy
    u. pancreatoscope

ultratome
    U. double-lumen sphincterotome
    Microvasive u.
    U. XL triple-lumen sphincterotome

ultraviolet irradiation

Ultravist
    U. 300

Ultrex
    U. cylinder
    U. Plus penile prosthesis

Ultroid

Ultzmann test

umbilical
    u. artery
    u. cord
    u. fissure
    u. fistula
    u. granuloma
    u. hernia
    u. hernia rupture
    u. ligament
    u. port
    u. port grasper
    u. portography
    u. region
    u. scissors

u. tape
u. vein
u. vein catheterization
u. vein recanalization
umbilicalis
plica u.
umbilicated angioma
umbilication
umbilicoplasty
umbilicovesical fascia
umbilicus
everted u.
Richet fascia u.
umbrella
Mobin-Uddin u.
UMCL
upper midclavicular line
UN
urea nitrogen
Unasyn
UNaV
urinary sodium excretion
unbanded gastroplasty
UNC
urine net charge
unciform pancreas
uncinate
u. process
u. process of pancreas
uncoated mesh stent
uncomplicated
u. cystitis
u. urinary tract infection
unconjugated
u. bilirubin (UCB)
u. hyperbilirubinemia
unconscious incontinence
uncorrected
u. maternal morbidity
u. reflux morbidity
undecapeptide
amino-terminal u.
undecenoate of testosterone
underactivity
detrusor muscle u.
underdosing
underfilling
arterial u.
undersurface of liver
underwater spark gap
underwear
Prevail protective u.

undescended testis
undifferentiated
u. adenoma
u. cell
u. embryonal sarcoma of liver
u. malignant teratoma
u. structure
undigested food in stool
undiversion
urinary u.
unenhanced
u. helical computed tomography
u. helical CT
unequal calf diameter
unextractable gallstone
unformed stool
unguliformis
ren u.
unicameral cyst
unicornuate uterus
unidirectional transfer
Uni-Flate 1000 penile prosthesis
uniformis
Bacteroides u.
uniform loading
Uni-Gold *Helicobacter pylori* **test**
unilateral
u. fused kidney
u. megaureter
u. nephrectomy
u. periorbital emphysema
u. renal artery stenosis
u. renal hypoplasia
u. renin production
u. subcostal incision
u. ureteral obstruction (UUO)
unilobular cirrhosis
unilocular
u. hydatid disease
u. ovarian cyst
uninhibited
u. neurogenic bladder
u. overactive bladder
union
anomalous pancreaticobiliary u.
(APBU)
anomalous pancreaticobiliary
ductal u. (APBDU)
U. Internationale Contre le Cancer
(UICC)
unipapillary kidney
uniplanar imaging

U

NOTES

unipolar
 u. glass electrode
 u. neuron
unit
 amylase u.
 arbitrary u. (AU)
 biceps femoris musculocutaneous u.
 Bodansky u.
 Bovie electrocoagulation u.
 Cameron electrosurgical u.
 Cameron-Miller electrocoagulation u.
 Century bicarbonate dialysis
  control u.
 colony-forming u. (CFU)
 crypt-villus u.
 densitometric u.
 Diasonics DRF ultrasound u.
 duodenal cluster u.
 electrosurgical u. (ESU)
 Erbotom F2 electrocoagulation u.
 good performance u.
 GPL u.
 gracilis musculocutaneous u.
 Grass Model SIU5A stimulation
  isolation u.
 HemoTherapies liver dialysis u.
 Hounsfield u. (HU)
 image-processing u.
 international androgen u.
 Karmen u.
 KeyMed u.
 King-Armstrong u.
 5-15 King Armstrong u.
 liver dialysis u.
 OSMO reverse osmosis u.
 u. of packed red blood cells
  (UPRBC)
 Proscan ultrasound u.
 QAD-1 sonography u.
 real-time sonographic u.
 Siemens MRI u.
 Siemens Somatom DRH CT
  analyzer u.
 Somogyi u.
 SSE2-L electrosurgical u.
 TENS u.
 ThermoFlex thermotherapy u.
 UroCystom u.
 Valleylab E3B cautery u.
 Valleylab SSE-2 cautery u.
Unitary inflatable penile prosthesis
United
 U. Bongort Life-style pouch
 U. Kingdom Transplant Support
  Service Authority (UKTSSA)
 U. Max-E drainable pouch
 U. Network for Organ Sharing
  (UNOS)

 U. Ostomy Association (UOA)
 U. Ostomy irrigation set
 U. Skin Prep
 U. States Renal Data System
  (USRDS)
 U. Surgical Bongort Life-style
  pouch
 U. Surgical Convex insert
 U. Surgical Featherlite ileostomy
  pouch
 U. Surgical Hypalon faceplate
 U. Surgical Seal Tite gasket
 U. Surgical Shear Plus drainable
  pouch
 U. Surgical Soft & Secure pouch
 U. XL 14 skin barrier
univariate analysis
Universal
 U. esophagoscope
 U. gastroscope
 U. sheath
 U. sheath system
 U. stent
universale
 angiokeratoma corporis diffusum u.
University
 U. of Wisconsin fluid
 U. of Wisconsin solution
UNOS
 United Network for Organ Sharing
**unreconstructable obstructive
  azoospermia**
unrelenting
 u. diarrhea
 u. pain
unrelieved pain
unremitting pain
unresectable hepatocellular carcinoma
unresolved urinary tract infection
unrest
 peristaltic u.
unroofing
 u. of diverticulum
 transurethral u.
unsaturated fatty acid
unsporulated coccidian
unstable
 u. bladder
 u. colon
 u. urethra
unsteady gait
untethering procedure
UOA
 United Ostomy Association
Uosm
 urine osmolarity
U/P
 urine-plasma ratio

UPEP
 urine protein electrophoresis
UPJ
 ureteropelvic junction
uPM3 urine test
U pouch
U-pouch construction
UPP
 urethral pressure profile
upper
 u. alimentary endoscopy
 u. arm flap
 u. endoscopy and colonoscopy
 u. esophageal sphincter (UES)
 u. esophageal sphincter relaxation
 (UESR)
 u. gastrointestinal (UGI)
 u. gastrointestinal angioma
 u. gastrointestinal barium
 roentgenographic study
 u. gastrointestinal bleeding (UGIB)
 u. gastrointestinal endoscopy
 (UGIE)
 u. gastrointestinal panendoscopy
 u. gastrointestinal procedure
 u. gastrointestinal tract
 u. GI endoscope
 u. GI hemorrhage
 u. GI series
 u. GI tract foreign body
 U. Hands retractor
 u. midclavicular line (UMCL)
 u. motor neuron
 u. tract dilation
 u. tract disease
 u. tract stricture
 u. tract urothelial tumor
 u. ureter
 u. urinary tract calculus
UPRBC
 unit of packed red blood cells
upregulation
Uprima
upsaliensis
 Campylobacter u.
upset stomach
upside down stomach
upstream pancreatic duct
upstroke
 delayed u.
uptake
 glucose u.

 hepatic u.
 [^{3}H]thymidine u.
URA
 urethral resistance factor
Urabeth tabs
urachal
 u. abscess
 u. adenocarcinoma
 u. cyst
 u. disorder
 u. diverticulum
 u. fistula
 u. sinus
urachus
 patent u.
uracil/tegafur
uragogue
uranyl
 u. acetate
 u. acetate stain
urate
 u. calculus
 u. crystal
 monosodium u.
 u. nephropathy
 u. renal excretion
 sodium acid u.
uraturia
urea
 u. adequacy
 u. breath test (UBT)
 u. breath testing
 u. channel
 u. clearance
 u. cycle
 u. distribution volume
 hepatic u.
 u. hydrolysis
 u. kinetic modeling (UKM)
 u. kinetics
 Kt/V u.
 u. nitrogen (UN)
 u. nitrogen test
 percent reduction in u. (PRU)
 u. permeability
 plasma u.
 u. reduction ratio (URR)
 u. synthesis
urea-derived cyanate
urea-impermeable membrane

U

NOTES

urealyticum
    Ureaplasma u.
Ureaplasma
    U. urealyticum
    U. urethritis
urease
    cytoplasmic u.
    mucosal u.
    u. test
urea-splitting organism
urecchysis
Urecholine
urecholine supersensitivity test
uredema, uroedema
Urelief
uremia
    extrarenal u.
    retention u.
uremic
    u. acidosis
    u. breath
    u. cardiomyopathy
    u. colitis
    u. encephalopathy
    u. gastritis
    u. gastrointestinal lesion
    u. medullary cystic disease
    u. PMN
    u. pruritus
    u. serositis
    u. serum subfraction
    u. syndrome
ureolyticus
    Bacteroides u.
ureter
    abdominal u.
    aberrant u.
    bifid u.
    circumcaval u.
    u. contractility
    u. creep
    u. duplication anomaly
    ectopic u.
    en bloc u.
    extraperitoneal excision of lower
      one-third of u.
    ileal u.
    impassable u.
    u. implantation
    intramural u.
    juxtavesical u.
    left u.
    lower u.
    middle u.
    pelvic u.
    pelvis of u.
    postcaval u.
    retrocaval u.

retroiliac u.
right u.
tortuous u.
torus u.
upper u.
ureteral
    u. anastomosis
    u. atony
    u. bladder augmentation
    u. bud
    u. calculi in pregnancy
    u. *Candida*
    u. carcinoma
    u. catheterization
    u. colic
    u. dissection
    u. ectopia
    u. electromyography
    u. encasement
    u. endoscopic disconnection
    u. hernia
    u. injury
    u. intestinal implantation
    u. jet
    u. jet into bladder
    u. meatoscopy
    u. meatotomy
    u. muscle cell
    u. neocystostomy
    u. obstruction
    u. occlusion balloon catheter
    u. orifice
    u. patch procedure
    u. peristalsis second messenger
    u. pressure
    u. reimplantation
    u. reimplantation stenosis
    u. schistosomiasis
    u. scoping basketing
    u. spatulation
    u. split-cuff nipple
    u. stent
    u. stenting
    u. stent placement
    u. stoma
    u. stoma removal
    u. stone
    u. stricture
    u. torsion
    u. tuberculosis
    u. tumor
    u. tunnel
ureteralgia
uretercystoscope
ureterectasia
ureterectomy
    distal u.
    segmental u.

ureteric
- u. bud
- u. calcification
- u. calculus
- u. diverticulum
- u. obstruction
- u. plexus
- u. reimplantation
- u. retrieval net
- u. ridge
- u. stoma
- u. stone

uretericus
- plexus u.

ureteritis
- u. cystica
- u. cystica calcinosa
- u. glandularis

ureterocalicostomy

ureterocele
- u. cobra-head deformity
- u. drooping lily sign
- ectopic u.
- intravesical u.
- orthotopic u.
- u. prolapse
- single-system u.

ureterocelectomy
ureterocelorraphy
ureterocervical
ureterocolic
- u. fistula
- u. stricture

ureterocolonic anastomosis
ureterocolostomy
ureterocutaneostomy
ureterocutaneous fistula
ureterocystanastomosis
ureterocystography
ureterocystoneostomy
ureterocystoplasty
ureterocystoscope
ureterocystostomy
ureteroduodenal
ureteroendoscopy
ureteroenteric
- u. status
- u. stricture

ureteroenteroanastomosis
ureteroenterostomy
ureterogram
- bulb-tip retrograde u.

ureterography
ureteroheminephrectomy
ureterohydronephrosis
ureteroileal
- u. anastomosis
- u. neocystostomy
- u. stenosis
- u. stricture

ureteroileocecoproctostomy
ureteroileoneocystostomy
ureteroileostomy
- Bricker u.

ureterointestinal anastomosis
ureterolith
ureterolithiasis
ureterolithotomy
- laparoscopic u.

ureterolysis
- combined u.
- extravesical u.
- intravesical u.
- laparoscopic u.
- Lich-Gregoire u.
- Pacquin u.
- Politano-Leadbetter u.

ureteromeatotomy
ureteroneocystostomy
- Cohen u.
- Glenn-Anderson u.
- u. herniation
- Leadbetter-Politano u.
- modified Lich-Gregoir u.
- Politano-Leadbetter u.
- reoperative u.

ureteroneopyelostomy
ureteronephrectomy
ureteronephrosis
ureteropathy
ureteropelvic
- u. fungus ball
- u. junction (UPJ)
- u. junction obstruction

ureteropelvioneostomy
ureteropelvioplasty
- Culp u.
- Culp-DeWeerd u.
- Foley Y-type u.
- Foley Y-V u.
- Scardino u.
- Scardino-Prince u.

ureterophlegma

U

NOTES

ureteroplasty
    ileal patch u.
ureteroproctostomy
ureteropyelitis
ureteropyelogram
    retrograde u.
ureteropyelography
    retrograde u.
ureteropyeloneostomy
ureteropyelonephritis
ureteropyelonephrostomy
ureteropyeloplasty
ureteropyeloscope
    Karl Storz flexible u.
ureteropyeloscopy
    flexible u.
ureteropyelostomy
ureteropyosis
ureterorectostomy
ureterorenal reflux
ureterorenoscope procedure sheath
ureterorenoscopy
    flexible u.
    transurethral u. (URS)
ureterorrhagia
ureterorrhaphy
ureteroscope
    Circon-ACMI (MR-6, MR-9) u.
    flexible u.
    Gautier u.
    Micro-6 u.
    offset lens u.
    Olympus URF type P2 flexible u.
    Panoview rod-lens u.
    rigid u.
    semirigid fiberoptic u.
    u. sheath
    Storz 27022 SK u.
    Wolf u.
    working port u.
ureteroscopic
    u. endopyelotomy
    u. intracorporeal electrohydraulic
      lithotripsy
ureteroscopy
    rigid u.
ureterosigmoid anastomosis
ureterosigmoidostomy
    ileocecal u.
    Mainz-type u.
    Maydl u.
ureterostegnosis
ureterostenoma
ureterostenosis
ureterostoma
ureterostomosis
ureterostomy
    cutaneous loop u.

    Davis intubated u.
    high-loop cutaneous u.
    low-loop cutaneous u.
    retroperitoneal cutaneous u.
ureterotome
    optical u.
ureterotomy
    Davis intubated u.
    intubated u.
ureterotrigonoenterostomy
ureterotrigonosigmoidostomy
ureterotubal anastomosis
ureteroureteral anastomosis
ureteroureterostomy
ureterouterine fistula
ureterovaginal fistula
ureterovesical
    u. junction (UVJ)
    ureterovesical obstruction
ureterovesicoplasty
    Leadbetter-Politano u.
ureterovesicostomy
urethra, pl. **urethrae**
    accessory phallic u.
    anterior u.
    AS-800 male bulbous u.
    u. blowout injury
    bulbar u.
    bulbomembranous u.
    bulbus urethrae
    compressor u.
    devastated u.
    u. duplication
    u. feminina
    fixed drain pipe u.
    fossa of male u.
    fossa navicularis u.
    hemispherium bulbi u.
    intrinsic striated muscle of the u.
    isthmus u.
    labium u.
    lacuna of u.
    membranous u.
    u. muliebris
    native u.
    pendulous u.
    penile u.
    posterior u.
    preprostatic u.
    prostatic u.
    septum bulbi u.
    short u.
    spinning top u.
    unstable u.
    u. virilis
urethral
    u. abscess
    u. apoplexy

u. artery
u. arthritis
u. atresia
u. calculus
u. cancer
u. carcinoma
u. caruncle
u. catheterization (UC)
u. closure mechanism
u. closure pressure
u. closure pressure profile
u. cooling
u. crest
u. cyst
u. dilation
u. discharge (UD)
u. diverticulectomy
u. diverticulum
u. electrical conductance
u. feedback trigger
u. fistula
u. gland
u. hemangioma
u. hematuria
u. hemi-Kock
u. hypermobility
u. lacuna
u. meatal erythema
u. meatus
u. obstruction
u. occlusion
u. plate
u. plate division
u. plug
u. pressure measurement
u. pressure profile (UPP)
u. pressure profilometry
u. prolapse
u. pseudodiverticulum
u. pseudotumor
u. reconstruction complication
u. resistance
u. resistance factor (URA)
u. sarcoidosis
u. sensory threshold
u. sphincter
u. sphincterotomy
u. sphincter recruitment reflex
u. stenosis
u. stent
u. stent prosthesis
u. stricture

u. stripping
u. surgical reconstruction
u. suspension
u. swab
u. syndrome
u. temperature
u. tuberculosis
u. tumor
u. valve
u. vein
urethral-cooling surface
urethralgia
urethralis
   annulus u.
   crista u.
urethrameter
urethratresia
urethrectomy
urethremorrhagia
urethremphraxis
urethreurynter
Urethrin
urethrism, urethrismus
urethritis
   acute u.
   atrophic u.
   chlamydia u.
   u. cystica
   u. glandularis
   gonococcal u. (GU)
   gonorrheal u.
   gouty u.
   u. granulosa
   hypoestrogenic u.
   mycoplasma u.
   nongonococcal u.
   nonspecific u. (NSU)
   u. orificii externi
   u. petrificans
   polypoid u.
   prophylactic u.
   specific u.
   u. syndrome
   Ureaplasma u.
   u. venerea
urethrobalanoplasty
urethroblennorrhea
urethrocavernous fistula
urethrocele
urethrocutaneous fistula
urethrocystitis
urethrocystocele

U

NOTES

urethrocystography
urethrocystometrography
urethrocystometry
urethrocystopexy
urethrocystoplasty
urethrocystoscopy
urethrodetrusor facilitative reflex
urethrodynia
urethrogram
    ascending u.
    retrograde u. (RUG)
urethrograph
urethrography
    positive-pressure u.
    retrograde u. (RUG)
urethrohymenal fusion
urethrolysis
    retropubic u.
    transvaginal u.
urethrometer
urethrometry
urethropelvic ligament
urethropenile
urethroperineal
urethroperineoscrotal
urethropexy
    Gittes u.
    laparoscopic Burch u.
    Lapides-Ball u.
    Marshall-Marchetti-Krantz u.
    Stamey u.
    transabdominal Burch u.
urethrophraxis
urethrophyma
urethroplasty
    anastomotic u.
    buccal mucosal substitution u.
    Cantwell-Ransley u.
    Cecil u.
    modified Young u.
    onlay island flap u.
    patch graft u.
    pedicled penile skin u.
    pedicle flap u.
    substitution u.
    Tanagho bladder flap u.
    Thiersch-Duplay u.
    tubed u.
    Turner-Warwick u.
urethroprostatic
urethrorectal fistula
urethrorrhagia
urethrorrhaphy
urethrorrhea
urethroscope
    Robertson TM u.
urethroscopic

urethroscopy
    retropubic u.
urethroscrotal
urethrospasm
urethrosphincteric
    u. guarding reflex
    u. inhibitory reflex
urethrostaxis
urethrostenosis
urethrostomy
    perineal u.
urethrotome
    u. knife
    Otis u.
    Sachse u.
    Storz u.
urethrotomy
    core-through optical u.
    direct vision internal u. (DVIU)
    endoscopic optical u.
    external u.
    internal u.
    Otis u.
    perineal u.
    Sachse u.
    Syme external u.
urethrotrigonitis
urethrovaginal
    u. fistula
    u. septum
    u. sphincter
urethrovesical anastomosis
urethrovesicopexy
urethrovesiculodifferential reflux
uretic
Urex Tablets
URF-P2 choledochoscope
urge
    u. to defecate
    u. incontinence
    u. syndrome
urgency
    defecatory u.
    u. incontinence
    motor u.
    sensory u.
    urinary u.
uric
    u. acid
    u. acid calculus
    u. acid crystal
    u. acid infarct
    u. acid level
    u. acid nephropathy
    u. acid shower
    u. acid stone
    u. acid test
    u. acid urinary lithiasis

uricaciduria
uricometer
uricosuria
uricosuric
Uricult dipslide
uridine
  u. 5′-diphosphate (UDP)
  u. diphosphate
    glucuronosyltransferase (UDPGT)
  u. diphosphate
    glucuronosyltransferase deficiency
  u. phosphorylase
  u. rescue
Uridium
uridyltransferase
  galactose-1-phosphate u.
Urifon-Forte
Urigen
Uri-Kit culture kit
Urimar-T
urina
  u. chyli
  u. cibi
  u. galactodes
  u. jumentosa
  u. spastica
urinable
urinacidometer
urinae
  ardor u.
  detrusor u.
  incontinentia u.
urinal
  condom u.
  Millie female u.
  Uro-Tex McGuire male u.
  URSEC u.
urinalysis (UA)
  chemical u.
  u. color
  u. dipstick
  midstream u.
  u. pH
  u. sediment microscopy
  u. sediment microscopy bacteria
  u. sediment microscopy cast
  u. sediment microscopy cell
  u. sediment microscopy crystal
  u. sediment microscopy parasite
  u. sediment microscopy prostatic
    secretion
  u. sediment microscopy yeast

  u. specific gravity
  u. turbidity
urinaria, pl. urinariae
  fundus vesicae u.
  tela subserosa vesicae u.
  vertex vesicae u.
  vesica u.
urinarius
  meatus u.
urinary
  u. abscess
  u. acidity
  u. albumin to creatinine (UA/C)
  u. alkalinization
  u. amylase
  u. anion gap
  u. ascites
  u. bicarbonate
  u. bilirubin
  u. bladder
  u. cachexia
  u. calcium
  u. calculus
  u. catecholamine
  u. catheterization
  u. cGMP level
  u. chloride
  u. chloride excretion
  u. citrate
  u. composition
  u. conduit
  u. continence
  u. continence reflex
  u. continuity
  u. control urethral insert
  u. cortisol
  u. crystal
  u. cyclic AMP
  u. cyst
  u. diversion
  u. dribbling
  u. exertional incontinence
  u. extravasation
  u. extraversion
  u. fibronectin
  u. flow
  u. frequency
  u. glucose
  u. hesitancy
  u. indican
  u. kallikrein
  u. kallikrein excretion

U

NOTES

urinary *(continued)*
  u. ketone
  u. leukocyte esterase
  u. lithiasis
  u. lithogenesis
  u. marker protein
  u. 3-methylhistidine
  u. nitrite test
  u. obstruction
  u. output
  u. oxalate
  u. pH
  u. protein excretion
  u. protein-urinary creatinine ratio
  u. retention
  u. sand
  u. schistosomiasis
  u. sediment
  u. sediment cast
  u. sediment yeast
  u. sodium excretion (UNaV)
  u. specific gravity
  u. stone
  u. stress incontinence
  u. stuttering
  u. tract
  u. tract anomaly
  u. tract disease
  u. tract four-glass evaluation
  u. tract infection (UTI)
  u. tract infection suppression
  u. trypsin inhibitor
  u. umbilical fistula
  u. undiversion
  u. urea nitrogen excretion (UUN)
  u. urgency
  u. urge symptom
  u. urobilinogen
urination
  precipitant u.
  straining for u.
  stuttering u.
urine
  u. acidification
  anemic u.
  u. ascites
  barium sediment in u.
  Bence Jones u.
  u. bilirubin
  black u.
  u. chloride test
  chylous u.
  u. color
  concentrated u.
  u. concentration
  u. concentration test
  crude u.
  u. culture

  u. cytokine analysis
  u. cytology
  dark concentrated u.
  diabetic u.
  u. dipstick
  dyspeptic u.
  u. electrophoresis
  u. extravasation
  febrile u.
  u. flow rate
  u. glitter cell
  gouty u.
  hyperosmotic u.
  hypoosmotic u.
  U. Meter Foley tray
  midstream specimen of u. (MSU)
  milky u.
  nebulous u.
  nervous u.
  u. net charge (UNC)
  u. osmolality
  u. osmolarity (Uosm)
  postvoid dribbling of u.
  postvoid residual u.
  u. protein electrophoresis (UPEP)
  residual u.
  u. sample
  u. specific gravity
  u. supersaturation
  u. transport
  u. turbidity
  u. urea nitrogen (UUN)
  u. urobilinogen
  voided u.
urine-based enzyme linked
  immunosorbent assay
urine-collecting tubule
urinemia
urine-plasma ratio (U/P)
uriniferous
  u. pseudocyst
  u. tubule
uriniparous tubule
urinocryoscopy
urinogenous
urinoglucosometer
urinologist
urinology
urinoma
urinometer
urinometry
urinosexual
urinous abscess
Uriscreen test
Urised
Urisedamine
UriSite urine collection kit
Urispas

Uri-Three culture kit
Uritrol
Urizole
uroanthelone
Urobak
urobilin complex
urobilinogen
      fecal u.
      urinary u.
      urine u.
urobilinogenuria
urobilinuria
Uro-Bond skin adhesive
Urocam video camera
Urocath external catheter
urocele
urocheras
urochesia
urochezia
urochrome
urochromogen
Urocit
Urocit-K
uroclepsia
UroCoil self-expanding stent
urocortin
urocrisis
urocriterion
urocyanogen
urocyst
Urocystin
urocystitis
UroCystom unit
Urocyte diagnostic cytometry system
urocytogram
UROD
      uroporphyrinogen decarboxylase
urodeum
Urodiagnost x-ray table
urodialysis
urodochium
urodynamic
      u. assessment
      u. catheter
      u. dysfunction
      u. evaluation
      u. flow study
      u. obstruction
      u. testing
urodynamics
      ambulatory u.
urodynia

urodysfunction
uroedema (*var. of* uredema)
uroenterone
uroepithelial glycoid receptor
uroerythrin
urofacial syndrome
uroflavin
uroflow
      u. index
      peak u.
uroflowmeter
      Dantec Urodyn 1000 u.
      Drake u.
      Etude cystometer u.
      Synectics-Dantec Flo-Lab II u.
      Synectics-Dantec UD10000 u.
uroflowmetry
      Bristol nomogram for u.
      home u.
      Siroky nomogram for u.
urofuscin
urofuscohematin
urogastrone
urogenital (UG)
      u. diaphragm
      U. Distress Inventory (UDI)
      u. fistula
      u. prolapse
      u. region
      u. sinus
      u. sinus anomaly
      u. sphincter muscle
      u. triangle
urogenitale
      trigonum u.
urogenous pyelitis
Urogesic
uroglaucin
Urografin 290 contrast medium
urogram
      constant infusion excretory u.
        (CIXU)
      excretory u. (XU)
      intravenous u. (IVU)
      retrograde u. (RU)
urograph
      Disa 5500 u.
urography
      antegrade u.
      cystoscopic u.
      descending u.
      excretory u. (EU, EXU)

U

NOTES

urography *(continued)*
    high-dose intravenous u.
    intravenous u. (IVU)
    magnetic resonance u. (MRU)
    one-shot intravenous u.
    percutaneous antegrade u.
    retrograde u.
Uro-Guide stent
urogynecologist
urohematin
urohematonephrosis
urohematoporphyrin
urohypertensin
Uro-jet delivery system
urokinase plasminogen activator
urokinetic
Uro-KP-Neutral
urokymography
Urolab Janus System III
Urolase
    Bard U.
    CR Bard U.
    U. laser
    U. neodymium:YAG laser fiber
Urolene Blue
urolith
urolithiasis
    asymptomatic u.
    recurrent calcium u. (RCU)
urolithic
urolithology
urolithotomy
urologic, urological
    u. condition
    u. disease
    u. drug compendium
    u. surgery
    u. symptom
    u. system cancer
urologist
urology
    Brief Male Sexual Function
      Inventory for U.
    u. clinic
    geriatric u.
    pediatric u.
    perinatal u.
    u. set
Uroloop
UroLume
    U. endoprosthesis
    U. Endourethral Wallstent prosthesis
    U. prostate stent
    U. urethral prosthesis
    U. urethral stent
    U. Wallstent stent
urolutein
Uro-Mag

uromancy
uromantia
Uromat dilation
UroMax II high-pressure balloon
    catheter
uromelanin
urometer
uromodulin gene
uromucoid
uronate
    glycosaminoglycan u. (GAGUA)
    macromolecular u. (MMUA)
uroncus
uronephrosis
uronic acid-rich protein
uronology
urononcometry
uronophile
uronoscopy
Uro-Pak system
uropathogen
uropathologist
uropathy
    chronic obstructive u.
    congenital u.
    obstructive u.
    positional obstructive u.
uropenia
uropepsinogen
urophanic
urophein
urophosphometer
uroplania
Uroplus DS, SS
uropoiesis
uropoietic
uropontin
uroporphyria
uroporphyrinogen decarboxylase (UROD)
uropsammus
uropterin
uropyonephrosis
uropyoureter
Uroquid-Acid
uroradiology
    diagnostic u.
    interventional u.
urorectal septum
urorhythmography
urorubin
urorubrohematin
Uro-San Plus external catheter
uroscheocele
uroschesis
urosemiology
urosepsin
urosepsis
uroseptic

UROS infuser
urosis
UroSnare cystoscopic tumor snare
Urosoft stent
urospectrin
Urospiral urethral stent
urostalagmometry
urostealith calculus
urostomy
Uro-Tex McGuire male urinal
urothelial
    u. basement membrane (UBM)
    u. cancer
    u. carcinoma
    u. dysplasia
    u. mucosa
    u. neoplasm
    u. tumor
urothelium
    seromuscular enterocystoplasty lined
      with u. (SELU)
urotherapy
urotoxia
Urotract x-ray system
uroureter
Urovac bladder evacuator
Urovision ultrasound imaging system
Urovist
    U. Cysto
    U. Meglumine
    U. Sodium 300
UroVive self-contained balloon system
UroVysion assay
Urowave thermotherapy
uroxanthin
URR
    urea reduction ratio
URS
    transurethral ureterorenoscopy
URSEC urinal
Ursinus Inlay-Tabs
Urso 250
ursodeoxycholate (UDC)
ursodeoxycholic acid (UDCA)
ursodiol
urticarial
    u. fever
    u. reaction
urticaria pigmentosa
URYS 800 nerve stimulator
U.S. Army double-ended retractor

use
    long-term catheter u.
U-shaped skin flap
USPIO
    ultrasmall superparamagnetic iron oxide
USRDS
    United States Renal Data System
Ussing
    U. chamber
    U. chamber technique
U-stitch reimplantation technique
uteri (pl. of uterus)
uterine
    u. artery
    u. colic
    u. coring
    u. enlargement
    u. fibroid
    u. lateral fusion defect
    u. rupture
    u. size
    u. tenderness
    u. tympanites
utero
    hydronephrosis in u.
uterocele
uterolysis
    laparoscopic u.
uterosacral ligament
uteroscope
    Circon-ACMI u.
uterus, pl. uteri
    anteflexed u.
    anteverted u.
    bicornuate u.
    descensus uteri
    u. didelphys
    double u.
    duplicate u.
    enlarged u.
    gravid u.
    u. masculinus
    pregnant u.
    retroflexed u.
    retroverted u.
    unicornuate u.
UTI
    urinary tract infection
utricle
    prostatic u.
utriculitis
utriculocele

U

NOTES

utriculus
    u. masculinus
    u. prostaticus
    u. vestibuli
U-tube
    U-t. stent
U-turn maneuver
UUN
   urinary urea nitrogen excretion
   urine urea nitrogen
UUO
   unilateral ureteral obstruction
uveitis
UV-Flash ultraviolet germicidal exchange device

UVJ
   ureterovesical junction
UV-linked
uvomorulin
UV transilluminator
uvula, pl. **uvulae**
    u. of bladder
    Lieutaud u.
    u. vesica
uvular
    u. deviation
    u. swelling
uvularis
UW solution

299v
   Lactobacillus plantarum 299v
V33W high-density endocavity probe
V8 protease
VAB
   Velban, actinomycin-D, bleomycin
VAB-6 chemotherapy protocol
VABES
   vasoablative endothelial sarcoma
VAB-II
   Velban, actinomycin-D, bleomycin,
     platinum
VAB-VI
   cyclophosphamide, Velban, actinomycin-
     D, bleomycin, platinum
VAC
   vincristine, Adriamycin,
     cyclophosphamide
VacA
   vacuolating toxin gene A
     VacA cytotoxin
     VacA toxin
vaccination
   T-cell v.
vaccine
   V. Adverse Event Reporting
     System
   BCG v.
   edible v.
   hepatitis A v.
   hepatitis A inactivated and hepatitis
     B (recombinant) v.
   hepatitis B v.
   hepatitis B virus v. (HBVV)
   irradiated tumor v.
   JT1001 prostate cancer v.
   mucosal v.
   OraVax v.
   rhesus rotavirus-tetravalent v.
     (RRV-TV)
   rotavirus tetravalent v.
   tumor v.
   yeast-recombinant hepatitis B v.
VACTERL
   vertebral, anal, cardiac,
     tracheoesophageal fistula, renal, limb
     VACTERL syndrome
vacuolar
   v. H+-ATPase
   v. nephrosis
   v. type proton pump
     immunocytochemistry
vacuolating toxin gene A (VacA)
vacuolating toxin gene A cytotoxin

vacuole
   pinocytosis v.
   testicular adenomatoid tumor v.
vacuolization
   isometric tubular v.
Vacutainer
   V. bag
   V. bottle
vacuum
   v. constriction device (VCD)
   v. constriction erection
   v. entrapment device
   v. erection device (VED)
   v. erection technology
   v. extraction device
   v. tumescence device
VAD
   vincristine, doxorubicin, dexamethasone
VAG
   vascular access graft
vagal
   v. efferent outflow
   v. input neuron
   v. preganglionic neuron
   v. stimulation
vagina
   atrophic v.
   high-ending v.
   passage of flatus per v.
   septate v.
vaginal
   v. atresia
   v. bleeding
   v. *Candida*
   v. celiotomy
   v. cone
   v. cone biopsy
   v. cone for pelvic floor exercises
   v. construction
   v. cuff cellulitis
   v. cutback
   v. descent
   v. discharge
   v. electrical stimulation
   v. eversion
   v. fistula
   v. fistula cup
   v. flap
   v. flap reconstruction and
     pubovaginal sling procedure
   v. foreign body
   v. inflammation
   v. lithotomy
   v. mass
   v. morcellation

V

vaginal *(continued)*
v. mucosa
v. needle suspension procedure
v. suppository
v. trichomoniasis
v. ulcer
v. vesicostomy
v. wall approach
v. wall sling procedure
vaginalis
Gardnerella v.
patent processus v.
processus v.
Trichomonas v.
tunica v.
vestigium processus v.
vaginalitis
vaginate
vaginectomy
vaginoplasty
cutback type v.
posterior flap v.
tissue expansion v.
vaginoscopy
vaginosis
bacterial v.
vaginourethroplasty
vagosympathetic balance
vagotomy
bilateral v.
hemigastrectomy and v. (H&V)
highly selective v.
laparoscopic v.
laser laparoscopic v.
medical v.
parietal cell v. (PCV)
proximal gastric v. (PGV)
v. and pyloroplasty (V&P)
pyloroplasty and v. (P&V)
Roux-en-Y procedure with v.
selective v.
selective proximal v. (SPV)
superselective v.
surgical v.
total bilateral v.
truncal v.
**vagovagally mediated receptive
relaxation**
vagus nerve
valacyclovir
valerian
valethamate bromide
valganciclovir
valine
Valium
vallate papilla
vallecula, pl. **valleculae**

vallecular
v. dysphagia
v. pooling
Valleylab
V. E3B cautery unit
V. SSE-2 cautery unit
V. SSE2L generator
V-alpha gene
Valpin
V. 50
valproate
sodium v.
valproic
v. acid
v. acid hepatotoxicity
v. acid therapy
Valsalva
V. leak point pressure (VLPP)
V. leak point pressure concept
V. maneuver
V. ratio
taeniae of V.
valsalviana
dysphagia v.
Valtrac BAR
value
F v.
negative predictive v. (NPV)
positive predictive v. (PPV)
predictive v.
reference v.
therapeutic v.
valva
v. ilealis
v. ileocaecalis
valve
v. ablation
Amussat v.
anal v.
anterior urethral v.
antireflux v.
Ball v.
Bauhin v.
v. of Bauhin
Benchekroun hydraulic ileal v.
v. bladder
blunting of v.
Braune v.
v. of colon
competent ileocecal v.
continent v.
esophageal v. (ESV)
failed nipple v.
flap v.
frenulum of ileocolic v.
Gerlach v.
gonadal vein v.
v. of Guerin

Heister v.
Holter v.
Houston v.
v. of Houston
ileal intestinal antireflux v.
ileal nipple v.
ileocecal intestinal antireflux v.
incompetent ileocecal v.
intestinal antireflux v.
intussuscepted nipple v.
v. of Kerckring
Kock nipple v.
Kohlrausch v.
LeVeen v.
lipomatous ileocecal v.
Lopez enteral v.
v. of Macalister
Mitrofanoff v.
modified ileocecal v.
Morgagni v.
nipple v.
nonintussuscepted v.
posterior urethral v. (type I–IV)
  (PUV)
v. prolapse
rectal v.
Setguard antireflux v.
sigmoid v.
spiral v.
Spivack v.
urethral v.
v. of Varolius
valved
v. rectum
v. voice prosthesis
valvotomy
rectal v.
valvula
Amussat v.
v. fossae navicularis
v. processus vermiformis
v. spiralis
valvulae
v. anales
v. conniventes
valvular
v. heart disease
valvule
valvulectomy
Vamin amino acid solution
van
V. Bogaert disease

v. Buren disease
v. Buren sound
V. de Kramer fecal fat procedure
v. den Bergh disease
v. den Bergh test
v. der Bergh reaction
v. Hansemann cell
V. Hees index
v. Hook operation
v. Slyke formula
v. Sonnenberg gallbladder catheter
v. Sonnenberg sump drain
Vanceril inhaler
Vancocin HCl
vancomycin hydrochloride
vancomycin/nalidixic acid agar
vancomycin-resistant enterococcus (VRE)
vanillacetic acid (VLA)
vanilloid agent
vanillylmandelic acid (VMA)
vanished testis syndrome
vanishing
v. bile duct syndrome
v. bile duct system
v. gonad
v. testis
Vanquish Analgesic Caplets
Vansil
Vantin
Vapor Cut loop
vaporization
benign prostatic hyperplasia
  transurethral v.
Contact Laser v.
laser v.
VaporTome
VaporTrode electrode
Varco gallbladder forceps
vardenafil
variability
variable
v. nuclear crowding
time-dependent v.
variance
geographic v.
hypovolemic v.
isovolemic v.
Kruskal-Wallis analysis of v.
Varian model 3600 gas chromatography
variant
kidney v.
trifurcation v.

V

NOTES

variant *(continued)*
    Wilms tumor clear cell sarcoma v.
    Wilms tumor multilocular cyst v.
    Wilms tumor rhabdomyosarcoma v.
variation
    coefficient of v.
    diurnal v.
    phasic-free tone v.
variceal
    v. banding
    v. band ligation
    v. bleeding
    v. column
    v. decompression
    v. hemorrhage
    v. ligator
    v. pressure
    v. sclerosant
    v. sclerosis
    v. sclerotherapy
    v. sclerotherapy in esophagus
    v. size inclusion criteria
    v. wall
varicella-zoster
    v.-z. infection
    v.-z. virus (VZV)
varices (*pl. of* varix)
varicocele
    v. embolization
    symptomatic v.
varicocelectomy
    inguinal v.
    laparoscopic v.
    microsurgical inguinal v.
    v. recurrence
    retroperitoneal v.
    scrotal v.
    subinguinal microsurgical v.
varicole
Varicoscreen
varicosis coli totalis
varicosity
variegate
    v. coproporphyria
    v. porphyria (VP)
Variject needle
varioliform
    v. gastritis
    v. gastropathy
varioliformis
    gastritis v.
variolosa
    orchitis v.
varix, pl. **varices**
    actively bleeding v.
    alcoholic v.
    anorectal v.
    bar-type esophageal v.

    bleeding gastric v. (BGV)
    blue v.
    v. of colon
    colonic v.
    common bile duct v.
    downhill esophageal v.
    duodenal v.
    ectopic v.
    EEA stapling of v.
    endoscopic band ligation of v.
    esophageal v.
    esophagogastric v.
    familial colonic v.
    fundal v.
    fundic v.
    gallbladder v.
    gastric v.
    gastroesophageal v. (type 1, 2)
    v. grading system F1, F2, F3
    idiopathic v.
    ileal v.
    isolated gastric varices (type 1, 2)
      (IGV)
    jejunal v.
    v. ligation
    mesenteric v.
    obliterated v.
    Okuda transhepatic obliteration
      of v.
    paraesophageal v.
    percutaneous transhepatic
      obliteration of esophageal v.
    peristomal v.
    radius of v.
    rectal v.
    rectosigmoid v.
    transesophageal ligation of v.
Varolius
    valve of V.
vas, pl. **vasa**
    v. aberrans
    v. afferens glomeruli
    vasa afferentia
    v. deferens
    v. deferens obstruction
    v. deferens secretion
    v. deferens stricture
    v. efferens glomeruli
    v. epididymidis
    vasa recta
    vasa recta bundles
    vasa vasorum
vasalgia
vasal pedicle orchiopexy
Vas-Cath
vascular
    v. abnormality
    v. access

v. access complication
v. access failure
v. access graft (VAG)
v. access site
v. anastomosis
v. bruit
v. cachexia
v. cecal fold
v. cell adhesion molecule-1 (VCAM-1)
v. cirrhosis
v. clamp
v. coat of stomach
v. collateral network
v. compromise
v. disease
v. ectasia
v. endothelial growth factor (VEGF)
v. hemangioma
v. injury
v. insufficiency
v. invasion
v. laceration
v. laceration repair
v. lamina
v. lesion
v. malformation
v. neoplasm
v. nephritis
v. nephropathy
v. pattern
v. pedicle
peripheral v.
v. permeability factor (VPF)
v. permeation of tumor cell
v. plasminogen activator (v-PA)
v. plexus
v. rejection
v. renal mass
v. smooth muscle
v. smooth muscle cell (VSMC)
v. stapler
v. steal syndrome
v. surgery
v. suture
v. tuft

vascularity
vasculature
intraprostatic v.
kidney v.

preglomerular v.
v. responsiveness

vasculitic
v. lesion
v. neuropathy

vasculitis
allergic v.
ANCA-associated systemic v.
antineutrophilic cytoplasmic autoantibody-small vessel v. (ANCA-SVV)
extrarenal v.
leukocytoclastic v.
lymphocytic v.
mesenteric v.
necrotizing bowel v.
renal v.
rheumatoid v.
systemic lupus erythematosus v.
visceral v.

vasculogenic impotence
vasculopathy
acute renal transplant v.
noncerebral v.
portal hypertensive intestinal v. (PHIV)

vasculosa
tunica v.

vasculum aberrans
vasectomized
vasectomy
crossover v.
no-scalpel v.
open-ended v.
percutaneous v.
v. reversal
reversible v.

Vaseline gauze
vasiform
vasitis
v. nodosa

vasoablative endothelial sarcoma (VABES)
vasoactive
v. drug
v. intestinal peptide (VIP)
v. intestinal peptide distribution
v. intestinal polypeptide (VIP)
v. intestinal polypeptide binding
v. intestinal polypeptide immunoreactivity (VIP-IR)
v. intestinal polypeptide stain

NOTES

vasoactive *(continued)*
    v. intestinal polypeptide tumor
      (VIPoma, vipoma)
    v. peptide-cytokine interaction
vasoconstriction
    afferent arteriolar v.
    baroreceptor-mediated mesenteric
      arterial v.
    radiocontrast-induced renal v.
    reflex splanchnic v.
    renal v.
    splanchnic v.
vasoconstrictor peptide
vasocutaneous fistula
vasodilatation
    peripheral v.
vasodilation
    endothelium-dependent v.
    v. of portasystemic collateral
    renal v.
    sympathetic response to v.
vasodilator
    renal v.
vasoepididymography
vasoepididymostomy
    ASSI METE-5168 (end-to-end) v.
    Silber v.
vasoformative
vasography
    fine needle v.
    percutaneous v.
    transrectal v.
vasoligation
Vasomax
vasomotor disorder
vasoorchidostomy
vasopressin
    arginine v. (AVP)
    1-deamino-8-d-arginine v.
    fetal arginine v.
    v. infusion
    neonatal arginine v.
    v. type 2 receptor
    v. with nitroglycerin
vasopressinase
vasopressin-induced cAMP
vasopuncture
vasorelaxation
vasoresection
vasorrhaphy
vasorum
    vasa v.
vasosection
vasospasm
vasospasmolytic
vasospastic
vasostomy
Vasotec

vasotomy
vasovagal reflex
vasovasostomy
vasovasotomy
    cross v.
    multiple v.
vasovesiculectomy
vasovesiculitis
vasovesiculography
Vasoxyl
vastomy
vastus lateralis muscle flap
VATER
    vertebral, anal, tracheoesophageal fistula,
    renal
      VATER syndrome
Vater
    ampulla of V.
    invaginating ampulla of V.
    papilla of V.
VATS
    video-assisted thoracic surgery
vault
    rectal v.
V-beta gene
VBG
    vertical banded gastroplasty
VCA
    antiviral capsid antigen
VCAM-1
    vascular cell adhesion molecule-1
VCD
    vacuum constriction device
      Dacomed Catalyst VCD
      Mentor-Piston VCD
      Mentor Response VCD
      Mentor-Touch VCD
      Mission VCD
      Osbon ErecAid VCD
      Pos-T-Vac VCD
VCG
    voiding cystogram
VCR
    vincristine
VCUG
    vesicoureterogram
    voiding cystourethrogram
Vd
    volume of distribution
VDR
    vitamin D receptor
VDRL
    Venereal Disease Research Laboratory
Vectastain ABC kit
vector
    amplitude-acrophase v.
    bacterial v.
vectorial delivery

Vector volume measurement
Vectra hemodialysis access graft
vecuronium
VED
    vacuum erection device
      Mission VED
Veetids
vegetable
    allium v.
    cruciferous v.
vegetans
    pyostomatitis v.
vegetarian diet
vegetative lesion
VEGF
    vascular endothelial growth factor
veil
    Jackson v.
vein
    aberrant obturator v.
    adrenal v.
    arcuate v.
    arterialization of portal v.
    azygos v.
    bladder v.
    Burow v.
    cardinal v.
    cavernosal v.
    cavernous v.
    cavernous transformation of the
      portal v. (CTPV)
    circumflex v.
    common iliac v.
    crural v.
    deep dorsal v.
    dilated v.
    dorsal v.
    esophageal collateral v. (ECV)
    external spermatic v.
    extrahepatic portal v.
    gastric v.
    gonadal v.
    gubernacular v.
    hepatic v. (HV)
    iliac v.
    inferior adrenal v.
    inferior mesenteric v. (IMV)
    inferior rectal v.
    interlobar v.
    internal iliac v.
    internal pudendal v.
    left hepatic v. (LHV)

    lumbar v.
    mesenteric v.
    middle hepatic v. (MHV)
    middle rectal v.
    muscularization of v.
    North American Medical
      Incorporated deep dorsal v.
    obturator v.
    omental v.
    palisade-type v.
    pancreaticoduodenal v.
    paraesophageal collateral v.
    paraumbilical v.
    v. patch
    periesophageal collateral v.
    peripheral acinar v.
    peritoneal v.
    periurethral v.
    portal v. (PV)
    pudendal v.
    rectal v.
    renal v.
    v. retractor
    Retzius v.
    right hepatic v. (RHV)
    Ruysch v.
    sacral v.
    saphenous v.
    shunt index via the inferior
      mesenteric v. (SI-I)
    shunt index via the superior
      mesenteric v. (SI-S)
    spermatic v.
    splanchnic v.
    splenic v.
    subclavian v.
    sulcus of umbilical v.
    superior mesenteric v. (SMV)
    superior rectal v.
    tangle of hemorrhoidal v.'s
    thoracoabdominal collateral v.
    umbilical v.
    urethral v.
    vesical v.
veins
    Krukenberg v.
Velban
    V., actinomycin-D, bleomycin
     (VAB)
    V., actinomycin-D, bleomycin,
     platinum (VAB-II)
    cisplatin, methotrexate, V. (CMV)

V

NOTES

Vella fistula
velocimetry
    laser Doppler v.
velocity
    angular v.
    dorsal nerve conduction v.
    v. measurement
    portal blood v.
    portal-vein blood flow v. (PFV)
    portal venous v. (PVV)
    prostate-specific antigen v. (PSAV)
    tumor peak systolic v. (TPSV)
Velosef
Velpeau hernia
vena, pl. **venae**
    vena cava
    vena cava hiatus
    venae cavernosae penis
    vena cavography
    vena marginalis epididymis of
      Haberer
venacavogram
venacavography
venae (*pl. of* vena)
venerea
    urethritis v.
venereal
    v. bubo
    v. disease
    V. Disease Research Laboratory
      (VDRL)
    v. proctocolitis
    v. sore
    v. wart
venereum
    lymphogranuloma v. (LGV)
    papilloma v.
veneris
    mons v.
venezuelensis
    Strongyloides v.
venlafaxine
venodilation
    nitrate-induced v.
    systemic v.
Venofer
venogenic impotence
venogram
    hepatic v.
    renal v.
    weeping willow appearance on v.
venography
    adrenal v.
    hepatic v.
    pedal control v.
    renal v.
    splenic v.

    splenoportal v.
    transjugular portal v.
venoocclusive
    v. dysfunction
    v. liver disease
venoperitoneostomy
venosi
    fissura ligamenti v.
venosum
    fissure for ligamentum v.
    ligamentum v.
venosus
    plexus v.
venous
    v. blood sample
    v. circulation
    v. ectasia
    v. engorgement
    v. hum
    v. invasion
    v. leakage
    v. leak impotence
    v. leak syndrome
    v. outflow obstructive disease
    v. pattern
    v. pooling
    v. stasis
    v. thromboembolism (VTE)
    v. thrombosis
    v. web
    v. web disease
venovenous
    v. bypass
    v. continuous hemodialysis
    v. hemofiltration
venter propendens
ventilation
    mechanical v.
venting
    v. percutaneous gastrostomy (VPG)
    v. percutaneous gastrostomy tube
Ventolin
ventral
    v. apron prepuce
    v. bending technique
    v. bud
    v. celiotomy
    v. chronic calcific pancreatitis
    v. hernia
    v. herniorrhaphy
    v. meatotomy
    v. mesogastrium
    v. sacral rootlet
    v. surface
    v. transperitoneal laparoscopic
      approach
ventralis
ventricle

ventricular
    v. canal
    v. tachycardia
ventriculare
    corpus v.
ventricularis
    fundus v.
ventriculi
    caecus minor v.
    corpus v.
    fibrae oblique v.
    fibromatosis v.
    fundus v.
    polyposis v.
    ulcus v.
ventriculoperitoneal (VP)
    v. shunt
ventrocystorrhaphy
ventroscopy
ventrotomy
ventrum
    v. of penis
    v. penis flap
venulae rectae renis
venular
venule
    collecting v.
    hepatic v.
    portal v.
    stellate v.
    straight v.
    subtunical v.
VePesid, ifosfamide (with mesna rescue), Platinol (VIP)
vera
    hemospermia v.
    melena v.
    polycythemia v.
verapamil
Veratrum alkaloid
Veress
    V. cannula
    V. needle
verge
    anal v.
veritas
    in vivo v.
vermicular
    v. appendage
    v. colic
    v. movement

vermicularis
    Enterobius v.
vermiform
    v. appendix
    v. body
vermiformis
    ostium appendicis v.
    valvula processus v.
verminous
    v. appendicitis
    v. colic
    v. ileus
Vermox
Verner-Morrison syndrome
Vernon-David
    V.-D. proctoscope
    V.-D. rectal speculum
    V.-D. sigmoidoscope
verruca vulgaris
verruciform xanthoma
verrucous
    v. carcinoma
    v. gastritis
Versabran
    Modane V.
Versa-PEG gastrostomy kit
VersaPulse Select laser
Versed
vertebra, pl. **vertebrae**
    picture-frame v.
vertebral
    v., anal, cardiac, tracheoesophageal fistula, renal, limb (VACTERL)
    v., anal, cardiac, tracheoesophageal fistula, renal, limb syndrome
    v., anal, tracheoesophageal fistula, renal (VATER)
    v., anal, tracheoesophageal fistula, renal syndrome
vertex
    v. of urinary bladder
    v. vesicae urinaria
vertical
    v. banded gastroplasty (VBG)
    v. fold
    v. mattress suture
    v. midline incision
    v. plication suture
    v. reduction rectoplasty
    v. ring gastroplasty (VRG)
    v. Silastic ring gastroplasty
    v strip pattern breast examination

NOTES

vertical *(continued)*
    v. transmission
    v. vesicomyotomy (VVM)
vertigo
    gastric v.
    objective v.
    subjective v.
verum
    diverticulum ilei v.
verumontanitis
verumontanum
very
    v. late activation (VLA)
    v. low birth weight infant
    v. low calorie diet (VLCD)
    v. low density lipoprotein (VLDL)
    v. low density lipoprotein
      cholesterol
Vesica
    V. percutaneous bladder neck
      stabilization
    V. percutaneous bladder neck
      suspension kit
    V. sling
    V. sling procedure
vesica, pl. **vesicae**
    v. biliaris
    bullous edema v.
    ectopia v.
    endometriosis v.
    v. fellea
    v. ileale pouch
    malacoplakia v.
    v. prostatica
    trigonum v.
    ulcus simplex v.
    v. urinaria
    uvula v.
vesical
    v. artery
    v. calculus
    v. compliance
    v. diverticulectomy
    v. diverticulum
    v. exstrophy
    v. external sphincter dyssynergia
      (VSD)
    v. fibrosis
    v. fistula
    v. hematuria
    v. ligament
    v. lithotomy
    v. neck
    v. neck resistance
    v. neck stenosis
    v. plexus
    v. prostatism

    v. schistosomiasis
    v. vein
vesicale
    plexus v.
vesicalis
    anus v.
    plexus v.
vesical-sacral-sphincter loop
vesicle
    brush-border membrane v. (BBMV)
    endocytotic v.
    v. hernia
    leiomyoma of seminal v.
    metanephric v.
    prechylomicron transport v.
    seminal v.
    spermatic v.
vesicoamniotic shunt
vesicoanal reflex
vesicocavernous
vesicocele
vesicocervical
vesicoclysis
vesicocolic fistula
vesicocolonic fistula
vesicocutaneous fistula
vesicoenteric fistula
vesicofixation
vesicoileal reflux
vesicointestinal
    v. fistula
    v. reflex
vesicolithiasis
vesicomyectomy
vesicomyotomy
    circular v. (CVM)
    vertical v. (VVM)
vesicopelvic fascia
vesicoperineal
vesicoprostatic
    v. calculus
    v. plexus
vesicopubic
vesicopustule
vesicorectal fistula
vesicorectostomy
vesicorenal
vesicosalpingovaginal fistula
vesicosigmoid
vesicosigmoidostomy
vesicosphincteric dyssynergia
vesicospinal
vesicostomy
    Blocksom v.
vesicostomy
    cutaneous v.
    Lapides v.

preputial continent v.
vaginal v.
vesicotomy
vesicoumbilical fistula
vesicourachal diverticulum
vesicoureteral
v. reflux (VUR)
v. regurgitation
v. suspension
vesicoureteric
v. reflux
v. stenosis
vesicoureterogram (VCUG)
vesicourethral
v. anastomosis
v. anastomotic stricture
v. canal
v. reflux
v. suspension
vesicouterina
excavatio v.
vesicouterine
v. fistula
v. pouch
vesicouterinum
cavum v.
vesicouterovaginal
vesicovaginal
v. fistula (VVF)
v. Holter
v. lithotomy
v. space
vesicovaginorectal fistula
vesicovaginostomy
vesicula
v. bilis
v. fellea
v. seminalis
vesiculase
vesiculectomy
prostatoseminal v.
retrovesical v.
total prostatoseminal v.
transcoccygeal v.
transperineal v.
transvesical v.
vesiculitis
vesiculobullous disorder
vesiculocavernous
vesiculodeferential artery
vesiculogram

vesiculography
seminal v. (SVG)
vesiculoprostatitis
vesiculotomy
seminal v.
vesiculotubular
vesiculotympanitic resonance
Vespore disinfectant
Vesprin
VESS
videoendoscopic swallowing study
Vess chair
vessel
accessory v.
blood v.
caliber-persistent v.
capsular blood v.
chyliferous v.
cremasteric v.
v. dilator
dysmorphic v.
ectatic v.
feeding v.
gastroepiploic blood v.
gonadal v.
hypogastric v.
hypoplastic blind-ending
spermatic v.
ileal blood v.
ileocolic v.
internal spermatic v.
lacteal v.
lymphatic v.
mesocolonic v.
nonbleeding visible v. (NBVV)
pudendal v.
replaced hepatic v.
serosal blood v.
telangiectatic v.
v. tip
ulcer v.
visible v.
visible ulcer v.
vestibular gland
vestibularis
anus v.
vestibule
laryngeal v.
vestibuli
utriculus v.
vestibulourethral
vestige

V

NOTES

vestigial
vestigium processus vaginalis
vest-over-pants
    v.-o.-p. hernial repair
    v.-o.-p. herniorrhaphy
VET-CO vacuum system
Vezien abdominal scissors
VFC
    Actis venous flow controller
V-flap meatoplasty
VGTT
    video graphic tool technology
VHL gene
viability
    intestinal v.
    v. testing
Viadur
Viagra
    esprolol plus V.
vial
    Port-A-Germ anaerobic transport v.
    scintillation v.
Vibramycin
Vibrio
    V. *alginolyticus*
    V. *cholerae*
    V. *cholerae* biotype *albensis*
    V. *cholerae* biotype *eltor*
    V. *cholerae* biotype *proteus*
    V. *eltor*
    V. *fetus* infection
    V. *fluvialis*
    V. *furnissii*
    V. *hollisae*
    V. *metschnikovii*
    V. *parahaemolyticus*
    V. *vulnificus*
vibriocidal
Vibrionaceae species
vibrotactile stimulation testing
Vickers M85a microdensitometer
Vicodin
Vicryl
    V. mesh
    V. suture
VID
    vitellointestinal duct
Vidal operation
vidarabine
video
    v. colonoscope
    v. densitometry
    v. duodenoscope
    v. endoscope
    v. endoscopy
    v. esophagoscopy
    v. graphic tool technology (VGTT)

V. Image Processor model 450
v. monitor
v. monitored TUR
v. pressure flow electromyography
v. processor
v. push enteroscope
v. recorder
v. small bowel enteroscopy
v. timer
v. transurethral resection technique
video-assisted thoracic surgery (VATS)
videocolonoscope
    EVE Fujinon v.
videocystourethrography
videoelectroscope
    Fujinon CEG-FP-series v.
videoendoscope
    double-channel v.
    JF-200 side-viewing v.
    Olympus GIF-series double-channel
      therapeutic v.
    Olympus GIF-SQ-series v.
    Olympus GIF-T-series v.
videoendoscopic swallowing study
  (VESS)
videoendoscopy
    Lugol-combined upper
      gastrointestinal v.
    zoom v.
videoesophagram
videofluoroscopic
    v. swallow study
    v. technique
videofluoroscopy
videofluorourodynamic study
videogastroscope
    Pentax EG-2900 v.
videolaseroscopy cholecystectomy
videoproctography
videoscope
    SlimSIGHT gastrointestinal v.
videosigmoidoscope
videourodynamic
    v. evaluation
    v. testing
view
    en face v.
    longitudinal v.
    postevacuation v.
    retroflexed v.
    slide-by v.
    transverse v.
vigabatrin
vigorous achalasia
VIGOR trial
villi (*pl. of* villus)
villiferous

villoglandular
    v. adenoma
    v. polyp
villous, villose
    v. arteritis
    v. arthritis
    v. atrophy
    v. coat of small intestine
    v. colorectal adenoma
    v. effacement
    v. epithelium
    v. folds of stomach
    v. papilloma
    v. polyp
    v. tip cell
    v. tumor
villus, pl. villi
    v. cell
    colonic v.
    duodenal v.
    fingerlike v.
    intestinal v.
    jejunal v.
    leaflike v.
    ridged-convoluted v.
    small intestinal v.
    v. tip
    tongue-shaped v.
vimentin staining
Vim-Silverman
    V.-S. biopsy needle
    V.-S. technique
    V.-S. technique for liver biopsy
vinblastine
    v., actinomycin D, bleomycin
      (mini-VAB)
    cisplatin, methotrexate, v. (CMV)
    doxorubicin, bleomycin sulfate, v.
      (ABV)
    methotrexate, cisplatin, v. (MCV)
Vincent curtsy
vincristine (VCR)
    v., Adriamycin, cyclophosphamide
      (VAC)
    v., doxorubicin, dexamethasone
      (VAD)
Vindelov method flow cytometry
  analysis
vinorelbine
Vinson syndrome
Viokase

violaceous
violation
    scrotal v.
violet
    gentian v.
violin-string adhesion
Vioxx Gastrointestinal Outcomes
  Research trial (VIGOR trial)
VIP
    vasoactive intestinal peptide
    vasoactive intestinal polypeptide
    VePesid, ifosfamide (with mesna rescue),
      Platinol
    voluntary interruption of pregnancy
      VIP antiserum
      VIP stain
VIP-IR
    vasoactive intestinal polypeptide
      immunoreactivity
VIPoma, vipoma
    vasoactive intestinal polypeptide tumor
      VIPoma syndrome
VIP-secreting neuronoma
Virag
    V. injector
    V. operation
viral
    v. cholangitis
    v. colitis
    v. culture
    v. cystitis
    v. diarrhea
    v. dysentery
    v. enteritis
    v. gastritis
    v. gastroenteritis
    v. hemorrhagic fever
    v. hepatitis
    v. hepatitis marker
    v. hepatitis type A, B
    v. inclusion body
    v. infection
    v. membrane fusion
    v. replication
    v. serologic titer
ViraPap HPV dot blot hybridization
  test
Virchow sentinel node
Virchow-Troisier node
viremia
    hepatitis C v.

V

NOTES

virgin
  v. lymphocyte
  v. ulcer
viridans
  Staphylococcus v.
  Streptococcus v.
virile
  membrum v.
  v. reflex
virilis
  crista urethralis v.
  orificium urethrae externum v.
  urethra v.
virilism
  adrenal v.
virilization
virilizing tumor
Virilon
virological
virology
virtual
  V. Biopsy system
  v. cystoscopy
  v. endoscopy
  v. enteroscopy
  v. focus shock wave
  v. nephroureteroscopy
  V. Vision
  V. Vision audiovisual system for
    EGD and colonoscopy
virucidal agent
virulent diarrhea
virus
  adenoassociated v. (AAV)
  antibody to hepatitis A v. (anti-
    HAV)
  antibody to hepatitis C v. (anti-
    HCV)
  antibody to hepatitis D v. (anti-
    HDV)
  delta v.
  dengue v.
  Epstein-Barr v. (EBV)
  esophageal condyloma v.
  GB virus C/hepatitis G v. (GBV-
    C/HGV)
  Hanta v.
  Hawaii v.
  hepatitis A v. (HAV)
  hepatitis B v. (HBV)
  hepatitis B-like DNA v.
  hepatitis C v. (HCV)
  hepatitis D v. (HDV)
  hepatitis delta v. (HDV)
  hepatitis E v. (HEV)
  hepatitis G v. (HGV)
  herpes simplex v. (HSV)
  herpes zoster v.

human immunodeficiency v. (HIV)
human T-cell leukemia v. of type
  I (HTLV-I)
human T-cell lymphotrophic v.
  (type I, II)
influenza v.
live attenuated v.
v. load
Manchester v.
Marburg v.
molluscum contagiosum v. (MCV)
mother-to-infant transmission of
  hepatitis C v.
neutropic v.
Norwalk v.
Norwalk-like v. (NLV)
recombinant capsid protein of
  Norwalk v. (rNV)
Sapporo v.
v. shedding
transfusion-transmitted v. (TTV)
TT v. (TTV)
varicella-zoster v. (VZV)
virus-like
  v.-l. action (VLA)
  v.-l. particle (VLP)
Viruzilin
viscera (*pl. of* viscus)
visceral
  v. angiography
  v. arteriography
  v. dysfunction
  v. hyperalgesia
  v. hypersensitivity
  v. ischemia
  v. larva migrans
  v. leishmaniasis
  v. muscle
  v. neuropathy
  v. pain
  v. peritoneum
  v. traction reflex
  v. vasculitis
visceralgia
visceralis
  fascia pelvis v.
visceromegaly
visceromotor
visceroparietal
visceroptosis, visceroptosia
viscerosensory reflex
viscerotomy
viscerotrophic
viscerotropic
viscerum
  situs inversus v.
viscid bile
viscidosis

viscoelastic
  v. collagen fiber
  v. gel
viscoelasticity
  bladder v.
viscometer
viscosity
  plasma v.
  semen v.
viscous
  v. bile
  v. lidocaine
  v. lidocaine premedication
  v. Xylocaine gargle
viscus, pl. **viscera**
  abdominal v.
  hollow v.
  intraabdominal v.
  intraperitoneal v.
  perforated v.
  strangulated v.
vise
  torque v.
visible
  v. abdominal distention
  v. peristalsis
  v. ulcer vessel
  v. vessel
  v. vessel significance
visible-light lithotripsy
visibly normal
Visicath endoscope
Visick
  V. dysphagia classification
  V. gastric cancer grading system
Visicol tablet
Visilex mesh
vision
  direct v.
  V. Sciences VSI 2000 flexible
    sigmoidoscope system
  V. System EndoSheath
  V. System sigmoidoscope
  tunnel v.
  Virtual V.
Visiport device
Visken
Vistaflex biliary stent
Vistaril
visual
  v. endoscopically controlled laser
  v. evoked potential

  v. laser ablation
  v. laser ablation of prostate
    (VLAP)
  v. laser-assisted prostatectomy
    (VLAP)
  v. sexual stimulation testing
visualization
vital
  V. feeding
  v. sign
  v. staining
vitamin
  v. A, B_{12} absorption test
  v. A deficiency
  v. Λ toxicity
  v. B_{12}
  v. B_6
  v. B_{12} malabsorption
  v. C
  v. D deficiency
  v. D-dependent calbindin-D9k
  v. D receptor (VDR)
  v. D resistance
  v. D supplementation
  v. E
  fat-soluble v.
  v. K2
  water-soluble v.
vitamin-D-binding protein (DBP)
Vitaneed
  V. feeding
  V. tube feeding formula
vitelline
  v. duct
  v. duct anomaly
vitellointestinal
  v. cyst
  v. duct (VID)
vitiligo
vitro
  in v.
vitronectin inhibiting HGF-induced
  tubulogenesis
Vittaforma corneae
Vivactil
viverrini
  Opisthorchis v.
vividialysis
vividiffusion
vivo
  ex v.
  in v.

V

NOTES

Vivonex
    V. Acutrol Enteral Feeding System
    V. HN powdered feeding
    V. Moss tube
    V. TEN
    V. TEN feeding
VLA
    vanillacetic acid
    very late activation
    virus-like action
VLAP
    visual laser ablation of prostate
    visual laser-assisted prostatectomy
VLCD
    very low calorie diet
VLDL
    very low density lipoprotein
        VLDL cholesterol
        VLDL triglyceride
VLP
    virus-like particle
VLPP
    Valsalva leak point pressure
VM-26
    teniposide
VMA
    vanillylmandelic acid
VMC
    von Meyenburg complex
vocal cord
Vocare bladder system
Vogel operation
Voges-Proskauer test
voice restoration
voided
    v. urine
    v. volume
voiding
    alarm clock v.
    v. biofeedback
    v. cystogram (VCG)
    v. cystometrography
    v. cystometry
    v. cystourethrogram (VCUG)
    v. cystourethrography
    v. diary
    dysfunctional v.
    v. dysfunction classification
    v. flow rate
    fractionated v.
    incomplete v.
    v. initiation
    orthotopic v.
    reflex v.
    staccato v.
    v. study
    timed v.
    trigger v.

    v. urethral pressure measurement (VUPM)
    v. urine cytology (VUC)
Voillemier point
vol
    volume
volar
Volhard-Fahr method
Volhard nephritis
Volkmann
    V. operation
    V. pancreatic calculus spoon
    V. rake retractor
    V. spoon for pancreatic calculus
voltage
    RMS v.
    root mean square v.
voltage-gated channel
Voltaren
volume (vol)
    bladder v.
    v. displacement transducer
    v. of distribution (Vd)
    drain v.
    effective arterial blood v. (EABV)
    emptying delta v.
    v. expansion
    extracellular fluid v. (ECV)
    fiber bundle v. (FBV)
    flow v.
    functional hepatic v.
    gallbladder v.
    gastric v.
    interstitial v.
    intragastric v.
    intraperitoneal v.
    intravascular v.
    liver v.
    maximal toleration v. (MTV)
    maximum tolerable v. (MTV)
    mean corpuscular v. (MCV)
    mean prostatic v.
    mean renal v.
    v. overload
    pelvic ileal reservoir v.
    PET dialysate v.
    plasma v.
    prostate v.
    prostatic v.
    renal v.
    v. replacement
    residual urine v. (RUV)
    semen v.
    spermatozoon v.
    target v. (TV)
    transition zone v.
    urea distribution v.

voided v.
weight-based peritoneal exchange v.
voluminous hiatus hernia
voluntarily stopping eating and
  drinking (VSED)
voluntary
  v. guarding
  v. interruption of pregnancy (VIP)
  v. sphincter contraction
volvulated Meckel diverticulum
volvulus
  cecal v.
  v. of colon
  colonic v.
  gastric v.
  idiopathic v.
  intestinal v.
  mesenteroaxial gastric v.
  midgut v.
  v. neonatorum
  nongangrenous sigmoid v.
  Onchocerca v.
  organoaxial gastric v.
  v. reduction
  secondary v.
  sigmoid colon v.
vomica
  nux v.
vomicus
vomiting
  bilious v.
  v. center
  chemotherapy-induced v.
  concealed v.
  cyclic v.
  cyclical v.
  diarrhea and v. (D&V)
  dry v.
  epidemic v.
  episodic v.
  erotic v.
  explosive v.
  fecal v.
  hysterical v.
  intractable v.
  ipecac-induced v.
  nausea and v. (N&V)
  nervous v.
  periodic v.
  perioperative v.
  periotic v.
  pernicious v.

persistent v.
postoperative v.
postprandial v.
posttussive v.
profuse v.
projectile v.
psychogenic v.
recurrent bouts of v.
retention v.
Rhodes Inventory of Nausea
  and V.
self-induced v.
stercoraceous v.
surreptitious v.
winter v.
vomition
vomitive
vomito negro
vomitory
vomiturition
vomitus
  Barcoo v.
  bile-stained v.
  black v.
  bloody v.
  bright red v.
  coffee-ground v.
  v. cruentes
  feculent v.
  v. marinus
  v. matutinus
  v. niger
  nonbilious v.
  stercoraceous v.
Von
  V. Andel dilating catheter
  V. Ebner gland
  V. Haberer-Finney anastomosis
  V. Petz suturing apparatus
von
  v. Brunn epithelial nest
  v. Gierke disease
  v. Haberer-Aguirre gastrectomy
  v. Hanseman cell
  v. Hippel-Lindau cerebellar
    hemangioblastomatosis
  v. Hippel-Lindau disease
  v. Hippel Lindau gene
  v. Hippel-Lindau syndrome
  v. Jaksch test
  v. Kossa stain
  v. Kupffer cell

V

NOTES

von *(continued)*
    v. Mering reflex
    v. Meyenburg complex (VMC)
    v. Petz clamp
    v. Petz suture clip
    v. Recklinghausen disease
    v. Recklinghausen neurofibromatosis
    v. Rokitansky disease
    v. Willebrand disease
    v. Willebrand factor
voracious appetite
Voronoff operation
VP
    variegate porphyria
    ventriculoperitoneal
    VP shunt
VP-16
V&P
    vagotomy and pyloroplasty
v-PA
    vascular plasminogen activator
VPF
    vascular permeability factor
VPG
    venting percutaneous gastrostomy
VPI
    Coloscreen VPI
    VPI nonadhesive open-end pouch
V/Q mismatch
VRE
    vancomycin-resistant enterococcus
VRG
    vertical ring gastroplasty
VSD
    vesical external sphincter dyssynergia
VSED
    voluntarily stopping eating and drinking
V-shaped ulcer
V sign of Naclerio
VSI 2000 sigmoidoscope
VSMC
    vascular smooth muscle cell
VTC biliary catheter

VTE
    venous thromboembolism
VTR-300 enteral feeding pump
VTU-1 vacuum erection device
VUC
    voiding urine cytology
vulgaris
    acne v.
    pemphigus v.
    Proteus v.
    verruca v.
vulgatus
    Bacteroides v.
vulnificus
    Vibrio v.
vulva, pl. **vulvae**
    rima v.
vulvar
    v. carcinoma
    v. vestibulitis syndrome
vulvitis
vulvoplasty
vulvorectal fistula
vulvovaginal
    v. anus
    v. candidiasis
vulvovaginoplasty
    Williams v.
VUPM
    voiding urethral pressure measurement
VUR
    vesicoureteral reflux
VVF
    vesicovaginal fistula
    VVF repair
VVM
    vertical vesicomyotomy
V-Y
    V-Y plasty
    V-Y sliding skin graft
Vygon Nutricath S catheter
VZV
    varicella-zoster virus

W

W pelvic ileal pouch
W pouch

Wacker Sil-Gel 604 silicone cement

wafer

Stomahesive skin barrier w.

Wagner test

WAGR syndrome

wait-and-see approach

wake reflex

Waldenström macroglobulinemia

Waldeyer

W. fascia
pelvic colon of W.
W. sheath

Wales rectal bougie

Walker gallbladder retractor

walking stick phenomenon

wall

abdominal w.
anterior abdominal w.
bowel w.
capillary w.
colonic w.
esophageal w.
gallbladder w.
gas-forming organism in bowel w.
glomerular capillary w. (GCW)
hydrocele w.
midabdominal w.
pharyngeal w.
posterior abdominal w.
sinusoidal w.
w. tension
thickened gallbladder w.
w. thickening
variceal w.

Wallace

W. anastomosis
W. technique
W. technique urinary diversion

Wallstent

W. delivery device
W. endoprosthesis
W. esophageal prosthesis
W. stent

Wallstent-covered SEM stent

Wallstent-I

Walsh

W. procedure
W. radical retropubic prostatectomy
W. surgical modification

Walther

W. dilator
W. sound

Waltz endoscopic lithotriptor

wand

ultrasound w.

wandering

w. gallbladder
w. liver

Wangensteen

W. anastomosis clamp
W. colostomy
W. drain
W. drainage
W. incision
W. operation
W. suction
W. suction apparatus
W. suction tube

Wappler

W. cystoscope with microlens optics
W. microlens cystourethroscope

warfarin

warfarin-associated subcapsular hematoma

warm

w. ischemia
w. ischemia time
w. saline solution

war nephritis

Warren splenorenal shunt

wart

anal w.
cervical w.
exophytic w.
genital w.
intraanal w.
perianal w.
venereal w.

Warthen spur crusher

Warthin-Starry

W.-S. method
W.-S. silver stain

Warwick and Ashken technique

wash

povidone-iodine w.

washer

Olympus Europe ETD automated endoscope w.

washing

bladder w.
w. catheter

washout

w. cannula
w. factor
high rectal w.
mucosal w.

W

827

washout *(continued)*
    w. pyelography
    seminal tract w.
    w. test
Wassilieff disease
wastage
    pregnancy w.
waste
    w. nitrogen excretion
    nitrogenous w.
wastebasket
    w. diagnosis
    w. pouchitis
wasting
    muscle w.
    renal sodium w.
    w. syndrome
water
    w. balance
    body w.
    w. brash
    w. channel
    contamination of w.
    w. cushion lithotriptor
    w. cystometry
    degassed w.
    w. displacing balloon
    w. diuresis
    w. excretion
    fecal contamination of w.
    w. immersion
    insensible loss of w.
    w. loading
    w. permeability
    w. pot perineum
    w. probe
    total body w. (TBW)
water-filled balloon sheath
water-gurgle test
Waterhouse-Friderichsen syndrome
water-induced thermotherapy (WIT)
water-infusion esophageal manometry catheter
watering-can
    w.-c. perineum
    w.-c. scrotum
water-losing nephritis
watermelon
    w. cecum
    w. rectum
    w. stomach (WS)
water-nutrient test
water-perfused catheter
Waterpik
    endoscopic W.
    W. lavage
water-recovery test
water-restriction test

watershed area
water-sipping test
water-soluble
    w.-s. bilirubin
    w.-s. contrast
    w.-s. contrast enema
    w.-s. contrast esophageal swallow
    w.-s. contrast esophageal swallow test
    w.-s. contrast medium
    w.-s. vitamin
Waterston method
water-trap stomach
watery
    w. diarrhea
    w. diarrhea, hypokalemia, achlorhydria (WDHA)
    w. diarrhea, hypokalemia, and hypovolemia (WDHH)
    w. diarrhea syndrome
    w. diarrhea with hypokalemic alkalosis (WDHA)
    w. stool
Watson
    W. capsule
    W. capsule biopsy
Watson-Alagille syndrome
Watson-Schwartz test
wattage
Watzki sleeve
Waugh-Clagett
    W.-C. operation
    W.-C. pancreaticoduodenostomy
wave
    abdominal fluid w.
    clustered w.'s (CW)
    clustered jejunal w.'s
    double-peaked w.
    duodenal pressure w.
    extracorporeal shock w.
    flipped T w.
    fluid w.
    focused shock w.
    mechanical stress w.
    peristaltic w.
    primary peristaltic w.
    propulsive w.
    pyloric pressure w.
    real focus shock w.
    secondary peristaltic w.
    shock w.
    simultaneous bilateral extracorporeal shock w.'s
    slow w.
    T w.
    virtual focus shock w.
waveform
    blend w.

coagulase w.
cut w.
electrical w.
low-pulsatility arterial w.
waveguide
quartz w.
wavelength
Wavicide disinfectant
wax-matrix
w.-m. slow-release form
w.-m. tablet
wax-tipped bougie
WBC
white blood cell
WBC band
WBC basophil
WBC differential
elevated WBC
WBC immature forms
WBC leukocyte
WBC lymphocyte
WBC monocyte
WBC neutrophil
WD
Whipple disease
Wilson disease
WDHA
watery diarrhea, hypokalemia,
achlorhydria
watery diarrhea with hypokalemic
alkalosis
WDHA syndrome
WDHH
watery diarrhea, hypokalemia, and
hypovolemia
WDPM
well-differentiated papillary
mesothelioma
weakness
extremity w.
proximal muscle w.
weaning brash
web
antral w.
duodenal w.
endoscopic resection of antral w.
esophageal w.
hepatic w.
intestinal w.
mucosal w.
postcricoid w.
venous w.

Webb-Balfour abdominal retractor
webbed penis
webbing
penoscrotal w.
Weber-Christian disease
Weck
W. clip
W. high flow laparator
Weck-cel sponge
weddellite calculus
wedge
W. electrosurgical resection device
w. hepatic biopsy
W. loop
w. pressure
w. resection
wedged hepatic venous pressure
(WHVP)
weeping willow appearance on
venogram
Weerda endoscope
Wegener granulomatosis
Weibel-Palade granule
Weigert-Meyer
W.-M. law
W.-M. rule
weighing
gravimetric w.
weight (wt)
actual w. (AW)
actual body w. (ABW)
body w. (BW)
desirable body w. (DBW)
dry w.
Femina vaginal w.
w. gain
ideal body w. (IBW)
kidney w. (KW)
w. loss
w. loss with hyperphagia
low molecular w. (LMW)
molecular w. (mol wt)
w. reduction surgery
seminal vesicle w.
weight-based peritoneal exchange
volume
weighted tip
Weight Watchers diet
Weil
W. disease
W. syndrome

W

NOTES

Weinberg
    W. modification of pyloroplasty
    W. vagotomy retractor
Weinstein syndrome
Weiss reaction
Weitlaner retractor
Welch
    W. Allyn flexible sigmoidoscope
    W. Allyn video colonoscope 8451
    W. Allyn video endoscope
    W. Allyn video endoscopy system
welchii
    Clostridium w.
weld
    laser tissue w.
welding
    chromophore enhanced laser w.
    laser w.
    laser tissue w.
well-defined anatomical entry criteria
well-differentiated
    w.-d. adenoma
    w.-d. papillary mesothelioma
    (WDPM)
Wellferon
well-matched organ
Wells posterior rectopexy
Welt syndrome
Werdnig-Hoffman disease
Wermer syndrome
Wernicke
    W. encephalopathy
    W. syndrome
Wernicke-Korsakoff syndrome
Wesson perineal retractor
Westcott tenotomy scissors
Western
    W. blot
    W. blot analysis
    W. blotting
    W. diet
Weston rectal snare
Westphal
    W. gall duct forceps
    W. hemostat
Westphal-Strümpell disease
wet
    w. colostomy
    w. swallow
Wexler retractor
WGTS
    whole-gut transit scintigraphy
Wharton duct
wheal
wheat
    w. amylase inhibitor
    w. gluten
    w. starch

Wheelhouse operation
whewellite calculus
whiff test
Whipple
    W. disease (WD)
    W. operation
    W. pancreatectomy
    W. pancreaticoduodenectomy
    W. pancreaticoduodenostomy
    W. procedure
    W. resection
    W. syndrome
    W. triad
    W. triad test
whipplei
    Trophermyma w.
whipworm infection
whispered pectoriloquy
whistle stent
whistle-tip ureteral catheter
Whitaker
    W. hook
    W. perfusion pressure
    W. pressure-perfusion test
white
    w. anococcygeal line
    w. atrophy
    w. ball sign
    w. bile
    w. blood cell (WBC)
    w. blood cell blast
    w. blood cell cast
    w. blood cell count
    w. blood count differential
    w. diarrhea
    w. line of Toldt
    w. nipple sign
    W. operation
    w. patch
    w. thrombus
Whitehead
    W. classification
    W. deformity
    W. operation
whitish exudate
Whitmore
    W. bag
    W. classification prostate cancer
Whitmore-Jewitt prostate cancer classification system
WHO
    World Health Organization
    WHO gastric carcinoma
    classification
whole
    w. blood
    w. blood clearance and blood-water
    clearance

w. crypt mitotic count
w. gut transit
whole-blood trough level
whole-body cooling
whole-cell oxygen consumption
whole-grain
rye w.-g. (RWG)
whole-gut
w.-g. irrigation
w.-g. lavage solution
w.-g. transit scintigraphy (WGTS)
whole-kidney fractional excretion
WHVP
wedged hepatic venous pressure
Wickham
W. retractor
W. technique
wide
w. albumin gradient ascites
w. elliptical anastomosis
w. pubic diastasis
wide-angled loupe
wide-lumen stapled anastomosis
wide-mouth sac
widening
mediastinal w.
width
red cell distribution w. (RDW)
Wiedemann-Beckwith syndrome
Wilkie disease
Wilkins-Chalgren agar
Wilkinson abdominal retractor
Willauer thoracic scissors
Williams
W. intestinal forceps
W. needle
W. overtube sleeve
W. syndrome
W. varix injection overtube
W. vulvovaginoplasty
Willis
antrum of W.
W. pancreas
W. pouch
Willscher
W. catheter
W. tube
Wilms
W. tumor
W. tumor angiography
W. tumor capsule invasion

W. tumor clear cell sarcoma
variant
W. tumorlet
W. tumor multilocular cyst variant
W. tumor recurrence
W. tumor rhabdomyosarcoma
variant
W. tumor tubuloglomerular pattern
Wilpowr
Wilson
W. disease (WD)
W. muscle
Wilson-Cook
W.-C. dilating balloon
W.-C. double-channel
sphincterotome
W.-C. endoprosthesis
W.-C. esophageal balloon
W.-C. feeding tube kit
W.-C. fine-needle-aspiration catheter
W.-C. French stent
W.-C. gastric balloon
W.-C. ligator (4, 6, 10 band)
W.-C. mechanical lithotriptor
W.-C. (modified) wire-guided
sphincterotome
W.-C. nasobiliary tube
W.-C. NJFT-series feeding tube
W.-C. papillotome
W.-C. plastic prosthesis
W.-C. prosthesis introducer
W.-C. Protector guidewire
W.-C. Quantum TTC esophageal
balloon dilatation catheter
W.-C. 6-shooter
W.-C. 10-shooter
W.-C. THSF-series guidewire
W.-C. Tracer guidewire
Wilson disease (WD)
Wiltek papillotome
Winckler test
wind colic
window
w. of Deaver
gastric w.
mesenteric w.
peritoneal w.
zinc selenide w.
windowed esophageal balloon
wind-sock appearance

W

NOTES

winged
  w. catheter
  w. steel needle
wink
  anal w.
  w. reflex
Winslow
  foramen of W.
  W. pancreas
winter
  w. acidosis
  w. gastroenteritis
  W. procedure
  W. shunt
  W. shunt for priapism
  w. vomiting
wire (*See also* guidewire)
  bypass w.
  cesium-137 w.
  Cope w.
  cutting w.
  diathermy w.
  w. electrode
  Extra Stiff Amplatz w.
  glide w.
  hydrophilic w.
  ^{192}Ir w.
  J w.
  lead w.
  w. loop connector
  memory w.
  monofilament snare w.
  needle-knife w.
  nitinol w.
  Pathfinder w.
  protector plus w.
  Roadrunner w.
  safety w.
  w. snare
  stiffening w.
  torque w.
  Tracer ST w.
  trip w.
  ultrastiff w.
wire-guided
  w.-g. balloon-assisted endoscopic
    biliary stent exchange
  w.-g. cytology
  w.-g. hydrostatic balloon
  w.-g. J-tube
  w.-g. metal spiral retrieval device
  w.-g. placement
  w.-g. polyvinyl bougie
  w.-g. sphincterotome
wireless capsule endoscopy
wire-loop lesion
Wire-Wrap

wiring
  jaw w.
Wirsung
  canal of W.
  W. dilation
  duct of W.
  W. sphincter
Wirthlin splenorenal clamp
Wisconsin solution
Wishbone Omni-Track retractor
Wiskott-Aldrich syndrome
WIT
  water-induced thermotherapy
withdrawal
  steroid w.
Witzel
  W. closure
  W. dilator
  W. duodenostomy
  W. enterostomy
  W. enterostomy catheter
  W. feeding jejunostomy tunnel
  W. gastrostomy
  W. jejunostomy
Witz test
Woldman test
Wolf
  W. aspiration/injection system
  W. delivery system
  W. lithotrite
  W. percutaneous universal
    nephroscope
  W. Piezolith 2300 lithotripsy
    device
  W. Piezolith 2300 lithotriptor
  W. resectoscope
  W. rigid panendoscope
  W. Sonolith lithotriptor
  W. ureteroscope
Wolfe miniscope
Wolff
  duct of W.
  W. syringe
  W. telescope
wolffi
  corpus w.
  ductus w.
wolffian
  w. duct
  w. ductal system
Wolff-Junghans test
Wolf-Henning gastroscope
Wolf-Knittlingen gastroscope
Wolfram syndrome
Wolf-Schindler semiflexible gastroscope
Wolfson
  W. gallbladder retractor
  W. intestinal clamp

Wolinella
Wolman
W. disease
W. xanthomatosis
Womack procedure
Wood
W. lamp
W. operation
wooden
w. belly
w. resonance
Woodward
W. esophagogastroscopy
W. esophagogastrostomy
Wookey skin tube
wool ball
Woolf
W. method
W. test
working
w. port ureteroscope
w. sheath
workload
emergency-to-elective w.
workstation
Dornier MFL 5000 urological w.
World Health Organization (WHO)
worm
bilharzial w.
bladder w.
w. colic
herring w.
kidney w.
wort
St. John's w.
wound
anal w.
w. approximation
aseptic w.
w. closure
w. dehiscence
w. drainage
w. healing
w. healing disorder
w. hematoma
w. infection
open w.
penetrating w.
renal stab w.
septic w.
stab w.
submucosal w.

woven Dacron tube
W-pouch configuration
wrap
antireflux w.
double gracilis w.
floppy Nissen fundic w.
gamma split-sling w.
gastric fundus w.
Kerlix w.
Nissen fundoplication w.
rectus fascial w.
single gamma w.
slipped fundoplication w.
total gastric w.
tunica vaginalis blanket w.
wrapping
fat w.
omental w.
Wright
W. stain
W. stain of stool
Wright-Giemsa stain
writer
laser w.
WS
watermelon stomach
W-shaped
W-s. forceps
W-s. ileal pouch-anal anastomosis
W-s. pouch
W-stapled
W-s. ileal neobladder
W-s. urinary reservoir
wt
weight
mol wt
molecular weight
WTI gene
Wuchereria bancrofti
Wurbs-type nasobiliary tube
Wyamine
Wyamycin
W. E
W. S
Wyanoids Relief Factor
Wylie
W. hypogastric clamp
W. splanchnic retractor
Wymox

W

NOTES

Xanax
xanthelasma
xanthic calculus
xanthine
    x. calculus
    x. oxidase
    x. oxidation
    x. urinary lithiasis
xanthinuria
xanthogranuloma
    juvenile x.
xanthogranulomatous
    x. cholecystitis
    x. cystitis
    x. pyelonephritis (XGP)
xanthoma
    bladder x.
    x. cell
    gastric x.
    planar x.
    skin x.
    tendon x.
    verruciform x.
xanthomatosis
    biliary hypercholesterolemia x.
    cerebrotendinous x.
    familial hypercholesteremic x.
    Wolman x.
Xanthomonas maltophilia
XC
    excretory cystogram
Xc
    reactance
X chromosome
Xc/R
    reactance and resistance
    Xc/R ratio
Xenical
xenoantigen
xenobiotic
    x. absorption
    x. glutathione conjugate
    x. pump
xenograft
    x. rejection
    x. transplantation
xenon
    x. lamp
    x. light source
xenon-washout technique
xenopi
    Mycobacterium x.
xenoreactive antibody
xenotransplantation
Xeroform gauze

xerophthalmia
xerostomia
xerotica
    balanitis x.
XGIF-MR30
    nonferromagnetic MR
      endoscope X.-M.
XGP
    xanthogranulomatous pyelonephritis
Xillix LIFE-Lung system
xiphisternum
xiphoid appendix
xiphoid-to-pubis midline abdominal
  incision
xiphoid-to-umbilicus incision
XL
    Ditropan XL
    Procardia XL
XL1-Blue cell
XLAS
    X-linked Alport syndrome
XLH
    X-linked hypophosphatemia
X-linked
    X-l. Alport syndrome (XLAS)
    X-l. hypophosphatemia (XLH)
    X-l. infantile agammaglobulinemia
    X-l. recessive NDI
    X-l. recessive nephrolithiasis (XRN)
    X-l. recessive trait
Xpeedior catheter
X-Prep
    X-P. bowel preparation
    Senokot X-P.
XQ230 Olympus gastroscope
XQ video instrument
XR
    Pyridorin XR
x-ray
    x.-r. analysis
    x.-r. beam
    x.-r. crystallography
    x.-r. diffractometry
    x.-r. photoelectron spectroscopy
XRN
    X-linked recessive nephrolithiasis
XU
    excretory urogram
XX
    XX male mosaicism
    XX male syndrome
xylene
Xylocaine
    X. jelly

X

Xylocaine *(continued)*
    topical X.
    X. topical anesthetic
xylometazoline

xylose
    x. absorption test
    x. tolerance test
XYY male syndrome

Y
Y adapter
Y chromosome
YAG
yttrium-aluminum-garnet
YAG 1064
YAG laser
Laserscope YAG 1064
YAG laser therapy
Yang
Y. needle
Y. polyclonal assay
Y. Pros-Check PSA assay
Y. Pros-Check PSA test
Y. PSA radioimmunoassay
Yang-Monti ileovesicostomy
Yangtze Valley fever
Yankauer
Y. esophagoscope
Y. suction tube
yarn-collected specimen
Yates correction
Y-connecting tubing
90Y-CYT-356
yeast
y. balanitis
y. overgrowth
y. saccharomyces
y. strain mannan
urinalysis sediment microscopy y.
urinary sediment y.
yeast-recombinant hepatitis B vaccine
Yellolax
yellow
y. atrophy of the liver
y. nodule
y. phosphorus hepatotoxicity
Yeoman rectal biopsy forceps
Yeoman-Wittner rectal forceps
Yersinia
Y. enteritis
Y. enterocolitica
Y. enterocolitica colitis
Y. frederiksenii
Y. intermedia
Y. kristensenii
Y. pestis
Y. pseudotuberculosis
yersiniosis
yield
sperm y.
Yocon
yogurt
Trial Using Medicinal
Microbiotic Y. (TUMMY)

yohimbine hydrochloride
Yohimex
yokogawai
Metagonimus y.
yolk
y. sac
y. sac carcinoma
y. sac tumor
York-Mason procedure
Yoshi-864
Young
Y. cystoscope
Y. enucleator
Y. epispadias repair
Y. intestinal forceps
Y. needle holder
Y. operation
Y. prostatic retractor
Y. prostatic tractor
Y. syndrome
Y. technique
young
maturity-onset diabetes of the y.
(MODY)
Young-Dees
Y.-D. bladder neck reconstruction
Y.-D. operation
Y.-D. procedure
Y.-D. technique
Y.-D. tube
Young-Dees-Leadbetter
Y.-D.-L. bladder neck
reconstruction
Y.-D.-L. operation
Youssef syndrome
yo-yo weight fluctuation phenomenon
Y-plasty
Foley Y-p.
Schweizer-Foley Y-p.
Y-port connector
Y-set system
Y-shaped incision
yttrium-90
yttrium-aluminum-garnet (YAG)
Y-type Dianeal peritoneal dialysis solution
Yu-Holtgrewe prostatic retractor
Y-V
Y-V anoplasty
Y-V meatotomy
Y-V plasty
Y-V sliding skin graft
YY
beta-endorphin peptide YY
peptide YY (PYY)

Y

Z

Z line
Z stent
Z suture
Z tract
Zachary Cope-DeMartel clamp
zacopride
Zacutex
Zadaxin
zafirlukast
Zahn

anomaly of Z.
Z. infarct
zalcitabine
Zamboni fixative
Zanca syndrome
Zanosar
zanoterone
Zantac

Z. EITERdose
Z. GELdose
Zappacosta test
Zaroxolyn
Za-Stent endoscopic biliary stent
ZCE 025 antibody
ZE

Zollinger-Ellison
ZE Caps
ZE syndrome
Zebra exchange guidewire
Zebrax
Zefazone
Zeiss

Z. IDO3 phase-contrast microscope
Z. morphomate M30
Z. S9 electron microscope
Zellweger syndrome
Zelmac
Zenapax
Zenith

Z. AAA endovascular graft system
Z. abdominal aortic aneurysm
endovascular graft system
Zenker

Z. diverticulum
Z. leiomyoma
Z. pouch
Zeppelin clamp
ZES

Zollinger-Ellison syndrome
Zestril
Zeta probe nylon filter
zidovudine
Ziehl-Neelsen stain

Zieve

Z. syndrome
Z. system
zileuton
Zimmon

Z. biliary stent
Z. papillotome/sphincterotome
zinc

z. colic
z. deficiency
z. finger
z. selenide window
zinc-requiring enzyme
zipper

leucine z.
Zipser penile clamp
Zixoryn
Z-line
Z-Med catheter
Zn-alpha-2-glycoprotein

seminal plasma Z.-g.
Zocor
Zoladex implant
Zolicef
Zollinger-Ellison (ZE)

Z.-E. syndrome (ZES)
Z.-E. tumor
zomepirac
zona

z. fasciculata
z. glomerulosa
z. hamster egg test
z. occludens
z. pellucida (ZP)
z. reticularis
zonal gastritis
zone

abdominal z.
adrenal cortex z.
anal transitional z. (ATZ)
border z.
calcified z.
cooled antenna z.
Daseler z.
electric z.
epigastric z.
hemorrhoidal z.
high-pressure z. (HPZ)
hyperemic border z.
hypogastric papillary z.
nephrogenic z.
peripheral z.
portal z.
prostate gland peripheral z.
prostate gland periurethral z.

Z

zone *(continued)*
    prostate gland transition z.
    prostate-specific antigen density of
      the transition z. (PSA-TZ)
    rugae z.
    transformation z.
    transitional z.
    Türck z.
zonulae occludens
zoom videoendoscopy
Zoon
    balanitis of Z.
    Z. erythroplasia
zoospermia
zoster
    herpes z.
Zovirax
ZP
  zona pellucida
Z-plasty anastomosis
Z-stent
    Z-s. esophageal endoprosthesis
     system
    Gianturco Z-s.

    Gianturco-Rosch biliary Z-s.
    modified Z-s.
Z-stitch
Z-test
Z-type deformity
Zuckerkandl
    organ of Z.
Zugsmith sign
Zyderm
Zygomycetes
zygomycosis
zygote
Zyloprim
Zymase
zymogen
    z. granule
    lab z.
zymogenic cell
zymosan
    opsonized z.
zymosis gastrica
Zypan
ZZ phenotype

Appendix 1
Anatomical Illustrations

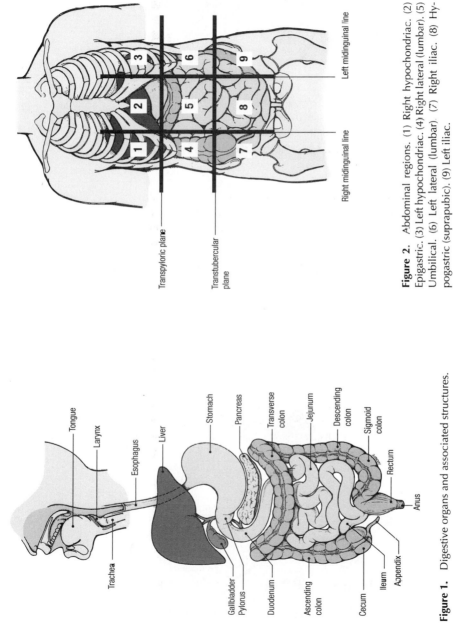

Figure 2. Abdominal regions. (1) Right hypochondriac. (2) Epigastric. (3) Left hypochondriac. (4) Right lateral (lumbar). (5) Umbilical. (6) Left lateral (lumbar). (7) Right iliac. (8) Hypogastric (suprapubic). (9) Left iliac.

Figure 1. Digestive organs and associated structures.

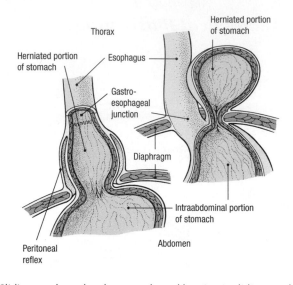

Figure 3. Sliding esophageal and paraesophageal hernias. In sliding esophageal hernias (left), the upper stomach and cardioesophageal junction slide in and out of the thorax; in paraesophageal hernias (right), all or part of the stomach pushes through diaphragm next to gastroesophageal junction. This image, created by Michael Schenk for *Stedman's Medical Dictionary, 27th Edition,* Baltimore, Lippincott Williams & Wilkins, 2000, p. 812, appears here with permission and courtesy of Lippincott Williams & Wilkins.

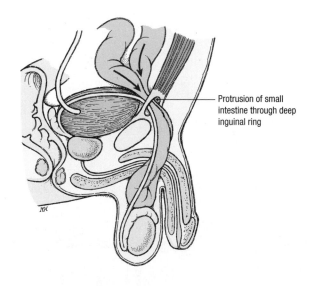

Figure 4. Indirect inguinal hernia.

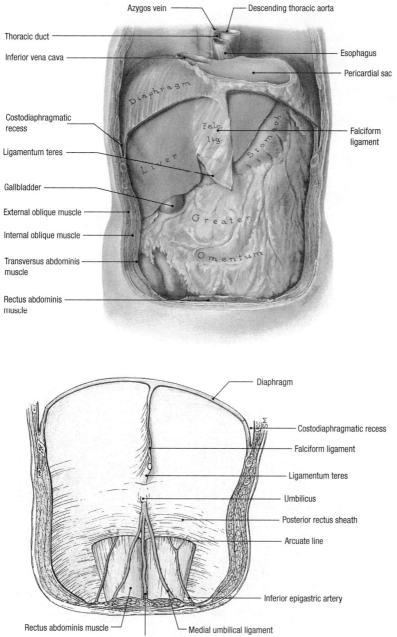

Azygos vein
Descending thoracic aorta
Thoracic duct
Esophagus
Inferior vena cava
Pericardial sac
Diaphragm
Costodiaphragmatic recess
Falc. lig.
Stomach
Falciform ligament
Ligamentum teres
Liver
Gallblader
External oblique muscle
Greater
Internal oblique muscle
Omentum
Transversus abdominis muscle
Rectus abdominis muscle

Diaphragm
Costodiaphragmatic recess
Falciform ligament
Ligamentum teres
Umbilicus
Posterior rectus sheath
Arcuate line
Inferior epigastric artery
Rectus abdominis muscle
Medial umbilical ligament
Median umbilical ligament

Figure 5. Abdominal contents, undisturbed, anterior view (top). Posterior aspect of anterior abdominal wall, cut from top (bottom).

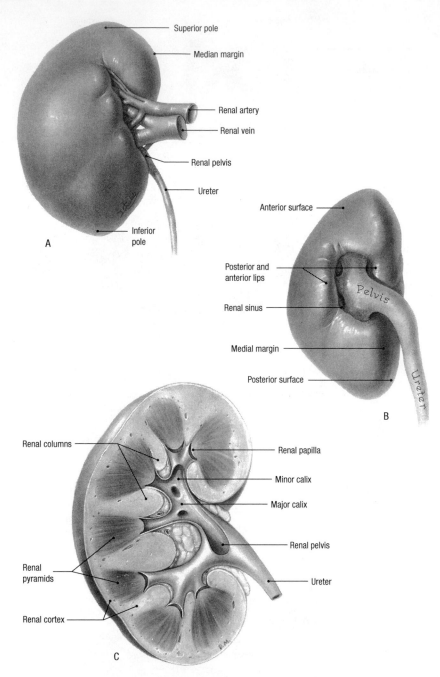

Figure 6. Kidney. (A) Right kidney, anterior view. (B) Sinus of kidney, anteromedial view. (C) Kidney, coronal view.

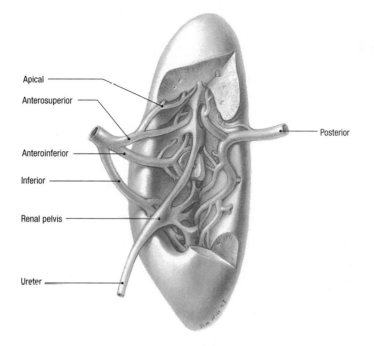

Apical

Anterosuperior

Posterior

Anteroinferior

Inferior

Renal pelvis

Ureter

Figure 7. Branches of renal artery within renal sinus, medial view.

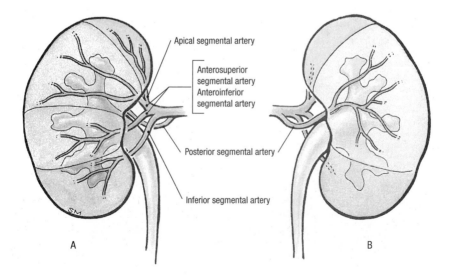

Apical segmental artery

Anterosuperior
segmental artery
Anteroinferior
segmental artery

Posterior segmental artery

Inferior segmental artery

A

B

Figure 8. Segmental arteries. (A) Anterior View, (B) Posterior view.

A5

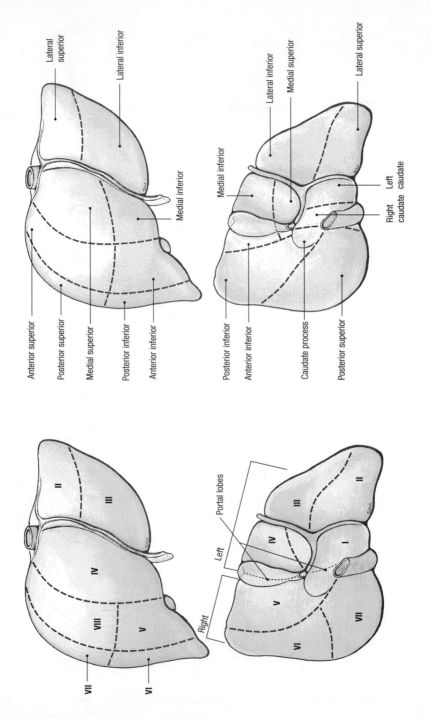

Figure 9. Segments of liver. Each of the lobes is divided into segments that can be numerically identified, as shown (left).

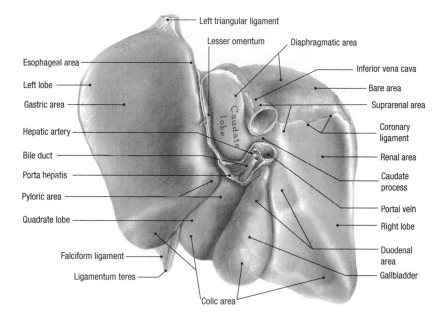

Left triangular ligament

Lesser omentum   Diaphragmatic area

Esophageal area

Left lobe

Gastric area

Hepatic artery

Bile duct

Porta hepatis

Pyloric area

Quadrate lobe

Falciform ligament

Ligamentum teres

Colic area

Inferior vena cava

Bare area

Suprarenal area

Coronary ligament

Renal area

Caudate process

Portal vein

Right lobe

Duodenal area

Gallbladder

Figure 10.   Inferior and posterior surfaces of liver.

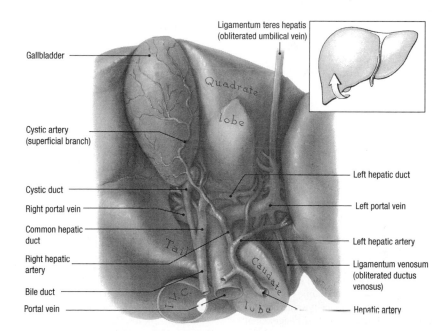

Ligamentum teres hepatis (obliterated umbilical vein)

Gallbladder

Cystic artery (superficial branch)

Cystic duct

Right portal vein

Common hepatic duct

Right hepatic artery

Bile duct

Portal vein

Left hepatic duct

Left portal vein

Left hepatic artery

Ligamentum venosum (obliterated ductus venosus)

Hepatic artery

Figure 11.   Porta hepatis and cystic artery, posterior view.

A7

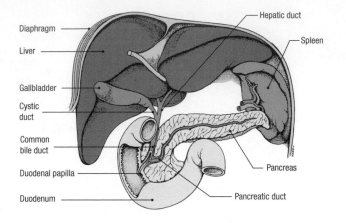

Figure 12. Gallbladder, liver, and biliary system.

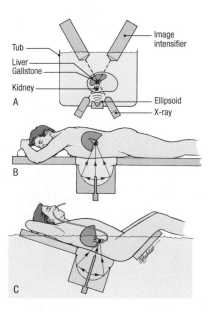

Figure 13. Extracorporeal shock wave lithotripsy. (A) Gallbladder stone is localized by imaging; shock waves are generated in ellipsoid reflector and transmitted through water to stone. (B) Positioning of patient for treatment of stones located in gallbladder; fluid-filled bag is recessed in table and transmits shock wave from generator to patient's skin. (C) Positioning of patient for treatment of stones located in common bile duct; the patient is partially submerged in a water bath; nasobiliary tube is used to introduce contrast material to permit visualization and localization of stone and to decompress biliary tree. This image, created by Mikki Senkarik for *Stedman's Medical Dictionary, 27th Edition,* Baltimore, Lippincott Williams & Wilkins, 2000, p. 1025, appears here with permission and courtesy of Lippincott Williams & Wilkins.

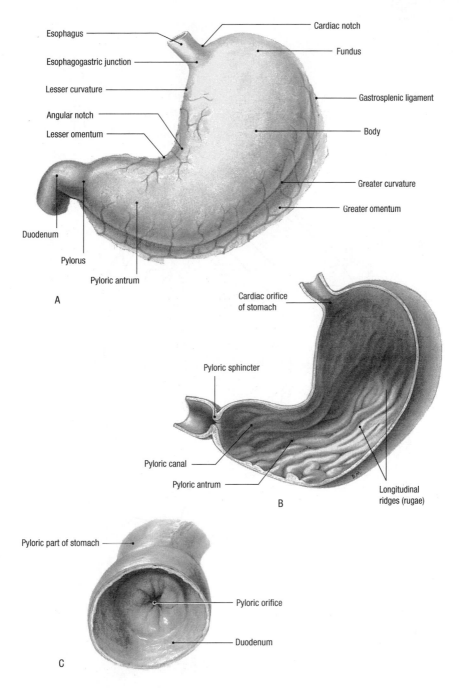

Figure 14. Stomach. (A) External surface, anterior view. (B) Internal surface (mucous membrane), anterior wall removed. (C) Pylorus, viewed from the duodenum.

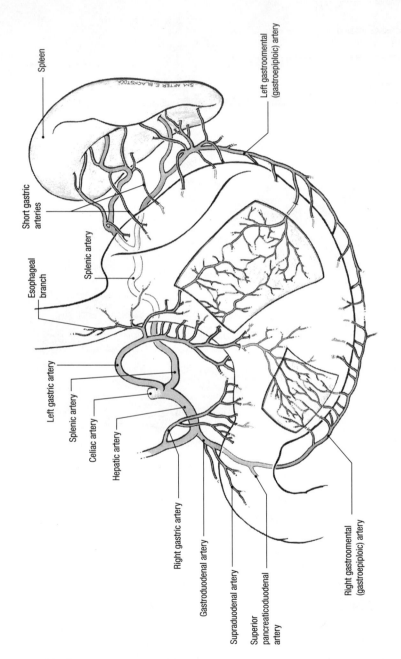

Figure 15. Arteries of stomach and spleen, anterior view.

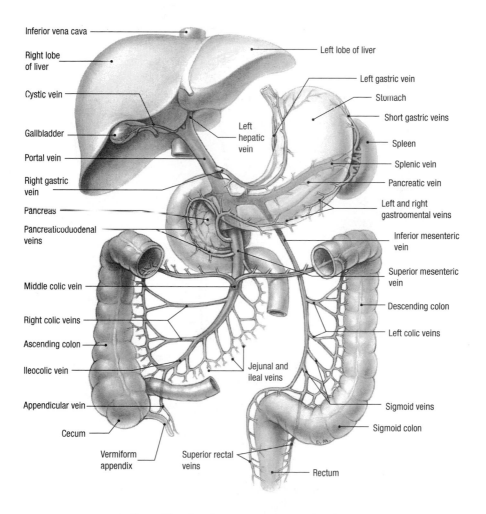

Inferior vena cava

Right lobe of liver

Cystic vein

Gallbladder

Portal vein

Right gastric vein

Pancreas

Pancreaticoduodenal veins

Middle colic vein

Right colic veins

Ascending colon

Ileocolic vein

Appendicular vein

Cecum

Vermiform appendix

Left hepatic vein

Left lobe of liver

Left gastric vein

Stomach

Short gastric veins

Spleen

Splenic vein

Pancreatic vein

Left and right gastroomental veins

Inferior mesenteric vein

Superior mesenteric vein

Descending colon

Left colic veins

Jejunal and ileal veins

Sigmoid veins

Sigmoid colon

Superior rectal veins

Rectum

Figure 16. Portal venous system, anterior view.

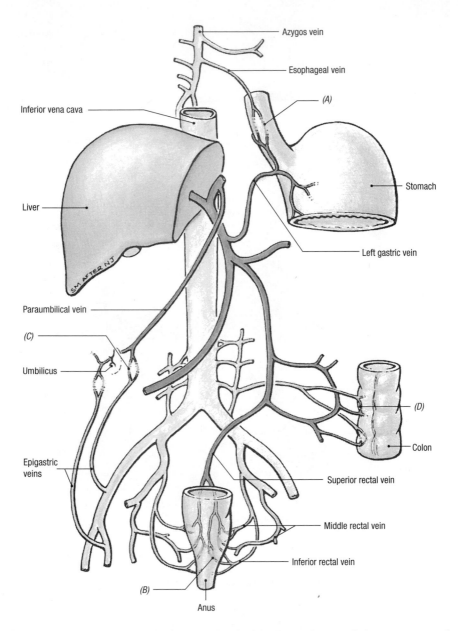

Azygos vein

Esophageal vein

(A)

Inferior vena cava

Stomach

Liver

Left gastric vein

Paraumbilical vein

(C)

Umbilicus

(D)

Colon

Epigastric
veins

Superior rectal vein

Middle rectal vein

Inferior rectal vein

(B)

Anus

Figure 17. Portacaval system, anterior view. Portal tributaries are shown in dark gray; systemic tributaries and communicating veins are shown in light gray. Sites of anastomosis (A, B, C, and D).

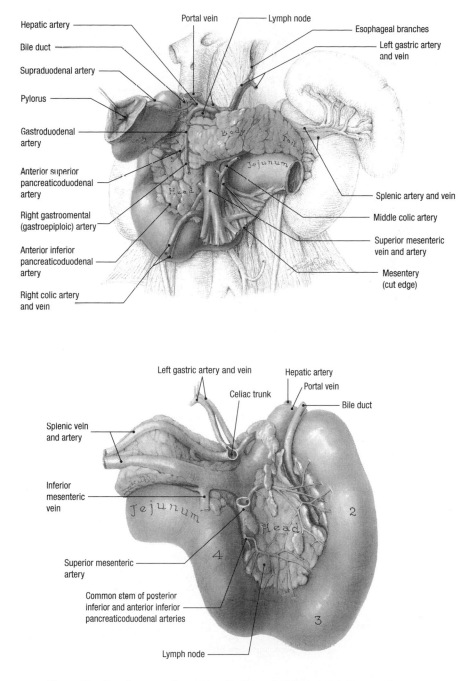

Hepatic artery

Bile duct

Supraduodenal artery

Pylorus

Gastroduodenal artery

Anterior superior pancreaticoduodenal artery

Right gastroomental (gastroepiploic) artery

Anterior inferior pancreaticoduodenal artery

Right colic artery and vein

Portal vein

Lymph node

Esophageal branches

Left gastric artery and vein

Splenic artery and vein

Middle colic artery

Superior mesenteric vein and artery

Mesentery (cut edge)

Left gastric artery and vein

Celiac trunk

Hepatic artery

Portal vein

Bile duct

Splenic vein and artery

Inferior mesenteric vein

Superior mesenteric artery

Common stem of posterior inferior and anterior inferior pancreaticoduodenal arteries

Lymph node

Figure 18. Duodenum and pancreas. Anterior view (top). Posterior view (bottom).

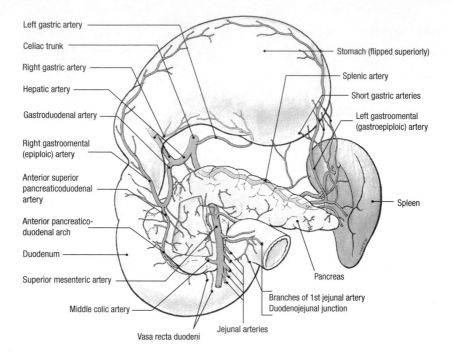

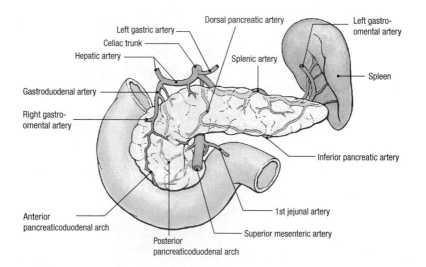

Figure 19. Blood supply to the pancreas, duodenum, and spleen, anterior views. Celiac trunk and superior mesenteric artery (top). Pancreatic and pancreaticoduodenal arteries (bottom).

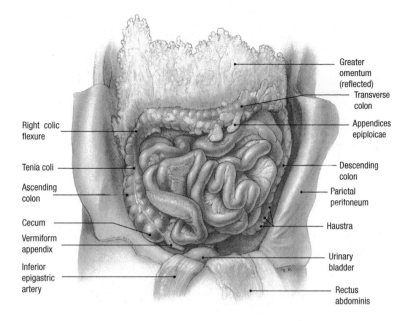

Greater
omentum
(reflected)

Transverse
colon

Right colic
flexure

Appendices
epiploicae

Tenia coli

Descending
colon

Ascending
colon

Parietal
peritoneum

Cecum

Haustra

Vermiform
appendix

Urinary
bladder

Inferior
epigastric
artery

Rectus
abdominis

Figure 20. Small and large intestine. Greater omentum reflected, anterior views.

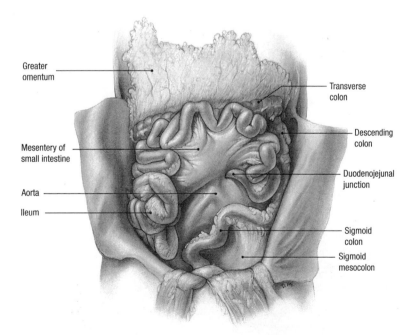

Greater
omentum

Transverse
colon

Descending
colon

Mesentery of
small intestine

Duodenojejunal
junction

Aorta

Ileum

Sigmoid
colon

Sigmoid
mesocolon

Figure 21. Descending and sigmoid colon and mesentery of small intestine.

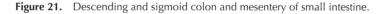

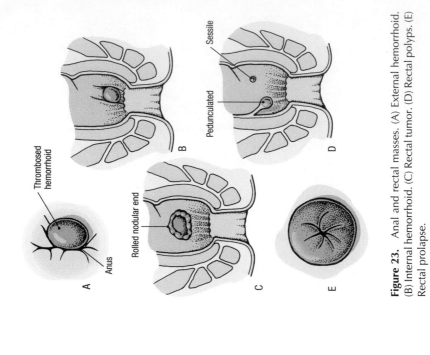

Figure 23. Anal and rectal masses. (A) External hemorrhoid. (B) Internal hemorrhoid. (C) Rectal tumor. (D) Rectal polyps. (E) Rectal prolapse.

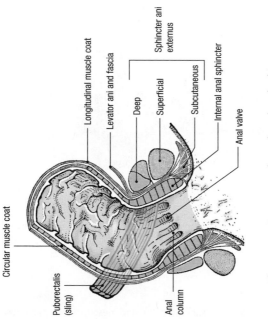

Figure 22. Rectum, anal canal, and anal sphincter.

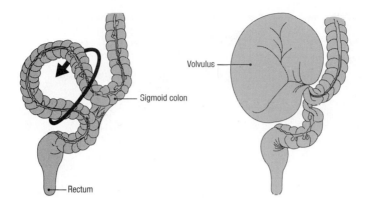

Figure 24. Volvulus of sigmoid colon. The unattached loop of bowel twists (left image), causing the bowel lumen to become obstructed (right image), which leads to the inability of stool to pass and compression of the blood supply to the looped bowel segment.

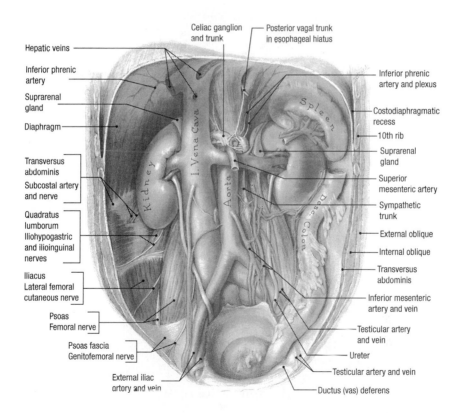

Figure 25. Viscera and vessels of posterior abdominal wall. Great vessels, kidneys, and suprarenal glands, anterior view.

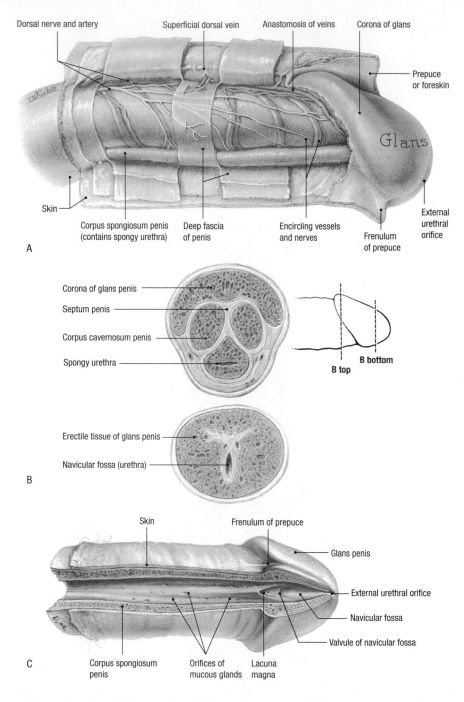

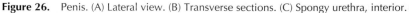

Figure 26. Penis. (A) Lateral view. (B) Transverse sections. (C) Spongy urethra, interior.

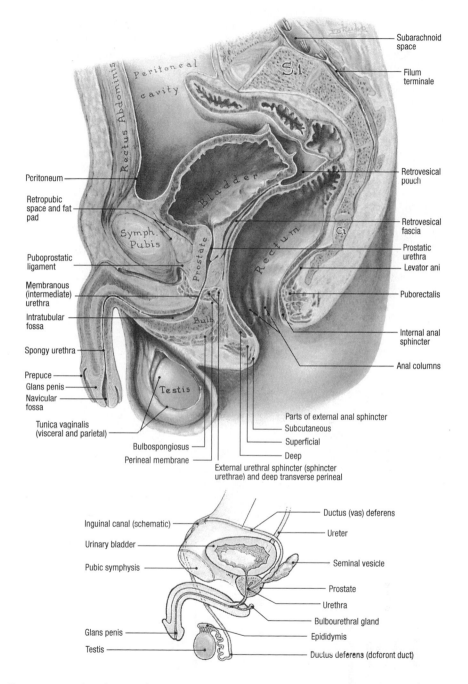

Figure 27. Male pelvis. Median section (top). Overview of urogenital system, median section (bottom).

A19

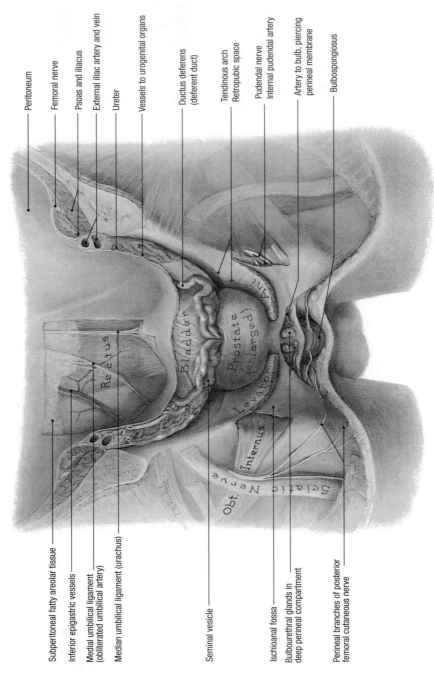

Peritoneum

Femoral nerve

Psoas and iliacus

External iliac artery and vein

Ureter

Vessels to urogenital organs

Ductus deferens
(deferent duct)

Tendinous arch

Retropubic space

Pudendal nerve

Internal pudendal artery

Artery to bulb, piercing
perineal membrane

Bulbospongiosus

Rectus

Bladder

Ant.

Prostate
(enlarged)

Levator

Internus

Obt.

Sciatic Nerve

Subperitoneal fatty areolar tissue

Inferior epigastric vessels

Medial umbilical ligament
(obliterated umbilical artery)

Median umbilical ligament (urachus)

Seminal vesicle

Ischioanal fossa

Bulbourethral glands in
deep perineal compartment

Perineal branches of posterior
femoral cutaneous nerve

Figure 28. Male pelvis, view of anterior portion from behind.

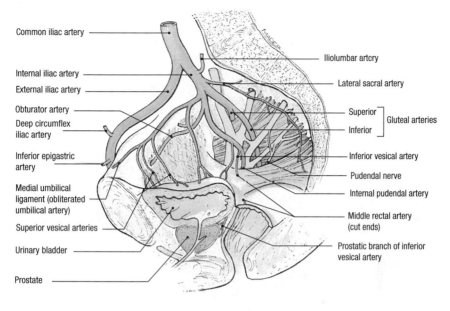

Common iliac artery

Internal iliac artery

External iliac artery

Obturator artery

Deep circumflex iliac artery

Inferior epigastric artery

Medial umbilical ligament (obliterated umbilical artery)

Superior vesical arteries

Urinary bladder

Prostate

Iliolumbar artery

Lateral sacral artery

Superior ⎤
         ⎦ Gluteal arteries
Inferior

Inferior vesical artery

Pudendal nerve

Internal pudendal artery

Middle rectal artery (cut ends)

Prostatic branch of inferior vesical artery

Figure 29. Arteries of the pelvis. Male pelvis, median section.

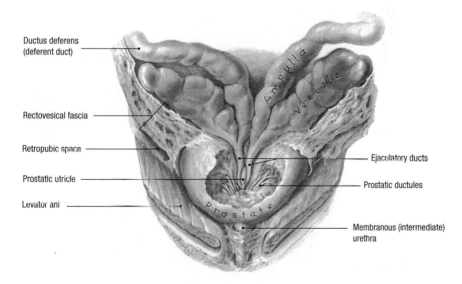

Ductus deferens (deferent duct)

Rectovesical fascia

Retropubic space

Prostatic utricle

Levator ani

Ejaculatory ducts

Prostatic ductules

Membranous (intermediate) urethra

Figure 30. Prostate, posterior view.

A21

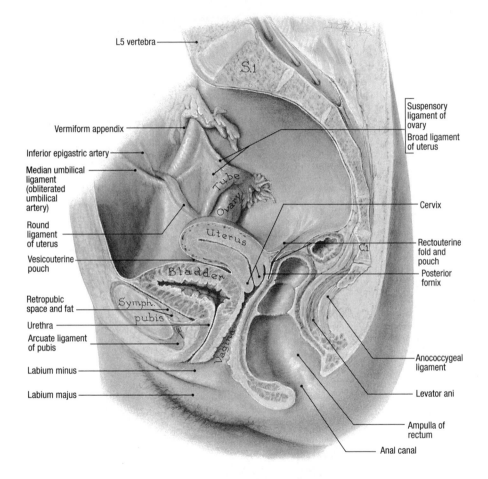

Figure 31. Female pelvis, median section.

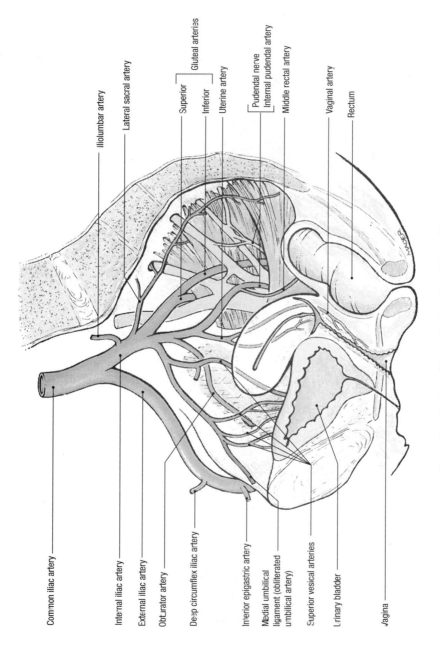

Figure 32. Arteries of the pelvis. Female pelvis, median section.

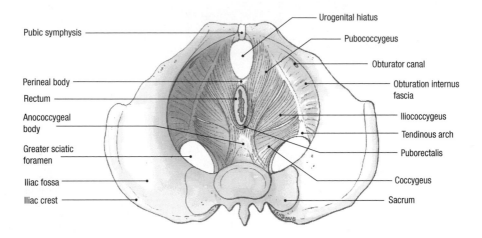

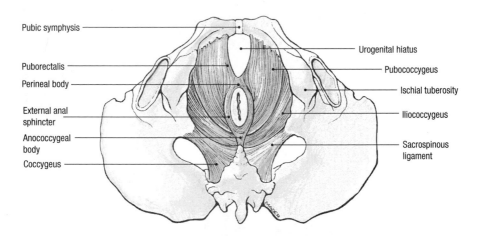

Figure 33. Muscles of pelvic walls and floors. Superior view (top) and inferior view (bottom).

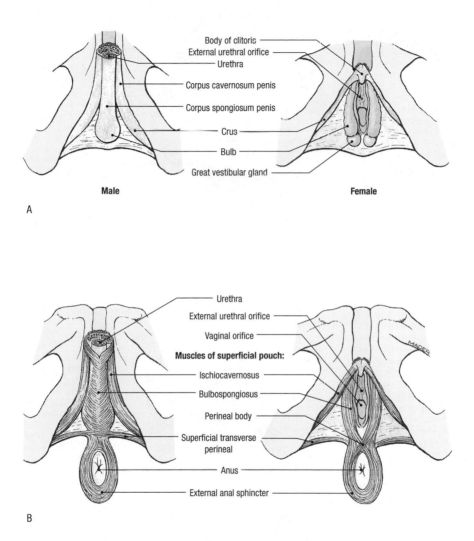

Figure 34. Male and female perineum, inferior views. (A) Crura and bulb of penis and clitoris. (B) Muscles of superficial perineal compartment.

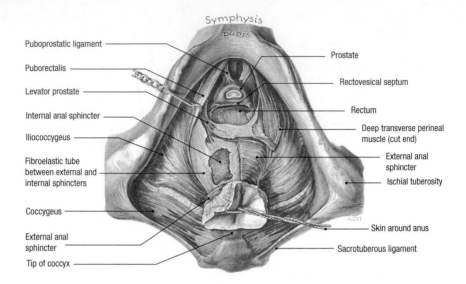

Figure 35. Dissection of male perineum. Levator ani and coccygeus muscles, and exposure of prostate, inferior view.

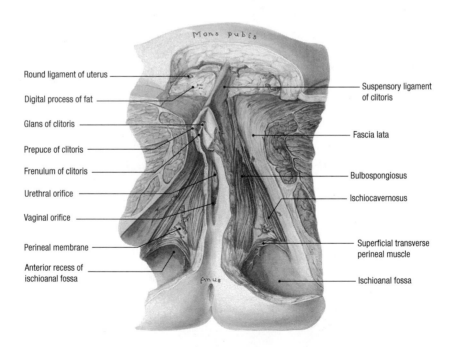

Figure 36. Female perineum, inferior view.

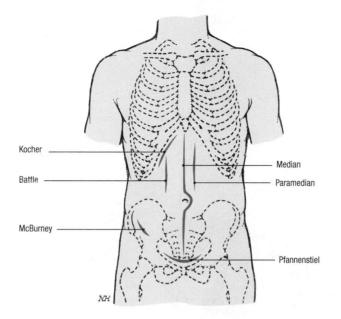
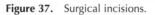

Kocher

Battle

McBurney

Median

Paramedian

Pfannenstiel

Figure 37. Surgical incisions.

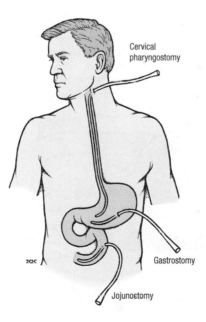

Cervical
pharyngostomy

Gastrostomy

Jojunostomy

Figure 38. Enterostomy tubes. Flexible tubes passing through surgical openings into selected portions of gastrointestinal tract, providing access for liquid food.

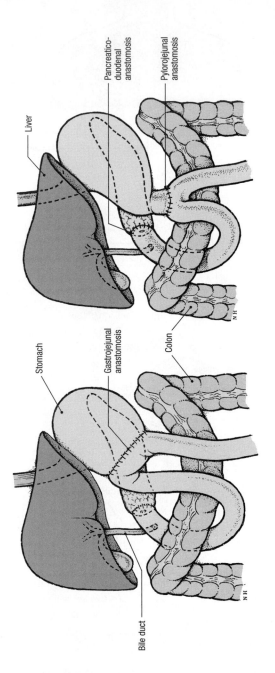

Figure 39. Pancreatoduodenectomy. Excision of all or part of the pancreas together with the duodenum and usually the distal stomach. Whipple operation (left). Pylorus-saving Whipple procedure (right).

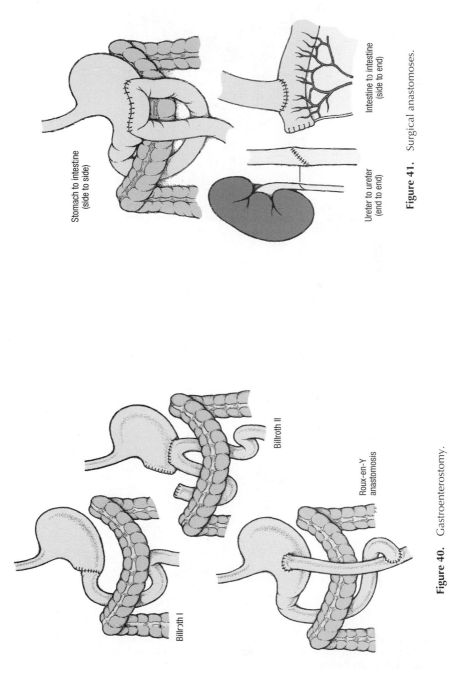

Stomach to intestine (side to side)

Intestine to intestine (side to end)

Ureter to ureter (end to end)

Figure 41. Surgical anastomoses.

Billroth I

Billroth II

Roux-en-Y anastomosis

Figure 40. Gastroenterostomy.

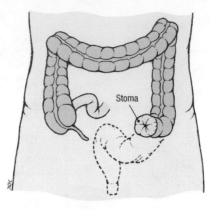

Figure 42. Colostomy. Stoma opens on anterior abdominal wall.

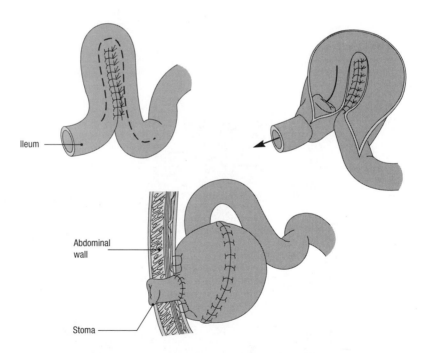

Figure 43. Three-part illustration showing section of intestine undergoing procedure for creating a continent ileostomy. Bowel segment anastomosed (top). Pouch is formed (center.) Pouch shown in place with stoma (bottom).

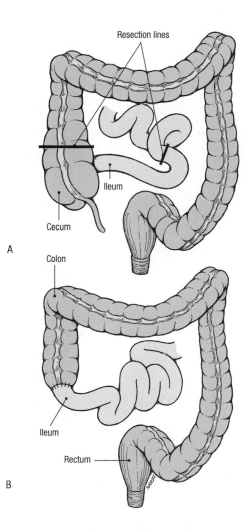

Resection lines

Ileum

Cecum

A

Colon

Ileum

Rectum

B

Figure 44. Ileocolostomy. (A) Diseased portion of ileum and cecum resected. (B) Resected ends anastomosed.

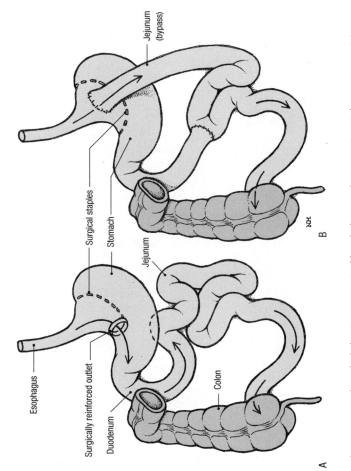

Figure 45. Surgical procedures to control morbid obesity. (A) Vertical banded gastroplasty. (B) Gastric bypass (gastrojejunostomy). In both procedures, the reduction in gastric capacity leads to early satiety and, thus, favors consumption of smaller meals.

Normal Lab Values

Tests	Conventional Units	SI Units
*bilirubin		
serum		
adult		
conjugated	0.0–0.3 mg/dL	0–5 μmol/L
unconjugated	0.1–1.1 mg/dL	1.7–19 μmol/L
delta	0–0.2 mg/dL	0–3 μmol/L
total	0.2–1.3 mg/L	3–22 μmol/L
neonates		
conjugated	0–0.6 mg/dL	0–10 μmol/L
unconjugated	0.6–10.5 mg/dL	10–180 μmol/L
total	1.5–12 mg/dL	1.7–180 μmol/L
urine, qualitative	negative	negative
calcium, urine		
low calcium diet	50–150 mg/24 h	1.25–3.75 mmol/24 h
usual diet; trough	100–300 mg/24 h	2.50–7.50 mmol/24 h
catecholamines, urine		
dopamine	65–400 μg/24 h	425–2610 nmol/24 h
epinephrine	0–20 μg/24 h	0–109 nmol/24 h
norepinephrine	15–80 μg/24 h	89–473 nmol/24 h
*creatinine clearance, serum		
or plasma and urine		
male	94–140 mL/min/1.73 m^2	0.91–1.35 mL/s/m^2
female	72–110 mL/min/1.73 m^2	0.69–1.06 mL/s/m^2
cyclic AMP		
plasma (EDTA)		
male	4.6–8.6 ng/mL	14–26 nmol/L
female	4.3–7.6 ng/mL	13–23 nmol/L
urine, 24 h	0.3–3.6 mg/d or 0.29–2.1 mg/g creatinine	100–723 μmol/d or 100–723 μmol/mol creatinine
cystine or cysteine, urine, qualitative	negative	negative
phosphorus, urine	0.4–1.3 g/24 h	12.9–42 mmol/24 h
porphobilinogen, urine		
qualitative	negative	negative
quantitative	<2.0 mg/24 h	<9 μmol/24 h
porphyrins, urine		
coproporphyrin	34–230 μg/24 h	52–351 nmol/ 24 h
uroporphyrin	27–52 μg/24 h	32–63 nmol/ 24 h
potassium		
urine, 24 h	25–125 mmol/d; varies with diet	25–125 mmol/d; varies with diet

continued

Tests	Conventional Units	SI Units
*prostate-specific antigen (PSA), serum		
male	<4.0 ng/mL	<4.0 µg/L
*protein, serum		
total	6.4–8.3 g/dL	64–83 g/L
albumin	3.9–5.1 g/dL	39–51 g/L
globulin		
α_1	0.2–0.4 g/dL	2–4 g/L
α_2	0.4–0.8 g/dL	4–8 g/L
β	0.5–1.0 g/dL	5–10 g/L
γ	0.6–1.3 g/dL	6–13 g/L
urine		
qualitative	negative	negative
quantitative	50–80 mg/24 h (at rest)	50–80 mg/24 h (at rest)
sodium		
urine, 24 h	40–220 mEq/d (diet dependent)	40–220 mmol/d (diet dependent)
urea nitrogen, serum	6–20 mg/dL	2.1–7.1 mmol urea/L
urea nitrogen/creatinine ratio, serum	12:1 to 20:1	48–80
urea/creatinine mole ratio		
*uric acid		
serum, enzymatic		
male	4.5–8.0 mg/dL	0.27–0.47 mmol/L
female	2.5–6.2 mg/dL	0.15–0.37 mmol/L
child	2.0–5.5 mg/dL	0.12–0.32 mmol/L
urine	250–750 mg/24 h (with normal diet)	1.48–4.43 mmol/24 h (with normal diet)
urobilinogen, urine	0.1–0.8 EU/2 h 0.5–4.0 EU/d	0.1–0.8 EU/2 h 0.5–4.0 EU/d

*Test values are method dependent.

Appendix 3
Herbs Used to Treat GI/GU Conditions

Herb	Condition
African plum	Benign prostatic hyperplasia.
alder buckthorn	See buckthorn bark.
aloe	Short-term treatment of occasional constipation.
angelica root	Loss of appetite, peptic discomforts such as mild spasms of the gastrointestinal tract, feeling of fullness, and flatulence.
artichoke leaf	Liver dysfunction, bloating, nausea, and impairment of digestion; lipid-lowering agent.
asparagus root	Irrigation therapy for inflammatory diseases of the urinary tract and for prevention of kidney stones; also used as a diuretic and laxative.
bazoton	Intravesical treatment for overactive bladder.
bilberry fruit	Nonspecific, acute diarrhea and local therapy for mild inflammation of the mucous membranes of the mouth and throat.
blessed thistle	Loss of appetite, dyspepsia, and used to increase gastric juice secretion.
boldo leaf	Mild dyspepsia and spastic gastrointestinal complaints, gallstones, liver ailments, and cystitis.
bottlebrush	See horsetail.
box holly	See butcher's broom.
brewer's yeast Hansen CBS 5926	Symptomatic treatment of acute diarrhea; prophylactic and symptomatic treatment of traveler's diarrhea; diarrhea occurring while tube feeding.
bromelain	In combination with pancreatic extracts of titrated trypsin; suggested as treatment for dyspepsia symptoms and exocrine hepatic insufficiency.
buckthorn bark	Stool softener.
butcher's broom	Itching and burning of hemorrhoids.
cascara	Constipation; stool softener.
cassia (cassia cinnamon)	See Chinese cinnamon bark.
cascara sagrada bark	See cascara.
cranberry	Treatment of urinary tract infection.
Ceylon cinnamon	See cinnamon bark.

Herb	Condition
chamomile flower	Used internally as symptomatic treatment of digestive ailments such as dyspepsia, epigastric bloating, impaired digestion, and flatulence. Used externally for irritation of the mouth and gums, and for hemorrhoids.
Chinese cinnamon bark	Loss of appetite, gastrointestinal tract spasm, bloating, flatulence, colic or dyspepsia.
chittem bark	See cascara.
cinnamon bark	Loss of appetite, dyspeptic complaints such as mild spastic conditions of the gastrointestinal tract, bloating, and flatulence.
coriander seed/fruit	Dyspeptic complaints and loss of appetite.
dandelion	Loss of appetite, dyspepsia, constipation, cholecystitis, and prevention of renal gravel.
dandelion root	Disturbances in bile flow, stimulation of diuresis, loss of appetite, and dyspepsia.
devil's claw root	Loss of appetite and dyspepsia.
Echinacea purpurea (herb and root)	Administered orally in supportive therapy for infections of the urinary tract.
fennel oil/seed	Dyspepsia, fullness, and flatulence.
fenugreek seed	Anorexia, dyspepsia, gastritis.
flaxseed/flax	Chronic constipation, colon damage from laxative abuse, irritable colon, diverticulitis; mucilage for gastritis and enteritis.
frangula	See buckthorn bark.
garlic	As an adjuvant to dietetic management in treatment of hyperlipidemia.
gentian root	Loss of appetite, fullness, and flatulence.
ginger	Prophylaxis of nausea and vomiting associated with motion sickness, postoperative nausea, and seasickness.
goldenrod/European goldenrod	Irrigation therapy for inflammatory diseases of the lower urinary tract, urinary calculi, and kidney gravel; prophylaxis for urinary calculi and kidney gravel.
holy thistle	See blessed thistle
horehound/white horehound	Loss of appetite, bloating, and flatulence.
horsetail	Inflammation of the lower urinary tract and renal gravel.
huckleberry	See bilberry fruit.
juniper berry/common juniper	Bladder and kidney conditions.

Herb	Condition
lemon balm/common balm	Gastrointestinal complaints.
licorice root	Gastric or duodenal ulcers.
linseed	See flaxseed/flax.
melissa	See lemon balm.
milk thistle fruit/St. Mary's thistle	Chronic inflammatory liver disease and hepatic cirrhosis.
mint oil	Flatulence, as well as functional gastro-intestinal and gallbladder disorders.
oak bark	Nonspecific, acute diarrhea and local treatment of mild inflammation of the genital and anal area.
orange peel, bitter	Loss of appetite and dyspeptic ailments.
onion	Loss of appetite.
parsley herb and root	Flushing out the urinary tract and preventing and treating kidney gravel, dysuria, and flatulent dyspepsia.
peppermint leaf	Spastic complaints of the gastrointestinal tract, gallbladder, and bile ducts.
peppermint oil	Spastic discomfort of the upper gastrointestinal tract and bile ducts; irritable colon.
Permixon	Brand name version of saw palmetto. Used in treatment of benign prostatic hyperplasia or lower urinary tract symptoms.
psyllium seed	Bulk-forming laxative used for treatment of chronic and temporary constipation, irritable bowel syndrome, and constipation related to duodenal ulcer or diverticulitis. Also used as a stool softener after anorectal surgery and for patients with hemorrhoids.
pumpkin seed	Irritable bladder and micturition problems of benign prostatic hyperplasia stages 1 and 2, functional disorders of the bladder, difficult urination, childhood enuresis nocturna, and irritable bladder; also used successfully to eradicate tapeworms.
rhubarb root	Short-term treatment of occasional constipation.
rye pollen	Treatment of outflow tract obstruction due to benign prostatic hyperplasia.
sacred bark	See cascara.
sage leaf	Dyspeptic symptoms, stomatitis.

Herb	Condition
saw palmetto berry	Urinary problems in benign prostatic hyperplasia stages 1 and 2, testicular atrophy, sex hormone disorders, and prostatic enlargement.
senna leaf/fruit	Short-term treatment of occasional constipation.
shave grass/shavetail grass	See horsetail.
South African star grass	Benign prostatic hyperplasia.
soy lecithin/phospholipid	Hypercholesterolemia.
sparrowgrass	See asparagus root.
stinging nettle herb/leaf	Irrigation therapy for inflammatory diseases of the lower urinary tract; prevention and treatment of kidney gravel.
sweet balm	See lemon balm.
turmeric root	Treatment of acid, flatulent, or atonic dyspepsia.
uva ursi leaf	Inflammatory disorders of the efferent urinary tract.
wild gentian	See gentian root.
witch hazel	Local inflammation of hemorrhoids.
whortleberry	See bilberry fruit.
yarrow	Mild spastic discomforts of the gastrointestinal tract.
yellow gentian	See gentian root.
yohimbine	Erectile dysfunction.

Sample Reports and Dictation

BILATERAL PELVIC LYMPHADENECTOMY AND RADICAL RETROPUBIC PROSTATOVESICULECTOMY

DIAGNOSIS: Carcinoma of the prostate.

DESCRIPTION OF PROCEDURE: In the supine position, after endotracheal anesthesia, the abdomen and genitalia were prepped and draped in the usual fashion. A midline incision was made from the symphysis pubis towards the umbilicus for about 5 inches, deepened through the subcutaneous tissues down to the fascial layer, which was incised. Retropubic exposure was accomplished, exposing the iliopsoas fossa, and this was retracted with the Bookwalter retractor to expose and allow the lymphadenectomy.

The lymphadenectomy was done in limited fashion by mobilizing the fibroareolar tissue on both sides (anterior medial and inferior to the iliac vein into the obturator fossa off the obturator nerve vessels) using medium or large hemoclips as appropriate. Frozen section revealed these to be negative. The procedure was continued by mobilizing the endopelvic fascia and incising it posteriorly to anteriorly. At the anterior portion, we incised the puboprostatic ligaments. Triple ligation of the dorsal vein complex was accomplished. Dividing between the second and third cephalad sutures, we identified the urethroprostatic angle, at which point the lateral exposure was accomplished by dividing the fascia again to drop the neurovascular bundle posterolaterally.

The posterior urethra was now incised. The catheter was removed. Dissection of the prostate off the rectum was done through Denonvilliers fascia. Proximally we were able to mobilize the lateral aspects of the pedicles between hemoclips. Seminal vesicles were exposed through incision of Denonvilliers fascia again and division of pedicles between hemoclips. The pedicles to the seminal vesicles and ejaculatory ducts were divided between Ligaclips. A portion of this ejaculatory duct was removed with the seminal vesicles, and the bladder neck was mobilized against some mild traction of the Foley, sparing about a 1-cm section of prostatic urethra. This was everted with 3–0 chromic sutures on the seromuscular layer and anastomosed to the urethra using the Greenfield suture guide. Irrigation revealed no leaks or bleeding after thorough irrigation of the pelvis. All counts were correct.

Insertion of the J-P drain was accomplished through a separate stab incision on the right side and secured using 3–0 nylon. Closure was done with a running Dexon, with subcutaneous tissues anastomosed with 3–0 Dexon and a subcuticular 3–0 Dexon suture. Steri-Strips and OpSite dressing was applied. The patient tolerated the procedure well with no complications encountered and was sent to the recovery room in stable and satisfactory condition.

IMPRESSION: Carcinoma of the prostate.

COLONOSCOPY WITH POLYPECTOMY BY HOT BIOPSY ABLATION

PREPROCEDURE DIAGNOSIS: Unexplained gastrointestinal bleeding.

POSTPROCEDURE DIAGNOSES
1. Two small sessile polyps in the sigmoid colon. Hot biopsy ablation performed.
2. Internal hemorrhoids.

PROCEDURE PERFORMED: Colonoscopy with polypectomy using hot biopsy forceps.

DESCRIPTION OF PROCEDURE: After obtaining informed consent, the patient was placed in the left lateral position. Medications were given to achieve and maintain optimal sedation. The video colonoscope was introduced through the anal opening into the rectum and was advanced up to the cecum. The appendiceal opening and ileocecal valve were identified. The colonoscope was withdrawn. The only significant findings were two small sessile polyps in the sigmoid colon. These were removed using hot biopsy forceps. Internal hemorrhoids were noted. The rest of the exam was unremarkable. The colonoscope was withdrawn. The patient was transferred to the recovery room in stable condition.

IMPRESSION: No significant pathology that can explain gastrointestinal bleeding.

PLAN: Transfuse two units of packed red blood cells since the hematocrit is 25; maintain the hematocrit and consider further gastrointestinal evaluation if the gastrointestinal bleeding persists.

CYSTOSCOPY, LEFT URETEROSCOPY, AND INSERTION OF A DOUBLE-J STENT

DIAGNOSIS: Left distal ureteral calculus.

PROCEDURES PERFORMED
1. Cystoscopy.
2. Left ureteroscopy.
3. Insertion of a double-J stent.

DESCRIPTION OF PROCEDURE: After spinal anesthesia, the abdomen and genitalia were prepped and draped in the usual fashion. Endoscopic evaluation failed to reveal any abnormalities of the bladder. Bimanual pelvic examination revealed a very small cystic change in the apex. Retrograde pyelogram revealed the distal ureteral calculus to be on the edge of the distal ureter. Endoscopically this was most likely a phlebolith as it was not intramural and intramucosal. The distal ureteral stricture was dilated to 15 French with a 4-cm balloon at 17 atmospheres. A double-J stent was inserted and secured in place to prepare for left ESWL of the patient's 1-cm stone in the lower pole of the left kidney. The patient tolerated the procedure well and was sent to the recovery room in stable condition.

CYSTOSCOPY AND TRANSURETHRAL RESECTION OF THE PROSTATE WITH VAPORIZATION

DIAGNOSIS: Benign prostatic hypertrophy.

PROCEDURE PERFORMED: Cystoscopy and transurethral resection of the prostate with vaporization.

DESCRIPTION OF PROCEDURE: In the dorsal lithotomy position after spinal anesthesia, the abdomen and genitalia were prepped and draped in the usual fashion. Endoscopic evaluation demonstrated that the patient had no significant urethral abnormalities. The prostate revealed two visual fields of significant intravesical components with median lobe type of hypertrophy and 3+ trabeculation of the bladder muscle without significant other pathology. Resection was carried out using the Iglesias rectoscope element with continued monitoring, continued Sorbitol irrigation, and video monitoring. Resection was done to the median lobe components to the circular capsule of fibers of the bladder neck floor, lateral lobes, anterior tissue and apically, circumferentially removing all of the obstructive tissue down to the level of the verumontanum. Irrigation was done and all chips were removed. Fulguration was done with a VaporTrode electrode and VaporTrode ball at a setting of 250 watts for complete hemostasis. At the end of the procedure, no injuries to the bladder, trigone, ureteral orifices, prostatic fossa, external sphincter, verumontanum, or urethra were noted. The patient tolerated the procedure well and was taken to the recovery room in stable and satisfactory condition.

ESOPHAGOGASTRODUODENOSCOPY WITH RANDOM BIOPSIES AND ESOPHAGEAL DILATATION

PREOPERATIVE DIAGNOSES
1. Foreign body of the esophagus.
2. Dysphagia

POSTOPERATIVE DIAGNOSES
1. Foreign body of the esophagus.
2. Dysphagia
3. Esophagitis and Schatzki ring of the distal esophagus with stricture.

PROCEDURE PERFORMED: Esophagogastroduodenoscopy with random biopsies and esophageal dilatation.

DESCRIPTION OF PROCEDURE: After satisfactory IV analgesia with Versed and Sublimaze and topical anesthesia with viscous Xylocaine and Hurricaine spray, the procedure was performed without incident. The GIF video endoscope was inserted under direct vision. The patient was found to have a meat bolus in the distal esophagus. The patient was found to have a Schatzki ring and diffuse inflammation. The bolus was displaced into the stomach. The stomach itself had an inflamed gastric mucosa with linear streaking and superficial erosions in the antrum and prepyloric region. The first segment of the duodenum also had inflammation. The remainder was normal. The patient had no evidence of ulcerative, neoplastic, or polypoid lesions. I randomly biopsied the antral and prepyloric areas to exclude Helicobacter pylori and randomly biopsied the EG junction. I then did an esophageal dilatation using the balloon, without incident. I visualized the EG junction, and it seemed that the ring had been fractured, but I did not see any significant bleeding. The patient tolerated all of these procedures well and was returned to the recovery room in stable condition.

EXPLORATORY LAPAROTOMY AND SPLENECTOMY

PREOPERATIVE DIAGNOSIS: Blunt abdominal trauma.

POSTOPERATIVE DIAGNOSIS: Splenic laceration and hemoperitoneum.

PROCEDURE PERFORMED: Exploratory laparotomy and splenectomy.

FINDINGS
1. Hemoperitoneum, about 1000 cc.
2. Splenic laceration, grade 3.

DESCRIPTION OF PROCEDURE: The patient was taken to the operating room where a Foley bladder catheter was placed using a sterile technique. The patient had two large-bore IVs and was given high-rate boluses of IV fluids and blood. The abdomen and upper thighs were prepped from the nipples to the knees. The patient was sterilely draped. The anesthetist then put the patient to sleep, and the incision was made nearly simultaneously. The blood pressure did remain stable with the administration of blood.

The subcutaneous tissues were opened sharply to the fascia, which was also opened sharply. The peritoneum was grasped and carefully opened. The incision was opened along its length, which extended from the xiphoid to the infraumbilical region. A large amount of hemoperitoneum, mainly in the left hemiabdomen, was evacuated. Packs were placed in all four quadrants, starting with left upper quadrant and then the right upper quadrant. There was a large gush of blood in the right upper quadrant, somewhat concerning for a liver injury. Once all four quadrants were packed and the patient remained stable, the packs were removed initially from the lower quadrants, revealing no injuries but adhesions and scarring around the cecum. Then packs were removed from around the liver, and careful inspection of the right and left lobes of the liver revealed no injury to the liver. The packs were gradually removed from the left upper quadrant, and it was found that the spleen was indeed lacerated in the lower half, fairly significantly. This was definitely the source of the bleeding. The peritoneal attachments were quickly divided bluntly. The hilum was isolated. The splenic vessels were divided between straight clamps, and the spleen was removed. Packs were held over the area until hemodynamic stability could again be confirmed. The blood vessels were then controlled with suture ligatures of 0 Vicryl. Short gastric vessels were also ligated. A pack was placed, and again the rest of the abdomen was explored. The adhesions in the right lower quadrant were divided so that the omentum could be freed up. Once this was done, the small bowel was run from the ligament of Treitz to the cecum, and no injury was noted. The entire colon was inspected, and again no injury was noted. The left upper quadrant was again inspected, and another 3–0 silk suture ligature was used to complete the hemostasis. Hemostasis was good. An NG tube was positioned in good location. All of the packs were removed.

The fascia was closed with running 0 Vicryl suture. Given the large amount of laps used, abdominal films were taken, which revealed no evidence of retained lap sponges. Subcutaneous tissues were irrigated, and the skin was closed with staples. The patient tolerated the procedure and was transported to the ICU postoperatively in good condition.

HEMICOLECTOMY AND PANCREATICODUODENECTOMY (WHIPPLE PROCEDURE)

PROCEDURES PERFORMED
1. Partial colectomy with anastomosis (right hemicolectomy).
2. Pancreaticoduodenectomy (Whipple procedure).

DESCRIPTION OF PROCEDURE: The patient was brought to the operating suite and was administered a general intubation anesthetic. Foley catheter was placed to gravity drainage. The abdomen was prepped with Betadine and sterilely draped.

A midline incision was made with a scalpel and electrocautery through the subcutaneous fat and then through the rectus fascia. The peritoneal cavity was entered above the level of the umbilicus. The lower abdomen and pelvis were obliterated, with adhesions involving the omentum. These omental adhesions involved the entire lower abdomen and pelvis. Dissection was carried out with electrocautery and Metzenbaum scissors to free up the omentum and to free up multiple loops of small bowel which were adherent to each other. There were noted to be sutures from a previous surgery in what appeared to be the sigmoid colon. The patient also had sutures in the distal small bowel, about 6 to 8 cm from the ileocecal valve, also consistent with what appeared to be some type of small bowel resection.

The ascending colon was mobilized with sharp dissection, and palpation revealed a soft mass within the proximal ascending colon. Dissection was carried around the hepatic flexure, incising the peritoneum, separating it into pedicles, which were clipped and then divided. Dissection was carried around and through the gastrocolic tissue. Again, this tissue was either divided between large Weck clips or between clamps, and the tissue was tied with 2–0 silk. It was at this point that a mass was noted in the head of the pancreas that measured about 3 cm x 4 cm. The remainder of the pancreas was smooth with only one or two other areas of slight induration, one in the body and one in the tail.

There were enlarged lymph nodes around the common bile duct. These were soft. One of these was removed and sent for frozen section. Meanwhile, dissection was carried out to complete mobilization of the terminal small bowel and the ascending colon over to the mid transverse colon. The omentum was divided up to the midpoint of the transverse colon. The vessels along the right side of the middle colic artery and vein were sacrificed after the bowel had been divided between a bowel clamp and a Kocher. The dissection extended to the origin of the right colic and ileocolic vessels, and these vessels were divided between clamps and tied with 0 silk. There were small palpable nodes evident in the proximal mesocolon. These nodes were included as much as possible. The duodenum was dissected away from the mesocolon to allow for proximal ligation of the respective vessels. The distal small bowel was divided between a Kocher clamp and a bowel clamp. This was just proximal to the area of the previous anastomosis. The remaining mesentery of the terminal ileum and cecum was divided between clamps and tied with 2–0 silk.

The bowel was then prepared for an end-to-end anastomosis. This was carried out in two layers with the outer layer of interrupted seromuscular 3–0 silk and an inner layer of continuous interlocking 3–0 chromic. The mesenteric defect was closed with interrupted 3–0 silk. By this time I received word that the lymph node removed from the common bile duct area did not show any evidence of malignancy. Both right and left lobes of the liver were unremarkable to palpation. The gallbladder was moderately distended. The stomach was unremarkable. There was no evidence of any tumor studding the peritoneum. There was no free fluid within the peritoneal cavity. At this point, I went out and spoke with the patient's family and apprised them of the situation involving the pancreas. After discussion, it was decided to proceed at this time with the pancreaticoduodenectomy for the suspected neoplasm at the head of the pancreas.

The midline incision was extended up to the xiphoid. The self-retaining Bookwalter retractor was used, and the mobilization of the duodenum was completed to the inferior vena cava. The ligament of Treitz was mobilized by incising the peritoneum there. Gastroepiploic vessels were divided near their origin at the region of the head of the pancreas, and the head of the pancreas and duodenum were mobilized. The dissection was carried along the middle colic vein to the identified superior mesenteric vein, which then led into the identification of the portal vein. Blunt dissection was carried out easily over the portal vein behind the neck of the pancreas. The neck of the pancreas was totally normal. Dissection was then carried out in the lesser curvature area of the stomach over the duodenum to identify the gastroduodenal vessel. This was identified as being separate from the hepatic artery. The gastroduodenal vessel was encircled with a vessel loop. The opening was made in the lesser sac, and dissection was carried out over the superior aspect of the pancreas to allow for passage of a large Kelly clamp behind the neck of the pancreas. Again, a vessel loop was wrapped around the neck of the pancreas. Dissection was then carried out over the common bile duct, separated from the hepatic artery and the portal vein. The common bile duct appeared to be about 8 mm to 9 mm in diameter. It was encircled again with a vessel loop. At this point another enlarged node was located just above the neck of the pancreas near the celiac access. This lymph node was not hard, but it was enlarged and appeared to be slightly discolored. At this point there was no evidence of any extension of the tumor beyond the region of the head of the pancreas. It was elected then to proceed with the pancreaticoduodenectomy.

The pancreas was divided over its neck, with the TA-55 stapler applied across the proximal portion. The severed neck of the pancreas had bleeding, which was controlled easily with several 3–0 silk sutures. The pancreatic duct was found to lie in the posterior portion of the gland, and it measured perhaps 3 mm to 4 mm. Dissection was carried along the lateral aspect, right along the portal vein. The pancreaticoduodenal arteries were divided between clamps. The tissue along here was separated into small pedicles, and these were divided between clamps and tied with 2–0 silk. In this fashion, the head of the pancreas and the uncinate process were removed and dissection carried up towards the gastroduodenal vessel, which was then divided between clamps and tied with 2–0 silk. The distal common bile duct was also subsequently divided, and this allowed resection of the head of the pancreas along with the uncinate process.

The duodenum was divided between clamps just distal to the pylorus, and the small bowel at the duodenojejunal junction was divided as well, with a TA-55 stapler being applied distally, and then the bowel transected. The resected specimen, then, was the head of the pancreas, duodenum and distal common bile duct. Later inspection revealed that the preserved pylorus and 3 cm of duodenum appeared a bit dusky, and so I elected to resect the distal half of the stomach as well. The antrectomy was carried out by dividing the gastric vessels and ligating them with 0 silk.

The pancreaticojejunostomy anastomosis was carried out. This was an end-to-side fashion. The outer layer of the pancreaticojejunostomy was interrupted 3–0 silk. The inner layer was mucosa to mucosa with interrupted 4–0 silk, and the anterior outer layer was interrupted 3–0 silk in two layers. Approximately 8 cm distal to this anastomosis, the site was selected for the choledochojejunostomy. Before this was accomplished, the gallbladder was resected. The gallbladder was taken down from the fundus to the cystic duct in the usual fashion with electrocautery and also in some areas tissue divided between clamps, tied, and divided with 2–0 silk. Weck clips were also used in these areas. The dissection was carried down to identify the cystic artery, which was ligated with 2–0 silk and divided. The cystic duct was dissected down and then divided and ligated with 2–0 silk. The choledochojejunostomy was an end-to-side anastomosis. This was carried out in essentially one layer with interrupted 3–0 Vicryl, although 3–0 silk was used on either side of the anastomosis. The loop of jejunum was then brought around so that a gastrojejunostomy could be performed. This again was an end-to-side anastomosis. The midpoint of the stomach was divided between a ball clamp, which was applied along the greater curvature for about 4 cm, and then the medial half of the stomach was closed with a TA-90 stapler, 4.8 staple height. Again the anastomosis was carried out in two layers. An outer layer was interrupted 3–0 seromuscular silk, and the inner layer was continuous interlocking 3–0 chromic. All three anastomoses were accomplished with excellent blood supply to the respective organs and without any tension.

Irrigation of the abdominal cavity was carried out. Inspection revealed good hemostasis. Some of the omentum over the transverse colon appeared to be dusky, so this was resected. Next, two Jackson-Pratt drains were brought through the abdominal wall, one on the right side and one on the left side. One was placed near the area of the choledochojejunostomy, and the other one was located near the pancreaticojejunostomy. These were secured to the skin using 2–0 nylon. After an accurate sponge, instrument, and needle count was conducted, the abdomen was closed with continuous 1–0 Panacryl. The skin was approximated with skin staples. The patient was subsequently transferred to a cart and taken to recovery in good condition.

LAPAROSCOPIC CHOLECYSTECTOMY

PREOPERATIVE DIAGNOSES
1. Cholelithiasis.
2. History of paroxysmal atrial tachycardia.

POSTOPERATIVE DIAGNOSES
1. Cholelithiasis.
2. History of paroxysmal atrial tachycardia.

PROCEDURES PERFORMED
1. Laparoscopic cholecystectomy.
2. Hasson cannula insertion.

ANESTHESIA: General endotracheal.

DESCRIPTION OF PROCEDURE: The patient was taken to the operating room, placed in the supine position. After placement of pneumatic compression devices, a Foley catheter, and orogastric tube, the patient had undergone satisfactory induction of general endotracheal anesthesia. The abdomen was prepped and draped using a Betadine preparation and sterile drapes. The patient had had a previous TAH/BSO and had a very long vertical midline incision. A cutdown was, therefore, performed at the infraumbilical position. Significant scar tissue was entered. The peritoneum was entered between hemostats, and finger dissection freed any intraabdominal adhesions. Then 0 Vicryl was placed for tacking sutures, and a Hasson cannula was inserted. A pneumoperitoneum was created without difficulty.

At this point, the 10-mm, 0-degree laparoscope was inserted. Two 5-mm trocars were placed under direct vision, one in the right anterior axillary line and one in the right midclavicular line. A second Veress port was placed in the left midline subxiphoid position. Gallbladder grasping forceps were used to grasp Hartmann pouch and the fundus of the gallbladder. A Maryland dissector was used to identify the gallbladder-cystic junction. No palpable stones were noted. The cystic duct appeared to be quite small. This was then doubly clipped and singly clipped proximally, and the cystic artery was similarly dealt with. The gallbladder was removed from the liver bed with electrocautery dissection. No spillage of bile or blood was appreciated.

The camera was applied to the subxiphoid port. The gallbladder was grasped with forceps and delivered through the umbilical wound without any contamination. The trocars were removed under direct vision, without evidence of bleeding.

The umbilicus was closed with interrupted sutures of 0 Vicryl. The skin was closed with 4–0 Vicryl in a similar fashion.

All sponge and needle counts were correct. The patient tolerated the procedure well and left the operating room in satisfactory condition.

LAPAROSCOPIC NISSEN FUNDOPLICATION

PREOPERATIVE DIAGNOSIS: Refractory gastroesophageal reflux disease.

POSTOPERATIVE DIAGNOSIS: Refractory gastroesophageal reflux disease.

PROCEDURE PERFORMED: Laparoscopic Nissen fundoplication.

ANESTHESIA: General.

DESCRIPTION OF PROCEDURE: With the patient in the supine position with his legs in the stirrups, initially an abdominal puncture was made for a Veress needle. After inflating the abdomen, a 10-mm port was placed approximately 5 cm above the umbilicus. Under direct vision, additional ports were placed in the right and left subcostal areas in the upper midline to facilitate dissection.

The liver was distracted superiorly using liver retractor, and this exposed the esophageal hiatus. There was a moderate-sized paraesophageal hernia, which was reduced. The crura were then dissected until the esophagus was freed from the crura circumferentially. Care was taken to preserve the vagus nerve trunk.

Once the crural area was well dissected, attention was turned to the fundus, which was mobilized by taking down the short gastric using a Harmonic scalpel. One of the short gastrics had some brisk bleeding which was controlled readily, again, with the Harmonic scalpel. Approximately 75 cc of blood was lost during the course of controlling that small short gastric bleeder. Once the fundus was completely freed, the crural repair was accomplished with interrupted sutures of 0 Ethibond placed with an EndoStitch device. The wrap was then passed posterior to the esophagus and held in place while a 50-French bougie was passed. With the bougie in place, the fundoplication was accomplished using interrupted sutures of 2–0 Ethibond, taking care to get the sutures through the medial and lateral portions of the fundus for the plication as well as the anterior surface of the esophagus. The most superior sutures were placed between the esophageal crura and the apex of the wrap.

Being satisfied with the wrap, the area of dissection was irrigated. Hemostasis was assured, and the ports were then removed under direct vision. The port sites were closed with 0 Vicryl interrupted for the fascia and 3–0 Vicryl subcuticular, with benzoin and Steri-Strips for the skin. The patient tolerated the procedure well.

LEFT EXTRACORPOREAL SHOCK WAVE LITHOTRIPSY

DIAGNOSIS: Left renal calculi.

PROCEDURE PERFORMED: Left extracorporeal shock wave lithotripsy.

DESCRIPTION OF PROCEDURE: After the patient was placed in the supine position and in the F2 focus of the MSL 5000 lithotriptor, shock wave lithotripsy was started at 17 kV and went up to 23, where a total of 3000 shocks were given to the stone with fragmentation of this left renal calculi. No complications were encountered. The patient was sent to the recovery room in stable and satisfactory condition.

LEFT HEMICOLECTOMY AND TRANSVERSE COLORECTAL ANASTOMOSIS

PREOPERATIVE DIAGNOSIS: Refractory inflammatory bowel disease.

POSTOPERATIVE DIAGNOSIS: Refractory inflammatory bowel disease

PROCEDURE PERFORMED: Left hemicolectomy with transverse colorectal anastomosis.

FINDINGS: A few small plaques on the transverse colon (one excised for biopsy).

DESCRIPTION OF PROCEDURE: The patient was taken to the operating room where general anesthesia was introduced. Her abdomen was prepped and draped in the usual sterile fashion with the patient in the modified lithotomy position. The previous midline scar was excised. The midline vertical scar was excised using a 10-blade scalpel. The subcutaneous tissues were divided with electrocautery. The fascia was also opened with electrocautery. The peritoneum was carefully grasped and entered. The incision was opened up along its length that extended from about 3 cm supraumbilical down to a few centimeters from the pubis. Gross peritoneal exploration was done. In the cul-de-sac, there was some fluid, which was submitted for cytology. There were a few plaques on the transverse colon. The liver was normal. I could not really evaluate the previous Nissen fundoplication from the lower abdominal incision. The colon looked normal. There was surgical absence of appendix.

The left colon was then dissected from the retroperitoneum. There was a fair amount of scar tissue, and this dissection took some time. The ureter was identified and was kept well out of the field of dissection. The greater omentum was dissected off the transverse colon to mobilize the splenic flexure. Resection was done by dividing the colon at the distal aspect of the transverse colon. I could see that there was essentially a branching blood vessel, probably the original middle colic artery, right at the area of the bowel I divided. I did take the left branch of the middle colic vessel and resect the mesentery. Vessels were ligated with clamps. This was done to where the rectum had been mobilized. The previous anastomosis was intact and widely patent.

A49

A TA-55 stapler was applied across the rectum, about 3 cm below the previous anastomosis. Once the mesentery was divided, the TA stapler was fired. Attempts were made to save the superior hemorrhoidal vessels. The specimen was submitted to pathology. The transverse colon was then prepared for anastomosis. The staple line was excised, and a sizer was used to confirm that a 31-mm sizer fit easily within the lumen, secured with a pursestring suture. The remaining stapler was then passed up through the anus in the usual fashion and the spike advanced to the TA-55 staple line. This was fired, creating an anastomosis in the usual fashion. This was reinforced in a few areas using 3–0 silk popoffs. The TA-55 staple line outside of the anastomosis was also reinforced using interrupted 3–0 Lembert sutures. The anastomosis was then tested by placing it underwater and insufflating through the anus. This confirmed that the anastomosis was patent, and there was no evidence of bubbles or a leak. The water was evacuated. The mesenteric defect was then closed to prevent internal hernias. The small bowel was run from the ligament of Treitz to the cecum, and there were no abnormalities noted.

Attention was then turned towards closure. The fascia was reapproximated using a running 0 Vicryl suture. The skin edges were then approximated using skin clips. A sterile dressing was applied. The patient was extubated and an epidural catheter was placed. The patient was taken to the recovery room in stable condition.

LIMITED COLONOSCOPY

INDICATIONS: Heme-positive stool with anemia of unclear origin.

PROCEDURE PERFORMED: Limited colonoscopy.

PREMEDICATION: Demerol 50 mg IV, Versed 3 mg IV, and glucagon 1 mg IV.

DESCRIPTION OF PROCEDURE: The video colonoscope was only able to be passed to approximately 40 cm. Because of intense spasm in the midst of innumerable diverticula along with some stool, it was felt that the scope could not be safely advanced further. The procedure was therefor terminated, despite trying to advance the scope in both left and right lateral decubitus positions.

IMPRESSION: Severe narrowing/spasm of the midsigmoid colon in the midst of diverticulosis, otherwise unremarkable distal 40 cm.

PUBOVAGINAL SLING

PROCEDURE PERFORMED: Pubovaginal sling.

DETAILS OF PROCEDURE: In lithotomy position, the patient was prepped and draped in sterile fashion. A 16-French Foley catheter was placed initially into the bladder. An Allis clamp was placed on the vaginal mucosa. The bladder neck was then identified and marked using a sterile marking pencil. The vaginal mucosa was then infiltrated using 1% Xylocaine with epinephrine to help aid in hydrodissection. Following this, Malis scissors were then used to dissect the vaginal flap, which was in the shape of an inverted U. Dissection was performed laterally to the pelvic side-walls and in the retropubic space bilaterally. Following this, a transverse incision was made in the suprapubic region down to the level of the rectus fascia. Stamey needles were then placed on either side of the bladder neck.

Following this, the fascia lata graft was then prepared using a mattress suture of 0 Prolene on either side. Having marked the midline, the 0 Prolene suture was then placed through either eye of the Stamey needles, and the sutures were brought out through the abdominal wall. Cystoscopy was then performed, which was within normal limits. A 4-French open-ended catheter was placed up each ureteric orifice and easily passed, and normal efflux of urine could be seen from each ureteral orifice. The midline of the fascia lata flap was then attached to the underlying vaginal wall in the midline using 4–0 Vicryl. A running suture of 2–0 chromic was used to approximate the vaginal incisions. The sutures of 0 Prolene were then tied across each other along the anterior rectus fascia and allowed good suspension of the bladder neck. The subcutaneous tissue in the abdominal incision was then approximated using interrupted sutures of 3–0 chromic. The skin edges were approximated using a running suture of 4–0 Vicryl. The patient tolerated the procedure well.

Bilateral Pelvic Lymphadenectomy and Radical Retropubic Prostatovesiculectomy

Bookwalter retractor
cephalad suture
Denonvilliers fascia
dorsal vein complex
ejaculatory duct
endopelvic fascia
fibroareolar tissue
genitalia
Greenfield suture guide
hemoclip
iliopsoas fossa
lymphadenectomy
neurovascular bundle
obturator fossa
obturator nerve
OpSite dressing
prostatic urethra
retropubic exposure
seminal vesicle
seromuscular layer
symphysis pubis
umbilicus
urethroprostatic angle

Colonoscopy with Polypectomy by Hot Biopsy Ablation

appendiceal opening
cecum
colonoscopy
gastrointestinal bleeding
hematocrit
hot biopsy ablation
hot biopsy forceps
ileocecal valve
internal hemorrhoid

packed red blood cells
polypectomy
sessile polyp
sigmoid colon
video colonoscope

Cystoscopy, Left Ureteroscopy, and Insertion of a Double-J Stent

apex
atmosphere
balloon
bimanual pelvic examination
cystoscopy
distal ureteral calculus
double-J stent
extracorporeal shock wave lithotripsy (ESWL)
endoscopically
genitalia
intramucosal
intramural
lower pole
phlebolith
retrograde pyelogram
ureter
ureteroscopy

Cystoscopy and Transurethral Resection of the Prostate with Vaporization

benign prostatic hypertrophy
bladder neck floor
circumferential
cystoscopy
dorsal lithotomy position
endoscopic evaluation
external sphincter
fulguration
hemostasis

hypertrophy
Iglesias rectoscope element
intravesical component
lateral lobe
median lobe
prostatic fossa
resection
Sorbitol irrigation
spinal anesthesia
trabeculation
transurethral resection of the prostate
trigone
ureteral orifice
urethra
vaporization
VaporTrode ball
VaporTrode electrode
verumontanum
video monitoring

Esophagogastroduodenoscopy with Random Biopsies and Esophageal Dilatation

antrum
balloon
bolus
distal esophagus
dysphagia
esophagogastric (EG) junction
esophageal dilatation
esophagitis
first segment of the duodenum
foreign body
GIF video endoscope
Helicobacter pylori
Hurricaine spray
linear streaking
neoplastic
polypoid lesion
prepyloric region
random biopsy
Schatzki ring
stricture
Sublimaze

topical anesthesia
ulcerative
Versed
viscous Xylocaine

Exploratory Laparotomy and Splenectomy

adhesion
blunt abdominal trauma
cecum
evacuated
exploratory laparotomy
fascia
hemiabdomen
hemodynamic stability
hemoperitoneum
hilum
infraumbilical region
lap sponge
large-bore IV
ligament of Treitz
ligature
left upper quadrant (LUQ)
nasogastric (NG) tube
omentum
peritoneal attachment
peritoneum
quadrant
right upper quadrant (RUQ)
short gastric vessel
small bowel
splenectomy
splenic laceration
subcutaneous tissue

Hemicolectomy and Pancreaticoduodenectomy (Whipple Procedure)

adhesion
anastomosis
antrectomy
blunt dissection
Bookwalter retractor
cecum

choledochojejunostomy
colic vessel
common bile duct
dissection
electrocautery
end-to-end anastomosis
Foley catheter
frozen section
gastroduodenal area
gastroepiploic vessel
gastrojejunostomy
gravity drainage
head of the pancreas
hemicolectomy
ileocolic vessels
induration
jejunum
Jackson-Pratt drain
Kocher clamp
lesser curvature
ligament of Treitz
mesentery
mesocolon
Metzenbaum scissors
middle colic artery
middle colic vein
neoplasm
omentum
palpable node
Panacryl
pancreaticoduodenectomy
partial colectomy
pedicle
peritoneal cavity
portal vein
pylorus
rectus fascia
seromuscular
small bowel
subcutaneous fat
superior mesenteric vein
TA-55 stapler

tail of the pancreas
terminal ileum
tumor studding
umbilicus
uncinate process
Weck clip
Whipple procedure
xiphoid

Laparoscopic Cholecystectomy

Betadine preparation
bile
cholecystectomy
cholelithiasis
cystic artery
cystic duct
electrocautery dissection
finger dissection
Foley catheter
fundus of the gallbladder
gallbladder-cystic junction
gallbladder grasping forceps
general endotracheal anesthesia
Hartmann pouch
Hasson cannula
hemostat
infraumbilical position
intraabdominal adhesions
laparoscope
liver bed
Maryland dissector
midclavicular line
midline subxiphoid position
orogastric tube
peritoneum
pneumatic compression device
pneumoperitoneum
trocar
umbilical wound
umbilicus
Veress port

Laparoscopic Nissen Fundoplication
benzoin
crura
EndoStitch device
esophageal hiatus
Ethibond
50-French bougie
fundus
Harmonic scalpel
hemostasis
laparoscopic Nissen fundoplication
liver retractor
paraesophageal hernia
refractory gastroesophageal reflux disease
short gastric
Steri-Strips
vagus nerve trunk
Veress needle
subcuticular

Left Extracorporeal Shock-Wave Lithotripsy (ESWL)
F2 focus
fragmentation
kilovolt (kV)
MSL 5000 lithotriptor
renal calculi
shock wave lithotripsy
supine position

Left Hemicolectomy and Transverse Colorectal Anastomosis
biopsy
cecum
colorectal anastomosis
electrocautery
epidural catheter
extubated

fascia
field of dissection
greater omentum
hemicolectomy
Lembert suture
ligament of Treitz
mesentery
middle colic artery
modified lithotomy position
patent
peritoneum
plaque
popoff suture
resection
refractory inflammatory bowel disease
retroperitoneum
sizer
splenic flexure
subcutaneous tissue
supraumbilical
TA-55 stapler
10-blade scalpel
transverse colon
Vicryl suture

Limited Colonoscopy
colonoscopy
Demerol
diverticula
diverticulosis
glucagon
heme-positive stool
midsigmoid colon
left lateral decubitus position
right lateral decubitus position
spasm
Versed

Pubovaginal Sling
Allis clamp
bladder neck
cystoscopy

efflux of urine
fascia lata graft
4-French open-ended catheter
hydrodissection
inverted U
lithotomy position
Malis scissors
mattress suture
Prolene suture
pubovaginal sling

rectus fascia
16-French Foley catheter
Stamey needle
suprapubic region
ureteric orifice
vaginal flap
vaginal mucosa
vaginal wall
Xylocaine with epinephrine

Appendix 6

Drugs by Indication

ACHALASIA

Adrenergic Agonist Agent

- Brethaire®
- Brethine®
- Bricanyl®
- terbutaline

Calcium Channel Blocker

- Adalat®
- Adalat® CC
- Adalat PA® (Can)
- Apo®-Nifed (Can)
- Gen-Nifedipine (Can)
- nifedipine
- Novo-Nifedin (Can)
- Nu-Nifed (Can)
- Nu-Nifedin (Can)
- Procardia®
- Procardia XL®

Vasodilator

- Apo®-ISDN (Can)
- Cedocard (Can)
- Cedocard®-SR (Can)
- Coradur® (Can)
- Coronex (Can)
- Deponit® Patch
- Dilatrate®-SR
- Isordil®
- isosorbide dinitrate
- Minitran® Patch
- Nitro-Bid® I.V. Injection
- Nitro-Bid® Ointment
- Nitro-Dur® Patch
- Nitrogard® Buccal
- nitroglycerin
- Nitroglyn® Oral
- Nitroject (Can)
- Nitrolingual® Translingual Spray
- Nitrol® Ointment
- Nitrong® Oral Tablet
- Nitrostat® Sublingual
- Novo-Sorbide (Can)
- Sorbitrate®
- Transdermal-NTG® Patch
- Transderm-Nitro® Patch
- Tridil® Injection

ACHLORHYDRIA

- Acidulin (Can)
- glutamic acid

AMEBIASIS

Amebicide

- Apo®-Metronidazole (Can)
- Diodoquin® (Can)
- Flagyl® Oral
- Humatin®
- iodoquinol
- Metrocream (Can)
- MetroGel® Topical
- MetroGel®-Vaginal
- Metro I.V.® Injection
- metronidazole
- Neo-Metric (Can)
- NidaGel (Can)
- Noritate (Can)
- Novo-Nidazol (Can)
- paromomycin
- Protostat® Oral
- Trikacide (Can)
- Yodoxin®

Aminoquinoline (Antimalarial)

- Aralen® Phosphate
- chloroquine phosphate

ANTICHOLINERGIC DRUG POISONING

Cholinesterase Inhibitor

- Physostigmine

ASCARIASIS

Anthelmintic

albendazole
Albenza®

ASCITES
Diuretic, Loop
  Apo®-Furosemide (Can)
  bumetanide
  Bumex®
  Burinex® (Can)
  Demadex®
  Edecrin®
  ethacrynic acid
  furosemide
  Furoside® (Can)
  Lasix®
  Novo-Semide (Can)
  torsemide
  Uritol® (Can)
Diuretic, Miscellaneous
  Apo®-Chlorthalidone (Can)
  Apo®-Indapadmide (Can)
  chlorthalidone
  Hygroton®
  indapamide
  Lozide® (Can)
  Lozol®
  metolazone
  Mykrox®
  Novo-Thalidone (Can)
  PMS-Indapamide (Can)
  Thalitone®
  Uridon® (Can)
  Zaroxolyn®
Diuretic, Potassium Sparing
  Aldactone®
  Novo-Spiroton (Can)
  spironolactone
Diuretic, Thiazide
  Apo®-Hydro (Can)
  Aquatensen®
  bendroflumethiazide
  chlorothiazide
  Diucardin®

Diuchlor® (Can)
Diuchlor H (Can)
Diurigen®
Diuril®
Duretic (Can)
Enduron®
Esidrix®
Ezide®
hydrochlorothiazide
HydroDIURIL®
hydroflumethiazide
Hydro-Par®
Metahydrin®
methyclothiazide
Microzide™
Naqua®
Naturetin®
Neo-Codema® (Can)
Novo-Hydrazide (Can)
Oretic®
polythiazide
Renese®
Saluron®
trichlormethiazide
Urozide® (Can)

BEDWETTING (SEE ENURESIS)

BENIGN PROSTATIC HYPERPLASIA (BPH)
Alpha-Adrenergic Blocking Agent
  Apo®-Prazo (Can)
  Cardura®
  doxazosin
  Flomax®
  Hytrin®
  Minipress®
  Novo-Prazin (Can)
  Nu-Prazo (Can)
  prazosin
  tamsulosin
  terazosin

Antiandrogen
  finasteride
  Proscar®

BLADDER IRRIGATION
  acetic acid
  Midol Douche (Can)

CACHEXIA
Antihistamine
  cyproheptadine
  Gen-Cyproterone (Can)
  Periactin®
  PMS-Cyproheptadine (Can)
Progestin
  Megace®
  megestrol acetate

CELIAC DISEASE
Electrolyte Supplement, Oral
  Alka-Mints® [OTC]
  Amitone® [OTC]
  Apo®-Cal® (Can)
  Biocal (Can)
  Cal-500 (Can)
  Cal Carb-HD® [OTC]
  Calci-Chew™ [OTC]
  Calciday-667® [OTC]
  Calcimax (Can)
  Calci-Mix™ [OTC]
  Calcite (Can)
  calcium carbonate
  calcium citrate
  calcium glubionate
  calcium lactate
  Calcium-Sandoz (Can)
  Cal-Plus® [OTC]
  Calsan (Can)
  Caltrate® 600 [OTC]
  Caltrate, Jr.® [OTC]
  Chooz® [OTC]
  Citracal® [OTC]
  Dicarbosil® [OTC]
  Equilet® [OTC]

Femiron® [OTC]
Feosol® [OTC]
Feostat® [OTC]
Feratab® [OTC]
Fergon® [OTC]
Fer-In-Sol® Drops [OTC]
Fer-Iron® [OTC]
Ferodan (Can)
Fero-Grad (Can)
Fero-Gradumet® [OTC]
Ferospace® [OTC]
Ferralet® [OTC]
Ferralyn® Lanacaps® [OTC]
Ferra-TD® [OTC]
Ferro-Sequels® [OTC]
ferrous fumarate
ferrous gluconate
ferrous sulfate
Fertinic® (Can)
Florical® [OTC]
Fumasorb® [OTC]
Fumerin® [OTC]
Gencalc® 600 [OTC]
Hemocyte® [OTC]
Hi Potency Cal (Can)
Ircon® [OTC]
Maalox Quick Dissolve (Can)
Mallamint® [OTC]
Mega-Cal (Can)
Mol-Iron® [OTC]
Neo Cal (Can)
Neo-Calglucon® [OTC]
Neo-Fer (Can)
Nephro-Calci® [OTC]
Nephro-Fer™ [OTC]
Novo-Ferrogluc (Can)
Novo-Ferrosulfate (Can)
Novo-Fumar (Can)
Os-Cal® 500 [OTC]
Oyst-Cal 500 [OTC]
Oystercal® 500
Palafer® (Can)
Pharmacal (Can)

Rolaids® Calcium Rich [OTC]
Simron® [OTC]
Slow FE® [OTC]
Span-FF® [OTC]
Titralac (Can)
Tums® [OTC]
Tums® E-X Extra Strength Tablet [OTC]
Tums® Extra Strength Liquid [OTC]
Vitamin
  Ferancee® [OTC]
  Fero-Grad 500® [OTC]
  ferrous salt and ascorbic acid
  ferrous sulfate, ascorbic acid, and vitamin B-complex
  ferrous sulfate, ascorbic acid, vitamin B-complex, and folic acid
  Iberet-Folic-500®
  Iberet®-Liquid [OTC]
Vitamin, Fat Soluble
  AquaMEPHYTON® Injection
  Konakion® Injection
  Mephyton® Oral
  Phytonadione

CHOLELITHIASIS

Actigall™
Moctanin®
monoctanoin
Urso®
Ursodiol

CHOLESTASIS

AquaMEPHYTON® Injection
Konakion® Injection
Mephyton® Oral
Phytonadione

CIRRHOSIS

Bile Acid Sequestrant
  cholestyramine resin
  LoCHOLEST®
  LoCHOLEST® Light
  Novo-Cholamine (Can)

PMS-Cholestyramine (Can)
Prevalite®
Questran®
Questran® Light
Chelating Agent
  Cuprimine®
  Depen®
  penicillamine
Electrolyte Supplement, Oral
  Alka-Mints® [OTC]
  Amitone® [OTC]
  Apo®-Cal® (Can)
  Biocal (Can)
  Cal-500 (Can)
  Cal Carb-HD® [OTC]
  Calci-Chew™ [OTC]
  Calciday-667® [OTC]
  Calcimax (Can)
  Calci-Mix™ [OTC]
  Calcite (Can)
  calcium carbonate
  calcium citrate
  calcium glubionate
  calcium lactate
  Calcium-Sandoz (Can)
  Cal-Plus® [OTC]
  Calsan (Can)
  Caltrate® 600 [OTC]
  Caltrate, Jr.® [OTC]
  Chooz® [OTC]
  Citracal® [OTC]
  Dicarbosil® [OTC]
  Equilet® [OTC]
  Florical® [OTC]
  Gencalc® 600 [OTC]
  Hi Potency Cal (Can)
  Maalox Quick Dissolve (Can)
  Mallamint® [OTC]
  Mega-Cal (Can)
  Neo Cal (Can)
  Neo-Calglucon® [OTC]
  Nephro-Calci® [OTC]
  Os-Cal® 500 [OTC]

Oyst-Cal 500 [OTC]
Oystercal® 500
Pharmacal (Can)
Rolaids® Calcium Rich [OTC]
Titralac (Can)
Tums® [OTC]
Tums® E-X Extra Strength Tablet
    [OTC]
Tums® Extra Strength Liquid [OTC]
Immunosuppressant Agent
    azathioprine
    Imuran®
Vitamin D Analog
    Calciferol™
    Drisdol®
    ergocalciferol
    Ostoforte® (Can)
    Radiostol® (Can)
Vitamin, Fat Soluble
    AquaMEPHYTON® Injection
    Aquasol A®
    Arovit (Can)
    Del-Vi-A®
    Konakion® Injection
    Mephyton® Oral
    Palmitate-A® 5000 [OTC]
    phytonadione
    vitamin A

COLITIS (ULCERATIVE)

Adrenal Corticosteroid
    Cortenema® Rectal
    hydrocortisone (rectal)
5-Aminosalicylic Acid Derivative
    Apo®-Sulfasalazine (Can)
    Asacol® Oral
    Azulfidine®
    Azulfidine® EN-tabs®
    balsalazide
    Colazal™
    Dipentum®
    mesalamine
    Mesasal (Can)

olsalazine
Pentasa® Oral
PMS-Sulfasa (Can)
Quintasa (Can)
Rowasa® Rectal
Salazopyrin (Can)
Salofalk (Can)
sulfasalazine
Antiinflammatory Agent
    balsalazide
    Colazal™

CONSTIPATION

Laxative
    Acilac (Can)
    Alpha Keri (Can)
    Alpha-Lac (Can)
    Alphamul® [OTC]
    Arlex® Liquid
    Bisac-Evac® [OTC]
    bisacodyl
    Bisacodyl Uniserts®
    Bisco-Lax® [OTC]
    Black Draught® [OTC]
    calcium polycarbophil
    Carter's Little Pills® [OTC]
    cascara sagrada
    castor oil
    Cephulac®
    Cholac®
    Cholan-HMB®
    Chronulac®
    Citrucel® [OTC]
    Clysodrast®
    Comalose-R (Can)
    Constilac®
    Constulose®
    Correctol (Can)
    Dacodyl® [OTC]
    Decholin®
    Deficol® [OTC]
    dehydrocholic acid
    Dulcolax® [OTC]

Duphalac®
Dycholium (Can)
Effer-Syllium® [OTC]
Emulsoil® [OTC]
Enemol™ (Can)
Enulose®
Epsal®
Equalactin® Chewable Tablet [OTC]
Evalose®
Feen-A-Mint (Can)
Fiberall® Chewable Tablet [OTC]
Fiberall® Powder [OTC]
Fiberall® Wafer [OTC]
FiberCon® Tablet [OTC]
Fiber-Lax® Tablet [OTC]
Fibrepur® (Can)
Fleet® Babylax® Rectal [OTC]
Fleet® Bisacodyl [OTC]
Fleet® Enema [OTC]
Fleet® Flavored Castor Oil [OTC]
Fleet® Laxative [OTC]
Fleet® Phospho®-Soda [OTC]
Gel-Ose (Can)
Gen-Lac (Can)
glycerin
Gly-Rectal (Can)
Haley's M-O® [OTC]
Heptalac®
Hydrocil® [OTC]
Konsyl® [OTC]
Konsyl-D® [OTC]
Kristalose®
Lactulax (Can)
lactulose
Lactulose PSE®
Laxilose (Can)
Le 500 D (Can)
magnesium hydroxide
magnesium hydroxide and mineral
  oil emulsion
magnesium oxide
magnesium sulfate
Magnolax (Can)

Mag-Ox® 400 [OTC]
malt soup extract
Maltsupex® [OTC]
Maox® [OTC]
Metamucil® [OTC]
Metamucil® Instant Mix [OTC]
methylcellulose
Mitrolan® Chewable Tablet [OTC]
Modane® Bulk [OTC]
Mucinum Herbal (Can)
Neoloid® [OTC]
Novo-Mucilax (Can)
Osmoglyn®
Perdiem® Plain [OTC]
Pharmalose (Can)
Phillips'® Milk of Magnesia [OTC]
psyllium
Purge® [OTC]
Reguloid® [OTC]
Rhodialax (Can)
Rhodialose (Can)
Ricifruit (Can)
Sani-Supp® Suppository [OTC]
senna
Senna-Gen® [OTC]
Senokot® [OTC]
Serutan® [OTC]
sodium phosphates
sorbitol
Syllact® [OTC]
Unisoil (Can)
Uro-Mag® [OTC]
V-Lax® [OTC]
X-Prep® Liquid [OTC]

Laxative/Stool Softener
Dialose® Plus Capsule [OTC]
Diocto C® [OTC]
Diocto-K Plus® [OTC]
Dioctolose Plus® [OTC]
Disanthrol® [OTC]
docusate and casanthranol
DSMC Plus® [OTC]
Genasoft® Plus [OTC]

Peri-Colace® [OTC]
Pro-Sof® Plus [OTC]
Regulace® [OTC]
Silace-C® [OTC]
Stool Softener
Albert® Docusate (Can)
Calax (Can)
Colace® [OTC]
Colax-C® (Can)
Colax-S (Can)
Correctol Stool Softener (Can)
DC 240® Softgel® [OTC]
Dialose® Tablet [OTC]
Diocto® [OTC]
Diocto-K® [OTC]
Dioctyl (Can)
Dioeze® [OTC]
Disonate® [OTC]
docusate
DOK® [OTC]
DOS® Softgel® [OTC]
Doxate-C (Can)
Doxate-S (Can)
D-S-S® [OTC]
Ex-Lax Stool Softener (Can)
Kasof® [OTC]
Laxagel (Can)
Modane® Soft [OTC]
Pharmalax (Can)
PMS-Docusate Calcium (Can)
Pro-Cal-Sof® [OTC]
Regulax SS® [OTC]
Regulex® (Can)
Selax® (Can)
Silace (Can)
SoFlax® (Can)
Sulfalax® [OTC]
Surfak® [OTC]

COPROPORPHYRIA
Apo®-Propranolol (Can)
Betachron®
Detensol® (Can)

Inderal®
Inderal® LA
Novo-Pranol (Can)
Nu-Propranolol (Can)
Propranolol

CROHN DISEASE
5-Aminosalicylic Acid Derivative
Apo®-Sulfasalazine (Can)
Asacol® Oral
Azulfidine®
Azulfidine® EN-tabs®
Dipentum®
mesalamine
Mesasal (Can)
olsalazine
Pentasa® Oral
PMS Sulfasa (Can)
Quintasa (Can)
Rowasa® Rectal
Salazopyrin (Can)
Salofalk (Can)
sulfasalazine
Gastrointestinal Agent, Miscellaneous
infliximab
Remicade®

CRYPTORCHIDISM
A.P.L.®
Chorex®
chorionic gonadotropin
Choron®
Corgonject®
Follutein®
Glukor®
Gonic®
Pregnyl®
Profasi® HP

CYSTINURIA
Cuprimine®
Depen®
Penicillamine

CYSTITIS (HEMORRHAGIC)
mesna
Mesnex™
Uromitexan (Can)

DIABETIC GASTRIC STASIS
Apo®-Metoclop (Can)
Clopra®
Emex (Can)
Maxeran® (Can)
Maxolon®
metoclopramide
Octamide®
Reglan®

DIARRHEA
Analgesic, Narcotic
  opium tincture
  paregoric
Anticholinergic Agent
  Donnagel® (Can)
  Donnapectolin-PG®
  hyoscyamine, atropine, scopolamine, kaolin, and pectin
  hyoscyamine, atropine, scopolamine, kaolin, pectin, and opium
  Kapectolin PG®
Antidiarrheal
  Anti-Diarrheal (Can)
  attapulgite
  Children's Kaopectate® [OTC]
  Diar-aid® [OTC]
  Diarex (Can)
  Diarrhea Relief (Can)
  Diasorb® [OTC]
  difenoxin and atropine
  diphenoxylate and atropine
  Donnagel®-MB (Can)
  Donnagel®-PG Capsule (Can)
  Donnagel®-PG Suspension (Can)
  Fowlers Diarrhea Tablet (Can)
  Fowlers Oral Suspension (Can)
  Imodium®
  Imodium® A-D [OTC]
  Imodium® Advanced
  Kaodene® [OTC]
  kaolin and pectin
  kaolin and pectin with opium
  Kaopectate® Advanced Formula [OTC]
  Kaopectate® II [OTC]
  Kaopectate® Maximum Strength Caplets
  Kao-Spen® [OTC]
  Kapectolin® [OTC]
  Logen®
  Lomanate®
  Lomotil®
  Lonox®
  Loperacap (Can)
  loperamide
  Motofen®
  Parepectolin®
  Pepto® Diarrhea Control [OTC]
  PMS-Loperamine (Can)
  Rheaban® [OTC]
Gastrointestinal Agent, Miscellaneous
  Bacid® [OTC]
  Bismatrol® [OTC]
  Bismed (Can)
  bismuth subgallate
  bismuth subsalicylate
  Bismylate (Can)
  calcium polycarbophil
  Devrom® [OTC]
  Equalactin® Chewable Tablet [OTC]
  Fermalac® (Can)
  Fiberall® Chewable Tablet [OTC]
  FiberCon® Tablet [OTC]
  Fiber-Lax® Tablet [OTC]
  Lactinex® [OTC]
  Lactobacillus
  Mitrolan® Chewable Tablet [OTC]
  More-Dophilus® [OTC]
  Pepto-Bismol® [OTC]

Somatostatin Analog
  octreotide
  Sandostatin®
  Sandostatin LAR®

DIARRHEA (BACTERIAL)
  Mycifradin® Sulfate
  Myciguent (Can)
  Neo-fradin®
  neomycin
  Neo-Tabs®

DIARRHEA (BILE ACIDS)
Bile Acid Sequestrant
  cholestyramine resin
  LoCHOLEST®
  LoCHOLEST® Light
  Novo-Cholamine (Can)
  PMS-Cholestyramine (Can)
  Prevalite®
  Questran®
  Questran® Light

DIARRHEA (TRAVELER'S)
  Bismatrol® [OTC]
  Bismed (Can)
  bismuth subsalicylate
  Bismylate (Can)
  Pepto-Bismol® [OTC]

DIVERTICULITIS
Aminoglycoside (Antibiotic)
  Alcomicin (Can)
  Cidomycin (Can)
  Diogent (Can)
  Garamycin®
  Garatec (Can)
  Genoptic®
  Gentacidin®
  gentamicin
  Gentrasul®
  G-myticin®
  Jenamicin®
  Nebcin® Injection

Ocugram (Can)
PMS-Tobramycin (Can)
RO-Gentycin (Can)
TOBI™ Inhalation Solution
tobramycin
Antibiotic, Miscellaneous
  Apo®-Metronidazole (Can)
  Azactam®
  aztreonam
  Cleocin HCl® Oral
  Cleocin Pediatric® Oral
  Cleocin Phosphate® Injection
  Cleocin® Vaginal
  Clinda-Derm® Topical
  clindamycin
  Dalacin® C (Can)
  Dalacin T (Can)
  Flagyl® Oral
  Metro I.V.® Injection
  metronidazole
  Neo-Metric (Can)
  NidaGel (Can)
  Noritate (Can)
  Novo-Nidazol (Can)
  Protostat® Oral
  Trikacide (Can)
Carbapenem (Antibiotic)
  imipenem and cilastatin
  Primaxin®
Cephalosporin (Second Generation)
  cefmetazole
  Cefotan®
  cefotetan
  cefoxitin
  Mefoxin®
  Zefazone®
Penicillin
  ampicillin
  ampicillin and sulbactam
  Ampicin (Can)
  Ampicin® Sodium (Can)
  Ampilean (Can)
  Apo®-Ampi (Can)

bacampicillin
Jaa Amp® (Can)
Marcillin®
Nu-Ampi (Can)
Omnipen®
Omnipen®-N
Penglobe (Can)
piperacillin and tazobactam sodium
Principen®
Spectrobid® Tablet
Tazocin (Can)
ticarcillin and clavulanate potassium
Timentin®
Totacillin®
Unasyn®
Zosyn™

DUODENAL ULCER
Antacid
  calcium carbonate and simethicone
  magaldrate
  magaldrate and simethicone
  magnesium hydroxide
  magnesium oxide
  Mag-Ox® 400 [OTC]
  Maox® [OTC]
  Phillips'® Milk of Magnesia
    [OTC]
  Riopan® [OTC]
  Riopan Plus® [OTC]
  Titralac® Plus Liquid [OTC]
  Uro-Mag® [OTC]
Diagnostic Agent
  pentagastrin
  Peptavlon®
Gastric Acid Secretion Inhibitor
  Aciphex™
  lansoprazole
  Losec® (Can)
  omeprazole
  Prevacid®
  Prilosec™
  rabeprazole

Gastrointestinal Agent, Gastric or
  Duodenal Ulcer Treatment
  Carafate®
  Novo-Sucralate (Can)
  PMS-Sucralfate (Can)
  ranitidine bismuth citrate
  sucralfate
  Sulcrate®
  Tritec®
Histamine H$_2$ Antagonist
  Apo®-Cimetidine (Can)
  Apo®-Famotidine (Can)
  Apo®-Nizatidine (Can)
  Apo®-Ranitidine (Can)
  Axid®
  Axid® AR [OTC]
  cimetidine
  famotidine
  Gaviscon Prevent (Can)
  Maalox H2 Acid Controller (Can)
  nizatidine
  Novo-Cimetine (Can)
  Novo-Famotidine (Can)
  Novo-Ranidine (Can)
  Nu-Cimet (Can)
  Nu-Famotidine (Can)
  Nu-Ranit (Can)
  Pepcid®
  Pepcid® AC Acid Controller [OTC]
  Pepcid RPD®
  Peptol® (Can)
  ranitidine hydrochloride
  Tagamet®
  Tagamet-HB® [OTC]
  Zantac®
  Zantac® 75 [OTC]

DYSURIA
Analgesic, Urinary
  Azo-Dine®
  Azo-Gesic®
  Azo-Natural®
  Azo-Standard®

Baridium®
Geridium®
Phenazo (Can)
phenazopyridine
Prodium™ [OTC]
Pyridiate®
Pyridium®
Pyronium® (Can)
Re-Azo®
Uristat® [OTC]
Urodine®
Urodol®
Urofemme® [OTC]
Urogesic®
UTI Relief® [OTC]
Vito Reins® (Can)
Antispasmodic Agent, Urinary
flavoxate
Urispas®
Sulfonamide
Azo Gantrisin (Can)
sulfisoxazole and phenazopyridine

ENURESIS
Anticholinergic Agent
belladonna
Antidepressant, Tricyclic (Tertiary Amine)
Apo®-Imipramine (Can)
imipramine
Impril (Can)
Janimine®
Novo-Pramine (Can)
PMS-Imipramine (Can)
Tofranil®
Tofranil-PM®
Antispasmodic Agent, Urinary
Albert® Oxybutynin (Can)
Ditropan®
Ditropan® XL
Nu-Oxybutyn (Can)
Oxybutyn (Can)
oxybutynin

Vasopressin Analog, Synthetic
DDAVP®
desmopressin acetate
Octostim® (Can)
Stimate®

ERECTILE DYSFUNCTION (ED)
sildenafil
Viagra®

ESOPHAGEAL VARIX
Hormone, Posterior Pituitary
Pitressin®
Pressyn® (Can)
vasopressin
Sclerosing Agent
Ethamolin®
ethanolamine oleate
sodium tetradecyl
Sotradecol®
Tromboject (Can)
Trombovar (Can)

ESOPHAGITIS
lansoprazole
Losec® (Can)
omeprazole
Prevacid®
Prilosec™

FAMILIAL ADENOMATOUS POLYPOSIS
Celebrex™
Celecoxib

FLATULENCE (SEE GAS PAINS)

GAG REFLEX SUPPRESSION
Analgesic, Topical
Anestacon® Topical Solution
Dilocaine® Injection

Duo-Trach® Injection
lidocaine
Lidodan (Can)
LidoPen® I.M. Injection Auto-
Injector
Nervocaine® Injection
Octocaine (Can)
PMS-Lidocaine Viscous (Can)
Solarcaine® Topical
Xylocaine® HCl I.V. Injection for
   Cardiac Arrhythmias
Xylocaine® Oral
Xylocaine® Topical Ointment
Xylocaine® Topical Solution
Xylocaine® Topical Spray
Xylocard® (Can)
Local Anesthetic
Americaine® [OTC]
Ametop® (Can)
Anbesol® [OTC]
Anbesol Baby (Can)
Anbesol® Maximum Strength [OTC]
Babee® Teething® [OTC]
Baby Liquid (Can)
Baby Nighttime (Can)
Baby Orajel (Can)
benzocaine
benzocaine, butyl aminobenzoate,
   tetracaine, and benzalkonium
   chloride
Benzocol® [OTC]
Benzodent® [OTC]
Cepacol Sore Throat (Can)
Cepacol Viractin (Can)
Cetacaine®
Chiggertox® [OTC]
Cylex® [OTC]
Dermoplast® [OTC]
Detane (Can)
Dyclone®
dyclonine
Foille® [OTC]
Foille® Medicated First Aid [OTC]

Hurricaine®
Lanacane® [OTC]
Maximum Strength Anbesol® [OTC]
Maximum Strength Orajel® [OTC]
Mycinettes® [OTC]
Numzitdent® [OTC]
Numzit Teething® [OTC]
Orabase®-B [OTC]
Orabase®-O [OTC]
Orajel® Brace-Aid Oral Anesthetic
   [OTC]
Orajel® Maximum Strength [OTC]
Orajel® Mouth-Aid [OTC]
Orasept® [OTC]
Orasol® [OTC]
Pontocaine®
Rhulicaine® [OTC]
Rid-A-Pain® [OTC]
Sirop Dentition (Can)
Slim-Mint® [OTC]
Solarcaine® [OTC]
Spec-T® [OTC]
Sucrets® [OTC]
Sucrets® for Kids (Can)
Supracaine (Can)
Tanac® [OTC]
Teething Syrup (Can)
tetracaine
Topicaine (Can)
Trocaine® [OTC]
Unguentine® [OTC]
Vicks Children's Chloraseptic®
   [OTC]
Vicks Chloraseptic® Sore Throat
   [OTC]
Zilactin®-B Medicated [OTC]

GAS PAIN

aluminum hydroxide, magnesium
   hydroxide, and simethicone
Amphojel Plus (Can)
Antacide Suspension avec
   Antiflatulent (Can)

Antacid Liquid (Can)
Antacid Plus Antiflatulant (Can)
Antacid Tablet (Can)
Baby's Own Infant Drops (Can)
calcium carbonate and simethicone
Centra Acid Plus (Can)
Degas® [OTC]
Di-Gel® [OTC]
Diovol Plus (Can)
Flatulex® [OTC]
Gas-Ban DS® [OTC]
Gas-X® [OTC]
Maalox Anti-Gas® [OTC]
Maalox GRF (Can)
Maalox® Plus [OTC]
magaldrate and simethicone
Magalox Plus® [OTC]
Mylanta® [OTC]
Mylanta Gas® [OTC]
Mylanta®-II [OTC]
Mylicon® [OTC]
Ovol (Can)
Phazyme® [OTC]
Riopan Plus® [OTC]
Silain® [OTC]
Siligaz (Can)
simethicone
Stomaax Plus (Can)
Titralac® Plus Liquid [OTC]

GASTRIC ULCER
Antacid
calcium carbonate and simethicone
magaldrate
magaldrate and simethicone
magnesium hydroxide
magnesium oxide
Mag-Ox® 400 [OTC]
Maox® [OTC]
Phillips'® Milk of Magnesia [OTC]
Riopan® [OTC]
Riopan Plus® [OTC]
Titralac® Plus Liquid [OTC]

Uro-Mag® [OTC]
Histamine H 2 Antagonist
Apo®-Cimetidine (Can)
Apo®-Famotidine (Can)
Apo®-Nizatidine (Can)
Apo®-Ranitidine (Can)
Axid®
Axid® AR [OTC]
cimetidine
famotidine
Gaviscon Prevent (Can)
Maalox H2 Acid Controller (Can)
nizatidine
Novo-Cimetine (Can)
Novo-Famotidine (Can)
Novo-Ranidine (Can)
Nu-Cimet (Can)
Nu-Famotidine (Can)
Nu-Ranit (Can)
Pepcid®
Pepcid® AC Acid Controller [OTC]
Pepcid RPD®
Peptol® (Can)
ranitidine hydrochloride
Tagamet®
Tagamet-HB® [OTC]
Zantac®
Zantac® 75 [OTC]
Prostaglandin
Cytotec®
Misoprostol

GASTRITIS
Antacid
Almagel (Can)
Aludrox® [OTC]
Alumag (Can)
aluminum hydroxide and magnesium
hydroxide
Amphojel 500 (Can)
Antacide Suspension (Can)
Antacid Suspension (Can)
Antiacide (Can)

Centra Acid (Can)
Diovol (Can)
Diovol EX (Can)
Gelusil® (Can)
Maalox® [OTC]
Maalox TC (Can)
Maalox® Therapeutic Concentrate
[OTC]
Mylanta® Plain (Can)
Neutralca-S (Can)
Stomaax (Can)
Univol (Can)
Histamine H 2 Antagonist
Apo®-Cimetidine (Can)
Apo®-Ranitidine (Can)
cimetidine
Gaviscon Prevent (Can)
Novo-Cimetine (Can)
Novo-Ranidine (Can)
Nu-Cimet (Can)
Nu-Ranit (Can)
Peptol® (Can)
ranitidine hydrochloride
Tagamet®
Tagamet-HB® [OTC]
Zantac®
Zantac® 75 [OTC]

GASTROESOPHAGEAL
REFLUX DISEASE (GERD)

Antacid
aluminum hydroxide and magnesium
trisilicate
Gasulsol (Can)
Gasva (Can)
Gaviscon®-2 Tablet [OTC]
Gaviscon® Tablet [OTC]
Cholinergic Agent
bethanechol
Duvoid®
Myotonachol™
PMS-Bethanechol Chloride (Can)

Urabeth®
Urecholine®
Gastric Acid Secretion Inhibitor
Aciphex™
lansoprazole
Losec® (Can)
omeprazole
Prevacid®
Prilosec™
rabeprazole
Gastrointestinal Agent, Prokinetic
Apo®-Metoclop (Can)
cisapride
Clopra®
Emex (Can)
Maxeran® (Can)
Maxolon®
metoclopramide
Octamide®
Prepulsid® (Can)
Propulsid®
Reglan®
Histamine H 2 Antagonist
Apo®-Cimetidine (Can)
Apo®-Famotidine (Can)
Apo®-Nizatidine (Can)
Apo®-Ranitidine (Can)
Axid®
Axid® AR [OTC]
cimetidine
famotidine
Gaviscon Prevent (Can)
Maalox H2 Acid Controller (Can)
nizatidine
Novo-Cimetine (Can)
Novo-Famotidine (Can)
Novo-Ranidine (Can)
Nu-Cimet (Can)
Nu-Famotidine (Can)
Nu-Ranit (Can)
Pepcid®
Pepcid® AC Acid Controller [OTC]

Pepcid RPD®
Peptol® (Can)
ranitidine hydrochloride
Tagamet®
Tagamet-HB® [OTC]
Zantac®
Zantac® 75 [OTC]
Proton Pump Inhibitor
Panto™ I.V. (Can)
Pantoloc™ (Can)
pantoprazole
Protonix®

GASTROINTESTINAL DISORDERS

Acthar®
Actharn (Can)
Adlone® Injection
Ak-Tate (Can)
Amcort® Injection
A-methaPred® Injection
Apo®-Prednisone (Can)
Aristocort® Forte Injection
Aristocort® Intralesional Injection
Aristocort® Oral
Aristospan® Intra-articular Injection
Aristospan® Intralesional Injection
Atolone® Oral
Balpred (Can)
betamethasone (systemic)
Celestone® Oral
Celestone® Phosphate Injection
Celestone® Soluspan®
Cel-U-Jec® Injection
Cortef®
corticotropin
cortisone acetate
Cortone® Acetate
Decadron® Injection
Decadron®-LA
Decadron® Oral
Decaject®

Decaject-LA®
Delta-Cortef® Oral
Deltasone®
depMedalone® Injection
Depoject® Injection
Depo-Medrol® Injection
Depopred® Injection
dexamethasone (systemic)
Dexasone®
Dexasone® L.A.
Dexone®
Dexone® LA
Diopred (Can)
D-Med® Injection
Duralone® Injection
Haldrone®
Hexadrol®
H.P. Acthar® Gel
hydrocortisone (systemic)
Hydrocortone® Acetate
Inflamase (Can)
Jaa-Prednisone® (Can)
Kenacort® Oral
Kenaject® Injection
Kenalog® Injection
Key-Pred® Injection
Key-Pred-SP® Injection
Liquid Pred®
Medralone® Injection
Medrol® Oral
Medrol Veriderm (Can)
methylprednisolone
Meticorten®
M-Prednisol® Injection
Novo-Prednisolone (Can)
Orasone®
paramethasone acetate
Pediapred® Oral
PMS-Dexamethasone (Can)
Prednicen-M®
prednisolone (systemic)
Prednisol® TBA Injection

prednisone
Prelone® Oral
RO-Predphate (Can)
Scheinpharm Triamcine-A (Can)
Solu-Cortef®
Solu-Medrol® Injection
Solurex L.A.®
Stemex®
Tac™-3 Injection
Tac™-40 Injection
Triam-A® Injection
triamcinolone (systemic)
Triam Forte® Injection
Triamonide® Injection
Tri-Kort® Injection
Trilog® Injection
Trilone® Injection
Trisoject® Injection
Ultracortenol (Can)
Winpred (Can)

GENITAL HERPES
famciclovir
Famvir™
valacyclovir
Valtrex®

GENITAL WART
Aldara™
Imiquimod

GIARDIASIS
Amebicide
Apo®-Metronidazole (Can)
Flagyl® Oral
Humatin®
Metrocream (Can)
Metro I.V.® Injection
metronidazole
Neo-Metric (Can)
NidaGel (Can)
Noritate (Can)
Novo-Nidazol (Can)
paromomycin

Protostat® Oral
Trikacide (Can)
Anthelmintic
albendazole
Albenza®
Antiprotozoal
furazolidone
Furoxone®

GINGIVITIS
BactoShield® [OTC]
Baxedin (Can)
Betasept® [OTC]
chlorhexidine gluconate
Chlorhexseptic (Can)
Dyna-Hex® [OTC]
Exidine® Scrub [OTC]
Hexifoam (Can)
Hibidil (Can)
Hibitane (Can)
Oro-Clense (Can)
Peridex®
Periochip®
PerioGard®
Rouhex-G (Can)
Spectro Gram (Can)

GONORRHEA
Antibiotic, Macrolide
Rovamycine® (Can)
spiramycin (Canada only)
Antibiotic, Miscellaneous
spectinomycin
Trobicin®
Antibiotic, Quinolone
gatifloxacin
Tequin™
Cephalosporin (Second Generation)
cefoxitin
Ceftin® Oral
cefuroxime
Kefurox® Injection
Mefoxin®
Zinacef® Injection

Cephalosporin (Third Generation)
  cefixime
  ceftriaxone
  Rocephin®
  Suprax®
Quinolone
  Apo®-Oflox (Can)
  Ciloxan™ Ophthalmic
  Cipro®
  ciprofloxacin
  Floxin®
  Ocuflox™ Ophthalmic
  ofloxacin
Tetracycline Derivative
  Achromycin® Ophthalmic
  Achromycin® Topical
  Achromycin V (Can)
  Apo®-Doxy Tabs (Can)
  Apo®-Tetra (Can)
  Bio-Tab®
  Doryx®
  Doxy-200®
  Doxy-Caps®
  Doxychel®
  Doxycin (Can)
  doxycycline
  Doxy-Tabs®
  Doxytec (Can)
  Monodox®
  Nor-tet® Oral
  Novo-Doxylin (Can)
  Novo-Tetra (Can)
  Nu-Doxycycline (Can)
  Nu-Tetra (Can)
  Panmycin® Oral
  Robitet® Oral
  Sumycin® Oral
  Tetracap® Oral
  tetracycline
  Tetracyn (Can)
  Topicycline® Topical
  Vibramycin®
  Vibra-Tabs®

HELICOBACTER PYLORI INFECTION
Antibiotic, Miscellaneous
  Apo®-Metronidazole (Can)
  Flagyl® Oral
  Metrocream (Can)
  Metro I.V.® Injection
  metronidazole
  Neo-Metric (Can)
  NidaGel (Can)
  Noritate (Can)
  Novo-Nidazol (Can)
  Protostat® Oral
  Trikacide (Can)
Antidiarrheal
  bismuth subsalicylate, metronidazole, and tetracycline
  Helidac™
Gastrointestinal Agent, Gastric or Duodenal Ulcer Treatment
  ranitidine bismuth citrate
  Tritec®
Gastrointestinal Agent, Miscellaneous
  Bismatrol® [OTC]
  Bismed (Can)
  bismuth subsalicylate
  Bismylate (Can)
  Pepto-Bismol® [OTC]
Macrolide (Antibiotic)
  Biaxin®
  Biaxin® XL
  clarithromycin
Penicillin
  amoxicillin
  Amoxil®
  Apo®-Amoxi (Can)
  Gen-Amoxicillin (Can)
  Novamoxin® (Can)
  Nu-Amoxi (Can)
  Pro-Amox® (Can)
  Trimox®
  Wymox®

Tetracycline Derivative
  Achromycin V (Can)
  Apo®-Tetra (Can)
  Nor-tet® Oral
  Novo-Tetra (Can)
  Nu-Tetra (Can)
  Panmycin® Oral
  Robitet® Oral
  Sumycin® Oral
  Tetracap® Oral
  tetracycline
  Tetracyn (Can)

HEMORRHOID
Adrenal Corticosteroid
  Anusol-HC® Suppository
  Colocort™
  Cortenema® Rectal
  Corticreme (Can)
  Cortifoam® Rectal
  Cortiment (Can)
  hydrocortisone (rectal)
  Proctocort™ Rectal
  ProctoCream ® HC Cream
  Rectocort (Can)
Anesthetic/Corticosteroid
  Corticaine® Topical
  dibucaine and hydrocortisone
  Enzone®
  Pramosone®
  Pramox HC (Can)
  pramoxine and hydrocortisone
  ProctoFoam®-HC
  Zone-A Forte®
Astringent
  Preparation H® Cleansing Pads (Can)
  Tucks® [OTC]
  witch hazel
Local Anesthetic
  Americaine® [OTC]
  Anusol® Ointment [OTC]
  benzocaine
  Dermoplast® [OTC]

dibucaine
Foille® [OTC]
Foille® Medicated First Aid [OTC]
Hurricaine®
Lanacane® [OTC]
Nupercainal® [OTC]
pramoxine
Prax® [OTC]
ProctoFoam® NS [OTC]
tetracaine
Tronolane® [OTC]
Tronothane® [OTC]

HEPATIC CIRRHOSIS
amiloride
Midamor®

HEPATITIS A
Gammabulin Immuno (Can)
immune globulin (intramuscular)

HEPATITIS B
Antiviral Agent
  Epivir®
  Epivir®-HBV™
  Heptovir® (Can)
  interferon alfa-2b and ribavirin
    combination pack
  lamivudine
  Rebetron™
  3TC® (Can)
Biological Response Modulator
  interferon alfa-2b
  interferon alfa-2b and ribavirin
    combination pack
  Intron® A
  Rebetron™
Reverse Transcriptase Inhibitor
  adefovir
  Preveon®

HEPATITIS C
Antiviral Agent
  interferon alfa-2b and ribavirin
    combination pack

Rebetron™
Biological Response Modulator
  interferon alfa-2b
  interferon alfa-2b and ribavirin
    combination pack
  Intron® A
  Rebetron™
Interferon
  Infergen®
  interferon alfacon-1

HERPES SIMPLEX

Antiviral Agent
  acyclovir
  Avirax® (Can)
  Cytovene®
  famciclovir
  Famvir™
  foscarnet
  Foscavir®
  ganciclovir
  trifluridine
  vidarabine
  Vira-A® Ophthalmic
  Viroptic® Ophthalmic
  Vitrasert®
  Zovirax®

HIATAL HERNIA

calcium carbonate and simethicone
magaldrate
magaldrate and simethicone
Riopan® [OTC]
Riopan Plus® [OTC]
Titralac® Plus Liquid [OTC]

HICCUPS

Apo®-Chlorpromazine (Can)
Chlorpromanyl (Can)
chlorpromazine
Chlorprom® (Can)
Largactil (Can)
Ormazine®
Thorazine®

triflupromazine
Vesprin®

HOOKWORM

albendazole
Albenza®
Antiminth® [OTC]
Combantrin (Can)
Jaa Pyral® (Can)
mebendazole
Pin-Rid® [OTC]
Pin-X® [OTC]
pyrantel pamoate
Reese's® Pinworm Medicine [OTC]
Vermox®

HYPERACIDITY

Antacid
  Alka-Mints® [OTC]
  Almagel (Can)
  ALternaGEL® [OTC]
  Alu-Cap® [OTC]
  Aludrox® [OTC]
  Alugel (Can)
  Alumag (Can)
  aluminum carbonate
  aluminum hydroxide
  aluminum hydroxide and magnesium
    carbonate
  aluminum hydroxide and magnesium
    hydroxide
  aluminum hydroxide and magnesium
    trisilicate
  aluminum hydroxide, magnesium
    hydroxide, and simethicone
  Alu-Tab® [OTC]
  Amitone® [OTC]
  Amphojel® [OTC]
  Amphojel 500 (Can)
  Amphojel Plus (Can)
  Antacide Suspension avec
    Antiflatulent (Can)
  Antacide Suspension (Can)
  Antacid Liquid (Can)

Antacid Plus Antiflatulant (Can)
Antacid Suspension (Can)
Antacid Tablet (Can)
Antiacide (Can)
Apo®-Cal® (Can)
Basaljel® [OTC]
Basaljel (Can)
Biocal (Can)
Brioschi (Can)
Cal-500 (Can)
Cal Carb-HD® [OTC]
Calci-Chew™ [OTC]
Calciday-667® [OTC]
Calci-Mix™ [OTC]
Calcite (Can)
calcium carbonate
Calcium Carbonate and Magnesium
   Hydroxide
calcium carbonate and simethicone
Cal-Plus® [OTC]
Calsan (Can)
Caltrate® 600 [OTC]
Caltrate, Jr.® [OTC]
Centra Acid (Can)
Centra Acid Plus (Can)
Chooz® [OTC]
Dialume® [OTC]
Dicarbosil® [OTC]
Di-Gel® [OTC]
dihydroxyaluminum sodium
   carbonate
Diovol (Can)
Diovol EX (Can)
Diovol Plus (Can)
Equilet® [OTC]
Florical® [OTC]
Gas-Ban DS® [OTC]
Gasulsol (Can)
Gasva (Can)
Gaviscon®-2 Tablet [OTC]
Gaviscon® Liquid [OTC]
Gaviscon® Tablet [OTC]
Gelusil® (Can)

Gencalc® 600 [OTC]
Hi Potency Cal (Can)
Maalox® [OTC]
Maalox® Plus [OTC]
Maalox Quick Dissolve (Can)
Maalox TC (Can)
Maalox® Therapeutic Concentrate
   [OTC]
magaldrate
magaldrate and simethicone
Magalox Plus® [OTC]
magnesium hydroxide
magnesium oxide
Mag-Ox® 400 [OTC]
Mallamint® [OTC]
Maox® [OTC]
Mega-Cal (Can)
Mylanta® [OTC]
Mylanta® Gelcaps® [OTC]
Mylanta®-II [OTC]
Mylanta® Plain (Can)
Mylanta® Tablets [OTC]
Mylanta® Ultra Tablet [OTC]
Neo Cal (Can)
Nephro-Calci® [OTC]
Nephrox Suspension [OTC]
Neut®
Neutralca-S (Can)
Os-Cal® 500 [OTC]
Oyst-Cal 500 [OTC]
Oystercal® 500
Pharmacal (Can)
Phillips'® Milk of Magnesia [OTC]
Riopan® [OTC]
Riopan Plus® [OTC]
Rolaids® [OTC]
Rolaids® Calcium Rich [OTC]
sodium bicarbonate
Stomaax (Can)
Stomaax Plus (Can)
Titralac (Can)
Titralac® Plus Liquid [OTC]
Tums® [OTC]

Tums® E-X Extra Strength Tablet
[OTC]
Tums® Extra Strength Liquid [OTC]
Univol (Can)
Uro-Mag® [OTC]
Electrolyte Supplement, Oral
Calcimax (Can)
calcium lactate
Calcium-Sandoz (Can)

HYPOGONADISM

Androgen
Andriol (Can)
Androderm® Transdermal System
Android®
Andro-L.A.® Injection
Andropository® Injection
Delatest® Injection
Delatestryl® Injection
depAndro® Injection
Depotest® Injection
Depo®-Testosterone Injection
Duratest® Injection
Durathate® Injection
Everone® Injection
Histerone® Injection
Malogen Aqueous (Can)
Malogen in Oil (Can)
Malogex (Can)
Metandren (Can)
methyltestosterone
Oreton® Methyl
Scheinpharm Testone-Cyp (Can)
Tesamone® Injection
Testoderm®
Testoderm® TTS
Testoderm® with Adhesive
Testopel® Pellet
testosterone
Tcstrcd®
Virilon®
Diagnostic Agent
Factrel®

gonadorelin
Lutrepulse®
Relisorm (Can)

HYPONATREMIA

Electrolyte Supplement, Oral
sodium acetate
sodium bicarbonate
sodium chloride
sodium phosphates

IMPOTENCY

Androgen
Android®
Metandren (Can)
methyltestosterone
Oreton® Methyl
Testred®
Virilon®
Miscellaneous Product
Aphrodyne™
Dayto Himbin®
Yocon®
yohimbine
Yohimex™
Vasodilator
ethaverine
Ethavex-100®

INFERTILITY

Antigonadotropic Agent
Antagon™
Ganirelix

INFERTILITY (MALE)

Gonadotropin
A.P.L.®
Chorex®
chorionic gonadotropin
Choron®
Corgonject®
Follutein®
Glukor®
Gonic®
Humegon™

menotropins
Pergonal®
Pregnyl®
Profasi® HP
Repronex™

INFLAMMATORY BOWEL DISEASE
Apo®-Sulfasalazine (Can)
Asacol® Oral
Azulfidine®
Azulfidine® EN-tabs®
Dipentum®
mesalamine
Mesasal (Can)
olsalazine
Pentasa® Oral
PMS-Sulfasa (Can)
Quintasa (Can)
Rowasa® Rectal
Salazopyrin (Can)
Salofalk (Can)
Sulfasalazine

INTERSTITIAL CYSTITIS
Analgesic, Urinary
Elmiron®
pentosan polysulfate sodium
Urinary Tract Product
dimethyl sulfoxide
Kemsol (Can)
Rimso®-50

INTESTINAL ABSORPTION (DIAGNOSTIC)
d-xylose
Xylo-Pfan® [OTC]

IRRITABLE BOWEL SYNDROME (IBS)
Antispasmodic Agent, Gastrointestinal
Modulon® (Can)
trimebutine (Canada only)
Gastrointestinal Agent, Miscellaneous

Dicetel® (Can)
pinaverium (Canada only)
5-HT3 Receptor Antagonist
alosetron
Lotronex®

KIDNEY STONE
Alkalinizing Agent
Polycitra®
potassium citrate
sodium citrate and potassium citrate
mixture
Urocit®-K
Chelating Agent
Cuprimine®
Depen®
penicillamine
Electrolyte Supplement, Oral
K-Phos® Neutral
Neutra-Phos®-K
potassium phosphate
potassium phosphate and sodium
phosphate
Uro-KP-Neutral®
Irrigating Solution
citric acid bladder mixture
Renacidin®
Urinary Tract Product
Calcibind®
cellulose sodium phosphate
Thiola™
tiopronin
Xanthine Oxidase Inhibitor
Alloprim™ Injection
Alloprin (Can)
allopurinol
Apo®-Allopurinol (Can)
Novo-Purol (Can)
Purinol® (Can)
Zyloprim®

LACTOSE INTOLERANCE
Dairyaid (Can)
Dairy Ease® [OTC]

LactAid® [OTC]
lactase
Lactrase® [OTC]
PMS-Prolactase (Can)
Prolactase (Can)

MALABSORPTION

Trace Element
  Chroma-Pak®
  Iodopen®
  Molypen®
  M.T.E.-4®
  M.T.E.-5®
  M.T.E.-6®
  MulTE-PAK-4®
  MulTE-PAK-5®
  Neotrace-4®
  PedTE-PAK-4®
  Pedtrace-4®
  P.T.E.-4®
  P.T.E.-5®
  Sele-Pak®
  Selepen®
  Trace-4®
  trace metals
  Zinca-Pak®
Vitamin, Fat Soluble
  Aquasol A®
  Arovit (Can)
  Del-Vi-A®
  Palmitate-A® 5000 [OTC]
  vitamin A

MALNUTRITION

Electrolyte Supplement, Oral
  Anusol (Can)
  Anuzinc (Can)
  Eye-Sed® Ophthalmic [OTC]
  Micro Zn (Can)
  Orazinc® Oral [OTC]
  PMS-Egozinc (Can)
  Verazinc® Oral [OTC]
  Zincate® Oral
  zinc sulfate

Nutritional Supplement
  cysteine
  glucose polymers
  Moducal® [OTC]
  Polycose® [OTC]
  Sumacal® [OTC]
Trace Element
  Chroma-Pak®
  Iodopen®
  Molypen®
  M.T.E.-4®
  M.T.E.-5®
  M.T.E.-6®
  MulTE-PAK-4®
  MulTE-PAK-5®
  Neotrace-4®
  PedTE-PAK-4®
  Pedtrace-4®
  P.T.E.-4®
  P.T.E.-5®
  Sele-Pak®
  Selepen®
  Trace-4®
  trace metals
  Zinca-Pak®
  zinc chloride
Vitamin
  Adeflor®
  ADEKs® Pediatric Drops
  Becotin® Pulvules®
  Cefol® Filmtab®
  Chromagen® OB [OTC]
  Eldercaps® [OTC]
  Icaps® (Can)
  Infantol® (Can)
  LKV-Drops® [OTC]
  Maltlevol® (Can)
  Materna® (Can)
  Multi Vit® Drops [OTC]
  M.V.C.® 9 + 3
  M.V.I.®-12
  M.V.I.® Concentrate
  M.V.I.® Pediatric

Natabec® [OTC]
Natabec® FA [OTC]
Natabec® Rx
Natalins® [OTC]
Natalins® Rx
NeoVadrin® [OTC]
Niferex®-PN
Ocuvite™ (Can)
Orifer® F (Can)
Penta/3B® Plus (Can)
Poly-Vi-Flor®
Poly-Vi-Sol® [OTC]
Pramet® FA
Pramilet® FA
Prenavite® [OTC]
Prenavite® Forte (Can)
Secran®
Sopalamine/3B Plus C (Can)
Spectrum™ Forte 29 (Can)
Stresstabs® 600 Advanced Formula
    Tablets [OTC]
Stuartnatal® 1 + 1
Stuart Prenatal® [OTC]
Therabid® [OTC]
Theragran® [OTC]
Theragran® Hematinic®
Theragran® Liquid [OTC]
Theragran-M® [OTC]
Tri-Vi-Flor®
Tri-Vi-Sol® [OTC]
Unicap® [OTC]
Vicon Forte®
Vicon® Plus [OTC]
Vi-Daylin® [OTC]
Vi-Daylin/F®
vitamin (multiple/injectable)
vitamin (multiple/oral)
vitamin (multiple/pediatric)
vitamin (multiple/prenatal)
Vitamin, Fat Soluble
    Amino-Opti-E® [OTC]
    Aquasol A®
    Aquasol E® [OTC]

Arovit (Can)
Del-Vi-A®
E-Complex-600® [OTC]
E-Vitamin® [OTC]
Novo E (Can)
Organex (Can)
Palmitate-A® 5000 [OTC]
Vita-E (Can)
vitamin A
vitamin E
Vita-Plus® E Softgels® [OTC]
Vitec® [OTC]
Vite E® Creme [OTC]
Vitamin, Water Soluble
    Apatate® [OTC]
    B6–250 (Can)
    Betalin®S
    Betaxin® (Can)
    Bewon® (Can)
    Gevrabon® [OTC]
    Hexa-Betalin (Can)
    Lederplex® [OTC]
    Lipovite® [OTC]
    Mega B® [OTC]
    Megaton™ [OTC]
    Mucoplex® [OTC]
    NeoVadrin® B Complex [OTC]
    Nestrex®
    Orexin® [OTC]
    pyridoxine
    Surbex® [OTC]
    thiamine
    vitamin B complex

MAPLE SYRUP URINE DISEASE
Betalin®S
Betaxin® (Can)
Bewon® (Can)
Thiamine

MASTOCYTOSIS
Apo®-Cimetidine (Can)
Apo®-Famotidine (Can)

Apo®-Ranitidine (Can)
cimetidine
famotidine
Gaviscon Prevent (Can)
Maalox H2 Acid Controller (Can)
Novo-Cimetinc (Can)
Novo-Famotidine (Can)
Novo-Ranidine (Can)
Nu-Cimet (Can)
Nu-Famotidine (Can)
Nu-Ranit (Can)
Pepcid®
Pepcid® AC Acid Controller [OTC]
Pepcid RPD®
Peptol® (Can)
ranitidine hydrochloride
Tagamet®
Tagamet-HB® [OTC]
Zantac®
Zantac® 75 [OTC]

MECONIUM ILEUS
acetylcysteine
Airbron (Can)
Mucomyst®
Mucosil™
Parvolex (Can)

MOUTH INFECTION
Dequadin® (Can)
dequalinium (Canada only)

NAUSEA (ALSO SEE VOMITING)
Anticholinergic Agent
Buscopan (Can)
Isopto® Hyoscine
Scopace® Tablet
scopolamine
Transderm Scop®
Transderm-V (Can)
Antiemetic
Benzacot® Injection
Cesamet®
dronabinol
droperidol
Emecheck® [OTC]
Emetrol® [OTC]
Inapsine®
Marinol®
nabilone
Naus-A-Way® [OTC]
Nausetrol® [OTC]
phosphorated carbohydrate solution
Tigan®
trimethobenzamide
Antihistamine
Calm-X® Oral [OTC]
Children's Motion Sickness Liquid (Can)
cyclizine
dimenhydrinate
Dimetabs® Oral
Dinate® Injection
Dramamine® Oral [OTC]
Dramilin® Injection
Dymenate® Injection
Gravol (Can)
Hydrate® Injection
Marezine® Oral [OTC]
Marmine® Injection
Marmine® Oral [OTC]
Nauseatol (Can)
Nausex (Can)
Novo-Dimenate (Can)
Tega-Vert® Oral
Travamine (Can)
Travel Aid (Can)
Travelmate (Can)
Travel Tabs (Can)
TripTone® Caplets® [OTC]
Gastrointestinal Agent, Prokinetic
Apo®-Metoclop (Can)
Clopra®
Emex (Can)
Maxeran® (Can)
Maxolon®

metoclopramide
Octamide®
Reglan®
Phenothiazine Derivative
  Apo®-Chlorpromazine (Can)
  Apo®-Perphenazine (Can)
  Chlorpromanyl (Can)
  chlorpromazine
  Chlorprom® (Can)
  Compazine®
  Histantil (Can)
  Largactil (Can)
  Nu-Prochlor (Can)
  Ormazine®
  perphenazine
  Phenazine® Injection
  Phenergan® Injection
  Phenergan® Oral
  Phenergan® Rectal
  PMS-Perphenazine (Can)
  PMS-Prochlorperazine (Can)
  prochlorperazine
  promethazine
  Prorazin® (Can)
  Prorex® Injection
  Stemetil (Can)
  thiethylperazine
  Thorazine®
  Torecan (Can)
  triflupromazine
  Trilafon®
  Vesprin®
Selective 5-HT 3 Receptor
    Antagonist
  granisetron
  Kytril™
  ondansetron
  Zofran®
  Zofran® ODT

NEPHROLITHIASIS
  potassium citrate
  Urocit®-K

NEPHROPATHIC CYSTINOSIS
  Cystagon®
  Cysteamine

NEPHROTIC SYNDROME
Adrenal Corticosteroid
  Acthar®
  Actharn (Can)
  Adlone® Injection
  Ak-Tate (Can)
  Amcort® Injection
  A-methaPred® Injection
  Apo®-Prednisone (Can)
  Aristocort® Forte Injection
  Aristocort® Oral
  Aristospan® Intra-articular Injection
  Atolone® Oral
  Balpred (Can)
  betamethasone (systemic)
  Celestone® Oral
  Celestone® Phosphate Injection
  Celestone® Soluspan®
  Cel-U-Jec® Injection
  Cortef®
  corticotropin
  cortisone acetate
  Cortone® Acetate
  Decadron® Injection
  Decadron®-LA
  Decadron® Oral
  Decaject®
  Decaject-LA®
  Delta-Cortef® Oral
  Deltasone®
  depMedalone® Injection
  Depoject® Injection
  Depo-Medrol® Injection
  Depopred® Injection
  dexamethasone (systemic)
  Dexasone®
  Dexasone® L.A.
  Dexone®

Dexone® LA
Diopred (Can)
D-Med® Injection
Duralone® Injection
Haldrone®
Hexadrol®
H.P. Acthar® Gel
hydrocortisone (systemic)
Hydrocortone® Acetate
Inflamase (Can)
Jaa-Prednisone® (Can)
Kenacort® Oral
Kenaject® Injection
Kenalog® Injection
Key-Pred® Injection
Key-Pred-SP® Injection
Liquid Pred®
Medralone® Injection
Medrol® Oral
Medrol Veriderm (Can)
methylprednisolone
Meticorten®
M-Prednisol® Injection
Novo-Prednisolone (Can)
Orasone®
paramethasone acetate
Pediapred® Oral
PMS-Dexamethasone (Can)
Prednicen-M®
prednisolone (systemic)
Prednisol® TBA Injection
prednisone
Prelone® Oral
RO-Predphate (Can)
Scheinpharm Triamcine-A (Can)
Solu-Cortef®
Solu-Medrol® Injection
Solurex L.A.®
Stemex®
Tac™-3 Injection
Tac™-40 Injection
Triam-A® Injection
triamcinolone (systemic)

Triam Forte® Injection
Triamonide® Injection
Tri-Kort® Injection
Trilog® Injection
Trilone® Injection
Trisoject® Injection
Ultracortenol (Can)
Winpred (Can)
Antihypertensive Agent, Combination
Alazide®
Aldactazide®
Apo®-Spirozide (Can)
Apo®-Triazide (Can)
Dyazide®
hydrochlorothiazide and
    spironolactone
hydrochlorothiazide and triamterene
Maxzide®
Novo-Spirozine (Can)
Novo-Triamzide (Can)
Nu-Triazide (Can)
Spironazide®
Spirozide®
Diuretic, Loop
Apo®-Furosemide (Can)
bumetanide
Bumex®
Burinex® (Can)
Demadex®
furosemide
Furoside® (Can)
Lasix®
Novo-Semide (Can)
torsemide
Uritol® (Can)
Diuretic, Miscellaneous
Apo®-Chlorthalidone (Can)
Apo®-Indapadmide (Can)
chlorthalidone
Hygroton®
indapamide
Lozide® (Can)
Lozol®

metolazone
Mykrox®
Novo-Thalidone (Can)
PMS-Indapamide (Can)
Thalitone®
Uridon® (Can)
Zaroxolyn®
Diuretic, Thiazide
Apo®-Hydro (Can)
Aquatensen®
bendroflumethiazide
benzthiazide
chlorothiazide
Diucardin®
Diuchlor® (Can)
Diuchlor H (Can)
Diurigen®
Diuril®
Duretic (Can)
Enduron®
Esidrix®
Exna®
Ezide®
hydrochlorothiazide
HydroDIURIL®
hydroflumethiazide
Hydro-Par®
Metahydrin®
methyclothiazide
Microzide™
Naqua®
Naturetin®
Neo-Codema® (Can)
Novo-Hydrazide (Can)
Oretic®
Saluron®
trichlormethiazide
Urozide® (Can)
Immunosuppressant Agent
azathioprine
cyclosporine
Imuran®
Neoral®

Sandimmune®
SangCya™

NEPHROTOXICITY (CISPLATIN-INDUCED)
amifostine
Ethyol®

NEUROGENIC BLADDER
Anticholinergic Agent
Banthine®
methantheline
Antispasmodic Agent, Urinary
Albert® Oxybutynin (Can)
Ditropan®
Ditropan® XL
Nu-Oxybutyn (Can)
Oxybutyn (Can)
Oxybutynin

NOCTURIA
Antispasmodic Agent, Urinary
flavoxate
Urispas®

ORAL LESION
benzocaine, gelatin, pectin, and
sodium carboxymethylcellulose
Orabase® With Benzocaine [OTC]

OSTOMY CARE
A and D™ Ointment [OTC]
Aquasol A & D (Can)
Nutrol A D (Can)
vitamin A and vitamin D

OVERACTIVE BLADDER
Detrol™
Tolterodine

PANCREATIC EXOCRINE INSUFFICIENCY
Cotazym®
Cotazym-S®

Creon®
Creon® 5
Creon® 10
Creon® 20
Digepepsin®
Digcss (Can)
Donnazyme®
Hi-Vegi-Lip®
Ilozyme®
Ku-Zyme® HP
Lipram®
Opti-Zyme (Can)
Pancrease®
Pancrease® MT 4
Pancrease® MT 10
Pancrease® MT 16
Pancrease® MT 20
pancreatin
Pancrecarb MS-4®
Pancrecarb MS-8®
pancrelipase
Pancrex (Can)
Protilase®
Ultrase®
Ultrase® MT12
Ultrase® MT18
Ultrase® MT20
Viokase®
Zymase®

PANCREATIC EXOCRINE INSUFFICIENCY (DIAGNOSTIC)
secretin
Secretin-Ferring Powder

PANCREATITIS
Anticholinergic Agent
Banthine®
methantheline
Pro-Banthine®
Propanthel (Can)
propantheline

PARALYTIC ILEUS (PROPHYLAXIS)
Gastrointestinal Agent, Stimulant
dexpanthenol
Ilopan-Choline® Oral
Ilopan® Injection
Panthoderm® Cream [OTC]

PEPTIC ULCER
Antibiotic, Miscellaneous
Apo®-Metronidazole (Can)
Flagyl® Oral
Metro I.V.® Injection
metronidazole
Neo-Metric (Can)
NidaGel (Can)
Noritate (Can)
Novo-Nidazol (Can)
Protostat® Oral
Trikacide (Can)
Anticholinergic Agent
Anaspaz®
Apo®-Chlorax (Can)
A-Spas® S/L
atropine
Banthine®
Barbidonna®
belladonna
Bellatal®
Cantil®
clidinium and chlordiazepoxide
Clindex®
Corium® (Can)
Cystospaz®
Cystospaz-M®
Donnamar®
Donnatal®
ED-SPAZ®
Gastrosed™
glycopyrrolate
hyoscyamine
hyoscyamine, atropine, scopolamine, and phenobarbital

Hyosophen®
Levbid®
Levsin®
Levsinex®
Levsin/SL®
Librax®
mepenzolate
methantheline
methscopolamine
Pamine®
Pathilon®
Pro-Banthine®
ProChlorax (Can)
Propanthel (Can)
propantheline
Robinul®
Robinul® Forte
Spasmolin®
tridihexethyl
Antidiarrheal
bismuth subsalicylate, metronidazole,
and tetracycline
Helidac™
Gastric Acid Secretion Inhibitor
lansoprazole
Losec® (Can)
omeprazole
Prevacid®
Prilosec™
Gastrointestinal Agent, Gastric or
Duodenal Ulcer Treatment
Carafate®
Novo-Sucralate (Can)
PMS-Sucralfate (Can)
sucralfate
Sulcrate®
Gastrointestinal Agent, Miscellaneous
Bismatrol® [OTC]
Bismed (Can)
bismuth subsalicylate
Bismylate (Can)
Pepto-Bismol® [OTC]
Histamine H$_2$ Antagonist

Apo®-Cimetidine (Can)
Apo®-Famotidine (Can)
Apo®-Nizatidine (Can)
Apo®-Ranitidine (Can)
Axid®
Axid® AR [OTC]
cimetidine
famotidine
Gaviscon Prevent (Can)
Maalox H2 Acid Controller (Can)
nizatidine
Novo-Cimetine (Can)
Novo-Famotidine (Can)
Novo-Ranidine (Can)
Nu-Cimet (Can)
Nu-Famotidine (Can)
Nu-Ranit (Can)
Pepcid®
Pepcid® AC Acid Controller [OTC]
Pepcid RPD®
Peptol® (Can)
ranitidine hydrochloride
Tagamet®
Tagamet-HB® [OTC]
Zantac®
Zantac® 75 [OTC]
Macrolide (Antibiotic)
Biaxin®
Biaxin® XL
clarithromycin
Penicillin
amoxicillin
Amoxil®
Apo®-Amoxi (Can)
Gen-Amoxicillin (Can)
Novamoxin® (Can)
Nu-Amoxi (Can)
Pro-Amox® (Can)
Trimox®
Wymox®

PERIANAL WART
Immune Response Modifier

Aldara™
imiquimod

PINWORM
Antiminth® [OTC]
Combantrin (Can)
Jaa Pyral® (Can)
mebendazole
Pin-Rid® [OTC]
Pin-X® [OTC]
pyrantel pamoate
Reese's® Pinworm Medicine [OTC]
Vermox®

PROCTITIS
Asacol® Oral
mesalamine
Mesasal (Can)
Pentasa® Oral
Quintasa (Can)
Rowasa® Rectal
Salofalk (Can)

PROCTOSIGMOIDITIS
Asacol® Oral
mesalamine
Mesasal (Can)
Pentasa® Oral
Quintasa (Can)
Rowasa® Rectal
Salofalk (Can)

PROSTATIC HYPERPLASIA (SEE BENIGN PROSTATIC HYPERPLASIA [BPH])

PROSTATITIS
Quinolone
Apo®-Oflox (Can)
Floxin®
ofloxacin
Sulfonamide
Apo®-Sulfatrim (Can)
Bactrim™

Bactrim™ DS
Cotrim®
Cotrim® DS
co-trimoxazole
Novo-Trimel (Can)
Nu-Cotrimox (Can)
Protrin (Can)
Roubac® (Can)
Septra®
Septra® DS
Sulfamethoprim®
Sulfatrim®
Sulfatrim® DS
Trisulfa® (Can)
Trisulfa-S® (Can)
Uroplus® DS
Uroplus® SS

PROTEIN UTILIZATION
Enisyl® [OTC]
l-lysine
Lycolan® Elixir [OTC]

PROTOZOAL INFECTION
Apo®-Metronidazole (Can)
Flagyl® Oral
furazolidone
Furoxone®
Metrocream (Can)
MetroGel® Topical
MetroGel®-Vaginal
Metro I.V.® Injection
metronidazole
NebuPent™ Inhalation
Neo-Metric (Can)
NidaGel (Can)
Noritate (Can)
Novo-Nidazol (Can)
Pentacarinat® Injection
Pentam-300® Injection
pentamidine
Pneumopent (Can)
Protostat® Oral
Trikacide (Can)

PYELONEPHRITIS
gatifloxacin
Tequin™

REGIONAL ENTERITIS (SEE GASTROINTESTINAL DISORDERS)

RENAL ALLOGRAFT REJECTION
antithymocyte globulin (rabbit)
Thymoglobulin®

RENAL COLIC
Analgesic, Non-narcotic
Apo®-Ketorolac (Can)
ketorolac tromethamine
Toradol®
Anticholinergic Agent
Barbidonna®
Bellatal®
Donnatal®
hyoscyamine, atropine, scopolamine, and phenobarbital
Hyosophen®
Spasmolin®

ROUNDWORM
Antiminth® [OTC]
Combantrin (Can)
Jaa Pyral® (Can)
mebendazole
Pin-Rid® [OTC]
Pin-X® [OTC]
pyrantel pamoate
Reese's® Pinworm Medicine [OTC]
Vermox®

SALIVATION (EXCESSIVE)
Anaspaz®
A-Spas® S/L
atropine
Cantil®
Cystospaz®

Cystospaz-M®
Donnamar®
ED-SPAZ®
Gastrosed™
glycopyrrolate
hyoscyamine
Levbid®
Levsin®
Levsinex®
Levsin/SL®
mepenzolate
Robinul®
Robinul® Forte
Scopace® Tablet
scopolamine

SYPHILIS
Antibiotic, Miscellaneous
chloramphenicol
Chloromycetin® Injection
Diochloram (Can)
Fenicol (Can)
Novo-Chlorocap (Can)
Ophtho-Chloram (Can)
Pentamycetin® (Can)
Sopamycetin (Can)
Spersanicol (Can)
Penicillin
Ayercillin® (Can)
Bicillin® L-A
Crysticillin® A.S.
Megacillin (Can)
penicillin G benzathine
penicillin G (parenteral/aqueous)
penicillin G procaine
Permapen®
Pfizerpen®
Wycillin®
Tetracycline Derivative
Achromycin® Ophthalmic
Achromycin® Topical
Achromycin V (Can)
Apo®-Doxy Tabs (Can)

Apo®-Tetra (Can)
Bio-Tab®
Doryx®
Doxy-200®
Doxy-Caps®
Doxychel®
Doxycin (Can)
doxycycline
Doxy-Tabs®
Doxytec (Can)
Monodox®
Nor-tet® Oral
Novo-Doxylin (Can)
Novo-Tetra (Can)
Nu-Doxycycline (Can)
Nu-Tetra (Can)
Panmycin® Oral
Robitet® Oral
Sumycin® Oral
Tetracap® Oral
tetracycline
Tetracyn (Can)
Topicycline® Topical
Vibramycin®
Vibra-Tabs®

TAPEWORM
Amebicide
Humatin®
paromomycin
Anthelmintic
Biltricide®
praziquantel

TENESMUS
belladonna and opium
B&O Supprettes®
PMS-Opium & Beladonna (Can)

TETANY
Electrolyte Supplement, Oral
calcium gluconate
H-F Antidote (Can)
Kalcinate®

Vitamin D Analog
DHT™
dihydrotachysterol
Hytakerol®

THREADWORM (NONDISSEMINATED INTESTINAL)
ivermectin
Stromectol®

UPPER GASTROINTESTINAL MOTILITY DISORDERS
domperidone (Canada only)
Motilium® (Can)

URINARY BLADDER SPASM
Banthine®
methantheline
Pro-Banthine®
Propanthel (Can)
propantheline

URINARY RETENTION
Antispasmodic Agent, Urinary
Albert® Oxybutynin (Can)
Ditropan®
Ditropan® XL
Nu-Oxybutyn (Can)
Oxybutyn (Can)
oxybutynin
Cholinergic Agent
bethanechol
Duvoid®
Myotonachol™
neostigmine
PMS-Bethanechol Chloride (Can)
Prostigmin®
Urabeth®
Urecholine®

URINARY TRACT INFECTION

Antibiotic, Carbacephem
  Lorabid™
  loracarbef
Antibiotic, Miscellaneous
  Apo®-Nitrofurantoin (Can)
  Azactam®
  aztreonam
  Dehydral® (Can)
  fosfomycin
  Furadantin®
  Furalan®
  Furan®
  Furanite®
  Hiprex®
  Lyphocin® Injection
  Macrobid®
  Macrodantin®
  Mandelamine®
  methenamine
  Monurol™
  Nephronex® (Can)
  nitrofurantoin
  Novo-Furan (Can)
  Primsol®
  Proloprim®
  trimethoprim
  Trimpex®
  Urasal® (Can)
  Urex®
  Vancocin® CP (Can)
  Vancocin® Injection
  Vancocin® Oral
  Vancoled® Injection
  vancomycin
Antibiotic, Penicillin
  pivampicillin (Canada only)
  Pondocillin® (Can)
Antibiotic, Quinolone
  gatifloxacin
  Levaquin™
  levofloxacin
  Tequin™
Antibiotic, Urinary Antiinfective
  Atrosept®
  Dolsed®
  methenamine, phenyl salicylate,
    atropine, hyoscyamine, benzoic
    acid, and methylene blue
  UAA®
  Uridon Modified®
  Urised®
  Uritin®
Cephalosporin (First Generation)
  Ancef®
  Apo®-Cephalex (Can)
  Biocef®
  cefadroxil
  Cefadyl®
  Cefanex®
  cefazolin
  cephalexin
  cephalothin
  cephapirin
  cephradine
  Ceporacin (Can)
  Ceporex (Can)
  Duricef®
  Keflex®
  Keflin (Can)
  Keftab®
  Kefzol®
  Novo-Lexin (Can)
  Nu-Cephalex (Can)
  Velosef®
  Zartan®
  Zolicef®
Cephalosporin (Second Generation)
  Apo®-Cefaclor (Can)
  Ceclor®
  Ceclor® CD
  cefaclor
  cefamandole
  cefmetazole
  cefonicid

Cefotan®
cefotetan
cefoxitin
cefpodoxime
cefprozil
Ceftin® Oral
cefuroxime
Cefzil®
Kefurox® Injection
Mandol®
Mefoxin®
Monocid®
Novo-Cefaclor (Can)
Vantin®
Zefazone®
Zinacef® Injection
Cephalosporin (Third Generation)
   Cedax®
   cefixime
   Cefizox®
   Cefobid®
   cefoperazone
   cefotaxime
   ceftazidime
   ceftibuten
   ceftizoxime
   ceftriaxone
   Ceptaz™
   Claforan®
   Fortaz®
   Rocephin®
   Suprax®
   Tazicef®
   Tazidime®
Cephalosporin (Fourth Generation)
   cefepime
   Maxipime®
Genitourinary Irrigant
   neomycin and polymyxin B
   Neosporin® Cream [OTC]
   Neosporin® G.U. Irrigant
Irrigating Solution
   citric acid bladder mixture

   Renacidin®
Penicillin
   amoxicillin
   amoxicillin and clavulanate
     potassium
   Amoxil®
   ampicillin
   ampicillin and sulbactam
   Ampicin (Can)
   Ampicin® Sodium (Can)
   Ampilean (Can)
   Apo®-Amoxi (Can)
   Apo®-Ampi (Can)
   Apo®-Cloxi (Can)
   Apo®-Pen VK (Can)
   Augmentin®
   Ayercillin® (Can)
   bacampicillin
   Bactopen (Can)
   Bicillin® C-R
   Bicillin® C-R 900/300
   Bicillin® L-A
   carbenicillin
   Clavulin® (Can)
   cloxacillin
   Cloxapen®
   Crysticillin® A.S.
   dicloxacillin
   Dycill®
   Dynapen®
   Gen-Amoxicillin (Can)
   Geocillin®
   Geopen® (Can)
   Jaa Amp® (Can)
   Marcillin®
   Megacillin (Can)
   Mezlin®
   mezlocillin
   Nadopen-V® (Can)
   nafcillin
   Nallpen®
   Novamoxin® (Can)
   Novo-Cloxin (Can)

Novo-Pen-VK® (Can)
Nu-Amoxi (Can)
Nu-Ampi (Can)
Nu-Cloxi (Can)
Nu-Pen-VK (Can)
Omnipen®
Omnipen®-N
Orbenin® (Can)
oxacillin
Pathocil®
Penglobe (Can)
penicillin G benzathine
penicillin G benzathine and procaine
   combined
penicillin G (parenteral/aqueous)
penicillin G procaine
penicillin V potassium
Permapen®
Pfizerpen®
piperacillin
piperacillin and tazobactam sodium
Pipracil®
Principen®
Pro-Amox® (Can)
Pyopen (Can)
Spectrobid® Tablet
Taro-Cloxacillin® (Can)
Tazocin (Can)
Tegopen (Can)
ticarcillin and clavulanate potassium
Timentin®
Totacillin®
Trimox®
Truxcillin®
Unasyn®
Unipen® (Can)
Veetids®
Wycillin®
Wymox®
Zosyn™
Quinolone
   Apo®-Norflox (Can)
   Apo®-Oflox (Can)

Chibroxin™ Ophthalmic
Cinobac® Pulvules®
cinoxacin
enoxacin
Floxin®
lomefloxacin
Maxaquin®
nalidixic acid
NegGram®
norfloxacin
Noroxin® Oral
Novo-Norfloxacin (Can)
Ocuflox™ Ophthalmic
ofloxacin
Penetrex™
sparfloxacin
Zagam®
Sulfonamide
   Apo®-Sulfamethoxazole (Can)
   Apo®-Sulfatrim (Can)
   Azo Gantrisin (Can)
   Bactrim™
   Bactrim™ DS
   Coptin® (Can)
   Cotrim®
   Cotrim® DS
   co-trimoxazole
   Gantrisin®
   Novo-Soxazole (Can)
   Novo-Trimel (Can)
   Nu-Cotrimox (Can)
   Protrin (Can)
   Renoquid®
   Roubac® (Can)
   Septra®
   Septra® DS
   SSD (Can)
   sulfacytine
   sulfadiazine
   Sulfamethoprim®
   sulfamethoxazole
   Sulfatrim®
   Sulfatrim® DS

sulfisoxazole
sulfisoxazole and phenazopyridine
Sulfizole® (Can)
Trisulfa® (Can)
Trisulfa-S® (Can)
Uroplus® DS
Uroplus® SS
Urinary Tract Product
  acetohydroxamic acid
  Atrosept®
  Dolsed®
  Lithostat®
  methenamine, phenyl salicylate,
    atropine, hyoscyamine, benzoic
    acid, and methylene blue
  UAA®
  Uridon Modified®
  Urised®
  Uritin®

VENEREAL WART
  Alferon® N
  interferon alfa-n3

VOMITING
Anticholinergic Agent
  Buscopan (Can)
  Isopto® Hyoscine
  Scopace® Tablet
  scopolamine
  Transderm Scop®
  Transderm-V (Can)
Antiemetic
  Anxanil® Oral
  Apo®-Hydroxyzine (Can)
  Atarax® Oral
  Atozine® Oral
  Benzacot® Injection
  Cesamet®
  dronabinol
  droperidol
  Durrax® Oral
  Histantil (Can)
  hydroxyzine

Hy-Pam® Oral
Hyzine-50® Injection
Inapsine®
Marinol®
Multipax® (Can)
nabilone
Neucalm-50® Injection
Phenazine® Injection
Phenergan® Injection
Phenergan® Oral
Phenergan® Rectal
promethazine
Prorex® Injection
Quiess® Injection
Tigan®
trimethobenzamide
Vamate® Oral
Vistacon-50® Injection
Vistaquel® Injection
Vistaril® Injection
Vistaril® Oral
Vistazine® Injection
Antihistamine
  Calm-X® Oral [OTC]
  Children's Motion Sickness Liquid
    (Can)
  dimenhydrinate
  Dimetabs® Oral
  Dinate® Injection
  Dramamine® Oral [OTC]
  Dramilin® Injection
  Dymenate® Injection
  Gravol (Can)
  Hydrate® Injection
  Marmine® Injection
  Marmine® Oral [OTC]
  Nauseatol (Can)
  Nausex (Can)
  Novo-Dimenate (Can)
  Tega-Vert® Oral
  Travamine (Can)
  Travel Aid (Can)
  Travelmate (Can)

Travel Tabs (Can)
TripTone® Caplets® [OTC]
Phenothiazine Derivative
  Apo®-Chlorpromazine (Can)
  Apo®-Perphenazine (Can)
  Chlorpromanyl (Can)
  chlorpromazine
  Chlorprom® (Can)
  Compazine®
  Largactil (Can)
  Nu-Prochlor (Can)
  Ormazine®
  perphenazine
  PMS-Perphenazine (Can)
  PMS-Prochlorperazine (Can)
  prochlorperazine
  Prorazin® (Can)
  Stemetil (Can)
  thiethylperazine
  Thorazine®
  Torecan (Can)
  triflupromazine
  Trilafon®
  Vesprin®

WHIPWORM

Anthelmintic
  mebendazole
  Vermox®

ZOLLINGER-ELLISON SYNDROME

Antacid
  calcium carbonate and simethicone
  magaldrate
  magaldrate and simethicone
  magnesium hydroxide
  magnesium oxide
  Mag-Ox® 400 [OTC]
  Maox® [OTC]
  Phillips'® Milk of Magnesia [OTC]
  Riopan® [OTC]
  Riopan Plus® [OTC]
  Titralac® Plus Liquid [OTC]

Uro-Mag® [OTC]
Diagnostic Agent
  pentagastrin
  Peptavlon®
Gastric Acid Secretion Inhibitor
  Aciphex™
  lansoprazole
  Losec® (Can)
  omeprazole
  Prevacid®
  Prilosec™
  rabeprazole
Histamine H 2 Antagonist
  Apo®-Cimetidine (Can)
  Apo®-Famotidine (Can)
  Apo®-Ranitidine (Can)
  cimetidine
  famotidine
  Gaviscon Prevent (Can)
  Maalox H2 Acid Controller (Can)
  Novo-Cimetine (Can)
  Novo-Famotidine (Can)
  Novo-Ranidine (Can)
  Nu-Cimet (Can)
  Nu-Famotidine (Can)
  Nu-Ranit (Can)
  Pepcid®
  Pepcid® AC Acid Controller [OTC]
  Pepcid RPD®
  Peptol® (Can)
  ranitidine hydrochloride
  Tagamet®
  Tagamet-HB® [OTC]
  Zantac®
  Zantac® 75 [OTC]
Prostaglandin
  Cytotec®
  misoprostol

ZOLLINGER-ELLISON SYNDROME (DIAGNOSTIC)

secretin
Secretin-Ferring Powder